PRINCIPLES OF
MEDICAL
STATISTICS

Alvan R. Feinstein, M.D.

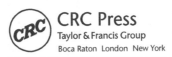

CRC Press
Taylor & Francis Group
Boca Raton London New York

CRC Press is an imprint of the
Taylor & Francis Group, an **informa** business

A CHAPMAN & HALL BOOK

CRC Press
Taylor & Francis Group
6000 Broken Sound Parkway NW, Suite 300
Boca Raton, FL 33487-2742

First issued in paperback 2022

© 2002 by Taylor & Francis Group, LLC
CRC Press is an imprint of Taylor & Francis Group, an Informa business

No claim to original U.S. Government works

Version Date: 20170126

ISBN 13: 978-1-03-247794-7 (pbk)
ISBN 13: 978-1-58488-216-9 (hbk)
ISBN 13: 978-0-429-11597-4 (ebk)

Publisher's Note
The publisher has gone to great lengths to ensure the quality of this reprint but points out that some imperfections in the original copies may be apparent.

Library of Congress Cataloging-in-Publication Data

Feinstein, Alvan R., 1925–
    Principles of medical statistics / Alvan R. Feinstein.
    p. ; cm.
    Includes bibliographical references and index.
    ISBN 1-58488-216-6 (alk. paper)
    1. Medicine--Statistical methods.
    [DNLM: 1. Statistics--methods. 2. Data Interpretation, Statistical. WA 950 F299p 2001] I. Title.

R853.S7 F45 2001
610'.7'27--dc21   2001001794

Visit the Taylor & Francis Web site at
http://www.taylorandfrancis.com

and the CRC Press Web site at
http://www.crcpress.com

Preface

What! Yet another book on medical biostatistics! Why? What for?

The purpose of this preface is to answer those questions and to add a few other pertinent remarks. The sections that follow describe a series of distinctions, some of them unique, that make this book different from other texts.

Goals and Objectives

The goal of the text is to get biomedical readers to think about data and statistical procedures, rather than learn a set of "cook-book recipes." In many statistics books aimed at medical students or biomedical researchers, the readers are believed to have either little interest or limited attention. They are then offered a simple, superficial account of the most common doctrines and applications of statistical theory. The "get-it-over-with-quickly" approach has been encouraged and often necessitated by the short time given to statistics in modern biomedical education. The curriculum is supposed to provide fundamental background for the later careers of medical and other graduate students, but the heavily stressed "basic science" topics are usually cellular and molecular biology. If included at all, statistics is usually presented briefly, as a drudgery to be endured mainly because pertinent questions may appear in subsequent examinations for licensure or other certifications.

Nevertheless, in later professional activities, practicing clinicians and biomedical researchers will constantly be confronted with reports containing statistical expressions and analyses. The practitioners will regularly see and use statistical results when making clinical decisions in patient care; and the researchers will regularly be challenged by statistical methods when planning investigations and appraising data. For these activities, readers who respect their own intellects, and who want to understand and interpret the statistical procedures, cannot be merely passive learners and compliant appliers of doctrinaire customs. The readers should think about what they want, need, and receive. They should also recognize that their knowledge of the substantive biomedical phenomena is a major strength and dominant factor in determining how to get, organize, and evaluate the data. This book is aimed at stimulating and contributing to those thoughts.

Another distinction of the text is that the author is a physician with intimate and extensive experience in both patient care and biomedical investigation. I had obtained a master's degree in mathematics before entering medical school, but thereafter my roots were firmly and irrevocably grounded in clinical medicine. When I later began doing clinical research and encountering statistical strategies, my old mathematical background saved me from being intimidated by established theories and dogmas. Although not all statisticians will approve the temerity of an "unauthorized" writer who dares to compose a text in which the fundamental basis of old statistical traditions is sometimes questioned, other statisticians may be happy to know more about the substantive issues contained in biomedical research, to learn what their clients are (or should be) thinking about, and to lead or collaborate in developing the new methods that are sometimes needed.

New Methods and Approaches

The text contains many new methods and approaches that have been made possible by advances in statistical strategy for both analytic description and inferential decisions.

Statistical description has traditionally relied on certain mathematical models, such as the Gaussian distribution of a "normal" curve, that summarize data with means, standard deviations, and arbitrarily constructed histograms. Readers who begin to think about what they really want, however, may no longer happily accept what is offered by those old models. For example, because biomedical data seldom have a Guassian distribution, the *median* is usually a much better summary value than the *mean*; and new forms of data display — the stem-and-leaf plot and the box plot — not only are superior to histograms, but are more natural forms of expression.

Another descriptive distinction, which is omitted or blurred in many text books, is the difference between a trend (for citing correlation or regression) and a concordance (for citing agreement). Investigators who study variability in observers or in laboratory procedures have usually been taught to express results with the conventional indexes of "association" that denote trend, but not concordance. This text emphasizes the difference between correlation and agreement; and separate chapters are devoted to both "nondirectional" concordance (for observer variability) and "directional" concordance (for accuracy of marker tests).

In statistical inference for decisions about probability, the customary approach has used hard-to-understand mathematical theories and hypothetical assumptions that were developed, established, and entrenched (for topics such as t tests and chi-square tests), because they led to standard formulas for relatively simple calculations. During the past few decades, however, the elaborate mathematical theories and assumptions have been augmented, and sometimes replaced, by easy-to-understand new methods, which use rearrangements or resamplings of the observed data. The new methods often require formidable calculations that were not practical in the pre-computer era; but today, the "computer-intensive" work can be done quickly and easily, requiring no more effort than pushing the right "button" for an appropriate program. The new methods, which may eventually replace the old ones, are discussed here as additional procedures that involve no complicated mathematical backgrounds or unrealistic assumptions about "parametric" sampling from a theoretical population. In the new methods — which have such names as *Fisher exact test*, *bootstrap*, and *jackknife* — all of the rearrangements, resamplings, and statistical decisions about probability come directly from the empirical real-world data. Another departure from tradition is a reappraisal of the use of probability itself, with discussions of what a reader really wants to know, which is *stability* of the numbers, not just probabilistic assessments.

The text also has sections that encourage methods of "physical diagnosis" to examine the data with procedures using only common sense and in-the-head-without-a-calculator appraisals. From appropriate summary statistics and such graphic tactics as box-plot displays, a reader can promptly see what is in the data and can then make some simple, effective, mental calculations. The results will often offer a crude but powerful check on more complex mathematical computations.

A particularly novel and valuable approach is the careful dissection (and proposed elimination) of the term *statistical significance*, which has been a source of major confusion and intellectual pathogenicity throughout 20th-century science. *Statistical significance* is an ambiguous term, because it does not distinguish between the theoretical stochastic significance of calculated probabilities (expressed as P values and confidence intervals) and the pragmatic quantitative significance or clinical importance of the "effect sizes" found in the observed results. Not only is the crucial difference between stochastic and quantitative significance emphasized and thoroughly discussed, but also a special chapter, absent from conventional texts, is devoted to the indexes of contrast used for expressing and evaluating the "effect size" of quantitative distinctions.

Two other unique features of this text are the following:

- Two chapters on the display of statistical data in tables, charts, and graphs contain good and bad examples that can be helpful to readers, investigators, and the artists who prepare medical illustrations.
- A chapter that discusses the challenges of evaluating "equivalence" rather than "superiority" also considers the management of problems that arise when discordance arises in what the investigator wants, what the results show, and what the statistical tests produce.

Sequence, Scope, Rigor, and Orientation

The text is arranged in a logical sequence of basic principles that advance from simple to more elaborate activities. It moves from evaluating one group of data to comparing two groups and then associating two variables. Thereafter, the scope extends into more complex but important topics that frequently appear as challenges in biomedical literature: controversies about stochastic issues in choosing one- or two-tailed tests, the graphic patterns of survival analysis, and the problems of appraising "power," determining "equivalence," and adjudicating "multiple hypotheses."

Nevertheless, despite some of the cited deviations from customary biostatistical discourse, the text describes all the conventional statistical procedures and offers reasonably rigorous accounts of many of their mathematical justifications. Whether retaining or rejecting the conventional procedures, a reader should know what they do, how they do it, and why they have been chosen to do it. Besides, the conventional procedures will continue to appear in biomedical literature for many years. Learning the mechanisms (and limitations) of the traditional tactics will be an enlightened act of self-defense.

Finally, although the conventional mathematical principles are given a respectful account, the book has a distinctly clinical orientation. The literary style is aimed at biomedical readers; and the examples and teaching exercises all come from the real-world medical phenomena. The readers are not expected to become statisticians, although appropriate historical events are sometimes cited and occasional mathematical challenges are sometimes offered. Clinical and biomedical investigators have made many contributions to other "basic" domains, such as cell and molecular biology, and should not be discouraged from helping the development of another "basic" domain, particularly the *bio*-portion of biostatistics. As preparation for a future medical career, such basic tools as the methods of history taking, auscultation, imaging, catheterization, and laboratory tests are almost always taught with a clinical orientation. As another important basic tool, statistics receives that same orientation here.

Containing much more than most "elementary" books, this text can help repair the current curricular imbalance that gives so little attention to the role of statistics as a prime component of "basic" biomedical education. Statistical procedures are a vital, integral part of the "basic" background for clinical or biomedical careers, and are essential for readers and investigators who want to be at least as thoughtful in analyzing results as in planning and doing the research. The biomedical readers, however, are asked to read the text rather than race through it. What they learn will help them think for themselves when evaluating various statistical claims in the future. They can then use their own minds rather than depending on editorial decisions, authoritarian pronouncements, or the blandishments of various medical, commercial, or political entrepreneurs.

Before concluding, I want to thank various faculty colleagues — (alphabetically) Domenic Cicchetti, John Concato, Theodore Holford, Ralph Horwitz, James Jekel, Harlan Krumholz, Robert Makuch, Peter Peduzzi, and Carolyn Wells—who have contributed to my own statistical education. I also want to acknowledge the late Donald Mainland, whose writings made me realize that statistics could be profound but comprehensible while also being fun, and who launched my career in statistics when he invited me to succeed him in writing a bimonthly set of journal essays on biostatistical topics. I am immensely grateful to the post-residency physicians who have been research fellows in the Yale Clinical Scholar Program, sponsored by the Robert Wood Johnson Foundation and also supported by the U.S. Department of Veterans Affairs. The Clinical Scholars are the people who inspired the writing of this text, who have received and worked through its many drafts, whose comments and suggestions have produced worthwhile improvements, and who helped create an intellectual atmosphere that I hope will be reflected and preserved. While I was trying to prod the group into learning and thinking, their responses gave me the stimuli and pleasures of additional learning and thinking.

My last set of acknowledgments contains thanks to people whose contributions were essential for the text itself. Donna Cavaliere and many other persons — now too numerous to all be named — did the hard, heroic work of preparing everything on a word processor. Robert Stern, of Chapman and Hall publishers, has been an excellent and constructive editor. Carole Gustafson, also of Chapman and Hall, has done a magnificent job of checking everything in the text for logic, consistency, and even grammar. I am grateful to Sam Feinstein for esthetic advice and to Yale's Biomedical Communications department for preparing many of the illustrations. And finally, my wife Lilli, has been a constant source of patience, encouragement, and joy.

Alvan R. Feinstein
New Haven
July, 2001

Biographical Sketch

Alvan R. Feinstein was born in Philadelphia and went to schools in that city before attending the University of Chicago, from which he received a bachelor's degree, a master's degree in mathematics, and his doctor of medicine degree. After residency training in internal medicine at Yale and at Columbia-Presbyterian Hospital in New York, and after a research fellowship at Rockefeller Institute, he became medical director at Irvington House, just outside New York City, where he studied a large population of patients with rheumatic fever. In this research, he began developing new clinical investigative techniques that were eventually expanded beyond rheumatic fever into many other activities, particularly work on the prognosis and therapy of cancer.

His new clinical epidemiologic approaches and methods have been reported in three books, *Clinical Judgment, Clinical Epidemiology,* and *Clinimetrics,* which describe the goals and methods of clinical reasoning, the structure and contents of clinical research with groups, and the strategy used to form clinical indexes and rating scales for important human clinical phenomena — such as pain, distress, and disability — that have not received adequate attention in an age of technologic data. His clinical orientation to quantitative data has been presented in two previous books, *Clinical Biostatistics* and *Multivariable Analysis,* and now in the current text.

To supplement the current biomedical forms of "basic science" that are used for explanatory decisions about pathophysiologic mechanisms of disease, Feinstein has vigorously advocated that clinical epidemiology and clinimetrics be developed as an additional humanistic "basic science" for the managerial decisions of clinical practice.

He is Sterling Professor of Medicine and Epidemiology at the Yale University School of Medicine, where he is also Director of the Clinical Epidemiology Unit and Director Emeritus of the Robert Wood Johnson Clinical Scholars Program. For many years he also directed the Clinical Examination Course (for second-year students).

Table of Contents

Part III Evaluating Associations

Part IV Additional Activities

1

Introduction

CONTENTS

Suppose you have just read a report in your favorite medical journal. The success rates were said to be 50% with a new treatment for Disease D, and 33% in the control group, receiving the customary old treatment. You now have a clinical challenge: Should you beginning the new treatment instead of the old one for patients with Disease D?

Decisions of this type are constantly provoked by claims that appear in the medical literature or in other media, such as teaching rounds, professional meetings, conferences, newspapers, magazines, and television. In the example just cited, the relative merits were compared for two treatments, but many other medical decisions involve appraisals of therapeutic hazards or comparisons of new technologic procedures for diagnosis. In other instances, the questions are issues in public and personal health, rather than the clinical decisions in diagnosis or treatment. These additional questions usually require evaluations for the medical risks or benefits of phenomena that occur in everyday life: the food we eat; the water we drink; the air we breathe; the chemicals we encounter at work or elsewhere; the exercise we take (or avoid); and the diverse patterns of behavior that are often called "life style."

If not provoked by statistics about therapeutic agents or the hazards of daily life, the questions may arise from claims made when investigators report the results of laboratory research. A set of points that looks like scattered buckshot on a graph may have been fitted with a straight line and accompanied by a statement that they show a "significant" relationship. The mean values for results in two compared groups may not seem far apart, but may be presented with the claim that they are distinctively different.

Either these contentions can be accepted in the assumption that they were verified by the wisdom of the journal's referees and editors, or — mindful of the long history of erroneous doctrines that were accepted and promulgated by the medical "establishment" in different eras — we can try to evaluate things ourselves. To do these evaluations, we need some type of rational mechanism. What kinds of things shall we think about? What should we look for? How should we analyze what we find? How do we interpret the results of the analysis?

The final *conclusions* drawn from the evaluations are seldom expressed in statistical terms. We conclude that treatment A is preferable to treatment B, that diagnostic procedure C is better than diagnostic procedure E, that treatment F is too hazardous to use, or that G is a risk factor for disease H. Before we reach these nonstatistical conclusions, however, the things that begin the thought process are often statistical expressions, such as success rates of 50% vs. 33%.

The statistical citation of results has become one of the most common, striking phenomena of modern medical literature. No matter what topic is under investigation, and no matter how the data have been collected, the results are constantly presented in statistical "wrappings." To evaluate the results scientifically, we need to look beneath the wrapping to determine the scientific quality of the contents. This look inside may not occur, however, if a reader is too flustered or uncomfortable with the exterior statistical covering. Someone familiar with medical science might easily understand the interior contents, but can seldom reach them if the statistical material becomes an obscure or intimidating barrier.

The frequent need to appraise numerical information creates an intriguing irony in the professional lives of workers in the field of medicine or public health. Many clinicians and public-health personnel entered those fields because they liked people and liked science, but hated mathematics. After the basic professional education is completed, the subsequent careers may bring the anticipated pleasure of working in a humanistic science, but the pleasure is often mitigated by the oppression of having to think about statistics.

This book is intended to reduce or eliminate that oppression, and even perhaps to show that statistical thinking can be intellectually attractive. The main point to recognize is that the primary base of statistical thinking is not statistical. It requires no particular knowledge or talent in mathematics; and it involves only the use of enlightened common sense — acquired as ordinary common sense plus professional knowledge and experience. Somewhat like a "review of systems" in examining patients, a statistical evaluation can be divided into several distinctive components. Some of the components involve arithmetic or mathematics, but most of them require only the ability to think effectively about what we already know.

1.1 Components of a Statistical Evaluation

The six main components of a statistical "review of systems" can be illustrated with examples of the way they might occur for the decision described at the start of this chapter.

1.1.1 Summary Expressions

The first component we usually meet in statistical data is a summary expression, such as a *50% success rate*. The statistical appraisal begins with the adequacy of this expression. Is it a satisfactory way of summarizing results for the observed group? Suppose the goal of treatment was to lower blood pressure. Are you satisfied with a summary in which the results are expressed as success rates of 50% or 33%? Would you have wanted, instead, to know the average amount by which blood pressure was lowered in each group? Would some other quantitative expression, such as the average weekly change in blood pressure, be a preferable way of summarizing each set of data?

1.1.2 Quantitative Contrasts

Assuming that you are satisfied with whatever quantitative summary was used to express the individual results for each group, the second component of evaluation is a contrast of the two summaries. Are you impressed with the comparative distinction noted in the two groups? Does a 17% difference in success rates of 50% and 33% seem big enough to be important? Suppose the difference of 17% occurred as a contrast of 95% vs. 78%, or as 20% vs. 3%. Would these values make you more impressed or less impressed by the distinction? If you were impressed not by the 17% difference in the two numbers, but by their ratio of 1.5 (50/33), would you still be impressed if the same ratio were obtained from the contrast of 6% vs. 4% or from .0039 vs. 0026? What, in fact, is the strategy you use for deciding that a distinction in two contrasted numbers has an "impressive" magnitude?

1.1.3   Stochastic Contrasts

If you decided that the 50% vs. 33% distinction was impressive, the next step is to look at the numerical sources of the compared percentages. This component of evaluation contains the type of statistics that may be particularly distressing for medical people. It often involves appraising the stochastic (or probabilistic) role of random chance in the observed numerical results. Although the quantitative contrast of 50% vs. 33% may have seemed impressive, suppose the results came from only five patients. The 50% and 33% values may have emerged, respectively, as one success in two patients and one success in three patients. With constituent numbers as small as 1/2 and 1/3, you would sense intuitively that results such as 50% vs. 33% could easily occur by chance alone, even if the two treatments were identical.

Suppose, however, that the two percentages (50% vs. 33%) were based on such numbers as 150/300 vs. 100/300? Would you now worry about chance possibilities? Probably not, because the contrast in these large numbers seems distinctive by what Joseph Berkson has called the traumatic interocular test. (The difference hits you between the eyes.) Now suppose that the difference of 50% and 33% came from numbers lying somewhere between the two extremes of 1/2 vs. 1/3 and 150/300 vs. 100/300. If the results were 8/16 vs. 6/18, the decision would not be so obvious. These numbers are neither small enough to be dismissed immediately as "chancy" nor large enough to be accepted promptly as "intuitively evident."

The main role of the third component of statistical evaluation is to deal with this type of problem. The process uses mathematical methods to evaluate the "stability" of numerical results. The methods produce the P values, confidence intervals, and other probabilistic expressions for which statistics has become famous (or infamous).

1.1.4   Architectural Structure

Suppose you felt satisfied after all the numerical thinking in the first three steps. You accepted the expression of "success"; you were impressed by the quantitative distinction of 50% vs. 33%; and the numbers of patients were large enough to convince you that the differences were not likely to arise by chance. Are you now ready to start using the new treatment instead of the old one? If you respect your own common sense, the answer to this question should be a resounding NO. At this point in the evaluation, you have thought only about the statistics, but you have not yet given any attention to the science that lies behind the statistics. You have no idea of how the research was done, and what kind of architectural structure was used to produce the compared results of 50% and 33%.

The architectural structure of a research project refers to the scientific arrangement of persons and circumstances in which the research was carried out. The ability to evaluate the scientific architecture requires no knowledge of statistics and is the most powerful analytic skill at your disposal. You can use this skill to answer the following kinds of architectural questions: Under what clinical conditions were the two treatments compared? Were the patients' conditions reasonably similar in the two groups, and are they the kind of conditions in which you would want to use the treatment? Were the treatments administered in an appropriate dosage and in a similar manner for the patients in the two groups. Was "success" observed and determined in the same way for both groups?

If you are not happy with the answers to these questions, all of the preceding numerical appraisals may become unimportant. No matter how statistically impressive, the results may be unacceptable because of their architectural flaws. The comparison may have been done with biases that destroy the scientific credibility of the results; or the results, even if scientifically credible, may not be pertinent for the particular kinds of patients you treat and the way you give the treatment.

1.1.5   Data Acquisition

The process of acquiring data involves two crucial activities: observation and classification. For clinical work, the observation process involves listening, looking, touching, smelling, and sometimes tasting. The observations are then described in various informal or formal ways. For example, the observer might see a 5 mm. cutaneous red zone that blanches with pressure, surrounding a smaller darker-red zone that does not blanch. For classification, the observer chooses a category from an available taxonomy of cutaneous lesions. In this instance, the entity might be called a *petechia*. If the detailed description is not fully recorded, the entry of "petechia" may become the basic item of data. Analogously, a specimen of serum may be "observed" with a technologic process, and then "classified" as sodium, 120 meq/dl. Sometimes, the classification process may go a step further, to report the foregoing sodium value as *hyponatremia*.

Because the available data will have been acquired with diverse methods of observation and classification, these methods will need separate scientific attention beyond the basic plan of the research itself. What procedures (history taking, self-administered questionnaire, blood pressure measurements, laboratory tests, biopsy specimens, etc.) were used to make and record the basic observations that produced the raw data? How was each patient's original condition identified, and how was each post-therapeutic response observed and classified as success or no success? Was "success" defined according to achievement of normotension, or an arbitrary magnitude of reduction in blood pressure? What kind of "quality control" or criteria for classification were used to make the basic raw data trustworthy?

The answers to these questions may reveal that the basic data are too fallible or unsatisfactory to be accepted, even if all other elements of the research architecture seem satisfactory.

1.1.6   Data Processing

To be analyzed statistically, the categories of classification must be transformed into coded digits that become the entities receiving data processing. This last step in the activities is particularly vital in an era of electronic analysis. Because the transformed data become the basic entities that are processed, we need to know how well the transformation was done. What arrangements were used to convert the raw data into designated categories, to convert the categories into coded digits, and to convert those digits into magnetized disks or diverse other media that became the analyzed information? What mechanisms were used to check the accuracy of the conversions?

The transformation from raw data into processed data must be suitably evaluated to demonstrate that the collected basic information was correctly converted into the analyzed information.

1.2   Statistical and Nonstatistical Judgments

Of the six activities just cited, the last three involve no knowledge of mathematics, and they also have prime importance in the scientific evaluation. During the actual research, these three activities all occur before any statistical expressions are produced. The architectural structure of the research, the quality of the basic data, and the quality of the processed data are the fundamental scientific issues that underlie the statistical results. If the basic scientific structure and data are inadequate, the numbers that emerge as results will be unsatisfactory no matter how "significant" they may seem statistically. Because no mathematical talent is needed to judge those three fundamental components, an intelligent reader who recognizes their primacy will have won at least half the battle of statistical evaluation before it begins.

Many readers of the medical literature, however, may not recognize this crucial role of nonstatistical judgment, because they do not get past the first three statistical components. If the summary expressions and quantitative contrasts are presented in unfamiliar terms, such as an odds ratio or a multivariable coefficient of association, the reader may not understand what is being said. Even if the summaries and contrasts are readily understood, the reader may be baffled by the P values or confidence intervals used in the stochastic evaluations. Flustered or awed by these uncertainties, a medically oriented reader may not penetrate beyond the outside statistics to reach the inside place where enlightened common sense and scientific judgment are powerful and paramount.

Because this book is about statistics, it will emphasize the three specifically statistical aspects of evaluation. The three sets of scientific issues in architecture and data will be outlined only briefly; and readers who want to know more about them can find extensive discussions elsewhere.[1-3] Despite the statistical focus, however, most of the text relies on enlightened judgment rather than mathematical reasoning. Once you have learned the strategy of the descriptive expressions used in the first two parts of the statistical evaluation, you will discover that their appraisal is usually an act of common sense. Except for some of the complicated multivariable descriptions that appear much later in the text, no mathematical prowess is needed to understand the descriptive statistical expressions used for summaries, contrasts, and simple associations. Only the third statistical activity — concerned with probabilities and other stochastic expressions — involves distinctively mathematical ideas; and many of them are presented here with modern approaches (such as permutation tests) that are much easier to understand than the traditional (parametric) theories used in most elementary instruction.

1.3   Arrangement of the Text

This book has been prepared for readers who have some form of "medical" interest. The interest can be clinical medicine, nursing, medical biology, epidemiology, dentistry, personal or public health, or health-care administration. All of the illustrations and examples are drawn from those fields, and the text has been written with the assumption that the reader is becoming (or has already become) knowledgeable about activities in those fields.

A major challenge for any writer on statistical topics is to keep things simple, without oversimplifying and without becoming too superficial. The achievement of these goals is particularly difficult if the writer wants to respect the basic intellectual traditions of both science and mathematics. In both fields, the traditions involve processes of assertion and documentation. In science, the assertion is called a *hypothesis*, and the documentation is called *supporting evidence*. In mathematics, the assertion is called a *theorem* or *operating principle*, and the documentation is called a *proof*.

To make things attractive or more palatable, however, many of the assertions in conventional statistical textbooks are presented without documentation. For example, a reader may be told, without explanation or justification, to divide something by $n - 1$, although intuition suggests that the division should be done with n. Many medical readers are delighted to accept the simple "recipes" and to avoid details of their justification. Other readers, however, may be distressed when the documentary traditions of both science and mathematics are violated by the absence of justifying evidence for assertions. If documentary details are included in an effort to avoid such distress, however, readers who want only "the beef" may become bored, confused by the complexity, or harassed by the struggle to understand the details.

The compromise solution for this dilemma is to use both approaches. The main body of the text has been kept relatively simple. Many of the sustaining mathematical explanations and proofs have been included, but they are relegated to the Appendixes in the back of the pertinent chapters. The additional details are thus available for readers who want them and readily skipped for those who do not.

1.4   A Note about References

The references for each chapter are numbered sequentially as they appear. At the end of each chapter, they are cited by first author and year of publication (and by other features that may be needed to avoid ambiguity). The complete references for all chapters are listed alphabetically at the end of the text; and each reference is accompanied by an indication of the chapter(s) in which it appeared.

For the first chapter, the references are as follows:

1. Feinstein, 1985; 2. Sackett, 1991; 3. Hulley, 2000.

1.5   A Note about "Exercises"

The list of references for each chapter is followed by a set of exercises that can be used as "homework." The end of the text contains a list of the official answers to many of the exercises, usually those with odd numbers. The other answers are available in an "Instructor's Manual." You may not always agree that the answers are right or wrong, but they are "official."

1.6 A Note about Computation

Statistics books today may contain instructions and illustrations for exercises to be managed with the computer programs of a particular commercial system, such as BMDP, Excel, Minitab, SAS, or SPSS. Such exercises have been omitted here, for two reasons. First, the specific system chosen for the illustrations may differ from what is available to, or preferred by, individual readers. Second, and more importantly, your understanding and familiarity with the procedures will be greatly increased if you "get into their guts" and see exactly how the computations are done with an electronic hand calculator. You may want to use a computer program in the future, but learning to do the calculations yourself is a valuable introduction. Besides, unlike a computer, a hand calculator is easily portable and always accessible. Furthermore, the results obtained with the calculator can be used to check the results of the computer programs, which sometimes do the procedures erroneously because of wrong formulas or strategies.

Nevertheless, a few illustrations in the text show printouts from the SAS system, which happens to be the one most often used at my location.

Exercises

1.1 Six types of "evaluation" were described in this chapter. In which of those categories would you classify appraisals of the following statements? [All that is needed for each answer is a number from 1–6, corresponding to the six parts of Section 1.1]

1.1.1. "The controls are inadequate."

1.1.2. "The data were punched and verified."

1.1.3. "Statistical analyses of categorical data were performed with a chi-square test."

1.1.4. "Compared with non-potato eaters, potato eaters had a risk ratio of 2.4 for developing omphalosis."

1.1.5. "The patient had a normal glucose tolerance test."

1.1.6. "The trial was performed with double-blind procedures."

1.1.7. "Newborn babies were regarded as sick if the Apgar Score was ≤6."

1.1.8. "The rate of recurrent myocardial infarction was significantly lower in patients treated with excellitol than in the placebo group."

1.1.9. "The reports obtained in the interviews had an 85% agreement with what was noted in the medical records."

1.1.10. "The small confidence interval suggests that the difference cannot be large, despite the relatively small sample sizes."

1.1.11. "The compared treatments were assigned by randomization."

1.1.12. "We are distressed by the apparent slowing of the annual decline in infant mortality rates."

2

Formation, Expression, and Coding of Data

During the 17th and 18th centuries, nations began assembling quantitative information, called *Political Arithmetic*, about their wealth. It was counted with economic data for imports, exports, and agriculture, and with demographic data for population census, births, and deaths. The people who collected and tabulated these descriptions for the state were called *statists*; and the items of information were called *statistics*.

Later in the 18th century, the royalty who amused themselves in gambling gave "grants" to develop ideas that could help guide the betting. The research produced a "calculus of probabilities" that became eventually applied beyond the world of gambling. The application occurred when smaller "samples" rather than the entire large population were studied to answer descriptive questions about regional statistics. The theory that had been developed for the probabilities of bets in gambling became an effective mechanism to make inferential decisions from the descriptive attributes found in the samples. Those theories and decisions thus brought together the two statistical worlds of description and probability, while also bringing P values, confidence intervals, and other mathematical inferences into modern "statistical analysis."

The descriptive origin of statistics is still retained as a job title, however, when "statisticians" collect and analyze data about sports, economics, and demography. The descriptive statistics can be examined by sports fans for the performances of teams or individual players; by economists for stock market indexes, gross national product, and trade imbalances; and by demographers for changes in geographic distribution of population and mortality rates. The descriptive origin of statistics is also the fundamental basis for all the numerical expressions and quantitative tabulations that appear as evidence in modern biologic science. The evidence may often be analyzed with inferential "tests of significance," but the inferences are a secondary activity. The primary information is the descriptive numerical evidence.

The numbers come from even more basic elements, which have the same role in statistics that molecules have in biology. The basic molecular elements of statistics are items of data. To understand fundamental biologic structures, we need to know about molecules; to understand the fundamentals of statistics, we need to know about data.

In biology, most of the studied molecules exist in nature, but some of them are made by humans. No data, however, exist in nature. All items of data are artifacts produced when something has been observed and described. The observed entity can be a landscape, a person, a conversation, a set of noises, a specimen of tissue, a graphic tracing, or the events that occur in a person's life. The medical observations can be done by simple clinical examination or with technologic procedures. The description can be expressed in letters, symbols, numbers, or words; and the words can occupy a phrase, a sentence, a paragraph, or an entire book.

The scientific quality of basic observations and descriptions depends on whether the process is suitable, reproducible, and accurate. Is the score on a set of multiple-choice examination questions a suitable description of a person's intelligence? Would several clinicians, each taking a history from the same patient, emerge with the same collection of information? Would several histopathologists, reviewing the same specimen of tissue, all give the same reading? If serum cholesterol is measured in several different laboratories, would the results — even if similar — agree with a measurement performed by the National Bureau of Standards?

2.1   Scientific Quality of Data

Suitability, reproducibility, and accuracy are the attributes of scientific quality. For *reproducibility*, the same result should be obtained consistently when the measurement process is repeated. For *accuracy*, the result should be similar to what is obtained with a "gold-standard" measurement. For *suitability*, which is sometimes called *sensibility* or *face validity*, the measurement process and its result should be appropriate according to both scientific and ordinary standards of "common sense."

These three attributes determine whether the raw data are trustworthy enough to receive serious attention when converted into statistics, statistical analyses, and subsequent conclusions. Of the three attributes, *accuracy* may often be difficult or impossible to check, because a "gold standard" may not exist for the definitive measurement of such entities as pain, discomfort, or gratification. *Reproducibility* can always be checked, however. Even if it was not specifically tested in the original work, a reader can get an excellent idea about reproducibility by noting the guidelines or criteria used for pertinent decisions. *Suitability* can also be checked if the reader thinks about it and knows enough about the subject matter to apply enlightened common sense.

The foregoing comments should demonstrate that the production of trustworthy data is a scientific rather than statistical challenge. The challenge requires scientific attention to the purpose of the observations, the setting in which they occurred, the way they were made, the process that transformed observed phenomena into descriptive expressions, the people who were included or excluded in the observed groups, and many other considerations that are issues in science rather than mathematics.

These issues in scientific architecture are the basic "molecular" elements that lie behind the assembled statistics. The issues have paramount importance whenever statistical work is done or evaluated — but the issues themselves are not an inherent part of the statistical activities. The data constitute the basic scientific evidence available as "news"; statistical procedures help provide summaries of the news and help lead to the "editorials" and other conclusions.

To give adequate attention to what makes the basic data scientifically trustworthy and credible, however, would require too many digressions from the statistical procedures. A reader who wants to learn mainly about the statistics would become distressed by the constant diversions into scientific priorities. Therefore, to allow the statistical discourse to proceed, many of the fundamental scientific issues receive little or no attention in this text. This neglect does not alter their primacy, but relies on the assumption that they will be known, recognized, and suitably considered by readers whose minds are liberated from mathematical confusion.

For the statistical discussion, the raw descriptive information and groups will be accepted here as satisfactory scientific evidence. This acceptance, an *ad hoc* literary convenience, is never warranted in the real world, where scientific credibility leads to the most important, but commonly overlooked, problems in statistical analyses. In fundamental scientific thinking, the focus is on what the information represents, how it got there, and how good it is. Accepting the underlying scientific process as adequate, however, we can turn to the statistical process discussed in this and the subsequent 27 chapters. The next level of thinking begins with conversion of the raw data to statistics.

2.2 Formation of Variables

The available raw information can be called *data*, but the data can seldom be analyzed statistically. For example, statements such as "John Doe is a 37-year-old man" and "Mary Smith is a 31-year-old woman" contain specific data about specific persons, but the information is not arranged in a manner suitable for statistical analysis. To get the data into an appropriate format, the first statement can be converted to "*Name*: **John Doe**; *Age in years*: **37**; *Sex*: **male**." The second statement would become "*Name*: **Mary Smith**; *Age in years*: **31**; *Sex*: **female**.

In the format just cited, specific attributes such as *name*, *age*, and *sex* were chosen as labels for each citation. Analogous attributes and formats would be needed to express details of the medical information contained in a patient's history, an account of a surgical operation, or a description of a pathologic specimen. Many other types of raw information, however, receive expressions that are immediately suitable for analysis. Examples are the laboratory report, *hematocrit*: **47%**, or the clinical description of *systolic blood pressure* as **125 mm Hg**.

Each of these formats refers to a selected attribute, cited in an available set of expressions. In the parlance of mathematics or statistics, the attributes are called *variables*, and the expressions available for citation are called a *scale*.

2.2.1 Definition of a Variable

A *variable* is a class of data in which different distinctions can be expressed. A person's *age*, *height*, *sex*, *diagnosis*, and *therapy* are all variables. Their distinctions might be cited respectively for a particular person as **52 years, 69 inches, male, peptic ulcer,** and **antacid tablets**. Although not particularly desirable as a scientific term, the word *variable* has become firmly entrenched in its mathematical role. You can think of it not as something that denotes diversity or change — in the sense of *variation* or *variability* — but simply as the name used for a class of data that can be cited differently for different people.

The expression of eight variables for six individual persons could be shown in a "matrix" table that has the following skeleton structure:

Identity of Person	Age	Height	Sex	Diagnosis	Therapy	Systolic Blood Pressure Before Treatment	Systolic Blood Pressure During Treatment	Systolic Blood Pressure After Treatment
A.B.								
C.D.								
E.F.								
G.H.								
I.J.								
K.L.								

Names of Variables

The interior "cells" of this table would contain the assembled citations of each variable for each person. (Exercises will use different ways and the additional categories for analyzing these data.)

2.2.2   Scales, Categories, and Values

The *scale* of a variable contains the available *categories* for its expression. The scale for the variable *sex* usually has two categories: **male** and **female**. The scale for *age in years* has the categories **1, 2, 3, 4, ..., 99, 100, ...** . (In statistics, as in literature, the symbol "..." indicates that certain items in a sequence have been omitted.)

For a particular person, the pertinent category of a scale is called the *value* of the variable. Thus, a 52-year-old man with peptic ulcer has 52 as the value of *age in years*, **male** as the value of *sex*, and **peptic ulcer** as the value of *diagnosis*. The word *value* is another entrenched mathematical term that has nothing to do with judgments or beliefs about such "values" as importance, worth, or merit. The value of a variable is the *result* of an observational process that assigns to a particular person the appropriate category of the variable's scale.

Any descriptive account of a person can be converted into an organized array of data using variables, scales, categories, and values.

2.3   Classification of Scales and Variables

Scales and variables can be classified in various ways. The most common and useful classification depends on the precision of ranking for the constituent categories.

2.3.1   Precision of Rankings

A 31-year-old person is 14 years younger than someone who is 45. A person with severe dyspnea is more short of breath than someone with mild dyspnea, but we cannot measure the exact difference. In both these examples, definite ranks of magnitude were present in the values of **31** and **45** for *age*, and in the values of **severe** and **mild** for *severity* of dyspnea. The ranks were distinct for both variables, but the magnitudes were more precise for *age* than for *severity of dyspnea*.

Certain other variables, however, are expressed in categories that have no magnitudes and cannot be ranked. Thus, no obvious rankings seem possible if *history of myocardial infarction* is **present** in one patient and **absent** in another; or if one patient has an **anterior** and another has a **posterior** *location of myocardial infarction*. We might want to regard **present** as being "more" than absent, but we cannot rank the magnitude of such locations as **anterior** or **posterior**.

The four examples just cited illustrate patterns of precision in ranking for the *dimensional, ordinal, binary,* and *nominal* variables that were used, respectively, to denote age, severity, existence, and location. These four patterns, together with *quasi-dimensional* scales, are the basic arrangements for categories in the scales of variables. The patterns are further discussed in the sections that follow.

2.3.1.1   Dimensional Scales — In a dimensional scale, the successive categories are monotonic and equi-interval. In the directional sequence of a monotonic ranking, each category is progressively either greater or smaller than the preceding adjacent category. For equi-interval ranks, a measurably equal interval can be demarcated between any two adjacent monotonic categories.

Thus, in the scale for *age in years*, a measurably equal interval of 1 year separates each of the successive categories **1, 2, 3, 4, ..., 99, 100, ...** . Similarly, for the variable *height in inches*, each of the successive categories **..., 59, 60, 61, 62, ..., 74, 75, ...** has an incremental interval of 1 inch.

Many alternative terms have been used as names for a dimensional scale, which is now the traditional form of scientific measurement. Psychologists and sociologists often refer to *interval scales*, but the word *interval* is often used medically for a period of time. The term *metric* might be a satisfactory name, but it regularly connotes a particular system of measurement (in meters, liters, etc.).

Mathematicians sometimes talk about *continuous* scales, but many dimensional categories cannot be divided into the smaller and smaller units that occur in continuous variables. For example, *age* and *height* are continuous variables. We could express age in finer and finer units such as years, months, days, hours, seconds, and fractions of seconds since birth. Similarly, with a suitably precise measuring system, we could express height not merely in inches but also in tenths, hundredths, thousandths, or millionths of an inch. On the other hand, *number of children* or *highest grade completed in school* are dimensional variables that are discrete rather than continuous. Their scale of successive integers has equi-interval characteristics, but the integers cannot be reduced to smaller units.

Psychologists sometimes use *ratio scale* for a dimensional scale that has an absolute zero point, allowing ratio comparisons of the categories. Thus, *age in years* has a ratio scale: a 24-year-old person is twice as old as someone who is 12. *Fahrenheit temperature* does not have a ratio scale: 68°F is not twice as warm as 34°F.

Although these distinctions are sometimes regarded as important,[1] they can generally be ignored. Any type of scale that has equi-interval monotonic categories can be called *dimensional*.

2.3.1.2 Ordinal Scales

2.3.1.2 Ordinal Scales — In an ordinal scale, the successive categories can be ranked monotonically, but the ranks have arbitrary magnitudes, without measurably equal intervals between every two adjacent categories.

Clinicians constantly use ordinal scales to express such variables as *briskness of reflexes* in the graded categories of *0, 1+, 2+, 3+, 4+. Severity of pain* is a variable often cited as **none, mild, moderate,** or **severe.** Although *age* can be expressed in dimensional data, it is sometimes converted to an ordinal scale with citations such as **neonatal, infant, child, adolescent, young adult, middle-aged adult, … .**

An ordinal scale can have either *unlimited ranks* or a *limited* number of *grades*. Most ordinal scales in medical activities have a finite group of grades, such as **0, 1+, …, 4+** or **none, mild, …, severe.** If we wanted to rank the people who have applied for admission to a medical school, however, we could use an unlimited-rank scale to arrange the applicants with ratings such as **1, 2, 3, 4, 5, …, 147, 148, … .** In this limitless scale, the lowest ranked person might be rated as **238** or **964,** according to the number of applicants. Scales with unlimited ranks seldom appear in medical research, but have been used (as discussed much later) for the mathematical reasoning with which certain types of statistical tests were developed.

2.3.1.3 Quasi-Dimensional Scales

2.3.1.3 Quasi-Dimensional Scales — A quasi-dimensional scale seems to be dimensional, but does not really have measurably equal intervals between categories. Quasi-dimensional scales can be formed in two ways. In one technique, the scale is the sum of arbitrary ratings from several ordinal scales. For example, a licensure examination might contain 50 questions, for which each answer is regarded as a separate variable and scored as **0** for *wrong*, **1** for *partially correct*, and **2** for *completely correct*. Despite the arbitrary ordinal values, which have none of the equi-interval characteristics of dimensional data, the candidate's scores on each question can be added to form a total score, such as **46, 78, 85,** or **100.** The arbitrary result looks dimensional and is often manipulated mathematically as though it were truly dimensional.

A second source of quasi-dimensional data is a graphic rating technique called a *visual analog scale*. The respondent rates the magnitude of a feeling, opinion, or attitude by placing a mark on a line that is usually 100 mm. long. The measured location of the mark then becomes converted to an apparently dimensional rating. For example, someone might be asked to mark the following line in response to a question such as "How bad is your pain?"

|———————————————————————————————————|

None   Worst
Ever

If the mark is placed as follows,

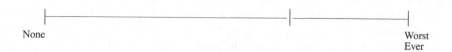

the measured distance could represent 67 "pain units." Despite the dimensional expression, such scales are not truly dimensional because adjacent categories — such as **70, 71,** and **72** — in the arbitrary graphic ratings are not accompanied by criteria that demarcate equal intervals.

2.3.1.4 *Binary (Dichotomous) Scales* —

A binary or dichotomous scale has two categories, such as **male** and **female** for the variable *sex.* Other common scales with two categories are **alive/dead, success/failure,** and **case/control.** In medical research, many binary scales refer to entities, such as chest pain, that can be classified as **present** or **absent**, or to a variable such as *previous pregnancy* that can be cited as **yes** or **no.** When used to represent existence or nonexistence, a binary scale is sometimes called an *existential scale.*

Although apparently binary, existential data can often be regarded as a subset of ordinal data. The ordinal ranking becomes apparent if gradations of probability are added to the scale. Thus, when *existence of acute myocardial infarction* is expressed as likelihood of existence, the available scale is ordinally expanded to include the categories of **definitely present, probably present, uncertain whether present or absent, probably absent**, and **definitely absent.**

2.3.1.5 *Nominal Scales* —

In a nominal scale, the unranked categories have no magnitudes. Nominal scales would express such variables as a person's name, address, color of eyes, birthplace, religion, diagnosis, or type of therapy.

Nominal characteristics can sometimes receive implicit ranks based on cultural, social, political, or even clinical preferences. Thus, a short name might be preferred to a long one; certain addresses might be regarded as being in better neighborhoods than others; someone might like blue eyes better than brown (or vice versa); a person raised in Alabama might be more accustomed to social patterns in Mississippi than someone from Maine; and a diagnosis of acute pancreatitis might be more desirable than pancreatic carcinoma. When such rankings occur, however, the variable is no longer nominal and needs a different title for its expression. For example, if the variable is designated as *desirability of diagnosis* rather than *diagnosis*, the previously nominal categories **acute pancreatitis, gallstone obstructive jaundice,** and **pancreatic carcinoma** might become an ordinal scale.

For analytic purposes, the individual categories of a nominal scale are often decomposed and converted into a set of "dummy" binary variables, each rated as **present** or **absent.** For example, suppose *current occupation* is expressed in the nominal categories **doctor, merchant,** or **other**. The categories can be converted into three binary variables: *occupation as a doctor, occupation as a merchant*, and *occupation as neither a doctor nor a merchant.* (The three variables could be suitably condensed into only the first two, because someone whose values are **no** for both *occupation as a doctor* and *occupation as a merchant* would have to be rated as **yes** for *occupation as neither a doctor nor a merchant.*)

2.3.2 Other Forms of Nomenclature

Because of their fundamental roles in scientific information, the five types of scales and data have received considerable attention from statisticians and psychosocial scientists, who have labeled the scales with many different titles. For dimensional data, we have already met the terms *interval* and *ratio*, which are used by psychologists, and *continuous*, used by statisticians. To distinguish the arbitrary non-dimensional categories, ordinal, binary, or nominal data are sometimes called *attribute data, categorical data*, or *discrete data* (although the last term is ambiguous, because integer dimensions are also discrete).

Being readily added, multiplied, and otherwise manipulated mathematically, dimensional data are sometimes called *quantitative data*, whereas categorical data, which can only be enumerated and cited as frequency counts, are sometimes called *qualitative* or *quantal data*.

For practical purposes as well as simplicity, we can escape all of the possible jargon by using five main terms: *dimensional, quasi-dimensional, ordinal, binary,* and *nominal*. To indicate the arbitrary categories of non-dimensional scales, they are sometimes here called *categorical*, although the term *non-dimensional* will usually convey the desired distinction.

2.4   Multi-Component Variables

Variables can also be classified according to their number of components and timing of component states. Regardless of the type of scale, a single variable can contain one component or more than one. A *simple* variable has only one main component; a *multi-component* or *composite* variable has more than one. A variable can also refer to only one stated condition, or to two or more states.

2.4.1   Composite Variables

A composite variable contains a combination of data from two or more component variables. Each component variable, expressed in its own scale, is "input" that is aggregated to form a separate "output" scale. For example, the *Apgar Score* for the condition of a newborn baby is a composite variable. Its output scale, ranging from **0** to **10**, is a sum of ratings for five simple variables — representing *heart rate, respiration, skin color, muscle tone,* and *reflex response* — each cited in its input scale of **0, 1,** or **2**. Although the aggregation can be an "additive score," some composite variables are formed as "Boolean clusters." A Boolean cluster contains a combination of categories joined in logical unions or intersections. For example, the TNM staging system for cancer contains categorical ratings for three component variables representing *Tumor, Nodes,* and *Metastases*. The individual ratings, which might be cited as **T5N1M0** or **T2N0M2**, are often combined into an ordinal set of clustered categories called *stages*. In one common pattern, **Stage III** represents patients who have distant metastases, regardless of the ratings for tumor and regional nodes. **Stage II** represents patients with involvement of regional nodes *and* no evidence of distant metastases, regardless of the ratings for tumor. **Stage I** represents patients with no evidence of either regional node or distant metastatic involvement.

A composite variable can also be formed from dimensional components. For example, for the variable called *anion gap*, the sum of serum chloride and bicarbonate concentrations is subtracted from the serum sodium concentration. The *Quetelet index* is the quotient of *weight* (in kg.) divided by the square of *height* (in cm.).

Composite variables have many different names. They are sometimes called *indexes, factors, stages, systems, classes, scales, ratings, criteria, multi-dimensional scales,* or *clinimetric indexes*. Although composite variables are usually expressed in dimensional or ordinal scales, some of the most complex constructions have binary existential citations. They occur for variables formed as diagnostic criteria for presence or absence of a particular disease. Thus, in the clinical diagnostic criteria for tuberculosis, rheumatic fever, rheumatoid arthritis, or myocardial infarction, the output scale is a simple binary expression such as **yes** or **no** (or **present** or **absent**). The input, however, consists of multiple variables, arranged in complex patterns, that often form intermediate axes or "subscales" before everything is ultimately aggregated into the binary output rating.

2.4.2   Component States

All of the variables described thus far refer to the *single-state* condition of a particular person at a single point in time. A single variable, however, can also express the comparison of results for two or more states. They can be the single-state condition of two persons, the change noted in a person's single state on several occasions, or descriptions of the same state by several independent observers.

In these situations, the comparative result is often cited as a separate variable, having its own scale for denoting an increment, decrement, or some other comparative distinction in the linked values. For example, if **70 kg** and **68 kg** are the values for two people "matched" in a particular study of weight, the difference between the two single-state values could be cited in a separate variable as **+2 kg** (or **–2 kg**). Alternatively, using a separate ordinal scale, one person could be regarded as **slightly** heavier than the other. In another study, a particular person's single-state values of serum cholesterol might have been **261** before treatment and **218** afterward. The change could be recorded in a separate variable as *fall in cholesterol*: **43**. In a study of observer variability, the S-T wave depression in the same electrocardiogram might be reported as **2.0 mm** by one electrocardiographer and as **2.4 mm** by another. The difference in the two measurements could be expressed in a separate variable as **0.4 mm**.

For the three foregoing examples, the value of the additional variable was calculated from values of the original single-state variables. In other circumstances, however, the change can be rated directly, without specific reference to single-state values. For example, a patient might express *response to treatment* in a rating scale such as **excellent, good, fair, poor** or in specifically comparative terms such as **much better, somewhat better, same, somewhat worse, much worse.** When a comparative change is cited without reference to single-state components, the expression is called a *transition variable.*

The total effect of more than two states in the same person often cannot be expressed in simple comparative terms, such as **larger, smaller,** or **same.** The expressions may therefore describe the *trend* in the entire series of values. Thus, the pattern of successive blood pressure measurements for a particular person might be cited in a scale such as **rising, stable,** or **falling.** Sometimes the general pattern of trend is categorized for its *average value, desirability,* or *diagnostic features.* For example, a set of successive daily values for post-therapeutic pain might be cited for their mean value, or in ratings of the total *response* as **excellent, good, ..., poor.** The set of successive dimensional values in a glucose tolerance curve might be classified as **normal, diabetic,** or **hypoglycemic.**

2.4.3   Scales for Multi-Component Variables

Regardless of how the components are expressed and assembled, multi-component variables are cited in the same types of dimensional, ordinal, binary, or other scales used for single-component variables. Thus, an *Apgar Score* of **10**, a *TNM Stage* of **III**, an *anion gap* of **9**, a *diagnosis* of **acute myocardial infarction**, or a *post-treatment response* of **much improved** could all come from multi-component variables, but could all be analyzed as values in individual variables.

To evaluate the scientific quality of the multi-component expression, however, we would need to consider not only the quality of each component, but also the suitability and effectiveness of the way they have been put together. For example, suppose a composite scale to indicate *satisfaction with life* contained certain weighted ratings for age, occupation, and income. Each of the components might be scientifically measured, but the combination would be an unsatisfactory expression for *satisfaction with life.* As another example, each of the components of the Apgar score might be suitably chosen and appraised, but their aggregate would be unsuitable if reflex responses were rated on a scale of **0, 5, 10** while the other four variables were rated as **0, 1, 2.**

2.5   Problems and Customs in "Precision"

The idea of *precision* is a fundamental concept in both science and statistics, but the concept is used with different meanings in the two domains. Furthermore, the attribute of *numerical precision* is different from ordinary *precision* and is usually a matter of arbitrary custom.

2.5.1   Concepts of Precision

Scientists use *precision* to denote "the quality of being exactly or sharply defined or stated."[2] Thus, the phrase "cachectic, dyspneic, anemic old man" is more precise than the phrase "sick patient." The numerical expression **3.14159** is a more precise value for π than **3.1**. Statisticians, however, use *precision* to refer to "the way in which repeated observations" conform to themselves and ... to the dispersion of the observations."[3] In this idea, a series of repeated measurements of the same entity, or individual measurements of multiple entities, is statistically precise if the spread of values is small relative to the average value. To a scientist, therefore, precision refers to increased detail and is an attribute of a *single* measurement. To a statistician, precision refers to a small spread or range in a *group* of measurements.

This fundamental difference in concepts may cause confusion when scientists and statisticians communicate with one another, using the same word for two different ideas. Furthermore, the difference in concepts leads to different goals in measurement. A prominent aim of scientific measurement is to increase precision by increasing details. Statistics does not have a word to indicate "detail," however, and many statistical activities are deliberately aimed at "data reduction,"[4] which helps eliminate details.

Doing studies of quality control or observer variability in a measurement process, regardless of its precision in detail, the scientist may be surprised to discover that excellent *reproducibility* for the process is regarded by the statistician as *precision*. The scientist may also be chagrined to find that the hard work of developing instruments to measure with high precision may be regarded statistically as producing excessive details to be reduced.

The two sets of concepts can readily be reconciled by recognizing that scientific *precision* refers to individual items of data, whereas statistical *precision* refers to a group of data. In trying to understand or summarize meaning for a group of data, both the scientist and the statistician will reduce the amount of detail conveyed by the *collection* of individual values. This reduction occurs with the formation of statistical indexes that denote the average value, spread, or other attributes of the collective group. Before or while the reduction occurs, however, the individual items of data will require certain policies or customs about the management of numerical precision.

2.5.2 Strategies in Numerical Precision

The idea of numerical precision involves concepts and customs for "significant figures" or "significant digits." In the decimal system of notation, any number can be converted to a standard numerical expression by moving the decimal point so that the number is cited as a value between 0 and 10, multiplied by a power of 10. Thus, .01072 becomes 1.072×10^{-2} and 1072 becomes 1.072×10^{3}. With this convention, a significant figure occurs at the left of the decimal point and the other significant figures occur at the right. The number 15,000 becomes 1.5000×10^{4} and 14,999 becomes 1.4999×10^{4}. Each number has five significant figures.

A prominent challenge in data reduction—at the level of individual values of data—is the decision about how many significant figures (or digits) to retain in each number. The decision will depend on how the number was obtained and how it will be used.

2.5.2.1 *Production of Numbers* — Numbers can be produced by measurement or by calculation, but there are two forms of measurement: mensuration and enumeration.

2.5.2.1.1 Mensuration. This unfamiliar term refers to the most familiar form of scientific measurement: identifying the magnitude of an entity on a calibrated scale. *Mensuration* is used to distinguish this type of measurement from the other type, *enumeration*, which is discussed in the next subsection. In the customary form of mensuration, the scale contains dimensional values, and the number is a measured amount, such as **137** meq/dl for serum sodium concentration or **15.2** units of hemoglobin. With more precise systems of measurement and calibration, sodium might be determined as **137.419** or hemoglobin as **15.23**, but such systems are rarely used because the extra precision is seldom necessary or helpful.

Because precision will depend on the "refinement" of the dimensional scale, decisions must be made about how to report results (i.e., how many significant figures to include) that lie between the two finest units of calibration. For example, if an ordinary ruler is marked at intervals of 1 mm, magnitudes that lie between two marks are often cited at the midpoint and expressed as 1.5 mm., 2.5 mm., etc.

Note that mensurations do not always produce dimensional numbers. With an ordinal, binary, or nominal scale, the result of the mensuration process may be values such as **3+, yes**, or **hepatitis**. The foregoing discussion of mensuration, however, was confined to dimensional numbers.

2.5.2.1.2   Enumeration. This fancy word for counting is often used because it refers to both the process and result and, therefore, offers a single term for the two words, *frequency count*. An enumeration has unlimited precision because the number of significant digits continues to increase as more entities are counted. For example, the census bureau can report counts of 1873 or 2,194,876 people in different regions.

2.5.2.1.3   Calculation. Most of the main numbers used in statistics are calculated from the basic results obtained with mensuration and/or enumeration. For example, as noted later, a *mean* is constructed when a sum of mensurations or enumerations is divided by another enumeration.

During the calculations, numerical precision can be altered in ways that no longer reflect the original precision of measurement. Addition and multiplication may increase the original number of significant digits; subtraction can decrease them; and division can produce either increases or decreases. For example, if one hematocrit is measured with high precision as **23.091** and another as **46,** the sum of **69.091** suggests that both measurements have 5 significant digits. Multiplication of the two numbers would produce the 7 significant digits of **1062.186.** For the three-digit serum calcium values of **11.3** and **10.9,** subtraction loses two digits, yielding **.4.** With division, the ratio of the two-digit ages **84** and **42** produces the one-digit **2,** but the ratio of **56/32** produces the three-digit **1.75.** In some instances, calculation can produce a "repeating" or "unending" decimal having as many significant digits as desired. Thus, 2/3 = .66666666… and 1/22 = .0454545… .

2.5.2.2   Transformations — Some variables are regularly transformed either as raw data or for analytic purposes. The raw-data transformations, often done for scientific custom, can express weight as **kg** rather than **lb**, height in **cm** rather than **in.**, and temperature in °**C** rather than °**F**. Many chemical concentrations today are transformed into standard international units from their original measurements in **mgm** or **Gm.** Other raw-data transformations, done for scientific convenience, will express hydrogen ion concentration as its negative logarithm, called **pH**.

In yet other transformations, used for analytic purposes discussed later, values of *survival time in months* or *bacterial counts* might be converted to logarithms. A series of dimensional values for *hemoglobin* might be compressed into an ordinal array such as **≤8, 9–11, 12–13, 14–15, 16–17,** and **≥18.** A series of values for *serum calcium* might be compressed into the categorical zones **low, normal,** and **high**. These transformations, however, usually occur during the statistical analyses, not in the original expression of the data.

2.5.2.3   Customs in Management — Certain customs have been established to achieve consistency in managing the diverse possibilities for computational alteration of numerical precision. Each custom depends on whether the number is being understood, reported, or formally calculated.

2.5.2.3.1   Understanding. For understanding what the numbers imply, and for doing certain mental or in-the-head calculations that can facilitate comprehension, most people are accustomed to using two significant digits. For example, if two percentages are reported as 49.63% and 24.87%, you may not immediately perceive their comparative relationship. The relationship is promptly apparent, however, when the numbers are "rounded" to 50% and 25%. Because most people have become accustomed to dealing with percentages, which range from 0 to 100 while usually having two digits, the process of comprehension usually requires no more than *two* significant digits.

Furthermore, the digits are usually most rapidly understood when presented in a range of 0 to 100. Thus, the proportions .50 and .25 are easier to compare when expressed in percentages as 50% and 25%. This custom is responsible for the frequency with which proportions are multiplied by 100 and expressed as percentages. The custom is also responsible for the epidemiologic tactic, discussed later, of expressing populational rates in unit values per 10,000 or per 100,000. Thus, an occurrence rate of 217/86,034 might be cited as 25.2×10^{-4} or 252 per hundred thousand rather than .00252.

(Certain tactics in prompt understanding will work with "convenient" numbers rather than significant digits. For example, if you see a number such as $\sqrt{157}$, you can almost immediately recognize that the result lies between 12 and 13 because $12^2 = 144$ and $13^2 = 169$.)

2.5.2.3.2 Reporting. In reporting numbers for readers, three significant digits are usually listed for measured amounts, and two digits for most percentages. The "rules" may be altered, however, if they produce ambiguous discriminations or misleading impressions. For example, two baseball players with "rounded" averages of .333 after the last day of the season may be tied for the batting championship. The winner, determined with extra decimal places, will be the batter with 216/648 = .3333 rather than 217/652 = .3328. Among a series of percentages, one member of the group may be listed as 0% because the proportion 2/483 = .00414 was rounded to 0 when converted to integers between 0 and 100. To avoid confusion between this 0 and another that arises as 0/512, the first one can be cited as 0.4%.

An unresolved custom in reporting is whether to use a "leading" **0** before the decimal point in numbers such as **.183**. Frequently seen expressions such as **P < .05** need not be reported as **P < 0.05,** but some writers believe that the leading zero, as in **0.183**, helps improve clarity in both typing and reporting. Other writers believe the leading **0** is a waste of space. In computer or other printouts of integer digits, numbers such as 01 or 08 look peculiar, but are increasingly used and accepted. (In this text, the leading zeros will be omitted except when needed to avoid ambiguity.)

2.5.2.3.3 Calculating. In contrast to the truncated two or three digits used for understanding and reporting, calculations should always be done with all pertinent digits retained during the calculation. Any truncation (or "rounding") of "trailing" digits on the right should be reserved until everything is done, when the final result is reported. The rule to follow is "Round at the end." Keep all numbers as intact as possible throughout the calculation and save any rounding until all the work is completed.

The rule is particularly important if you use an electronic hand calculator that can store no more than 9 digits. Many personal digital computers work in "single precision" with 6 digits or in "double precision" with 12. In the latter situation, or when a mainframe computer works with 24 significant digits in "extended precision," the computer seldom has problems in rounding. The reader of the printout may then be suffused with an excess of trailing digits, however, when the computer displays results such as ".04545454545" for divisions such as 1/22.

2.5.3 Rounding

Many people in the world of medicine learned about mathematical *rounding* long before the same word was applied in patient care. In mathematics, rounding consists of eliminating trailing digits at the right end of a number. The excess digits are those beyond the stipulated boundary of two, three, or sometimes more "significant figures."

With simple truncation, the trailing digits are chopped off directly with no "adjustment" of previous digits. With rounding, the previous adjacent digits are adjusted; and the adjustment may involve more than one digit. Thus, **19.09** might be rounded to **19** for two digits and **19.1** for three, but **19.99** would become **20** or **20.0.**

The rounding process is simple and straightforward if the terminal digits are between 0–4 and 6–9. If <5, the candidate digit is dropped without further action. If the candidate is >5, the preceding digit is incremented one unit. Thus, 42.7 becomes 43; 42.4 becomes 42; and 5378 becomes 5380 (or 5400 with more drastic rounding).

The only pertinent problem is what to do when the terminal digit is exactly 5 or has the sequence of 5000... . In many branches of science (and in most hand-held calculators), the rule is simple: If the last digit is ≥5, round upward. With this rule, 42.5 would become 43. A statistical argument has been offered, however, that the strategy is biased. Of the ten candidate digits, four (1, 2, 3, 4) are rounded down; four (6, 7, 8, 9) are rounded up; and one (0) has no effect. Therefore, a bias toward higher values will occur if all terminal 5's are rounded upward. To avoid this problem, terminal 5's are rounded to the preceding even digit. Thus, 17.5, having an odd digit before the 5, is rounded upward to 18; but 16.5, with an even digit before the 5, is rounded down to 16. With this tactic, the *preceding* digits of 0, 2, 4, 6, 8 are left intact, but 1, 3, 5, 7, 9 are rounded upward.

You may now want to argue that the procedure produces a bias toward getting *even* terminal digits. This bias might be a problem for betting in roulette, but should not be a difficulty in quantitative calculations. In fact, the rule would work just as well and the results would be just as "unbiased" if rounding were aimed toward a preceding odd rather than even digit. The *even* direction is probably maintained because rounding toward an even number is easier to remember than rounding "odd." If you (or your calculator) happen to neglect the rule, and if terminal 5's are routinely rounded upward, however, no great disasters are likely to occur.

Bear in mind that the round-even strategy applies only when the terminal nonzero digit is 5 (or 50000...). Otherwise, use the simple rule of rounding up for > 5 and down for < 5.

Like any other set of rules, the foregoing recommendations have exceptions that occur for discrimination, identification, and decrementation.

2.5.3.1   *Discrimination* — If the relative magnitude of two numbers must be discriminated, rounding can be counterproductive, as in the previous illustration of ranking baseball players. If the extra digits are needed to discriminate distinctions, do not round.

2.5.3.2   *Identification* — Among a series of percentages ranging from 1% to 99%, one member of the group may have the proportion 2/483 = 0.4%. If listed with no more than two integer digits, this result would be a misleading 0%. To avoid the problem, the rule can be "bent" for an exception listing the result as 0.4%.

2.5.3.3   *Decrementation* — Trailing digits are particularly important when two numbers are subtracted, because the size of the decrement may be determined entirely from distinctions in last few digits. A disastrous statistical syndrome, called *premature rounding*, occurs when trailing digits are "ejaculated" too soon. The malady can occur with hand-calculator determination of an entity called *group variance*, which precedes the determination of a standard deviation in Chapter 4.

2.6   Tallying

Despite the advances of electronic computation, you may sometimes (or often) find yourself doing enumeration by counting the frequency of data in a set of nominal, ordinal, or binary categories. Doing it manually can save a great deal of effort if you have a relatively small amount of data. By the time everything gets punched and verified for electronic processing, the manual tally can be long done, checked, and tabulated. For example, suppose a questionnaire returned by 150 people contains ratings of 1, 2, 3, 4, or 5 for each of 4 statements, A, B, C, and D. You want to know and summarize the distribution of frequency counts for the ratings. The rapid manual way to do this job is to prepare a "tally box" or "tally table" that has the skeleton shown in Figure 2.1.

The next step is to go through the questionnaires, one at a time, putting an appropriate tally in the columns for the rating given to A, B, C, and D by each person. With a convenient method of tallying, the frequency counts are evident as soon as you have completed the last questionnaire.

2.6.1   Conventional Methods

The conventional method of tallying uses a vertical slash or up-and-down mark for each of four tallies, then a diagonal mark through the fifth. The first two marks would be | |, the first four would be | | | |; the fifth would be ⫴. With this tactic, the tally ⫴ ⫴ ⫴ | | | would promptly be identified as 18.

Complete 'cheng'	Writing Sequence				
	(1)	(2)	(3)	(4)	(5)
正	一	丁	千	疔	正

The Chinese Character Cheng

Age in Years	Tally Mark	Frequency in Group
5	正 下	8
6	正 正 丁	12
7	正 正 正 一	16
8	正 正 正 丁	17
9	正 正 丁	12
10	正	5
Total		70

FIGURE 2.1
Illustration of a "Tally box" with five possible ratings for four statements.

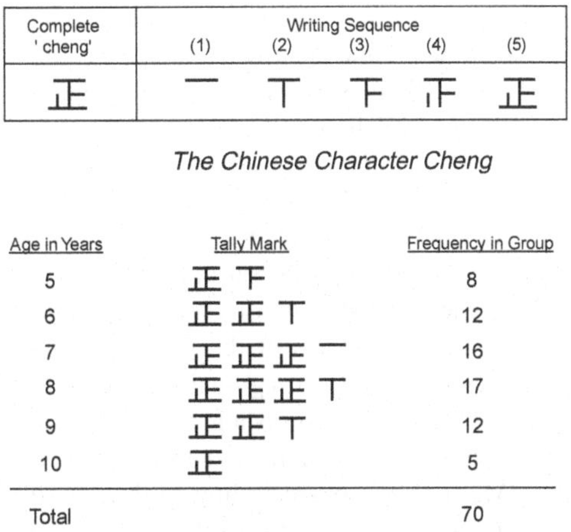

FIGURE 2.2
Alternative approach for tallying. [Taken from Chapter Reference 5.].

2.6.2 Alternative Methods

An alternative way of bunching groups of five, proposed by K. H. Hsieh,[5] is the Chinese tally count, which is based on the five strokes used in the Chinese character *cheng*. According to Hsieh, the result is "neater and easier to read than a series of slashes"; and because "an incomplete character can be identified at a glance," the method avoids having "to count carefully to see if four slashes have been recorded" before crossing the fifth. The upper part of Figure 2.2 shows the writing sequence for forming *cheng*, and the lower part illustrates its application in a tally table.

John Tukey[6] has proposed a system of dots and lines that shows 10, rather than 5, for each completed visual group. In the Tukey system, : : is 4, then lines are drawn around the periphery to form a box (so that ⊓ is 7). Diagonal lines are then drawn so that ⊠ is 10.

Any of the tally methods will work well if you become familiar and comfortable with it, and use it carefully. The Tukey method has the advantage of saving space if only a small area is available for the tally box.

References

1. Stevens, 1946; 2. Lapedes, 1974; 3. Kendall, 1971; 4. Ehrenberg, 1975; 5. Hsieh, 1981; 6. Tukey, 1977.

Exercises

2.1. The skeleton table in Section 2.2 contains variables for age, height, sex, diagnosis, treatment, and three values of blood pressure.

2.1.1. Identify the scale of each of those variables according to the classifications listed in Section 2.3.1.

2.1.2. You have been asked to prepare an analysis of the response of blood pressure to treatment. You can use the three cited values of blood pressure to form any additional variables you might wish to analyze. Indicate what those variables might be and how they would be formed.

2.2. The variable age is almost always expressed in a dimensional scale. Prepare transformations of the data that will express age in three different scales that are ordinal, binary, and nominal. Cite the contents of the categories that form the new scales.

2.3. The value of a variable expressing a change in state is usually determined by direct comparison of results in two single-state variables. Occasionally, however, a transition variable is created during clinical activities without specifically establishing two individual single-state values. Give an example of a question you might ask a patient (or about a patient) in which the answer would produce data that can be directly classified as a transition variable.

2.4. In Section 2.4.1, a composite variable was created by combining two or more separate variables. Can you give at least one example of a nonmedical phenomenon, occurring in daily life, that is regularly expressed as a composite variable?

2.5. In the TNM system for classifying patients with cancer, the *T* is expressed in 4 or 5 categories for rating certain attributes of the primary tumor. The *N* contains three ordinal categories for rating the spread of the tumor to regional lymph nodes. The *M* contains three ordinal categories for rating the spread of the tumor to distant metastatic sites. With numerical ratings assigned to each category, the results for a particular patient may be cited in such TNM index expressions as T3N1M0, T2N0M1, T1N2M2, and so on. According to the classifications you have learned in this chapter, what kind of a scale is this? Give the reasons for your decision.

2.6. Using the five types of classification listed in Section 2.3.1, what kind of scales are formed by the Apgar Score, TNM Stage, anion gap, and Quetelet index?

2.7. In extracting data from medical records, an investigator decides to cite *age in years* according to decade. The scale of categories will be **0, 1, 2, 3, ..., 8, 9** according to ages **0–9, 10–19, 20–29, 30–39, ..., 80–89,** and **≥ 90.** What do you foresee as the advantages and disadvantages of this scale when the extracted data are later analyzed statistically?

2.8. Find a set of diagnostic criteria for any disease in which you are interested. *Briefly* outline the construction of the criteria and classify the scale used to express the result.

2.9. From any literature at your disposal, find a variable that has been reported with what you regard as unsatisfactory precision, or that seems to have been categorized or coded in an unsatisfactory manner. The categorization or coding is "unsatisfactory" if you do not like the chosen categories, cannot determine how they were identified or demarcated, or believe that the selected codes were inadequate. For example, you might complain about a component of the Apgar Score if you think that heart rate should have been divided into four categories rather than three, if you cannot decide where to assign a baby with a heart rate of 100, if you would have difficulty using the stated criteria for scoring *muscle tone*, or if you think that *muscle tone* is not a "sensible" or sufficiently important variable to be included in the total score.

All that is needed for the answer here is one complaint. You need not identify or include a copy of the source publication, but please say enough about the topic or circumstances for your complaint to be clearly understood and justified.

Part I

Evaluating a Single Group of Data

If individual items of data are the statistical counterpart of biologic "molecules," groups of data are the "cells." In fact, the word *cell* is regularly used in statistics to denote the particular group of data in each location of the basic entity called a *table*. Just as cells are the smallest viable structure in biology, a group of data for a single variable—containing information such as each person's diastolic blood pressure, sex, clinical stage, or principal diagnosis—is the smallest analyzable structure in statistics.

The next seven chapters describe the many things that might be done with such a "univariate" group of data. The activities extend all the way from simple descriptive summary indexes, such as medians and standard deviations, to more complicated inferential calculations, such as standard errors, confidence intervals, and a "one-sample" t-test. This long tour through a single group of data will also include the main conventional activities of statistical inference — probabilities and parametric sampling — and some attractive new procedures made possible by modern computers: jackknife analyses and bootstrap resampling.

If you become impatient with the amount of attention being given to a single group, please bear in mind that (1) as a counterpart of the cells of biology, the phenomena have fundamental importance in statistics; and (2) all the activities of "advanced" statistics are essentially an extension of what can happen for a single group. If you understand the univarate descriptions and inferences, the rest is relatively easy.

Part 1

Evaluating a Single Group of Data

3

Central Index of a Group

CONTENTS

The items in a large collection of data can always be examined individually, but the collection cannot be interpreted until it receives a meaningful summary. To "make sense" of a collection of individual items of data, we begin by forming groups, inspecting the spectrum of data in each group, and choosing appropriate summaries for each spectrum. This chapter is concerned with the crucial first choice in that summary: a central index.

3.1 Formation of a Group

Most statistical discussions begin with the idea that a "sample" has been obtained and is about to be analyzed. In most medical activities, however, the idea of a sample is often misleading because a process of "sampling" did not occur.

Instead, the investigator usually collects data from conveniently available groups of people. Sometimes the group is "natural," consisting of everyone who came to the emergency room or received a particular treatment during a specified interval of time. Often the group is more "artificial," containing the individual persons who decided to respond to a mailed questionnaire or who volunteered for a special test. Sometimes the group may contain not individual people but a set of observations obtained repeatedly for the same person.

The way that groups are chosen and formed is an important scientific issue that is commonly overlooked when statistical procedures are applied. As an arbitrarily defined collection of conveniently available people, most groups are usually biased either for representing a larger population or for being compared with one another. The prevention, evaluation, and management of these biases are prime challenges in scientific architecture, but the statistical discussion here will proceed with the assumption that the groups have been suitably formed. The statistical goals are to prepare a "univariate" summary of the data for each variable in a group.

3.2   Role of Summary Indexes

The summary of a group is used for both internal and external purposes. *Internally*, it is a reference point for locating the relative status of individual members within the group. Is a particular person much older or much younger than the other people? *Externally*, the summary index locates the group for comparison with the outside general world or with some other selected group. Thus, we might want to know whether a particular collection of people contains mainly children or octogenarians or whether the group is generally older than a compared group. In other external activities, we may examine the relationship of one variable, such as *age*, to other variables, such as *serum cholesterol* and *survival time*.

The formation of a summary often receives perfunctory statistical attention. After a description of the *means* that offer an "index of central tendency" and the *standard deviations* that offer an "index of spread," the discourse promptly advances to more "interesting" topics: the inferential statistical procedures used for analyzing the summarized data. If the descriptive data have prime scientific importance, however, the choice of summary expressions is a key decision, requiring substantial thought and attention.

At least three major problems can arise if we merely calculate means and standard deviations, while ignoring the main scientific goals and the other statistical options:

1. *Representation:* The mean or other value chosen as a central index becomes the one single number that repeatedly represents the group thereafter, in all of the internal and external comparisons. If this central index is unsatisfactory, the group will not be adequately represented.

2. *Distortion:* If the spread of the data in the group's spectrum is denoted by the standard deviation, and if the standard deviation is not an effective index of spread, the data will be inadequately represented and possibly distorted for internal placement of relative locations, for various external comparisons, and for analytic correlations with other variables.

3. *Omission:* Many important clinical phenomena are expressed in categorical data, which cannot be summarized with means and standard deviations. Consequently, a focus on only the latter two indexes will omit the challenge of getting suitable summaries for non-dimensional variables.

For all these reasons, the role and choice of summary indexes require careful attention. The rest of this chapter is devoted to indexes of central tendency. The next two chapters are concerned with indexes of internal location and spread.

3.3   Spectrum (Distribution) of a Group

To choose appropriate summary indexes, the first step is to see what is in the data. The collection of values in the group form what is usually called a *spectrum* by biologic scientists and a *distribution* by statisticians. The contents and "shape" of the spectrum will indicate how best to summarize the results.

3.3.1 Displaying the Spectrum

A spectrum is arranged, displayed, and summarized differently for non-dimensional and dimensional data.

3.3.1.1 One-Way Frequency Tabulations — Non-dimensional data are usually displayed in a "one-way table" showing frequency counts and the relative frequencies (or proportions) for each categorical value. The results are called "one-way tables" because only a single variable is tabulated. Figure 3.1 shows the contents of such a table for the ordinal variable, *TNM stage*, in a group of 200 patients with lung cancer. The distribution has its highest individual proportions (25.5 and 34.0 percent) at the two "ends" of the data. The lowest proportion (9.0 percent) is in the "middle." (The "cumulative" frequencies marked in Figure 3.1 will be discussed in Chapter 4.)

TNM STAGE

TNM STAGE	Frequency	Percent	Cumulative Frequency	Cumulative Percent
I	51	25.5	51	25.5
II	27	13.5	78	39.0
IIIA	18	9.0	96	48.0
IIIB	36	18.0	132	66.0
IV	68	34.0	200	100.0

FIGURE 3.1
Distribution of TNM stages in 200 patients with lung cancer.

Dimensional data can also be displayed in one-way tables, but a "pattern" may not become apparent if the spectrum contains too many individual values.

3.3.1.2 Stem-Leaf Plots — To show the pattern of dimensional data, John Tukey[1] introduced the display called a *stem-leaf plot*. For this plot, each numerical value of data is split into two parts: the left side becomes a *stem*, and the right side, a *leaf*. For example, the numbers 114, 120, 93, 107, 128, 99, and 121 might be split as 11|4, 12|0, 9|3, 10|7, 12|8, 9|9, and 12|1. In the tabulated plot, the leaves are listed consecutively next to each common stem. In the foregoing group of values, which has three 12 stems and two 9 stems, the plot would be

```
12|081
11|4
10|7
 9|39
```

The number of digits in the available values will determine where to place the splits that separate stems and leaves. The subsequent plot can then be constructed simply and rapidly to show the spread, concentration, and shape of the data.

Figure 3.2 shows a stem-leaf plot for the values of hematocrit in 200 patients with lung cancer. The stems extend from **24** to **56**; and most of the leaves are **0** because hematocrit values are usually recorded as integers. The column on the right shows the number of leaves at each stem.

3.3.1.3 Histograms — Before stem-leaf plots were invented and became generally available via commercial computer programs, dimensional data were often displayed with histograms. (The term is a reduced combination of history-gram; it has nothing to do with histology.)

Instead of demarcations formed by the stems of leading digits, the data are divided into a series of intervals. Instead of showing the trailing digit(s) as leaves, the number of items are counted as frequencies for each interval. When placed on a graph, the X-axis for the results indicates the boundaries of each interval, and the Y-axis, the associated frequency counts or their relative proportional frequencies. The graph forms a *frequency polygon*, if shown with points, and a *histogram*, if shown with bars.

Stem	Leaf	#
56	0	1
55		
54	0	1
53	00	2
52	0	1
51	00	2
50	000000	6
49	000	3
48	000009	6
47	0001	4
46	0000000	8
45	00000000000006	15
44	000000000000	12
43	00000000000555	15
42	000000000000000009	19
41	00000000047	11
40	0000000000000005	16
39	00000000000003399	18
38	00000000004	11
37	0000000000558	13
36	000033	6
35	0000000	7
34	000000255	9
33	0000003	7
32	07	2
31	00	2
30	0	1
29		
28	0	1
27		
26		
25		
24	0	1

FIGURE 3.2
Stem-leaf plot for values of hematocrit in 200 patients with lung cancer.

To illustrate the procedures, consider the data of Table 3.1. For the raw values of data in the left-hand column, the boundaries of intervals are chosen arbitrarily. In one common approach, at least seven intervals are used for the spread of the data; in another approach each interval spans 5 dimensional units. Both tactics can be used to divide the data of Table 3.1 into seven intervals: **10–14, 15–19, ...,** and **40–44** units. The results for relative frequency are graphed in Figure 3.3 as both a frequency polygon and a histogram.

Table 3.2 shows a stem-leaf plot, prepared with an ordinary typewriter, for the data of Table 3.1. (Each digit must be given equal width if a stem-leaf plot is prepared by hand or by a typewriter that ordinarily shortens the width of the digit 1.) The horizontal pattern shown in Table 3.2 is essentially identical to the vertical pattern in Figure 3.3.

3.3.2 Inspection of Shape

The *shape* of a distribution is the pattern formed by the frequencies (or relative frequencies) displayed at each of the categorical values, stems, or demarcated intervals. For non-dimensional data, the shape is not particularly important because, as noted later, it does not affect the choice of summary indexes. For dimensional data, however, the patterns — when arranged vertically rather than in horizontal stem-leaf plots — can form the series of shapes shown in Figure 3.4.

TABLE 3.1

Raw Data, Interval Values, and Relative Frequencies

Raw Data	Demarcated Intervals	Frequency Count	Relative Frequency (%)
12,14,12,11,13	10–14	5	9
15,18,17,17,16,19,19,18,15 17,16,16,17,19,15,17,19,16,18	15–19	19	34
21,24,20,22,22,21,24,20 23,21,22,24,21	20–24	13	23
28,26,29,28,28,25 29,26,28,29	25–29	10	18
33,30,34,33	30–34	4	7
36,39,37	35–39	3	5
41,43	40–44	2	4
TOTAL		56	100

TABLE 3.2

Stem-Leaf Plot for Data in Table 3.1

4*	13
3•	697
3*	3043
2•	8698859689
2*	1402214031241
1•	5877699857667957968
1*	24213

Note: The symbol * is used for leaves having values of 0–4; the • symbol is for values of 5–9.

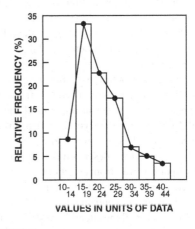

FIGURE 3.3

Histogram (*rectangles*) and frequency polygon (*dots and lines*) for data contained in Table 3.1.

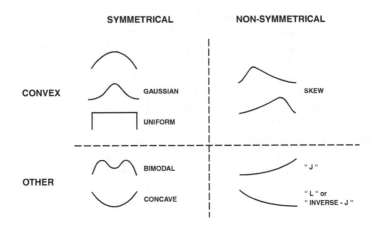

FIGURE 3.4

Shapes of different distributions of data. The vertical axes for each shape are relative frequencies of occurrence for the values (or intervals) in the horizontal axes.

These univariate patterns are sometimes mistakenly regarded as bivariate, because the graphs seem to have two variables, placed along an X- and Y-axis. The entity on the Y-axis, however, is not a variable. It is a statistic determined from counting the available values, not from acts of individual measurement. The Y-axis shows frequency counts or relative proportions for each category of the single variable on the X-axis.

3.3.2.1   Catalog of Shapes — The shapes in Figure 3.4 can be catalogued as convex or other, and as symmetrical and non-symmetrical.

Most patterns have one or more crests that form a basically *convex* shape, with small relative frequencies at one end of the distribution, rising toward one or more crests in the interior and falling toward the other end. With a single crest at the center of the curve, the convex shape is also *symmetrical*. The famous "bell" or "cocked-hat" shape of the Gaussian (or "normal") distribution has an essentially symmetrical convex pattern. (The distribution will be called Gaussian throughout this text to avoid the medical ambiguity produced when statistical jargon refers to this shape as "normal"). Another shape that can be regarded as symmetrically convex is a *uniform* (or rectangular) distribution. When the single crest is asymmetrically off-center, located toward one of the exterior ends, the distribution is called *skew*. The frequency polygon in Figure 3.3 has a right skew pattern.

A symmetrical distribution need not be convex. Symmetrical shapes can also be produced by a *bimodal* distribution with two distinctive crests and by a *concave* distribution with a U-shaped trough. (The latter type of shape would be produced by the data in Figure 3.1.) Bimodal and concave distributions can also be asymmetrical, according to the location of the crests and troughs.

A *sloping* distribution does not have the fall-rise-fall or rise-fall-rise pattern of any of the previous shapes. Instead, the curve of relative frequencies is "monotonic," continuously rising toward (or falling from) a crest that occurs at one end of the distribution. One type of sloping distribution is sometimes called *J-shaped*; another type is called *inverse-J-shaped*, or *L-shaped*. Statisticians often use the word *exponential* for these sloping shapes.

Shapes can also be described as *centripetal* if their crest (or crests) are somewhere near the center of the distribution away from either end. All basically convex shapes are centripetal. The shape is *centrifugal* if the crests are located at the ends, or if no specific crest occurs. The uniform, concave, and sloping distributions are all centrifugal.

The reason for all the attention to shape is that symmetrical distributions — whether convex or concave, centripetal or centrifugal — can be well represented by the means and standard deviations discussed later. All other distributions are eccentric and may require other types of summary indexes to avoid distortions.

3.3.2.2   Outliers — When arranged in ascending or descending order of magnitude, the items of a dimensional distribution are usually close to one another, forming a shape that seems well "connected" from its lowest to highest values. Sometimes, however, a large gap may occur between the main bulk of the data and one or more values at the extreme ends.

The extreme values, called *outliers*, create two types of problems. First, they may sometimes arise as errors in observing or transferring data. The error can be immediately detected if it represents an impossible value. For example, values of **–21** or **275** for *age in years* are obviously erroneous. A value of **275** for *weight in kg.* is unusual but not necessarily an error. (A complex *scientific* decision is whether to accept an outlier value as unusual or to discard it as erroneous.)

The second problem arises if non-symmetrical outlier values, which produce an eccentric shape, are accepted and included in the data. To avoid the possible distortion of summary indexes calculated as means and standard deviations, the raw data may be transformed (as noted in Section 3.8.1) into scales that reduce the impact of outliers, or the summary indexes can be chosen with methods that are unaffected by outliers.

3.4 Types of Summary Indexes

At least two types of *indexes of location* are used to summarize a set of data. For external comparisons, an *index of central tendency*, or *central index*, will represent the entire group of data when it is referred to the outside world. For this purpose, we want something that represents the group by being particularly typical, common, or central in the distribution. For internal comparisons, an *index of cumulative relative frequency* (or *percentile*) will locate the items of data with reference to one another. These (and other) indexes of inner location can also indicate the spread or dispersion of the data around the central index.

3.5 Indexes of Central Tendency

Although no single index can perfectly represent an array of values, we want something that will do the best possible job. The job will vary for non-dimensional or dimensional data.

3.5.1 Indexes for Non-Dimensional Data

Non-dimensional data are often summarized not with a single central index, but with an apportionment that shows the relative frequencies of each category. This type of expression, marked "percent," was used to summarize the five categories listed in Figure 3.1.

If a group has c categories, and if n_i represents the number of members in category i, the total size of the group will be $N = n_1 + n_2 + n_3 + ... + n_c$. The Greek symbol Σ is regularly used to show these summations. Thus, $N = \Sigma n_i = n_1 + n_2 + ... + n_c$. [In strict mathematical usage, the Σ is accompanied by upper and lower symbols that indicate exactly where the summation begins and ends. For the complete collection of data, the result here would be shown as $N = \sum_{i=1}^{c} n_i$. In pragmatic usage, however, the sum almost always extends from the first to the last items. The upper and lower symbols are therefore omitted from the Σ sign.]

The actual frequencies are converted to relative frequencies when cited as proportions of the total group. Thus, the relative proportion of the ith category is $p_i = n_i/N$. In Figure 3.1, which shows 5 categories, the third category has $n_3 = 18$ and N is 200, so that $p_3 = 18/200 = .09$ or 9%.

3.5.1.1   Binary Data — For binary data, only two proportions can be cited. If 35 people have lived and 15 have died in a group of 50, the survival proportion is p = 35/50 = .70 or 70%. The fatality proportion is q = 15/50 = .30 or 30%. Similarly, if a group of 60 people contains 21 women, the proportions are p = .35 for women and q = .65 for men, or vice versa.

Because q = 1 − p as a proportion (and 100 − p as a percentage), each of the two proportions (or percentages) is called the *complement* of the other. The complete spectrum of binary data is effectively summarized with either proportion. The choice of whether to use p or q usually depends on the item of interest, rather than the item that is most common. Thus, the summary of a group might say that 14% of its members have coronary disease, rather than 86% do not.

3.5.1.2   Nominal Data — Suppose a group of patients on a medical service has the following spectrum of nominal diagnoses: **pneumonia**, 8; **myocardial infarction**, 5; **ulcerative colitis**, 1; **stroke**, 4; **cancer**, 6; and **renal failure**, 2. In these 26 people, the relative frequencies of each diagnosis are **pneumonia**, .31 (or 31%) calculated as 8/26; **myocardial infarction**, .19; **ulcerative colitis**, .04; **stroke**, .15; **cancer**, .23; and **renal failure**, .08. To summarize a nominal spectrum, the relatively uncommon items of data are often consolidated into a single category called **other** or **miscellaneous**. Thus, the **ulcerative colitis** and **renal failure** diagnoses might be combined into an **other** category, with frequency of 3 and a relative frequency of .12. For the total spectrum, the individual proportions will add up to 1 (or 100%).

The spread of the spectrum is shown in the array of proportions for each cited category, but a single central index is difficult to choose for nominal data. The best single choice is usually the proportion of the most common item, which is called the *mode*. For the spectrum of the preceding 26 diagnoses, *pneumonia = 31%* would be the best single central index.

Alternatively, certain categories may be consolidated and expressed accordingly. Thus, *myocardial infarction* and *stroke* might be combined, and the central index listed as *cardiovascular = 34%* [= (5 + 4)/26].

3.5.1.3   Ordinal Data — For grades of ordinal data, the central index can come from the proportion of the most common category or from two or more consolidated categories. Suppose *response to treatment* is rated as **poor** in 6 people, **fair** in 12, **good** in 11, and **excellent** in 10. A single summary index could be formed from the mode of **fair** in 31% (= 12/39) or from the consolidated category, **good or excellent,** in 54% (= 21/39). The data in Figure 3.1 could be summarized with the statement that 61% (= 9% + 18% + 34%) of the patients are in the **metastatic** stages of **IIIA, IIIB,** or **IV.**

Because ordinal data can be ranked, the results can be summarized with a *median*, which is the middle value in the ranked grades. In the preceding 39 people, the 20th rank has the middle position. Counting the 20th rank from either end of the data, **good** is the median value. For the 200 people in Figure 3.1, the middle ranks are 100 and 101. **Stage IIIB,** the value at both those ranks, is the median. (Medians are more thoroughly discussed in the next section.)

In some instances, ordinal grades are given arbitrary numerical values, which are then treated as though they were dimensional. Thus, if the foregoing responses were rated as **1** = poor, **2** = fair, **3** = good, and **4** = excellent, the individual ratings might be added and averaged in the same manner shown in the next section for dimensional data. Although the propriety is often disputed, this additive procedure is often applied to ordinal data.

3.5.2   Indexes for Dimensional Data

For dimensional data, three different contenders are immediately available as an index of central tendency: the mode, the median, and the mean. The *mode* is the most common value in the data. It can be determined for any type of data — dimensional or non-dimensional. The *median* is the value that occupies the middle rank when the data are arrayed monotonically in ascending or descending magnitudes. A median can be determined for ordinal as well as dimensional data. The *mean*, as an arithmetical average of the added values, is most properly used only for the equi-interval data of dimensional variables.

Consider the group of data {13, 7, 1, 15, 22, 7, 21}. For these 7 items, the mean is produced with the formula $\Sigma X_i/n = \bar{X}$, when their sum, 86, is divided by the number of items to yield 86/7 = 12.3. The mode is 7, which happens to be the only value that appears more than once in this group. To find the median, we rearrange the values according to their ranks as 1, 7, 7, 13, 15, 21, and 22. The middle-ranked number, 13, is the median.

The mode can be determined, without any calculations, from a simple count of frequencies in the data. The median can also be determined without any substantial calculations. We simply rank the data and count the ranks until reaching the middle one. For N items of data, the median is the value of the item of data that has rank (N + 1)/2 if N is odd. If N is even, (N + 1)/2 is not an integer; and the median occurs between the values in ranks N/2 and (N + 2)/2. By custom, the median is assumed to be midway between them. Thus, in the foregoing array of 7 items, the median was at the rank of (7 + 1)/2 = 4. If the data contained 8 items — arranged as 1, 7, 7, 13, 15, 21, 22, and 25 — the median would be midway between the 4th and 5th items, at the value whose rank is (N + 1)/2 = (8 + 1)/2 = 4.5. There is a 2-unit distance between 13 (the 4th ranked value) and 15, the 5th ranked value. Half of this distance is 1 unit, and so the median would be 13 + 1 = 14.

Each of the three contenders has a reasonable claim for selection as the central index. The *mode* has the right of popularity: it is the most common occurrence. The *median* can argue that its central position is literally in the exact middle (or center) of the array. Half of the items are on one side of the median; half are on the other. The *mean* has the centrality of a fulcrum. It is the point that divides the data by weight. Half of the summed amounts (or weights) of the values are on one side of the mean; half are on the other.

Given these three reasonable options, which should be chosen as the index of central tendency? For people with commercial marketing interests, the best choice is often the *mode*. It lets the vendor know where to find the largest audience of potential buyers for a product. In medical research, however, the mode is generally not a good central index because the data may contain either no naturally occurring mode or several widely separated modal values.

3.5.3 Choice of Median or Mean

With the mode eliminated as a contender, the choice is between the mean or median. For this decision, we need to examine the pattern (or "shape") of the dimensional distribution.

The shapes of the diverse spectrums in Figure 3.4 demonstrate the problems of making a suitable choice. A centripetal distribution can be reasonably represented by a central index, but a centrifugal distribution does not have a central tendency; and any efforts to create one will inevitably be undesirable compromises.

For a symmetrical convex distribution, the mean and median will occur at essentially the same crest of the curve, and so no major decision is necessary. Either choice will give the same value. For a symmetrical distribution that is concave, bimodal, or even multi-modal, no central index can be really satisfactory. Citing a mode would be inadequate, since two or more modes would be needed to represent the two "crests" on either side of the center. The mean and median will have essentially similar values, but neither one will be "typical" of the main bulk of the data, which occurs on both sides of the center. Nevertheless, for lack of anything better, either the mean or the median would seem to be a reasonable compromise in these circumstances.

The main problems and challenges occur for the many medical distributions that are eccentric. Their shape can be overtly centrifugal, or centripetal but non-symmetric, or basically symmetric with distinctive outlier values at the low or high ends of the spectrum. Figure 3.5 illustrates the different locations of the mode, median, and mean in a common type of right-skewed non-symmetrical distribution that creates difficult decisions in choosing a single central index. [A simple mnemonic for remembering the location of the three indexes in a skewed distribution is that they are arranged both statistically and alphabetically starting at the skewed end of the data. Mean precedes median, which precedes mode.]

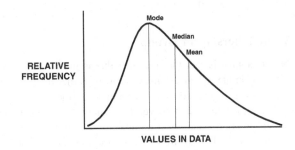

FIGURE 3.5
Customary location of mode, median, and mean in a right-skewed distribution.

3.6 Advantages of the Median

The median has four main descriptive advantages as an index of central tendency. It is better than the mean for summarizing eccentric distributions; it can also be properly used, unlike the mean, for ordinal data; it is often, unlike the mean, an actual member of the data set; and it can be applied, also unlike the mean, to sets containing incomplete longitudinal data.

3.6.1 Eccentric Distributions

The median is preferable to the mean for avoiding problems in summarizing eccentric distributions created by outliers or by asymmetrical (skew) patterns.

3.6.1.1 Avoidance of "Outlier" Distortions — Consider a group of eleven people aged 1, 2, 4, 4, 5, 5, 5, 6, 6, 8, and 97 years. Except for the first and last members of the group, all other values are arranged symmetrically around a central value of 5. If the last value were 9 rather than 97, the entire distribution would be symmetrical, with the mean and median each being 5. The outlier value of 97 substantially distorts the symmetry, however, and raises the mean to a value of 13.0 — an index that misrepresents the group's central location for age and that is not typical for any member of the group. The median, on the other hand, has the advantage of being unaffected by extreme outliers. For the eleven people just listed, the median value would be 5, regardless of what the highest value may be.

3.6.1.2 Use in Asymmetrical (Skew) Distributions — The virtues just cited for the median become more apparent when a distribution is overtly asymmetrical. For a convex skew distribution or for a sloping distribution, the crest of relative frequencies, the median, and the mean will each usually be located at different sites. For example, for the raw data listed in Table 3.1, the mode is 17, the median is 21, and the mean is 22.7. The shape of these data, as shown in Figure 3.3, is skewed to the right — a pattern that commonly occurs in medical data.

The more general pattern of a right-skewed distribution is shown in Figure 3.5. The most "typical" or common values of skew distributions will occur at their crests, which are the modal values that are unsatisfactory as indexes of central tendency. In choosing an alternative central index, the median seems preferable because the outlier values that create the skew will also move the mean far from the crest, leaving the median to fall between the crest and the mean.

The median thus has two advantages over the mean for summarizing an eccentric distribution. Being unaffected by the impact of outlier values, the median will always be consistently located in the central rank of the distribution; and the median will also be closer than the mean to the "popular" values in the crest.

3.6.2 Application to Ordinal Data

Another advantage of the median is that it can readily be applied to ordinal data because its proper calculation does not require dimensional values. In Section 3.5.1.3, the median produced **good** as a central index for 39 ordinal ratings of *response to therapy*, and **Stage IIIB** for 200 cases of lung cancer.

3.6.3 Membership in Group

Another advantage is that the median value is particularly likely to occur in an actual member of the group. For example, when a census report says that the average American family contains **2.3** children (calculated as a mean), you may wonder what the family does with the 0.3 child. If the average is reported as a median of **2**, however, the statement is immediately plausible.

If the group contains an even number of people, however, the median is calculated as an average of two middle values. If they are different, the median will not be a member of the group. Thus, for six people whose ages are 7, 9, 10, 28, 37, and 43, the two middle values would be 10 and 28. The median would be cited as halfway between them, or 19. Although not found in any member of the group, this median value seems reasonable as a central index. (The alternative choice would be a mean of 22.3.)

3.6.4 Application to Incomplete Longitudinal Data

Finally, the median is particularly valuable for expressing results of longitudinal data (such as *length of survival*) in groups where the *mean* value cannot be calculated because some of the people have not yet died (or otherwise ended the follow-up period). For example, suppose 17 patients followed for 3 years after treatment of a particular cancer have survival times that are **1, 2, 2, 3, 3, 3, 4, 4, 5, 6, 6, 7, 12, 17,** and **25** months, and **unknown** for two patients who are still alive after 36 months. The mean survival time cannot be calculated yet for this group; and the result will vary according to whether the two survivors die soon after 36 months or live much longer. The median survival, however, can be determined now. It is 5 months, and will remain at 5 months no matter how long the last two people live.

The median is also helpful as a *single* summary for survival of the group. The survival rates might be reported for individual time points such as 65% (=11/17) at three months, 35% (=6/17) at six months, and 24% (=4/17) at one year; and a survival curve could be drawn to show each temporal rate. To summarize survival with a single quantitative value, however, the best of the available options would be the median of 5 months.

3.7 Disadvantages of the Median

In view of all these advantages of the median, you may wonder why the mean is so commonly used in reports of medical research.

3.7.1 Symbolic

A trivial reason for preferring the mean is that it has a standard symbol, $\overline{X}$, but the median does not. It is sometimes labeled as X_m, M, or X_{med}. This problem can readily be solved, particularly with modern typewriter symbols, by using $\tilde{X}$ for a median.

3.7.2 Computational

A more substantive disadvantage of the median is the enumerative challenge of finding it. The data must be arranged in ranked order and the ranks must be counted to find the middle one. In the days before computers and programmable electronic hand calculators, this ranking procedure could be a nuisance, requiring considerable time to get all the numerical values ranked and then counted for a large group. A mean was easily determined, however, by the simple act of pushing buttons in a mechanical calculator, which would do the adding and dividing.

Today, this disadvantage has little pertinence. With modern computational devices, the median can often be determined just as easily as the mean; and, in fact, with a suitably programmed calculator, both values can emerge from the same act of button pushing.

3.7.3 "Elitist"

With the problem in counting eliminated, the only remaining objections to the median are conceptual. One conceptual complaint is that the median is somewhat "elitist." It is determined from only the middle or the two middlemost values in the data. The rest of the data are used as ranks and counts in finding the median, but do not participate as actual values. Since the choice of a central index is intended to provide intellectual communication rather than participatory populism, this objection does not seem cogent. Besides, a value that denotes "mediocrity" can hardly be regarded as "elitist."

3.7.4 Inferential

The most important conceptual objection to the median is that it seldom appears in the probabilistic reasoning and calculations of inferential statistics.

After being chosen for a group, the central index is often used for inferences about a "parent population," or for stochastic contrasts of "statistical significance" in two groups. The various strategies (confidence intervals, P values, etc.) used for these statistical inferences, as discussed later, have traditionally been developed with concepts that depend on means, rather than medians. Consequently, the mean is usually preferred because it can be analyzed for both descriptive and inferential statistics. Even if a median were used for description, we might still need the mean for inference.

This point is true, but not germane to the main descriptive issues; and the point may eventually become irrelevant for the inferential issues. In description, we want a summary that will communicate as effectively as possible. The median usually offers more effective communication than the mean. In the inferential activities, if a data set is poorly represented by the mean, its use is scientifically unattractive, regardless of whatever traditional mathematical theory may be associated. Most importantly, however, modern computational devices have allowed inferential statistical work to be done with new strategies called *non-parametric, permutation,* or *resampling procedures,* which do not require a mean for the calculations. As these new procedures become more popular and eventually replace the older ones (such as t or Z tests), the communicative advantages of the median will no longer be inhibited by extraneous features of statistical inference.

Until that time arrives, however, you will often see the mean, rather than the median, in most summaries of dimensional data.

3.8   Alternative Approaches

The descriptive problems of using the mean as a central index have led to many proposed substitutions and adjustments, having diverse titles or eponyms. Among the many proposed alternatives, only two are likely to appear in current medical literature: transformations of data and geometric means.

3.8.1   Transformations of Data

Various mathematical transformations have been used to convert non-symmetrical distributions into more symmetrical shapes, from which the mean is then calculated. After the raw data are changed into their square roots, logarithms, or some other suitably chosen value that will produce a "better" pattern, an additive mean is calculated for the transformed data. The result is then converted back to the original units of expression.

For example, in a study of antibody levels to poliomyelitis vaccine, the following values were found in 17 persons: 4, 4, 8, 8, 16, 16, 32, 64, 64, 256, 256, 256, 512, 512, 512, 1024, and 2048. For these skewed data, the median is 64, but the arithmetic mean is the unrepresentative value of 328.9. The data would become more symmetrical (or "Gaussian") if transformed to their logarithmic values (base 10). The logarithms of the 17 antibody values are respectively .60, .60, .90, .90, 1.20, 1.20, 1.51, 1.81, 1.81, 2.41, 2.41, 2.41, 2.71, 2.71, 2.71, 3.01, and 3.31. This distribution seems reasonably symmetrical, and its mean is 1.89. To convert the "log mean" back to the original values, we calculate $10^{1.89}$ and get 78.47. (Note that the reconverted log mean is reasonably close to the median value of 64.)

The logarithmic transformation is particularly useful (and common) for data that have a right skew or high-value outliers. A square root transformation is sometimes applied to help "adjust" data that have a left skew or low-value outliers. A transformation having the delightful eponym of Box-Cox[2] is often mentioned in statistical literature, but rarely (if ever) receives medical usage.

Two other seldom-used transformations are applied for their logical rather than "Gaussianizing" virtues. The *harmonic mean,* calculated from the reciprocals $(1/X_i)$ of the observed values, is often used for averaging rates of speed. The *quadratic mean* or *root mean square,* calculated from the squares of the observed values as $\sqrt{\sum X_i^2/n}$, appears later in the text here as a mechanism for summarizing a set of differences in two measurements of the same entities.

3.8.2   The Geometric Mean

The log-mean transformation was popular in the days before modern electronic calculators. Today, the same result can be calculated directly as an entity called the *geometric mean.* It is obtained by multiplying the N values of observed data and then taking the Nth root of their product. (The advantage of modern calculators is the "y^x" function that allows an easy computation of the Nth root, where y = product of the values and x = 1/N.)

The direct product of the 17 previous antibody values is $4 \times 4 \times 8 \times \ldots \times 512 \times 1024 \times 2048 = 1.622592769 \times 10^{32}$. The 17th (or 1/17) root of this number is 78.47, which is the same as the reconverted log-mean value.

The logarithmic transformation was popular for many years because it could often "Gaussianize" skew data and provide the numerical precursor of the geometric mean. Today, with the ease and rapidity permitted by electronic calculators, the geometric mean can be determined directly with hardly more effort than what is needed to obtain an arithmetic mean.

For people who want a "populist" index of central tendency, the geometric mean has the advantage of including all the values of data in the calculation, but the result is often close to the "elitist" median. This advantage of the geometric mean is lost, however, in several important situations. If any of the data values is 0, the entire product is 0, and the geometric mean must be 0. If the product of the data values is negative, a logarithm cannot be determined and the Nth root of the product (even if calculatable) may be meaningless. A different kind of problem occurs if the data are skewed to the left, rather than rightward. For example, suppose the data set contains the values 1, 62, 67, 67, and 75. The arithmetic mean of this group is 54.4 and the median is 67, but the geometric mean is 29.1, which is farther from the median than the arithmetic mean. On the other hand, if the data set were skewed right, with values of 62, 67, 67, 75, and 200, the arithmetic mean would be 94.2 and the geometric mean of 83.97 would be closer to the median of 67. For these reasons, except perhaps in an all-positive skewed-right distribution, the median is a better general index of central tendency than the geometric mean.

The geometric mean is often preferred, however, if the basic data are expressed "exponentially" in powers of 10 (or some other number) for such entities as bacterial counts and antibody titers. In the earlier example (Section 3.8.1) of 17 antibody levels to poliomyelitis vaccine, all of the values were expressed in exponential powers of 2, and the geometric mean was much better than the arithmetic mean as an index of central tendency. The geometric mean has also been used to summarize the "skewed distribution" of plasma prolactin concentrations[3] and the "log normal distribution" of blood-lead values.[4]

3.8.3   The Midrange

A particularly simple index, the *midrange*, is half of the sum of the minimum and maximum items in the data set. The *midrange* is a good "screening clue" for discerning an asymmetrical distribution, which probably exists if the midrange differs substantially from the ordinary additive mean, $\overline{X}$. In Table 3.1, the midrange of (12 + 43)/2 = 27.5 immediately indicates the asymmetry of the data set, for which the mean is 22.7.

3.8.4   "Robust" Means

In modern new approaches, called Exploratory Data Analysis (EDA),[5] the mean is still determined by addition, but is made more "robust" by different methods of thwarting the effect of outliers. The calculations use various tactics to eliminate or "trim" the extremes of the data. The results have names such as trimmed mean, Tukey's tri-mean, Studentized mean, Windsorized mean, and Hempel adjusted mean; and new suggestions are constantly proposed in the literature of statistics and data processing.

The mathematical attraction of the "robust means" seldom overcomes both their unfamiliarity and their inapplicability for inferential (rather than descriptive) statistics. The median seems much simpler and more intuitively appealing as a descriptive mechanism for avoiding the effects of outliers.

References

1. Tukey, 1972; 2. Sakia, 1992; 3. Baron, 1986; 4. Fulton, 1987; 5. Tukey, 1977.

Exercises

3.1. Which of the three central indexes — mean, median, and mode — would you choose to summarize the central tendency of the data in Table 3.1 and Figure 3.3? Why?

3.2. The results of a clinical trial are presented in a two-way table as follows:

Outcome	Number of Patients Who Received		
	Treatment A	Treatment B	Treatment C
Success	40	70	50
Failure	320	280	295

3.2.1. Classify the types of variables under assessment in this table.

3.2.2. What proportion of patients received Treatment A?

3.2.3. How would you summarize the results for success with Treatment C?

3.2.4. If you had to give a single index for the success achieved in this entire trial, what would you choose?

3.3. A group of patients on a medical service shows the following values for fasting blood sugar: 62, 78, 79, 80, 82, 82, 83, 85, 87, 91, 96, 97, 97, 97, 101, 120, 135, 180, 270, and 400. Calculate or demonstrate the following indexes for these data: mean, median, mode, geometric mean.

3.4. Using any method you want to apply for estimating shape, classify the shape of the distribution of data in Exercise 3.3.

4

Indexes of Inner Location

CONTENTS

For the *external* role of showing an "average" general location, the central index lets us know whether the members of a group are mainly children or octogenarians, fat or thin, rich or poor, high or low achievers — or somewhere in between. The central index also represents each group when it is compared to decide whether some other group is older, fatter, richer, or more achieving.

An index of inner location has a different job. It shows the relative position of individual members internally within the group. If told that someone had the 10th highest score in a certification test, we might be impressed if the group contained 273 people, and unimpressed if it contained 11. In another group with a central index of **80,** a value of **75** seems relatively close to the center — only 5 units away. The actual closeness of the **75** item, however, depends on all the other items of data. In the data set {75, 77, 77, 79, 79, 79, 81, 81, 81, 83, 83, 85} the **75** is relatively far away, separated by five intermediate items.

4.1   Analytic Roles of Inner Locations

An index of inner location can have four important roles in description and subsequent analysis.

1. The most obvious role is to identify members of a group as being relatively near or far from the center.
2. In a subsequent role, indexes of inner location can demarcate boundaries for *inner zones* that contain selected proportions of the data.
3. The size of the inner zones can indicate the data set's relative compactness or dispersion.
4. The relative dispersion of the data can then be used to assess the adequacy and (later) the stability of the central index itself.

The last three roles of indexes of inner location will be discussed in subsequent chapters. The rest of this chapter is concerned with the indexes themselves. The two most commonly used expressions are *percentiles* and *standard deviations*. The *percentile* index is simple, obvious, and direct: it relies on counting the relative "depth" of ranked items in the observed distribution. The *standard deviation*, as a calculated entity, is more complex, but is currently more popular because it has become a traditional statistical custom.

4.2   Percentiles

Percentiles are points that divide a set of ranked (dimensional or ordinal) data into proportions. At the 25th percentile point, .25 or 25% of the data are below the cited value, and 75% are above. The 50th percentile point divides the data into two equal halves.

The proportions are easy to determine because each member of a set of n items occupies a 1/n proportion of the data. The ranking can be done in either direction — from low values toward high, or vice versa — but as the ranks ascend (or descend), the proportions accumulate so that the first r ranks will occupy r/n of the data. For example, in the 56-item data set of Table 3.1, each item occupies 1/56 = .018 of the data. At the 39th rank, the first 39 items will occupy 39/56 = .696 of the data.

4.2.1   Problems in Identification

The concept is easy to describe and understand, but its application produces three tricky problems: shared boundaries, intra-item percentiles, and shared ranks.

4.2.1.1   *Shared Boundaries* — The proportions occupied by two adjacent members of a data set have boundaries that "touch" or are shared by the upper end of the first and the lower end of the second. For example, in a five-item data set, the first item occupies the proportions 0–.20; the second item

occupies .20–.40; the fifth occupies .80–1.00. To do the demarcation properly, the corresponding percentile point is located between the two items that might claim it. Thus, in the five-item data set, the 20th percentile would be placed between the first and second items, and the 80th percentile would be between the fourth and fifth.

When adjacent items "touch" the pertinent proportions, the in-between location allows the percentile to be additively reciprocal. Thus, the percentile point, P, when counted in one direction, will be $100-P$ when counted in the opposite direction. If we went from high to low ranks instead of from low to high in the five-item data set, the 20th percentile would become the 80th, and vice versa. The direction of counting ranks is unimportant as long as it is used consistently, because the percentile in one direction is always the additive reciprocal of the percentile in the other.

4.2.1.2   *Intra-Item Percentiles* —
In mathematical theories for "continuous" data, each value is a point of infinitesimal width on a curve. In pragmatic reality, however, each item of data occupies its own zonal proportion of the total collection. This attribute creates problems in the small data sets that are commonly analyzed in biomedical research, because certain percentiles may be contained *within* an item of data.

For example, in a five-item data set, the first item occupies the proportions 0–.20; and any of the percentiles from 1 to 19 would be contained within this item. Similarly, the fifth item of data would contain any of the percentiles from 81 to 99. The 50th percentile or median of the data set would pass through the third item, which occupies the proportions from .40 to .60.

This distinction of small data sets is responsible for the use of two different methods (discussed later) for determining percentiles. The pragmatic-reality method uses proportions of the discrete data; the mathematical-theory method relies on interval divisions for a continuous curve.

4.2.1.3   *Shared (Tied) Ranks* —
When two or more items have the same value in a data set, they are "tied" and will share the same ranks. To preserve the correct sums and proportions for the total of ranks, each tied value is assigned the same *average* rank. For example, in Table 3.1, the two values of **12** would occupy ranks 2 and 3. They are each assigned rank 2.5. (The next value, **13**, becomes rank 4.) The four values of **21** would occupy ranks 27, 28, 29, and 30. Their average rank can be determined as $(27 + 28 + 29 + 30)/4 = 28.5$, or, more simply, as the first plus last divided by 2. Thus, $(27 + 30)/2 = 28.5$. (The proper management of tied ranks is an important challenge that is further discussed for Rank Tests in Chapter 15.)

Tied ranks are seldom a substantial problem in determining percentiles, particularly if the same values "compete" for the location of a particular percentile point. For example, in the 56-item data set of Table 3.1, the first 28 items occupy the proportions 0–.50 and the last 28 items occupy .50 – 1. Because the .50 value is shared by ranks 28 and 29, the 50th percentile, or median, is placed between them. Since these ranks, as noted in the foregoing paragraph, are occupied by the same value, i.e., **21**, the value of the 50th percentile is **21**.

4.2.2   General Procedure

Each of the 56 items in the data set of Table 3.1 will have two ranks — one counted from each end. Thus, **11** is the first rank counting in one direction, and the 56th rank in the other; and **43** would correspondingly be either the 56th or the first rank.

As just noted, the middle rank or *median* for this distribution would be at the rank of $(56 + 1)/2 = 28.5$. Counting from low to high values, this rank occurs among the four values of **21** that occupy ranks 27 through 30. Going in the other direction, if **43** is counted as the first rank, the values of **24** occupy ranks 20–22; **23** has rank 23; values of **22** occupy ranks 24–26; and values of **21** occupy ranks 27–30.

Since the number of ranks will vary as n changes from one data set to another, the counted ranks are standardized by citation as proportions or relative frequencies of the data. The cumulative relative frequency or cumulative proportions will be 2/n after the second ranked item, 3/n after the third, and r/n after the rth ranked item.

In the ordinal data of Figure 3.1, the two rightmost columns show the cumulative count of frequencies as the categories ascend, and the associated cumulative relative frequency is marked cumulative percent. After the last category in any array, the cumulative count is always N (the total size of the group), and the cumulative percent is always 100%.

4.2.3   Points and Zones

The first percentile point demarcates a zone of cumulative relative frequency that includes 1/100 of the data. The second percentile point demarcates a zone for 2/100 of the data, and so on. Note that percentile points demarcate the boundaries of zones, whereas cumulative proportions refer to the amounts of data contained in each zone. Thus, the 50th percentile point demarcates two zones, each containing a .50 cumulative proportion, or half the data in the set. The 25th, 50th, and 75th percentile points demarcate four zones, each containing one fourth of the data.

The distinction is shown in Figure 4.1. The upper part of the figure indicates the percentile points for values of the data. The lower part shows the proportionate amount of the items of data located in each zone demarcated by the percentiles.

Figure 4.2 shows the location of the 25th, 50th, and 75th percentiles in a Gaussian distribution. Because the distribution is much denser near the center than at the edges, the zones containing the second and

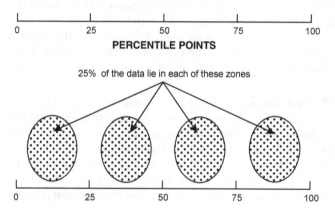

FIGURE 4.1
Distinction between percentile points (upper) and the corresponding zones of demarcated data (lower).

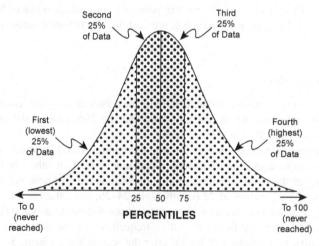

FIGURE 4.2
Location of 25th, 50th, and 75th percentiles, and associated zones in a Gaussian distribution.

third "quarters" of the data are taller and thinner than the zones for the first and fourth quarters. Despite the symmetrical shape of the Gaussian curve around its center, the distances between adjacent percentile points are not symmetrical. Thus, the distance from the 0th percentile (which is never quite reached) to the 25th percentile is much larger than the distance from the 25th to the 50th percentile. On the other hand, on the two sides of the curve, the *interpercentile* distances are symmetrical between the 25th to 50th and 50th to 75th percentiles, and between the 0th to 25th and 75th to 100th percentiles.

4.2.4   Tabular Illustration of Cumulative Frequencies

An empirical display of frequencies, relative frequencies, and cumulative relative frequencies is shown in Table 4.1, which contains the observed serum chloride values and the frequency of each value in 2039 consecutive patients tested at a university hospital's laboratory. The relative frequencies of each value, which are shown in the third column of the table, are plotted as a frequency polygon in Figure 4.3. The shape of the spectrum seems reasonably symmetrical, with the crest of the "curve" at the mode of 103.

TABLE 4.1

Serum Chloride Values for a Population of about 2,000 People (Courtesy of laboratory service, Yale-New Haven Hospital.)

Serum Chloride Concentration* mEq/dl)	Observed Frequency	Relative Frequency	Ascending Cumulative Relative Frequency	Descending Cumulative Relative Frequency	Z Scores
75–83	8	.0039	.0039	1.0000	—
84–85	12	.0059	.0098	.9961	—
86–87	12	.0059	.0157	.9902	—
88	10	.0049	.0206	.9843	−2.611
89	10	.0049	.0255	.9794	−2.418
90	28	.0137	.0392	.9745	−2.226
91	20	.0098	.0490	.9608	−2.034
92	22	.0108	.0598	.9510	−1.842
93	18	.0088	.0687	.9402	−1.649
94	32	.0157	.0844	.9313	−1.457
95	43	.0211	.1054	.9156	−1.264
96	51	.0250	.1305	.8946	−1.072
97	76	.0372	.1677	.8695	−0.879
98	96	.0471	.2148	.8322	−0.687
99	125	.0613	.2761	.7852	−0.495
100	146	.0716	.3477	.7239	−0.302
101	159	.0780	.4256	.6523	−0.110
102	204	.1000	.5257	.5743	0.082
103	222	.1089	.6346	.4743	−0.275
104	195	.0956	.7303	.3654	0.467
105	167	.0819	.8122	.2697	0.659
106	136	.0667	.8789	.1878	0.852
107	83	.0407	.9196	.1211	1.044
108	49	.0240	.9436	.0804	1.237
109	41	.0201	.9637	.0564	1.429
110	26	.0128	.9765	.0363	1.621
111	13	.0064	.9828	.0235	1.813
112	15	.0074	.9902	.0172	2.006
113–114	10	.0049	.9951	.0098	—
115–127	10	.0049	1.0000	.0049	—
TOTAL	2,039	1.0000	—	—	

Note: Mean = μ = 101.572; standard deviation = σ = 5.199; the Z score values are described in Chapter 5 of the text.

* At the top and bottom of this table, certain extreme values have been compressed to save space. The individual values and their observed frequencies are as follows: 75–1; 76–1; 77–1; 80–2; 82–1; 83–2; 84–5; 85–7; 86–7; 87–5; 113–4; 114–6; 115–1; 116–3; 117–1; 118–1; 120–1; 123–2; 127–1.

The relative frequencies of the chloride values can be cumulated in either an ascending or descending direction, as shown in the fourth and fifth columns of Table 4.1. In the ascending direction, starting with the lowest chloride value, each successive chloride value (or interval) adds its own relative frequency to what was previously cumulated. The cumulative results continue to increase until they reach their final total of 1.000 after the highest chloride value is added. In the descending direction, starting with the highest chloride value, the process is similar but opposite.

Figure 4.4 shows the relative *cumulative* frequencies in an ascending direction for each chloride value. The S-shaped or sigmoidal curve is called an *ogive*. The shape is characteristic of cumulative frequencies in a Gaussian distribution.

The data in Table 4.1 (or in Figure 4.4) allow any cited chloride value to be immediately located in the spectrum. The value of 94 occurs near the lower end, as shown by its ascending cumulative relative frequency of .0844. The chloride value of 108, with an analogous proportion of .9436, is located near the upper end. The value of 102, with an ascending cumulative relative frequency of .5257, is close to the middle.

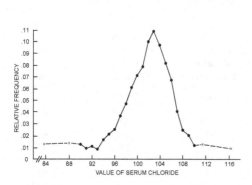

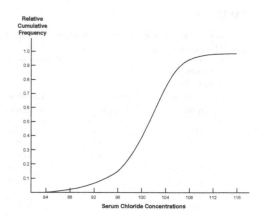

FIGURE 4.3

Frequency polygon showing the relative frequencies associated with the observed values of serum chloride listed in Table 4.1. The two extreme "tails" of the curve are shown with dotted lines because the points marked "×" are a composite of several values, as noted in Table 4.1.

FIGURE 4.4

Ogive curve of ascending relative cumulative frequencies for the chloride concentrations shown in Table 4.1 and Figure 4.3.

With either Table 4.1 or Figure 4.4, we can immediately find the chloride value that corresponds to a selected percentile, and vice versa. In an ascending direction, the value of **102** occupies the cumulative proportions from .4256 to .5257. In a descending direction, **102** occupies the cumulative proportions from .4743 to .5743. In either direction, the cumulative proportion of .50 is passed within the value of 102, which is therefore the 50th percentile point or median. With a similar inspection, the chloride value of **99** contains the 25th percentile point in an ascending direction and the 75th percentile point in a descending direction.

4.2.5   Nomenclature

When a set is divided into hundredths, the demarcations can properly be called either *centiles* or *percentiles*. The former term is preferred by some writers, but the latter (employed throughout this text) is more commonly used and seems to be preferred in both ordinary and statistical dictionaries.

The percentile (or centile, if you wish) is regularly used to denote the inner location of an item of data in a dimensional spectrum. If a particular item occupies several percentiles, it is commonly cited with the "esthetic" or "conventional" demarcations that end in (or near) the digits 0 or 5. Thus, the chloride value of 95, which occupies the ascending cumulative relative frequencies between .0844 and .1054 in Table 4.1, could be called the 9th percentile, but would usually be called the 10th.

4.2.5.1 Quantiles — Certain percentiles are given special names, called *quantiles*. The *tertiles* are the 33rd and 67th percentiles. The *quintiles* are the 20th, 40th, 60th, and 80th percentiles. The frequently used *quartiles* are the 25th, 50th, and 75th percentile points. These three quartiles are also respectively called the *lower quartile, median,* and *upper quartile*. The lower and upper quartiles are often symbolized as Q_1 and Q_3. (The median would be Q_2, but is usually shown with $\tilde{X}$ or some other special symbol.) The percentiles set at 2.5, 5.0, 7.5, …, 92.5, 95, 97.5, 100 each demarcate zones containing 1/40 of the distribution. Henrik Wulff[1] has proposed that they be called *quadragintiles*.

4.2.5.2 Quantile Zones — The names of certain percentiles are regularly applied erroneously to the demarcated zones as well as the boundary points. A set of k quantiles will demarcate $k + 1$ zones. Thus, the four quintile points demarcate five zones, each containing one fifth of the data. The three quartile points demarcate four zones, each containing one fourth of the data. These *zones* are really fifths and fourths, but they are often mislabeled as quintiles or quartiles.

4.2.5.3 Points, Ranks, and Values — An important distinction in nomenclature is the points, ranks, and values of percentiles.

A percentile *point* is a general location. Among 100 such points, it is regularly set (or found to be) at 20, 25, 50, 70, 75, or some other percentage of 100. In demarcating cumulative proportions of the data, these points would be denoted as .20, .25, .50, .70, and .75. When the term *percentile* is used without further specification, the reference is almost always to the point.

Percentile points will have different *ranks* within a set of data, according to the number of members in the distribution. The 50th percentile point (or median) occurs at rank 5 in a group of 9 items and at rank 14 in a group of 27.

A percentile *value* is the actual value of the particular item (or interpolated item) of data that is located at the percentile rank. This value will be 0.6, −12, 78.3, 1.9×10^6 or whatever occurs at that rank in the observed collection of data.

The following statement indicates all three uses of the terms: "He scored 786, which placed him in the 95th percentile, because he ranked 60th among the 1206 candidates who took the test." In this instance, the percentile *value* is 786, which is the actual score in the test. The percentile *rank* is cited directly as 60. The percentile *point* is determined from the proportion 60/1206 = .0498. Since high scores are usually reported with reciprocal percentiles, this proportion becomes converted to 1 − .0498 = .9502, or the 95th percentile.

4.3 Calculating Ranks, Zones, and Percentile Points

If r is the rank of an item in an n-item data set, the percentile point, P, occurs when the cumulative proportion, r/n, just exceeds P; i.e., (r/n) > P or r > Pn. Consequently, if the product Pn = r is exactly an integer, the selected rank must exceed Pn. It will have an intermediate rank that lies between r = Pn and the next rank, r + 1. For example, the formula Pn = r for the 25th percentile point of a 28-item data set yields (.25)(28) = 7; and the point will lie between the 7th and 8th ranks. Similarly, for the median or 50th percentile in that set, Pn = r is (.50)(28) = 14, and the point occurs between the 14th and 15th ranks.

On the other hand, if Pn = r is not an integer, the rank is *within* the next item. Thus, for the 5th percentile in a set of 28 items, Pn = r = (.05)(28) = 1.4. The 5th percentile is within the second rank.

This process will produce symmetrical results, working from either end of the data. With the proportion formula for the 95th percentile in a set of 28 items, we get r = (.95)(28) = 26.6, which becomes the 27th ranked item, counting from the lower end. This item will correspond to the 2nd ranked item (i.e., 5th percentile) counting from the upper end.

4.3.1 Calculating Ranks from Percentile Points

To calculate a rank from a percentile point, the simplest approach is to use the $r = Pn$ formula. If the result is not an integer, the rank is the next higher item. If the result is an integer, the rank lies between the surrounding items. Thus, if $Pn = 8$, the rank is between 8 and 9. If $Pn = 8.3$, the rank is within the 9th item.

4.3.2 Calculating Percentile Points from Ranks

Going in the other direction is not as easy because you start with a ranked integer, r, and cannot promptly use the foregoing rule to calculate $r = Pn$. After getting the value of $P = r/n$, however, you can use $r = Pn$ to see whether an integer emerges. Thus, for the 12th rank in a 37 item data set, $P = 12/37 = .32$ and $r = (.32)(37) = 11.8$, which confirms that the 32nd percentile is within rank 12. For the 14th item in a 28 item data set, $P = 14/28 = .5$, and $r = (.5)(28) = 14$, which is an integer. Therefore the 50th percentile must lie between ranks 14 and 15. In zones, the cumulative proportions end at .464 (=13/28) for the 13th rank, at .500 (=14/28) for the 14th rank, and at .536 (=15/28) for the 15th. The individual zones are from .464 to .500 for the 14th rank and .500 to .536 for the 15th. Because the 14th and 15th ranks share the "edges" of the .500 cumulative proportion, the percentile point must lie between them.

4.3.3 Alternative "Statistical Method"

The foregoing discussion is straightforward and direct, and the proposed method will always do the correct job. This method, however, is not what is offered in most conventional statistical discussions of percentiles. Accustomed to the theoretical collection of "continuous" data in Gaussian curves, the statistical approach does not deal with the problems of data sets that contain a finite number of individual items. Accordingly, in most statistical discussions, percentiles are used to demarcate intervals and interval boundaries, rather than the zones demarcated by those boundaries.

For large data sets (e.g., $n > 100$) or for the continuous curves that seldom occur in medicine but that are a common substrate in statistical reasoning, no real distinctions arise between the interval and the zonal approaches. In small data sets, however, where each item can occupy a substantial zone, the customary statistical approach will sometimes give slightly different (and erroneous) results. The next few subsections describe the statistical concepts and the reasons why the statistical formula usually appears as $r = P(n + 1)$ rather than $r = Pn$. If you are content with what you already know about percentiles, skip to section 4.4. If you want to know about the customary statistical reasoning, read on.

4.3.3.1 Concept of Intervals — A data set containing n members will have $n + 1$ interval boundaries. Consider the alphabet as a 26-member data set symbolized as

$$a, b, c, d,..., w, x, y, z.$$

There are 25 or $n - 1$ interval boundaries between each pair of adjacent members; and there are 2 boundaries at each end, separating the first and last members from the outside world. Thus, the total number of interval boundaries is 27, or $n - 1 + 2 = n + 1$. The first of these boundaries is the 0th percentile, which never actually occurs. Each letter then occupies 1/26 or .038 of the zones of this data set, and so the sequence of cumulative proportions is .038, .076, .115,... until 1 is reached after the letter z.

4.3.3.2 Use of n + 1 Formula — To convert back and forth from ranks to percentile points, the interval-based formula is $r = P(n + 1)$, where n is the number of items in the data set, P is the percentile point (expressed in hundredths), and r is the corresponding rank.

With this approach, if $P(n + 1)$ is an integer, it is the rank. Thus, the median (or 50th percentile) rank in a set of 29 items is $r = (.50)(30) = 15$. If $P(n + 1)$ is not an integer, the percentile lies between the two surrounding ranks. Thus, for the lower quartile in a set of 40 items, $(.25)(41) = 10.25$, and so Q_1 will lie between the 10th and 11th ranks.

The location of ranks for the two methods of calculations are shown in Table 4.2. For the two examples just cited, the results are the same with either formula. Thus, the proportion formula, r = Pn, yields (.50)(30) = 14.5, which becomes 15 for the median of a set of 29 items, and (.25)(40) = 10, which places Q_1 between ranks 10 and 11 for a set of 40 items.

TABLE 4.2

Location of Rank with Two Formula for Percentiles

Result of Calculation	Proportion: r = Pn	Interval: r = P(n + 1)
Integer (exactly r)	Between r and r + 1	r
Non-integer (r +...)	r + 1	Between r and r + 1

4.3.3.3   *Problems in Small Data Sets* — The r = P(n + 1) formula will work well for finding percentile ranks in large data sets, but can lead to difficulties in small data sets where the cumulative proportions and boundaries of intervals are not always the same.

For example, consider the five ranked items in the data set {a, b, c, d, e}, which has 6 interval boundaries, numbered as

$$\begin{array}{cccccc} 1 & 2 & 3 & 4 & 5 & 6 \\ |\ a\ | & b\ | & c\ | & d\ | & e\ | \end{array}$$

The median item, c, contains the .50 cumulative proportion; and it also will split the six interval boundaries evenly so that three of them are on each side of c. With the interval P(n +1) formula the ranked location of c is (.50)(6) = 3. The rank of the 25th percentile point, or lower quartile, however, would be (.25)(6) = 1.5, which suggests a location between the first and second ranks, which in this instance are the items a and b. In reality, however, the cumulative portion of .25 in a five-item data set occurs *within* the second item of data, which occupies the proportions from .20 to .40. Thus, the P(n + 1) calculation yields something between a and b for the lower quartile, but the cumulative proportion shows that it actually occurs within b.

Correspondingly, the upper quartile, determined for the cumulative proportion of .75, will lie within d, which occupies .60 to .80 of the data. If the percentile is calculated as a split interval, however, the upper quartile will lie between d and e.

4.3.3.4   *No Problem in Large Data Sets* — For large data sets, the difference in interval vs. proportion methods of calculation becomes trivial because the results will usually be the same whether the data are apportioned as n items or split into n + 1 intervals. Consequently, the P(n + 1) method is often preferred because it seems easier to work with.

For example, the 5th percentile value for the 2039 items in Table 4.1 is in the 102nd rank whether calculated as a cumulative proportion, (.05)(2039) = 101.95, or as an interval marker, (.05)(2040) = 102. In the table itself, the serum chloride values from 75 to 91 occupy 100 observed frequencies (=8 + 12 + 12 + 12 + 10 + 10 + 28 + 20), which are the ranks from 1 to 100. The chloride level of **92** has 22 observed frequencies, which occupy the ranks from 101 to 122. Thus, the 102nd rank occurs at a chloride level of **92**.

Analogously, to get the 2.5 percentile value for the 2039 items in Table 4.1, P(n) would produce 50.975 and P(n + 1) would produce 51. With either calculation, the percentile value would occur in the 51st rank. As shown in the table, the chloride levels from **75** to **88** occupy the first 42 ranks (=8 + 12 + 12 + 10). The chloride level of **89** occupies the next 10 ranks, from 43 to 52, and so the 2.5 percentile is at the chloride level of **89**.

In small data sets, however, the results of the two methods may differ. Being immediately anchored to the data, the proportion technique is always preferable for small data sets.

4.3.4   Management of Values for Inter-Rank Points

If the calculated rank lies between two integer ranks, the easiest way to choose the appropriate percentile value is to split the difference in values at those two ranks. Thus, if the calculated rank lies between the two values of **a** and **b,** the percentile value can be set at $(a + b)/2$. This result is equivalent to calculating $a + .5[(b - a)]$.

A preferable method of getting the inter-rank value, however, is to adjust the difference according to the "weight" of the percentile. With this technique, the inter-item value for the 20th percentile would be $a + .20(b - a) = .80a + .20b$. The calculation is $a + P(b - a)$ where P is the percentile in hundredths. In the opposite direction, if the 80th percentile lies between a and b, the formula for its value would be $b - .80(b - a) = .80a + .20b$, which produces the same result as before. Thus, if the lower quartile lies between the values of 31 and 37, the quartile value will be $(.75)(31) + (.25)(37) = 32.5$. The alternative formula for the calculation would be $31 + (.25)(6) = 32.5$.

This method of calculating the inter-rank values can be used regardless of whether the ranks are determined with the zonal formula $r = Pn$ or with the interval formula $r = P(n + 1)$. On the other hand, no great harm will be done if you ignore the distinction and simply split the value as $(a + b)/2$ rather than as $a + P(b - a)$.

4.3.5   Choice of Methods

Because of the possible disparities, data analysts are sometimes advised not to use percentiles unless the data set contains at least 100 members. Because this advice would eliminate a valuable index for the many small data sets that constantly occur in medical research, a better approach is to recognize that the $r = P(n)$ method is always more accurate for demarcating the *zones* that are usually a prime focus of analytic attention. The only disadvantages of the $r = P(n)$ method are the need to remember (1) that an integer result implies an intermediate rank, (2) that a non-integer result implies the next higher rank and (3) that most statistical textbooks (ignoring the challenges of small data sets) cite $r = P(n + 1)$ as a routine method of calculation. If in doubt about whether the data set is large enough, always use the $r = P(n)$ method. It will be correct for small data sets, and should agree with the $r = P(n + 1)$ result for large data sets.

Regardless of which method is used, the same percentile value should emerge for the rank calculated in both directions. Thus, the 2.5th, 5th, and 25th percentile values in one direction should be identical to the corresponding values that emerge, respectively, for the 97.5th, 95th, and 75th percentile ranks in the opposite direction.

4.4   Percentiles as Indexes of Inner Location

Despite the ambiguities of calculation for small data sets, the percentile technique is a simple method of immediately locating an item within a distribution. Low percentile points will denote a location at one end of the distribution; high percentiles will denote the other end; and the 40–60 region of percentile points will denote values near the middle.

4.4.1   Identifying Remoteness from Central Index

The percentile technique can be used to illustrate earlier comments (on the first page of this chapter) about two data sets, each containing 13 members, in which the value of **75** seemed close to or far away from the median of **80**.

Using the proportional technique to calculate percentiles for the small data sets, each item contains the proportions of $1/13 = .077$ of the data. The first item occupies percentiles from 0 to 7.7. The fourth ranked item occupies the percentiles from 3/13 to 4/13, which contains the proportions from .231 to .308. The sixth ranked item occupies the percentiles from 5/13 to 6/13, containing .385 to .462 of the cumulative proportions. Using customary expressions, we could say that the first item is at the 5th, the fourth item is at the 25th, and the sixth item is at the 40th percentile. Thus, in the first data set, **75** (as the sixth ranked item) is roughly at the 40th percentile, and in the second data set, **75** (as the first ranked item) is roughly at the 5th percentile.

[With the customary statistical (interval) method of calculation, the $r = P(n + 1)$ formula would produce the percentile point as $P = r/(n + 1)$. In the first data set, **75** is the sixth ranked member, and its percentile point would be $6/(13 + 1) = .43$. In the second data set, **75** is the first ranked member; and its percentile would be $P = 1/(13 + 1) = .07$. With either technique of calculation, the value of **75** is relatively close to the median of **80** in the first data set and relatively distant in the second.]

The percentile-point index shows where an item lies in the total distribution, but does not specifically designate distance from the center. Because the central percentile is at 50, the subtraction of $P - 50$ can promptly indicate remoteness from the center. The absolute size of the $P - 50$ difference, which can extend from 0 to 50, will indicate increasing remoteness, with negative values being below the center, and positive values above it.

4.4.2 Clinical Applications

Percentiles are commonly used by practicing pediatricians as a method for checking a child's growth. The patient's actual height and weight are located in a chart that shows the percentile distributions of these values in "standard" groups of normal children at different ages. If the child's percentile location for height and weight seems satisfactory for the age, the child is regarded as having normal development (at least in these two variables).

The height–weight percentiles can also be used for certain descriptive comparisons. If a child is at the 20th percentile for height and 80th percentile for weight, each percentile is within the limits of normal, but their relationship suggests that the child may be relatively too fat.

Percentiles are commonly used (as noted in a previous example) to rank candidates in a certifying examination, and can also be employed (as noted later) to compare the similarity or differences in data for two groups.

Some of the most valuable statistical applications of percentiles, however, are discussed in Chapter 5, where they are used to form zones of data.

4.5 Percentiles as Probabilities

Beyond their role in describing inner locations, percentiles can indicate probabilities for what might happen if members were randomly chosen from a distribution. For example, in the earlier data of Table 4.1, a chloride value of 99 has an ascending cumulative relative frequency of .2761; and 100 has a descending cumulative relative frequency of .7239. Therefore, if someone were randomly chosen from this distribution, the probability would be .2761, or about 28%, for getting a chloride value of ≤ 99 and about 72% for getting a chloride value of ≥ 100.

These probability values, as discussed later, have prime importance in the statistical applications of percentiles. In *descriptive* statistics, percentile boundaries are used to demarcate a range of "customary" or "normal" values. In *inferential* statistics, percentile zones of probability are used for decisions about "significant" distinctions.

4.6 Standard Deviation

The statistical entity called the "standard deviation" was originally devised and is best known for its role (discussed later in Chapter 5) as an index of dispersion. With certain mathematical principles, however, the standard deviation can become an index of inner location.

4.6.1   Definitions, Symbols, and Calculations

Usually symbolized as *s*, the standard deviation denotes the average deviation between the individual items of data and the mean. The ideas require some new symbols and terms. If X_i is a member of a data set having n members, with ΣX_i as the sum of values in the set, the mean is calculated as $\bar{X} = \Sigma X_i/n$. Each member of the data set deviates from the mean by the amount $X_i - \bar{X}$.

The obvious way to get the average of the deviations is to take their sum and divide it by n, the number of items in the data. Since some of the deviations in a set of data will lie above and others below the mean, however, the sum of the deviations, $\Sigma(X_i - \bar{X})$, will always be zero.

To avoid this problem, we can find the average deviation by eliminating the positive or negative signs, determining the sum of each absolute deviation, $\Sigma|X_i - \bar{X}|$, and then calculating the average absolute deviation as $\Sigma|X_i - \bar{X}|/n$. Although an excellent way to get average deviations, this method has not become statistically popular because the calculations were difficult in the days before electronic computation.

To escape from absolute values, and from positive and negative signs, the deviations are squared, as $(X_i - \bar{X})^2$. Their sum, which is always a positive number, is expressed symbolically as

$$S_{xx} = \Sigma(X_i - \bar{X})^2$$

[The reason for the xx subscript is that the calculation is really $\Sigma(X_i - \bar{X})(X_i - \bar{X})$. Later on, in Chapter 19, the calculation of $\Sigma(X_i - \bar{X})(Y_i - \bar{Y})$ for co-deviations between two variables is symbolized as S_{xy}.] S_{xx} has many synonymous names: *deviance, group variance, system variance,* and *sum of squares.* In strict statistical concepts, S_{xx} is the sum of squares in a "sample," and is used to estimate group variance in the parent population. This distinction is commonly neglected, however, in many discussions and computer printouts. Because both deviance and sum of squares can pertain to diverse computational arrangements, the calculation using the original mean of the data ($\bar{X}$) is easily and unambiguously cited as *group variance*—the term commonly used in this text.

In its role now, S_{xx} is merely an entity calculated enroute to a standard deviation. In many subsequent statistical activities, however, S_{xx} has an important job of its own.

4.6.2   Calculation of Group Variance: S_{xx}

The computation of S_{xx} can be simplified for hand calculators by using an algebraic expansion and reformulation of $\Sigma(X_i - \bar{X})^2$. It becomes

$$S_{xx} = \Sigma X_i^2 - n\bar{X}^2$$

or

$$S_{xx} = \Sigma X_i^2 - [(\Sigma X_i)^2/n]$$

The latter formula is preferable for hand calculation because "rounding" is avoided until the end of the calculations.

To illustrate the calculations of S_{xx}, consider three data sets, each containing three items, with **30** as the mean for each set. The calculations are as follows:

Data set	ΣX_i^2	$\bar{X}$	$n\bar{X}^2 = (\Sigma X_i)^2/n$	$S_{xx} = \Sigma X_i^2 - n\bar{X}^2 =$ $\Sigma X_i^2 - [(\Sigma X_i)^2/n]$
29, 30, 31	$29^2 + 30^2 + 31^2 = 2702$	30	$(90)^2/3 = 2700$	2
25, 30, 35	$25^2 + 30^2 + 35^2 = 2750$	30	2700	50
1, 30, 59	$1^2 + 30^2 + 59^2 = 4382$	30	2700	1682

These results immediately show the important role of the squared original observations, ΣX_i^2, in contributing to the group variance. Each of the three cited data sets had the same mean, and hence the same values of $\overline{X}$, ΣX_i and $(\Sigma X_i)^2/n$. The source of the differences in the S_{xx} values was the value of ΣX_i^2.

Each of the original values, X_i, contributes X_i^2 to the sum ΣX_i^2, which is sometimes called the "original" or "uncorrected" sum of squares. If each value of X_i were replaced by the mean, $\overline{X}$, the new square for each value would be $\overline{X}^2$, and the sum of the n squared values would be $n\overline{X}^2$. The difference in the two sums of squares, i.e., $\Sigma X_i^2 - n\overline{X}^2$, represents the reduction or "correction" achieved in the original sum of squares when each of the original values is replaced by a "fitted model." In this instance, the fitted model is the mean.

An advantage of using the mean as an index of central tendency is that the sum of squared deviations, S_{xx}, is smaller with the mean than with any other "model" (such as the median) that might have been chosen as a central index. (The median, $\tilde{X}$, is best for minimizing the sum of absolute deviations as $\Sigma |X_i - \tilde{X}|$, but not for sums of squared deviations.) The idea of a smallest value for sums of squares may not seem particularly impressive now, but it becomes important later on, when we fit data with other models and evaluate the achievement by noting the reductions produced in sums of squared deviations from the model.

4.6.3   Formula for Repeated Frequencies

If each value of the data, X_i, occurs repeatedly with a frequency of f_i, the formula for calculating S_{xx} is

$$\Sigma f_i(X_i)^2 - (\Sigma f_i X_i)^2/N$$

where $N = \Sigma f_i$. For the data in Table 3.1, the group variance calculated in the usual manner is 3255. If each interval in Table 3.1 is replaced by its midpoint (so that **10–14** is represented by **12, 15 – 19** by **17**, etc.), the result could be approximated as $5(12)^2 + 19(17)^2 + 13(22)^2 + 4(32)^2 + 3(37)^2 + 2(42)^2 - [5(12) + 19(17) + 13(22) + 10(27) + 4(32) + 3(37) + 2(42)]^2/56$. The result is $31524 - (1262)^2/56 = 31524 - 28440 = 3084$, and is not too different from the more accurate calculation of S_{xx}.

4.6.4   Calculation of Variance

With S_{xx} as the group variance for the total of n members, we want an average value that is "standardized" for the size of the group. For this purpose, S_{xx} is divided either by n or by $n - 1$ to produce a result called the *variance*, which is symbolized as s^2. The square root of the variance is s, the *standard deviation*.

In the three sets of data in Section 4.6.2, dividing each S_{xx} value by $n = 3$ produces the respective variances of .67, 16.67, and 560.67. The square roots of these variances are the respective standard deviations of .82, 4.08, and 23.68. If S_{xx} had been divided by $n - 1$, which is 2 in this instance, the respective standard deviations would be 1, 5, and 29.

4.6.5   Choice of Division by n or n − 1

A subtle issue in calculating the variance is whether to use n or $n - 1$ in the denominator. Because ordinary intuition suggests the use of n, you may wonder why $n - 1$ becomes a tenable or even desirable candidate for the divisor. The reason, as noted later when we consider the inferential strategies of statistics, is that division by $n - 1$ generally provides a better or allegedly "unbiased" estimate of variance in the hypothetical population from which the observed group is thought to have been "sampled."

For the moment, you can use the rule that if the data set is complete and is being summarized for purely descriptive purposes, S_{xx} is divided by n to yield the variance. On the other hand, if the standard deviation is going to be used for anything inferential — such as calculating the standard errors, confidence intervals, or P values discussed later in the text — S_{xx} is divided by $n - 1$.

If you are not sure about whether to use n or $n - 1$ in a particular situation, use $n - 1$. With a large data set, the results will be hardly affected. With a small data set, your statistical colleagues are more likely to feel comfortable and to approve. For most purposes, therefore, the formula for calculating the standard deviation is

$$s = \sqrt{\frac{S_{xx}}{n-1}} = \sqrt{\frac{\Sigma X_i^2 - [(\Sigma X_i)^2/n]}{n-1}}$$

If n is used as divisor, the variance becomes

$$S_{xx}/n = (\Sigma X_i^2 - n\overline{X}^2)/n = \Sigma(X_i^2/n) - \overline{X}^2$$

The latter (descriptive) formula is responsible for the statement that the variance is the "mean of the squares minus the square of the mean." With this formula, the standard deviation is

$$s = \sqrt{(\Sigma X_i^2/n) - \overline{X}^2}$$

4.6.6 Other Approaches

Calculations that use a central index can be avoided if an average deviation is determined for all possible pairs of values in the data set. If X_i and X_j are any two members in the data set, this average can be calculated from the squares of all differences, $(X_i - X_j)^2$, or from the absolute differences $|X_i - X_j|$. The latter approach is called *Gini's mean difference*. Although available and interesting, these "pairing" approaches are hardly ever used.

A different pairing tactic, called *Walsh averages*, can be applied for descriptions of non-Gaussian data sets. An array of means is calculated as $(X_i - X_j)/2$ for each pair of data, including each value paired with itself. For n items of data, there will be $n(n + 1)/2$ Walsh averages. The median of the array can be used as a central index, and the range of values above and below the median can help denote (as discussed later) the stability of the central index.

4.7 Standardized Z-Score

The inner location of any item in a distribution of data can be cited with a standardized Z-score, which is calculated as

$$Z_i = \frac{X_i - \overline{X}}{s}$$

and sometimes called a *standardized deviate*. The division by s produces a "standardization" that is unit-free, because Z_i is expressed in magnitudes of the standard deviation. The positive or negative value of each Z_i indicates whether the item lies above or below the mean.

To illustrate the standardizing effect, consider $\{9, 12, 17, 18, 21\}$ as a data set for *age in years*. This 5-item set of data has $\overline{X} = 15.4$ and $s = 4.827$. If age were expressed in months, however, the same set of data would be $\{108, 144, 204, 216, 252\}$. For the latter expression, $\overline{X} = 184.8$ and $s = 57.924$. Thus, with a simple change in units of measurement, the same set of data can have strikingly different values for $\overline{X}$, s, and the deviations, $X_i - \overline{X}$. The values of Z_i, however, will be identical in the two sets. In the first set, Z_i for the first item will be $(9 - 15.4)/4.827 = -1.326$. In the second set, Z_1 for the first item will be $Z_1 = (108 - 184.8)/57.924 = -1.326$. Identical Z_i values will also occur for all other corresponding items in the two data sets.

4.7.1 Distribution of Z-Scores

In the two foregoing sets of data, the Z-scores for age are {−1.326, −.704, .331, .539, 1.160}. The scores have a mean of 0 and a standard deviation of 1. This attribute of any set of Z-scores is inherent in their calculation and has nothing to do with the shape of the distribution of data. Regardless of whether a distribution is symmetrical or skew, convex or concave, the Z-scores will have a mean of 0 and a standard deviation of 1. (A proof of this statement appears in Appendixes 4.1 and 4.2.) This remarkable feature gives Z-scores many statistical advantages.

4.7.2 Z-Scores as Indexes of Inner Location

The main advantage to be discussed now is that Z-scores can be used as indexes of inner location. An item's Z-score of −0.6, 1.2, 0, −2.3, etc. will immediately indicate how relatively far (in standard deviation units) the item lies above or below the mean.

The rightmost column of Table 4.1 shows the Z scores calculated as $Z_i = (X_i - 101.572)/5.199$ for each item of the chloride data, using their mean and standard deviation. These Z-scores, rather than percentiles, could cite the relative inner location of any item in the data. Note that most of the items are included in a zone of Z-scores that extends from −2 to +2. If values of Z $>|2|$ are excluded, the Z-score zone from −2 to +2 in Table 4.1 contains the chloride values from **92** to **111**. The zone will contain about 93% of the data, excluding .049 of the data at the low end and .0172 of the data at the high end.

4.7.3 Application of Z-Scores

The ability of a Z-score to denote inner location is exploited in diverse ways. A common procedure, which you have probably already encountered in previous scholastic adventures, is the use of Z-scores for educational tests, where the process is sometimes called "grading on a curve." The Z-scores can avoid calculation of percentiles for small data sets, and can immediately be used to rank the test takers for performance in tests that have different scoring systems.

Standard reference Z-scores[2] were used in a recent study of zinc vs. placebo supplements in breastfed infants[3] to compare each infant's status for length and weight before and after treatments. Z-scores have also been advocated[4] as a replacement for percentiles in determining the nutritional status of children, particularly in developing countries. The argument is that the rank of many malnourished children is difficult to establish as a percentile, because they are below the first percentile of the World Health Organization (WHO) reference population.[5] A "road to health" chart, shown in Figure 4.5, has been proposed as an illustration that can help health workers understand the Z-score procedure. Figure 4.6 illustrates the mean Z-scores of weight according to age in a population of children in a region of South Africa.[6]

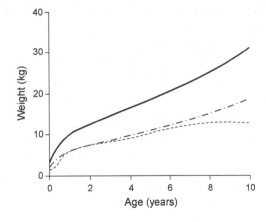

FIGURE 4.5
Z-scores for road-to-health charts. Comparison of 60% of median weight-for-age for males (−·−) with a 4 SD below the median (----); the bold line is the median. [Figure taken from Chapter Reference 4.]

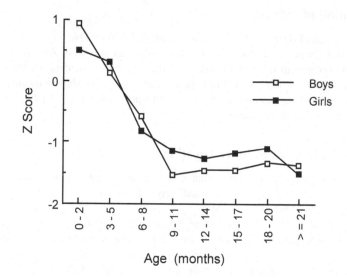

FIGURE 4.6

Mean weight-for-age Z-scores of 921 Basotho children by age and sex, Lesotho, 1985–1986. Z-scores were computed using the reference population of the National Center for Health Statistics. The child's weight was compared with the 50th percentile value of the reference populations and divided by the standard deviation of the references at that age. A Z-score of zero means that the child's weight is equal to the 50th percentile of the reference population. [Legend and figure taken from Chapter Reference 6.]

The use of Z-scores also avoids an undesirable technique, discussed in Chapter 5, which identifies inner locations according to the percentage by which each value is greater or less than the median value.

4.8   Conversion of Z-Scores to Probabilities

Compared with percentiles, Z-scores have one major disadvantage as indexes of inner location. By showing cumulative relative frequency, a percentile immediately denotes a specific location relative to other ranks; and the location can also be converted to a probability. Thus, a percentile of 95% tells us that only 5% of items have higher values and that the probability of getting one of those higher values is .05. A Z-score of 1.2, however, does not indicate either of these features. The array of Z-scores could be used to arrange a set of 5 items in ranked order as $\{-1.3, -.70, .33, .54, 1.2\}$, but we would not have known that 1.2 was the highest rank until we saw its location relative to the others.

This advantage can be overcome if the distributional shape of the data can be described with a conventional mathematical formula. When a suitable mathematical expression is available, each Z value can promptly be converted to a probability value for cumulative relative frequency. The eponymic mathematical distributions named after Gauss, Poisson, Bernouilli, etc. have been popular because of the correspondence between probability values and statistical indexes, such as Z.

4.8.1   Gaussian Distribution

The famous Gaussian distribution was promulgated in the 19th century by Carl Gauss, studying what today would be called "observer variability." As new technologic devices became available, the results found for repeated measurements of the same entity did not always agree. Confronted with the choice of which observation to accept, Gauss decided that their mean would be the correct value. He then noted that the deviations from the mean, called errors, were distributed around the mean in a symmetrical pattern that is today sometimes called *normal* by statisticians and *Gaussian* by people who want to avoid the medical connotations of *normal*.

Later in the 19th century, Adolphe Quetelet found that this same pattern occurred for the distribution of height in Belgian soldiers. This similarity of patterns helped give the Gaussian distribution its enthusiastic application in biostatistics of the 19th and early 20th centuries. The same pattern seemed to fit two different phenomena: multiple measurements of the same individual entity and individual measurements of multiple entities.

This dual accomplishment made the Gaussian distribution so mathematically attractive that Francis Galton, often regarded as the founder of modern biometry, believed it was a "Law of Frequency of Error." He expressed his admiration by saying, "the law would have been personified by the Greeks and deified, if they had known of it. It reigns with serenity and in complete self-effacement amidst the wildest confusion."[7]

The diverse technologic measurements of the 20th century, however, have demonstrated that most medical data do not have Gaussian distributions. Consequently, clinical investigators have had to think about other distributions and to use statistical strategies that do not depend on theoretical mathematical patterns. Nevertheless, despite the *descriptive* inadequacies, the Gaussian distribution remains valuable for *inferential* activities that will be discussed later.

4.8.2 Gaussian Mathematics

Although popularized by Gauss, the mathematical formula for the distributional pattern was actually discovered by Abraham DeMoivre. In that formula, the height of the curve shows the relative frequency, y, at each Z_i score. The mathematical expression is essentially

$$y = .4e^{-\frac{1}{2}Z_i^2}$$

where e is the well-known mathematical constant, 2.7183.... This formula describes a *standard* Gaussian curve, with mean = 0 and standard deviation = 1.

In the standard Gaussian curve, the height of the curve, y, is the relative frequency for each possible value of Z. Thus, when $Z = 0$, i.e., at the mean, $y = .4e^0 = .4$. When $Z = \pm.5$, $y = .4e^{-\frac{1}{2}(.25)} = .35$. When $Z = \pm2.0$, $y = .054$. The corresponding values of y and z are as follows:

Z	0	±.25	±.50	±.75	±1.0	±1.25	±1.50	±1.75	±2.0	±2.25	±2.5	±3.0	±3.5
y	.4	.39	.35	.30	.24	.18	.13	.087	.054	.032	.018	.004	.0009

The pattern of these points is shown in Figure 4.7. Note that the height of the curve becomes infinitesimal for Z values that exceed ±3, but the height never reaches zero. For example, if $Z = 6$, $y = 6.092 \times 10^{-9}$.

When Gaussian curves are expressed in values of X_i, rather than Z_i, their mean will be at $\overline{X}$ and their relative width will be determined by the size of the standard deviation, s. The value of Z_i in the foregoing Gaussian formula will be replaced by $(X_i - \overline{X})/s$ and the .4 factor will be divided by s, thus making the curve wider and shorter as s enlarges, and narrower and taller as s gets smaller.

4.8.3 Citation of Cumulative Probabilities

With integral calculus, the formula for the Gaussian curve can be converted to show the cumulative rather than individual relative frequencies at each value of Z_i. With this conversion, a specific probability value of cumulative relative frequency is associated for each of the possible negative and positive Z values.

The cumulative relative frequencies are usually expressed as proportions (or percentiles) that begin with 0 at $Z = 0$, and enlarge as Z becomes larger in either a positive or negative direction. In one mode of expression, the cumulative proportions on either side of 0 can be cited as follows:

Z	0	±.25	±.5	±.75	±1.0	±1.5	±2.0	±2.5	±3.0	±3.5
Cumulative Proportion	0	.099	.191	.27	.34	.43	.477	.494	.498	.499

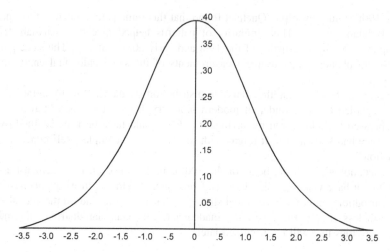

FIGURE 4.7
Values of y axis for Z-scores in Gaussian curve.

A more detailed account of the corresponding results is shown in Table 4.3. If you want to cumulate these proportions starting from the lower end of a Gaussian distribution and going upward, remember that the value of .5 should be added or subtracted appropriately for each of the foregoing values of the corresponding proportions. Thus, the Z value of –3.08, with a cumulative relative frequency of .4990 on the left side of the distribution, becomes .5 – .4990 = .001, which is the .1 percentile. The corresponding results for converting Z values to cumulative relative proportions are –.6 → .5 – .2257 = .2743, –.26 → .5 – .1026 = .3974, 0 → .5, .26 → .599, .6 → .7257, …, 2.0 → .9772, …, 3.6 → .999.

Although the cumulative proportions (and probabilities) can be used like percentiles merely to identify the inner locations of a distribution, their most frequent application occurs as P values in statistical inference. The P values are created when inner locations and probabilities for individual items in the data are demarcated into *zones* of location and probability. The demarcations and applications are discussed in the next chapter.

4.9   Inner Locations for Non-Dimensional Data

The percentiles and standard deviations that are pertinent for dimensional data cannot be used directly and must be modified to rank inner locations for the categories of non-dimensional data.

4.9.1   Nominal Data

Questions about the rank of an inner location do not arise for nominal data, which cannot be ranked.

4.9.2   Ordinal Data

Percentiles can easily be determined for ordinal data, although the same values will occupy many percentiles if the data are expressed in grades. For example, consider the 39 people whose therapeutic responses were rated as **poor**, 6; **fair**, 12; **good**, 11; and **excellent**, 10 in Section 3.5.1.3. Because each item occupies 1/39 = .026 of the data, the poor group would include the percentiles from 0 to 15 (since 6/39 = .154). The **fair** group occupies the subsequent percentiles up to 46 (since 18/39 = .462); the **good** group extends to the 74th percentile (since 29/39 = .744); and the **excellent** group occupies the rest.

Although not appropriate for ordinal data, standard deviations could be calculated if the four grades were regarded as dimensions (such as **1, 2, 3, 4**) and summarized with means.

TABLE 4.3

Cumulative Normal Frequency Distribution (Area under the standard normal curve from 0 to Z)

Z	0.00	0.02	0.04	0.06	0.08
0.0	0.0000	0.0080	0.0160	0.0239	0.0319
0.2	.0793	.0871	.0948	.1026	.1103
0.4	.1554	.1628	.1700	.1772	.1844
0.6	.2257	.2324	.2389	.2454	.2517
0.8	.2881	.2939	.2995	.3051	.3106
1.0	.3413	.3461	.3508	.3554	.3599
1.2	.3849	.3888	.3925	.3962	.3997
1.4	.4192	.4222	.4251	.4279	.4306
1.6	.4452	.4474	.4495	.4515	.4535
1.8	.4641	.4656	.4671	.4686	.4699
1.9	.4713	.4726	.4738	.4750	.4761
2.0	.4772	.4783	.4793	.4803	.4812
2.1	.4821	.4830	.4838	.4846	.4854
2.2	.4861	.4868	.4875	.4881	.4887
2.3	.4893	.4898	.4904	.4909	.4913
2.4	.4918	.4922	.4927	.4931	.4934
2.6	.4953	.4956	.4959	.4961	.4963
2.8	.4974	.4976	.4977	.4979	.4980
3.0	.4987	.4987	.4988	.4989	.4990
3.2	.4993	.4994	.4994	.4994	.4995
3.4	.4997	.4997	.4997	.4997	.4997
3.6	.4998	.4999	.4999	.4999	.4999
3.9	.5000				

Note: Abridged table showing correspondence of Z-scores (shown in first column, augmented by values in subsequent columns) and unilateral cumulative proportions (shown in cells) of Gaussian curve in zone from 0 to Z. Values not shown here can be obtained by interpolation.

4.9.3 Binary Data

A set of binary data, expressed as **yes/no, success/failure, alive/dead**, etc. can be coded as **1/0**. If the set contains n items, r items will be coded as **1** and n − r items will be coded as **0**. The binary proportion that summarizes the data will be either $p = r/n$ or $q = (n - r)/n$.

The percentiles of such a data set are relatively trivial. The first r values of **1** in the set **1, 1, 1, ..., 1, 0, 0, ..., 0** will occupy r/n = p or the first P percentiles. The standard deviation of the data set, however, is not trivial. It becomes particularly important later on when we consider the "standard error" of a proportion.

The standard deviation of a set of binary data can be calculated with the same formula used for dimensional data. In r items of the data, the deviation is $(1 - p)$ from the "mean" value, p; and n − r items will have the deviation $(0 - p)$. Thus, the group variance will be $r(1 - p)^2 + (n - r) \times (0 - p)^2$. Letting $1 - p = q$, $r = pn$, and $n - r = qn$, this expression becomes $pnq^2 + qnp^2 = npq(q + p) = npq$.

The group variance is customarily divided by n − 1 to form the variance of dimensional data, but by n for binary data. (The reason will be explained later.) Accordingly, the variance of a set of binary data is npq/n = pq, and the standard deviation is

$$s = \sqrt{pq}$$

Note that this remarkable formula refers to standard deviation of the data, not to variance of the binary proportion that is the central index. In other words, each of the **1** or **0** values in the data deviates from the central index, p, by an average of $\sqrt{pq}$. This same average deviation occurs if we express the central index as $q = 1 - p$, rather than p. Thus, for the 12 values of **1** and 7 values of **0** that are summarized as $p = 12/19 = .63$ or as $q = 7/19 = .37$, the standard deviation is $\sqrt{(12/19)(7/19)} = \sqrt{.233} = .48$. This same standard deviation would occur if the data set were three times larger, with p expressed as $36/57 = .63$.

Appendixes for Chapter 4

A.4.1 The Mean of a Set of Z-Scores is 0

Proof: If the original data are represented by $\{X_i\}$, $\overline{X}$, and s, each Z-score will be $Z_i = (X_i - \overline{X})/s$. Then $\Sigma Z_i = \Sigma(X_i - \overline{X})/s = (1/s)[\Sigma X_i - \Sigma \overline{X}] = (1/s)[N\overline{X} - N\overline{X}] = 0$.

A.4.2 The Standard Deviation of a Set of Z-Scores is 1

Proof: The group variance of the Z scores will be $\Sigma(Z_i - \overline{Z})^2 = \Sigma Z_i^2$, since $\overline{Z} = 0$. Since $Z_i = (X_i - \overline{X})/s$, each Z_i^2 will be $(X_i^2 - 2X_i\overline{X} + \overline{X}^2)/s^2$ and $\Sigma Z_i^2 = (\Sigma X_i^2 - n\overline{X}^2)/s^2$. If calculated with $n - 1$, the variance of the Z scores will be $\Sigma Z_i^2/(n - 1) = (\Sigma X_i^2 - n\overline{X}^2)/[(n-1)s^2]$. Since $(n - 1)s^2 = \Sigma X_i^2 - n\overline{X}^2$, the quotient for the variance is 1. Its square root, 1, will be the standard deviation.

References

1. Wulff, 1981; 2, Hall, 1993; 3. Walravens, 1992; 4. Shann, 1993; 5. WHO Working Group, 1986; 6. Ruel, 1992; 7. Galton, 1889.

Exercises

4.1. For the data in Table 3.1 (Chapter 3),

    4.1.1. What are the lower and upper quartile values?

    4.1.2. What values are at the 2.5 and 97.5 percentiles?

    4.1.3. In what percentile is the value of **30**?

4.2. For the data set in Exercise 3.3 (Chapter 3),

    4.2.1. What is the standard deviation calculated with n and with $n - 1$?

    4.2.2. Calculate the Z-scores for the two lowest and two highest items of the data. What do these Z-scores tell you about whether the distribution is Gaussian?

4.3. What feature of the Z values in Table 4.1 indicates that the chloride data do *not* have a Gaussian distribution?

4.4. Students graduating in the 25th percentile of "performance" at Medical School X had higher MCAT scores on admission than students graduating in the 75th percentile of performance at Institution Y. Assuming that performance has been determined and graded in the same way at both institutions, does this result indicate that MCAT scores are poor predictors of performance in medical school? If your answer is No, give an alternative possible explanation for the observed results.

4.5. In the certifying examination of American specialty boards (in Medicine, Pediatrics, Surgery, etc.), the candidates receive a total "raw" numerical score based on right and wrong answers to the questions. For psychometric purposes in the theory of educational testing, the Boards transform these results so that each group of candidates will have a mean score of 500, with a standard deviation of 100. How are the raw scores altered to accomplish this goal?

4.6. As the Dean of Students for your Medical School, you must prepare each student's class ranking in clinical work. The ranking, which will be used for internship and other recommendations, comes from a combination of grades for clinical clerkships in five departments. Each grade is given an equal weight in the student's "class standing." The five clinical departments express their individuality by using different scales for giving grades. The scales are as follows:

Internal Medicine: A,B,C,D,E, (with A = highest and E = lowest)
Obstetrics-Gynecology: A+, A, A−, B+, B, B−, C+, C, C−, D, and E
Pediatrics: Numerical examination grade from 100 (perfect) to 0 (terrible)
Psychiatry: Superior, Satisfactory, Fail
Surgery: High honors, Honors, Pass, Fail

How would you combine these non-commensurate scaling systems to form a composite score for class standing?

4.7. Please mark each of the following statements as true or false (correct or incorrect). If you disagree, indicate why.

4.7.1. Harry had a percentile score of 70 in a board certification test. The result implies that he correctly answered 70% of the items.

4.7.2. At the beginning of the year, Mary had a percentile score of 90 in class standing. By the end of the year, she had moved to a percentile score of 99. During the same period, John moved from the 50th to 59th percentile. The two students, therefore, made about equal progress.

4.7.3. There is little difference between Joan's score at the 98 percentile and Bob's score at the 99.9 percentile, but a large difference between Bill's 84th percentile and Joan's 98th.

4.7.4. Since Nancy scored at the 58th percentile and Dick at the 64th, Dick obviously did much better in the test.

4.7.5. The Dean of Students at Almamammy medical school wants to evaluate secular trend in the students' performance on National Board examinations. He believes the trend can be correctly determined if he forms an average of each student's overall percentile score for members of last year's class and uses it to compare this year's performance.

4.8. A pediatrician who likes to be different decides to use Z-scores rather than percentiles for characterizing the status of patients. What would be the approximate Z-scores associated with the following percentiles: 2.5, 25, 40, 50, 60, 75, 97.5?

4.9. Joe has brought a lawsuit against the American Board of Omphalology because he failed the certifying examination, although he knows (from information sent by the Board) that he correctly answered 72% of the items. What would your argument be if you were Joe's lawyer? If you were the Board's lawyer, how would you defend it?

4.10. If you enjoy playing with algebra, and want to check your ability to manipulate statistical symbols (and also have the available time), here are two interesting but optional assignments.

4.10.1. Show that $\Sigma(X_i - \overline{X})^2 = \Sigma X_i^2 - N\overline{X}^2$

4.10.2. A sum of squares or group variance can be calculated as $\Sigma(X_i - M)^2$ with any selected central index, M. Prove that this group variance is a minimum when $M = \overline{X}$ (the mean). (Hint: Let $M = \overline{X} \pm c$, where $c > 0$. Then see what happens. Another approach, if you know the calculus, is to differentiate this expression in search of a minimum.)

5

Inner Zones and Spreads

We now know how to indicate a group's external location and the relative internal location of individual members, but we do not yet have a way to denote a group's *spread*. This chapter is devoted to indexes of spread and to the demarcation of several valuable *inner zones* of spread. Their important roles are to denote the compactness of the group and the adequacy with which the group is represented by its central index.

5.1   The Range

A simple, obvious index of spread for a set of dimensional data is the range from the lowest to highest values. In Table 3.1, where the data extend from values of **11** to **43**, the range can be cited as **11–43**. For the chloride values in Table 4.1, the range (noted from the footnotes in that table) is **75–127**.

The two extreme boundaries of a range are usually listed individually and are seldom subtracted to produce such single values as **32** or **52**.

5.1.1   Non-Dimensional Ranges

With non-dimensional data, a formal expression is seldom needed, because the range is readily evident when the array of categories in each variable's distribution is summarized with frequency counts or relative frequencies.

For a binary variable, the range is obvious: it covers the two categories for **yes/no**, **present/absent**, **success/failure**, **0/1**, etc. For ordinal data, the range extends from the smallest to largest of the available grades or ranks. The ordinal grades would have ranges of **I–III** for the three TNM Stages **I, II,** or **III,** and **1–10** for the 10 values of the composite Apgar Score. If not expressed as a set of counted ranks, an ordinal variable seldom has more than ten grades.

Not having ranked magnitudes, the categories of nominal variables cannot be shown as a range. A nominal variable, such as *occupation*, might contain twelve categories arbitrarily coded as **01, 02, ...,** **12**, but would not be summarized as a range of **01–12**.

5.1.2   Problems in Dimensional Ranges

The main problem in using range for the spread of dimensional data is potential distortion by outliers. This problem, which keeps the mean from being an optimal central index, may also make the range an unsatisfactory index of spread. For example, a range that extends 12 units from **19 to 31** for an array of 200 items would suddenly have its spread become five times larger (from 12 units to 60) if the data set contains a single outlier value of **79**. The range thus offers a useful "quick and dirty" way to appraise the spread of the data, but some other index will be preferred to avoid the potential adverse effect of outliers.

5.2   Concept of an Inner Zone

To eliminate the problem of outliers, the spread of dimensional data can be truncated and converted to a smaller inner zone. The goal is to exclude the extreme values but to have the inner zone contain either most of the "bulk" of the data or a selected proportion thereof. [The "bulk" of the data refers to individual items, not the "weight" or "magnitude" of the values of those items. Thus, the data sets {1, 3, 6, 7} and {95, 108, 234, and 776} each have a bulk of four items.]

The location and magnitude of inner zones are chosen arbitrarily. Some of them can readily be demarcated in a relatively "natural" manner. For example, because 25% of the items of data are contained in each zone demarcated by the 25th, 50th, and 75th percentiles, the inner zone between the lower and upper quartiles will comprise 50% of the data, with each half of that zone containing 25%. With quartile demarcations, the **bulk** of items in the inner 50% zone is symmetrically distributed around the median, but in other circumstances, the selected inner zone may be located eccentrically, or may hold a much larger "bulk" than 50%.

The decisions about symmetry in location and quantity of "bulk" will depend on the purpose to be served by the inner zone.

5.2.1 Symmetry in Location

In many circumstances, the low and high values of a data set are relatively well balanced at the two ends of the spectrum. This reasonably symmetrical pattern, which occurs in the chloride data of Table 4.1, could allow bidirectional decisions that certain values are "too low" and others are "too high." An inner zone for the "range of normal" would therefore be located symmetrically (or concentrically) around the center of the data.

In other instances, however, the data may be overtly unbalanced or skewed, with most of the items occurring eccentrically at one end of the distribution. For example, in a large group of people examined routinely at a hospital emergency department, most of the levels of blood alcohol would be **0**. On various occasions, the patients' values would be high enough to make the mean for the total group exceed **0**, but the "range of normal" for blood alcohol would be placed eccentrically, beginning at the **0** end of the data.

Even if the spectrum is relatively symmetrical, however, we may sometimes be interested in only one side of the distribution. For example, we might want to know the probability of finding a person with hyperchloridemia in Table 4.1. For this purpose, the "inner zone" would be located eccentrically. It would extend from the lowest chloride value in the table to an upper boundary chosen as demarcating a "too high" chloride. If the latter boundary is set at **109**, the inner zone would start at **75** (the lowest chloride value in Table 4.1) and extend through **108**. The zone would include .9436 of all values in the data. The "outer zone," at chloride levels of **109** onward, would include the remaining .0564 proportion of the group. The probability would be .0564 that a particular person has a value in the zone denoted by chloride levels ≥ **109**.

Inner zones are most commonly set symmetrically with two boundaries that form an external zone at each end of the distribution. The two external zones beyond the boundaries are often called "tails" when the results are cited as probability values. Sometimes, however, the inner zone has only one demarcated boundary, and the result (as in the example just cited) is called "one-tailed" for probability.

5.2.2 Decisions about Magnitude of "Bulk"

A separate decision refers to the quantity of the distribution that will be regarded as the "bulk," "great bulk," or "most" of all the items in the data. For some comparative purposes, the "bulk" may be set at 50%, 80%, or 90%. For conclusions about uncommon, unusual, or "abnormal" members of a distribution, the bulk is often set at 95%.

The choice of 95% is completely arbitrary. It has no inherent biologic or logical virtue and could just as well have been set at 83%, 94%, 96%, or some other value. The current custom arose when R.A. Fisher, a prominent leader in 20th century statistics, noted that 95% of the data in a Gaussian distribution was contained in a symmetrical inner zone bounded by 1.96 standard deviations on both sides of the mean. Because the "1.96" could easily be remembered as "2," a convenient mnemonic symbol was constructed. With $\overline{X}$ as mean and s as standard deviation, $\overline{X} \pm 2s$ became the symbol that designated the 95% inner zone of a Gaussian distribution. Fisher then referred to the remaining values of data, located in the two segments of the outer zone, as highly uncommon or unusual.

5.3 Demarcation of Inner Zones

After the decisions about symmetrical location and magnitude of bulk, inner zones can be demarcated with three tactics: percentiles, standard deviations, or Gaussian Z-scores.

5.3.1 Percentile Demarcations

An inner zone demarcated with percentiles is called an *inner-percentile range*, abbreviated as **ipr**. It is centered at the median, and its bulk is indicated with a subscript, such as ipr_{95} for a zone covering 95%

of the data, which extends from the 2.5 to the 97.5 percentile. The ipr_{95} can also be called the *quadragintile range*, since each 2.5 percentile zone contains 1/40 of the data. The ipr_{50} contains 50% of the data and goes from the lower to upper quartile, i.e., the 25th and 75th percentiles. It is sometimes called the *interquartile range* or *spread*.

[In some of the modern tactics proposed as exploratory data analysis,[1] the bulk of data is first divided into two parts at the median. The upper and lower halves are then each divided into two parts by entities called the upper and lower *hinges*. The distance between the values of the two hinges is called the *H-spread*. Although the method of calculation is different, the values of the hinges are usually quite close to the corresponding quartiles. For most practical purposes, therefore, the H-spread and the interquartile range are identical.]

Inner-percentile ranges are always symmetrical around the median in their bulk, but not in their demarcating values of data. For example, in Table 3.1, the interquartile range has a symmetrical bulk, with 25% of data located on each side around the median value of **21**. The lower quartile boundary value of **17**, however, is nearer to the median than the upper quartile of **28**. Because the boundary values are often asymmetrical, both are usually listed when an inner percentile range is demarcated. Thus, for the data of Table 3.1, we could write "ipr_{50}: 17, 28" to denote the interquartile range.

Because the standard deviation (as noted shortly) is often used as a *single* value to denote spread, a counterpart single value can also be obtained from percentile demarcations. The most commonly used single entity, the *quartile deviation*, is half the distance from the lower to upper quartile values and is symbolized as $(Q_3 - Q_1)/2$. (Another name for this entity is the *semi-interquartile range*.) For the data in Table 3.1, the quartile deviation is $(28 - 17)/2 = 5.5$.

5.3.2   Standard-Deviation Demarcations

The standard deviation, s, is the most commonly used index of spread. The popularity comes from its symbolic economy and conceptual implication. Symbolically, the single s value is simpler and shorter to write than the two boundary values of an ipr. Conceptually, as noted earlier, a span of 1.96 standard deviations on both sides of the mean will include the inner 95% zone of data in a Gaussian distribution.

5.3.2.1   Apparent Notational Simplicity — Because the value of 1.96 is easily remembered as **2**, the inner 95% standard-deviation zone can be simply written with four symbols: $\overline{X} \pm 2s$. The apparent advantage of this simplicity, however, is somewhat illusory. As noted in Section 5.3.1, a single value, analogous to the standard deviation, could readily be obtained from the previously described quartile or quadragintile deviations. If $\tilde{X}$ represents the median, and q represents the percentile-based deviation, we could analogously write $\tilde{X} \pm 2q$.

The full scope of pertinent percentiles for an ipr_{95} zone could be written with three symbols within brackets: the 2.5 percentile, the median (in italics), and the 97.5 percentile. In Table 4.1, this zone would be shown as [92; *102*; 109]. The conventional standard-deviation inner 95% zone for the data would be cited as $101.572 \pm (2)(5.199)$. The ipr_{95} percentile notation is more accurate in showing the correct inner 95% zone; and the reader does not have to do the multiplication and addition that determine the two outer boundaries. Furthermore, because decimal results are not produced in the calculations for this example, the percentile notation here actually occupies less space.

5.3.2.2   Peculiar Symbolism — Although the main symbolic role of s is to denote the 95% inner zone implied by $\overline{X} \pm 2s$, many distributions are summarized in medical literature as "$\overline{X} \pm s$." The latter symbols save one digit in space, but they create a peculiar zone that has no intellectual, logical, or statistical advantages. The Gaussian zone that extends from $\overline{X} - s$ to $\overline{X} + s$ contains about 68% of the data — a proportion that seldom has any analytic merit. (Descriptively, however, the "passing score" for certain medical Board certification examinations is set at $\overline{X} - s$.)

For example, if the chloride data in Table 4.1 are summarized with the $\overline{X} \pm 2s$ formula as $101.6 \pm 2(5.2) = 101.6 \pm 10.4$, the "inner 95% zone" would extend from 91.2 to 112.0. As noted from the direct results in Table 4.1, this zone actually includes about 95% of the data; and we could justifiably conclude that the zone covers the great bulk of the data. We might even, if desired, try to demarcate the "range of normal" for chloride levels as extending from 91.2 to 112.0—or more realistically, from 91 to 112.

Because the data in Table 4.1 are discrete integers rather than continuous values, the size of the zone depends on whether the boundary values are included or excluded. In Section 4.7.2, when the boundaries were excluded, the proportion of data in the inner zone was $1 - (.049 + .0172) = .9338$. If the values of **91** and **112** are included in the zone, Table 4.1 shows that the cumulative frequencies ascend to .0392 at a value of **90** and descend from .0098 starting at a value of **113**. Thus, the inner zone from **91** to **112** would contain a proportion of $1 - (.0392 + .0098) = 0.951$.

When written in the $\overline{X} \pm s$ format as 101.6 ± 5.2, however, the conventional symbols would form an inner zone that extends from the values of **96.4** to **106.8**. In a Gaussian distribution, this zone, covering the 68% of data associated with one standard deviation around the mean, would have little or no analytic value. [If we let the zone extend from **96** to **107**, the appropriate cumulative frequencies in Table 4.1 are .1054 at **95** and .0804 at **108**. The zone from **96–107** would therefore include $1 - (.1054 + .0804) = .8142$ of the data. The theoretical and empirical values do not agree, because the chloride distribution, as shown in Figure 4.3, is not strictly Gaussian.]

5.3.2.3 *Distorted or Impossible Zones* — The main hazard of standard-deviation demarcations occurs when the inner 95% zone is calculated as $\overline{X} \pm 2s$ for distributions that are not Gaussian. If the distribution is either Gaussian or symmetrical without being exactly Gaussian, this inner zone will usually contain about 95% of the data. If the distribution is asymmetrical, however, the inner zone may be distorted or impossible.

When boundary values are placed symmetrically on either side of the mean by the $\overline{X} \pm 2s$ technique, the result does not correctly show the 95% inner zone for most eccentric distributions. Furthermore, if the data are highly skew or contain many outliers on one side of the distribution, the calculated 95% inner zone will yield an impossible result. For example, in a group of patients receiving non-steroidal anti-inflammatory therapy, the duration of "rheumatic activity" was reported as a mean of 37.6 days with a standard deviation of 21.4. The inner 95% zone, calculated as $37.6 \pm (2)(21.4)$, will be 37.6 ± 42.8. It will extend from −5.2 to 80.4 days. No matter how efficacious, the treatment cannot produce a retroactive inactivity of −5.2 days.

Figure 5.1 shows a dramatic illustration of the problem, constructed by W. S. Cleveland[2] in a drawing he called "Failure of means and sample standard deviations." The upper panel displays the strikingly

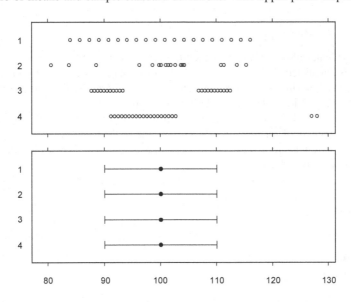

FIGURE 5.1
W. S. Cleveland's demonstration of identical means and standard deviations for four strikingly different distributions. For further details, see text. [Figure taken from Chapter Reference 2.]

different distributions of four sets of data, each with the same number of observations. The lower panel shows that despite the obvious differences, the four sets of data have identical means and standard deviations.

5.3.2.4 Reasons for Survival of Standard Deviation

— In view of the potential (and sometimes actual) major distortions produced when 95% inner zones are calculated from $\overline{X} \pm 2s$, you may wonder why the standard deviation has managed to survive so long and be used so often as a descriptive index.

Aside from the reasons already cited, an additional advantage of the standard deviation was computational. In the era before easy ubiquitous electronic calculation, the standard deviation was easier to determine, particularly for large data sets, than the locations of percentile ranks and values. With easy electronic calculation, this advantage no longer pertains today.

The main apparent remaining advantage of the standard deviation arises from *inferential* rather than *descriptive* statistics. The standard deviation is an integral part of the Z tests, t tests, and other activities that will be encountered later when we begin to consider P values, confidence intervals, and other inferential statistics. This inferential advantage, however, may also begin to disappear in the next few decades. Easy electronic calculation has facilitated different approaches — using permutations and other rearrangements of data — that allow inferential statistical decisions to be made without recourse to standard deviations.

Accordingly, if your career is now beginning, the standard deviation may have become obsolete by the time your career has ended.

5.3.3 Gaussian Z-score Demarcations

If a distribution is Gaussian, a cumulative probability will be associated with the Z-score calculated as $Z_i = (X_i - \overline{X})/s$. This probability can promptly be converted to the spans of inner and outer zones of data. In fact, the $\overline{X} \pm 2s$ principle discussed in Section 5.3.2 depends on the Gaussian idea that the interval will span about 95% of the data.

Since very few medical distributions are truly Gaussian, however, Z-score probabilities are seldom used *descriptively* as indexes of spread. The Z-score probabilities, however, will later become prominent and useful for the strategies of statistical *inference* in Chapter 6.

5.3.4 Multiples of Median

Multiples of the median, called **MoMs**, are sometimes proposed as a mechanism for replacing Z-scores. The MoM score is calculated as $X_i/\tilde{X}$ when each item of data X_i is divided by the median, $\tilde{X}$. The method is controversial, having both supporters[3] and detractors.[4] The MoM score produces a distinctive relative magnitude for each item of data, but the span of scores is grossly asymmetrical. The MoMs will range from 0 to 1 for X_i values below the median, but will extend from 1 to infinity for values above the median. Furthermore, unlike a percentile or Z-score, the MoM result is not a standardized location. A MoM score of .7 will indicate that the item's value is proportionately .7 of the median, but does not show the item's rank or inner location.

Lest mothers be upset by rejection of something called MoM, however, the technique, although unsatisfactory for denoting a standardized inner location or zone, may be a good way of denoting a "standardized" magnitude for individual items of data.

5.4 Indexes of Spread

The main role of an index of spread is to allow the prompt demarcation of either a suitable inner zone for the data or an index of relative spread, which will denote (as discussed in Section 5.5) the "compactness" of the data set.

5.4.1 Standard Deviation and Inner Percentile Range

For most practical purposes, indexes of spread are calculated and used only for dimensional data. Since the range, standard-deviation zones, and Z-score Gaussian demarcations have major disadvantages for eccentric data, the inner-percentile ranges would seem to be the best routine way to describe spread. Nevertheless, for reasons noted earlier, the standard deviation is the most popular expression today, usually shown in citations such as $\overline{X} \pm s$ or $\overline{X} \pm 2s$. If the goal is to demarcate a 95% inner zone that will always be both realistic and accurate, however, the ipr_{95} — extending from the 2.5 to 97.5 percentile values — is the best choice.

5.4.2 Ordinal Data

Since ordinal data can be ranked, their range can be reduced to a spread that is expressed (if desired) with an inner zone determined from percentiles. The quartile deviation (or semi-interquartile range) is commonly used for this purpose.

Although the mathematical propriety is disputed, ordinal data are sometimes managed as though they were dimensional, with means, standard deviations, and corresponding inner zones being calculated from the arbitrary digits assigned as ordinal codes.

5.4.3 Nominal Data

Since nominal data cannot be ranked, an inner zone cannot be demarcated. Several "indexes of diversity" have been proposed, however, to summarize the proportionate distribution of the nominal categories. Hardly ever appearing in medical literature, these indexes are briefly noted at the end of the chapter in Section 5.10.

5.5 Indexes of Relative Spread

For ranked dimensional or ordinal data, indexes of relative spread have two important roles: they indicate the compactness of the distribution and they will also help (as noted later in Chapter 6) indicate the stability of the central index.

An index of relative spread is calculated by dividing an index of spread, derived from standard deviations or percentiles, by a central index, such as a mean or median. The result indicates the relative density or compactness of the data.

5.5.1 Coefficient of Variation

The best known index of relative spread is the *coefficient of variation*, often abbreviated as *c.v.* It is calculated from the ratio of standard deviation and mean as

$$c.v. = s/\overline{X}$$

For example, the c.v. is $80.48/120.1 = .67$ for the data in Table 3.1 and $.05 \, (= 5.199/101.572)$ for Table 4.1. A compact distribution with a tall and narrow shape will have a relatively small standard deviation and therefore a relatively small c.v. For a short, wide shape, the c.v. will be relatively large.

As the external representative of the distribution, the mean cannot do a good job if the distribution is too widely spread, but no specific boundaries have been established for c.v.s that are "too large." Wallis and Roberts[5] have proposed a boundary of $\leq.10$. Snedecor and Cochran,[6] suggesting a zone between .05 and .15, say that higher values "cause the investigator to wonder if an error has been made in calculation, or if some unusual circumstances throw doubt on the validity of the experiment."

These proposed standards seem theoretically excellent, but they may be too strict for the kinds of variation found in medical data. If the results have doubtful validity when the c.v. exceeds .10 or .15, a great many medical research projects will be brought under an enormous cloud, and hundreds of published papers will have to be either disregarded or recalled for repairs.

5.5.2   Coefficient of Dispersion

Directly analogous to the coefficient of variation, the coefficient of dispersion, sometimes abbreviated as CD, is determined with absolute deviations from the median, rather than squared deviations from the mean. The average absolute deviation from the median, AAD, is calculated as $\Sigma|X_i - \tilde{X}|/n$. It is then divided by the median, $\tilde{X}$ to form $CD = (AAD)/\tilde{X}$. Because of the algebraic "awkwardness" of absolute deviations, this index is seldom used.

5.5.3   Percentile-Derived Indexes

Since neither the mean nor the standard deviation may be a good representative of a dimensional data set, the coefficient of variation might be replaced by percentile-derived values for indexes of relative dispersion. An index that corresponds directly to c.v. could be obtained by dividing the quartile deviation by the median.

A formal entity called the *quartile coefficient of variation* is calculated from the lower quartile value (Q_1) and the upper quartile value (Q_3) as $(Q_3 - Q_1)/(Q_3 + Q_1)$. Since $(Q_3 - Q_1)/2$ corresponds to a standard deviation, and $(Q_3 + Q_1)/2$ corresponds to a mean, this ratio is a counterpart of the result obtained with the c.v. For example, for the data in Table 4.1, the lower quartile is 99 and the upper quartile is 105. The quartile coefficient of variation is $(105 - 99)/(105 + 99) = .029$, which corresponds to the c.v. of .05 for those data.

5.5.4   Other Analytic Roles

Perhaps the most important statistical role of coefficients of variation (or other indexes of relative spread) occurs in subsequent decisions when we evaluate the stability of a central index, or when central indexes are compared for two groups. These decisions will be discussed in Chapter 7 and later in Part II of the text.

5.6   Searching for Outliers

Another reason for demarcating inner zones and indexes of relative spread is to play a fashionable indoor sport called "searching for outliers." The activity has scientific and statistical components.

5.6.1   Scientific Errors

Scientifically, the outlier may be a wrong result. The measurement system was not working properly; the observer may have used it incorrectly; or the information may have been recorded erroneously. For example, an obvious error has occurred if a person's age in years is recorded as 250. Outliers that represent obvious errors are usually removed from the data and replaced by blank or unknown values. Sometimes, however, the error can easily be corrected. Miller[9] gives an example of a data set {12.11, 12.27, 12.19, 21.21, and 12.18} in which "we can be fairly certain that a transcription error has occurred in the fourth result, which should be 12.21."

In laboratory work where substances are usually measured dimensionally, diverse statistical approaches are used to find suspicious values. One approach, cited by Miller[7] and called Dixon's Q, forms a ratio,

$$Q = |\text{suspect value} - \text{nearest value}|/\text{range}$$

If the value of Q is higher than the value authorized in a special statistical table, the result is deemed suspicious and probably erroneous.

5.6.2 Statistical Misfits

Outliers are commonly sought for statistical reasons, not to detect wrong values, but to remove "misfits." In many statistical procedures that involve fitting the data with a "model," such as a mean or an algebraic equation, the choice or fit of the model may be substantially impaired by outliers. The problem becomes more prominent later when we reach the algebraic models used for regressions and correlations, but we have already seen some examples in the way that outliers can alter the location of a mean or the magnitude of a standard deviation.

In the algebraic activities discussed later, the outlier is often removed from the data, which are then fitted into a new model. Most scientists, however, are not happy about removing *correct* items of data simply to improve the "feelings" of a mathematical model. Furthermore, if something is wrong with a system of measurement, why should we be suspicious only of the extreme values? Should not the interior values be viewed just as skeptically even if they do not stand out statistically?

5.6.3 Compromise or Alternative Approaches

The different motives in searching for outliers will often lead to different approaches for management.

In one tactic already mentioned (Section 3.8.4), the problem is avoided with "robust" methods that are relatively unaffected by outlier values. Thus, values of the median and inner percentile ranges, which are usually unaffected by outliers, are preferred to means and standard deviations. [Later on, when we reach issues in statistical inference, the "robustness" of "non-parametric" methods will often make them preferred over "parametric" methods.]

Nevertheless, in examining distributions of univariate data for a single group, we may want some sort of mechanism to make decisions about outliers, regardless of whether the main goal is to find scientifically wrong values or statistical misfits. To escape from outlier effects on means and standard deviations, the best tactics are to examine the data directly or to employ medians and inner-percentile ranges. Both these approaches can be used during the displays and examinations discussed in the next section.

5.7 Displays and Appraisals of Patterns

The stem-leaf plots discussed earlier in Section 3.3.1.2. have been replacing the histograms that were used for many years to display the shape and contents of dimensional data. Histograms are gradually becoming obsolete because they show results for arbitrary intervals of data rather than the actual values, and because the construction requires an artistry beyond the simple digits that can easily be shown with a typewriter or computer for a stem-leaf plot.

5.7.1 One-Way Graph

Data can always be displayed, particularly if the stem-leaf plot is too large, with a "one-way graph." The vertical array of points on the left of Figure 5.2 is a one-way graph for the data of Table 3.1. In this type of graph, multiple points at the same vertical level of location are spread horizontally close to one another around the central axis. A horizontal line is often drawn through the vertical array to indicate the location of the mean. The horizontal line is sometimes adorned with vertical flanges so that it appears as ⊢⊣ rather than — .The adornment is merely an artist's esthetic caprice and should be omitted because it can be confusing. The apparently demarcated length of the flange may suggest that something possibly useful is being displayed, such as a standard deviation or standard error.

5.7.2 Box Plot

If you want to see the *pattern* of dimensional data, the best thing to examine is a stem-leaf plot. To *summarize* the data, however, the best display is another mechanism: the box plot, which Tukey called a "box-and-whiskers plot." Based on quantiles rather than "parametric" indexes, the box plot is an excellent way to show the central index, interquartile (50%) zone, symmetry, spread, and outliers of a distribution. The "invention" of the box plot is regularly attributed to John Tukey, who proposed[1] it in 1977, but a similar device, called a *range bar*, was described in 1952 in a text by Mary Spear.[8] Spear's horizontal "range bar," reproduced here as Figure 5.3, shows the full range of the data, the upper and lower quartiles that demarcate the interquartile range, and the median.

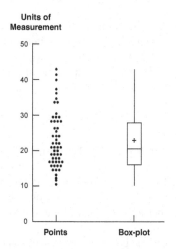

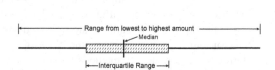

FIGURE 5.2
Display of data points and corresponding box-and-whiskers plot for data in Table 3.1.

FIGURE 5.3
Antecedent of box plot: the "range plot" proposed in 1952 by Spear. [Figure taken from Chapter Reference 8.].

5.7.2.1 *Construction of Box* —
In the customary box plots today, data are displayed vertically with horizontal lines drawn at the level of the median, and at the upper and lower quartiles (which Tukey calls "hinges"). The three horizontal lines are then connected with vertical lines to form the box. The interquartile spread of the box shows the segment containing 50% of the data, or the "H-spread." The box plot for the data of Table 3.1 is shown on the right side of Figure 5.2, using the same vertical units as the corresponding one-way graph on the left. For the boundaries of the box, the lower quartile is at **17** between the 14th and 15th rank, and the upper quartile is at **28** between the 41st and 42nd rank. The box thus has **28** as its top value, **21** as the median, and **17** at the bottom. The mean of **22.7** is shown with a + sign above the median bar.

The width of the horizontal lines in a box plot is an esthetic choice. They should be wide enough to show things clearly but the basic shape should be a vertical rectangle, rather than a square box. When box plots are compared for two or more groups, the horizontal widths are usually similar, but McGill et al.[9] have proposed that the widths vary according to the square root of each group's size.

5.7.2.2 *Construction of "Whiskers"* —
Two single lines are drawn above and below the box to form the "whiskers" that summarize the rest of the distribution beyond the quartiles. The length of the whiskers will vary according to the goal at which they are aimed.

If intended to show the ipr_{95}, the whiskers will extend up and down to the values at the 97.5 and 2.5 percentiles. For the 2.5 and 97.5 percentiles, calculated with the proportional method, the data of Table 3.1 have the respective values of **12** and **41**. Because the upper and lower quadragintile boundaries may not be located symmetrically around either the median or the corresponding quartiles, the whiskers may have unequal lengths. In another approach, the whiskers extend to the smallest and largest observations that are within an H-spread (i.e., interquartile distance) below and above the box.

For many analysts, however, the main goal is to let the whiskers include everything but the outliers. The egregious outliers can often be noted by eye, during examination of either the raw data or the stem-leaf plot. The box-plot summary, however, relies on a demarcating boundary that varies with different statisticians and computer programs. Tukey originally proposed that outliers be demarcated with an inner and outer set of boundaries that he called *fences*. For the *inner fences*, the ends of the whiskers are placed at 1.5 H-spreads (i.e., one and a half interquartile distances) above the upper hinge (i.e., upper quartile) and below the lower hinge (i.e., lower quartile). The *outer fences* are placed correspondingly at 3.0 H-spreads above and below the hinges. With this convention, the "mild" or "inner" outliers are between the inner and outer fences; the "extreme" or "outer" outliers are beyond the outer fence.

[Tukey's boundaries are used for box-plot displays in the SAS data management system,[10] where the inner outliers, marked 0, are located between 1.5 and 3 H-spreads; the more extreme outliers, marked *, occur beyond 3 H-spreads. In the SPSS system,[11] however, an "inner outlier" is in the zone between 1.0 and 1.5 H-spreads and is marked with an X; the "outer" (or extreme) outliers are beyond 1.5 H-spreads and are marked E.]

In the data of Table 3.1 and Figure 5.2, the spread between the hinges at the upper and lower quartiles is $28 - 17 = 11$. Using the 1.5 H-spread rule, the whiskers would each have a length of $1.5 \times 11 = 16.5$ units, extending from 0.5 (=17 − 16.5) to 43.5 (=28 + 16.5). Because the data in Table 3.1 have no major outliers, the whiskers can be shortened to show the entire range of data from 11 to 43. This shortening gives unequal lengths to the whiskers in Figure 5.2.

On the other hand, if boundaries are determined with the 1 H-spread rule, each whisker would be 11 units long, extending from a low of **6** (= 17 − 11) to a high of **39** (= 28 + 11). The lower value could be reduced, because the whisker need only reach the smallest value of data (**11**), but the upper whisker would not encompass the data values of **41** and **42,** which would then appear to be outliers.

5.7.2.3 *Immediate Interpretations* — The horizontal line of the median between the two quartiles divides the box plot into an upper and lower half. If the two halves have about the same size, the distribution is symmetrical around the central index. A substantial asymmetry in the box will promptly indicate that the distribution is not Gaussian.

The "top-heavy" asymmetry of the box in Figure 5.2 immediately shows that the distribution is skewed right (toward high values). Because the mean and median have the same location in a Gaussian distribution, the higher value of the mean here is consistent with the right skew. In most distributions, the mean is inside the box; and a location beyond the box will denote a particularly egregious skew.

5.8 "Diagnosis" of Eccentricity

The "diagnosis" of a non-Gaussian or eccentric distribution of data has several important purposes: (1) to warn that the distribution may not be properly represented by the mean and standard deviation; (2) to help identify outliers; (3) to suggest methods of "therapy," such as transformations, that may either cure the statistical ailment or reduce its severity.

The statistical methods of "diagnosis" are analogous to the tactics used in clinical medicine. Some of the procedures are done with simple "physical examination" of the data. Others use easy, routine ancillary tests that might correspond to a urinalysis or blood count. Yet others involve a more complex technologic "work-up."

The simple methods of "physical examination" will be recurrently emphasized in this text because they can be valuable "commonsense" procedures, often using nothing more than inspection or a simple in-the-head calculation. These "mental" methods, although seemingly analogous to screening tests, are actually different because a distinctive result is seldom false. Thus, in many of the mental methods to be discussed, a "positive" result is almost always a "true positive," but a "negative" result should seldom be accepted as truly negative without additional testing.

The methods for diagnosing eccentric distributions can be divided into the "mental" tactics, the simple ancillary test of examining the box plot, and the more elaborate tests available in a formal statistical "work-up."

5.8.1 "Mental" Methods

Three simple "mental" methods for determining eccentricity are to compare the mean with the standard deviation and with the mid-range index, and to see if $\overline{X} \pm 2s$ exceeds the limits of the range.

5.8.1.1 Mean vs. Standard Deviation

5.8.1.1 Mean vs. Standard Deviation — The coefficient of variation (see Section 5.5.1) is formally calculated as the standard deviation divided by the mean. An even simpler approach, however, is to compare the two values. In a symmetrical relatively compact data set, the standard deviation is substantially smaller than the mean. If the value of s is more than 25% of $\overline{X}$, something must be wrong. Either the distribution is eccentric, or it is highly dispersed. Thus, in Table 3.1, where s = 7.693 is about 1/3 of $\overline{X}$ = 22.732, eccentricity can promptly be suspected. In Table 4.1, however, where s = 5.199 and $\overline{X}$ = 101.572, the s vs. $\overline{X}$ comparison does not evoke suspicions. A non-Gaussian diagnosis for Table 4.1 requires more subtle testing.

5.8.1.2 Mean vs. Mid-Range Index

5.8.1.2 Mean vs. Mid-Range Index — The mid-range can easily be mentally calculated as half the distance between the maximum and minimum values of the data set. The formula is mid-range index = $(X_{max} + X_{min})/2$. If the mid-range differs substantially from the mean, the data have an eccentric distribution. In Table 3.1, the mid-range is (43 + 11)/2 = 27, which can produce a prompt diagnosis of eccentricity, because the mean is $\overline{X}$ = 22.7. In Table 4.1, however, the mid-range is (127 + 75)/2 = 101, which is quite close to the mean of 101.6.

5.8.1.3 Range vs. $\overline{X} \pm 2s$

5.8.1.3 Range vs. $\overline{X} \pm 2s$ — A third type of mental check is sometimes best done with a calculator to verify the arithmetic. In Table 3.1, the value of $\overline{X} \pm 2s$ is 22.7 ± 2(7.693). With a calculator, the spread is determined as 7.314 to 38.086. Without a calculator, however, you can approximate the data as 23 ± 2(8) and do the arithmetic mentally to get a spread that goes from 7 to 39. Because the actual range in that table is from 11 to 43, the lower value of the $\overline{X} \pm 2s$ spread — with either method of calculation — goes beyond the true limit. Therefore, the distribution is eccentric. In Table 4.1, however, $\overline{X} \pm 2s$ would be 101.6 ± 2(5.2) which can be calculated as going from 91.2 to 112.0, or 92 to 112. Either set of spreads lies within the true range of 75 to 127.

5.8.2 Examination of Box Plot

After a box plot has been drawn, its direct inspection is the simplest and easiest method for identifying eccentricity.

In a symmetrical or quasi-Gaussian distribution, the box plot will show three features of "normality": (1) the mean and median are relatively close to one another; (2) the two halves of the box, formed above and below by the location of the upper and lower quartiles, should be relatively symmetrical around the median; and (3) no egregious asymmetrical outliers should be present. Obvious violations of any of these three requirements can easily be discerned as an "abnormality" in the box plot, indicating an eccentric distribution. If all three requirements are fulfilled, the data are almost surely Gaussian or quite symmetrical.

The decisions about what is *relatively close, symmetrical,* or *egregious* will depend on the analyst's "statistical judgment."

5.8.3 Special Tests for Eccentricity

For analysts who prefer more precise "laboratory tests" rather than the simple judgments just discussed, diverse tactics have been devised to offer warnings about non-Gaussian distributions. The methods are automated and the results regularly appear, often without having been solicited, in computer programs that display summaries of univariate data.

The additional results can regularly be ignored, but are there if you want them. They include indexes of "normality" and various graphical plots. The procedures are briefly mentioned here to outline what they do, should you ever decide (or need) to use them. Further explanation of the strategies is usually offered in the associated manuals for the computer programs, and their interpretations can be found in various statistical textbooks.

5.8.3.1   Indexes of "Normality" — Two relatively simple tests produce an index of skewness, reflecting different locations for mean and median, and an index of kurtosis which denotes whether the distributional shape is leptokurtic (too tall and thin), platykurtic (too short and fat), or mesokurtic (just right). One of these calculations is called Geary's test of kurtosis.[12]

Royston has described computational[13] and graphical[14] methods that offer more sophisticated approaches for evaluating normality.

5.8.3.2   Graphical Plots — A different way of checking for normality is to do simple or complicated graphical plots. In a simple plot, which shows the residual values of $X_i - \overline{X}$ graphed against X_i, the results of a Gaussian curve should show nonspecific variations, with no evident pattern, around a horizontal line drawn at the mean of $\overline{X}$.

The more complicated plots compare the observed values of the data with the corresponding quantile or standard-deviation points calculated for a Gaussian distribution that has the observed $\overline{X}$ and s as its determining features.

5.8.3.3   Illustration of Univariate Print-Out — Figure 5.4 shows the univariate print-out produced by the SAS system for the 200 values of hematocrit whose stem-leaf plot was previously shown in Figure 3.2. The upper left corner shows the group size of N = 200, the mean of 41.09, and standard deviation of 5.179 (with $s^2 = 26.825$), with c.v. = $(s/\overline{X} \times 100)$ = 12.605 and standard error of the mean (marked "Std Mean") = .366. The uncorrected sum of squares (USS) for ΣX_i^2 is 343015.8 and the corrected sum of squares (CSS) for S_{xx} is 5338.32. The other data in the upper left corner show indexes of skewness and kurtosis and results for three other tests [T: mean; M(Sign); and Sgn Rank] that will be discussed later. The middle part of the upper half of the printout shows the various quantile values, and the far right upper section shows the five lowest and highest observed values in the data, together with their individual identification codes (marked "Obs") among the 200 members.

The stem-leaf plot on the lower left is a condensed version (marked for even-numbered stems only) of what was shown earlier in Figure 3.2. Next to it is the box plot, which is ordinarily the most useful part of the visual display. It shows the essentially similar values for mean and median in this set of data. The two halves of the box here falsely appear asymmetrical because of an artifact of the graphic plotting system, which contained no provision for odd values. Hence, the mean and median, with values of 41, were plotted at values of 40. [This graphic artifact should warn you always to check the actual values of the three quartiles before concluding that a box plot is asymmetrical.]

With an interquartile range of 6 (= 44 – 38), the two whiskers extend a distance of 9 (= 1.5 × 6) units above and below the margins of the box, leaving low outlier values (marked "0") at values of 28 and 24, with high outliers at 54 and 56.

The normal probability plot in the lower right corner of Figure 5.4 shows + marks to denote where points would be located if the distribution were perfectly Gaussian. Thus, the locations for − 0.5, −1, and −1.5 standard deviations below the mean for these data should be respectively at values of 41.09 − (0.5)(5.179) = 38.5; 41.09 − 5.179 = 35.9, and 41.09 − (1.5)(5.179) = 33.3. The asterisks (or "stars") show the actual locations of the points in the distribution. In this instance, they follow the Gaussian line of + marks fairly closely, but dip below it at the low end and extend above at the high end.

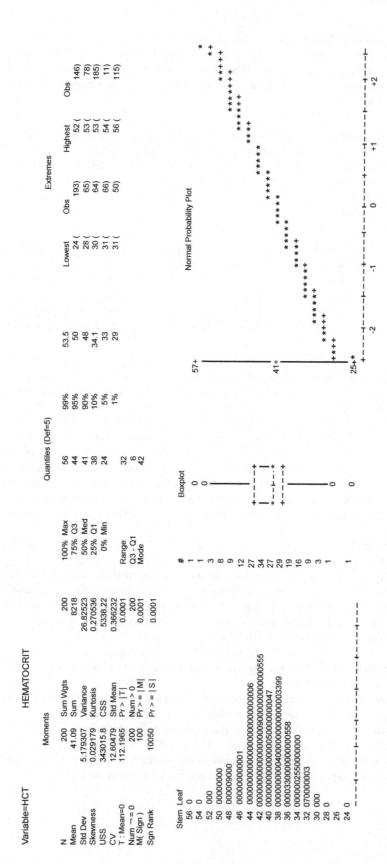

FIGURE 5.4

Printout of univariate display for group of 200 hematocrit values previously shown in Figure 3.2. The display was created by the PROC UNIVARIATE program of the SAS system. All results in the upper half of the display appear routinely. The stem-leaf, box, and normal probability plots are all requested options.

5.9 Transformations and Other "Therapy"

When worried about the misrepresentation that can occur if an eccentric distribution is externally represented by its mean and standard deviation, data analysts can use various tactics to discern and try to "repair" non-Gaussian distributions of dimensional data.

The usual mechanism of repair, as noted earlier, is to eliminate outliers from the data or to perform "Gaussianizing" transformations. The transformations were particularly popular during the pre-computer era of statistical analysis, but the tactic is used much less often today.

1. Many new forms of analysis, as noted in Parts II-IV of the text, do not depend on Gaussian (parametric) procedures. The data can be processed according to their ranks (or other arrangements) that do not rely on means and standard deviations. Having been automated in various "packaged" computer programs, the new methods are easy to use and readily available.

2. Many forms of medical data are not expressed in dimensional variables. They are cited in binary, ordinal, or nominal categories for which means and standard deviations are not pertinent.

3. Despite apparent contradictions of logic and violations of the basic mathematical assumptions, the parametric methods are quite "robust" not for *description* of eccentric data, but for inferences that will be discussed later. Without any transformations or alterations, the "unvarnished" methods often yield reasonably accurate inferential conclusions — i.e., the same conclusions about "statistical significance" that might come from transformed data or from the "gold standard" non-parametric methods.

For all these reasons, analysts today do not transform data as often as formerly. The univariate distributions should still be carefully inspected, however, to determine whether the dimensional data are so eccentric that they require non-parametric rather than parametric procedures.

5.10 Indexes of Diversity

Indexes of spread are seldom determined for categorical data, but the dispersion of frequency counts among the categories can be expressed, if desired, with statistical indexes of diversity.

Maximum diversity in any group occurs when its members are distributed equally among the available categories. Thus, with c categories for a group of N members, the group has maximum diversity if the frequency count, f_i, in each category is $f_i = N/c$. The various indexes of diversity differ in the way they express the distribution, but all of them compare the observed distribution score with the maximum possible score.

Although these indexes seldom appear in medical or biological literature, they can sometimes be used to describe the proportionate distribution of a set of categorical descriptions in ecologic studies of birds or animals, or even, in the first example cited here, for clinical "staging" of people.

5.10.1 Permutation Score for Distributions

One expression of diversity uses scores obtained from factorial permutations. The number of permutations of N items is $N! = 1 \times 2 \times 3 \times \ldots \times N$. If divided into c categories containing $f_1, f_2, \ldots, f_c$ members, the total number of permutations will be $N!/(f_1!\ f_2!\ \ldots f_c!)$. [We shall meet this same idea later when permutation procedures are discussed.]

Suppose a group of 21 patients contains 4 in Stage I, 6 in Stage II, and 11 in Stage III. The permutation score would be $21!/(4!\ 6!\ 11!) = 5.1091 \times 10^{19}/(24 \times 720 \times 39{,}916{,}800) = 7.4070358 \times 10^7$. If the group were perfectly divided into three parts, the maximum possible score would have been $21!/(7!\ 7!\ 7!) = 3.9907 \times 10^8$. The ratio of the actual and maximum scores would be $7.4070358 \times 10^7/3.9907 \times 10^8 = .186$.

The log-of-factorial-permutations score has been used clinically[15] for comparing different partitions of groups in the preparation of prognostic "staging" systems. For example, suppose a group of 200 people can be distributed as {19, 77, 82, 22} or as {20, 84, 72, 24}. The result of the log permutation score is 100.9 for the first partition and 102.4 for the second. If all other factors were equal, the second partition would be regarded as having a better (i.e., more diverse) distribution.

5.10.2   Shannon's H

An entity called Shannon's H[16] is derived from concepts of "entropy" in information theory. The idea refers to "uncertainty" in a distribution. If all cases are in the same category, there is no uncertainty. If the cases are equally divided across categories, the uncertainty is at a maximum.

The formula for Shannon's index of diversity is

$$H = -\Sigma p_i \log p_i$$

where p_i is the proportion of data in each category. For patients in the three categorical stages in the example of Section 5.10.1, the respective proportions are .190, .286, and .524. Shannon's index of diversity is

$$H = -[.190 \log .190 + .286 \log .286 + .524 \log .524] = -[-.4396] = .4396$$

The last index cited here expresses qualitative variation from a heterogeneity score calculated as the sum of the products of all pairs of frequency counts. For three categories, this sum will be $f_1 f_2 + f_1 f_3 + f_2 f_3$. In the example cited here, the score will be $(4 \times 6) + (4 \times 11) + (6 \times 11) = 134$. The maximum heterogeneity score — with equal distribution in all categories — would occur as $(7 \times 7) + (7 \times 7) + (7 \times 7) = 147$. The index of qualitative variation is the ratio of the observed and maximum scores. In this instance, it is $134/147 = .91$.

Indexes of diversity are probably most useful for comparing distributions among groups, rather than for giving an absolute rating. Because the scores depend on the number of categories, the comparisons are best restricted to groups divided into the same number of categories. For the two groups of 200 people cited at the end of Section 5.10.1, the observed heterogeneity scores would respectively be 13251 and 13392. The higher result for the second group would indicate that it is more heterogeneous than the first, as noted previously with the permutation score.

References

1. Tukey, 1977; 2. Cleveland, 1994; 3. Wald, 1993; 4. Reynolds, 1993; 5. Wallis, 1956; 6. Snedecor, 1980; 7. Miller, 1993; 8. Spear, 1952; 9. McGill, 1978; 10. SAS Procedures Guide, 1990; 11. SPSS^x User's Guide, 1986; 12. Geary, 1936; 13. Royston, 1993a; 14. Royston, 1993b; 15. Feinstein, 1972; 16. Shannon, 1948.

Exercises

5.1. In one mechanism of constructing a "range of normal," the values of the selected variable are obtained for a group of apparently healthy people. The inner 95% of the data is then called the "range of normal." Do you agree with this tactic? If not, why not — and what alternative would you offer?

5.2. At many medical laboratories, the "range of normal" is determined from results obtained in a consecutive series of routine specimens, which will include tests on sick as well as healthy people. What would you propose as a pragmatically feasible method for determining the "range of normal" for this type of data?

5.3. A "range of normal" can be demarcated with a Gaussian inner zone around the mean, with an inner percentile zone, or with a zone eccentrically placed at one end of the data. Each of these methods will be good for certain variables, and not good for others. Name two medical variables for which each of these three methods would be the best statistical strategy of establishing a "range of normal." Offer a brief justification for your choices. (Total of six variables to be named. Please avoid any already cited as illustrations.)

5.4. The quartile deviation is almost always smaller than the corresponding standard deviation. Why do you think this happens?

5.5. For the data in Table 3.1, the mean is 22.732 and the standard deviation (calculated with $n - 1$) is 7.693.

    5.5.1. What would have been the standard deviation if calculated with n?

    5.5.2. What is the coefficient of variation for the data?

    5.5.3. What is the quartile coefficient of variation?

5.6. What corresponding values do you get when an inner 95% zone is determined by percentiles and by a Gaussian demarcation in the data of Table 3.1? Why do the results differ?

5.7. Using whatever medical journal you would like, find three sets of data (each describing one variable in one group) that have been summarized with an index of central tendency and an index of spread. From what you know or have been shown about the data, are you content with these summary values? Mention what they are, and why you are content or discontent. Be sure to find at least one data set for which the published summary indexes have evoked your displeasure, and indicate why you are unhappy. As you read more of the published report where those indexes appeared, do you think they have led to any serious distortions in the authors' conclusions? If so, outline the problem.

5.8. A colleague who wants to analyze categories rather than dimensional values has asked you to divide the data of Table 3.1 into five categories. What partition would you choose? How would you demonstrate its effectiveness?

6

Probabilities and Standardized Indexes

CONTENTS

We now have methods to summarize a group of data by citing indexes of central location and spread. We can also examine box plots and relative spreads to indicate whether the data have a symmetric distribution, and whether the central index does a satisfactory job of representing the group. For decisions that one group is taller, heavier, or wealthier than another, the central indexes can be compared directly if they are satisfactory. If not, additional mechanisms will be needed for the comparison.

The foregoing approach seems reasonable and straightforward, but it does not take care of a major problem that has not yet been considered: the stability of the indexes. When we compared 50% vs. 33% back in Chapter 1, each group was suitably represented by the proportions of 50% and 33%, but we were uneasy about the comparison if the actual numbers were 1/2 vs. 1/3, and relatively comfortable if they were 150/300 vs. 100/300.

6.1 Stability, Inference, and Probability

The comparison of 1/2 vs. 1/3 left us uneasy because the summary indexes were unstable. If the first group had one more member, its result could be 1/3, producing the same 33% as in the second group. If the second group had one more member, its result might be 2/4, producing the same 50% as in the first group. On the other hand, the original comparison of 50% vs. 33% would hardly be changed if one more person were added to (or removed from) groups with results of 150/300 vs. 100/300.

Even if the groups are large, stability of the indexes is not always assured. For example, in two groups that each contain 1000 people, a ratio indicating that one group has twice the mortality rate of the other might seem impressive if the rates are 200/1000 vs. 100/1000, but not if they are 2/1000 vs. 1/1000.

For these reasons, statistical decisions require attention to yet another component — stability of the central index — that is not denoted merely by the index itself or by the spread of the data. The evaluation of stability involves concepts of probability and inference that will be discussed in this chapter before we turn to the mechanisms of evaluation in Chapters 7 and 8.

6.1.1 "Perturbation" and Inference

Stability of a central index is tested with various methods of "perturbing" the data. The methods, which are discussed in Chapters 7 and 8, include such tactics as "jackknife" removal of individual items, "bootstrap" resampling from an empirical group, and "parametric" sampling from a theoretical population to determine a "confidence interval."

The perturbations are used to answer the question, "What would happen if…?" Each set of results allows us to estimate both a range of possible values for the central index, and also a probability that the values will be attained. All of these estimates represent *inference*, rather than evidence, because they are derived from the observed data but are not themselves directly observed.

6.1.2 Probability and Sampling

If a set of data has already been collected, it can be "perturbed" in various ways to make inferences about the probability of what might happen. A different and particularly important role of probability, however, occurs when we do not yet have any data, but plan to get some by a sampling process. For example, suppose we want to conduct a political poll to determine the preferences of a group of voters. How large a sample would make us feel confident about the results? The latter question cannot be answered with the tactic of perturbing an observed group of data, because we do not yet have any data available. The decision about the size of the sample can be made, however, with principles of probability that will be cited later.

Because probability has many other roles in statistics, this chapter offers an introductory discussion of its concepts and application. The idea of probability usually appears in statistics not for descriptive summaries of observed data, but in reference to inferential decisions. Nevertheless, *probability* has already been mentioned several times (in Sections 4.5 and 4.8) in connection with such descriptive indexes as percentiles and Z-scores. In addition, all of the inner zones discussed in Chapter 5 describe proportions of the observed data; and each proportion can be regarded as the probability that a randomly chosen item of data would come from the designated zone.

A particularly valuable attribute of zones of probability is their role as the main intellectual "bridge" between the descriptive and inferential strategies of statistical reasoning. An internal zone of probability is used, as noted later in Chapter 7, to construct boundaries for a *confidence interval* that shows possible variations in the location of a central index. An external zone of probability is used, as discussed here and in many subsequent chapters, to establish P values for the possibility that important distinctions in the observed results arose by chance alone.

6.2 Why Learn about Probability?

Mathematical discussions of probability are usually the place at which most non-statisticians lose interest in statistics. The reader (or student) usually wants to learn about quantitative distinctions: how to examine the magnitudes of observed data in a group; how to contrast the results in two (or more) groups; how to check the associations among two (or more) variables. Seeking enlightenment about these pragmatic activities in the real world of statistical description, the reader wonders why the discussion has entered the theoretical world of probabilities and statistical inference. When the discussion begins to include long mathematical details about the "laws of probability," principles of sampling, and other theoretical background, the reader is usually bored, repelled, or confused beyond redemption.

The purpose of these remarks is to indicate why probability is important, and to assure you that the forthcoming discussion will try to avoid many of the unattractive mathematical details.

The prime reason for being concerned about probability is that medical research often involves small groups and data that create uncertainty about unstable numerical results, such as those discussed at the beginning of this chapter. The instabilities can lead to potentially troublesome events. A political candidate who discovers she is favored by 67% of the voters may reduce her campaigning efforts because she feels sure of winning the election. If the value of 67% reflects the preference of only 4 of 6 people, however, the decision might be disastrous. If we conclude that treatment A is definitely better than treatment B because the respective success rates are 50% vs. 33%, the conclusion might be dramatically wrong if the actual observed numbers were only 4/8 vs. 2/6.

In considering the consequences of numerical instability, we use probabilities to determine the chance of occurrence for potentially distressing events. If the probability is small enough, we might stop worrying. Thus, if the political poll in a properly conducted survey shows that the candidate is favored by 40 of 60 voters, the probability is about one in a hundred (as is demonstrated later) that the observed result of .67 represents a voting population whose preference for that candidate might actually be as low as .51. With this small a chance of losing, the candidate — particularly if running out of funds — may decide to reduce campaign efforts.

Not all statistical decisions involve appraisals of probability. When the first heart was successfully transplanted, or the first traumatically severed limb was successfully reattached, neither statistics nor probabilities were needed to prove that the surgery could work. No control groups or statistical tabulations were necessary to demonstrate success on the initial occasions when diabetic acidosis was promptly reversed by insulin, when bacterial endocarditis was cured by penicillin, or when a fertilized embryo was produced outside the uterus. No calculations of probability are used when a baseball team wins the pennant with a success proportion of 99/162 = .611, although this result seems but trivially larger than the 98/162 = .605 result for the team that finishes in second place.

Many eminent scientists have said, "If you have to prove it with statistics, your experiment isn't very good," and the statement is true for many types of research. If the experiment always produces the same "deterministic" result, no statistics are needed. The entity under study always happens or it does not; and the probability of occurrence is either 100% or 0%. For example, if we mix equal amounts of the colors blue and yellow, the result should always be green. If the color that emerges is purple, statistics are not needed to prove that something must have gone wrong.

If the anticipated results are not "deterministic," however, probabilities will always be produced by the uncertainties. If told there is a 38% chance of rain today, we have to decide whether to take an umbrella. If told that a particular treatment usually has 80% failure, we might wonder about believing a clinician who claims three consecutive successes.

The probabilities that can often be valuable for these decisions are also often abused. A surgeon is said to have told a patient, "The usual mortality rate for this operation is 90%; and my last nine patients all died. You are very lucky because you are the tenth."

Many (if not most) decisions in the world of public health, clinical practice, and medical research involve statistical information that has an inevitable numerical uncertainty. The groups were relatively small or the data (even if the groups were large) had variations that were nondeterministic. In these circumstances, wrong decisions can be made if we fail to anticipate the effects of numerical instability.

The world of probabilistic inference joins the world of descriptive statistics, therefore, because decisions are regularly made amid numerical instability, and because citations of probability are invaluable components of the decisions. The discussion of probability in this chapter has three main goals:

1. To acquaint you with the basic principles and the way they are used;
2. To emphasize what is actually useful, avoiding details of the mathematical "ethos" that underlies the principles; and
3. To make you aware of what you need to know, and wary of unjustified tactics or erroneous claims that sometimes appear in medical literature.

Finally, if you start to wonder whether all this attention to probability is warranted for a *single group* of data, you can be reassured that all decisions about probability are based on a single group of data. When two or more groups are compared, or when two or more variables are associated, the probabilistic decisions are all referred to the distribution of a single group of data. That single group can be constructed in an empirical or theoretical manner, but its distribution becomes the basis for evaluating the role of probability in comparing the observations made in several groups or several variables. Thus, if you understand the appropriate characteristics of a single group of data, you will be ready for all the other probabilistic decisions that come later.

6.3   Concepts of Probability

In many fields of science, the most fundamental ideas are often difficult to define. What should be intellectual bedrock may emerge on closer examination to resemble a swamp. This type of problem can be noted in medicine if you try to give unassailable, non-controversial definitions for such ideas as *health*, *disease*, and *normal*. In statistics, the same problem arises for *probability*. It can represent many different ideas, definitions, and applications.

6.3.1   Subjective Probabilities

In one concept, *probability* represents a subjective impression that depends on feelings rather than specific data. This type of subjective guess determines the odds given for bets on a sporting event. The odds may be affected by previous data about each team's past performance, but the current estimate is always a hunch. Similarly, if you take a guess about the likelihood that you will enjoy learning statistics, you might express the chance as a probability, but the expression is subjective, without any direct, quantitative background data as its basis.

6.3.2   Frequentist Probabilities

In most statistical situations, *probability* represents an estimate based on the known frequency characteristics of a particular distribution of events or possibilities. These estimates, which are called *frequentist* probabilities, are the customary concept when the idea of "probability" appears in medical literature. The results depend on frequency counts in a distribution of data.

If the data are binary, and the results show 81 successes and 22 failures for a particular treatment, the success proportion of $81/103 = .79$ would lead to 79% as the probability estimate of success. If the data are dimensional, as in the chloride information of Table 4.1 in Chapter 4, the distribution of results can lead to diverse probabilities based on relative and cumulative relative frequencies. If we randomly selected one chloride value from the series of items in that table, the chances (or probabilities) are .0780 that the item will be exactly **101**, .0598 that it will lie below **93**, .8598 (= .9196 − .0598) that it will lie between **93–107**, and .0804 that it will be above **107**.

Frequentist probabilities need not come from an actual distribution of data, however. They can also be obtained theoretically from the structure of a particular device, mechanism, or model. Knowing the structure of a fair coin, we would expect the chance to be 1/2 for getting a head when the coin is tossed. Similarly, a standard deck of 52 playing cards has a structure that would make us estimate 13/52 or 1/4 for the chance of getting a spade if one card is chosen randomly from the deck. The chance of getting a "picture card" (Jack, Queen, or King) is (4 + 4 + 4)/52 = 12/52 = .23.

Frequentist probabilities can also be constructed, as noted later, from modern new tactics that create empirical redistributions or resamplings from an observed set of data.

6.3.3 Other Approaches

Just as human illness can be approached with the concepts of "orthodox" medicine, chiropractic, naturopathy, witchcraft, and other schools of "healing," statistical approaches to probability have different schools of thought. The conventional, customary approach — which employs frequentist probability — will be used throughout this text. Another school of thought, however, has attracted the creative imagination of capable statisticians. The alternative approach, called *Bayesian inference*, often appears in statistical literature and is sometimes used in sophisticated discussions of statistical issues in medical research. Bayesian inference shares an eponym with Bayes theorem, which is medically familiar from its often proposed application in the analysis of diagnostic tests. Bayes *theorem*, however, is a relatively simple algebraic truism (see Chapter 21), whereas Bayesian *inference* is a highly complex system of reasoning, involving subjective as well as frequentist probabilities.

Yet another complex system for making estimates and expressing probabilities is the likelihood method which relies on various arrangements for multiplying or dividing "conditional" probabilities. Its most simple applications are illustrated later in the text as the *likelihood ratios* that sometimes express results of diagnostic tests, and as the *maximum likelihood* strategy used to find regression coefficients when the conventional "least squares" method is not employed in statistical associations.

6.4 Empirical Redistributions

The frequentist probabilities discussed in Section 6.3.2 were obtained in at least three ways. One of them is empirical, from a distribution of observed data, such as the success proportion of .79 (=81/103), or the different values and frequencies in the chloride data of Table 4.1. The other two methods rely on theoretical expectations from either a device, such as a coin or a deck of cards, or from the "model" structure of a mathematical distribution, such as a Gaussian curve. Mathematical models, which will be discussed later, have become a traditional basis for the probabilities used in statistical inference.

The rest of this section is devoted to a fourth (and new) method, made possible by modern computation, that determines probabilities and uncertainties from redistributions or "resamplings" of the observed, empirical data.

6.4.1 Principles of Resampling

The great virtue of a theoretical distribution is that it saves work. If we did not know whether a coin was "fair," i.e., suitably balanced, we would have to toss it over and over repeatedly to tabulate the numbers of heads and tails before concluding that the probability of getting a head was 1/2. If we were asked to estimate the chance of drawing a spade from 100 well shuffled decks of cards, we could promptly guess 1/4. Without the theoretical "model," however, we might have to count all 5200 cards or check results in repeated smaller samplings.

The Gaussian distribution discussed in Section 4.8.3 has a similar virtue. If we know that a particular distribution of data is Gaussian and if we are given a particular member's Z-score, we can promptly use the Gaussian attributes of Z-scores to determine the corresponding percentile and probability values. If we could not assume that the data were Gaussian, however, we would have to determine the desired probabilites either by examining the entire group of data or by taking repeated samplings.

The repeated-sampling process, in fact, was the way in which certain mathematical model distributions were discovered. For example, the t-distribution (discussed later) was found when W. S. Gosset, who published his results under the pseudonym of "Student," took repeated small samples from a large collection of measurements describing finger lengths and other attributes of criminals.[1]

With the modern availability of easy electronic computation, new methods have been developed to create distributions empirically as resampled rearrangements of an observed set of data. The method of forming these ad hoc empirical redistributions, without recourse to any theoretical mathematical models, uses *bootstrap* and *jackknife* strategies that will be briefly described here and further discussed in Chapter 7.

6.4.1.1   *Illustrative Example* —

To illustrate the resampling process, suppose we want to assess the stability of the mean in the three-member data set $\{1, 6, 9\}$, for which $\overline{X} = 16/3 = 5.33$. We know that the three items of data have come from somewhere, and that the source included items whose values were 1, 6, and 9. As discussed later, we can try to construct a hypothetical population that might be the source, and we can contemplate theoretical samples that might be drawn from that population. Alternatively, however, we can work with the real data that have actually been observed. We can regard the values of **1**, **6**, and **9** as the entire "parent population." We can then take repeated samples of 3 members from this "population," being careful to replace each member after it is drawn. We determine the mean of each sample and then note the distribution of those means. The variations in the array of means can then help answer the question about stability of the original mean.

To construct each sample, we randomly draw one member from the set of data $\{1, 6, 9\}$. After replacing it, we randomly draw a second member. We replace it and then randomly draw a third member. We then calculate the mean for those three values. The process is repeated for the next sample. As the sampling process continues, it will yield a series of means for each of the three-member sets of data. To denote variation in the distribution, we can determine the standard deviation and other features of that series of means.

6.4.1.2   *Mechanism of Redistribution* —

The sampling process itself can be avoided if we work out the specific details of what might happen. Since three possibilities exist for each choice of a member from the 3-item data set, there will be $3^3 = 27$ possible samples of three members. Those samples, and their means, are shown in Table 6.1.

Table 6.2 shows the frequency distribution of the 27 means in Table 6.1. The distribution has a mode of 5.33, which is the same as the original mean of 5.33. The mean of the 27 means is also 5.33, calculated as $[(1 \times 1.00) + (3 \times 2.67) + (3 \times 3.67) + \ldots + (3 \times 8.00) + (1 \times 9.00)]/27 = 143.98/27 = 5.33$. The group variance, using the formula $\Sigma X_i^2 - [(\Sigma X_i)^2/n]$, is $[(1 \times 1.00^2) + (3 \times 2.67^2) + (3 \times 3.67^2) + \ldots + (3 \times 8.00^2) + (1 \times 9.00^2)] - [(143.98)^2/27] = 865.700 - 767.787 = 97.913$. For this complete set of 27 samples, the group variance is divided by n to calculate variance, which becomes $92.913/27 = 3.626$. The square root of the variance is the standard deviation, 1.904.

6.4.2   Standard Error, Coefficient of Stability, and Zones of Probability

The term *standard error* of the mean refers to the standard deviation found in the means of an array of repeated samples. In resamplings of the data set $\{1, 6, 9\}$, the mean value of 5.33 will have a standard deviation, i.e., standard error, of 1.904.

The more customary method of determining standard error is with theoretical principles discussed later. According to those principles, however, the standard error in a sample containing n members is $\sigma/\sqrt{n}$,

TABLE 6.1

All Possible Samples and Corresponding Means in a
3-Member Complete Resampling of the Set of Data {1, 6, 9}

Sample	Mean	Sample	Mean	Sample	Mean
{1, 1, 1} :	1.00	{6, 1, 1} :	2.67	{9, 1, 1} :	3.67
{1, 1, 6} :	2.67	{6, 1, 6} :	4.33	{9, 1, 6} :	5.33
{1, 1, 9} :	3.67	{6, 1, 9} :	5.33	{9, 1, 9} :	6.33
{1, 6, 1} :	2.67	{6, 6, 1} :	4.33	{9, 6, 1} :	5.33
{1, 6, 6} :	4.33	{6, 6, 6} :	6.00	{9, 6, 6} :	7.00
{1, 6, 9} :	5.33	{6, 6, 9} :	7.00	{9, 6, 9} :	8.00
{1, 9, 1} :	3.67	{6, 9, 1} :	5.33	{9, 9, 1} :	6.33
{1, 9, 6} :	5.33	{6, 9, 6} :	7.00	{9, 9, 6} :	8.00
{1, 9, 9} :	6.33	{6, 9, 9} :	8.00	{9, 9, 9} :	9.00

where σ is the standard deviation of the parent population. In this instance, the group of data {1, 6, 9} is a complete population, rather than a sample, and its standard deviation is calculated with n rather than n − 1. Thus $\sigma^2 = [(1^2 + 6^2 + 9^2) - (16^2/3)]/3 = 10.89$ and $\sigma = 3.30$. The value of $\sigma/\sqrt{n}$ will be $3.30/\sqrt{3} = 1.905$, which is essentially identical to the result obtained with resampling.

To evaluate stability, we can examine the ratio of standard error/mean. This ratio, which might be called the *coefficient of stability*, is a counterpart of the coefficient of variation, calculated as c.v. = standard deviation/mean. In this instance, the coefficient of stability (c.s.) will be 1.905/5.33 = .36. The interpretation of this index will be discussed later. Intuitively, however, we can immediately regard the value of .36 as indicating an unstable mean. We would expect a "stable" coefficient of stability for the mean to be substantially smaller than an adequate coefficient of variation for the data. Yet the value of .36 for c.s. is much larger than the values of .10 or .15 proposed in Section 5.5.1 as a standard of adequacy for the c.v.

Another approach to the array of resampled means in Table 6.2 is to note that the value of the mean will range from **2.67** to **8.00** in 25 (92.6%) of the 27 possible resamplings. Excluding the four most extreme values at each end of Table 6.2, we could state that the mean will range from **3.67** to **7.00** in 19/27 (=70.4%) of the resamplings. Expressed in probabilities, the chances are .704 that the mean would be in the range **3.67 − 7.00**, and .926 for the range of **2.67 − 8.00**. There is a chance of 1/27 = .04 that the mean would be either as high as **9.00** or as low as **1.00**.

TABLE 6.2

Frequency Distribution
of Means in Table 6.1

Value	Frequency
1.00	1
2.67	3
3.67	3
4.33	3
5.33	6
6.00	1
6.33	3
7.00	3
8.00	3
9.00	1
Total	27

This resampling activity may seem like a lot of needless work to get the same standard error of 1.904 that could have been found so easily with the theoretical $\sigma/\sqrt{n}$ formula. The resampling process, however, has several major advantages that will be discussed later. Two virtues that are already apparent are (1) it helps confirm the accuracy of the $\sigma/\sqrt{n}$ formula, which we would otherwise have to accept without proof; and (2) it offers an accurate account of the inner zone of possible variations for the resampled means. The inner zone from 2.67 to 8.00, which contains 92.6% of the possible values, is something we shall meet later, called a *confidence interval* for the mean. The range of this interval can also be determined with the theoretical tactics discussed later (Chapter 7), but the resampling process offers an exact demonstration.

6.4.3 Bootstrap Procedure

The strategy of examining samples constructed directly from members of an observed distribution is called the *bootstrap* procedure. If the original group contains m members, each one is eligible to be a member of the resampled group. If each resampled group has n members, there will be m^n possible samples. Thus, there were $3^3 = 27$ arrangements of resamples containing 3 members from the three-member group. If each of the resampled groups contained only two members, there would be a total of $3^2 = 9$ groups.

In a complete resampling, as in Section 6.4.1.2, all possible arrangements are considered — so that m^m samples are produced. Thus, a complete resampling from the 20 items of data in Exercise 3.3 would produce $20^{20} = 1.05 \times 10^{26}$ arrangements. A properly programmed computer could slog through all of them, but a great deal of time would be required. Consequently, the bootstrap approach seldom uses a complete resampling. Instead, the computer constructs a large set (somewhere between 500 and 10,000) of random samples, each taken from the original group of n members, with each member suitably replaced each time. The name *Monte Carlo* is sometimes used for the process of taking multiple random samples from an observed collection of data. The Monte Carlo resamples are then checked for the distributional patterns of means (or any other desired attributes) in the collection of samples.

With dimensional data, the bootstrap procedure is often applied for a limited rather than complete resampling of the original data, but the complete procedure is relatively easy to do if the data have binary values of **0/1**. For binary data, mathematical formulas (discussed later in Chapter 8) can be used to anticipate the complete bootstrapped results.

6.4.4   Jackknife Procedure

An even simpler method of determining the stability of the mean for the set of data $\{1, 6, 9\}$ is to use a sequential removal (and restoration) strategy. For the three-item data set, the removal of the first member produces $\{6, 9\}$, with a mean of 7.5. After the first member is restored, removal of the second member produces $\{1, 9\}$, with a mean of 5.0. Removal of the third member leads to $\{1, 6\}$, with a mean of 3.5. Thus, removal of a single member can make the original mean of 5.33 change to values that range from 3.5 to 7.5. [Note that the mean of the rearrangements is $(7.5 + 5.0 + 3.5)/3 = 16/3 = 5.33$, which is again the value of the original mean.]

The strategy of forming rearrangements by successively removing (and then later restoring) each member of the data set is called the *jackknife procedure*. In a data set containing n members, the procedure produces n rearranged groups, each containing $n - 1$ members.

The jackknife procedure, which will later be used here to evaluate the "fragility" of a comparison of two groups of data, is particularly valuable in certain multivariable analyses. At the moment, however, the main value of the jackknife is its use as a "screening" procedure for the stability of a mean. In the data set of $\{1, 6, 9\}$ we might want to avoid calculating standard errors with either a theoretical formula or a bootstrap resampling. If the jackknife possibilities show that a mean of 5.33 can drop to 3.5 or rise to 7.5 with removal of only 1 member, the mean is obviously unstable. This type of "screening" examination, like various other tactics discussed later, offers a simple "commonsense" approach for making statistical decisions without getting immersed in mathematical formulas or doctrines.

6.4.5   "Computer-Intensive" Statistics

The *bootstrap* and *jackknife* procedures are examples of a "revolution," made possible by computers, that is now occurring in the world of statistics. An analogous revolution, which has caused *diagnostic radiology* to change its name to *imaging*, has already been facilitated by computers in the world of medicine.

The jackknife procedure was first proposed by Quenouille[2] and later advocated by Tukey.[3] An analog of resampling was developed many years ago by R. A. Fisher[4] to construct a special permutation test discussed in Chapter 12, but the modern approaches to resampling methods were developed by Julian Simon[5] and independently by Bradley Efron[6]. Efron introduced the term *bootstrap* and later gave the name *computer-intensive*[7] to both types of new procedures, because they could not be used regularly or easily until computers were available to do the necessary calculations.

In the "revolution" produced by the new procedures, statistical inference with probabilities can be done in an entirely new manner, without relying on any of the theoretical "parametric" mathematical models that have become the traditional custom during the past century. The revolution has not yet become widespread, however, and most elementary statistical instruction, as well as a large amount of discourse in this text, still employs the traditional "parametric" statistical strategies.

Nevertheless, the revolution is happening, and you should be prepared for its eventual results. Respectable statisticians today are even proposing such heresies as, "All techniques designed before the advent of automatic computing must be abandoned."[8] Until the revolution becomes totally established, however, the traditional statistical strategies will continue to be used and published. Consequently, the traditional strategies will be discussed here to prepare you for today's realities. The new strategies will regularly be mentioned, however, to indicate things that can not only be done today, but routinely expected within the foreseeable future.

6.5   Demarcating Zones of Probability

Regardless of whether a sample is constructed empirically or theoretically, zones of probability in the distribution have a particularly important role in both statistical description and statistical inference. Descriptively, the zones are used to demarcate the "bulk" of a set of data or to form a "range of normal." Inferentially, analogous zones lead to decisions that a particular observation is too "uncommon" or "far out" to be accepted as a regular part of the distribution. For these purposes, boundary markers must be set for zones of probability.

6.5.1   Choosing Zones

In gambling, we may want to know the probabilities for a single event, such as drawing a spade in cards or tossing a **7** in dice. In statistical activities, however, we often want to know the probabilities for a *zone* of events or values. We would seldom ask about the probability that a single chloride value will be exactly **101**, but we might regularly want to know the chances that the value will lie in a zone below **93** or above **107**.

A *zone* almost always refers to a series of directly contiguous dimensional (or ordinal) values in a distribution. In the chloride example just cited, the selected zone would extend from **93** to **107**. Sometimes, however, a zone can be a cluster of selected noncontiguous values. For example, when you make a "field" bet in tosses of two dice, the successful zone consists of any member of the items 2, 3, 4, 9, 10, 11, or 12.

6.5.2   Setting Markers

One way to set markers for a zone is from the cumulative relative frequencies associated with an actual or resampled distribution. The array of frequencies could be examined to note the values that demarcate zones of either chloride measurements in Table 4.1 or resampled means in Table 6.1.

A direct check of individual frequencies can be avoided, however, if the distribution has certain mathematical characteristics, such as the distributions eponymically cited with such names as Gauss, "Student," and Bernouilli. If we know (or can assume) that a collection of data has one of these model distributions, we can easily find markers for the desired probabilities, without resorting to specific tabulations of frequencies.

This mathematical attribute has given the eponymic model distributions their statistical popularity. To determine probabilites, we first calculate a special index, called a "test statistic," from the observed data. We then assume, based on mathematical justifications discussed later, that the test statistic is associated with a particular mathematical model such as the standard Gaussian distribution. The value of the test statistic then becomes the marker for a zone of probability. For example, the Z-score is often used as a test statistic that has specific probability values, shown in Section 4.8.3, for each of its locations in a standard Gaussian distribution. [Other well-known test statistics are referred to a t (or "Student") distribution or to a chi-square distribution.]

The percentiles and standard deviations discussed in Chapters 4 and 5 can thus be used in two ways: descriptively, to indicate specific zones for an empirical set of data, and inferentially, to demarcate zones of probability in a mathematical model.

6.5.3   Internal and External Zones

The total cumulative probability in any distribution always has a sum of 1. This total can be divided into different sets of zones. An *internal* zone of data contains values that are within or smaller than the demarcated boundary. An *external* zone contains values that are outside or beyond the demarcated boundary. For example, the ipr_{95} has an internal cumulative probability of .95 and an external cumulative probability of .05. At the 97.5 percentile point, the internal cumulative probability is .975 (for values of data smaller than the associated percentile value), and the external cumulative probability is .025.

6.5.4   Two-Zone and Three-Zone Boundaries

A single percentile point, such as P_{95}, demarcates two zones — one internal and the other external. Boundaries established by two percentiles, such as the 2.5 and 97.5 percentile points that form the ipr_{95}, will demarcate three zones of cumulative probability: a central internal zone, surrounded by two external zones. The distinctions are shown in Figure 6.1.

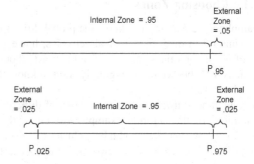

FIGURE 6.1

Cumulative probability zones for ipr_{95}. Upper drawing shows the 95 percentile point as one boundary with two zones. Lower drawing shows the 2.5 and 97.5 percentile points as two boundaries with three zones.

6.5.5   P-Values and Tails of Probability

In many appraisals of probability, the focus is on the external zone, i.e., the chance of observing something more extreme than what is contained within the selected boundary. This external zone of cumulative probability is called a *P-value*. The external zone is often demarcated as the *area* located in the "tail" of the curve of relative frequencies for a mathematical model.

The cumulative aspect of the frequencies is omitted when the P-values or other cumulative results are cited as *probabilities*, but the cumulative feature is implicit in the word *tail*, which describes the location of the zone. Thus, if only two zones have been demarcated with a single boundary, the single external zone is called a *one-tailed probability*. A key distinction in one-tailed probabilities is stipulating a direction to indicate whether the focus of the external zone is on values that are above or below the selected boundary. If three zones have been formed from two boundaries, the two external zones are called a *two-tailed probability*. Two-tailed probabilities are always bi-directional, demarcating external zones that occupy both extremes of the distribution.

6.5.6   Confidence Intervals and Internal Zones

For the entity called the *confidence interval* for a central index, the focus is on an internal zone of probability. It usually has two boundaries, set around the proposed location of the central index, for a zone within which the location might vary under circumstances discussed earlier and also later in Chapter 7.

6.5.7 To-and-from Conversions for Observations and Probabilities

Observations in a set of data can readily be converted to probabilities, and vice versa. Beginning with observed (or cited) values of data, we can find probabilities; or beginning with probabilities, we can find observed values.

6.5.7.1 From Observations to Probabilities — For the data of Table 4.1, suppose we want to know the probability that a chloride value is below **93**. The single cited boundary of **93** establishes a directional two-zone arrangement. For the extreme values *below* **93**, the cumulative relative frequency is external to the boundary. For values of **93** *or higher*, the cumulative relative frequency is internal. In Table 4.1, the external probability for values **below 93** is .0598 and the internal probability is .9402 (= 1 – .0598).

For chloride levels bounded by values of **93** and **107**, the three zones have an internal probability for the zone of **93–107**, an external probability for the zone below **93**, and another external probability for the zone above **107**. The respective values for these three probabilities in Table 4.1 are .0598, .8598, and .0804.

Note that the internal and external probabilities in a frequency distribution always have a sum of 1. This important distinction is often disregarded, however, when people make *subjective* estimates about probabilities for a particular choice (such as a diagnosis or murder suspect) among a series of candidates.[10] The total of the probability values estimated for individual candidates may exceed 1. Other human inconsistencies in using probabilities (and magnitudes) are discussed in Section 6.8.

6.5.7.2 From Probabilities to Observed Values — To determine cumulative relative frequencies or probabilities, we read horizontally rightward in Table 4.1 beginning with the observed chloride values. We could also, however, go leftward, from cumulative frequencies toward chloride values. For example, from the definition of percentiles, we know that the 25th percentile occurs where the ascending cumulative frequency (or lower external probability) passes 0.25. Table 4.1 shows that the 25th percentile occurs at the chloride level of **99**. The table also shows that the 50th percentile is at the chloride level of **102**, and the 75th percentile at **105**. An ipr$_{95}$, extending from the 2.5 to the 97.5 percentile in Table 4.1, could be marked by the chloride levels of **89** to **110**.

6.6 Gaussian Z-Score Demarcations

Despite all the difficulties in *non*-Gaussian distributions, the standard deviation is a splendid way of demarcating inner zones when a distribution is truly Gaussian. In particular, the Z-scores determined from the standard deviation of Gaussian data will correspond directly to probability values discerned from the mathematical formula for the Gaussian curve.

One of these probability values, often called a *probability density*, is the height of the curve at a particular value, i.e., the relative frequency of items having the individually cited Z-score. These were the probability values shown with the Gaussian formula and small table in Section 4.8.2. (In a *tabulation* of either dimensional or categorical data, the probability density represents the proportion or relative frequency of the distribution occurring at a particular individual value.)

A different set of probability values refers to *cumulative* relative frequencies rather than the focal density at a cited value of Z. These cumulative proportions were shown for one side of the curve in Table 4.3 and for both sides in the in-text table in Section 4.8.3. Because of the symmetry and versatility of the Gaussian curve, a single value of Z can be associated with probabilities that represent several different zones of cumulative relative frequencies. These cumulative relative frequencies are the *areas* formed under the Gaussian curve.

6.6.1   One-Tailed Probabilities

A percentile value demarcates a one-tailed probability for
the zone of data spanned as the distribution moves upward
from its lowest value.

The top part of Figure 6.2 shows the demarcation for a
positive value of Z. The zone of internal probability is the
percentile value associated with Z, counting from the lower
end of the distribution. The rest of the distribution contains
the zone of external probability. As shown in the middle part
of Figure 6.2, if Z has the same but negative value, the zone
of internal probability again starts from the lower end of the
distribution, but is smaller than in the first situation. The
zones of internal and external probability in each situation
are opposite counterparts.

In many appraisals, however, the data analyst is interested
in external probabilities for values of Z that are more
extreme, *in the same direction*, than the observed value.
Thus, if Z = 1.3, we want external probabilities for values
of Z that are ≥ 1.3. If Z is −1.3, we want external probabilities
for values of Z that are ≤ −1.3. In the latter situation, therefore, the external probability would be redesignated on the
lower side of the Gaussian curve, as shown in the bottom
part of Figure 6.2. The upper and lower figures become mirror images around the central value where Z = 0.

If the external one-tailed probability value is called P, it
corresponds to a percentile value of 1 − P. For example, a
Z-score of 1.0 in a Gaussian curve represents a one-tailed
exterior probability (or P value) of .16. The corresponding
interior probability or percentile point is 1 − .16 = .84. This
same result can be obtained by noting in Table 4.3 that a
Z-score of 1.0 has a cumulative relative probability of .34
on the right side of the curve. Because the left side of the
curve contains a cumulative probability of .50, the total will
produce an interior probability of .84 for the percentile point.

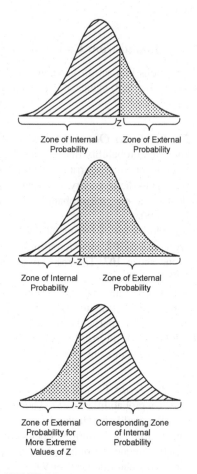

FIGURE 6.2
Zones of internal and external probability for a
single value of Z in a Gaussian curve.

6.6.2   Two-Tailed Probabilities

The proportion of data contained in the symmetrical inner
zone formed between the positive and negative values of
a Gaussian Z has an inner probability. The remaining data,
on the two outside portions beyond the inner zone, have
a total external probability, which is called a *two-tailed
P value*.

The distinction is shown in Figure 6.3. In this instance,
if the Z-score is ±1, the external probability is .16 on one
side of the curve and .16 on the other, so that the two-tailed
P value is .32. The inner zone of probability is 1 − .32 =
.68. (The latter value should look familiar. It was mentioned
in Section 5.3.2.2 with the statement that a zone of $\overline{X} \pm s$,
i.e., one standard deviation around the mean, occupies 68%
of a set of Gaussian data.)

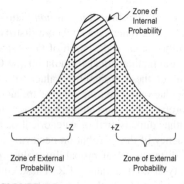

FIGURE 6.3
Zones of internal and external probability for
the customary value of ±Z in a Gaussian curve.

6.6.3 Distinctions in Cumulative Probabilities for Z-Scores

In special tables or in computer print-outs for a Gaussian distribution, the Z-scores and the corresponding cumulative probabilities are almost always shown as two-tailed (external) P values. These can easily be halved to denote the one-tailed P values, but the distinctions must be carefully considered if you want to determine percentiles, to find internal rather than external probabilities, or to go back and forth from Z values to P values. Table 6.3 shows the corresponding one-tailed and two-tailed cumulative probability values of Z-scores in a standard Gaussian distribution.

To find internal probabilities or percentiles, the cited external probabilities must be suitably subtracted. With a two-tailed P value, symbolized as 2P, the internal probability (for the zone of inner values) is 1 − 2P. For a one-tailed inner zone of probability, however, the two-tailed P value must be halved before it is subtracted from 1. Because percentile points represent one-tailed probability values, the Z-score corresponding to the 95th percentile would be 1.645, because it has an external one-tailed probability of .05.

TABLE 6.3

Cumulative Relative Frequencies and P Values Associated with Z Values
in a Standard Gaussian Distribution

Z	One-Tailed External Probability*	Two-Tailed External Probability	Two-Tailed Internal Probability
0	.5000	1	0
±0.500	.3090	.6170	.3830
±0.674	.2500	.5000	.5000
±1.000	.1585	.3170	.6830
±1.282	.1000	.2000	.8000
±1.500	.0670	.1340	.8660
±1.645	.0500	.1000	.9000
±1.960	.0250	.0500	.9500
±2.000	.0230	.0460	.9540
±2.240	.0125	.0250	.9750
±2.500	.0060	.0120	.9880
±2.576	.0050	.0100	.9900
±3.000	.0073	.0027	.9973
±3.290	.0005	.0010	.9990

* For positive Z values only. For negative Z values, the external probability (for values higher than −Z) is 1 minus the cited result. For example, at Z = − 1.282, the one-tailed external probability is 1 − .1 = .9.

6.6.3.1 *"Decreasing Exponential" Z/P Relationship* — As Z gets larger, the external two-tailed P values get smaller. Since P is an area under the curve, the Z and P values have a "decreasing exponential" rather than linear relationship in Gaussian curves. The distinctions are shown in Figure 6.4. A 19% increase in Z, from 1.645 to 1.96, will halve the two-tailed P value, from .1 to .05. A 40% decrease in Z, from 3.29 to 1.96, will produce a 50-fold increase in the two-tailed P, from .001 to .05. Consequently, whenever Z exceeds 1, small changes in Z can have a major proportionate impact on P in the zones used for critical decisions about "significance."

If interested in *one-tailed* P values, we would find the Z-score associated with twice the one-tailed P. This one-tailed value for Z will be smaller, but not half as small, as the two-tailed value. Thus, for a two-tailed P of .025, Z is 2.24; but for a one-tailed P of .025, Z is 1.96, which corresponds to a two-tailed P of .05. A Z-score of 1.645 has a P of .1 when two-tailed and .05 when one-tailed.

6.6.3.2 *Ambiguous Interpretations* — These Z/P relationships are particularly noteworthy when external probabilites are cited for P values that represent statistical inferences rather than direct descriptions. In tests of statistical inference, as noted later, many investigators prefer to use one-tailed

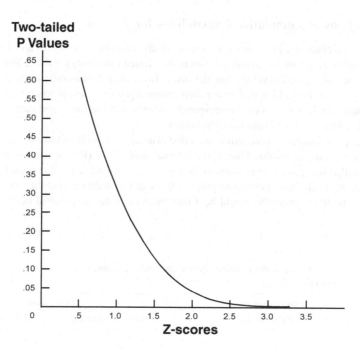

FIGURE 6.4
Relationship of 2- tailed P values and Z-Scores in a Gaussian curve.

P values because, for the same value of Z, the one-tailed P will be lower (and hence more "significant") than the two-tailed value. A currently unresolved dispute, discussed later in Chapter 11, has arisen between advocates of the two opposing policies: to always demand 2-tailed or sometimes accept 1-tailed P values for expressing "significance." Regardless of which policy is adopted, however, a reader will need to know how the decisions were made by the investigator (or editor).

If the inferential result is merely cited as "P < .05," however, the reader will not know whether it is one-tailed or two-tailed. To avoid ambiguity, P values can be reported as "2P < .05" when two-tailed and "P < .05" when one-tailed. This convention has begun to appear in published medical literature, but is not yet common. Until it becomes universal, writers should specify (in the associated text) whether P values are one-tailed or two-tailed.

6.6.4   Designated and Observed Zones of Probability

Special symbols are used to distinguish a previously designated zone of probability from zones that are observed in the data. For example, we might decide to give the accolade of **high honors** to anyone who ranks in or above the 95th percentile in a certification test. Someone who scores in the 97th percentile would receive this acclaim, but not someone who is in the 89th.

The Greek symbol α is used for designated levels of these zones. For the preceding percentile example, P_α was set at $\geq .95$. In many statistical decisions, $\alpha \leq .05$ is commonly set as the boundary level for P values that will be called "significant." In statistical decisions, the Z value that corresponds to α is marked Z_α. For a two-tailed $\alpha = .05$, $Z_{.05} = 1.96$.

6.6.4.1   *Inner Percentile Zones and Symbols* — For inner percentile ranges, the corresponding zones are based on two-tailed *internal* probabilities. If α represents the two-tailed *external* probability, the inner zone is determined as $1 - \alpha$.

To find an ipr_{95}, the corresponding zone is $1 - \alpha = .95$, and the two-tailed α is .05. If you want an ipr_{90}, $\alpha = .1$ and the Gaussian $Z_{.1} = 1.645$. For an ipr_{50}, or interquartile range, $\alpha = .5$ and $Z_{.5} = .674$.

6.6.4.2   *Observed (Calculated) Values* — If we start with observed data and want to determine probabilities, no Greek symbols are used. The value of Z is calculated as $(X_i - \bar{X})/s$, and is simply marked Z or Z_i. We then find the probability (or P value) associated with that value of Z. (Later in the text, to distinguish the observed value of Z from other possibilities, it will be cited as Z_0 and the corresponding P value will be P_0.)

6.6.4.3   *Limited Tables of Z/P Values* — With modern computer programs, a precise value of P, such as .086, is printed for each calculated Z value, such as 1.716. Before this computational convenience became available, however, Z values had to be interpreted with published tables showing the P values that correspond to selected values of Z_α. These tables, which resemble Table 4.3, are still needed and used if Z is determined with a hand calculator or other apparatus that does not immediately produce the corresponding P value.

If the available tables do not show all possibilities, the observed Z value will often lie between the tabular values for cited levels of Z_α. Consequently, a Z value such as 1.716 is often reported with the interpolated statement .05 < P < .1, indicating that P lies between two pertinent Z_α values, which in this instance are $Z_{.05} = 1.96$ and $Z_{.1} = 1.645$. If a particular boundary of Z_α has been set for "statistical significance," as discussed later, only the most pertinent level of α is usually indicated, with statements such as P < .1 or P > .05.

6.6.4.4   *Wrong Expression of Intermediate Values* — When a P value lies between two values of α, such as .1 and .05, the > and < signs are sometimes placed incorrectly, so that the expression becomes an impossible .1 < P < .05. To avoid this problem, always put the lowest value on the left, as it would appear on a graph. The best expression for the intermediate P is then .05 < P < .1.

6.6.5   Problems and Inconsistencies in Symbols

As long as α, Z_α, and P always represent two-tailed values and selections, the symbols are clear and unambiguous. The α, Z_α, and P symbols, however, traditionally refer to two-tailed probabilities. When the symbols (as well as the corresponding values) are modified for one-tailed applications, confusion can be produced by the inverse relationship that makes Z and P go in opposite directions. If 2P and P respectively represent two-tailed and one-tailed external probabilities determined from the data, the modified symbols are clear, except perhaps for readers who do not realize that P (alone) will then specifically represent one tail rather than the conventional two. To avoid this problem, the solo P can be modified with the parenthetical remark "(one-tailed)."

The big problems arise in choosing subscripts for Z, particularly when it demarcates boundaries against which the values of P or 2P will be compared for decisions about "statistical significance." In most special tabulations of Z values, the associated P values are two-tailed. For a two-tailed α, the total external zone of α is split into two parts, each containing $\alpha/2$, as shown in Figure 6.5. A 2P value is therefore compared against a boundary that has $\alpha/2$ externally on each side.

In a one-tailed procedure, all of the external probability is unilateral, occupying the full value of α rather than $\alpha/2$. To allow the external probability on one side of the curve to be α, the selected demarcation point for the ordinarily two-tailed Z would be $Z_{2\alpha}$. With this demarcation in Figure 6.6, an $\alpha/2$ probability zone is transferred from the left to the right side of the curve. Having been placed under a higher point in the curve, the additional $\alpha/2$ area is achieved with a smaller horizontal distance for Z than was previously needed at the other end of the curve. Thus, the values for Z_α and $Z_{2\alpha}$ do not correspond proportionately to the relative magnitudes of α and $\alpha/2$.

The probability zones, demarcations, and symbols can be cited as follows for two-tailed and one-tailed decisions:

Decisions	Probability in Pertinent Zones	Demarcation Point	Symbol for P Value
Two-tailed	$\alpha/2$	Z_α	2P
One-tailed	α	$Z_{2\alpha}$	P (one-tailed)

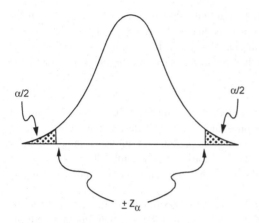

FIGURE 6.5

Demarcation of two $\alpha/2$ zones of probability by $\pm Z_\alpha$.

FIGURE 6.6

Demarcation of a one-tailed probability zone for α.

For two-tailed decisions with $\alpha = .05$, $Z_{.05}$ is set at 1.96; the inner 95% zone has two exterior zones that each have a probability of .025; and the corresponding internal probability is $1 - \alpha = .95$. For one-tailed decisions with $\alpha = .05$, the 2α demarcation point is set at $Z_{.10} = 1.645$; the one-tailed external probability is .05, and the internal probability is still $1 - \alpha = .95$.

A reasonably complete set of values in a Z/P tabulation is shown in Table 6.4, where values of 2P are shown for positive values of Z extending from 0 to about 3.9. Because almost all published tables of probability show two-tailed values, the Z boundaries are sometimes labelled as $Z_{\alpha/2}$, to clarify their connotation. Regardless of the label used for Z, however, the corresponding value of P in any two-tailed Z/P table is halved to get the one-tailed P value.

To try to avoid confusion, the symbols P, α, and Z_α will be used here in an uncommitted general way to denote observed or specified levels of probability. Most discussions will refer to the conventional two-tailed approach, but one-tailed directions will often be considered. To allow this flexibility, the symbols will be "P" for the general probability, "2P" when it is specifically two-tailed, and "(one-tailed) P" when it is one-tailed. The α and Z_α symbols will be used as such, without recourse to the confusing forms of $\alpha/2$, 2α, $Z_{\alpha/2}$ or $Z_{2\alpha}$. The one- or two-tailed direction of α or Z_α will always be cited in the associated text. Although perhaps undesirable for mathematical rigor, the apparent inconsistency has the pedagogic advantage of being reasonably clear and permitting an unconstrained discussion. If not otherwise specified, P and Z_α can be considered as two-tailed.

6.6.6 Determining Gaussian Zones

After Z_α is chosen, Gaussian zones of data are easy to determine when Z_α is multiplied by the observed standard deviation, s, to form Z_αs. The latter value is then added and subtracted from the mean, $\overline{X}$, to form $\overline{X} \pm Z_\alpha$s. In Chapter 4, the value of **2** was used instead of the more precise **1.96** to produce an inner 95% Gaussian zone as $\overline{X} \pm 2$s. The Z_α multiplying factor can be changed, when desired, to form Gaussian zones of different sizes, such as ipr_{90} or ipr_{50}. The corresponding values of α will be **.10** and **.50**; and the corresponding values of Z_α (derived from Table 6.4) will be **1.645** and **.674**.

With smaller values of Z_α, the inner zones will shrink as $1 - \alpha$ gets smaller. Thus, in a set of data where $\overline{X} = 10$ and s = 3, the corresponding Gaussian zones will be as follows:

ipr	α	Z_α	Z_αs	Extent of $\overline{X} \pm Z_\alpha$s
95	.05	1.906	5.880	4.120 to 15.880
90	.10	1.645	4.935	5.065 to 14.935
50	.50	.674	2.022	7.978 to 12.022

TABLE 6.4

Values of 2P for Positive Values of Z

Z	0.000	0.002	0.004	0.006	0.008
0.00	•	99840	99681	99521	99362
0.04	98609	96650	96490	96331	96172
0.08	93624	93465	93306	93147	92988
0.12	90448	90290	90132	89974	89815
0.16	87288	87131	86973	86816	86658
0.20	84148	83992	83835	83679	83523
0.24	81033	80878	80723	80568	80413
0.28	77948	77794	77641	77488	77335
0.32	74897	74745	74594	74442	74291
0.36	71885	71735	71586	71437	71287
0.38	70395	70246	70098	69950	69802
0.40	68916	68768	68621	68474	68327
0.42	67449	67303	67157	67011	66865
0.44	65994	65849	65704	65560	65415
0.46	64552	64408	64265	64122	63978
0.48	63123	62981	62839	62697	62555
0.50	61708	61567	61426	61286	61145
0.52	60306	60167	60028	59889	59750
0.54	58920	58782	58644	58507	58369
0.56	57548	57412	57275	57139	57003
0.58	56191	56057	55922	55788	55653
0.60	54851	54717	54584	54451	54319
0.62	53526	53394	53263	53131	53000
0.64	52217	52087	51958	51828	51698
0.66	50925	50797	50669	50541	50413
0.68	49650	49524	49398	49271	49145
0.7	48393	47152	45930	44725	43539
0.8	42371	41222	40091	38979	37886
0.9	36812	35757	34722	33706	32709
1.0	31731	30773	29834	28914	28014
1.1	27133	26271	25429	24605	23800
1.2	23014	22246	21498	20767	20055
1.3	19360	18684	18025	17383	16759
1.4	16151	15561	14987	14429	13887
1.5	13361	12851	12356	11876	11411
1.6	10960	10523	10101	09691	09296
1.7	08913	08543	08186	07841	07508
1.8	07186	06876	06577	06289	06011
1.9	05743	05486	05238	05000	04770
2.0	04550	04338	04135	03940	03753
2.1	03573	03401	03235	03077	02926
2.2	02781	02642	02509	02382	02261
2.3	02145	02034	01928	01827	01731
2.4	01640	01552	01469	01389	01314
2.5	01242	01174	01109	01047	00988
2.6	00932	00879	00829	00781	00736
2.7	00693	00653	00614	00578	00544
2.8	00511	00480	00451	00424	00398
2.9	00373	00350	00328	00308	00288
3.0	00270	00253	00237	00221	00207
3.2	00137	00128	00120	00111	00104

3.4: 00067	3.5: 00047	3.6: 00032	3.7: 00022	3.8: 00014	3.891: 00010

Note: The three decimal places in the top headings become reduced to two when Z reaches 0.7. Thus, for Z = .82, the 2P value is found as .41222 in the column marked 0.002. For Z = 1.96, the value of 2P in the 0.006 column is 0.5000. [Table derived from page 28 of Geigy Scientific Tables, Vol. 2, ed. by C. Lentner, 1982. Ciba-Geigy Limited. Basle, Switzerland.]

6.7   Disparities Between Theory and Reality

In a Gaussian distribution, the two sides of the curve are symmetrical around the center. No matter what boundary is chosen, the external two-tailed probabilities will be identical and equally divided. Thus, if a boundary of Z_α is set at 1.96 for 2P = .05, the internal probability contains .475 of the data in the inner zone from $Z = 0$ to $Z = 1.96$, and .475 of the data in the zone from $Z = 0$ to $Z = -1.96$. The total inner probability is $.475 + .475 = .95$. The external probability is .05, representing the sum of the upper zone of .025 beyond $Z = 1.96$, and the lower zone of .025 below $Z = -1.96$.

If only a one-tailed probability is desired, however, the internal probability contains the entire 50% of items in the zone below the mean, plus the demarcated group in the corresponding zone above the mean. Thus, for a one-tailed probability with Z_α set at 1.96, the internal probability is 0.975, calculated as 0.5 (for the lower half of the data) + 0.475 for the zone from $Z = 0$ to $Z = 1.96$. The external probability is 0.025 for the zone beyond $Z = 1.96$.

This perfect symmetry is seldom present, alas, in the empirical data of the real world. For example, the values in Table 4.1 show ascending cumulative frequencies of 0.0255 when the chloride level is **89** and .9765 when the level is **110**. These two chloride boundaries would offer a reasonably symmetrical inner zone (the ipr$_{95}$) for the inner 95% of the data, but the chloride levels of **89** and **110** are *not* symmetrically located around either the median of **102** or the mean of **101.6**.

The chloride values of Table 4.1 appear in this text by courtesy of the laboratories of Yale-New Haven Hospital. In response to a request seeking a Gaussian set of data, the laboratory produced a print-out of distributions for about 30 of the many chemical substances it measures. To ensure that the "sample size" would be large enough to show the true shape of the distribution, at least 2000 measurements were included in the set of data for each variable. The main point of this story is that *none* of the distributions was Gaussian. The chloride values were chosen for display here because they had the most "Gaussianoid" appearance of all the examined results.

The moral of the story is a warning to beware of using Gaussian statistics to *describe* medical data. The mean may be dislocated from the center of the distribution; the standard deviations may be affected by outliers or asymmetrical distributions; and the Gaussian Z-scores may yield misleading values for percentiles. The absence of a truly Gaussian pattern in most biologic data has been entertainingly described by Micceri[9] as "the unicorn, the normal curve, and other improbable creatures."

Gaussian statistics are most effectively used, as discussed later, for roles in statistical inference, not description. Gaussian confidence intervals can be employed for inferences about possible *variation in a central index*, but not for describing the data set itself. For the variations in a central index, as we shall see in the next two chapters, a reasonable mathematical justification can be offered for using the Gaussian strategy.

6.8   Verbal Estimates of Magnitudes

The last aspect of probability to be considered in this chapter is the quantitative inconsistency with which different people attach numbers to verbal terms describing magnitudes such as amounts, frequencies, and probabilities. In 1976, after consulting with various authorities, U.S. President Gerald R. Ford said that a swine flu epidemic in the next winter was "a very real possibility." When asked by a science writer,[11] four experts estimated this probability as 2%, 10%, 35%, and "less than even." Ever since this revelation, disagreement has often been studied for the quantitites implied when people use such verbal terms as *a little, a lot, often, unlikely,* and *usually.*

6.8.1   Poetic License

One of the earliest recorded complaints about verbal imprecision was made by Charles Babbage, renowned as the inventor of a 19th century "calculating engine" that is often regarded as the earliest ancestor of today's digital computers.

After reading Alfred Tennyson's poem "The Vision of Sin," Babbage is said to have written the following letter to the poet:

> In your otherwise beautiful poem, there is a verse which reads:
>
> > "Every moment dies a man
> > Every moment one is born."
>
> It must be manifest that, were this true, the population of the world would be at a standstill. In truth the rate of birth is slightly in excess of that of death. I would suggest that in the next edition of your poem you have it read:
>
> > "Every moment dies a man
> > Every moment $1\frac{1}{16}$ is born."
>
> Strictly speaking this is not correct. The actual figure is a decimal so long that I cannot get it in the line, but I believe $1\frac{1}{16}$ will be sufficiently accurate for poetry. I am etc.[12]

6.8.2   Estimates of Amounts

After hearing reports that a child "throws up a lot" or " throws up the whole feed," Pillo-Blocka et al.[13] asked 58 mothers of children less than 2 years old to estimate "two volumes of standard formula — 5 ml. and 10 ml. — which had been spilled uniformly over a baby's wash cloth, with the mother out of sight." The median estimates were 30 ml. for the smaller spill and 50 ml. for the larger. Only 1 of the 58 mothers underestimated the spill, and only two mothers were close to correct. All the other mothers "grossly" overestimated the emesis volumes, and the degree of accuracy had no correlation with the mothers' educational status or age.

6.8.3   Estimates of Frequencies and Probabilities

In the foregoing example, the observers responded to a direct visual challenge. In the other investigations cited here, the research subjects were asked conceptually to quantify the meaning of words for frequency and/or probability. Different subjects and research structures were used for the projects. The number of verbal terms to be quantified ranged from a few (i.e., 5) to many (i.e., 41). The quantitative expressions could be chosen from the following citations: dimensional selections on an unmarked continuum from 0 to 1; choices in increments of .05 or .1 extending from 0 to 1; "percentages" for each term; and four formats of quantitative expressions that contained special zones for "high probability" and "low probability," as well as a "uniform" ordinal scale, and a "free choice" between 0 and 100. The research subjects included different groups of medical personnel (nurses, house officers, students, laboratory technologists, hospital-based physicians in various specialties) as well as members of a hospital Board of Trustees. The nonmedical participants included graduate students at a school of business administration, highly skilled or professional workers (secondary school teachers, engineers), an otherwise unidentified group of "nonphysicians," and a set of male employees of the "System Development Corporation."

With these diverse designs and approaches, the investigators then proceeded to analyze and report the inconsistencies.

6.8.3.1   Frequencies — Figure 6.7 shows Robertson's summary[14] of four studies that included ratings for five categories ranging from *always* to *rarely*. Although the mean values were reasonably consistent (except for a Board of Trustees mean estimate that *rarely* had a frequency of 23%), the most noteworthy results were the wide range of individual responses. In the conclusion of the review, physicians were urged to use precise percentages instead of "shooting from the mouth."

Analogous results were obtained when 94 physicians and 94 non-physicians responded to a similar challenge that contained 22 verbal modifiers.[15] The investigators concluded that physicians had a better

Quantifying Word Meanings				
Sample Term	N Engl J Med Study, % (n=32)	Seattle Physicians, % (n=53)	University of Washington MBAs, % (n=80)	Children's Orthopedic Hospital, Board of Trustees, % (n=40)
Always				
$\bar{x} \pm$ SD	99 ± 2	98 ± 6	98 ± 3	100 ± 0
Range	90-100	60-100	80-100	100
Often				
$\bar{x} \pm$ SD	61 ± 13	59 ± 17	61 ± 16	57 ± 13
Range	30-80	20-90	20-90	20-90
Sometimes				
$\bar{x} \pm$ SD	33 ± 17	34 ± 16	38 ± 12	37 ± 21
Range	10-60	0-90	10-60	10-70
On occasion				
$\bar{x} \pm$ SD	12 ± 7	20 ± 16	20 ± 10	18 ± 21
Range	0-20	0-70	5-50	10-60
Rarely				
$\bar{x} \pm$ SD	5 ± 4	15 ± 34	12 ± 20	23 ± 36
Range	0-10	0-95	0-90	0-60

FIGURE 6.7

Summary of results in four studies of quantification for five terms referring to frequency. [Figure adapted from Chapter Reference 14.]

consensus on meaning of the verbal expressions than laymen, but that physicians should take "no consolation" from the apparent superiority. According to the authors, the results "highlight the folly of assuming that any two randomly chosen physicians are likely to have similar percentages in mind" when these terms are used and that laymen have an "even greater likelihood of misunderstanding" when the terms are communicated. The authors' main recommendation was the subtitle of their paper: "Verbal specifications of frequency have no place in medicine."

This argument was reinforced in a study[16] showing that endoscopists had major differences, unrelated to experience or site of training, in the number of cm. intended when the size of a gastric ulcer was described as *small, medium,* or *large.* With this variation, an ulcer called *large* in a first examination and *small* in a second may actually have increased in size.

6.8.3.2   Probabilities — In other investigations of medical personnel, diverse ranks and ranges of values were obtained for 30 "probability estimates" in a study[17] of 16 physicians; the magnitude of "rare" seemed to change with the pharmaceutical agent for which side effects were being estimated;[18] different medical professionals were found[19] to have relatively good agreement in quantitative beliefs about 12 expressions ranging from *certain* to *never.* In the last study, the numerical estimates were reasonably consistent within groups studied in different eras, and clinical context influenced the values but not the order of the quantitative ratings. Although recommending development of a "codification based on common usage," Kong et al.[19] wanted to do additional research (apparently not yet reported) "before proposing an overall scheme." The summary results were regarded as possibly "adequate for codifying usage for physicians speaking to physicians," but the authors believed that a formal code could not be enforced, because physicians and patients may want "to use qualitative expressions and some people are more comfortable with them than with exact values. Sometimes we want to be vague."

6.8.4 Virtues of Imprecision

The virtues of preserving certain forms of "vagueness" have been noted by several commentators, including Mosteller and Youtz,[20] who presented a meta-analysis of 20 studies of quantification for verbal expressions of probability. According to Clark,[21] quantitative studies often fail to distinguish between "word meaning" and "word use." Cliff[22] argued that "words are inherently fuzzy and communicating degree of fuzziness is a significant aspect of communication ... (I)f boundaries were not vague, there would be endless debates about where such boundaries should lie." Wallsten and Budescu [23] stated that "probability phrases should not be made to appear more precise than they really are" and that sometimes an "imprecise judgment is useful information in and of itself."

The imprecise qualitative terms have survived in human communication because they are necessary and desirable. Such terms are often used when an exact number is either unknown or not needed, or when the precise quantity, after being determined with a great deal of effort, might be misleading. For example, the word *often* was used in the preceding sentence because I would not want to identify or count all the possible occasions on which an exact quantity is best replaced with an imprecise term; and I doubt that citing proportions such as 8/21 or 37/112 would convey the idea better than *often*. The term *a great deal* was also used in that sentence because I have no data — and have no intention of getting the data — on how much effort was spent when the investigators did the cited research projects. At best, the amount of *time* might be measured or estimated, but no suitable rating scale exists for this type of *effort*. I feel sure, i.e., 100% certain, that the total research took more than a few days, but the term *a great deal* suitably conveys the idea.

When doctors communicate with one another or with patients, the exchanged words must be clearly and mutually understood. This understanding can be thwarted by both quantitative and nonquantitative features of the communication: an inadequate scale may be used to express risk;[24] the doctor may be too busy or imperceptive; the patient may be too frightened or intimidated; the patient may have answered a self-administered questionnaire containing ambiguous phrases and concepts. In clinical practice, the direct personal exchange called *history taking* can help prevent or remedy the misunderstandings if both doctors and patients are aware of the possibilities and if both groups are constantly encouraged to ask, "What do you mean by that?"

Some of the desired quantifications may be statistically precise but clinically wrong. For example, prognosis in patients with cancer is commonly estimated from statistical results for morphologic categories of the TNM staging system. A patient in TNM Stage III, with an "inoperable" metastasized cancer, might be told, "Your chance of 6-month survival is 57%." Nevertheless, with additional clinical classifications based on functional severity of illness,[25] the TNM stage III can be divided into distinct clinical subgroups with prognoses for 6-month survival ranging from 5% to 85%. A physician who uses the 57% estimate may be given credit for being a good quantifier, but the patient is poorly served by statistically average results that may not pertain to individual clinical distinctions.

Efforts to quantify the unquantifiable have produced currently fashionable mathematical models, such as decision analysis and quality-adjusted-life years (QALYs), that have all the virtues of precision, quantitative analysis, economic comparisons, successful grant requests, and multiple academic publications, but none of the virtues of a realistic portrait of clinical decisions and human aspirations.[26]

Having made many efforts to improve quantification in clinical medicine, including the construction of specific rating scales for clinimetric phenomena[27] that are now identified imprecisely or not at all, and being now engaged in further quantitative advocacy by writing a book on statistics, I trust that the foregoing comments will not be misunderstood. Workers in the field of health need quantitative information for its many invaluable and irreplaceable contributions to communication, reasoning, and human life. The rest of this text is devoted to the ways of analyzing that information. We also, however, need qualitative terms and quantitatively imprecise words for all the human phenomena and ideas that cannot or should not be subjugated into quantitative rigidity. Like workers in fireworks factories, we should remember that it is sometimes better to curse the darkness than to light the wrong candle.

I shall not demand that a great chef quantify a "pinch" of salt, that a superb violinist indicate the Hertzian frequency of a splendid vibrato, or that an excellent artist specify wave length or area for a "dab" of color. Trying to do a good job of writing, I hope you will let me end this chapter here. If so, I shall thank you very much, unless you insist on .863 units of gratitude.

References

1. Student, 1908; 2. Quenouille, 1949; 3. Tukey, 1958; 4. Fisher, 1925; 5. Simon, 1969; 6. Efron, 1979; 7. Efron, 1983; 8. De Leeuw, 1993; 9. Micceri, 1989; 10. Teigen, 1983; 11. Boffey, 1976; 12. Babbage, 1956; 13. Pillo-Blocka, 1991; 14. Robertson, 1983; 15. Nakao, 1983; 16. Moorman, 1995; 17. Bryant, 1980; 18. Mapes, 1979; 19. Kong, 1986; 20. Mosteller, 1990; 21. Clark, 1990; 22. Cliff, 1990; 23. Wallsten, 1990; 24. Mazur, 1994; 25. Feinstein, 1990d; 26. Feinstein, 1994; 27. Feinstein, 1987a.

Exercises

6.1. Here is a set of questions that will help prepare you for your next visit to the statistical citadels of Atlantic City, Las Vegas, or perhaps Ledyard, Connecticut:

6.1.1. A relatively famous error in the history of statistics was committed in the 18th century by d'Alembert. He stated that the toss of two coins could produce three possible outcomes: two heads, two tails, or a head and a tail. Therefore, the probability of occurrence was 1/3 for each outcome. What do you think was wrong with his reasoning?

6.1.2. The probability of tossing a 7 with two dice is 1/6. Show how this probability is determined.

6.1.3. The probability of getting a 7 on two consecutive tosses of dice is $(1/6)(1/6) = 1/36 = .03$ — a value smaller than the .05 level often set for "uncommon" or "unusual" events. If this event occurred while you were at the dice table of a casino, would you conclude that the dice were "loaded" or otherwise distorted? If not, why not?

6.1.4. The shooter at the dice table has just tossed a **6**. What is the probability that his next toss will also be a **6**?

6.1.5. At regular intervals (such as every 30 minutes) at many casinos, each of the identical-looking roulette wheels is physically lifted from its current location and is exchanged with a roulette wheel from some other location. The process is done to thwart the "system" of betting used by certain gamblers. What do you think that system is?

6.2. Using the chloride data of Table 4.1, please answer or do the following:

6.2.1. What is the probability that a particular person has a chloride level that lies at or within the boundaries of 94 and 104?

6.2.2. What interval of chloride values contains approximately the central 90% of the data?

6.2.3. Assume that the data have a Gaussian pattern with mean = 101.572 and standard deviation = 5.199. Using Table 6.4 and the mathematical formula for Gaussian Z-scores, answer the same question asked in 6.2.1.

6.2.4. Using the same Gaussian assumption and basic methods of 6.2.3, answer the same question asked in 6.2.2.

6.3. We know that a particular set of data has a Gaussian distribution with a standard deviation of 12.3. A single randomly chosen item of data has the value of 40. What would you do if asked to estimate the location of the mean for this data set?

6.4. An investigator has drawn a random sample of 25 items of dimensional data from a data bank. They have a mean of 20 with a standard deviation of 5. What mental screening process can you use (without any overt calculations) to determine whether the data are Gaussian and whether the mean is stable?

6.5. A political candidate feels confident of victory because he is favored by 67% (= 6/9) of potential voters in a political poll.

6.5.1. What simple calculations would you do — with pencil and paper, without using a calculator — to find the standard deviation, standard error, and coefficient of stability for this proportion? Do you regard it as stable?

6.5.2. Suppose the same proportion is found in a poll of 900 voters. Would you now regard the result as stable? What nonstatistical question would you ask before drawing any conclusions?

6.6. "Statistical significance" is usually declared at $\alpha = .05$, i.e., for 2P values at or below .05. A group of investigators has done a randomized clinical trial to test whether a new active drug is better than placebo. When appropriately calculated, by methods discussed later in Chapter 13, the results show a Gaussian Z-score of 1.72 for a difference in favor of the active drug. Because the corresponding one-tailed P value is <.05, the investigators claim that the difference is "statistically significant." The statistical reviewers, however, reject this claim. They say that the result is not significant, because the P value should be two-tailed. For Z = 1.72, the two-tailed P is >.05. What arguments can be offered on behalf of both sides of this dispute?

6.7. Find a published report — not one already cited in the text — in which an important variable was cited in a verbal scale of magnitude, i.e., an ordinal scale. Comment on what the investigators did to ensure or check that the scale would be used with reproducible precision. Do you approve of what they did? If not, what should they have done?

6.8. Here is a chance to demonstrate your own "quantitative" concepts of "uncertainty," and for the class convener to tabulate observer variability in the ratings.

Please rank the following verbal expressions from 1 to 12, with 1 indicating the highest degree of assurance for definite occurrence and 12 the lowest.

Probable	Uncertain	Expected	Possible
Credible	Impossible	Likely	Certain
Doubtful	Hoped	Unlikely	Conceivable

7

![section rule]

Confidence Intervals and Stability:
Means and Medians

The concepts of probability discussed in Chapter 6 can now be used for their critical role in evaluating the stability of a central index. For the evaluation, we want to determine not only the magnitude of possible variations when the index is "perturbed," but also the probability of occurrence for each variation.

The perturbations that produce the magnitudes and probabilities can be done with modern methods of empirical reconstruction, such as the jackknife and bootstrap, or with the traditional parametric-sampling strategy.

7.1   Traditional Strategy

The traditional statistical strategy — which constantly appears in modern literature — is complicated, making its discussion particularly difficult to read and understand. The reason for the difficulty is that the customary statistical approach involves hypothetical entities such as standard errors and confidence intervals, and uses an array of mathematical theories that do not correspond to reality or to anything that might actually be done by a pragmatic medical investigator.

The theories were originally developed to deal with a real-world challenge called *parametric sampling*; and they have worked well for that challenge. The mathematical strategy behind the theories was then applied, however, for a quite different challenge in *evaluating stability*. The same parametric theories thus became used in two very different situations. For parametric sampling, the theories involve the hypothetical possibility of repeatedly taking an infinite number of samples from an unknown population that is seldom actually observed. For evaluating stability, however, we examine what was found in a single group of data.

7.1.1   Goals of Sampling

In a sampling process, we determine the mean, standard deviation, or other attributes, called *parameters*, of a large entity, called the *parent population*, that would be too difficult or costly to examine completely. For example, in industrial work, such as mining gold or making beer, the chemical testing of quality takes time and destroys the material being analyzed. We therefore use samples (often called *aliquots*) to save time and to avoid losing too much gold or beer. In marketing activities, the makers of a new product will examine samples of potential purchasers to appraise its possible public reception, because a test of the total population would be unfeasible and too expensive. The sampling activity called *poll-taking* is constantly used by political or social scientists to determine beliefs or opinions in a much larger public than the people included in the sample. On election night, a sampling process is used when the media try to forecast the winner before all the precincts have been reported.

The sampling activities are not always successful; and the failures have become legendary examples of errors to be avoided or corrected. In the United States, many older persons still remember the fallacious marketing research that led to the Edsel automobile and to the (temporary) removal of classic Coca Cola from the market; and almost everyone can give an example of blunders in political polls or in election-night forecasts. In general, i.e., "on average," however, the pragmatic results have confirmed (or "validated") what was found with the theoretical sampling strategy.

7.1.2   Random Sampling

An important basis for the theoretical strategy is that the sampling be done randomly. The term *random* is not easy to define, but it requires that every member of the target or parent population have an equal chance of being selected for inclusion in the sample. This requirement is not fulfilled if the sample is chosen haphazardly (e.g., without a specific plan) or conveniently (e.g., whatever happens to be available in the persons who came to the clinic today or who mailed back a questionnaire). To get a truly random sample from a parent population requires special maneuvers, such as making selections by tossing a coin or using either a random-number generator or table of random numbers.

Many sampling activities fail not because the mathematical theory was flawed, but because the sample was not a representative random choice. The material may not have been well mixed before the tested aliquots were removed. The group of people who mailed back the questionnaire may have been a relatively extreme sector of the target population. (Another nonmathematical source of error is the way the questions were asked. The inadequate wording or superficial probing of the questions is now regarded as the source of the marketing disasters associated with the Edsel and with "New Coke.")

The necessity for random sampling is another problem that makes the parametric theory seem strange when used in medical research. Random sampling almost never occurs in clinical investigation, where the investigators study the groups who happen to be available. In a randomized trial, the treatments are assigned with a random process, but the patients who enter the trial were almost never obtained as a random sample of all pertinent patients. A random sampling may be attempted for the household surveys of public-health research or in the "random-digit dialing" sometimes used to obtain "control" groups in case-control studies. Even these activities are not perfectly random, however, because the results usually depend on whoever may be home when the doorbell or telephone rings and on the willingness of that person to participate in the study. Consequently, medical investigators, knowing that they work with potentially biased groups, not with random samples, are often uncomfortable with statistical theories that usually ignore sources of bias and that assume the groups were randomly chosen.

7.1.3 Reasons for Learning about Parametric Sampling

Despite these scientific problems and discomforts, the theory of parametric sampling is a dominant factor in statistical analysis today. The theory has been the basic intellectual "ethos" of statistical reasoning for more than a century. If you want to communicate with your statistical consultant, this theory is where the consultant usually "comes from." The parametric-sampling theory is also important because it has been extended and applied in many other commonly used statistical procedures that involve neither sampling nor estimation of parameters. One of these roles, discussed in this chapter, is evaluating the stability of a central index. Other roles, discussed in later chapters, produce the Z, t, and chi-square tests frequently used for statistical comparisons of two groups. As noted earlier and later, however, the parametric theory may be replaced in the future by "computer-intensive" statistical methods for evaluating stability and comparing groups.

Even if this replacement occurs, however, the parametric theory is still an effective (and generally unthreatened) method for the challenge of determining an adequate sample size *before* a research project begins. Furthermore, despite the complicated mathematical background, the parametric methods lead to relatively simple statistical formulas and calculations. This computational ease has probably been responsible for the popularity of parametric procedures during most of the 20th century, and will continue to make them useful in circumstances where computers or the appropriate computer programs are not available.

For all these reasons, the parametric theory is worth learning. Before it arrives, however, we shall first examine two relatively simple methods — the jackknife and bootstrap procedures introduced in Chapter 6 — that can yield appraisals of stability without the need for complex mathematical reasoning. The intellectual ardors of parametric theory will begin in Section 7.3, and will eventually be followed by a pragmatic reward: the application of your new parametric knowledge to construct a common statistical procedure called a *one-group t test*.

7.2 Empirical Reconstructions

A parametric sampling, such as a political poll, must be planned "prospectively" *before* any data are available for analysis. Consequently, the strategy must be based on theoretical principles. If data have already been obtained, however, the stability of the central index can be evaluated "retrospectively" with an empirical reconstruction of the observed results.

The various empirical rearrangements are based on what was actually observed and do not require theoretical reasoning about a larger, parametric population. Like the parametric approach, the empirical strategy depends on distributions, but each distribution is generated in an *ad hoc* manner from the observed set of data. Furthermore, the empirical strategies — applied to data obtained without a sampling process — are used only for drawing conclusions about the observed group. The conclusions are not expected or intended to refer to a larger parametric population.

The *jackknife* reconstruction technique, as shown in Section 7.2.1, determines what would happen to the "unit fragility" of the central index (or some other selected value) if a member is successively removed from (and then returned to) the data set. The *bootstrap* reconstruction technique, as shown earlier in Section 6.4.3 and here in Section 7.2.2, is a resampling process that determines what would happen in samples prepared as rearrangements of all or some of the observed members of the data.

7.2.1 Jackknifed Reconstruction

The jackknife method, which is seldom formally used for checking the stability of a central index, is presented here mainly to give you an idea of how it works and to indicate the kinds of things that can be done when investigators become "liberated" from parametric doctrines. You need not remember any of the details, but one aspect of the process, discussed in Sections 7.2.1.2 and 7.2.1.3, offers a particularly simple "screening test" for stability of a central index.

7.2.1.1   Set of Reduced Means — The jackknife process works by examining the variations that occur when one member is successively removed (and then restored) in the data set. If the data set has n members, each symbolized as X_i, the mean value is $\overline{X}$, calculated as $\Sigma X_i / n$. If one member of the set, X_i, is removed, the reduced set of data will have $n-1$ members, and the "reduced" mean in the smaller data set will be $\overline{X}_i = (\Sigma X_i - X_i)/(n-1) = (n\overline{X} - X_i)/(n-1)$. As each X_i is successively removed, a total of n reduced groups and n reduced means will be created.

For example, consider the group of blood sugar values that appeared in Exercise 3.3. Table 7.1 shows what would happen successively as one member of the group is removed. Because the reduced means range from values of **105.37** to **123.16**, we can be completely (i.e., 100%) confident that any of the reduced means will lie in this zone. Because the reduced set of means has 20 values, we can exclude the two extreme values to obtain a 90% inner zone of 18 values whose ipr_{90} extends from **112.21** to **122.32**. If we want a narrower zone of values, but less confidence about the results, we can prepare an ipr_{80} by removing the two highest and two lowest values. With this demarcation, we could be 80% confident that the reduced mean lies between **116.95** and **122.26**.

7.2.1.2   Decisions about Stability — The jackknife procedure offers a particularly useful "screening" tactic for stability of a central index. The "screening" occurs when we consider both the "distress" that would be evoked by some of the extreme values that appear in the array of reduced jackknife means, and also the possibility that such extreme values might occur.

Thus, in the data of Table 7.1, the most extreme of the 20 values is **400**. Its removal, which has a random chance of 1 in 20, would lower the reduced mean to 105.37. This drop is a reduction of (120.1 − 105.37)/120.1 = 12.3% from the original value. How distressed would we be if **105.37** were the true mean of the data set, thereby making **120.1** a misrepresentation? Conversely, if the true mean is **120.1**, how seriously would the data be misrepresented if the last member (with a value of **400**) had been omitted, so that **105.37** were used as the observed mean?

In this data set, which has 20 members, the (one-tailed) probability is only 1/20 = .05 that **105.37** would become the reduced mean. The ipr_{90} mentioned earlier for the reduced mean denotes a probability of only .10 that the reduced mean would drop to **112.21** (a proportionate change of about 7%) or lower. Because the highest value (**123.16**) for the reduced mean is not too disparate from the original value, we would be concerned mainly about the removal of extreme individual values such as **270** or **400**. In highly skewed data sets, such as the blood sugar values in Table 7.1, the relative frequency of possible jackknife changes may therefore be appraised in a "one-tailed" rather than "two-tailed" direction.

TABLE 7.1

Formation of Reduced Means and Reduced Medians for Data Set in Exercise 3.3

Values of original group: 62, 78, 79, 80, 82, 82, 83, 85, 87, 91, 96, 97, 97, 97, 101, 120, 135, 180, 270, 400. $\Sigma x_i = 2402$; $\bar{X} = 120.10$.

Value Removed	Sum of Values in Reduced Group	Reduced Mean	Reduced Median
62	2340	123.16	96
78	2324	122.32	96
79	2323	122.26	96
80	2322	122.21	96
82	2320	122.11	96
82	2320	122.11	96
83	2319	122.05	96
85	2317	121.95	96
87	2315	121.84	96
91	2311	121.63	96
96	2306	121.37	91
97	2305	121.32	91
97	2305	121.32	91
97	2305	121.32	91
101	2301	121.11	91
120	2282	120.11	91
135	2267	119.32	91
180	2222	116.95	91
270	2132	112.21	91
400	2002	105.37	91

$$\bar{X} = 120.10$$
$$s = 4.128$$

Thus, with no special calculations except "screening" by the jackknife perturbation, there is a .05 chance that the mean might become proportionately 12% lower than its original value, and a .1 chance that it will be changed by 7% or more. If troubled by these possibilities, you will reject the observed mean as unstable. If untroubled, you will accept it. In the absence of standards and criteria, the decision is "dealer's choice."

The main virtue of this type of jackknife "screening" is that you can determine exactly what would happen if one person were removed at each extreme of the data set. You need not rely on an array of theoretical parametric samplings or empirical bootstrap resamplings to determine and then interpret a standard error and confidence interval.

7.2.1.3 Screening with the Jackknife — To evaluate stability of a central index, the jackknife tactic is valuable mainly for mental screening, aided by a simple calculation. For the procedure, remove one item from an extreme end of the dimensional data set and determine the reduced mean. If it is proportionately too different from the original mean, or if it takes on a value that extends beyond an acceptable external boundary, *and* if the data set is small enough for the event to be a reasonably frequent possibility, the original mean is too fragile to be regarded as stable. The internal and external criteria for stability will be further discussed in Section 7.4.

7.2.2 Bootstrap Resampling

Of the two empirical methods for checking the stability of a mean, the complete bootstrap tactic is easy to discuss but hard to demonstrate. Unless the bootstrapped samples are relatively small, a computer is required to do all the work. Furthermore, even with a computer, the complete bootstrap tactic becomes formidable as the basic group size enlarges. For example, as noted earlier in Section 6.4.3, the complete bootstrap resampling of a group with 20 members would require 1.05×10^{26} resampled arrangements. Consequently, a smaller resampling, consisting of perhaps 1000 randomly selected bootstrapped samples, is usually prepared. After the values of the means in those 1000 samples are ranked, an ipr_{95} interval would depend on the boundaries of the inner 950 values. This ipr_{95} is called a *95% confidence interval* for the range of possible variation of the observed mean.

7.2.2.1 Illustration of Bootstrap Process

— A complete bootstrap rearrangement was prepared earlier in Section 6.4.1.1, and in Tables 6.1 and 6.2. Another example of the process is shown now for all the samples of two items that can be drawn from the set of data {1, 2, 3, 4}. The number of samples is small enough to show everything easily, whereas 256 entries ($= 4^4$) would be needed for a complete bootstrap of all four items.

When considered as a parent population, this 4-item set of data has 2.5 as its mean, μ, and its group variance is $\Sigma X_i^2 - n \overline{X}^2 = 30 - 25 = 5$. Because the original data set is a parent population for the bootstrap procedure, its standard deviation is calculated with n, as $\sigma = \sqrt{5/4} = 1.118$.

With m members in the original data set, and n members in each sample, the number of possible bootstrap samples is m^n. In this instance, with $m = 4$ and $n = 2$, we can expect $4^2 = 16$ samples of two members each. Those 16 samples are shown in Table 7.2.

TABLE 7.2

Bootstrap Samples of Two Items Each from the Set of Data {1,2,3,4}

Sample of Two Items	Mean of This Sample	Deviation from μ	Squared Deviation from μ
1,1	1	−1.5	2.25
1,2	1.5	−1.0	1.00
1,3	2	−0.5	0.25
1,4	2.5	0	0
2,1	1.5	−1.0	1.00
2,2	2	−0.5	0.25
2,3	2.5	0	0
2,4	3	+0.5	0.25
3,1	2	−0.5	0.25
3,2	2.5	0	0
3,3	3	+0.5	0.25
3,4	3.5	+1.0	1.00
4,1	2.5	0	0
4,2	3	+0.5	0.25
4,3	3.5	+1.0	1.00
4,4	4	+1.5	2.25
Total of Foregoing Values	40	0	10
Mean of Foregoing Values	2.5	0	(10/16) = 0.625 = variance $\sqrt{0.625}$ = .791 = standard deviation

The distribution of means in those 16 samples is shown in Figure 7.1.

The next few sections contain a general discussion of the bootstrap results, with illustrations supplied from Table 7.2 and Figure 7.1.

7.2.2.2 Mean of the Resampled Means

— The mean of a collection of bootstrapped sample means is the same as the mean in the original set of data. In Table 7.2, the bootstrapped means extend, as expected, from 1 to 4, but their mean value is 2.5. (The same principle occurred for the complete resampling of means in Tables 6.1 and 6.2.)

7.2.2.3 Shape of the Distribution of Means

— Regardless of the shape of the original data set that becomes the parent population, the collection of means in a bootstrapped sample will have a

Gaussian distribution, provided that n is large enough. This assertion about a Gaussian distribution for resampled means is particularly crucial for parametric reasoning and will be discussed later in Section 7.3.6.

In Table 7.2, the array of means for samples where n = 2 obviously does not have enough items to produce a smooth curve, but the shape in Figure 7.1 clearly has the symmetry and convex central crest that are consistent with a Gaussian distribution. (The shape seen earlier in Table 6.2 is also "Gaussianoid.")

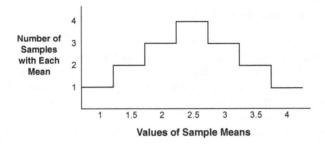

FIGURE 7.1
Distribution of means in bootstrapped samples shown in Table 7.2.

7.2.2.4 *Standard Deviation of the Sample Means* — In bootstrapped samples containing n members each, the standard deviation of the means is $\sigma/\sqrt{n}$. This formula, which is another basic concept discussed later in parametric reasoning, was illustrated earlier in Section 6.4.2. The formula is again confirmed in Table 7.2, where the variance of the 16 bootstrapped sample means is .625 and their standard deviation is .791. With $\sigma = 1.118$ in the parent population, the formula $\sigma/\sqrt{n}$ produces $1.118/\sqrt{2} = .791$.

7.2.2.5 *Inner Percentile Ranges for the Samples of Means* — We can determine certain ipr zones for the resampled means directly from the results shown in Table 7.2. Each of the 16 items occupies 1/16 or .0625 of the distribution. Consequently, the ipr_{95} and ipr_{90}, which respectively go from the 2.5 to 97.5 percentiles and from the 5 to 95 percentiles, will be bounded by the extreme values of 1 and 4. The interquartile range, from the 25 to 75 percentiles, will cover the inner 50% of the data. The lower quartile occurs at 2, and the upper quartile at 3, so that the ipr_{50} would be from 2 to 3. Actually, because 10 of the 16 sample means lie between the values of 2 and 3, this zone occupies 62.5% of the data. Because 14 of the 16 means lie between the values of 1.5 and 3.5, the inner zone from 1.5 to 3.5 will cover 14/16 (= 87.5%) of the data.

Thus, examining the data in Table 7.2, we can choose the size of the desired zone of confidence — 50%, 90%, 95%, etc. — and demarcate the corresponding boundaries of the confidence interval for the resampled means.

7.2.2.6 *Application of Bootstrap* — The foregoing illustration was intended merely to show how the bootstrap works. The method is seldom used or needed in determining a confidence interval for the mean of a single group of *dimensional* data. In fact, perhaps the main value of the bootstrap for such data is to offer empiric confirmation for the parametric theory, discussed later, that the standard error of a mean is $\sigma/\sqrt{n}$. Nevertheless, a bootstrap confidence interval can be valuable for small data sets that may not always comply with theoretical principles.

For example, for the 3-item data set {1, 6, 9} in Section 6.4.1.1, the mean was 5.33 and the standard error of the mean was 1.905. Using the parametric theory to be discussed shortly, a 70.4% confidence interval for the mean would be constructed with $\alpha = .296$ and $Z_\alpha = 1.04$. The interval would be placed symmetrically around the mean as $5.33 \pm (1.04)(1.905) = 5.33 \pm 1.98$, and would extend from 3.35 to 7.31. As shown in the bootstrap resampling in Table 6.2 and Section 6.4.2, however, the 70.4% confidence interval actually extends from 3.67 to 7.00.

The bootstrap method becomes particularly valuable when we turn to binary data in Chapter 8, because each item of data is coded as either **0** or **1**. The bootstrap is therefore relatively easy to use and display; and in fact, a mathematical model devised several centuries ago by Bernouilli can indicate exactly what would be produced by a complete bootstrap.

7.3 Theoretical Principles of Parametric Sampling

Although the jackknife and bootstrap methods seem easy to understand and were easy to illustrate in the deliberately simple foregoing examples, the "computer-intensive" calculations can become formidable for most of the groups of data collected in medical research. Consequently, in the era before ubiquitous availability of digital computers, the alternative approach, using parametric theories, became popular because the associated calculations were easy. The harder part, for nonmathematicians, was to understand the parametric reasoning.

The parametric sampling method begins with the idea that a group of n items has been randomly sampled from a parent population, which has its own correct values for such parameters as the mean and standard deviation. We do not know what those parameters are, and the goal is to estimate their values from the sample. To be distinguished from the corresponding results in the observed sample, the population parameters are designated with Greek symbols: μ for the mean and σ for the standard deviation in dimensional data and π for the (binary) proportion in binary data. The corresponding symbols for the sampled group would be $\overline{X}$, s, and p. The aim is to observe the results for $\overline{X}$, s, or p in the sample, and to use them for inferences about the unobserved populational parameters: μ, σ, or π.

The parametric process uses a sequence of reasoning that involves the following activities:

1. Repetitive sampling from the parent population.
2. Calculation of central index (or other anticipated parameters) in each sample.
3. Distribution of the central indexes of those samples.
4. Standard deviation, i.e., "standard error," of the central indexes.
5. Calculation of a "test statistic" for each sample.
6. Distribution of the test statistics.
7. Confidence interval for the population parameters.
8. Use of test statistics for an individual group.

These activities are described in the sections that follow. Note that the first four steps are exact counterparts of what occurred earlier in bootstrap resampling.

Figure 7.2 illustrates the difference between the theoretical and empirical methods of rearranging a group of data. In the theoretical method, a parametric population is inferred, from which theoretical repeated samplings are then taken. In the empirical method, specific groups or resamples are reconstructed from the observed data.

7.3.1 Repetitive Sampling

In the theoretical parametric process, we repeatedly take random samples of n members from a parent population. For this process, we assume that the parent population is infinitely (or at least very) large. In smaller or "finite" populations, the theory requires each sample member to be returned immediately afterward, so that the next sample member is obtained after the replacement. In the parametric process, however, we do not actually "take" each sample. The entire activity is theoretical.

7.3.2 Calculation of Anticipated Parameters

In each of the repeated (although theoretical) samples, we determine the observed values of the central indexes or other parameters that are being estimated. They would be the mean, $\overline{X}$, and standard deviation, s, for samples of dimensional data, and the binary proportion, p, in samples of binary data.

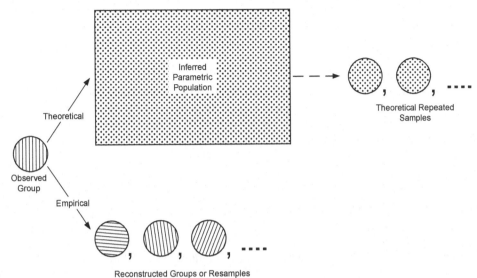

FIGURE 7.2
Theoretical and empirical methods of arrangement.

7.3.3   Distribution of Central Indexes

Each sample in the repetitive array can be denoted with the subscript j, and each has its own central index: a mean $\overline{X}_j$ or a binary proportion p_j. Thus, the first sample of n items has mean $\overline{X}_1$; the second sample of n items has mean $\overline{X}_2$; the third sample has mean $\overline{X}_3$, and so on. Each of those central indexes will have its own deviation from the parent population's parametric value. The deviations will be $\overline{X}_j - \mu$ for each mean or $p_j - \pi$ for each proportion. The parametric reasoning depends on the average results found in the deviations of those central indexes.

The pattern of deviations will turn out to have a mathematical distribution that allows decisions about stability, confidence intervals, and even a test of statistical hypothesis about zones of probability.

7.3.4   Standard Error of the Central Indexes

[The discussion that follows is confined to samples of dimensional data for which the central index is a mean. The process for binary data, summarized with proportions, will be considered in Chapter 8].

The series of means, $\{\overline{X}_1, \overline{X}_2, ..., \overline{X}_j, ...\}$, found in the repeated samples becomes a sample of its own, with its own mean, its own standard deviation, and its own pattern of distribution. The standard deviation of that series of means is the crucial entity called the *standard error of the mean*. A prime step in the parametric reasoning, therefore, is to estimate the standard deviation, i.e., standard error, of the hypothetical sample of sample means.

7.3.4.1   *Standard Deviation of the Means* — The *standard error of the mean*, which is the standard deviation in the theoretical sample of repetitive means, $\{\overline{X}_1, \overline{X}_2, ..., \overline{X}_j, ...\}$, is often abbreviated as s.e., s.e.m., or SEM, and is symbolized as $\sigma_{\bar{x}}$. Intuitively, you would expect the standard deviation of a set of means to be smaller than σ, the standard deviation in the parent population of data.

The actual value is

$$\text{standard error of mean} = \sigma_{\bar{x}} = \sigma / \sqrt{n}$$

The accuracy of this formula was confirmed with bootstrap sampling for a 3-item data set in Section 6.4.2 and for a 2-item data set in Section 7.2.2.4. A more formal and general proof of the formula requires a good deal of mathematics that has been relegated to the Appendix, which can be examined or omitted as you wish. The mathematics involves determining the variance in a sum or difference of two variables (Appendixes A.7.1 and A.7.2), the variance of a parametric distribution (Appendix A.7.3), and finally, the variance of a sample mean (Appendix A.7.4).

7.3.4.2   Estimation of σ with s — Because we do not know the parent population's value of σ, it must be estimated. Diverse candidates might be used from the available single sample of observed data, but the best "unbiased" estimate on average comes from the value of s produced when the observed sample's group variance is divided by n − 1. Thus, using the "^" (or "hat") symbol to indicate an estimated value, we decide that the best estimate (for dimensional data) is

$$\hat{\sigma} = s = \sqrt{S_{xx}/(n-1)}$$

This assertion is proved in Appendixes A.7.4 and A.7.5.

7.3.4.3   Estimation of Standard Error — Because $\sigma/\sqrt{n}$ is the standard error of the parametric data and σ is estimated with s for the sample, we can estimate the standard error of the mean as

$$s_{\bar{x}} = s/\sqrt{n}$$

For the set of dimensional data in Exercise 4.3, the standard deviation, s, was calculated with n − 1 to be 80.48. With n = 20, the standard error of the mean would be estimated as $80.48/\sqrt{20} = 18.0$.

With the standard error, we can eventually construct a zone of probable location, called a *confidence interval*, for the parametric mean, μ. We can also develop an index of stability for the observed mean, $\bar{X}$.

7.3.5   Calculation of Test Statistic

In Chapter 4, we constructed descriptive Z-scores as standard deviates formed in a set of data by the "critical ratio" of (observed value − mean value) divided by standard deviation of the data. These ratios, or other analogous entities, are regularly constructed for inferential activities as indexes that are called *test statistics* because they are often used for testing statistical hypotheses that are discussed later.

For descriptive Z-scores, we learned earlier that each score can be associated with a particular probability (or percentile) if the data come from a mathematical distribution that allows a correspondence between Z scores and probability values. This correspondence occurs with a Gaussian distribution, but other correspondences occur for the associated distributions of other test statistics. For example, probability values can be readily determined between values of a different test statistic (to be discussed later) and a distribution called *chi-square*.

For the sample of means we have been theoretically assembling, a Z_j test statistic can be determined for each mean, $\bar{X}_j$. A particular observed value in the sample of means will be $\bar{X}_j$; the mean value of the observed means will be the parametric mean, μ; and the standard deviation in the sample of means will be the standard error, $\sigma/\sqrt{n}$. Thus, as repetitive samples of means are drawn from the population with parameters μ and σ, each of the sampled means, $\bar{X}_j$, can be expressed in the Z-score format of a standardized deviate,

$$Z_j = \frac{\bar{X}_j - \mu}{\sigma/\sqrt{n}} \qquad [7.1]$$

If we had a mathematical model for the distribution of these Z_j values, each Z_j could be associated with a P value that indicates its percentile location.

7.3.6   Distribution of the Test Statistics

The distribution of the test statistic in Formula [7.1] is demonstrated by the *Central Limit Theorem*, which is one of the most majestic discoveries in statistics and in all of mathematics.[1] The proof of this theorem, which requires too many pages of higher mathematics to be shown here, received contributions from many stars in the firmament of statistics: DeMoivre, Gauss, Laplace, Legendre, Tchebyshev, Markov, and Lyapunov.

According to this theorem, repeated samples of means, each having sample size n, will have a Gaussian distribution, *regardless of the configuration of shape in the parent population*. Thus, if you take repeated samples from data having a Gaussian distribution, an exponential distribution, a uniform distribution, or any of the other shapes shown in Figure 3.4, the *means* of those repeated samples will have a Gaussian distribution. Consequently, the values of Z_j calculated with Formula [7.1] will also have a Gaussian distribution.

The crucial contribution of the Central Limit Theorem, therefore, is that it allows the use of Gaussian mathematical models for *inferences* about means, even when Gaussian models are unsatisfactory for *describing* an observed set of data.

7.3.7 Estimation of Confidence Interval

Once we know that Z_j has a Gaussian distribution for the samples of means, we can take care of the original challenge of finding a zone to locate the unobserved value of the parametric mean, μ. As the theoretical sampling process continues over and over, positive and negative values of Z_j will occur when calculated for each $\overline{X}_j$ found as the sampled mean. Because of the Gaussian distribution, Z_j will be a standard Gaussian deviate and can be used or interpreted with Gaussian P values. We can therefore solve Formula [7.1] for μ, substituting s for σ and bearing in mind that the Z_j values might be positive or negative. The result is

$$\mu = \overline{X}_j \pm Z_j(s/\sqrt{n}).$$ [7.2]

If we want to denote an inner probability zone for the location of μ, we replace Z_j by an assigned value of Z_α, using Gaussian levels of α for the size of the desired zone.

7.3.7.1 Choice of $\overline{X}_j$ — Formula [7.2] offers an excellent method for locating μ, but has one major problem. It is based on the array of theoretical means denoted as $\overline{X}_j$ and on each corresponding Z_j value. In reality, however, we shall obtain a single random sample and have to work with its results. The next section demonstrates that we use the observed sample's value of $\overline{X}$ to substitute for $\overline{X}_j$ in Formula [7.2].

7.3.7.2 Estimation of μ — In Chapter 6 and also in the current chapter, the bootstrap or jackknife resamples had a mean that was the same as the mean of the original group. An analogous event happens in the repetitive sampling now under discussion. The mean of the series of means will turn out to be μ, the parametric mean. In the bootstrap and jackknife procedures, however, the original observed group was the parent population used for the resampling procedures, but in the current activities, the parent population was not observed. Although the parametric reasoning allows us to contemplate a theoretical series of samples, the reality is that we obtain a single random sample from the parent population. We therefore have to estimate the value of μ from something noted in that single observed sample. The "something" might be the sample's mean or median or some other selected index. The best estimate of μ, according to a mathematical proof not shown here, is produced, on average, by the observed mean, $\overline{X}$. For example, if the twenty blood sugar measurements in Exercise 4.3 were a random sample from a larger population, its mean, μ, would be estimated from the sample mean as $\hat{\mu} = \overline{X} = 120.10$.

7.3.7.3 Choice of Z_α — If the observed $\overline{X}$ is used for $\overline{X}_j$, we can substitute a designated value of Z_α for Z_j, and Formula [7.2] will become

$$\mu = \overline{X} \pm Z_\alpha(s/\sqrt{n})$$ [7.3]

After choosing Z_α, we can promptly calculate a confidence interval for μ. For example, suppose we want an inner probability zone of 90% for an observed value of $\overline{X}$. In Table 6.3, the corresponding value of Z_α is 1.645. The corresponding zone for μ would be $\overline{X} \pm 1.645 \, (s/\sqrt{n})$. If we wanted an inner probability zone of 95%, the value of Z_α in Table 6.3 is 1.96, and the zone would be $\overline{X} \pm 1.96 \, (s/\sqrt{n})$.

The choice of α will affect the amount of confidence we can have that μ is truly located in the cited interval. The level of confidence is $1 - \alpha$. Thus, if $\alpha = .05$, $1 - \alpha = .95$, and the result is called a *95% confidence interval*. If $\alpha = .1$, $1 - \alpha = .90$, and the result is a *90% confidence interval*. Note that confidence increases as α gets smaller; but as α gets smaller, Z_α gets larger, so that the size of the confidence interval enlarges.

For example, suppose a particular random sample of 25 members produces $\overline{X} = 10$ and $s = 2$, so that $s/\sqrt{n} = 2/5 = .4$. With a 90% confidence interval, we can estimate $\hat{\mu} = \overline{X} \pm 1.645 \, s/\sqrt{n} = 10 \pm (1.645)(.4) = 10 \pm .658$. The interval extends from 9.342 to 10.658. With a 95% confidence interval, the estimate for $\hat{\mu}$ is $10 \pm (1.96)(.4) = 10 \pm .784$; and the interval extends from 9.218 to 10.784. We can be more confident that the true parametric mean, μ, will be contained in the larger interval (for 95%) than in the smaller interval (for 90%).

7.3.7.4   Contents of Confidence Interval

7.3.7.4   Contents of Confidence Interval — The usual way of expressing a confidence-interval estimate is to say that we are 95% (or whatever was chosen as $1 - \alpha$) confident of finding the correct value of μ in the calculated interval. Strictly speaking, however, the actual confidence is that μ will be included in 95% of the zones formed by calculations from all the potential values of $\overline{X}_j$ in the repeated samples. The reason for this distinction is that the confidence intervals are calculated around the observed values of $\overline{X}_j$, not the unobserved value of μ.

Suppose we took ten samples of means, each group having 25 members, from a parent population having $\mu = 36$ and $\sigma = 10$. The standard error of the mean will be $\sigma/\sqrt{n} = 10/\sqrt{25} = 2$. The 95% confidence interval around each sampled mean will be $\overline{X}_j \pm (1.96)(2) = \overline{X}_j \pm 3.92$. When each sampled mean is checked, we find the following:

Value of $\overline{X}_j$	Confidence Interval	Does This Interval Include 36?
40.2	36.28 to 44.12	No
39.7	35.78 to 43.62	Yes
38.2	34.28 to 42.12	Yes
37.1	33.18 to 41.02	Yes
36.3	32.38 to 40.22	Yes
35.4	31.48 to 39.32	Yes
34.6	30.68 to 38.52	Yes
33.5	29.58 to 37.42	Yes
32.7	28.78 to 36.62	Yes
31.8	27.88 to 35.72	No

In this instance, the true parametric value of the mean, 36, was included in 8 of the 10 confidence intervals calculated with $Z_{.05} = 1.96$, but in repetitive sampling, the parametric value would (or should) be included in 95% of those intervals.

7.3.8   Application of Statistics and Confidence Intervals

As a conventional method of denoting "stability," confidence intervals have two main applications: to estimate the zone of location for a parametric index and to indicate the extremes of potential variation for an *observed* central index.

7.3.8.1   Parametric Zones

7.3.8.1   Parametric Zones — The most obvious application of confidence intervals is in the role for which they were originally devised. In political polls, market research, or industrial testing, the goal is to infer the parametric attributes of a larger population by using what is found in a smaller random sample. The confidence interval indicates the zone in which the desired parameter (such as the mean) is likely to occur; and the selected value of Z_α increases or decreases the confidence by affecting the size of the zone and thus the probability that μ is located in that zone. The process will be further illustrated in Chapter 8, for political polls or election-night forecasting, when the sampled central index is a proportion, p, rather than a mean, $\overline{X}$.

7.3.8.2 Potential Extremes of Variation — In contrast to the process of parametric sampling, the observed group in most medical research is not chosen as a random sample, and a parameter is not being estimated. Nevertheless, because the group *is* a sample of something, the central index might have numerical variations arising merely from the few or many items that happen to be included. For example, a particular treatment might have a success rate of 50% in the "long run" of 200 patients, but might be successful in 75% of a "short run" of 4 patients. By making provision for numerical caprices that might occur in a group of size n, the confidence interval serves to warn or anticipate what could happen in the longer run.

For observed groups, the confidence interval is calculated from the $\pm$ contribution of Z_α ($s/\sqrt{n}$) and is placed symmetrically around the mean, $\overline{X}$. The two extreme ends of the interval will indicate how large or small $\overline{X}$ might really be. For example, if the mean weight of a group of adults is 110 pounds, we might conclude that they are relatively thin until we discover that the mean itself might vary, in an 80% confidence interval, from 50 to 170 pounds.

This role of confidence intervals becomes particularly important later for comparison of two groups in Chapter 13. Whether the observed difference between the two means is tiny or huge, the extremes of the confidence interval for the difference in means can be inspected, before any firm conclusions are drawn, to show how big that difference might really be.

7.3.9 Alternative Approaches

Despite the popularity and customary use of the foregoing procedures, they can often produce problems, particularly with the small data sets discussed in Section 7.2.2.6 and throughout Section 7.5. Many statisticians today may therefore advocate that parametric procedures be replaced and that confidence intervals be obtained with bootstrap methods.[2] They have the advantage of being applicable to any type of distribution and can also be used[3] for the ranked data discussed in Chapter 15.

7.4 Criteria for Interpreting Stability

Regardless of whether we use parametric theory or empirical resampling (with bootstraps or jackknives), the decision about stability of a central index can be made intrinsically, from its own potential variation, or extrinsically, in reference to a selected outer boundary of "tolerance."

7.4.1 Intrinsic Stability: Coefficient of Stability

In Section 5.5.1, the coefficient of variation (c.v.) was calculated as $s/\overline{X}$ to indicate the "effectiveness" with which the mean represents the individual items of data. If the coefficient was too large, the mean was not effective. This same approach, which was introduced in Section 6.4.2, can be used to denote the effectiveness or stability with which the observed mean, $\overline{X}$, represents the potential means $\overline{X}_1$, $\overline{X}_2$, ..., $\overline{X}_j$, ... that might have been obtained in the repetitive sampling.

Because $s/\sqrt{n}$ is the standard deviation, i.e., standard error, of the samples of means, the coefficient of stability for the mean can be calculated as

$$\frac{s/\sqrt{n}}{\overline{X}}$$

We would expect this coefficient to be much smaller than the ordinary c.v., which is multiplied by the factor $1/\sqrt{n}$ to form the c.s. (coefficient of stability); but specific standards have not been established for "stability." If .25 is used as a liberal upper boundary for $s/\overline{X}$ to be "effective" and if 20 is a typical sample size, then $\sqrt{20} = 4.47$ and $1/4.47 = .22$. A crude upper boundary for "stability" would therefore be $.25 \times .22 = .056$. Because the value of .05 has many other mnemonic stimuli in statistics, we might use it as a rough guide for intrinsic stability in considering the potential variation for a mean.

In the data set of Exercise 3.3, the mean was 120.10, and the standard error was 18.0. The value of $18.0/120.10 = .15$ would suggest that the mean in that set of data is *not* stable.

7.4.2 Extrinsic Boundary of "Tolerance"

A different approach to stability is to establish an extrinsic critical boundary of "tolerance" that should be avoided or exceeded by the observed results. For example, a political candidate might want to be sure that she is getting more than 50% of the votes; or we might want the mean value of blood lead in a group of children to be below 10 units. If the observed central index for the group is suitably above (or below) the selected boundary of tolerance, the confidence interval can be used to provide assurance that the boundary level is suitably avoided.

The multiplication by Z_α will make the size of the interval vary according to the "confidence" produced with the choice of α. We can make the interval small by choosing a relatively large α, such as .5, for a 50% confidence interval in which Z_α will be only .674. For greater confidence, with a 95% interval, α will be much smaller at .05, and Z_α will enlarge about three times to 1.96. If the confidence interval is small with a *large* Z_α, we can feel particularly confident about its stability in relation to the chosen boundary.

For example, suppose the mean blood level of lead in a group of children is 7.1 with an SEM of 2.2. With a 50% confidence interval, the potential spread will be $7.1 \pm (.674)(2.2)$, and will extend from 5.6 to 8.6. With a 95% confidence interval, however, the factor $(1.96)(2.2) = 4.3$ will make the interval extend from 2.8 to 11.4. Thus, we could be 50% confident that the mean lead level is below the tolerance boundary of 10, but not 95% confident. Similarly, a political candidate who is favored by 60% of a random sample of 30 voters might have different degrees of confidence that the percentage exceeds the tolerance level of >50% needed for winning the election. (The use of confidence intervals with binary data and the mechanisms used for "election night predictions" are discussed in Chapter 8.)

7.5   Adjustment for Small Groups

All of the foregoing ideas about the Gaussian distribution of sampled means and values of Z_j are splendid, but not strictly true. They pertain only if the group sizes, n, are suitably large (usually above 30). For smaller groups, the critical ratio calculated for Z_j as

$$\frac{\overline{X} - \mu}{\sigma/\sqrt{n}}$$

has a distribution that is not strictly Gaussian. By pointing out this distinction in a 1908 paper[4] published under the pseudonym of "Student," W. S. Gosset, a statistician working at the Guinness brewery, became a member of the statistical hall of fame.

7.5.1   The t Distribution

Gosset showed that for small samples of n, the ratio $(\overline{X} - \mu)/(\sigma/\sqrt{n})$ has a sampling-distribution that resembles the basic Gaussian curve, while differing at the peaks and tails. The sampling distribution is often called *t*, but you may prefer *Gossetian* if you like eponyms. Furthermore, the patterns of a t distribution have slight variations in shape according to the *degrees of freedom* (d.f.) in each sample. For a sample having n members, the value for degrees of freedom is

$$\nu = n - 1.$$

Figure 7.3 shows the basic resemblances and variations for a standard Gaussian distribution and for standard t distributions having 4 and 14 degrees of freedom. The same critical ratio, $(\overline{X} - \mu)/(\sigma/\sqrt{n})$, is used to calculate either Z or t; and the three curves in Figure 7.3 were plotted for critical ratio values at intervals of 0.5 from 0 to ± 3.0. The t curves are slightly shorter in the center and slightly taller in the tails than the Gaussian curve. The two curves become quite close, however, as group sizes (or degrees of freedom) increase.

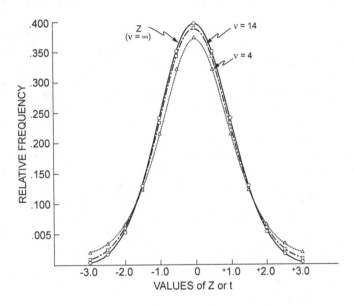

FIGURE 7.3
Relative frequencies associated with Z and with t distribution at 14 and 4 degrees of freedom.

7.5.2 Explanation of Degrees of Freedom

The term *degrees of freedom*, abbreviated as *d.f.*, appears so often in inferential statistics that it warrants a brief explanation.

In the actual data, we find $\overline{X}$ as the mean of a sample of n members. For inferential purposes thereafter, we use $\overline{X}$ to estimate μ, the population mean. When the repetitive theoretical sampling takes place, we assume that each of those samples also offers an estimate of μ. Consequently, when each sample is drawn from the parent population, the first $n - 1$ members can vary in any possible way, but the last member is constrained. For each sample to be an estimate of μ, with $\hat{\mu} = \overline{X}$, the sum of its values must be $\Sigma X_i = n\hat{\mu} = n\overline{X}$.

For example, suppose a group of 6 people have a mean of 73 units, so that $\Sigma X_i = 6 \times 73 = 438$. In repeated theoretical sampling thereafter from a parent population with $\hat{\mu} = 73$, the first five values of a sample might be 132, 63, 72, 52, and 91, with a sum of 410. To estimate $\hat{\mu}$ as 73, however, the total sum of the sample values should be 438. Therefore, the sixth member of the group must have a value of $438 - 410 = 28$.

This constraint removes one degree of freedom from the possible variations in X_i. Before the observed group was formed, n values could be chosen freely for any sample. Once that group has been formed, however, and after the parametric value of $\hat{\mu}$ has been estimated from $\overline{X}$, only $n - 1$ values can vary freely in each sample thereafter.

This idea is the source of the *degrees of freedom* concept. In general, a degree of freedom is lost for each parameter that has been estimated from a sample. Thus, when n − 1 is used in the calculation of $\hat{\sigma} = s = \sqrt{S_{xx}/(n-1)}$, the principle is that the best estimate of population variance comes from dividing the group variance (S_{xx}) by the degrees of freedom in the sample.

7.5.3   Using the t Distribution

For small samples, the critical ratio of $(\bar{X} - \mu)/(s/\sqrt{n})$ is interpreted not as Z_j, but as $t_{\nu,j}$, from a t distribution, using the appropriate value of ν. When confidence intervals are constructed, the value that corresponds to Z_α is $t_{\nu,j}$, selected from a table showing the P values associated with the degrees of freedom, ν, and with the assigned value of α for each $t_{\nu,j}$. The relationship of P values, t values, and degrees of freedom is shown in Table 7.3.

If you have calculated a t_j value as the critical ratio from data for a sample of size n, you enter the table at $\nu = n - 1$ degrees of freedom, and find the value of P. If you have designated a confidence interval of size $1 - \alpha$, you enter the table at $\nu = n - 1$, and find the value of $t_{\nu,\alpha}$ in the location where $P = \alpha$.

Near the end of Section 7.3.7.3, a 95% confidence interval for a data set of 25 members was calculated with $Z_\alpha = 1.96$. A more appropriate calculation, however, would use the corresponding value of t. Since $\nu = 25 - 1 = 24$ for those data, we would find the value for $t_{24,.05}$ in Table 7.3 to be 2.064. The 95% confidence interval would then be $10 \pm (2.064)(.4) = 10 \pm .83$. It would be slightly larger than before, extending from 9.17 to 10.83.

If you examine Table 7.3 closely, you will see that the t values become Z values as the sample sizes enlarge and become infinite. In particular, the t values are quite close to Z values for sample sizes ≥ 30. For example, at the external probability P value of .05, the critical ratios at 30 degrees of freedom are 1.960 for Z, and 2.042 for t. If the sample sizes are quite small, the critical ratios are more disparate. Thus, at the .05 level of P, the critical values of t increase to 2.365 and 2.776 for 7 and 4 degrees of freedom, respectively. When group sizes have these small values, however, decisions about external probability might preferably be made by a bootstrap resampling method as discussed earlier.

7.5.4   Distinctions of t vs. Z

The achievement that made W. S. Gosset a statistical immortal was his revelation, as "Student," that a t rather than Gaussian distribution should be used for inference with the means of small samples. For reasonably large samples (i.e., $\nu \geq 30$), however, the distinction makes relatively little difference; and for smaller samples, the theoretical inferential method may be replaced by a different (empirical) resampling technique in the foreseeable future.

Consequently, despite all of the fame and popularity of the t distribution and t test (to be discussed later), the t technique is not substantially different from the counterpart Z technique. Nevertheless, as long as the t test retains its current popularity, the medical literature will often contain results that were referred to a t distribution. Furthermore, you will keep your "orthodox" statistical colleagues happier if you use $t_{\nu,\alpha}$ or $t_{\nu,j}$ in most circumstances where you might have been tempted to use Z_α or Z_j.

7.6   Finite Population Correction for Unreplaced Samples

All of the discussion thus far in this chapter has been based either on an infinite parametric population or on resampling procedures in which each sampled item was replaced as soon as it was drawn. If the parent population is not enormous and the sampling is done *without* replacement, an important warning must be noted.

With random sampling from a parent population containing N items, the principles of probability depend on the idea that each item in the sample has a 1/N chance of being selected. If N is a very large number, or if the sampling is done *with* replacement, this principle holds true. When sampling is done *without* replacement in smaller populations, however, a correction must be made for the changes that occur in N as each member is removed. (This point is important to bear in mind when samples are taken from a roster of medical admissions, discharges, autopsies, etc.)

TABLE 7.3

Distribution of 2-Tailed P Values for Values of t at Different Degrees of Freedom*

Degrees of Freedom	Probability of a Larger Value, Positive or Negative								
	0.500	0.400	0.200	0.100	0.050	0.025	0.010	0.005	0.001
1	1.000	1.376	3.078	6.314	12.706	25.452	63.657		
2	0.816	1.061	1.886	2.920	4.303	6.205	9.925	14.089	31.598
3	.765	0.978	1.638	2.353	3.182	4.176	5.841	7.453	12.941
4	.741	.941	1.533	2.132	2.776	3.495	4.604	5.598	8.610
5	.727	.920	1.476	2.015	2.571	3.163	4.032	4.773	6.859
6	.718	.906	1.440	1.943	2.447	2.969	3.707	4.317	5.959
7	.711	.896	1.415	1.895	2.365	2.841	3.499	4.029	5.405
8	.706	.889	1.397	1.860	2.306	2.752	3.355	3.832	5.041
9	.703	.883	1.383	1.833	2.262	2.685	3.250	3.690	4.781
10	.700	.879	1.372	1.812	2.228	2.634	3.169	3.581	4.587
11	.697	.876	1.363	1.796	2.201	2.593	3.106	3.497	4.437
12	.695	.873	1.356	1.782	2.179	2.560	3.055	3.428	4.318
13	.694	.870	1.350	1.771	2.160	2.533	3.012	3.372	4.221
14	.692	.868	1.345	1.761	2.145	2.510	2.977	3.326	4.140
15	.691	.866	1.341	1.753	2.131	2.490	2.947	3.286	4.073
16	.690	.865	1.337	1.746	2.120	2.473	2.921	3.252	4.015
17	.689	.863	1.333	1.740	2.110	2.458	2.898	3.222	3.965
18	.688	.862	1.330	1.734	2.101	2.445	2.878	3.197	3.922
19	.688	.861	1.328	1.729	2.093	2.433	2.861	3.174	3.883
20	.687	.860	1.325	1.725	2.086	2.423	2.845	3.153	3.850
21	.686	.859	1.323	1.721	2.080	2.414	2.831	3.135	3.819
22	.686	.858	1.321	1.717	2.074	2.406	2.819	3.119	3.792
23	.685	.858	1.319	1.714	2.069	2.398	2.807	3.104	3.767
24	.685	.857	1.318	1.711	2.064	2.391	2.797	3.090	3.745
25	.684	.856	1.316	1.708	2.060	2.385	2.787	3.078	3.725
26	.684	.856	1.315	1.706	2.056	2.379	2.779	3.067	3.707
27	.684	.855	1.314	1.703	2.052	2.373	2.771	3.056	3.690
28	.683	.855	1.313	1.701	2.048	2.368	2.763	3.047	3.674
29	.683	.854	1.311	1.699	2.045	2.364	2.756	3.038	3.659
30	.683	.854	1.310	1.697	2.042	2.360	2.750	3.030	3.646
35	.682	.852	1.306	1.690	2.030	2.342	2.724	2.996	3.591
40	.681	.851	1.303	1.684	2.021	2.329	2.704	2.971	3.551
45	.680	.850	1.301	1.680	2.014	2.319	2.690	2.952	3.520
50	.680	.849	1.299	1.676	2.008	2.310	2.678	2.937	3.496
55	.679	.849	1.297	1.673	2.004	2.304	2.669	2.925	3.476
60	.679	.848	1.296	1.671	2.000	.299	2.660	2.915	3.460
70	.678	.847	1.294	1.667	1.994	2.290	2.648	2.899	3.435
80	.678	.847	1.293	1.665	1.989	2.284	2.638	2.887	3.416
90	.678	.846	1.291	1.662	1.986	2.279	2.631	.2878	3.402
100	.677	.846	1.290	1.661	1.982	2.276	2.625	2.871	3.390
120	.677	.845	1.289	1.658	1.980	2.270	2.617	2.860	3.373
(z)	.6745	.8416	1.2816	1.6448	1.9600	2.2414	2.5758	2.8070	3.2905

* This table has been adapted from diverse sources.

For example, the first card selected from a deck of 52 cards has a 13/52 chance of being a spade. If the card is not replaced, the denominator for selecting the next card will be 51; and the probability of the next card being a spade will be either 13/51 or 12/51, according to what was chosen in the first card. Thus, the probability that four consecutive unreplaced cards will all be spades is *not* $(13/52)^4 = .004$. It is $(13/52)(12/51)(11/50)(10/49) = .003$.

With the jackknife reconstruction technique, in contrast to the bootstrap resampling method, the sampling is done *without* replacement. Each jackknifed "sample" contains $n - 1$ persons taken, without replacement, from the "parent population" of n persons. A mathematical principle can be derived for the shifting probabilities and necessary corrections of variance that occur when samples of size n are drawn without replacement from a "finite" population of size N. We can expect those samples to have a smaller variance than what would be found if they were taken each time from the intact population, but we need a quantitative indication of how much smaller the variance might be.

If σ^2 is the variance of the total but finite population, the variance of the *means* in samples of size n can be called $\sigma^2_{\bar{x}_n}$. It can be calculated as

$$\sigma^2_{\bar{x}_n} = \frac{N-n}{N-1}(\sigma/\sqrt{n}).$$ [7.4]

Because $N - n$ is smaller than $N - 1$, this value will be smaller than $\sigma/\sqrt{n}$. To illustrate the calculation, the parent population of the data set in Table 7.1 has 20 members, and their variance (calculated with N, rather than $N - 1$) is $(78.44)^2$. [The variance calculated with $N - 1$ was $(80.48)^2$]. Because each of the jackknife samples has $n = 19$, the foregoing formula will produce

$$\sigma_{\bar{x}_n} = \frac{20-19}{20-1}(78.44/\sqrt{19}) = 4.128$$

This is the same result obtained in Table 7.1, when a standard deviation was calculated for the n reduced means produced by the jackknife procedure.

Note that if N is very large, the value of $(N - n)/(N - 1)$ in Formula [7.4] will be approximately 1. The standard deviation of means in general samples of size n will then be

$$\sigma_{\bar{x}_n} = \sigma/\sqrt{n}$$

This is the formula for the "standard error" or standard deviation of means when parametric sampling is done from a population of infinite size.

7.7   Confidence Intervals for Medians

Because the median is used so infrequently in current reports of medical research, most statistical texts give relatively little attention to finding a confidence interval for a median. The procedure is mentioned here because it may become more common when the median replaces the mean as a routine index of central tendency.

7.7.1   Parametric Method

With the parametric approach, the standard error of a median in a Gaussian distribution is mathematically cited as

$$s_{\bar{X}} = (\sqrt{\pi/2})(\sigma/\sqrt{n})$$

where π is the conventional 3.14159... . For an actual group (or "sample") of data, the value of σ would be approximated by the s calculated from the sample. Because $\sqrt{\pi/2} = 1.253$, this formula implies that the median is generally more unstable, i.e., has a larger standard error, than the mean. This distinction may be true for Gaussian distributions, but the median is particularly likely to be used as a central index for non-Gaussian data. Consequently, the formula has few practical merits to match its theoretical virtues.

7.7.2 Bootstrap Method

The bootstrap method could be applied, if desired, to produce a confidence interval for the stability of a median. The approach will not be further discussed, however, because currently it is almost never used for this purpose.

7.7.3 Jackknife Method

The jackknife process is particularly simple for medians. Because the original group in Table 7.1 contains 20 members, the reduced group will contain 19 members, and the reduced median will always be in the 10th rank of the group. This value will have been the 11th rank in the original group. Counting from the lower end of the original data, the 11th ranked value is 96. It will become the reduced median after removal of any original item that lies in the first 10 ranks, i.e., between 62 and 91. The value of **91** will become the reduced median after removal of any items that lie in the original ranks from 11 to 21, i.e., from 96 to 400.

Thus, the reduced median will be either **91** or **96**, as noted in the far right column of Table 7.1. We can also be 100% confident that the reduced median will lie in the zone from **91** to **96**. Because the original median in these data was $(91 + 96)/2 = $ **93.5**, the reduced median will always be 2.5 units lower or higher than before. The proportional change will be 2.5/93.5 = .027, which is a respectably small difference and also somewhat smaller than the coefficients of stability for the mean. Furthermore, the proportional change of 2.7% for higher or lower values will occur in all values and zones of the reduced median. Accordingly, with the jackknife method, we could conclude that the median of these data is quite stable.

If the data set has an even number of members, the jackknife removal of one member will make the median vary between some of the middlemost values from which it was originally calculated. For an odd number of members, most of the reduced medians will vary to values that are just above or below the original median and the values on either side of it. Thus, if the data set in Table 7.1 had an extra item of **94**, this value would be the median in the 21 items. When one member is removed from the data set, the reduced median would become either $(94 + 96)/2 = 95$, or $(91 + 94)/2 = 92.5$, according to whether the removed member is above the value of **96** or below **91**. The median would become $(87 + 94)/2 = 90.5$ with the removal of **91**, $(91 + 96)/2 = 93.5$ with the removal of **94**, and $(94 + 97)/2 = 95.5$ with the removal of **96**. Thus, if X_m is the value at the rank m of the median, the maximum range of variation for the reduced median will be from $(X_{m-2} + X_m)/2$ to $(X_{m+2} + X_m)/2$.

Although seldom discussed in most statistical texts, this type of appraisal is an excellent screening test for stability of a median.

7.8 Inferential Evaluation of a Single Group

A single group of data is often evaluated inferentially to determine whether the central index of the group differs from a value of μ that is specified in advance by a particular hypothesis about the data.

Although "hypothesis testing" will be extensively discussed in Chapter 11, the illustration here can be regarded either as a preview of coming attractions or as a "bonus" for your labors in coming so far in this chapter.

7.8.1   One-Group t or Z Test

The test-statistic ratios for Z or t can be applied stochastically for inferring whether the mean of a single set of data differs from a previously specified value of μ. The test-statistic is calculated as

$$\text{t or Z} = (\overline{X} - \mu)/(s/\sqrt{n})$$

and the result is interpreted as a value for Z_j or for $t_{v,j}$ according to the size of the group. The corresponding P value will denote the external probability that the observed or an even more extreme value of $\overline{X}$ would arise by chance from a parent population whose mean is μ. If we assume that $\mu = 0$, the test statistic becomes $\overline{X}/(s/\sqrt{n})$, which is also the inverse of the coefficient of stability for the mean.

   This application of the t or Z index produces what is called a *one-group* or *paired* "test of significance." It can be used to determine whether the mean of a group (or sample) differs from a previously specified value, which serves as μ. More commonly, however, the test is done with "paired" data, such as a set of before-and-after treatment values for a particular variable in a collection of n people. If we let w_i be the values *before* treatment and v_i be the paired values *after* treatment, they can be subtracted to form a single increment, $d_i = v_i - w_i$ for each person.

   The values of d_i will represent a single variable, with mean $\overline{d}$ and standard deviation

$$s_d = \sqrt{\Sigma(d_i - \overline{d})^2/(n-1)}$$

If we believe that the value of $\overline{d}$ is significantly different from 0 — i.e., that the *after*-treatment values are substantially different from the *before* values — we can establish the "null" hypothesis that the d_i values have been randomly sampled from a population for which $\mu = 0$. The critical ratio of

$$\frac{\overline{d} - 0}{s_d/\sqrt{n}} = \frac{\overline{d}}{s_d/\sqrt{n}}$$

can be converted to indicate the external probability, or P value, for the possibility that the observed value of $\overline{d}$, or a more extreme value, has occurred by chance under the null hypothesis. Using principles to be discussed later, we can then decide whether to reject or concede the null hypothesis that the true mean for the d_i data is 0.

   Note that the "one-group" procedure requires either a single group of data or two groups that can be "paired" to form the increments of a single sample.

7.8.2   Examples of Calculations

The one-group t test is illustrated here in application to a single group and to a set of paired data.

7.8.2.1   *Single-Group t (or Z) Test* — A clinical professor at our institution claims that the group of patients in Exercise 3.3 is highly atypical. She says that the customary mean of blood sugar values is **96**, and that the observed mean of **120.1** implies that the group must be inordinately diabetic.

   The claim can be stochastically evaluated using a one-group t test, with **96** assumed to be the parametric mean. We would calculate

$$= \frac{\overline{X} - \mu}{s/\sqrt{n}} = \frac{120.1 - 96}{18.0} = \frac{24.1}{18.0} = 1.339$$

In Table 7.3, at 19 degrees of freedom, the two-tailed P value associated with this value of t is close to .2, lying between .2 and .1.

This type of result is commonly symbolized, with the lower values coming first, as .1 < P < .2. To indicate the two tails, a better symbolism would be .1 < 2P < .2. The two-tailed P value indicates the possibility that a mean at least 24.1 units *higher or lower* than 96 could arise by chance in the observed group of 20 patients. Because the original conjecture was that **120.1** was too high (rather than merely atypical in either direction), we might be particularly interested in the one-tail rather than two-tail probability. We would therefore take half of the 2P value and state that the external probability is .05 < P < .1 for the chance that a mean of 120.1 or higher would be observed in the selected 20 people if the true mean is 96.

Chapter 11 contains a further discussion of one-tailed and two-tailed probabilities, and their use in rejecting or conceding assumed hypotheses about the observed data.

7.8.2.2 *Paired One-Group t Test* —

Suppose that the 20 patients in Exercise 3.3 were treated with various agents, including some aimed at reducing blood sugar. The values after treatment, shown in Table 7.4, have a mean of −23.3 for the average change in blood sugar. The standard deviation of the increments, however, is 65.6, suggesting that the data are extremely dispersed. This point is also evident from inspecting the wide range of values (going from −254 to +13) for the increments of paired results shown in Table 7.4.

The wide range might elicit strong suspicion that the observed distinction is unstable. Nevertheless, our main question here is not whether **−23.3** is a stable value, but whether the mean blood sugar was indeed lowered by more than the value of **0** that might occur by random chance alone. To answer the latter question, we can do a paired single-group t test on the incremental values. We assume the hypothesis that they came from a population of increments having 0 and 65.6 as the parameters for μ and σ respectively.

The calculation shows

$$t = \frac{d - \mu}{s_d/\sqrt{n}} = \frac{-23.3}{65.6/\sqrt{20}} = 1.588$$

Interpreted at 19 d.f. in Table 7.3, this value of t has an associated two-tailed P value that is between 0.1 and 0.2. If given a one-tail interpretation (because we expected blood sugars to go downward), the P value would be between 0.05 and 0.1. If this chance is small enough to impress you, you might reject the conjecture that the group of increments came from a population whose true mean is 0. This rejection would not make the mean of −23.4 become stable. The inference would be that no matter how unstable the mean may be, it is unlikely to have come from a parent population whose parametric mean is 0.

TABLE 7.4

Before and After Values of Treatment of Blood Sugar for 20 Patients in Table 7.1

Before	After	Increment
62	75	+13
78	82	+4
79	78	−1
80	91	+11
82	82	0
82	84	+2
83	80	−3
85	79	−6
87	94	17
91	90	−1
96	99	+3
97	91	−6
97	85	−12
97	98	+1
101	97	−4
120	112	−8
135	123	−12
180	140	−40
270	110	−160
400	146	−254

	Total	−468
	Mean	−23.3
	s.d.$_{n-1}$	65.6

7.8.2.3 *Confidence Interval for One-Group t Test* —

Another approach to the main question about changes in blood glucose is to calculate a parametric confidence interval for the observed mean of −23.4. Using $t_{19, .05} = 2.093$, the 95% confidence interval would be $-23.4 \pm (2.093)(65.5/\sqrt{20})$ $= -23.4 \pm 30.65$. Extending from −54.05 to 7.25, the interval includes **0**, thus suggesting that the observed results are consistent with a no-change hypothesis.

You may now want to argue, however, that the confidence interval should be one-tailed rather than two-tailed, because of the original assumption that blood sugar values were being lowered. With a one-tailed hypothesis, the appropriate value for a 95% confidence interval is $t_{19, .1} = 1.729$. With this approach, the interval is $-23.4 \pm (1.729)(65.5/\sqrt{20}) = -23.4 \pm 25.32$. Because the upper end of this interval also includes 0, we might feel more comfortable in acknowledging that the observed value of -23.4 is not unequivocally different from the hypothesized value of 0.

Appendixes: Documentation and Proofs for Parametric Sampling Theory

This appendix contains documentation and "proofs" for the assertions made in Chapter 7 about standard errors, estimation of σ, and other inferential strategies. Because the proofs have been kept relatively simple (avoiding such complexities as "expectation theory"), they are reasonable, but not always mathematically rigorous.

A.7.1   Determining the Variance of a Sum or Difference of Two Variables

This concept is needed in Chapter 7 to help determine the "standard error" of a mean, but is also used later in Chapter 13 to find the variance for a difference in two means.

To demonstrate the process, suppose we add or subtract the values of two independent variables, W_i and V_i, each containing n members, having the respective means, $\overline{W}$ and $\overline{V}$, with group variances S_{ww} and S_{vv}, and variances s_w^2 and s_v^2. The result will be a new variable, formed as $W_i + V_i$ or $W_i - V_i$, having n members and its own new mean and new variance.

It is easy to show that the new mean will be $\overline{W} + \overline{V}$ or $\overline{W} - \overline{V}$. A more striking point is that the new group variances and variances will be the same, $S_{ww} + S_{vv}$ and $s_w^2 + s_v^2$, regardless of whether we subtract or add the two variables.

The latter point can be proved with the following algebra: For the addition of the two variables, the new group variance will be $\Sigma[(W_i + V_i) - (\overline{W} + \overline{V})]^2 = \Sigma[(W_i - \overline{W}) + (V_i - \overline{V})]^2 = \Sigma(W_i - \overline{W})^2 + 2(W_i - \overline{W})(V_i - \overline{V}) + (V_i - \overline{V}^2)] = \Sigma(W_i - \overline{W})^2 + 2\Sigma(W_i - \overline{W})(V_i - \overline{V}) + \Sigma(V_i - \overline{V}^2)$. In the latter three expressions, the first and third are S_{ww} and S_{vv}. The middle term essentially vanishes because W_i and V_i are independent and because $\Sigma(W_i - \overline{W}) = 0$ and $\Sigma(V_i - \overline{V}) = 0$. Therefore, the group variance of $W_i + V_i$ will be $S_{ww} + S_{vv}$, and the variance will be $(S_{ww} + S_{vv})/(n - 1)$, which is $s_w^2 + s_v^2$.

If the two variables are subtracted rather than added, the new mean will be $\overline{W} - \overline{V}$. The new group variance will be $\Sigma[(W_i - V_i) - (\overline{W} - \overline{V})]^2 = \Sigma[(W_i - \overline{W}) - (V_i - \overline{V})]^2 = \Sigma[(W_i - \overline{W}) - 2(W_i - \overline{W})(V_i - \overline{V}) + (V_i - \overline{V})^2] = S_{ww} + S_{vv}$, when the middle term vanishes. Thus, when two independent variables, V_i and W_i, are either added or subtracted, the variance of the new variable is $s_w^2 + s_v^2$.

A.7.2   Illustration of Variance for a Difference of Two Variables

Table 7.4 can be used to illustrate this point if we regard the "Before" values as a sample, $\{W_i\}$, and the "After" values as another sample, $\{V_i\}$, each containing 20 items. The 20 items in the W_i and V_i groups can then be subtracted to form the $(W_i - V_i)$ group shown as the "increment" in Table 7.4. The results show means of 120.1, and V = 96.8. For the difference of the two variables, the mean is (as expected) 23.3 for $(\overline{W} - \overline{V})$.

The respective variances are 6477.35 and 403.95 for s_w^2 and s_v^2, with their sum being 6881.30. This sum is much larger than the variance of 4298.77 formed in the $(W_i - V_i)$ group. The reason for the difference in observed and expected variances is that $W_i - V_i$ are not independent samples. The basic principle demonstrated by the mathematics will hold true, on average, for samples that are not related. In this instance, however, the two sets of data are related. They are not really independent, and thus do *not* have a zero value for covariance. In other words, the statement in A.7.1 that "the middle term essentially vanishes" was not correct. The term vanishes in each instance only if $\Sigma(W_i - \overline{W})(V_i - \overline{V})$ is 0. A little algebra will show that this term becomes $\Sigma W_i V_i - N\overline{W}\,\overline{V}$. For samples that are not independent, this term is not zero. Thus, for the data in Table 7.4, $\Sigma W_i V_i = 257047$, and $N\overline{W}\,\overline{V} = 232513.6$. Consequently, $\Sigma(W_i - \overline{W})(V_i - \overline{V}) = 257047 - 232513.6 = 24533.4$, rather than 0. The value of 24533.4 is doubled to 49066.8 and then divided by $19(= n - 1)$ to produce 2582.46 as the incremental contribution of the WV covariance component. Accordingly, $6881.30 - 2582.4 = 4298.84$ for variance in the difference of the two variables.

A.7.3 Variance of a Parametric Distribution

By definition, the parametric population has mean μ and standard deviation σ. Any individual item, X_i, in that population will deviate from the parametric mean by the amount $X_i - \mu$. By definition of σ, the average of the $X_i - \mu$ values will be σ, and the average of the $(X_i - \mu)^2$ values for variance will be σ^2.

In any individual sample of n items, the sum of squared deviations will be $S_{xx} = \Sigma(X_i - \overline{X})^2$ from the sample mean, and $\Sigma(X_i - \mu)^2$ from the parametric mean. With σ as the average value of $X_i - \mu$, the average value of the squared deviations from the parametric mean will be $\Sigma\sigma^2 = n\sigma^2$.

Because $X_i - \mu = (X_i - \overline{X}) + (\overline{X} - \mu)$, the average value of $\overline{X} - \mu$ will be the difference between σ and the standard deviation, s, in the sample. We can square both sides of the foregoing expression to get

$$(X_i - \mu)^2 = (X_i - \overline{X})^2 + 2(X_i - \overline{X})(\overline{X} - \mu) + (\overline{X} - \mu)^2$$

Summing both sides we get

$$\Sigma(X_i - \mu)^2 = \Sigma(X_i - \overline{X})^2 + 2\Sigma(X_i - \overline{X})(\overline{X} - \mu) + \Sigma(\overline{X} - \mu)^2$$

For any individual sample, $\overline{X} - \mu$ is a fixed value, and $\Sigma(X_i - \overline{X}) = 0$. The middle term on the right side will therefore vanish, and we can substitute appropriately in the other terms to get the average expression:

$$n\sigma^2 = S_{XX} + n(\overline{X} - \mu)^2 \qquad [A.7.1]$$

This expression shows that in a sample of n members the average group variance will be larger around the parametric mean, μ, than around the sample mean, $\overline{X}$. The average parametric group variance, $n\sigma^2$, will exceed the sample group variance, S_{XX}, by the magnitude of $n(\overline{X} - \mu)^2$. This concept will be used later in Section A.7.5.

A.7.4 Variance of a Sample Mean

When n members, designated as $X_1, \ldots, X_n$, are sampled from a parametric distribution, their mean will be

$$\frac{X_1 + \ldots + X_n}{n} = \overline{X}$$

The deviation of this value from the parametric mean will be

$$\bar{X} - \mu = \frac{X_1 + \ldots + X_n}{n} - \mu = \frac{X_1 - \mu}{n} + \ldots + \frac{X_n - \mu}{n}$$

In repetitive samples, each constituent value of X_i will take on different values for X_1, X_2, X_3, etc. We can therefore regard each of the $(X_i - \mu)/n$ terms as though it were a variable, with the $\bar{X} - \mu$ term being a sum of the n constituent variables.

According to Section A.7.1, the average variance of $(\bar{X} - \mu)^2$ will be the sum of average variances for the constituent variables. Each constituent variable here has the variance

$$\left(\frac{X_i - \mu}{n}\right)^2$$

and the average value of $(X_i - \mu)^2$, by definition, is σ^2. Therefore, the average value of $(\bar{X} - \mu)^2$ can be cited as

$$(\bar{X} - \mu)^2 = \frac{\sigma^2}{n^2} + \ldots + \frac{\sigma^2}{n^2} = n\left(\frac{\sigma^2}{n^2}\right) = \frac{\sigma^2}{n}$$

Thus, the average variance of a sampled mean is σ^2/n. The square root of this value, $\sigma/\sqrt{n}$, is the special "standard deviation" that is called the "standard error" of the mean.

A.7.5 Estimation of σ

If you understand the mathematics of Appendixes A.7.3 and A.7.4, the procedure here is simple. In Appendix A.7.3, Formula [A.7.1] showed that $n\sigma^2 = S_{XX} + n(\bar{X} - \mu)^2$; and in Appendix A.7.4, we learned that σ^2/n was the average value of $(\bar{X} - \mu)^2$. When the latter value is substituted in Formula [A.7.1], we get

$$n\sigma^2 = S_{XX} + n(\sigma^2/n) = S_{XX} + \sigma^2$$

Therefore,

$$(n - 1)\sigma^2 = S_{XX.}$$

This result tells us that on average, the value of $S_{XX}/(n - 1)$ will be the value of σ^2. The result also explains why S_{XX} is divided by $n - 1$, rather than n, to form the variance of a sample. When the sample standard deviation is calculated as

$$s = \sqrt{S_{XX}/(n - 1)}$$

we get the best average "unbiased" estimate of the parametric standard deviation, σ.

References

1. Adams, 1974; 2. Carpenter, 2000; 3. Sanderson, 1998; 4. Student, 1908.

Exercises

7.1. The hematocrit values for a group of eight men are as follows:

$$\{31, 42, 37, 30, 29, 36, 39, 28\}$$

For this set of data, the mean is 34 with $s_{n-1} = 5.18$ and $s_n = 4.84$. The median is 33.5. [You should verify these statements before proceeding.]

    7.1.1. What are the boundaries of a parametric 95% confidence interval around the mean?

    7.1.2. What is the lower boundary of a parametric one-tailed 90% confidence interval around the mean?

    7.1.3. What are the extreme values and their potential proportionate variations for the jackknifed reduced means in this group?

    7.1.4. What are the extreme values and their potential proportionate variations for the reduced medians?

    7.1.5. Do you regard the mean of this group as stable? Why? Does it seem more stable than the median? Why?

7.2. One of your colleagues believes the group of men in Exercise 7.1 is anemic because the customary mean for hematocrit should be 40. How would you evaluate this belief?

7.3. A hospital laboratory reports that its customary values in healthy people for serum licorice concentration have a mean of 50 units with a standard deviation of 8 units. From these values, the laboratory calculates its "range of normal" as $50 \pm (2)(8)$, which yields the interval from 34 to 66. In the results sent to the practicing physicians, the laboratory says that 34–66 is the "95% confidence interval" for the range of normal. What is wrong with this statement?

7.4. Our clinic has an erratic weighing scale. When no one is being weighed, the scale should read 0, but it usually shows other values. During one set of observations, spread out over a period of time, the following values were noted with no weight on the scale: +2.1, –4.3, +3.5, +1.7, +4.2, 0, –0.8, +5.2, +1.3, +4.7. Two scholarly clinicians have been debating over the statistical diagnosis to be given to the scale's lesion. One of them says that the scale is inconsistent, i.e., its zero-point wavers about in a nonreproducible manner. The other clinician claims that the scale is biased upward, i.e., its zero point, on average, is significantly higher than the correct value of 0. As a new connoisseur of statistics, you have been asked to consult and to settle the dispute. With whom would you agree? What evidence would you offer to sustain your conclusion?

8

Confidence Intervals and Stability: Binary Proportions

The evaluation of stability and confidence intervals for binary proportions needs a separate chapter, because the methods will often differ from those discussed in Chapter 7 for dimensional means. The differences in basic structure of the binary data will make the methods sometimes similar, but other times either simpler or more complex.

Any proportion always has a binary structure, but the entities called *binary proportions* are the central indexes for a group of binary data, in which each item has one of two complementary categories, such as **yes/no, failure/success, dead/alive**. With the items coded as either **0** or **1**, the array of data will be $\{0, 1, ..., 0, 1, 0, ..., 1\}$. If the group contains n items, r will be coded as **1**, and $n - r$ as **0**. The central index can be chosen as either $p = r/n$ or $q = 1 - p = (n - r)/n$. Thus, if 15 people are alive and 27 are dead, the group's binary proportion can be the survival rate, 15/42 = .36, or the fatality rate, 27/42 = .64.

The binary proportions that commonly appear in medical statistics can describe diverse clinical entities, but can also refer to population "rates" (over intervals of time) for such demographic events as births, marriages, and deaths. The differences between *proportions* and *rates* are discussed in Chapter 17, but in pragmatic reporting, the two terms are often used interchangeably, and are also often cited with a third term, *percentages*. In the statistics of daily life, binary percentages can express baseball batting averages, weather forecasts, polls of public opinion, interest on bank accounts, discounts for sale merchandise, the composition of foods, and the concentration of atmospheric pollutants.

8.1 Sources of Complexity

Although stability and confidence zones can sometimes be evaluated with the same theoretical and empirical procedures used for a mean, the rearrangements of binary proportions have three important features that increase the complexity.

1. Because each proportion can be cited as either p or q, rather than with a unique single value, the proportionate changes and potential variation of a rearrangement can differ dramatically if referred to p or q. Thus, a 6% increment in rates will seem relatively large if divided by the observed success rate of 10%, but much smaller if divided by the corresponding failure rate of 90%.

2. The language and concepts can become tricky when an increment such as .06 or 6% in two proportions is divided by another proportion — such as the observed success rate of .10 or 10% — to form a third proportion, which is .06/.10 = .6 or 60%. If the published results mention an "improvement of 60%," you will not know whether the writers have cited a *proportionate* change (in which the compared values were 10% and 16%), or a direct *incremental* change in the observed success rate (which would have had to go from 10% to 70%). Furthermore, if someone wants to minimize rather than maximize the apparent accomplishment of a 6% increment between success rates of 10% and 16%, the change could be referred to the original failure rate of 90%. With the latter citation, the proportionate decline in the failure rate would be .06/.90 = .067 or 7%. Thus, the same observed change could be reported as 6%, 60%, or 7%, according to the choice made by the "seller." All three citations are legitimate and accurate, but the "buyer" will have to beware.

3. Stability and confidence intervals for binary proportions can often be well estimated with the Gaussian mathematics used for means. If the group size is small, however, or if the proportion is far below (or above) 50%, the Gaussian procedure may yield distorted results. A more accurate set of calculations can be obtained with binomial (or Bernouilli) distributions, discussed in Section 8.4, for the **0/1** structure of the data.

8.2 Jackknife Screening

The jackknife technique has already been illustrated at the beginning of Chapter 7 for examining stability in such proportions as 1/2, 1/3, 150/300, and 100/300.

A proportion constructed as r/n can change either to the smaller value of $(r - 1)/(n - 1)$ if the removed member is a **1**, or to the larger value of $r/(n - 1)$ if the removed member is a **0**. For example, if p = 2/7 = .2857, the reduced proportions will be either 1/6 = .1667 or 2/6 = .3333. The chance of getting the smaller value will be r/n, and the chance of getting the larger value will be $(n - r)/n$.

The strategy of examining the two extreme jackknife results (and the chances of getting those results) offers a quick, almost purely mental method of screening for the stability of a proportion. Regardless of how the potential values and chances are interpreted, the results here show that the 2/7 proportion is certainly unstable. Aside from a jackknife screening that shows obvious fragility, however, the stability of a proportion is usually evaluated with more formal mathematical methods.

8.3 Gaussian Confidence Intervals

The same parametric reasoning used in Chapter 7 can be applied to estimate the standard error of a proportion and to determine confidence intervals. We assume that the parent population contains binary data, with π as the parametric proportion. When repeated samples of size n are drawn from the parent population in the theoretical sampling process, each sample will have p_j as its central index. We can find the standard error of those sampled proportions by determing the average or "standard" deviation of $p_j - \pi$. We then use the standard error to calculate a confidence interval for the zone in which π is located.

8.3.1 Standard Error of a Proportion

The parametric strategy for determining standard error of a proportion is exactly analogous to what was done with a mean. You may recall, from Section 4.9.3, that the variance of an observed set of binary data was $s^2 = pq$, which will estimate the parametric variance as $\hat{\sigma}^2 = pq$. The standard error of the proportion will then be estimated as

$$\frac{\hat{\sigma}}{\sqrt{n}} = \sqrt{\frac{pq}{n}}$$

This simple formula is possible because npq, the group variance of the binary data, was divided by n to form the variance in Section 4.9.3. Now that the degrees-of-freedom concept has been discussed, the reason for this divisor can be explained. When group variance was calculated for dimensional data as $\Sigma X_i^2 - n\overline{X}^2$, there were n degrees of freedom in the choice of the X_i values, and 1 d.f. in the choice of $\overline{X}$. Thus, the value for d.f. was $n - 1$. When a binary proportion is determined as p, there are n degrees of freedom in choice of the **0** or **1** component values. As soon as p is known, however, the value of q is promptly found as $q = 1 - p$, and the group variance is also promptly found as npq, without any subtractions to reduce the n degrees of freedom. Accordingly, the group variance npq is divided by n to form the variance. The standard deviation, $\sqrt{pq}$, is then divided by $\sqrt{n}$ to determine the standard error.

For example, if a political candidate is favored by 60% of voters in a poll, the standard error of the proportion is $\sqrt{(.40)(.60)/10} = .155$ if the sample size was 10, and $\sqrt{(.40)(.60)/100} = .049$, if the size was 100.

A "short-cut" method for calculating the standard error of p = r/n is to use the formula $\sqrt{(r)(n-r)/n^3}$. For p = 4/10, the result would be $\sqrt{(4)(6)/10^3} = .155$; and for 40/100, the result is $\sqrt{(40)(60)/100^3} = .049$.

8.3.2 Confidence Interval for a Proportion

Another splendid attribute of Gaussian mathematics and binary proportions is that the values of Z_j calculated for p_j in repeated samplings will have a Gaussian distribution (if n is suitably large). With this principle, we can form the ratio

$$Z_j = \frac{p_j - \pi}{\sigma / \sqrt{n}} \qquad [8.1]$$

and interpret it as though it were a standard Gaussian deviate.

Using the observed value of p for p_j, and $\sqrt{pq}$ for σ, we can estimate boundaries for the location of the parametric π by choosing an appropriate value of Z_α for the desired $1 - \alpha$ level of the Gaussian confidence interval. After Formula [8.1] receives suitable substitution and conversion, the calculation becomes

$$\hat{\pi} = p \pm Z_\alpha \sqrt{\frac{pq}{n}} \qquad [8.2]$$

and is an exact counterpart of the confidence interval Formula [7.3] for a mean. To compare the observed p with a hypothesized π, Formula [8.1] becomes the critical ratio

$$Z = (p - \pi)/\sqrt{pq/n} \qquad [8.3]$$

8.3.2.1 *Example of Calculation* —

Suppose the observed proportion is $26/42 = .62$. The value of the standard error $\sqrt{pq/n} = \sqrt{(26/42)(16/42)/42} = \sqrt{.00561} = .075$. [With the short-cut formula, this calculation is $\sqrt{(26)(16)/42^3} = \sqrt{.00561} = .075$.] The 95% confidence interval will be

$$\pi = .62 \pm (1.96)(.075) = .62 \pm .147$$

and will extend from .473 to .767.

Suppose someone believes that this result, despite a group size of 42, is a "short-term fluke" and that the "long-run" parametric value in the population is actually $\pi = .50$. With Formula [8.3], we can calculate $Z = (.62 - .50)/.075 = 1.6$, for which $2P > .05$. As discussed later, we could have anticipated that this result would have $2P > .05$, because the 95% confidence interval included the parametric value of $\pi = .50$.

8.3.2.2 *Example of Practical Application* —

Confidence intervals for proportions are constantly used on election night when the media make forecasts about a winner. A particular voting precinct (or cluster of precincts) is chosen as a random (or at least trustworthy) representative of the political region under scrutiny. As increasing numbers of votes accrue from the selected precinct(s), confidence intervals are repeatedly calculated. When a high-level confidence interval excludes .50, a victor will be predicted.

When the forecasts go wrong, the error may have scientific or statistical sources. Scientifically, the selected precincts may have been poorly chosen. Because of population migration or some other reason, the precincts may no longer suitably represent the entire region. If the precincts have been well chosen, however, the source of wrong predictions can be two statistical factors: the value of Z_α chosen for the level of confidence, and the increment of tolerance by which the lower level of the estimate must exceed .50. With lower values of confidence level and higher tolerance, the forecasts can be made earlier on election night (i.e., with smaller numbers of precinct ballots), but will have a greater margin for error.

For example, suppose the early results show Candidate A ahead of Candidate B by 60 votes to 40. With a 90% confidence interval, the estimate is

$$\pi = (60/100) \pm 1.645 \sqrt{(.60)(.40)/100}$$
$$= .60 \pm (1.645)(.049) = .60 \pm .08.$$

The confidence interval extends from .52 to .68. Since the "tie" value of .50 is excluded, Candidate A might be proclaimed the winner. On the other hand, with a 99% confidence interval, Z_α will be 2.58. The interval will be $.60 \pm (2.58)(.049) = .60 \pm .126$ and extends from .484 to .726. With this result, Candidate A cannot yet be guaranteed victory. With Z_α set at 1.96, a 95% confidence interval could be calculated as $.6 \pm (1.96)(.049) = .6 \pm .096$, and would extend from .504 to .696. If the forecasters are content to regard 50.4% as a suitable margin of tolerance above 50%, they might issue a victory prediction.

8.3.2.3   Customary Applications and Abuses — In the foregoing discussion, we were trying to estimate a populational parameter from the results found in a sample; and a specific sampling process was either planned or had actually occurred. In most medical publications, however, the investigator has obtained results from an observed group of people (or other entities) who happened to be conveniently available for the research. For the binary proportion, p, that was found in these entities, the main goal is to determine the stability of the result, not to estimate a populational parameter.

Nevertheless, the goal of checking stability in convenient groups is almost always approached with the same strategy used for estimating parameters in random samples. A standard error and/or confidence interval, determined from the observed result, become used for appraising its stability. As the observed result is *not* a random sample, all of the mathematical reasoning based on randomness is not really appropriate or justified. To allow the reasoning to be used, however, the assumption is made that the observed group is indeed a random sample.

This abuse of the fundamental mathematics has persisted for about a century and has become sanctified by the recommendation and approbation received from authoritative statisticians and as well by constant appearance in medical publications. A major advantage of bootstrap (or Bernouilli) confidence intervals discussed in the next section is that they come only from the observed data, without making parametric estimates and without requiring mathematical assumptions about parametric sampling or distributional shapes.

8.4   Binomial (Bernouilli) Confidence Intervals

A different way to determine standard errors and confidence intervals for binary proportions is both empirical and theoretical. Empirically, the observed group of n members is used directly as a parent population in a bootstrap resampling procedure. Theoretically, the results of the binary sampling process can be exactly anticipated with a mathematical model. Applied to items having the binary or "binomial" values of **0** or **1**, the model is often called the *binomial distribution*.

8.4.1   Illustration of Bootstrap Procedure

Consider the binary proportion $6/10 = .60$. Because each of the ten people in this group can be rated as 0 or 1, success or failure, yes or no, the existing group of data can be depicted as a set of six members of one type and four of the other. One such depiction would be the data set {Y, Y, Y, Y, Y, Y, N, N, N, N}, where each Y = yes and each N = no.

8.4.1.1   Formation of Samples — To show each member in a complete bootstrap resampling would require 10^{10} samples. The process is therefore easier to demonstrate if we do the complete bootstrap for 5 items, which will involve only $10^5 = 100,000$ samples from the set of data.

Each time an item is chosen, there are 10 possibilities. For the first choice in the sample, we could get any one of the 6 Y items, or any one of the 4 N items. For the second choice, we could again get any one of the 6 Y items or any one of the 4 N items. The 100 possibilities in the first two choices would thus contain the patterns

YY: $6 \times 6 = 36$ possibilities

YN: $6 \times 4 = 24$ possibilities

NY: $4 \times 6 = 24$ possibilities

NN: $4 \times 4 = 16$ possibilities

These four patterns contain three sets of contents: YY, NN, and a set that has one N and one Y.

With 10 more chances in the third choice, the total number of possibilities would be expanded to 1000, the number of patterns to eight, and the number of different contents to four. Among the four sets of contents, one group would have 3 Y's; one would have 2 Y's and 1 N; one would have 1 Y and 2 N's;

and one would have 3 N's. The fourth and fifth choices would expand the number of possibilities to 10,000 and then to 100,000; the number of patterns would go to 16 and then to 32; the number of sets with different contents would go to five and then to six.

8.4.1.2   Summary of Results

— The sequence of possible patterns and contents for the foregoing choices is shown in Table 8.1.

The 100,000 possible patterns after five choices will be arranged in the six basic formats of: 5 Y's; 4 Y's and 1 N; 3 Y's and 2 N's; 2 Y's and 3 N's; 1 Y and 4 N's; and 5 Y's. Table 8.2 shows a summary of the patterns, frequencies, and relative frequencies of the contents in Table 8.1. For each set, the respective proportions, p_i, are 1.00, .80, .60, .40, .20, or 0. The relative frequency, f_i, of choices for each proportion, p_i, is shown in the sixth column of Table 8.2. [The far right column, binomial relative frequency, is explained in Section 8.4.2.3.]

8.4.1.3   Mean, Variance, and Standard Error

— To find the mean value for the proportion of Y's in the 100,000 bootstrapped samples of Table 8.2, we can multiply each value of p_i by its total number of choices, m_i, and then divide by 100,000. Alternatively, we can multiply each p_i by its relative frequency f_i and then take the sum of the products as

$$\Sigma p_i f_i$$

With the latter calculation, the bootstrap-sample mean is $(1.00)(.0778) + (.80)(.2592) + (.60)(.3456) + (.40)(.2304) + (.20)(.0768) + (0)(.0102) = .60$, which is the expected result for p.

For the variance of the bootstrapped samples, we can use the formula

$$\Sigma f_i (p_i - p)^2$$

which yields $(.0778)(1.00 - .60)^2 + .2592(.80 - .60)^2 + .3456(.60 - .60)^2 + .2304(.40 - 60)^2 + .0768 (.20 - .60)^2 + .0102(0 - .60)^2 = .048$.

The standard deviation of the bootstrapped proportions is $\sqrt{.048} = .219$. Note that this is the same standard error obtained for the binary data using the Gaussian formula of $\sqrt{pq/n} = \sqrt{(.60)(.40)/5} = .219$.

8.4.1.4   Confidence Intervals

— The main virtue of Tables 8.1 and 8.2 is that they show the exact distribution of proportions in the array of bootstrap samples. An important thing to note about this distribution is that the relative frequencies are *not* arranged symmetrically around the central index value of p = .60. This asymmetry will occur whenever the sample sizes are relatively small (i.e., n < 20 or 30) for any proportion in which p is not at the "meridian" value of **.50**. Consequently, the symmetrical confidence interval calculated with the component value, $\pm Z_\alpha \sqrt{pq/n}$, will not be wholly accurate with small sample sizes. Thus, just as the t distribution is best used for small samples of dimensional data, the Bernouilli binomial distribution (which is discussed shortly, and which provides the same results as the bootstrap) is best used for small samples of binary data.

From Table 8.2, we can demarcate a symmetrical confidence interval using the proportions .40 to .80. They would include $.2304 + .3456 + .2592 = .8352$ or 84% of the data. The proportions from .20 to 1.00 would create an asymmetrical interval that contains 99% of the data, with the 0 value of the proportion excluded.

As noted shortly, the Bernouilli or binomial distribution takes a Gaussian shape when n is large. (The relative frequencies in Table 8.2 already look somewhat Gaussian despite the small n of 5.) Accordingly, the Gaussian Z indexes are often applied to estimate confidence intervals for a proportion, using the standard error $\sqrt{pq/n}$. For example, $Z_{.16} = 1.41$ and $\sqrt{pq/n}$ for the data here is .219; thus, $1.41 \times .219 = .31$. With the Gaussian formula, the 84% confidence interval would be the zone of $.60 \pm .31$, which extends from .29 to .91. It approximates but is larger than the corresponding 84% zone of .40 to .80 found with the bootstrap.

TABLE 8.1

100,000 Possible Patterns in Five Selections from Population
with Binary Proportion of .6

1st Choice	2nd Choice	3rd Choice	4th Choice	5th Choice	Number of Patterns	Contents of Pattern	Proportion of Y's in Pattern
				Y(6)	7776	5Y	1.00
			Y(6)	N(4)	5184	4Y,1N	.80
		Y(6)	N(4)	Y(6)	5184	4Y,1N	.80
				N(4)	3456	3Y,2N	.60
	Y(6)		Y(6)	Y(6)	5184	4Y,1N	.80
		N(4)		N(4)	3456	3Y,2N	.60
			N(4)	Y(6)	3456	3Y,2N	.60
				N(4)	2304	2Y,3N	.40
Y(6)			Y(6)	Y(6)	5184	4Y,1N	.80
		Y(6)		N(4)	3456	3Y,2N	.60
			N(4)	Y(6)	3456	3Y,2N	.60
	N(4)			N(4)	2304	2Y,3N	.40
			Y(6)	Y(6)	3456	3Y,2N	.60
		N(4)		N(4)	2304	2Y,3N	.40
			N(4)	Y(6)	2304	2Y,3N	.40
				N(4)	1536	1Y,4N	.20
			Y(6)	Y(6)	5184	4Y,1N	.80
		Y(6)		N(4)	3456	3Y,2N	.60
			N(4)	Y(6)	3456	3Y,2N	.60
	Y(6)			N(4)	2304	2Y,3N	.40
			Y(6)	Y(6)	3456	3Y,2N	.60
		N(4)		N(4)	2304	2Y,3N	.40
			N(4)	Y(6)	2304	2Y,3N	.40
				N(4)	1536	1Y,4N	.20
N(4)			Y(6)	Y(6)	3456	3Y,2N	.60
		Y(6)		N(4)	2304	2Y,3N	.40
			N(4)	Y(6)	2304	2Y,3N	.40
	N(4)			N(4)	1536	1Y,4N	.20
			Y(6)	Y(6)	2304	2Y,3N	.40
		N(4)		N(4)	1536	1Y,4N	.20
			N(4)	Y(6)	1536	1Y,4N	.20
				N(4)	1024	5N	0

TABLE 8.2

Summary of Results in Table 8.1 for $p = .6$, $q = .4$

Contents	$p_i =$ Proportion of Y's	Number of Choices within This p_i	Number of Patterns within Each Choice	$m_i =$ Frequency of This p_i	$m_i/100,000 =$ $f_i =$ Relative Frequency	Binomial Relative Frequency
5Y	1.00	7776	1	7,776	.0778	$p^5 = .0778$
4Y,1N	.80	5184	5	25,920	.2592	$5p^4q = .2592$
3Y,2N	.60	3456	10	34,560	.3456	$10p^3 q^2 = .3456$
2Y,3N	.40	2304	10	23,040	.2304	$10p^2q^3 = .2304$
1Y,4N	.20	1536	5	7,680	.0768	$5pq^4 = .0768$
5N	0	1024	1	1,024	.0102	$q^5 = .0102$
			TOTAL	100,000	1.0000	1.0000

8.4.2 Bernouilli Procedure

The diverse possibilities in a bootstrap sampling of binary data were mathematically determined by Jacob Bernouilli more than three centuries ago. He formulated an elegant expression, called the *binomial expansion*, which is

$$(p + q)^n$$

You met the simple forms of this expansion in your elementary algebra as $(a + b)^2 = a^2 + 2ab + b^2$, and $(a + b)^3 = a^3 + 3a^2b + 3ab^2 + b^3$.

To illustrate how the expansion works, suppose we toss a coin three times. With H for head and T for tails, there are 8 possible outcomes: HHH, HHT, HTH, HTT, THH, THT, TTH, and TTT. One of these eight outcomes has all heads; three have two heads and one tail; three have one head and two tails; and one has all tails. This result could have been expected from the binomial expansion of $(p + q)^3$, if we let $p = $ probability of a head and $q = $ probability of a tail. The expansion is $p^3 + 3p^2q + 3pq^2 + q^3$. The probability of getting all heads is $p^3 = (1/2)^3 = 1/8$. The probability of getting two heads and a tail is $3p^2q = 3/8$. Correspondingly, $3pq^2 = 3/8$ and $q^3 = 1/8$ are the probabilities for the other two outcomes.

8.4.2.1 General Format of Binomial Terms — In general application, the binomial expansion for a sample of n items has $n + 1$ terms. They are p^n, $p^{n-1}q$, $p^{n-2}q^2$, ..., $p^{n-r}q^r$, ..., p^2q^{n-2}, pq^{n-1}, q^n. The values of r increase successively from 0 for the first term to n for the last. Each term will reflect a sampled proportion having the value $(n - r)/n$. For example, in Table 8.2, the sampled proportion associated with p^5 was $5/5 = 1$; the sampled proportion associated with p^2q^3 was $2/5 = .40$.

8.4.2.2 Binomial Coefficients — Each term will also have an associated binomial coefficient, which can be symbolized as $_nC_r$, C_r^n, or $\binom{n}{r}$. The $\binom{n}{r}$ symbol will be used here. It is calculated as

$$\binom{n}{r} = \frac{n!}{r!(n-r)!}$$

The binomial coefficient is particularly worth knowing about because it also plays an important role later in Chapter 12 when we meet the Fisher Exact Probability test for comparing two proportions. The coefficient represents the different number of individual combinations that can be formed when n things are taken r at a time. The first term can be chosen in n different ways. The next term can then be chosen from $n - 1$ items. The third term can come from $n - 2$ items, and so on. Thus, there are $n \times (n - 1) \times (n - 2) \times ... \times 2 \times 1 = n!$ sequences, called *permutations*, in which the n items could be arranged. If only r items are selected from the total group of n, the permutation will extend from n down to $n - r + 1$.

For example, suppose you are being dealt 13 consecutive cards from a well-shuffled deck of 52. The first card can be chosen in 52 ways, the second in 51, the third in 50, and so on down to the 13th in 40 ways. The value of 40 is $n - r + 1 = 52 - 13 + 1$. Accordingly, the sequence in which you get the cards has $52 \times 51 \times 50 \times \ldots \times 41 \times 40$ possibilities. This sequence can be expressed as $52!/39! = (52 \times 51 \times 50 \times \ldots \times 2 \times 1)/(39 \times 38 \times 37 \times \ldots \times 2 \times 1)$, because we divide by 39! to remove the remaining 39! possibilities from the original 52!. The general formula for the sequence of r things taken from a group of n is $n!/(n - r)!$.

In receiving the cards, however, you do not care about the sequence in which they arrive. What concerns you is the particular combination of 13 cards that constitutes your "hand." Because those 13 cards could themselves be permuted in 13! sequences, the combination in your particular hand could have been constructed in $(52!/39!) \div 13!$ ways. The latter expression is $52!/[(39!)(13!)]$. If you work out this calculation, the result turns out to be $8.0658 \times 10^{67}/[(2.0398 \times 10^{46})(6.227 \times 10^{9})] = 6.3501 \times 10^{11}$.

The general formula for the combination that forms your "hand" is therefore $n!/[(n-r)! \, (r!)]$. An important thing to know when working with factorials is that $0! = 1$. If you take all n things at once, there is only one possible combination. It is $n!/[(n!)(0!)] = 1$.

8.4.2.3 Application of Binomial Coefficients and Terms — The binomial expansion of $(p + q)^n$ can be expressed as

$$\Sigma \binom{n}{r} p^{n-r} q^r \qquad [8.4]$$

The first term, with $r = 0$, is $\{n!/[(n!)(0!)]\}p^n = p^n$. The second term, with $r = 1$, is $\{n!/[(n-1)! \, (1!)]\}p^{n-1}q = np^{n-1}q$. The third term with $r = 2$, is $\{n!/[(n-2)!(2!)]\}p^{n-2}q^2 = [n(n-1)/2]p^{n-2}q^2$, and so on down to q^n.

For example, the binomial expansion when $n = 5$ is $p^5 + 5p^4q + 10p^3q^2 + 10p^2q^3 + 5pq^4 + q^5$. The two coefficients of 5 came from $5!/(4!1!)$ and the two coefficients of 10 came from $5!/(3!2!)$. Each of these terms will indicate the relative frequency, i.e., the probability, of getting the particular arrangement of **1**'s, and **0**'s implied by the $p^{n-r}q^r$ part of the term. Thus, when $n = 5$ and $r = 2$, there would be three **1**'s and two **0**'s, producing the proportion 3/5 or $(n - r)/n$. The chance of occurrence for this proportion would be $10p^3q^2 = 10(3/5)^3 (2/5)^2 = .346$. Each of the $\binom{n}{r} p^{n-r}q^r$ terms represents the binomial relative frequency, cited in the far right column of Table 8.2, for the p_i proportion that is calculated as $(n - r)/n$.

8.4.2.4 Example of Application — In Table 8.2, the bootstrap sampling showed the possibilities occurring when samples of 5 members were taken from a population with π estimated to be .6. If we apply the Bernouilli process with $n = 5$, $p = .6$, and $q = 1 - .6 = .4$, we get the binomial relative frequencies shown in the far right column of Table 8.2. These relative frequencies are identical to those obtained previously as values of f_i with the bootstrap process.

As another example, suppose we want to evaluate the proportion of spades that would be obtained in five selections, each from a full deck of cards. Because $p = 1/4$, we obtain the possibilities are shown in Table 8.3.

TABLE 8.3

Bernouilli Distribution or Probability for Spades Found in 5 Selections Each from a Full Deck of Cards

Selection	Observed Proportion of Spades	Chance of Getting This Proportion	
All spades	1	$(1/4)^5$	= .0010
Four spades, one non-spade	.8	$5(1/4)^4(3/4)$	= .0146
Three spades, two non-spades	.6	$10(1/4)^3(3/4)^2$	= .0879
Two spades, three non-spades	.4	$10(1/4)^2(3/4)^3$	= .2637
One spade, four non-spades	.2	$5(1/4)(3/4)^4$	= .3955
No spades	0	$(3/4)^5$	= .2373
		TOTAL	= 1

In this instance, proportions of spades ranging from 0 to .6 would be found in $.2373 + .3955 + .2637 + .0879 = .9844$ of the selections. We could thus form a nonsymmetrical 98% confidence interval, demarcated by values from 0 to .6, for the expected proportions if five items were taken from a distribution with $\pi = .25$. Note that the interval of 0 to .6 is *not* symmetrical around the value of .25. Note also that the expected proportion of .25 was impossible to obtain in a sample of 5 members. The highest individual probabilities were .3955 for getting a proportion of .2 for the spades, and .2637 for a proportion of .4.

If we had tried to get this result with a Gaussian calculation, the closest approach would be with $Z_{.01} = 2.58$ for a 99% confidence level. The standard error would be $\sqrt{(1/4)(3/4)/5} = .194$ and the interval would be $.25 \pm (2.58)(.194) = .25 \pm .50$. It would extend from an impossible $-.25$ to .75. (In the binomial expansion, the interval from 0 to .8 would have covered 99.9% of the possibilities.)

8.4.2.5　Binomial Expansions for Confidence Intervals — Because of the possible asymmetries and unrealistic results, the confidence intervals for proportions are best determined with binomial expansions when the sample or group size, n, is small. As n enlarges, the binomial and Gaussian results become less disparate.

For example, suppose the proportion of .2 has been observed as 4 successes and 16 failures in a group of 20. The binomial expansion would contain 21 terms for possible proportions whose values would be 1, .95, .90, ..., .10, .05, 0. The binomial coefficients and terms would produce tiny values for the relative frequencies of the first ten terms with potential proportions of 1, .95, ... , .60, .55. For the remaining 11 terms, shown in Table 8.4, about 84% ($= .1090 + .1745 + ... + .1369$) of the possible proportions would be in the zone from .10 to .30. An additional 11% ($= .0545 + .0576$) would be included if the zone extends from .05 to .35. Thus, the interval from .05 to .35 would include 95% of the possible proportions if a sample of 20 members was drawn from a binary population with parameter $\pi = .20$. The tactic of getting the confidence interval by using the exact binomial formula and working toward the center from both ends is sometimes called the Clopper-Pearson method.[1]

TABLE 8.4

Demonstration of Bernouilli Probabilities for 11 terms of $p = 4/20 = .20$

Potential Proportion	Bernouilli Probability of Occurrence
$10/20 = .50$	$184756(.2)^{10}(.8)^{10} = .0020$
$9/20 = .45$	$167960(.2)^{9}(.8)^{11} = .0074$
$8/20 = .40$	$125970(.2)^{8}(.8)^{12} = .0222$
$7/20 = .35$	$77520(.2)^{7}(.8)^{13} = .0545$
$6/20 = .30$	$38760(.2)^{6}(.8)^{14} = .1090$
$5/20 = .25$	$15504(.2)^{5}(.8)^{15} = .1745$
$4/20 = .20$	$4845(.2)^{4}(.8)^{16} = .2182$
$3/20 = .15$	$1140(.2)^{3}(.8)^{17} = .2054$
$2/20 = .10$	$190(.2)^{2}(.8)^{18} = .1369$
$1/20 = .05$	$20(.2)(.8)^{19} = .0576$
$0/20 = 0$	$(.8)^{20} = .0116$

If this same 95% confidence interval were calculated with Gaussian arithmetic, the result would be $.20 \pm (1.96) \sqrt{(.2)(.8)/20} = .20 \pm .175$. The interval would extend from .025 to .375. [If you wanted to use a t-distribution approach for the small sample, the 95% confidence interval for 19 degrees of freedom would be $.20 \pm (2.093) \sqrt{(.2)(.8)/19} = .20 \pm .192$. This interval would extend from .008 to .392.]

Both of the Gaussian and t parametric calculations are now much closer to, but are still not quite the same as, the "gold standard" zone of .05 to .35 obtained with the binomial Clopper-Pearson method.

8.4.2.6　Binomial Tactics for Rare Events — A particularly valuable use of the binomial calculations occurs when claims are made about rare or uncommon events. For example, suppose an

investigator has observed that a particular treatment failed in only 1 (4%) of 23 patients. An evaluator who thinks that the true rate of failure should be 15% then suspects the investigator of either not telling the truth or having a peculiar group of patients. To determine whether the observed result is within the limits of chance, we can find the relative frequencies with which 1 failure would be expected in 23 treatments if the true rate of failure is 15%, with the success rate being .85 (= 85%).

If .85 is the success rate, the chance of observing no failures (i.e., all successes) in 23 patients would be $(.85)^{23} = .0238$. The chance of observing 1 failure in 23 patients would be $23(.85)^{22} (.15) = .0966$. Thus, if the true failure rate is 15%, there is a chance of $.0966 + .0238 = .1204$, or 12% of observing as few as 1 or no failures in 23 people. The decision about whether the investigator is telling the truth depends on how you interpret the chance of 12%.

8.4.2.7 Use of Reference Tables

— Because the Clopper-Pearson calculations are cumbersome (particularly for more than one or two events), they are seldom used routinely for determining Bernouilli confidence intervals. The main reason for discussing them is to let you know of their existence as the "gold standard" approach for small samples and for proportions that are remote from the meridian value of **.5**.

To save time and effort, special tables have been constructed to show "exact confidence limits" for events or proportions calculated with binomial distributions. For example, consider the observed value of $4/20 = .20$. In an "exact-confidence-limits" table for the binomial distribution (cf. page 89 of the Geigy Scientific Tables[2]), the 95% confidence interval for 4/20 is listed as extending from .0573 to .4366. Note that this result differs slightly from the exact boundary of .05 to .35 that was noted earlier for the Clopper-Pearson calculations shown here in Section 8.4.2.5. The reason for the disagreement is that the results in the Geigy tables are calculated with a complex iterative method for working with Formula [8.4]. The subsequent solutions can then produce values, such as .573 or .4366, that cannot be precisely achieved with a sample of exactly 20 members.

As another example, to answer the concern posed in Section 8.4.2.6 about a failure rate of 15% in 23 patients, page 103 of the Geigy tables shows that the 95% "Confidence limits for Np" extend from 0 to 8 persons if the true proportion is .15 in a group of 23 persons. Consequently, the observed failure of only 1 in 23 persons is within the 95% confidence interval for a .15 rate of failure.

The main point of this subsection is simply to let you know that appropriate tables exist for diverse attributes of binomial distributions. If you later find yourself in situations where the tables can be helpful, you can then learn the pertinent operational details and interpretations.

8.5   Mental and "No Events" Short-Cut Approximations

Two simple techniques are available as "screening" or short-cut methods for approximating the confidence interval of certain proportions. One technique can often be done mentally, without a calculator; the other offers a simple rule for the confidence interval around a proportion of 0, in circumstances where no events have been observed.

8.5.1   Mental Approximation

The standard deviation, $\sqrt{pq}$, is close to .5 for a wide span of proportions ranging from .3 to .7. For example, if $p = .4$, $pq = (.4)(.6) = .24$ and $\sqrt{pq} = .49$. If $p = .7$, $pq = .21$ and $\sqrt{pq} = .46$. For a 95% confidence interval, $Z_\alpha = 1.96$ can be approximated as 2. Consequently, in the span of proportions from .3 to .7, $Z_\alpha \sqrt{pq}$ can be approximated as $\sim(2)(.5) = 1$. Therefore, the confidence interval component $Z_\alpha \sqrt{pq/n}$ can be approximated as $\sqrt{1/n}$.

By estimating the square root of $1/n$ mentally, you can promptly get a good idea of the scope of the confidence interval component. If you feel insecure about this mental feat, bear in mind that when $n = 25$, $\sqrt{1/n} = 1/5 = .2$. When $n = 100$, $\sqrt{1/100} = .1$. Thus, for group sizes between 25 and 100, the confidence interval component will lie between .2 and .1. With this tactic, you can promptly get a reasonably good estimate of the confidence interval for any proportions ranging between .3 and .7. [For p or q = .2 or .8, $\sqrt{pq}$ = .4; and for p or q = .1 or .9, $\sqrt{pq}$ = .3. The corresponding estimates for the latter proportions will be 80% and 60%, respectively, of the foregoing results for $\sqrt{pq}$ ~.5.]

Examples: Suppose the observed proportion is 42/76 = .55. As 76 is close to 81, let $\sqrt{1/n}$ = 1/9 = .11. The approximate 95% confidence interval, calculated mentally becomes .55 ± .11 and goes from .44 to .66. The actual calculation for standard error here is $\sqrt{(42)(34)/76^3}$ = .057 and the actual $Z_\alpha \sqrt{pq/n}$ value is (1.96)(.057) = .11. If the observed proportion is 8/65 = .12, use $\sqrt{64}$ = 8, and 1/8 = .125, then multiply by .60 to get .075 as the approximate value. Its calculated result will be 1.96 $\sqrt{(8)(57)/65^3}$ = .080.

8.5.2 "Rumke's Rule" for "No Events"

If no adverse events occur in a clinical trial, the investigators may want assurance about the likelihood that no such events will occur in the future. At a scientific level, the assurance will depend on the types of future patients, dosage, and additional treatments. At a purely statistical level, however, numerical calculations are possible.

For example, suppose no side effects were observed in 40 patients. If the true rate of side effects is .01, the observed event has a chance probability of $(.99)^{40}$ = .67. If the true rate is .04, the probability is $(.96)^{40}$ = .20. For a rate of .07, the probability is $(.93)^{40}$ = .055; and for a rate of .08, the probability is $(.92)^{40}$ = .036. Thus, because .05 lies between the latter two probabilities, a one-sided 95% confidence interval could be estimated that the true rate is as high as something between 7% and 8%.

The calculations can be greatly simplified by a "rule of thumb" proposed by C. L. Rumke.[3] In Rumke's rule, if "nothing" has been observed in n patients, the one-sided upper 95% confidence limit is 3/n. Thus, for 40 patients, 3/40 = .075 = 7.5%. In a trial with 120 patients, the corresponding result is 3/120 = .025 = 2.5%. [To check this, note that $(.975)^{120}$ = .048, consistent with a 95% confidence interval.]

The formulas in Rumke's rule are changed to 4.61/n for a 99% confidence interval and 5.30/n for a 99.5% confidence interval.

8.6 "Continuity" and Other Corrections for Mathematical Formulas

For a binary proportion expressed as p = r/n, the commonly used Gaussian confidence interval is called a Wald-type interval, calculated with Formula [8.2] as

$$p \pm Z_\alpha \sqrt{pq/n}$$

where Z_α is chosen from a Gaussian distribution to provide a 100 $(1 - \alpha)$ percent level for the interval.

8.6.1 Customary "Continuity Correction"

Aside from the problems already noted in Section 8.4.2.4, this formula is inappropriate because a Gaussian curve is continuous, whereas a distribution of binomial proportions has the discrete "noncontinuous" values shown in Tables 8.1 through 8.4. The customary solution recommended for this problem is an incremental "continuity correction," $1/(2n)$, that reduces the size of Z and expands the width of the confidence interval. Thus, the critical ratio noted in Formula [8.3] would be corrected to

$$Z = \frac{|p - \pi| - (1/2n)}{\sqrt{\dfrac{pq}{n}}} \qquad [8.5]$$

The confidence interval around p would extend from

$$p - Z_\alpha \sqrt{pq/n} - (1/2n) \text{ to } p + Z_\alpha \sqrt{pq/n} + (1/2n) \qquad [8.6]$$

and the net effect is to widen the confidence interval by twice the value of 1/2n.

If we applied this correction factor to the proportion observed earlier as .6 in a group of 5 members. The 95% confidence interval would be

$$.60 \pm \left[(1.96) \sqrt{\frac{(.60)(.40)}{5}} + \frac{1}{10} \right] =$$
$$.60 \pm [.429 + .100] = .60 \pm .529$$

and would go from .071 to the impossible value of 1.129. [Without the correction, the interval would have been .60 ± .429, and would go from .171 to 1.029.]

Like many parametric "corrections" and "estimations," this one works better "on average" than in isolated individual instances. For example, in Section 8.4.2.5, the Bernouilli 95% confidence interval around the proportion 4/20 = .20 went from .05 to .35. The Gaussian interval was larger, going from .025 to .375. With the continuity correction, the Gaussian interval would become even larger and more disparate from the true result. On the other hand, an argument can be offered that the "true" result cited here is not strictly accurate. If you add the relative frequencies for the zone of proportions from .05 to .35 in Table 8.4, they occupy .9561 of the data, so that they slightly exceed a 95% confidence interval. If the Gaussian 95% interval of .025 to .375 is enlarged, things will be even less accurate.

Like many other "corrections," the customary continuity correction has relatively little effect at large sample sizes, where 1/2n becomes very small; but at small sample sizes, if accuracy is really important, the exact Bernouilli method is the "gold standard." Thus, the continuity correction is mentioned here mainly so you will have heard of it. You need not use it in any of the "homework" exercises, but you may sometimes meet it in the medical literature.

8.6.2 Other Corrections and Appraisals

In a modified continuity correction, proposed by Blyth and Still,[4] the $\sqrt{n}$ factor in the denominator of Formula [8.6] is replaced by a smaller term, which enlarges the size of the interval. Another modification, lauded in a thorough review by Vollset,[5] is a continuity-corrected "score interval," which involves "an approximation using the limit estimate instead of the point estimate in the standard error."

After carefully considering 13 mathematical methods for calculating the confidence interval of a binary (or "binomial") proportion, Vollset "strongly discouraged" both the usually recommended Gaussian formula and the customary continuity-corrected version. He concluded that the upper and lower limits are best obtained with an exact Clopper-Pearson computation, as demonstrated earlier in Section 8.4.2.5 and Table 8.4. Among mathematical formulas, Vollset preferred the continuity-corrected score interval and said that a formula for "Pratt's approximation" comes quite close to the Clopper-Pearson results and is easier to calculate.

8.7 Interpretation of Stability

In Chapter 7, the stability of a central index was evaluated in two ways. In one way, the coefficient of stability was checked as a ratio of the standard error divided by the central index. The other way relied on avoiding or including an extrinsic boundary value such as >50% in an election poll.

8.7.1 Impact of Directional Variations

The coefficient of stability is easy to determine for dimensional data as $(s/\sqrt{n})/\overline{X}$ because the central index has a unique, single value. With binary proportions, however, the central index is ambiguous: it can be either p or q; and the coefficient of stability can be dramatically different according to which value, p or q, is used as the reference.

With the standard error cited as $\sqrt{pq/n}$, the coefficient of stability will depend on whether it is referred to p or q. It will be $\sqrt{pq/n}/p = \sqrt{q/p}/\sqrt{n} = \sqrt{q/np} = \sqrt{q/r}$ if referred to p, and $\sqrt{pq/n}/q = \sqrt{p/nq} = \sqrt{p/(n-r)}$ if referred to q.

For example, the Gaussian standard error of $2/7 = .2857$ is $\sqrt{(2/7)(5/7)/7} = .1707$. The coefficient of stability will be $.1707/.2857 = .598$ if referred to p and $.1707/.7143 = .239$ if referred to q. An alternative way of getting these same results is with the $\sqrt{q/r}$ formula as $\sqrt{.7143/2} = .598$ and with $\sqrt{p/(n-r)}$ as $\sqrt{.2857/5} = .239$. With either coefficient of stability, the proportion 2/7 is highly unstable, but the existence of two possible values can be disconcerting.

[One way of trying to get around the problem is to use the geometric mean, $\sqrt{pq}$, of the two values for p and q. With $\sqrt{pq}$ as the denominator, the ratio for the coefficient of stability becomes $\sqrt{pq/n}/\sqrt{pq} = \sqrt{1/n}$, which is the same value used in Section 8.5.1 for mentally approximating the scope of a 95% confidence interval for proportions ranging from .3 to .7.]

8.7.2   Impact on Small Proportions

Ambiguous results for the coefficient of stability can create big problems for small proportions. A *small* proportion can be defined, according to many beliefs, as having a value below .1. You may want to set its upper boundary, however, at a smaller level such as .05. Most people would agree that .01 is a small proportion, and agreement would probably be unanimous if the level were set at .001.

To illustrate the problems of small proportions, suppose we evaluate the stability of the fatality proportion $4/100 = .04$. The Gaussian standard error for this proportion is $\sqrt{(.04)(.96)/100} = .0204$. When referred to $q = .96$, the coefficient of stability is $.0204/.96 = .021$ — a relatively small value. When referred to $p = .04$, however, the analogous result is $.0204/.04 = .5103$, which is 24 times larger.

Furthermore, if one of the four fatalities is removed by the jackknife procedure, the reduced proportion will be $3/99 = .0303$, which is a proportionate drop of $(.04 - .0303)/.04 = .24$, or almost 25% of the original value. This drastic change would occur, however, in only 4 of the 100 jackknife-reduced proportions. In the other 96 instances, the reduced proportion will be $4/99 = .0404$, which is only slightly altered from the original value of .04. Nevertheless, the potential for getting a drastically altered result might be too distressing to make us want to rely on the stability of 4/100. If the observed proportion has a value such as 2/1000, the potential instability of the reduced proportion would be even greater, although its probability of occurrence is even smaller.

8.7.3   Effect of Small Numerators

The impact of potentially drastic changes is responsible for the statistical doctrine that the trustworthiness of data for proportions (or rates) depends on the size of the *numerators*. If the numerators are small, as in 4/100, the results will be relatively unstable. The same proportion of .04, however, would be more stable if obtained from 40/1000 or from 400/10,000.

To illustrate the problem, suppose we arrange so that the smaller value of r or $n - r$ is used as r. The cited proportion (as is common in death rates) will be $p = r/n$. The coefficient of stability for p will be the formula demonstrated earlier (Section 8.7.1) as $\sqrt{q/r} = \sqrt{[(n-r)/n]/r}$. If $n - r$ is substantially larger than r, the factor $\sqrt{(n-r)/n}$ will be close to 1. The coefficient will then be essentially $1/\sqrt{r}$. Thus, if $r = 5$, the coefficient will be approximately $1/\sqrt{5} = 0.45$, which greatly exceeds the boundary of .05 for stability. A coefficient less than the .05 boundary will be achieved only if r exceeds 400, because $1/\sqrt{400} = .05$.

With the jackknife procedure, the main threat of instability occurs when the reduced value is $(r-1)/(n-1)$. In this instance, the proportionate change from the original value will be $[(r/n) - (r-1)/(n-1)]/[r/n] = [q/(n-1)]/[r/n]$. If n is large, $(n-1)/n$ approximates 1, and so the proportionate change will be essentially q/r. The q/r formula immediately shows the potential for a very large change if a small proportion, i.e., $p < .1$, also has a small numerator. For example, the potential for an almost 25% change in the 4/100 proportion can be determined rapidly as $.96/4 = .24$. If the proportion .04 came from 40/1000, however, the extreme jackknife instability would be only $.96/40 = .024$. On the other hand, with Gaussian calculations the standard error for 40/1000 would be $\sqrt{(.04)(.96)/1000} = .006197$, and its coefficient of stability will be the "unstable" value of $.006197/.04 = .155$. If the .04 came from 400/10,000, the standard error would be .00196 and the coefficient would be "stable," at a value of .049.

For this reason, calculations of sample size and subsequent determinations of stability will be strongly affected by the number of "events" that become the numerator value of r in the smaller complement of binary proportions.

8.7.4 Events-per-Variable Ratio

The instability produced by small numerators is worth remembering in statistical methods that use multivariable analysis. You become confronted with those problems when medical journals contain results published for binary data (such as survival rates) that were analyzed with such multivariable methods as logistic regression or proportional hazards (Cox) regression. Although you may not yet know how the latter methods work, you can already use the "small numerator" principle to evaluate the stability of the claimed results. If the multivariable procedure contains k variables and e events in the outcome variable, such as deaths, the ratio of e/k is called the *event-per-variable (epv) ratio*. Harrell et al.[6] have proposed, and Peduzzi et al.[7] have empirically demonstrated, that the analytic results are unstable if this ratio is ≤ 10.

Many published multivariable results contain an elaborate array of statistical statements, but give no attention to the importance of the epv ratio.[8] Thus, without knowing anything formal about multivariable procedures, you can easily look at the data, determine the values of k and e, and mentally calculate *epv* as e/k. If the result is too small, be skeptical of the authors' claims. (When you determine e, remember that it is the smaller of the two types of binary events. Thus, in a study of 4 predictor variables for 180 survivors in a total of 210 patients, $e = 210 - 180 = 30$ deaths, and $epv = 30/4 = 7.5$.)

8.8 Calculations of Sample Size

When sample size is calculated for a single group, the goal is to get a result having a specified zone of error, or tolerance. The easiest (and conventional) approach is to use the Gaussian technique cited here in Formula [8.2]. The calculated size of the sample should allow suitable confidence about the estimated value of π.

8.8.1 Political Polls

In political polls, the candidate's manager wants to spend the least amount of money that will yield a confident result. The required steps are to estimate the apparent value of p, choose a magnitude of tolerance, select a level of confidence, and apply the formula for $Z_\alpha \sqrt{pq/n}$. For example, suppose the manager, estimating that her candidate will receive 60% of the popular vote, wants 95% confidence (or assurance) that the actual vote is not below 51%. In this instance, the value of

$$.60 \pm 1.96 \sqrt{(.60)(.40)/n}$$

must not go below .51. The calculation would be

$$.60 - 1.96 \sqrt{(.60)(.40)/n} \geq .51$$

which becomes

$$(.60 - .51)/1.96 \geq \sqrt{(.60)(.40)/n}$$

After all the algebra is developed, and both sides are squared, this becomes

$$.0021085 \geq .24/n$$

and the result is

$$n \geq 114$$

The random sample for the poll should contain at least 114 persons.

8.8.2   General Formula

The general formula for sample size of a single group can be developed as follows: If $\hat{p}$ is the estimated proportion, with b as the lowest acceptable boundary and $1 - \alpha$ as the desired level of confidence, the formula will be

$$(\hat{p} - b)/Z_\alpha \geq \sqrt{\hat{p}\hat{q}/n}$$

The desired sample size is

$$n \geq \hat{p}\hat{q}\left(\frac{Z_\alpha}{\hat{p} - b}\right)^2 \qquad\qquad [8.7]$$

Formula [8.7] shows that n will increase for larger levels of confidence (where Z_α increases), and for smaller increments between the estimated $\hat{p}$ and the boundary it must exceed.

For example, suppose the candidate's apparent proportion of support was 53% rather than 60%. If the manager were content with a 90% confidence interval and 50.5% as the lower boundary of tolerance, the required sample size would be

$$n \geq (.53)(.47)\left(\frac{1.645}{.53 - .505}\right)^2 \sim 1079.$$

The calculations are sometimes simplified by assuming that $p = q = .5$, choosing a level of Z_α, and letting $Z_\alpha \sqrt{pq/n}$ be designated as a "margin of error." With this approach, if e is the margin of error, we want

$$Z_\alpha\sqrt{\frac{pq}{n}} \leq e$$

and so

$$n \geq \frac{pq\, Z_\alpha^2}{e^2} \qquad\qquad [8.8]$$

For a 95% confidence interval and a 2% margin of error, the sample size will be

$$n \geq \frac{(.5)(.5)(1.96)^2}{(.02)^2} \sim 2401.$$

These results help show why getting accurate political polls can be a costly activity. The formulas also show why a "tight race," with small values of $\hat{p} - b$, can be particularly expensive for accuracy in polling.

8.8.3 Sample Sizes in Medical Research

Medical investigators frequently ask statistical consultants for help in determining a suitable sample size. The calculations for comparing two groups will be discussed later. If only one group is being considered, however, the consultant trying to apply the foregoing formulas will have to know the estimated value of p, the desired boundary of b, and the level of α. A value of e could be used for margin of error instead of b.

When probing to get these values, the consultant is often frustrated by the investigator's inability (or unwillingness) to state them. The discourse sometimes resembles history taking from a patient who does not state a chief complaint or account of the present illness.

"What do you anticipate as the expected proportion?" asks the consultant.

"If I knew what it was, I wouldn't be doing the research," is the reply.

"What tolerance or margin of error do you want?"

"Whatever seems right."

"What level of confidence would you like?"

"That's your job."

"I can't determine a sample size unless you give me the necessary information."

"But I was told to consult a statistician. You're supposed to let me know what the sample size should be."

Eventually, if suitably pressed, the statistician will conjure up some guesses, plug them into the formula, and calculate a result. The investigator, having abandoned a primary role in stipulating the basic quantities, then happily departs after receiving all the guesswork as an exact number for the desired sample size.

8.8.4 Sample Size for Dimensional Data

If the data are dimensional rather than binary, the sample-size job is even harder. An estimated value of p for binary data can immediately be used to get the variance as pq, but with an estimated value of $\overline{X}$ for the mean of dimensional data, an additional separate estimate is needed for the variance, s^2. The calculation may require four rather than three previous decisions: for estimates of $\overline{X}$ and s, and for levels of α and b. The formula will be

$$n \geq s^2 \left(\frac{Z_\alpha}{\overline{X} - b} \right)^2 \tag{8.9}$$

If e is used as the margin of error for $\overline{X} - b$, only three decisions are needed in the formula

$$n \geq \left(\frac{sZ_\alpha}{e} \right)^2.$$

For example, suppose we expect a mean of 30 with a standard deviation of 6. We want a 95% confidence interval within a margin of 2. The sample size will be

$$n \geq \left(\frac{6 \times 1.96}{2} \right)^2 = 34.6$$

8.8.5   Checks on Calculations

To be sure the calculations are correct, it is helpful to try them in reverse and see what happens. In the research just described, suppose the investigator finds a mean of 30 and a standard deviation of 6 in 35 patients. The standard error of the mean will be $6/\sqrt{35} = 1.01$. A 95% confidence interval will depend on $Z_\alpha s_{\bar{x}}$, which will be $1.96 \times 1.01 = 1.99$. The margin around the observed mean of 30 will be 30 ± 1.99 and will just be within the desired boundary of 2.

Note that the foregoing calculation was done with Z_α rather than $t_{\nu,\alpha}$. Trying to use the t statistic would have created a "double bind." We need to know the value of ν (for degrees of freedom) to choose the right value of t, but we cannot know the value of ν until we find the value of n for which the calculation is intended. To avoid this problem, the calculation can be done with Z_α. If n turns out to be small, it can be used for choosing an appropriate value of $t_{\nu,\alpha}$ and then recalculating. The calculations can then be adjusted back and forth until the level of $t_{\nu,\alpha}$ produces the desired confidence level for the calculated level of n.

8.8.6   Enlargement for "Insurance"

Because any of these sample-size calculations will yield results that "just make it" if everything turns out perfectly, a certain amount of imperfection should be expected. The calculated sample size is enlarged as "insurance" against this imperfection. The amount of the enlargement is "dealer's choice." Some investigators or consultants will arbitrarily double the calculated size; others will raise it by 50%; still others will multiply it by a factor of 1.2 (for a 20% increase).

The "bottom line" of the discussion in this section is that a precisely quantitative sample size is regularly calculated from highly imprecise estimates. To avoid disappointment afterwards, whatever emerges from the advance calculations should be suitably enlarged.

8.9   Caveats and Precautions

For reasons discussed later in Chapter 13, confidence intervals are now being increasingly demanded by medical editors; the results regularly appear in medical publications; and an entire book[9] has been devoted to the available formulas for calculating the intervals for many statistical summary indexes.

For a single group, with $p = r/n$, the formula usually recommended for a 95% confidence interval is the Wald-type Gaussian expression, $p \pm 1.96\sqrt{pq/n}$, although authors are sometimes urged to use the customary continuity-corrected modification. These "conventional" formulas will usually allow a manuscript to pass scrutiny from most statistical reviewers in biomedical literature, but as noted in Section 8.6.2, "high-powered" statisticians may disagree about the best way to calculate a binomial confidence interval.

The main point of this comment is simply to warn you that you can usually "get away with" the Gaussian formula, but sometimes a statistical reviewer may object to it. If the boundaries of the confidence interval are *really* important (rather than merely serving as publicational "window dressing"), you may want to resort to a more exact method.

A more substantive (and substantial) problem in any confidence interval, regardless of the method used for its calculation, relies on the single value of p (or q) as being the central index for a homogeneous group of data. Because biomedical groups are seldom homogeneous, a cautious evaluator will want to know the proportions found in pertinent subgroups, not a single "average" value of p that is both scientifically and "politically" incorrect because it ignores diversity. Good clinicians are not content with a rate that cites 5-year survival for a particular cancer as 60%; the clinicians want to know the rates in pertinent subgroups such as stages for the spread of the cancer. Political managers want to know the proportion of voting preferences in different demographic subgroups (according to age, sex, gender, socio-economic status, and likelihood of actually voting), not for a single monolithic average proportion for the entire sample.

Even in sports such as baseball, the team managers will make decisions based on "situational variables," rather than a player's overall average performance. In an engaging paper in a prominent statistical journal, Albert[10] discussed about 20 of the situational variables (handedness of batter and pitcher, home or away games, day or night, grass or turf, time of season, etc.) that can affect a player's batting average. Thus, for Wade Boggs, the overall 1992 batting average was .259 (= 133/514). The 95% confidence interval component for this "average" would be $1.96 \sqrt{(133)(381)/514^3} = .038$, and so the statistically expected 95% range would be from .211 to .297. Nevertheless, in different batting situations, Boggs's batting average ranged from .197 to .322.

The moral of these stories is that you can calculate confidence intervals to pay appropriate homage to the statistical ritual. If you really want to know what's happening, however, check the results not for an overall "average," but for substantively pertinent subgroups.

References

1. Clopper, 1934; 2. Lentner, 1982; 3. Rumke, 1975; 4. Blyth, 1983; 5. Vollset, 1993; 6. Harrell, 1985; 7. Peduzzi, 1995; 8. Concato, 1993; 9. Gardner, 1989; 10. Albert, 1994.

Exercises

8.1. For many years in the United States, the proportion of women medical students was about 10%. At Almamammy medical school, however, 30 persons have already been accepted for admission to the next entering class. Of those 30 persons, 12 are women. What would you do to determine whether this 40% proportion of women is likely to continue in the long run, and whether it is compatible with the old "10%" policy or a substantial departure?

8.2. According to a statement near the middle of Section 6.2, if a political "candidate is favored by 40 of 60 voters, the probability is about one in a hundred ... that the ... voting population('s) ... preference for that candidate might actually be as low as .51." Verify that statement and show your calculation.

8.3. Another statement in Section 6.2 referred to our willingness to believe "a clinician who claims three consecutive successes" for "a particular treatment (that) usually has 80% failure." What would you do to decide whether this claim is credible? What is your conclusion?

8.4. In a clinical trial of a new pharmaceutical agent, no adverse reactions were found in 50 patients. Can the investigators confidently assume that the rate of adverse reaction is below 1/50? What evidence would you offer for your conclusion?

8.5. The state health commissioner, having a list of inhabitants of all nursing homes in your state, wants to examine their medical records to determine what proportion of the inhabitants are demented. Because the examination of records is costly, the commissioner wants to check the smallest sample that will give an accurate result within an error tolerance of 1%. When you ask about a level of confidence, the commissioner says, "Use whatever is needed to make the report acceptable."

> 8.5.1. What sample size would you choose if the commissioner also does not know the probable proportion of demented patients?
>
> 8.5.2. What size would you choose if the estimated proportion of dementia is 20%?
>
> 8.5.3. If the commissioner says funds are available to examine no more than 300 records, what would you propose?

8.6. A clinical epidemiologist wants to do a study to determine how often endometrial cancer is found at necropsy after having been undetected during life. In examining the diagnoses cited at 26,731 consecutive necropsies, he finds about 40 such undetected endometrial cancers, all of them occurring in women above age 50 with intact uteri.

He can use 40 as the numerator for a "rate of undetected cancer," but he needs an appropriate denominator for the eligible patient population. To determine the number of post-menopausal, uterus-possessing women who constitute the appropriate eligible denominator population in the necropsy group, he would prefer not to have to check these characteristics in the entire group of 26,731 people who received necropsy. He therefore decides to take a random sample that can be counted to give an accurate approximation of the number of women, above age 50, with intact uteri.

He estimates that the autopsy population contains 50% women, that 80% of the women have intact uteri, and that 70% of the women are above 50 years of age. Thus, the proportion of eligible women is estimated at $(.50)(.80)(.70) = 28\%$. The investigator wants to be able to confirm this estimated value with 95% confidence that the true value lies within 1% of the estimated result in either direction, i.e., between 27% and 29%. He calculates that 7745 people will be needed for the cited 95% confidence interval.

After checking with a statistician, however, the clinical epidemiologist learns something that reduces the sample size to 6005. What do you think was learned, and what was the appropriate calculation?

8.7. (**Optional exercise if you have time**) Using any literature at your disposal, find a published example of either logistic regression or proportional hazards (Cox) regression. [Note: Such papers appear about once a week on average in the *NEJM* or *Lancet*.] Determine the events per variable ratio and show the source of your calculation. Did the authors appear to pay any attention to this ratio?

9

Communication and Display of Univariate Data

CONTENTS

Before the statistical horizon expands from one group to two, the last topic to be discussed is the different ways in which a group's data can be communicated. A good picture is said to be worth a thousand words, but a good statistical portrait may sometimes be even more valuable, because the summary for a large group may reflect more than a thousand items of data. On the other hand, a few well chosen words (or numbers) of description can often be better than an unsatisfactory portrait.

Statistical information is communicated with tables, graphs, charts, and individual summary indexes. The rest of this chapter describes some of the "lesions" to be avoided and some useful things to consider when results are shown for *univariate data* of a single group. The catalog of visual challenges in statistical display will be augmented later after the subsequent discussion of data for two groups.

9.1 Construction of Visual Arrangements

The visual displays of tables, graphs, and charts can be made consistent and clear with some basic rules, cited in the next few sections.

9.1.1 Tables

Arranging tables creates a tricky problem because they are oriented differently from graphs. In a 2-dimensional graph, the examination usually goes in an upward diagonal direction ($\nearrow$) when the X and Y axes unfold as $\hookrightarrow$. A two-way table has the opposite direction ($\searrow$), however, as the columns and rows move rightward and down, $\swarrow$.

The cells of tables show frequency counts for the corresponding values of the data. These counts are commonly displayed for the categories of binary, ordinal, and nominal data, but dimensional data are usually shown as points in a graph. The main decisions about a table are the arrangement of orientation and sequence of categories.

9.1.1.1   *Orientation* — The difference in orientation can produce many inconsistencies, not only for two-way tables (which will be discussed later), but also for the one-way tables that display data for a single group. In general, because many readers are accustomed to comparing magnitudes in a vertical tier, a one-way table usually goes in a vertical direction as

Category	Frequency
A	21
B	82
C	38
D	67

rather than horizontally as

Category	A	B	C	D
Frequency	21	82	38	67

Editors usually prefer the horizontal arrangement, however, because it saves space.

9.1.1.2   *Sequence of Categories* — In the sequence of categories for binary variables, should **presence** precede **absence** or vice versa? For ordinal variables, should the sequence be **mild, moderate, severe** or **severe, moderate, mild**? And what should be done with nominal variables, which cannot be ranked? Should they be listed alphabetically, enabling easy identification of each category, or placed according to the magnitude of the frequency counts, allowing easy visualization of results? If frequency counts determine the orientation, should they go downward or upward in the sequence of categories?

The sequence of binary or ordinal categories within an arrangement is usually "dealer's choice." Remembering the analogous codes of **0/1** for binary data and **1, 2, 3, ...** for ordinal data, many readers prefer to see the sequence go from lower to higher "values" as

Absent		Mild
	or	Moderate
Present		Severe

rather than

Present		Severe
	or	Moderate
Absent		Mild

Either sequence is acceptable, but once chosen, it should be used consistently thereafter for all binary and ordinal variables. If the first tabulated ordinal variable is sequenced as **3, 2, 1,** all subsequent ordinal sequences should usually go the same way, not as **1, 2, 3** for some variables and **3, 2, 1** for others.

The sequencing of nominal categories depends on the purpose of the table. If it is an exhaustive presentation of details, such as the population of each of the 50 United States, the categories should be arranged alphabetically (or by region) so that individual states (or regions) can be easily identified. If the table will be used to compare frequencies among several but not a large number of categories, the sequence can be listed according to magnitude. The largest frequencies are usually shown first. Thus, the previous alphabetical arrangement would become

Category	Frequency
B	82
D	67
C	38
A	21

9.1.2 Graphs

Graphs are intended to show the individual points of the data. A one-way dimensional graph, as illustrated earlier in Figure 5.2 and here in section 9.1.2.1, is almost always oriented in a vertical direction. The main decision is how to display the scale. The conventional rules for this decision are discussed in the next few subsections.

9.1.2.1 Increments in Scale — The increments on the scale should be large enough to show the distinctions suitably. If the increments are too small, tiny distinctions will be excessively magnified into misleading comparisons. For example, the three numbers 103.1, 102.6, and 103.8 are all relatively close to one another. They might become quite distant, however, if the graph had increments of 0.1 unit, so that the separations become 5 units for the first and second numbers, and 7 units for the first and third. The left side of the vertical graph in Figure 9.1 shows the first distinction; the right side shows the second. If the graphic increments are too large, important distinctions may become trivialized. Thus, the numbers 4.3, 2.7, 1.8, and 3.1 might all seem to be in essentially the same place of the coarse graphic scale in Figure 9.2.

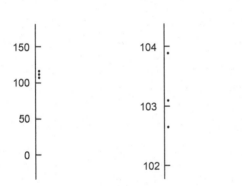

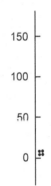

FIGURE 9.1
Excessively small (on left) and large (on right) scales for same three numbers.

FIGURE 9.2
Four numbers appearing in essentially the same location of a coarse scale.

9.1.2.2 Origin — The origin (0 point) of the scale should almost always be shown. This demand will avoid the misleading magnifications produced on the right side of Figure 9.1 when the origin was omitted and the scale ranged from 102 to 104. The 0 point can be avoided in situations where its display would be silly, as when one of the variables indicates calendar years, such as 1980, 1985, 1990, ..., or when a 0 value does not appear in the data, such as *height*.

9.1.2.3 Changes in Scale — If the points have a wide spread but several "modal" zones, the results may be bunched in an unsatisfactory way for each zone. One way to avoid this problem is to change the scale at different places in the graph. The changes should always be shown, however, with a clearly demarcated break in the identifying axis. Thus, the six points 129, 135, 140, 2051, 2059, and 2048 might appear in two ways as shown in Figure 9.3.

This same break-in-scale approach can be used whenever the data cover a wide range. To change scale in mid-graph without a clear identification of the change, however, is one of the cardinal sins of data display.

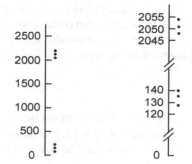

FIGURE 9.3
Crowded display on left converted to clear
display with changes in axis on right.

9.1.2.4 *Transformations of Scale* — Rather than breaking the scale for a wide range of data, the investigator can convert the results into some other continuous scale, such as the popular logarithmic transformation. For example, the six numbers of the foregoing section could easily be transformed to the base-10 logarithms of 2.11, 2.13, 2.15, 3.312, 3.314, and 3.311. The results could then be readily shown in a scale whose demarcations extend from 0 to 4.

Alternatively, the data could be plotted directly on graph paper that is calibrated in logarithmic units and that will show the same distinctions, without the need for calculating logarithmic values. In this type of scale, the value of 0 will represent 1, and the other values will be 1 (for 10), 2 (for 100), 3 (for 1000) and 4 (for 10,000).

Two important details to remember about logarithmic transformations are that they may sometimes be used merely to display data, not necessarily to analyze it, and that the logarithms are sometimes constructed with a "base" other than 10. Logarithms with base 2 can be used for showing antibody values; and "natural" logarithms, abbreviated with *ln* and constructed with e = 2.7183 as the base, are commonly used in certain types of multivariable analysis. In a graph scaled with natural logarithms, the correspondence of *ln* and original values would be 0 for 1, 1 for 2.72, 2 for 7.39, 3 for 20.1, 4 for 54.6, 5 for 148.4, etc. (This type of scale seems to have been used for values of *whole-body glucose disposal* in Figure E.19.4 of the Exercises in Chapter 19.)

9.1.3   Charts

The word *chart* can be used for any pictorial display of statistical data that does not involve the cells of a table or points of a graph. The pictogram charts that can be used to illustrate (or distort) comparisons will be further discussed in Chapter 16. Most other charts appear as bar graphs.

9.1.3.1   *Arrangement of Bars* — The frequency counts or relative frequencies of categories in a univariate group of data are often displayed in *bar charts* (also called *bar graphs*).

The bars are usually oriented vertically, showing the height of each corresponding magnitude for the category listed at the base of the bar. A histogram is a bar chart in which the horizontal categories are the ordinalized intervals of dimensional data. For example, age might be shown in intervals of **<10, 10–19, 20–29, 30–39,** etc.

In any bar chart, all the bars should have equal widths, but the basic width may vary to permit suitable labeling. For example, the bars may be narrow, as in the left of Figure 9.4, or wide as on the right.

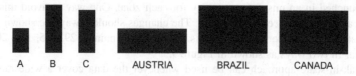

A   B   C   AUSTRIA   BRAZIL   CANADA

FIGURE 9.4
Narrow bars on left, enlarged on right to permit wider labels.

For dimensional and ordinal data, the bars can touch contiguously to represent the ranked arrangment. Thus, the bars might be shown as in Figure 9.5, but many artists and investigators prefer to leave small spaces between each bar. For unranked nominal data categories, the bars should be separated by spaces as in the foregoing **A, B, C** or **Austria, Brazil, Canada** illustrations in Figure 9.4. In a histogram, the bars always touch one another, but the bars at the two ends may be omitted if the extreme intervals are unbounded, as in the arrangement **<10, 10–19, 20–29, 30–39, 40–49, ..., 70–79, ≥80**. If the extreme intervals are bounded, with widths that differ from the equal-sized intervals in the interior, the outside intervals can have unequal widths, but the height of each bar should then be adjusted to represent the average value for the entire interval.

FIGURE 9.5

Contiguous arrangement of three ordinal categories in bar chart.

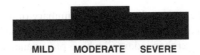

MILD   MODERATE   SEVERE

9.1.3.2 *Artistic Abuses* — Because each category has a single associated magnitude, the length of the bar is its only item of numerical communication. For this purpose, as discussed later, the bars could easily be replaced by simple lines. As an esthetic custom, however, the bars are usually made wide enough to allow suitable labels, but major distortions can be produced by esthetic manipulations done to make things look "interesting" or "pretty." For example, in certain pictograms, the bars may be replaced by drawings of persons, places, or things that have the same heights as the bars; but the different widths of the associated objects convert the visual image from a length to an area, thus creating deceptive impressions by magnifying the actual differences in size.

A particularly lamentable custom is "volumizing"—a tactic that converts the two-dimensional bar to a three-dimensional post. Since the second-dimension was needed only for labeling, the third-dimension is completely unnecessary. Its use is an act of "marketing," not scientific communication. (Examples of these abuses for contrasts of groups will be shown later in Chapter 16.)

9.1.4 Labels

Each axis of a table, graph, or bar chart must be clearly labeled or explained in each direction. The statements for the vertical magnitudes in graphs or bar charts are easier to read if presented horizontally as PROPORTIONS

rather than in vertical contiguity as

P
R
O
P
O
R
T
I
O
N
S

or in vertical re-orientation as

PROPORTIONS

The vertical labels are conventional and are usually preferred because they allegedly save space, but a well-placed horizontal label will not increase space and may actually reduce the total width of the graph or chart.

9.1.5   Legends

Each visual display — table, graph, or chart — should have a legend that describes the contents in a "stand-alone" manner, i.e., the reader should be able to understand the basic results without having to refer to the text. The legend need not repeat the details of criteria for categories such as **mild, moderate,** and **severe,** but should always indicate the name of the *variable* whose categories are being displayed.

9.2   Summary Indexes

For the reader as well as the author, the statistical summary of a group should always indicate the size of the group and the spread of data, not just the central index. The absence of the additional information for spread and size leads to "orphan indexes," whose provenance is unknown. The two main orphans in the statistical "family" are unidentified indexes of spread and groups of unknown size.

9.2.1   Nonplussed Minus

An orphan index of spread occurs when dimensional data are summarized in an expression such as 37.8 $\pm$ 1.9, without mentioning whether the 1.9 is a standard deviation or standard error. To avoid the "nonplussed minus" lesion, the entity that appears after the $\pm$ sign should always be identified as a standard error or standard deviation. A minor problem occurs when authors use the $\pm$ symbol to report "SE = $\pm$ 1.9" or "SD = $\pm$ 31.7," thus erroneously implying that the standard error or deviation (which is always positive) might be a negative number.

Arguments have been offered[1] that the $\pm$ display be abandoned and replaced by expressions such as **37.8 (SE 1.9)**, but many editors resist the proposal because it seems to involve extra spaces of type when $\pm$ **1.9** is replaced by **(SE 1.9)**. Trying to conserve space whenever possible, such as eliminating periods after abbreviations—making **mm.** become **mm** and **Dr.** become **Dr**—editors are unhappy about abbreviations that require more space. On the other hand, no ambiguity is created when **mm.** becomes **mm,** but the absence of an identifying SD or SE makes the solo **1.9** become a malcommunicated menace. If the preferred **(SE 1.9)** or **(SD 20.7)** notation is still regarded as too long, one space could be saved by eliminating the parentheses and using $\pm$ **SD 1.9**. The statement could then be **37.8 $\pm$ SD 1.9**.

9.2.2   Sizeless Group

Even if the $\pm$ entity is identified as SE or SD, however, the number of members in the group is often omitted. If SE is given, stability of the mean can readily be estimated from the coefficient of stability, as $SE/\overline{X}$. Thus, if 1.9 in the foregoing example is SE, the value of $1.9/37.8 = .05$ indicates that the mean itself is relatively stable. If SD is cited but not n, however, stability of the mean cannot be determined for the sizeless group.

On the other hand, when the mean seems stable from the $\overline{X} \pm SE$ values, a reader who does not know the size of the group cannot determine whether the "stable" mean is a suitable representative of the data. Thus, if $n = 279$ and $SE = 1.9$, the standard deviation in the foregoing data will be $1.9 \sqrt{279} = 31.7$. The coefficient of variation will be $31.7/37.8 = .84$, an excessively high value, indicating that the distribution is too eccentric (or diffuse) for the mean to be a satisfactory central index.

If not immediately adjacent to the central index and index of spread, the size of the group should always be cited somewhere in the neighboring text. A particularly important aspect of size is the "effective" number of persons contained in the analysis, not the original number in the group. For example, in a study of 279 people, the indexes of central location and spread may actually have been calculated with $n = 205$, because the variable had 72 items with unknown values. Failure to cite the "effective" rather than merely the original size of the group is a violation of "truth in advertising."

9.2.3   Unpropped Proportions

A different manifestation of the sizeless-group lesion occurs when proportions or percentages are recorded merely as a central index, such as **.37** or **37%**, without an indication of either numerator or denominator. Because the variance of binary data with the proportion p is $p(1 - p)$, the reader can immediately determine variance, but is deprived of a crucial prop of information: the group size needed to discern the stability or standard error of the proportion.

Although the denominator can always be cited in a format such as **.37 (82)**, the easiest-to-understand presentation would show both numerator and denominator as **.37 (30/82)**. This arrangement, which puts the central index first, seems preferable to the alternative arrangement, **30/82 (.37)**.

9.3   Alternative Symbols for Spread

In deciding whether to display SE or SD, the main question is: What does the reader want to know or what does the author want to show? If the goal is to determine the stability of the mean, SE is preferred, because it easily leads to the evaluation of $SE/\overline{X}$.

On the other hand, because the more common scientific goal is to communicate evidence rather than inference, the most desirable information is the spread of the data. For this purpose, the citation of $\pm$ **SD** is unsatisfactory for the several reasons noted throughout Section 5.3.2. (A spread of one standard deviation around the mean demarcates a relatively useless Gaussian inner zone of about 68%; and Gaussian descriptive summaries will be unwarranted and possibly misleading for the many sets of medical measurements that do *not* have Gaussian distributions.

For example, a Gaussian 95% zone for the data in Section 9.2.2 would be approximated as $37.8 \pm (2) (31.7) = \mathbf{37.8 \pm 63.4}$. The zone would extend to an upper level of **101.2**, but its lower level would be a negative value of **−25.6**, which might be impossible. This problem can be avoided by reporting medians and inner percentile ranges rather than means and standard deviations. The median and ipr_{95} zone for the foregoing data might be cited in symbols such as **32[2-96]** or **[2; 32; 96]**. The citation may occupy a bit more space than $\overline{X} \pm SD$, but decimal points may be saved if the original data are expressed in integer values.

Another example can come from the 56 integers that constitute the data set of Table 3.1, where $\overline{X} = 22.73$ and s (calculated with $n - 1$) is 7.69. The median in this instance falls between the 28th and 29th ranks, both of which have values of **21**. Calculated with the proportional method, the 2.5 percentile occurs at **11** and the 97.5 percentile occurs at **41**. The data set could thus be summarized with $\overline{X} \pm s$ as **22.73 ± 7.69** or with X and ipr_{95} as **21[11-41]**. The second citation actually occupies less space than the first unless you round the decimals to **22.7 ± 7.7**.

The preferred percentile method of descriptive citation will probably not come into general usage for many years, however, until the increased use of computer-intensive statistics begins to replace the parametric Gaussian paradigm.

9.4   Displays of Binary Data

A graph or chart is seldom necessary or even desirable for binary data. Nothing is gained by showing a large array of **1**'s and **0**'s (or whatever binary feature is being considered). Because the central index and spread of data are easily summarized with a single binary proportion, $p = r/n$ [or $q = (n - r)/n$], a simple citation of this proportion and its two constituent numbers will suffice to show what is happening.

9.4.1   Citations of Both p and q

In some presentations, the values of p and q are separated for individual citations such as *Success Rate* = 25% (*18/72*) and *Failure Rate* = 75% (*54/72*). The two entities are redundant because the complement of any binary proportion is readily apparent. If the success rate is 25%, the failure rate must be 100% $-25\% = 75\%$.

The only possible need for listing more than one proportion occurs when the binary central index represents a compressed summary for nominal or ordinal rather than binary data. For example, suppose we want a *single* central index to summarize the post-therapeutic state in 72 people whose results are: **improved**, 18; **no change**, 44; and **worse**, 10. The largest single value would be the proportion 61% (44/72) for the **no-change** group. If this result is regarded as too uninformative, the summary might be offered with two proportions for **improved**, 25% (= 18/72) and **worse**, 14% (= 10/72). To avoid the redundant citation of **72** in both denominators, the summary might be stated as follows: "Of 72 patients, 25% improved and 14% were worse. All others were unchanged."

Methods of displaying ordinal and nominal data are further discussed in Sections 9.5 and 9.6.

9.4.2   Comparisons of p vs. q

In certain portraits, the redundant complementary proportions are placed next to one another on a bar graph, as in Figure 9.6, which shows the percentage of rapid and slow acetylator phenotypes in each of three HIV stages (marked A,B,C). This type of display makes the two results in each stage look as though they arose from contrasted groups, rather than from a single group. All the expense and space of the picture for each stage communicates less effectively than single statements, such as Rapid Acetylator Phenotype in Stage HIV C: 55% (11/20).

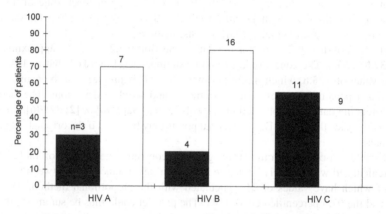

Distribution of rapid acetylator phenotypes *(solid bars)* and slow acetylator phenotypes *(open bars)* by HIV stages. Percentages are calculated for individual disease stages; absolute numbers are given on top of each *bar.*

FIGURE 9.6
Redundant bar graph showing proportions for both complementary percentages in each group. (Figure and attached legend taken from Figure 2 of Chapter Reference 2).

9.5   Displays of Nominal Data

Nominal data are particularly challenging to summarize and display. Because the data cannot be ranked, quantitative values cannot be calculated for a central index and index of spread. The only possible *single* central index is a modal or compressed binary proportion. For example, the illustrative set of nominal data in Section 9.1.1.1 had the following frequency counts for 208 persons: **A,** 21; **B,** 82; **C,** 38; **D,** 67. A single "plurality" central index could be obtained as the modal value = 82/208 = 39% for Category B. A "majority" central index could be produced by the compression of categories C and D to form the binary proportion 105/208 = 50.5%.

Visually, the frequencies or relative frequencies of nominal categories are often shown in bar charts, but the horizontal sequence of bars implies (incorrectly) that the categories are ranked. Accordingly, nominal data can be displayed in two other formats: pie graphs and dot charts.

9.5.1 Pie Graphs

The circular outline of a pie-graph can be divided into wedges that correspond to proportions of the nominal categories. If each category has the relative frequency, p_i, its angular slice is $p_i \times 360°$. For example, in the preceding data, the proportions are **A**, .10; **B**, .39; **C**, .18; and **D**, .32. The respective angles in the "pie" would be A, 36°; B, 140°; C, 65°, and D, 115°. The pie graph is usually constructed in a clockwise arrangement, starting at 12 o'clock, and the categories are usually sequenced with the largest coming first. Thus, the foregoing data would produce the pie graph shown in Figure 9.7.

An extraordinary pie graph, which may be among the worst ever constructed, is shown in Figure 9.8, for sources of income of a charity organization in the U.K.[3] The basic idea of a pie graph is abandoned because each category is given about the same angular slice, and the circular shape has been converted to a quasi-ellipse for portraying a third dimension. The extra dimension is height of the slices of pie, which act "volumetrically" to show the distinctions in magnitude.

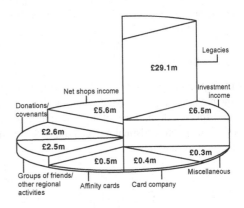

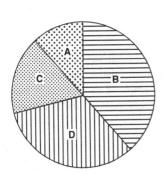

FIGURE 9.7

Pie graph for data in Section 9.5.1.

FIGURE 9.8

Pie-graph (? Edam-cheese graph) needlessly cast into three dimensions. [Figure taken from Chapter Reference 3.]

A useless pie graph is shown in Figure 9.9. Because only two categories are included, the authors are displaying both p and q for the same single binary proportion. Instead of appearing as two magnitudes in a redundant bar graph (as in Figure 9.6), however, these results are shown in a redundant pie graph.

9.5.2 Dot Charts

Pie graphs are difficult to draw, requiring a protractor or special paper for the angles, and are difficult to interpret, because most persons are not accustomed to assessing and comparing angular wedges. Although pie graphs continue to appear in published literature, the dot chart[5] is a preferred replacement that is easier to draw and interpret.

In a dot chart, the scale of values is placed horizontally and the categories are placed in rows that can be arranged in descending magnitudes or some other appropriate order (such as alphabetical). The dot chart for the data in Figure 9.7 is shown in Figure 9.10.

In addition to its other virtues, a dot chart has the advantage of easily showing magnitudes of 0, which cannot be readily displayed with bar charts or pie graphs.

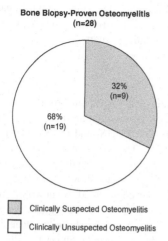

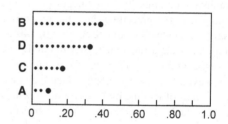

FIGURE 9.9
Redundant pie graph for "Relationship between clinical and bone biopsy diagnoses of osteomyelitis." [Figure taken from Chapter Reference 4.]

FIGURE 9.10
Dot chart corresponding to pie graph of Figure 9.7.

9.5.3 Bar Charts

Although a univariate distribution of unranked nominal categories should not be shown as a graph, the principle is regularly violated when the categories are ranked according to their relative frequencies and then displayed in the form of a bar graph or chart. Figure 9.11 shows an example of this approach, used by the American Statistical Association (ASA) to display[6] percentages for the categories of its "continuing education expenditures."

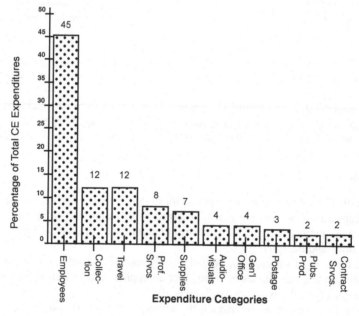

FIGURE 9.11
1992 Budgeted ASA continuing education expenditures. [Legend and figure derived from Chapter Reference 6.]

9.5.4   Hyperpropped Proportions

An opposite counterpart of unpropped proportions (in Section 9.2.3) is the hyperpropped proportions that occur when the same denominator is needlessly repeated in a tabulation of relative frequencies for categorical (nominal or ordinal) data.

For example, the relative frequencies of the nominal data in Section 9.1.1.1, can be shown in two ways as follows:

Category	Relative Frequency	Relative Frequency (N = 208)
A	21/208 (10%)	21 (10%)
B	82/208 (39%)	82 (39%)
C	38/208 (18%)	38 (18%)
D	67/208 (32%)	67 (32%)

The right-hand arrangement avoids the hyperpropping produced by the needless repetition of the "208" denominator in each row.

9.6   Displays of Ordinal Data

A central index for ordinal data can be expressed as a median or with the same plurality or compressed proportions used for nominal data. Sometimes an investigator will cite a mean value, using the ordinal

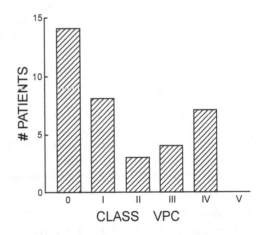

FIGURE 9.12
Bar graph of frequencies for an ordinal variable (Class of ventricular premature contractions). [Figure taken from Chapter Reference 7.]

codes of **1, 2, 3, 4,** ... as though they were dimensional data; and sometimes, particularly in clinical trials of analgesic agents, the ordinal pain scales are even expressed in standard deviations. A box plot could be used because it relies on quantiles that can be legitimately ranked, but the plot may not be particularly informative if the categorical grades have many frequencies that will be "tied" for the percentile values.

The usual display of ordinal data, therefore, is a bar chart or graph, as shown in Figure 9.12. Bar graphs can also be converted to dot charts, however, if desired for clarity. On the other hand, because the proportions of each category can easily be shown and understood in a simple one-way table, the virtues of a more formal visual display are often dubious.

9.7   Overlapping Multi-Binary Categories

A group of people may have a series of binary attributes, such as fever, chest pain, and sore throat, that are **present** or **absent** in different combinations. The proportionate *total* occurrence can easily be cited for each binary category; and a dot chart is the best way to display the individual proportions, which cannot be shown in a pie graph because they overlap, with a sum that exceeds 100%.

The investigator may also, however, want to display the spectrum of overlapping categories. Venn diagrams are excellent for this purpose. For example, Figure 9.13 shows the overlapping spectrum of different forms of new carditis in 54 recurrent episodes of rheumatic fever.[8]

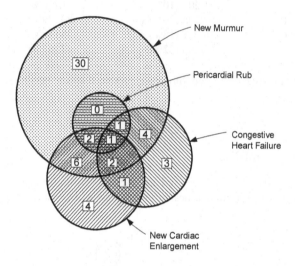

FIGURE 9.13
Incidence and types of different manifestations of new carditis in 54 recurrent episodes of rheumatic fever. [Figure taken from Chapter Reference 8.]

Sometimes the investigators (and artists) may get carried away to produce the exotic multi-binary portrait shown in Figure 9.14. For each of 232 "common congenital malformations,"[9] 17 lesions were identified as present or absent. A line was drawn between each two lesions present in the same patient. The lines get thicker as they are augmented for each identified pair. The resulting picture is probably more remarkable for its artistic imagery than for its statistical communication.

9.8   Gaussian Verbal Transformations

The fame of the Gaussian distribution has evoked efforts to display it in diverse ways. Among the most striking are "verbal transformations."

The first, shown in Figure 9.15, was prepared by the statisticican, W. J. Youden.[10] The second, shown in Figure 9.16, was done by John Hollander, a poet who is A. Bartlett Giamatti Professor of English at Yale University. Figure 9.16, which is taken from Hollander's book[11] on "Types of Shape," shows his poem for the "bell-shaped" Gaussian curve, together with additional exposition. If any of your molecular colleagues uses a new term you do not understand, you can now respond by asking what they know about *technopaignia, calligrammes,* or a *carmina figurata.* [You can act particularly superior if your colleagues say that these things are, respectively, an adverse reaction to a new imaging test, the weight gain avoided with non-metabolized sweeteners, or a stand-in for the female lead of an opera by Bizet.]

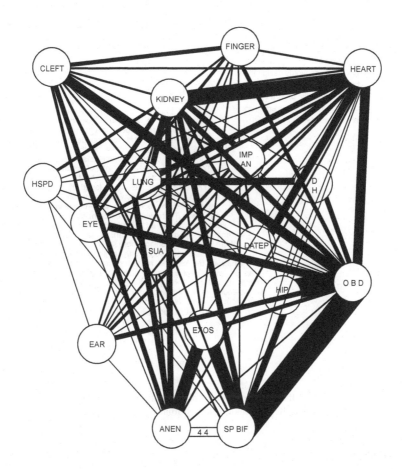

FIGURE 9.14
Interrelations of congential defects in 232 cases. HSPD: hypospadias; ANEN: anencephaly; EXOS; exomphalos; SP BIF: spina bifida; SUA: single umbilical artery; IMP AN: imperforate anus; OEATF: oesophageal atresia/tracheal fistula; DH: diaphragmatic hernia; OBD: other brain defects; etc. [Figure derived from Chapter Reference 9.]

THE
N O R M A L
LAW OF ERROR
STANDS OUT IN THE
EXPERIENCE OF MANKIND
AS ONE OF THE BROADEST
GENERALIZATIONS   OF   NATURAL
PHILOSOPHY   ◆ IT SERVES AS THE
GUIDING   INSTRUMENT   IN   RESEARCHES
IN THE PHYSICAL AND SOCIAL SCIENCES AND
IN MEDICINE AGRICULTURE   AND   ENGINEERING ◆
IT IS AN INDISPENSABLE   TOOL FOR THE ANALYSIS AND THE
INTERPRETATION   OF THE BASIC DATA OBTAINED BY OBSERVATION   AND   EXPERIMENT

FIGURE 9.15
W. J. Youden's verbal display of the Gaussian distribution. [Figure derived from Chapter Reference 10.]

"Pattern poems"; *technopaignia* (a game
of artifice); *carmina figurata*; shaped poems;
Guillaume Apollinaire's term *calligrammes*;
"figured poems"— these words designate a
kind of short poem whose inscribed or printed
format presents a schematic picture of some
familiar object that is itself the subject of some
kind of emblematic meditation by the text.

It is the
top which
seems to an
eye untorn by tears a
kind of base not from but
on which the whole sounding
body depends Up high the most
frequent the most ordinary will
bunch together there where mean
and mode unite At such a height a
tired watcher of bells might hope
for far more sound for rounder or
rarer tones O even there at the top
for bright clear fundamentals where
most normal noises are not of chiming
but of clonk and thunk But no for the
sound of ringing is only found in the
massed metal below down there where all
frequencies of bong bing and happenings
are lower There where the bronzed embrace
surrounds the heart of air the body sounder
and the deep pounding partials far more tidal
there at the widening there there the true bell
sings all ringed about with bell-shaped roundness
Whatever the pinched arch top may assert these wide
so generous depths affirm nothing and thereby never lie
Here at bell-level nearly at the lip of truth even a sigh
will resound and trembling will be a proclamation The sound
of an hour passing is that of another coming Unskewed by will
or cracked by what in fact the case may be in the surrounding
air and
all it is
ringing O
hear it
now

FIGURE 9.16
John Hollander's poetic portrait of "Bell curve: normal curve of distribution." Text on the left contains further description of this type of "emblematic meditation." [Figure and text derived from Chapter Reference 11.]

References

1. Altman, 1986; 2. Kauffman, 1996; 3. Copas, 1990; 4. Newman, 1991; 5. Singer, 1993; 6. Bailar, 1992; 7. Schulze, 1975; 8. Feinstein, 1967b; 9. Roberts, 1975; 10. Youden, 1983, p. 143; 11. Hollander, 1991, p. 10.

Exercises

The purpose of these assignments is to get you to find some things that are bad and to propose ways of improving them, and also to challenge you to create something new.

9.1. Using any published literature at your disposal, find a set of *univariate* data that has been summarized or displayed in an unsatisfactory way. (If univariate reports are difficult to find, you can use a section of a 2-way table, graph, or chart that involves two variables or two groups, but confine your comments to only one of the variables.) For each variable you choose, describe enough to indicate what is wrong and to justify your opinion. If the problem occurs in a visual display, attach a copy of the display. Please find one such example for a variable that is:

9.1.1.   Dimensional
9.1.2.   Binary
9.1.3.   Nominal
9.1.4.   Ordinal

9.2. For each problem that you describe in 9.1.1 through 9.1.4, propose the corresponding improvement or solution in Exercises 9.2.1, 9.2.2, 9.2.3, and 9.2.4.

9.3. What ideas do you have about how to improve any of the methods proposed in this chapter for summarizing and/or displaying data for a single variable? Because the need is particularly great for nominal, ordinal, or multi-binary variables, any suggestions about them will be particularly welcome.

Part II

Comparing Two Groups of Data

For almost a century, two groups of data have been compared with various "tests of statistical significance." The purpose of this part of the text is to describe those tests, but first to clarify and perhaps eliminate the confusion caused by the ambiguous meaning of *statistical significance*.

The confusion arises because the phrase *statistical significance* is usually applied to only one of the two evaluations needed for a numerical comparison. The first comparative evaluation refers to the quantitative magnitude of the observed distinction. Is a mean of 8.2 impressively larger than a mean of 6.7? Is a proportion of 25% substantially smaller than a proportion of 40%? This type of quantitative comparison evaluates what was descriptively observed in the data.

The second comparative evaluation looks at the stability of the central indexes. Are the means of 8.2 and 6.7 stable enough to be accepted as adequately representing their groups? Are the two means so fragile that their confidence intervals would have a large overlap? Do the proportions of 25% and 40% come from unstable numerical components, such as 1/4 vs. 2/5? These questions refer not to quantitative magnitudes, but to stability of the central indexes, and the comparison of stability involves stochastic inferences about what might happen if the indexes were perturbed or otherwise rearranged.

Of the two types of comparison, the quantitative decision requires *substantive* thought about the magnitudes of observed distinctions, whereas the inferential decision usually requires *mathematical* thought about stochastic probabilities and possibilities. Nevertheless, the inferential activities have been the main focus of attention during the statistical developments of the past century, and almost no emphasis has been given to intellectual mechanisms or criteria for the descriptive contrasts. With this monolithic concept, "statistical significance" has been restricted to the inferential procedures, and the descriptive evaluation has no name and no operational principles.

In statistical inference, the stability of two central indexes is usually contrasted with the t tests, chi-square tests, and other procedures that have become famous in decisions about "statistical significance." The quantitative contrast of magnitudes, however, is a different and even more fundamental statistical activity, but it is descriptive, not inferential. Lacking the mathematical panache of inference, the descriptive contrasts are hardly discussed in most textbooks and other accounts of statistical reasoning. *Descriptive* decisions about *quantitative* significance, however, are constantly made by investigators, reviewers, readers, and policy makers. As a former medical student, Gertrude Stein, once said, "A difference must make a difference to be a difference." A quantitative comparison may not be worthy of serious attention if the component numbers are too unstable to be statistically significant, but the real significance or importance of a comparative difference depends on the magnitude of what it shows and implies, not on its P value, confidence interval, or other calculation in a mathematical test of inference.

Several other crucial issues are also involved in making decisions about significance. As noted in Chapter 1, these issues are substantive—not an inherent part of the *statistical* reasoning. They refer to the architectural structure of the comparison and the quality of the raw data and processed data. Although paramount constituents of credibility for the data and the comparison, these substantive scientific issues are beyond the scope of discussion in the next eight chapters, which are concerned with exclusively statistical aspects of comparison.

The first topic will cover the methods of evaluating a quantitative contrast. The subsequent chapters will discuss the principles of forming and testing stochastic hypotheses, the different procedures used for testing different types of data, the mechanisms for displaying two-group contrasts, and the special epidemiologic tactics applied for comparing rates and proportions.

10

Quantitative Contrasts:
The Magnitude of Distinctions

CONTENTS

How would you decide that the difference between the two means of 8.2 and 6.4 is "impressive" or "unimpressive"? How would you make the same decision if asked to compare the two proportions, .25 and .40?

One manifestation of the customary inattention to quantitative contrasts is the uncertainty or even discomfort you might feel if asked these questions. What things would you look at or think about? What statistical indexes might you use to do the looking or thinking? For example, suppose you agree that the distinction is quantitatively impressive between the two means 11.3 and 25.6, but not between the two means 18.7 and 19.2. What particular statistical entities did you examine to make your decision? If you were reluctant to decide without getting some additional information, what kind of information did you want?

10.1 Nomenclature for Quantitative and Stochastic Significance

Decisions about quantitative magnitude and numerical stability are different statistical activities, but they are not clearly separated in traditional nomenclature. Both decisions involve thinking about significance for the observed distinction, and two different labels are needed for these two different ideas, but the commonly used term *statistical significance* is usually applied only to the appraisal of stability. The quantitative decision has no definite name.

In customary usage, *statistical significance* implies that the distinction is numerically stable and is not likely to arise from the random effects of chance variation. When someone wants to refer to an impressive magnitude, however, a specific title is not available for the quantitative distinction. It is sometimes given such labels as *clinical significance*, *biologic impressiveness*, or *substantive importance*. Lacking specific titles for the different decisions that distinguish quantitative contrasts from numerical stabilities, the two ideas become obfuscated and confused when the term *statistical significance* is restricted to only one of them. To escape the profound problems of this unsatisfactory nomenclature, the term *statistical significance* will generally be avoided hereafter in this text.

The term *quantitative significance* will refer to the magnitude of an impressive or important quantitative distinction. The term *stochastic significance* will denote the role of chance probabilities in the numerical stability of the observed distinction. [The word *stochastic*, which is easier to say than the alternative word, *probabilistic*, refers to random processes and comes from the Greek *stochastikos*, which means "proceeding by guesswork or conjecture in aiming at a target." Besides, not all stochastic appraisals involve a consideration of probabilities.]

The rest of this chapter is devoted to principles of *quantitative* significance in a contrast of two groups. The stochastic strategies for evaluating a two-group contrast are discussed in Chapters 11–16.

10.2 Context of Quantitative Decisions

Quantitative decisions always have two components. One of them is the magnitude of the observed distinction, such as the contrast of 11.3 vs. 25.6, or 19.2 vs. 18.7. The other component is the clinical, biologic, or other substantive context of the comparison. This context is responsible for such labels as *clinical significance*, *biologic impressiveness*, or *substantive importance* to describe a sufficiently large distinction.

For example, suppose .06 and .09 are the proportions of young patients who develop an adverse event after each of two treatments. If the adverse event is a transient, symptomless skin rash, the quantitative distinction will seem unimpressive. If the adverse event is permanent sterility, however, the same distinction will be important. In a different context, suppose the rate of occurrence for a rare but dreadful disease is .000004 after exposure to Agent A and .000003 in the unexposed general population. The incremental difference of .000001 in the two rates, or the ratio of $.000004/.000003 = 1.33$, may not seem impressive; but a nation that contains 50,000,000 people, half of whom are exposed to the agent, will have 25 (= 100 − 75) extra cases of the disease. As another example, an incremental rise of .0025 or

0.25% may seem like a trivial change in a proportion, but the change can have a major impact on the stock market if it represents an elevation in the Federal Reserve Board's prime lending rate.

Another issue in quantitative comparison is the variability of the measurement process. Suppose a patient's hematocrit rises from 10.2 to 10.4 after a blood transfusion, or suppose the diastolic blood pressure falls from 97 to 94 mm Hg after a particular treatment. Should these changes be ascribed to the effects of therapy, or could variations of 0.2 in hematocrit and 3 mm Hg in diastolic pressure occur simply as ordinary fluctuations in either the method of measurement or the patient's biologic state?

For all these reasons, quantitative contrasts must always be suitably considered within the context in which they occur. These contexts can include the severity of the observed phenomenon, the method of measurement, the immediately associated clinical or biologic factors, and the external social, regional, or national implications. These contextual features are always a crucial component of the total judgment used for decisions about quantitative significance in groups of people. The context may be less crucial if the compared phenomena refer to events in rodents or in inanimate systems. Even for nonhuman phenomena, however, the decisions may also be affected by important contextual features. An improvement of success rate from 90% to 95% may not seem immediately impressive, but may make the world beat a path to your door if you have built a better mousetrap (or a better computer mouse).

Aside from context, however, the other vital component of quantitative decisions is the numerical magnitude itself. Although the final judgment about quantitative significance will come from simultaneous consideration of both the numerical and contextual components, the numerical magnitude alone may sometimes suffice. For example, if a particular agent is suspected of causing a significant change in the potassium or calcium concentration of a rat's serum, we need not worry (at this point in the research) about the human clinical or populational implications of the change. We do need a way to decide, however, how much of a difference in the potassium or calcium level will be regarded as a "significant change."

Thus, although quantitative decisions are sometimes made without a concomitant evaluation of context, they always require an appraisal of magnitudes. The rest of this chapter is concerned with the principles that can be used for those appraisals.

10.3 Simple Indexes of Quantitative Contrast

When two groups are descriptively compared, their central indexes are converted into indexes of quantitative contrast.

(The magnitudes found in these contrasts are sometimes called *effect size*, a term that has two unattractive features. First, the entities being compared may be baseline states, such as age or weight, rather than the "effects" of an intervention, such as treatment. Second, many statisticians reserve *size* for the number of members in a group, e.g., "sample size.")

At least two simple indexes of contrast can be created immediately — a direct increment and a ratio — and the emerging results can have at least four different values.

10.3.1 Methods of Simple Expression

The four values for the simple indexes of contrast can come from two methods of calculation, each performed in two possible ways.

10.3.1.1 Direct Increments — A direct increment is the subtracted difference between the two values under comparison. If A and B represent the central indexes for Groups A and B, the direct increment can be calculated as $A - B$, or as $B - A$. For the two sets of means, 11.3 vs. 25.6 and 19.2 vs. 18.7, the respective increments are 14.3 units (= 25.6 −11.3) and 0.5 units (= 19.2 −18.7). Because the order of subtraction could have been reversed, these same values could have been expressed alternatively as −14.3 and −0.5. If $A - B$ yields a positive *increment*, the negative result of $B - A$ could be called a *decrement.* To avoid two words for this difference, the term *direct increment* will be used hereafter to represent either the positive or negative result of a subtraction.

10.3.1.2   Ratios — If the two central indexes are divided as *A/B* or as *B/A*, the index of contrast is called a *ratio.* For the two pairs of means under discussion, the respective ratios would be 0.44 (= 11.3/25.6) and 1.03 (= 19.2/18.7) if calculated as *A/B*, and 2.27 and 0.97 if calculated as *B/A*.

10.3.2   Orientation of Comparison

The four possible simple indexes of contrast for two central indexes, A and B, can promptly be reduced to two, if one of the two groups is used as a "reference" to orient the direction of the calculations. For example, if B represents the result of a control or placebo therapy, and if A represents an active treatment, the respective increment and ratio would be *A − B* and *A/B*. This same arrangement would also provide the desired indexes of contrast if *A* represents the observed value for a group and if *B* represents the expected value, or if *A* and *B* are the values *after* and *before* a particular treatment.

Because a reference group can be determined or inferred for almost any comparison of two groups, the decision about orientation is seldom difficult. If we assume that B is the basic or "control" group, B always becomes the subtractor or divisor. With this orientation, the choice of the appropriate simple index can be reduced to two candidates: *A − B* or *A/B*.

If a reference group is not obvious, as in a comparison of two standard active treatments, readers should remember that data analysts will usually choose a presentation that puts a "best foot forward" for the results. Thus, if the central indexes are 24.8 for Treatment C and 12.7 for Treatment D, the investigator may decide that a ratio of 1.95 for C/D is more "impressive" than the corresponding .51 for D/C. Both presentations are legitimate and honest, but their results seem quite different if inspected without further thought.

10.3.3   Customary Scientific Evaluations

If you had your first exposure to science in activities of physics or chemistry, you may recall that quantitative importance was often shown by the slope of a line on a graph. The effect of substance X on substance Y usually appeared in a plot of points such as in Figure 10.1. The larger the slope of the line that fit those points, the greater is the impact of X on Y.

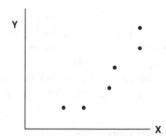

FIGURE 10.1
Impact of X and Y determined by
slope of bivariate curve.

If this principle is used to compare dimensional data for two groups, the two "one-way graphs" of points (recall Section 5.7.1) can be placed on a single graph if we regard the results as values of Y for an X-variable coded as 0 for group B and 1 for group A. Such a plot is shown in Figure 10.2. If a straight line is fitted to the two sets of points (by methods demonstrated later in Chapter 19), it will connect the two means, $\overline{Y}_A$ and $\overline{Y}_B$. With the 0/1 codes used for the X variable, the value of $\overline{X}_A - \overline{X}_B$ will be 1. The slope of the line will be $(\overline{Y}_A - \overline{Y}_B)/(\overline{X}_A - \overline{X}_B) = (\overline{Y}_A - \overline{Y}_B)/1$. Thus, the increment of two means, $\overline{Y}_A - \overline{Y}_B$, corresponds to the slope of the line connecting the two groups of data.

The same principle holds true for a comparison of two proportions, p_A and p_B. Their increment corresponds to the slope of the line connecting them. The individual values of 0 and 1 that are the constituents

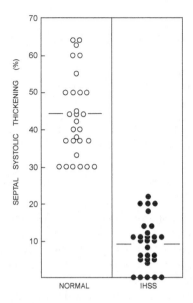

FIGURE 10.2

One-way graphs comparing two groups. Ordinates (Y-axis) show points of dimensional data for septal systolic thickening as percentage of diastolic thickness in two groups of 29 members each. The groups are "normal" on the left, and have idiopathic hypertrophic subaortic stenosis (IHSS) on the right. Horizontal line shows mean value for each set of points of the Y-axis. If the groups are respectively coded as **0** and **1** on the X-axis, the slope of the line joining the two means will be their increment. With the IHSS group coded as **1**, the slope will be an increment of about 10 − 43 = −33. [Figure taken from Chapter Reference 1.]

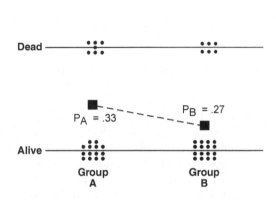

FIGURE 10.3

Binary points for two groups summarized in two proportions, p_A and p_B, and connecting line whose slope is the increment $p_A - p_B$. The proportions are $p_A = 7/21 = .33$ and $p_B = 6/22 = .27$.

of each proportion are shown as clusters of points in Figure 10.3. The proportions themselves are the "means" of each group, and the slope of the line that connects those means is the increment, $p_A - p_B$.

As the "natural" index of scientific comparison for two groups, the increment always takes precedence over the ratio, which is a mathematical artifact. The ratio was developed to help evaluate additional features of increments and is also popular in epidemiologic work (as discussed in Chapter 17), because the ratio allows two groups to be compared even when fundamental data are not available to determine the desired increment. Thus, if only a single index is to be used, it should be the increment, or some appropriately modified arrangement of the increment. Nevertheless, for an enlightened comparison, we usually examine the ratio as well as the increment.

10.3.4   Role of Two Indexes

For a contrast to be evaluated effectively, both the increment and the ratio should usually be considered simultaneously. If only one is examined, the result can be misleading.

Table 10.1 contains a set of examples to illustrate this point. The increment of 10 units, shown in the first row, might seem substantial if the contrast is between values of 12 and 2, but trivial if the comparison (as in the second row) is between values of 3952 and 3942. The feature that made the same increment seem "substantial" in one instance and "trivial" in the other was the ratio. In the first case, the associated ratio was 6, and in the second case, 1.003. An increment of 10 derived from the values of 10.2 and .2 in the third row of Table 10.1 might be even more impressive, because the associated ratio is 51.

TABLE 10.1

Different Ratios Associated with Same Increment and Different Increments Associated with Same Ratio

Value of A	Value of B	Value of Increment (A − B)	Value of Ratio (A/B)
12	2	10	6
3952	3942	10	1.003
10.2	.2	10	51
40	10	30	4
4	1	3	4
.060	.015	.045	4
.000008	.000002	.000006	4

Conversely, as shown in the last four rows of Table 10.1, a ratio of 4 might seem substantial if it represents an increment from 10% to 40% for therapeutic success, but not if the increase is from 1% to 4%. Similarly, if the ratio of 4 represents the increased chance of death associated with a "risk factor," an increment of 45 per thousand (representing death rates of .015 and .060) would be much more impressive than an increment of 6 per 10 million (from .000002 to .000008).

For these reasons, the quantitative distinction of a ratio can seldom be interpreted without simultaneous knowledge of the increment, and vice versa. The need to consider two indexes, rather than one, is another reason — beyond the problem of context — why scientists have been reluctant to set specific boundaries (analogous to "P < .05") for quantitative significance. What would be required is a demarcated zone that includes simultaneous levels of values for a ratio and an increment. The boundary chosen for this zone is not likely to evoke prompt consensus; and furthermore, particularly when the data under contrast are epidemiologic rather than clinical, substantial disagreements may arise between one evaluator and another.

10.4 Distinctions in Dimensional vs. Binary Data

Two mortality rates, .21 vs. .12, can be immediately compared because the units of expression are immediately evident. They are 21 per hundred and 12 per hundred. Two medians or means, 102.3 vs. 98.4, cannot be promptly compared, however, until we know the units of measurement. If they are degrees Fahrenheit, the two central indexes would become 39.1 vs. 36.9 when expressed in degrees Celsius.

Another distinction in dimensional vs. binary data is the connotation of stability for a central index. For dimensional data, the coefficient of stability, $(s/\sqrt{n})/\overline{X}$, will have the same value for the same set of data regardless of units of measurement. In the foregoing example, $(s/\sqrt{n})/\overline{X}$ would be the same for each group whether the temperature is measured as Fahrenheit or Celsius. For the proportions (or rates) that summarize binary data, however, the coefficient of stability and the connotation of a contrast will vary according to whether the results are expressed with p or with $q = 1 - p$. Thus, the increment of .09 in the foregoing mortality rates will seem more impressive if referred to a "control" mortality rate of .21 than to the equally correct but complementary survival rate of .79.

Binary proportions also have a unique attribute, discussed later in this chapter. They can be compared with a special index, called an odds ratio, which cannot be determined for the medians or means of dimensional data.

For all these reasons, the indexes of contrast are usually expressed (and interpreted) in different ways for dimensional data and for binary data.

10.5 Indexes for Contrasting Dimensional Data

Central indexes for two groups of dimensional data are seldom compared as direct ratios; but direct increments may be difficult to interpret because of the inconsistent effects of units of measurement.

Consequently, the direct increments are often converted into special expressions that are unit-free. According to the mode of construction, the unit-free expressions are called *standardized, proportionate,* or *common proportionate increments.*

10.5.1 Standardized Increment

The *standardized increment* is often used to compare two groups in the psychosocial sciences but is undeservedly neglected in medical publications. Sometimes called the *effect size,*[2] the standardized increment is a type of Z-score formed when the direct increment in the means of two groups, $\overline{X}_A$ and $\overline{X}_B$, is divided by their common standard deviation, s_p, to produce

$$SI = \frac{\overline{X}_A - \overline{X}_B}{s_p}$$

The *standardized increment* is particularly valuable because it is a unit-free expression and it also provides for variance in the data. It therefore becomes, as noted later, a direct connection between a descriptive contrast and the value of t or Z used in stochastic testing.

10.5.1.1 *Common Standard Deviation* — Calculating a standardized increment requires use of the common standard deviation that will be discussed in greater detail later when we consider stochastic tests. The symbol s_p is used, however, because the common standard deviation is found by pooling the group variances of each group. Their sum is

$$S_{XX_A} = \sum X_i^2 - n_A \overline{X}_A^2$$

for group A, plus

$$S_{XX_B} = \sum X_i^2 - n_B \overline{X}_B^2$$

for group B. Because each group has $n_A - 1$ and $n_B - 1$ degrees of freedom, the total degrees of freedom in the two groups is $n_A - 1 + n_B - 1 = N - 2$. Thus, the common pooled variance is calculated as $(S_{XX_A} + S_{XX_B})/(N - 2)$ and the common standard deviation is the square root of this value. If standard deviations have already been found as s_A and s_B for each group, the pooled group variance can be calculated as $S_{XX_A} + S_{XX_B} = (n_A - 1) s_A^2 + (n_B - 1) s_B^2$.

For example, suppose group A has $n_A = 6$, $\overline{X}_A = 25.6$, and $s_A = 7$, whereas group B has $n_B = 5$, $\overline{X}_B = 11.3$, and $s_B = 4$. The pooled group variance is $(6-1)(7)^2 + (5-1)(4)^2 = 309$. The total degrees of freedom is $6 - 1 + 5 - 1 = 9$, and the common variance is $s_p^2 = 309/9 = 34.33$. The common standard deviation is $\sqrt{34.33} = 5.86$. The standardized increment is

$$\frac{25.6 - 11.3}{5.86} = 2.44$$

To avoid calculating a common standard deviation, some investigators use the standard deviation of the "control" group rather than s_p for the denominator. If s_B is the standard deviation of the control group and SI represents standardized increment, the formula becomes

$$SI = (\overline{X}_A - \overline{X}_B)/s_B$$

10.5.1.2 *Applications of Standardized Increment* — As a unit-free ratio that is the counterpart of a Z-score, the standardized increment is an excellent method of comparing two means. Thus, if you recall the distribution of Z-scores from Chapter 6, the value of 2.44 in the previous subsection is relatively large, suggesting an impressive increment. In the social sciences, the standardized increment is frequently used as a conventional index of effect size for comparing results in any two groups.[2] The standardized increment has also been used in combining results of different studies in a meta-analysis.[3]

Unfortunately, because the magnitude of descriptive contrasts receives so little attention in medical literature, the standardized increment seldom appears in current publications. The infrequency of its usage thus gives medical investigators little or no experience with which to develop an "intuitive" feeling about boundaries (discussed later) for impressive or unimpressive magnitudes.

10.5.2   Conversion to Complex Increment

If both a ratio and increment are to be considered, their combination might allow two groups to be contrasted with a single complex increment. The two combinations that can be constructed are the proportionate increment and the common proportionate increment. They differ in the choice of a denominator for the comparison.

10.5.2.1   *Proportionate (Percentage) Increment* — The proportionate or percentage increment shows the relative incremental change from a baseline magnitude. For two groups A and B, the calculation is either $(A - B)/B$ or $(B - A)/A$; and the resulting proportion is customarily multiplied by 100 and expressed as a percentage. [This type of reference to a baseline was used earlier when the standard deviation, as the average change from the mean of a distribution, was divided by the mean to form the coefficient of variation.]

For a contrast of the two means, 11.3 and 25.6, the proportionate increment would be either $(11.3 - 25.6)/25.6 = -56\%$ or $(25.6 - 11.3)/11.3 = 127\%$.

If B is clearly the reference value, it is the obvious choice for denominator of the proportionate increment, but if C and D are both "active" treatments, the same problem arises that was noted for the ratio at the end of Section 10.3.2. If the central indexes are 24.8 for Treatment C and 12.7 for Treatment D, the results can be reported proportionately as a rise of 95% [= $(24.8 - 12.7)/12.7$] from Treatment D, or a fall of 49% [= $(12.7 - 24.8)/24.8$] from Treatment C. The investigator can legitimately present whichever value seems more "supportive," and the reader will have to beware that alternative presentations were possible.

10.5.2.2   *Redundancy of Simple Ratio and Proportionate Increment* — Despite its possible value for certain forms of "intuitive" understanding, the proportionate increment is really a redundant expression, because it can always be converted to the simple ratio. Algebraically, the proportionate increment, $(A - B)/B = (A/B) - 1$, is simply the ratio (A/B) minus 1. Analogously, $(B - A)/A = (B/A) - 1$. Consequently, the ratio and proportionate increment do not provide distinctively different items of information. A simple ratio can immediately be converted to a proportionate increment by subtracting 1 and then, if desired, multiplying by 100 to form a percentage. Conversely, a proportionate (or percentage) increment can immediately be converted to a ratio after division by 100 and the addition of 1. Thus, a proportionate increment of -15% becomes a ratio of .85.

On the other hand, the direct increment and the standardized increment are unique expressions. They cannot be determined from either the simple ratio or the proportionate increment.

10.5.2.3   *Common Proportionate Increment* — The problem of choosing a reference denominator can be avoided if the increment of A and B is divided by the *mean* of the two values. If group sizes are unequal, with $n_A + n_B = N$, the common mean will be $(n_A A + n_B B)/N$; and the common proportionate increment will be $N(A - B)/(n_A A + n_B B)$. For the two groups in Section 10.5.1.1, the common mean is $[(6)(25.6) + (5)(11.3)]/11 = 19.1$, and the common proportionate increment is $(25.6 - 11.3)/19.1 = .75$. If the group sizes are equal, the mean of the two values will be $(A + B)/2$, and the common proportionate increment will be $(A - B)/[(A + B)/2]$.

If A is larger than B, the simple ratio will be $r = (A/B)$. Replacing A by rB, the common proportionate increment (for equal group sizes, where $n_A = n_B = N/2$) will become $2(r - 1)/(r + 1)$. It will thus include contributions from the increment and the ratio. If the two means, 25.6 and 11.3, came from groups of equal size, the common proportionate increment would be $(25.6 - 11.3)/[(25.6 + 11.3)/2] = 14.3/18.45 = .78$. Alternatively, because $r = 25.6/11.3 = 2.265$, we could calculate $(2.265 - 1)/[(2.265 + 1)/2] = 1.265/1.632 = .78$.

A major advantage of the common (or any) proportionate increment is that it is unit-free. If the central indexes are 24 months and 12 months in two equal-sized groups of children, the direct increment is 12 months. If age were expressed in years, however, the direct increment would be 1 year. The proportionate increment in the two groups, however, would be 100% $[=(24 - 12)/12]$, and the common proportionate increment would be 67% $[= (24 - 12)/18]$, regardless of whether age is measured in months or years.

The main problem with the common proportionate increment is that it is seldom used. Consequently, it is unfamiliar and has no immediately intuitive meaning. The substantive experience that provides "intuition" for most biomedical scientists has usually come from direct increments, simple ratios, and ordinary proportionate increments.

10.6   Indexes for Contrasting Two Proportions

If the compared items are means or medians, only the two individual central indexes are available to form a direct index of contrast. If the two compared items are proportions or rates, however, *nine* numbers are available. When expressed in the form of $p = a/n$, any proportion (or rate) can be decomposed into three parts: n, the number of people in the denominator; a, the number of people in the category counted for the numerator; and (n −a), the number of people who are not in that category. When suitably arranged for each group and for the total, the three component parts produce nine numbers.

For example, suppose we want to contrast the two proportions, 33% and 50%, representing the respective rates of success with Treatments A and B. Each proportion comes from a numerator and denominator for which the underlying data might be 6/18 vs. 10/20. These data can be tabulated as the nine numbers shown in Table 10.2.

TABLE 10.2

Table with Nine Numbers Derived from the Four Numbers
of Two Proportions, 6/18 vs. 10/20.

	Success	Failure	Total
Treatment A	6	12	18
Treatment B	10	10	20
Total	16	22	38

10.6.1   General Symbols

In general symbols, data showing binary proportions for two groups can be expressed as $p_1 = a/n_1$ and $p_2 = c/n_2$. These proportions can be arranged to form the classical 2×2 or "fourfold" arrangement shown in Table 10.3. The additional five numbers that become available in Table 10.3 are $b = n_1 - a$, $d = n_2 - c$, and the totals $a + c$, $b + d$, and $N = n_1 + n_2$. Furthermore, in addition to the two stated proportions, p_1 and p_2, the two complementary proportions, q_1 and q_2, are also available for comparison. For example, if the stated proportion is a success rate of 33%, its complementary proportion is a failure rate of 67%. Thus, if $p_1 = a/n_1$, $q_1 = (n_1 - a)/n_1$.

TABLE 10.3

Classical 2×2 Table Formed from $p_1 = a/n_1$ vs. $p_2 = c/n_2$

	Number of People		
	In Category of Numerator	Not in Category	Total
Group 1	a	b	n_1
Group 2	c	d	n_2
Total	a + c	b + d	N

The two proportions, p_1 and p_2, could be contrasted in the usual two approaches as a direct increment $(p_2 - p_1)$ or as a simple ratio (p_2/p_1). We could also, however, contrast the complementary proportions $q_1 - q_2$ and q_1/q_2.

10.6.2   Increments

If the index of contrast is an increment, no problems are produced by comparing the complementary proportions, because $q_2 - q_1 = 1 - p_2 - (1 - p_1) = p_1 - p_2$. The increment for $p_2 - p_1$ will therefore be identical but opposite in sign to the increment $q_2 - q_1$. For example, with success rates of 55% and 33%, the increment is 22%; with the corresponding failure rates of 45% and 67%, the increment is −22%.

The increment in two proportions is usually expressed directly but can also be cited as a standardized increment.

10.6.2.1   Direct Increment — Since $p_1 - p_2$ and $q_1 - q_2$ will have equal but opposite values, negative signs can be avoided by citing the absolute direct increment as $|p_1 - p_2|$. The positive result will represent subtraction of the smaller from the larger value of the pair.

The direct increment is clear and never deceptive, but some people have difficulty interpreting increments cited in decimal proportions such as .17 or .0064.

10.6.2.2   Number Needed for One Extra Effect — To ease the interpretation of decimal proportions, Laupacis et al.[4] proposed that the increment be inverted into a reciprocal

$$1/|p_1 - p_2|$$

which they called NNT: the number needed to be treated.

For example, if the success rate is .61 for Treatment A and .44 for placebo, the incremental advantage for Treatment A is .61 − .44. = .17, which is 17 persons per hundred. The reciprocal, which is 1/.17 = 5.9, indicates that about six persons must receive Treatment A in order for one to have an incremental benefit that exceeds what would be produced by placebo. If the increment is .27 − .25 = .02, the value of NNT is 1/.02 = 50; and 50 persons must be treated for one to be incrementally benefited.

The result of the NNT is simple, direct, easy to understand, and applicable to many comparisons of proportions or rates. The nomenclature is somewhat confusing, however, because the compared entities are not always the effects of treatment. For example, suppose Disease D occurs at rate .01 in persons exposed to a particular "risk factor" and .0036 in persons who are not exposed. The incremental difference is .0064, and its reciprocal, 1/.0064 = 156, is an excellent way of expressing the contrast. Nevertheless, the result is not a number needed to be *treated* and is sometimes called NNH—the number needed to harm. To avoid several abbreviations and labels for the same basic idea, the Laupacis index can be called NNE, the number needed for one extra effect—a term applicable for comparing treatments, exposures, or other agents.

The NNE is a particularly valuable and effective way to express the apparent benefit of the therapeutic agents tested in clinical trials, but the expression is not enthusiastically accepted by public-health epidemiologists. One reason, noted later in Chapter 17, is that the available epidemiologic data may not contain the occurrence rates needed to construct and invert the increment. Another reason, discussed later in this chapter, is the very small proportions that become cited as rates of "risk" for etiologic agents. For example, the occurrence rates of disease D may be .005 in persons exposed to a "risk factor" and .001 in persons who are nonexposed. The ratio of .005/.001 is an impressive value of 5, but the direct increment of .004 is relatively unimpressive. Since the NNE of 1/.004 = 250 indicates that 250 persons must be exposed for one to become incrementally diseased, public-health campaigns and other efforts to impugn a "risk factor" are more likely to have an impact if the results are expressed in a "scary" ratio of 5 than in a less frightening NNE of 250.

After pointing out that "perceptions change when data are presented in a way that relates therapeutic efforts to clinical yields," Naylor et al.[5] suggest that "NNTs and similar measures relating efforts to yields dampen enthusiasm for drug therapy by offering a more clinically meaningful view of treatment effects." For an additional innovative expression, the Naylor group proposes the use of TNT, which is "tons needed to treat." According to Naylor et al., about "10.3 metric tons of cholestyramine were consumed for each definite coronary death prevented in the Lipid Research Clinics Coronary Primary Prevention Trial," and "about 200,000 doses of gemfibrozil were ingested in the Helsinki Heart Study per fatal or non-fatal myocardial infarction prevented."

10.6.2.3   *Standardized Increment* — If two proportions, p_1 and p_2, are expressed as a standardized increment, the common standard deviation is much simpler to determine than for two means. We first find the common proportion, which is $P = (n_1p_1 + n_2p_2)/N$. [If the groups have equal size, so that $n_1 = n_2$, $P = (p_1 + p_2)/2$.] The variance of the common proportion is PQ, where $Q = 1 - P$. The common standard deviation is then $\sqrt{PQ}$. The standardized increment becomes

$$\frac{p_1 - p_2}{\sqrt{PQ}}$$

Because both P and Q appear in the denominator, the standardized increment will produce the same absolute magnitude, whether the contrast is between $p_1 - p_2$ or $q_1 - q_2$.

For example, suppose we compare $p_1 = 10/20 = .50$ and $p_2 = 6/18 = .33$. The common proportion P is $(10 + 6)/(20 + 18) = .42$ and so $Q = 1 - .42 = .58$. The standardized increment is

$$\frac{.50 - .33}{\sqrt{(.42)(.58)}} = \frac{.17}{.49} = .35$$

For smaller proportions, such as the previous comparison of .01 vs. .0036, the common proportion (with equal group sizes) would be $P = .0068$, with $Q = .9932$. The standardized increment would be $(.01 - .0036)/\sqrt{(.0068)(.9932)} = .078$.

The main problem with the standardized increment is that using $\sqrt{PQ}$ in the denominator converts the result into the counterpart of a ratio. If P and Q are near the meridian value of .5, the value for $\sqrt{PQ}$ is also near .5. For example, if $P = .3$, $Q = .7$ and $\sqrt{PQ} = \sqrt{.21} = .46$. If P and Q are widely depart from the meridian value, however, $\sqrt{PQ}$ becomes increasingly close to the square root of the smaller value. The following table shows what happens as P decreases:

P	Q	PQ	$\sqrt{PQ}$
.1	.9	.09	.3
.01	.99	.0099	~.1
.001	.999	.000999	.032
.0001	.9999	.0001	~.01

Consequently, a tiny incremental change of .001 from .0005 to .0015, in two groups of equal size, will have $P = .001$ [$= (.0015 + .0005)/2$] and a standardized increment of $.001/.032 = .03$, which inflates the actual value of the increment. The NNE of 1000 [$= 1/.001$] will give a much better idea of the real comparison than the standardized increment.

10.6.3   Simple and Complex Ratios

Whenever one proportion is divided by another to form a ratio, the results can be correct but ambiguous or deceptive. Some of the problems, which have already been cited, will be briefly reviewed before we turn to a new complex index, the odds ratio.

10.6.3.1   *Ambiguity in Simple Ratios* — The simple ratio of two proportions, p_1 and p_2, can be an ambiguous index because it can also be formed from the complementary proportions, q_1 and q_2, and because p_2/p_1 does not necessarily equal q_2/q_1, which is $(1 - p_2)/(1 - p_1)$. Thus, a success ratio of

58%/33% = 1.76 (and its reciprocal 1/1.76 = .57) are not the same as the corresponding failure ratio of 42%/67% = .063 (and its reciprocal of 1.60).

10.6.3.2   Ambiguity in Proportionate Increments

— The proportionate increment for two proportions, p_1 and p_2, is a ratio that has two ambiguities. The first occurs when the numerator $|p_1 - p_2|$ is divided by a denominator that can be chosen from four possibilities: p_1, p_2, q_1, and q_2. The second ambiguity is in the nomenclature that expresses the result. For the two success percentages, 49% and 33%, the proportionate increment can be $(49 - 33)/33 = 48\%$ or $(33 - 49)/49 = -33\%$. Expressed for rates of failure, rather than success, the corresponding results would be $(51 - 67)/67 = -24\%$ and $(67 - 51)/51 = 31\%$. Aside from ambiguity in numerical constituents, the expressions themselves are potentially confusing, because two percentages are contrasted, but the contrast is expressed with a quite different percentage. Thus, 49% is 16% higher than 33% as a direct increment, but is 48% higher as a proportionate increment.

10.6.3.3   Possible Deception in Proportionate Increments

— Because investigators will always want to put a "best foot forward" in reporting results and because any of the cited statistical comparisons are correct and "legitimate," the proportionate increment is frequently (and sometimes deceptively) used to "magnify" the importance of a relatively small direct increment. For example, the mortality rate in a randomized trial may be 21% with placebo and 15% with active treatment. When the results are reported in prominent medical journals (and later in the public media), however, the investigators seldom emphasize the direct increment of 6%. Instead, they usually say that the active treatment lowered the mortality rate by 29% $[= (.21 - .15)/.21]$.

Furthermore, if we examine survival rather than death, the proportionate improvement in survival rates will be $(q_2 - q_1)/q_1 = (.85 - .79)/.79 = .06/.79 = .076 = 7.6\%$. Thus, the same treatment can paradoxically seem to produce an impressive reduction in mortality while simultaneously having relatively little effect on survival.

The problem is heightened when values of p_1 and p_2 are particularly small. For example, suppose the occurrence rate of Disease D is .005 after exposure to Agent X and .001 without exposure. The actual increment is $.005 - .001 = .004$ and the NNE is $1/.004 = 250$. The investigators will seldom use these unimpressive values, however, for citing their main results. Instead, the indexes of contrast will emphasize the direct ratio of 5, or the proportionate increment of $.004/.001$, which is a 400% rise from the rate in the unexposed group.

10.6.3.4   Relative Difference

— Another available but seldom used complex ratio for contrasting two proportions is the *relative difference* proposed by Sheps.[6] If p_A is the success rate for treatment A, and p_B is the success rate for treatment B, the proportion $1 - p_B$ indicates the "failures" with B who are available to become successes with A. The incremental accomplishment of A can then be proportionately expressed as the relative difference

$$\frac{p_A - p_B}{1 - p_B}$$

For example, if the success rates are $p_A = .53$ and $p_B = .43$, the proportion of failures in B is .57. The relative difference is $.10/.57 = .175$. In public-health risk results, such as $p_A = .005$ and $p_B = .001$, the relative difference would be $.004/.999 = .004$.

The relative difference is seldom used in public health statistics because $1 - p_B$ is often close to 1, so that the result is almost the same as the direct increment. For the larger rates that occur in clinical trials, investigators usually prefer to use the direct increment (which would be .10 for the comparison of .53 vs. .43), the NNT (which would be 10), or the proportionate increment (which would be $.10/.43 = .23$).

For small rates of success increments in clinical trials, the relative difference might be preferred *scientifically* as more overtly "honest" than the proportionate increment. For example, if the mortality rate is .02 with Treatment A and .04 with Treatment B, the relative difference is $(.02 - .04)/.96 = -.021$

or −2.1%. As a proportionate increment, however, the reduction is a much more "impressive" value of $(.02 − .04)/.04 = −.50$ or −50%.

10.6.4   Problems of Interpretation

Because indexes of contrast receive so little formal attention in statistical education, it is not surprising that physicians have great difficulty interpreting published results. In a series of special studies,[7–9] physicians were frequently deceived when the same set of results was compared in different ways. Treatment A was regularly preferred over Treatment B when the comparison was reported with a ratio or proportionate increment, but not when the same result was cited with a direct increment or as a number needed to treat.

What is more surprising, perhaps, is that the authors of medical publications are allowed "to get away with" misleading (although accurate) presentations of ratios and proportionate increments, without adequately emphasizing the alternative methods of citing and interpreting the same results. When historians of science review some of the medical and public-health errors of the second half of the 20th century, an interesting point of evaluation will be the vigilance (or lack thereof) with which editors and reviewers guarded the integrity of published literature and carried out the responsibility to prevent even inadvertent deception.

The problem will probably vanish or be greatly reduced in the 21st century when "statistical significance" is decomposed into its component parts, and when quantitative contrasts begin to receive the prime attention now diverted to stochastic inference.[10–12]

10.7   The Odds Ratio

The odds ratio gets special attention here because it is unique to binary data and is commonly used for contrasting two proportions.

10.7.1   Expression of Odds and Odds Ratio

The idea of odds is a classical concept in probability. If the probability that an event will happen is p, the probability that it will not happen is q. The odds of its occurrence are p/q. For example, in a toss of a coin, the chance of getting heads is 1/2 and the chance of tails is 1/2. The odds of getting heads (or tails) are therefore $(1/2)/(1/2) = 1$ — an "even money" bet. If the chance of failure with Treatment A is 12/18, the chance of success is 6/18, and the odds in favor of failure are $(12/18)/(6/18) = (12/6) = 2$, or 2 to 1.

Note the way in which the odds were constructed. If $a + b = n$, the odds in favor of b are $(b/n)/(a/n) = b/a$. The two probabilities, b/n and a/n, have n as a common denominator, which cancels out to allow the odds to be calculated simply as b/a.

With this tactic in mind, we can now re-examine the results for each treatment in the previous Table 10.2. The odds of success are $6/12 = .5$ (or 1 to 2) for Treatment A and $10/10 = 1$ (or 1 to 1) for Treatment B. These two sets of odds produce an odds ratio of $(6/12)/(10/10) = .5/1 = .5$, which expresses the relative odds of success for Treatment A vs. Treatment B.

We also could have formed the odds ratio in another way by asking: what are the odds that a successful patient received Treatment A vs. the odds that a failure received Treatment A? This odds ratio would be expressed as $(6/10)/(12/10) = .5$, and the result would be the same as before.

10.7.2   Odds Ratio as a Cross-Product Ratio

As a general algebraic principle, a fourfold table having the cellular structure $\left\{\begin{smallmatrix} a & b \\ c & d \end{smallmatrix}\right\}$ will have the odds ratio (a/b)/(c/d) or (a/c)/(b/d). With either algebraic arrangement, the calculation becomes ad/bc. Because the two opposing diagonal terms are multiplied and the two pairs of products are then divided, the odds ratio is sometimes called the *cross-product ratio*.

10.7.3   Attractions of Odds Ratio

The odds ratio has the statistical appeal of being "independent" of the group sizes expressed in the marginal totals of a 2×2 table. As long as the inner four components of the table remain proportionally similar, within each column (or row), the odds ratio will remain the same even if the marginal totals are substantially changed.

For example, suppose the question examined in Table 10.2 was answered from a case-control study, with 48 cases drawn from the "success" group and 110 controls drawn from the "failure" group. If treatment has the same effects as before, the new fourfold table will be $\left\{ \begin{smallmatrix} 18 & 60 \\ 30 & 50 \end{smallmatrix} \right\}$. Rates of success can no longer be calculated from this table, because the persons were "sampled" from the outcome events, rather than from the "exposure" to treatment. [If calculated, the "success rates" would be .23 (= 18/78) for Treatment A and .375 (= 30/80) for Treatment B, and would be much lower than the correct corresponding values of .33 and .50.] The odds ratio, however, calculated as $(18 \times 50)/(30 \times 60) = .5$ in the new table, will be identical to the .5 result obtained in Table 10.2.

This virtue of the odds ratio also leads to its two main epidemiologic attractions. One of them occurs in a multivariable analytic procedure called *multiple logistic regression*, where the coefficients that emerge for each variable can be interpreted as odds ratios. The most common appeal of the odds ratio, however, is that its result in a simple, inexpensive epidemiologic case-control study is often used as a surrogate for the risk ratio that would be obtained in a complex, expensive cohort study.

10.7.4   Approximation of Risk Ratio

The basic algebra that is briefly outlined here will be described and illustrated in greater detail in Chapter 17. Suppose a particular disease occurs at a very low rate, such as $p_2 = .0001$, in people who have not been exposed to a particular risk factor. Suppose the disease occurs at a higher but still low rate, such as $p_1 = .0004$, in people who have been exposed. The simple ratio, p_1/p_2, is called the *risk ratio*. In this instance, it would be $.0004/.0001 = 4$.

To determine this risk ratio in a cohort study of exposed and nonexposed people, we would have to assemble and follow thousands of persons for a protracted period of time and determine which ones do or do not develop the selected disease. Instead, with an epidemiologic case-control study, we begin at the end. We assemble a group of "cases," who already have the disease, and a group of "controls," who do not. We then ask each group about their antecedent exposure to the risk factor. The results are then manipulated as discussed in the next few subsections.

10.7.4.1   *Structure of 2 × 2 Table* — The fourfold (or 2×2) table in either a cohort or case-control study would have the following skeletal structure:

	Diseased Cases	Nondiseased Controls
Exposed	a	b
Nonexposed	c	d

In a cohort study, where we begin with exposed and nonexposed groups, they become the denominator for any calculations of rates of occurrence. Thus, $a + b = n_1$ is the denominator of exposed persons and $c + d = n_2$ is the denominator of unexposed persons.

In a case-control study, however, we assemble diseased and nondiseased groups. They consist of $a + c = f_1$ for the total of diseased cases, and $b + d = f_2$ for nondiseased controls. The values of $a + b$ and $c + d$ can be calculated, but they are not appropriate denominators for determining rates of disease occurrence. If any "rates" are to be calculated, they would have to be a/f_1 for rate (or proportion) of exposure in the cases and b/f_2 for the corresponding rate in the controls.

10.7.4.2   *Advantages of Case-Control Odds Ratio* — In a cohort study, the rate of occurrence for the disease in the exposed group would be $p_1 = a/(a + b) = a/n_1$. The corresponding rate in the unexposed group would be $p_2 = c/(c + d) = c/n_2$. The risk ratio would be $p_1/p_2 = (a/n_1)/(c/n_2)$.

In a case-control study, however, values of n_1 and n_2 in the exposed and nonexposed groups are not available to allow these calculations of p_1 and p_2. Nevertheless, if the cases and controls suitably represent the corresponding members of the cohort population, the odds of exposure should be the same in the two tables. Thus, the odds of a/c in the case group and b/d in the control group should have the same values as their counterpart odds in the cohort. The odds ratio, which is (a/c)/(b/d) = ad/bc, should be the same in both types of research.

In the cohort study, the odds ratio would be $(p_1/p_2)/(q_1/q_2) = (p_1/p_2)[(1 -p_2)/(1 - p_1)]$. It is the desired risk ratio, p_1/p_2, multiplied by $q_2/q_1 = (1 - p_2)/(1 -p_1)$. If the occurrence rates of disease are quite small, however, both $1 -p_2$ and $1 -p_1$ will be close to 1. The factor $(1 -p_2)/(1 - p_1)$ will then be approximately 1. Thus, in the foregoing example, $p_1 = .004$ and $p_2 = .001$. Because $1 -p_1 = .996$ and $1 -p_2 = .999$, the factor $.999/.996 = 1.003$. If we assume that this factor is essentially 1, the odds ratio will be $(p_1/p_2) \times$ (~1) and will approximate the risk ratio.[13]

A more formal algebraic proof of these relationships is provided in the Appendix to this chapter, and the topic is further discussed in Chapter 17. The main point to be noted now is that if the basic rate of disease is small and if the groups in the fourfold case-control table suitably represent their counterparts in the fourfold cohort-study table, the odds ratio in a relatively small case-control study should approximate the risk ratio produced by a much larger and elaborate cohort study.

This mathematical attribute of the odds ratio had made it (and case-control studies) so irresistibly appealing in epidemiologic research that the investigators regularly overlook the *scientific* criteria needed to accept the odds ratio as a credible scientific substitute for the risk ratio.[14]

10.8 Proportionate Reduction in System Variance (PRSV)

A descriptive index that is well known to statisticians, but not to most other readers, is the proportionate reduction that occurs in the total variance of a system when it is fitted with a "model." This index, which is particularly useful for describing the associations considered later in the text, is valuable now because it can be applied to contrasts of both dimensional and binary data, where the two compared groups form the "model."

For example, consider the two groups of binary data compared in Table 10.2. In the total data, before division into two groups, the system variance, using the formula NPQ, is (16/38) (22/38)(38) = 9.26. After the two-group split, the sum of group variances, using the formula $n_1p_1q_1 + n_2p_2q_2$, becomes (6/18)(12/18)(18) + (10/20)(10/20)(20) = 9.00. The proportionate reduction in system variance is (9.26 − 9.00)/9.26 = .028.

With dimensional data, as shown in the example in Section 10.5.1.1, the determination of system variance requires first that the grand mean of the system be identified as $G = (n_A\overline{X}_A + n_B\overline{X}_B)/N$. In the cited example, $G = [(6)(25.6) + 5(11.3)]/11 = 19.1$. Thus, the system variance will be $\Sigma X_A^2 + \Sigma X_B^2 - NG^2$, where $\Sigma X_A^2 = S_{XX_A} + n_A\overline{X}_A^2$ and $\Sigma X_B^2 = S_{XX_B} + n_B\overline{X}_B^2$. For the cited data, $\Sigma X_A^2 = (5)(7)^2 + 6(25.6)^2 = 4177.16$ and $\Sigma X_B^2 = 4(4)^2 + 5(11.3)^2 = 702.45$. Thus, the system variance is $4177.16 + 702.45 - 11(19.1)^2 = 866.7$. The sum of the two group variances is $S_{XX_A} + S_{XX_B} = 309$, so that the proportionate reduction in system variance is $(866.7 - 309)/866.7 = .64$.

The proportionate reduction in system variance (PRSV) is seldom considered in ordinary descriptive comparisons of two groups. It has three major advantages, however:

1. With some complex algebra not shown here, it can be demonstrated that the square of the standardized increment (or "effect size") — discussed in Sections 10.5.1 and 10.6.2.3 — is roughly 4 times the magnitude of the proportionate reduction in system variance, particularly if the two group sizes are reasonably large and relatively equal. Thus, in many situations, $(SI)^2 \sim 4(PRSV)$ and so $SI \sim 2\sqrt{PRSV}$. For example, for the two proportions 10/20 and 6/18, which have modestly sized groups, PSRV = .028 and $\sqrt{.028} = .167$ which is about half of the SI (.35) shown in Section 10.6.2.3. (For the very small groups of dimensional data in Section 10.5.1.1, the SI of 2.44 is about three times the $\sqrt{PRSV} = \sqrt{.64} = .8$.)*

---

* The actual formula, for two groups of dimensional data each having size n, is $SI = 2(\sqrt{PRSV}\sqrt{n-1})/[n(1-PRSV)]$. For two groups of binary data, the formula is $SI = 2\sqrt{PRSV}$.

2. Because PRSV can be determined for both dimensional and binary data and has a direct mathematical relationship to the standardized increment (or "effect size"), a single standard of evaluation can be used, if desired, for subsequent decisions about "quantitative significance" in contrasts of both types of data.

3. As will be noted later in Chapter 19, when we compare associations in two variables rather than contrasts in two groups, the value of $\sqrt{PRSV}$ is called the *correlation coefficient*. Therefore, the decisions discussed later for quantitative significance of a correlation coefficient can also be applied for evaluating SI and $\sqrt{PRSV}$ in a contrast of two groups.

10.9   Standards for Quantitative Significance

Although stochastic (or "statistical") significance is commonly proclaimed when a calculated P value is smaller than .05, no analogous boundary has been established for demarcating quantitative significance.

10.9.1   Reasons for Absence of Standards

Many excuses can be offered for the failure of biomedical scientists to set such a boundary.

10.9.1.1   *Substantive Context* — As noted in Section 10.2, quantitative contrasts always occur in a substantive context. The increment of $.03 = .09 − .06$ for two proportions of occurrence of an adverse drug reaction may be unimpressive if it refers to a minor skin rash, but important if it refers to sterility or death. Aside from the particular event being considered, the context also includes the size of the population "at risk" for the event. Suppose a skin cream that offers striking improvement in acne also raises the rate of fetal deformity from .010 to .011 if the cream is used by pregnant women. The increment of .001 seems tiny, but could lead to 2,000 unnecessarily deformed babies in a nation with 2,000,000 births. [One reason that public-health people often seem more "alarmed" than clinicians about "risks" is that the public-health denominator is so much larger than the clinical denominator. An obstetrician who delivers 200 women per year may not notice an adverse event that occurs at a rate of .005. In a community with 100,000 deliveries, however, the event will be much more apparent.]

Because the substantive context cannot be easily separated from the associated quantitative magnitude, biomedical scientists have often been reluctant to draw boundaries based on magnitude alone.

10.9.1.2   *Quantitative Complexity* — For the simple indexes of contrast, both a ratio and an increment must be considered. The demarcation of values for two indexes simultaneously is much more complicated than choosing a single boundary, such as .05, for "significance" of a stochastic probability.

For the other indexes discussed throughout Sections 10.5 and 10.6, neither the standardized increment nor the common proportionate increment is well known or frequently used for dimensional data. Consequently, neither index is accompanied by a "commonsense" background of analytic experience to aid in the interpretation. For binary data, the odds ratio is probably easy to interpret intuitively as a "risk ratio," but the odds ratio will falsely enlarge the "risk" ratio[15] if the compared proportions exceed values of .1. For example, if $p_1 = .04$ and $p_2 = .01$, the risk ratio is 4, and the odds ratio is $(.04/.01)(.99/.96) = 4.12$. If $p_1 = .84$ and $p_2 = .21$, however, the risk ratio is still 4, but the odds ratio is $(.84/.21)(.79/.16) = 19.75$.

10.9.1.3   *Intellectual Distraction* — In the fallacious belief that decisions about importance depend only on the P values (or confidence intervals) of stochastic significance, investigators may not feel that any boundaries are needed to demarcate quantitative significance. This intellectual distraction

has become untenable in recent years, however, because scientists have discovered two major circumstances in which quantitative boundaries must be demarcated.

10.9.2 Demand for Boundaries

Despite the inattention or efforts at avoidance, boundaries of quantitative significance are demanded and must be established in two common circumstances that occur before or after the research is done.

10.9.2.1 *Planning Sample Size* — In planning a research study, investigators will want to have a sample size that assures stochastic significance for the results. As noted later, the calculation requires establishment of a boundary for the contrasted magnitude that will be regarded as *quantitatively* significant.

10.9.2.2 *Checking for False Negative Results* — When a study has been completed and has yielded results that do *not* show an impressive quantitative distinction, the investigator may want to conclude that the compared groups do not have a major difference. To prevent this decision from being a "false negative" conclusion, certain stochastic calculations can be done to determine whether the group sizes were large enough to detect and confirm a "major difference." For the stochastic calculations to be interpreted, however, a boundary must be set for the magnitude of the "major difference."

10.9.3 Development of Standards

For both reasons just cited, modern investigators have been increasingly unable to escape the challenge of demarcating quantitative significance and have had to develop some methods for doing so.

10.9.3.1 *Sample Size in Clinical Trials* — One frequent challenge is to choose a magnitude of quantitative significance when sample size is calculated for a controlled clinical trial. The calculated formula (as discussed later) requires a demarcation for δ, the amount of a significant quantitative increment in the contrasted means or proportions. Thus, if $\hat{p}_A$ is the expected proportion of success in Group A, and if $\hat{p}_B$ is the corresponding proportion in Group B, the result is quantitatively significant in favor of Group A if

$$\hat{p}_A - \hat{p}_B \geq \delta$$

(The "^" or "hat" symbol indicates a result that is estimated or expected but not directly observed.)

In making decisions about δ, the investigators have seldom assigned a direct value for it. Instead, they usually choose a value for the proportionate increment, θ, that is to be regarded as quantitatively significant. Thus, $\theta = (\hat{p}_A - \hat{p}_B)/\hat{p}_B$. The value of δ is then found by anticipating a value of $\hat{p}_B$ for the reference group, and by applying the formula $\delta = \theta\hat{p}_B$. The customary choices of θ have been values of 25% or 50%. With these decisions, if the control group has had a success rate of 16%, a proportionate increment of 25% would require an actual increment of 4%, so that the treated group would need a success rate of 20%. If θ is 50% and the success rate is 16% in the control group, the treated group's success rate would have to rise to 24% to be quantitatively significant.

The proportionate increment θ has often been used for approaching decisions about quantitative significance, but it creates two problems. The first is that the choice of δ is left to depend entirely on the magnitude of $\hat{p}_B$ in the control group. Thus, if θ is 50% and the control group has a success rate of 2%, the rate of success required for a quantitatively significant difference in the treated group would be 3%. Despite the impressive value of 50% for θ, few commonsense evaluators would ordinarily be impressed either with a δ of 1% or with a "substantial improvement" that produces a success rate of only 3%.

The second problem is deciding which of the two complementary rates should be multiplied by θ. Thus, if $\theta = 50\%$ is applied to the control group's failure rate of $\hat{q}_B = 98\%$, the failure rate demanded for the new treatment will be $\hat{q}_A = 49\%$. This δ of 49% (= 98% − 49%) is substantially greater than the δ of 1% calculated when $\theta = 50\%$ was applied to the success rate of 2%.

For these reasons, the current concept of establishing quantitative significance with a θ value can be applauded because any clinical attempt to demarcate this type of significance is better than nothing. Nevertheless, because a thorough judgment requires a demarcation of two values — δ and θ — decisions based only on a θ value will inevitably be inadequate. Furthermore, such decisions perpetuate the custom of reporting results according to the somewhat misleading and occasionally deceptive proportionate increment.

10.9.3.2 *Importance of Epidemiologic Distinctions* —

In many epidemiologic studies of risk factors for disease, the proportions of people who become diseased is quite small. For example, in Doll and Hill's famous study[16] of smoking in British physicians, the occurrence rates of deaths ascribed to lung cancer were about 166 per hundred thousand in cigarette smokers and 7 per hundred thousand in non-smokers. These two values have an impressive ratio of 23.7 (= 166/7) but a highly unimpressive increment of .000159. Expressed in the NNE formula, an extra lung cancer would occur in one of 6289 (= 1/.000159) smokers.

For an *individual* smoker, the increased incremental risk of developing lung cancer may seem too small to warrant cessation of the habit. On the other hand, in a society that contains 200 million people, a small increment can have a large total impact. If half of those people are adults and if half of the adults are smokers, there would be 50,000,000 smokers. With an incremental risk of .000159, this group of smokers would develop 7950 cases of lung cancer that presumably would not have otherwise occurred. The increment in the two rates may seem unimpressive at an individual personal level, but be important at a societal level.

The importance of certain quantitative distinctions may sometimes depend on such external features as the frequency with which the cited issue occurs as a general or medical problem. The kinds of distinctions that might seem trivial in a clinical comparison of two treatments might thus become substantial in an epidemiologic contrast of risk factors for disease.

10.9.3.3 *Importance of Additional Clinical Distinctions* —

Finally, certain issues in the quantitative magnitude of significance will regularly be affected by associated clinical factors such as the costs of treatment and the type and risk of adverse reactions. If a particular drug is very expensive and has a high rate of untoward adverse reactions, we might demand that its efficacy exceed that of placebo by a greater amount than we might ask of a cheaper drug that is relatively risk-free.

10.10 Pragmatic Criteria

Because no formal criteria have been promulgated for quantitative significance, Burnand, Kernan, and Feinstein[17] investigated the boundaries that seemed to be used pragmatically for decisions about quantitative contrasts in a series of papers published in three general medical journals.

For comparisons of two means, the published reports did not always list the group sizes or standard deviations. Consequently, neither a standardized nor a common proportionate increment could regularly be determined. Accordingly, Burnand et al. examined the simple ratio, $\overline{X}_A / \overline{X}_B$, with $\overline{X}_A$ routinely chosen to be the larger mean, so that the ratio always exceeds 1. The investigators concluded that 1.2 was commonly used as a lower boundary for quantitative significance of the ratio in a contrast of two means. Thus, if $\overline{X}_A \geq 1.2 \, \overline{X}_B$, the value of $\overline{X}_A - \overline{X}_B$ will be $\geq .2 \, \overline{X}_B$. In other words, one mean must be proportionately at least 20% larger than the other. If $\overline{X}_A = 1.2 \, \overline{X}_B$ and if the two groups have equal size, the common proportionate increment will be (2)(.2)/(1 + 1.2) = .18. Thus, .18 might be regarded as a lower boundary for quantitative significance of the common proportionate increment.

To illustrate this process, suppose two compared groups have means of 18.9 and 10.1. The simple ratio is 18.9/10.1 = 1.87, which clearly exceeds the criterion boundary of 1.2. For this simple ratio, the common proportionate increment — for equal-sized groups — will be (2)(.87)/2.87 = .61.

For a contrast of two proportions, Burnand et al. found that 2.2 was a commonly used lower boundary for quantitative significance of the odds ratio. The odds ratio was chosen as a single index of contrast to avoid decisions based on increments alone in proportions that could range from very small values, such as .001 in public health rates, to much higher values, >.1, in clinical rates of "success." The odds ratio, which multiplies p_1/p_2 by q_2/q_1, also eliminated the ambiguity of deciding whether the compared ratio should be p_1/p_2 or q_2/q_1.

The boundaries of an impressive odds ratio, however, sometimes varied with the size of the groups under study. With the smaller groups and higher proportions (i.e., usually $\geq .01$) in most clinical studies, the published reports often used somewhat lower boundaries for "quantitative significance," than what appeared in the larger groups and lower proportions (i.e., $<.01$) of public-health research.

A value of .28 seemed to be a reasonable lower boundary for quantitative significance in a standardized increment of two proportions. This magnitude is slightly more than 1/4 of the common standard deviation between the two proportions. Thus, if $\sqrt{PQ} = .5$, the absolute increment between two proportions would have to exceed $(.28)(.5) = .14$. For comparisons of much smaller proportions, such as .01 vs. .07, where $P = .04$ and $\sqrt{PQ} = \sqrt{(.04)(.96)} = .196$, the absolute increment would have to exceed $(.28)(.196) = .055$.

Studying the "treatment effect size" in 21 trials of surfactant therapy for neonatal respiratory distress syndrome, Raju et al.[18] found that a median value of $\theta = 50\%$ had been used for the proportionate reduction expected in adverse outcomes after intervention. In most of the trials, however, the "observed treatment effect sizes were lower than the investigator-anticipated treatment effect sizes." Nevertheless, "all except 1 of 21 reports concluded that the therapy was useful, mostly based on subgroup analyses." [The phenomenon of clinical-trial distinctions that are unexpectedly small but nevertheless "significant" will be discussed later in several chapters.]

As noted later in Chapter 19, the variance of a system is not regarded as impressively altered unless the proportionate reduction is at least 10%. With this criterion for quantitative significance, $\sqrt{PSRV}$ must $\geq \sqrt{.1}$, which is about .3. If this criterion is extended to the "effect size," as discussed in Section 10.8, "quantitative significance" would require that $SI \geq .6$. This boundary is much higher than the value of .28 noted earlier for SI in two proportions, and some further thought will show why epidemiologists often avoid using the SI to present their results. For example, consider the "impressive" risk ratio of 5 for a disease having occurrence rates of .005 in exposed and .001 in nonexposed groups. When these rates are suitably expressed as $(.005 - .001)/\sqrt{(.003)(.997)}$, the SI has the unimpressive value of .07. If the occurrence rates are ten times higher, at .05 and .01, the SI is raised to the still unimpressive value of $(.05 - .01)/\sqrt{(.03)(.97)} = .23$. At the "clinical" rates of .5 and .1, however, the SI finally becomes impressive, reaching a value of $(.5 - .1)/\sqrt{(.3)(.7)} = .87$.

10.11 Contrasts of Ordinal and Nominal Data

In all of the two-group comparisons discussed so far, the data were either dimensional or binary. Ordinal and nominal data seldom receive descriptive comparisons because of the problem of choosing a single central index to compare, although the total distributions of data in the two groups can be contrasted *stochastically* with methods discussed for ordinal data in Chapter 15 and for nominal data in Chapter 27.

One common approach for descriptive comparisons in ordinal data is to assign arbitrary dimensional values to the categories, e.g., 0 = none; 1 = mild; 2 = moderate; 3 = severe. The results are then compared with means, medians, standard deviations, etc. as though the data were dimensional. The tactic is mathematically "shady," but has been repeatedly used and frequently accepted in studies where data for pain, anxiety, satisfaction, or other subjective feelings are expressed in ordinal scales. A mathematically proper descriptive index of contrast can be developed (see Chapter 15) for ordinal data, but the index is unfamiliar and seldom used.

For nominal data, which cannot be ranked, the most common descriptive approach is to summarize each group with a single binary proportion derived from the modal category of the total or from a compression of several categories. The selected binary proportions are then compared as though they were ordinary binary proportions.

10.12 Individual Transitions

All the discussion thus far has been concerned with comparing central indexes for two groups. A different type of quantitative contrast is appraised when an individual person's condition changes from one state to another. These transitions are easy to evaluate if graded (by patient or clinician) on a simple "transition scale" such as **better, same,** or **worse**.

A distinctive clinical change has also occurred if a single-state ordinal rating of **4**, on a pain scale of **0, 1, 2, 3, 4**, later declines to **2**. Changes of one category, from **4** to **3** or from **3** to **2**, are more difficult to evaluate unless accompanied by a separate transition rating such as **somewhat better**. A one-category single-state change from **1** (for slight pain) to **0** (for no pain), however, almost always represents a distinct clinical improvement.

The tricky problems in individual transitions arise for dimensional variables, where vicissitudes of the measuring system itself must also be considered. For example, a change of 0.2 units may represent measurement variations in hematocrit rather than a hematologic alteration; and a rise or fall in magnitude of at least two tube-dilutions is usually demanded to represent a change in Group A streptococcal antibody titers. Another problem in dimensional data is deciding whether to calculate direct or proportional increments from a person's baseline value for changes in such entities as blood pressure or weight.

In the absence of a clinically symptomatic observation to confirm the result of a laboratory test or physical measurement, the standard deviation of the group has been proposed as a basis for determining individual changes. Thus, a person may be rated as having a "significant" change if the direct increment exceeds one-fourth or one-half of the group's standard deviation in that variable.

The concepts and standards used for measuring individual transitions are now in a state of ferment, particularly as clinical investigators (and regulatory agencies) have begun giving increased attention to quantitative rather than merely stochastic accomplishments in therapeutic trials and other research.

10.13 Challenges for the Future

As a basic part of statistical appraisals, decisions about quantitative significance require intricate judgments for which a well-developed set of standards has not yet been established.

In the absence of standards, you will have to use your own judgment to determine whether a claim of "statistical significance" represents a truly important quantitative result or a stochastically low P-value obtained (as noted later) from a trivial difference with a large group size. If investigative judgments by you and your colleagues can lead to better general agreement about the strategies and boundaries, the results may produce desperately needed standards for quantitative significance. The new standards would allow the part of statistics that depends on substantive observation and analysis of quantitative significance to become at least as important as the stochastic significance that relies on mathematical theories of probability.

References

1. Rossen, 1974; 2. Cohen, 1977; 3. Glass, 1981; 4. Laupacis, 1988; 5. Naylor, 1992; 6. Sheps, 1958; 7. Forrow, 1992; 8. Bobbio, 1994; 9. Bucher, 1994; 10. Feinstein, 1992; 11. Sinclair, 1994; 12. Sackett, 1994; 13. Cornfield, 1951; 14. Feinstein, 1985; 15. Feinstein, 1986; 16. Doll, 1964; 17. Burnand, 1990; 18. Raju, 1993; 19. Steering Committee of the Physicians' Health Study Research Group, 1989; 20. Peto, 1988; 21. Boston Collaborative Drug Surveillance Program, 1974. 22. Stacpoole, 1992.

Appendix for Chapter 10

A.10.1   Algebraic Demonstration of Similarity for Cohort Risk Ratio and Case-Control Odds Ratio

In a cohort study, let e be the proportion of exposed persons in the total population, N. The size of the exposed group will be $n_1 = eN$; the unexposed group will have $n_2 = (1-e)N$ and $N = n_1 + n_2$. The occurrence rate of events in the exposed cohort will be p_1 and the number of events will be $a = p_1 n_1 = p_1 eN$. The number of persons without events will be $b = (1-p_1)n_1 = (1-p_1)eN$. The corresponding values in the nonexposed cohort will be p_2 for the occurrence rate, and $c = p_2 n_2 = p_2(1-e)N$ and $d = (1-p_2)(1-e)N$ for persons with and without events. The fourfold table for the cohort study will be as follows.

	Diseased Cases	Nondiseased Controls	Total
Exposed	$p_1 eN$	$(1-p_1)eN$	eN
Nonexposed	$p_2(1-e)N$	$(1-p_2)(1-e)N$	$(1-e)N$

When the odds ratio is calculated as ad/bc for this table, the factors of e, $1-e$, and N all cancel. The odds ratio becomes

$$\frac{p_1}{p_2} \times \frac{(1-p_2)}{(1-p_1)}$$

As noted in Section 10.7.4.2, this odds ratio is the risk ratio, p_1/p_2, multiplied by $(1-p_2)/(1-p_1)$, and the latter factor will approximate 1 if both p_2 and p_1 are relatively small.

In a case-control study, the "sampling" is done from the total of diseased cases and nondiseased controls. Suppose the sampling fractions are k for cases and k′ for controls. In other words, if we choose 50 of 1000 possible cases for the research, the sampling fraction is $k = 50/1000 = .05$. If we correspondingly choose 50 of 99,000 possible controls, the sampling fraction is $k′ = 50/99,000 = .000505$.

The fourfold table for the results of the case-control study will still appear as $\begin{Bmatrix} a & b \\ c & d \end{Bmatrix}$, but the data will actually represent the following:

	Diseased Cases	Nondiseased Controls
Exposed	$kp_1 eN$	$k′(1-p_1)eN$
Nonexposed	$kp_2(1-e)N$	$k′(1-p_2)(1-e)N$

When the odds ratio is calculated in the form of ad/bc for this table, the values of k and k′, as well as the values of e, $1-e$, and N, will cancel. The odds ratio will then represent $(p_1/p_2)[(1-p_2)/(1-p_1)]$. With the "uncommon" disease assumption that $1-p_1$ and $1-p_2$ are each ~ 1, this result will approximate p_1/p_2.

Exercises

10.1. Millions of persons in the U.K. and U.S. now take aspirin as daily (or every other day) "prophylaxis" against myocardial infarction. The therapy depends on results of a randomized trial of 22,071 male U.S. physicians, receiving aspirin 325 mgm every other day or a double-blind placebo, for an average of 60.2 months.[19] In summarizing the results, the investigators reported a "statistically significant" finding of a "44 percent reduction in the risk of myocardial infarction (relative risk 0.56…)" in men aged ≥ 50 years. In an analogous previous trial in the U.K.,[20] results for 5139 "healthy male doctors" receiving either no treatment or 500 mgm (or 300 mgm) of daily aspirin for an average of 6 years were somewhat "positive" but not "statistically significant." A summary of the pertinent data is in the following table.

	U.S. Study		U.K. Study	
	Aspirin	**Placebo**	**Aspirin**	**No Aspirin**
No. of participants	11,037	11,034	3429	1710
No. of subject years	54,560.0	54,355.7	18,820	9470
No. of:				
Total deaths (all causes)	217	227	270	151
Deaths from myocardial infarction	10	26	89	47
Nonfatal confirmed myocardial infarction	129	213	80	41
Fatal stroke	9	6	30	12
Nonfatal stroke	110	92	61	27

10.1.1. What results and indexes of descriptive comparison would you use to express the most cogent findings in the American trial?

10.1.2. What are the corresponding results in the U.K. trial?

10.1.3. What information was used by the U.S. investigators to calculate a "44 percent reduction" and "relative risk 0.56"?

10.1.4. Why do you think the total death rates were so much higher in the U.K. trial than in the U.S.?

10.1.5. How would you evaluate and compare the benefits of aspirin for MI versus its risk for stroke in the two trials?

10.1.6. Do the foregoing evaluations change your beliefs about the merits of daily or every-other-day aspirin prophylaxis? In other words, what did you think before you did this exercise, and what do you think now?

10.2. The following results were reported for two carefully conducted randomized trials of cholesterol-lowering treatment.

Trial A:

When 1,900 men receiving active treatment X were compared with 1,906 men given a placebo, the death rate from coronary heart disease after seven years was found to be 2.0% in the group given the placebo and 1.6% in the group given the active treatment, a reduction in the death rate from coronary heart disease of 0.4% over those seven years. (This difference was statistically significant.)

Trial B:

When active treatment Y was compared with placebo among almost 4000 middle-aged hyper-cholesterolemic men, a statistically significant 20% relative reduction was achieved in the 7-year rate of death from coronary heart disease.

Which of these two treatments would you prefer to offer your patients? Why?

10.3. In the first case-control study [21] that described an alleged relationship between reserpine and breast cancer, the data were as follows

	Breast Cancer Cases	"Control" Patients Without Breast Cancer	Total
Users of Reserpine	11	26	37
Nonusers of Reserpine	139	1174	1313
Total	150	1200	1350

10.3.1. What indexes would you use to contrast the risk of breast cancer in reserpine users vs. non-reserpine users?

10.3.2. What is the incremental risk of breast cancer in users of reserpine?

10.4. Here is a direct copy of the *Abstract* of a randomized trial in treatment of lactic acidosis.[22]

Abstract *Background.* Mortality is very high in lactic acidosis, and there is no satisfactory treatment other than treatment of the underlying cause. Uncontrolled studies have suggested that dichloroacetate, which stimulates the oxidation of lactate to acetyl-coenzyme A and carbon dioxide, might reduce morbidity and improve survival among patients with this condition.

Methods. We conducted a placebo-controlled, randomized trial of intravenous sodium dichloroacetate therapy in 252 patients with lactic acidosis; 126 were assigned to receive dichloroacetate and 126 to receive placebo. The entry criteria included an arterial-blood lactate concentration of ≥ 5.0 mmol per liter and either an arterial-blood pH of ≤ 7.35 or a base deficit of ≥ 6 mmol per liter. The mean ($\pm$ SD) arterial-blood lactate concentrations before treatment were 11.6. ± 7.0 mmol per liter in the dichloroacetate-treated patients and 10.4 ± 5.5 mmol per liter in the placebo group, and the mean initial arterial-blood pH values were 7.24 ± 0.12 and 7.24 ± 0.13, respectively. Eighty-six percent of the patients required mechanical ventilation, and 74 percent required pressor agents, inotropic drugs, or both because of hypotension.

Results. The arterial-blood lactate concentration decreased 20 percent or more in 83 (66 percent) of the 126 patients who received dichloroacetate and 45 (36 percent) of the 126 patients who received placebo ($P = 0.001$). The arterial-blood pH also increased more in the dichloroacetate-treated patients ($P = 0.005$). The absolute magnitude of the differences was small, however, and they were not associated with improvement in hemodynamics or survival. Only 12 percent of the dichloroacetate-treated patients and 17 percent of the placebo patients survived to be discharged from the hospital.

What conclusions would you draw about the value of dichloroacetate treatment?

10.5. Here is an opportunity for you to indicate what you mean by "quantitative significance" (and for the class convener to note observer variability in the decisions). You have been asked to choose a specific boundary point that will allow the following conclusions in quantitative contrasts. What boundaries would you choose for each decision? If you used specific increments and ratios in making the decisions, indicate what they were.

10.5.1. What value of the success rate for active treatment will make you decide that it is substantially better than a placebo success rate of 45%?

10.5.2. The mortality rate with placebo is 8%. What should this rate become to decide that the active treatment is worthwhile?

10.5.3. Short-term pain relief has been rated on a scale of 0 to 3, with 0 = no relief and 3 = complete relief. The mean rating for placebo is 1.3. What should the mean rating be for an effective active treatment?

10.5.4. The rate of endometrial carcinoma in postmenopausal women who do not use estrogens is .001. What rate, if correctly associated with estrogens, will alarm you enough to make you want to stop estrogen treatment in a patient whose distressing menopausal syndrome is under excellent control?

10.6. By now you should appreciate the point that decisions about quantitative and stochastic significance are not always concordant. A quantitatively significant difference, such as 75% vs. 25%, may not achieve stochastic significance if the sample sizes are too small, such as 3/4 vs. 1/4. Conversely, a quantitatively trivial difference, such as baseball batting averages of .333 vs. .332, can become stochastically significant if the group sizes are large enough. (The latter statement will be proved in Exercise 14.5.) Without going through an exhaustive search, can you find and cite an example of this discordance in published literature? In other words, you want to look for one of two situations. In one situation, the investigators claimed "statistical significance" for a contrast that you believe was *not* quantitatively significant. In the other situation, the investigators dismissed, as "not statistically significant," a contrast that you believe was important quantitatively and that should have received more serious attention.

One example — it can be either type — will suffice; but outline briefly what you found and why you disagree with the conclusion.

10.7. Find a published report of a randomized trial. It should be on a topic "important" enough to warrant advance calculation of sample size. Check to see what value of δ or θ (or any other demarcation of quantitative significance) was used for the sample-size calculation. Regardless of whether you can find this demarcation, note the results reported for the main outcome of the trial. Were they "statistically significant"? Do you regard them as quantitatively significant? (Give reasons and/or calculations for your answer.) Did the "significant" difference found in the actual results agree with the previously stated value of δ or θ?

11

Testing Stochastic Hypotheses

CONTENTS

Statistical inference was originally developed to estimate the parameters of a parent population by using the results found in a single random sample. As discussed in Chapters 7 and 8, the estimated parameters were the location of a point, such as the parametric mean or proportion, and the magnitude of a confidence interval surrounding the point. (In statistical parlance, these inferences are often called *point estimation* and *interval estimation*.) The inferential strategies were originally developed for use with random sampling only, but were later extended for their now common application to evaluate stability in single groups of data that were *not* obtained as random samples.

This chapter is devoted to another type of inference, particularly common in medical research and literature today, that is also an extension of the original methods for making estimates from a single random sample. The additional inferential activity, which is called *hypothesis testing*, uses the same basic strategy as before, but the "parameter" being estimated is the "value" of a mathematical hypothesis. The new process involves three main steps: (1) making a particular mathematical assumption, called a *null hypothesis*, about a parameter for the observed results; (2) appraising what happens when the observed results are rearranged under that hypothesis; and (3) deciding whether to reject or concede the hypothesis.

The process was illustrated (without being so identified) for the one-group t tests near the end of Chapter 7. In Section 7.8.2.2, we began with the null-hypothesis assumption that the observed data came from a parent population with mean $\mu = 0$. With that assumption, the "rearrangements" were done with theoretical repetitive sampling. Among the possible samples, the observed mean difference of -23.4 had a t-score of 1.598. The corresponding two-tailed P value was between .1 and .2 for the probability that the observed difference, or an even larger one in either direction, would emerge by chance from a parent population of sampled increments whose parametric mean was 0. After this P value was noted, however, the inferential process stopped, without a further decision. We are now ready to discuss how those decisions are made.

11.1   Principles of Statistical Hypotheses

In elementary geometry you probably engaged in the three-step process of forming, exploring, and deciding about hypotheses. To prove that two triangles were congruent, you formed the initial hypothesis that they were *not*. As the "proof" proceeded thereafter, various things happened that would lead to something impossible. If a hypothesis leads to impossible things, it cannot be maintained. You therefore rejected it and concluded that the triangles were congruent.

When the same type of reasoning is used in statistics, the basic strategy is similar. The initial hypothesis is stated as the *opposite* of what we want to prove. The "proof" occurs when an impossible consequence makes us reject the hypothesis. Unlike events in geometry, however, the things that might happen under a *statistical* hypothesis are never wholly impossible. There is always a chance, however tiny, that an extraordinary event might actually occur. Therefore, to reject a statistical hypothesis as incorrect or unacceptable, a boundary must be set for the level at which the chance possibility is too small to be taken seriously. The use of this *rejection boundary* is the main difference in the basic reasoning for evaluating mathematical hypotheses in geometry and in statistics.

The mathematical nomenclature, however, is used for a thought process that is drastically different from the often complex details and concepts of a *scientific* hypothesis. In science, the hypothesis is usually a specific substantive idea, such as "DNA is structured as a double helix" or "Vigorous control of elevated blood sugar will prevent vascular complications." In statistical inference, however, the hypotheses are strictly mathematical, and the conclusions refer not to anything substantive, but to the role of random-chance probability in the numerical results. The mathematical reasoning is the same, regardless of where the data come from and regardless of what they represent. The scientific hypothesis may be brilliant or foolish; the data may be accurate or wildly wrong; the comparison may be fair or grossly biased; but the statistical hypothesis does not know or care about these distinctions as it does its purely mathematical job.

The word *stochastic*, introduced in Section 10.1, is also a useful name for examining the possible events that might arise by chance under a mathematical hypothesis. Stochastic hypotheses are always stated in concise, simple mathematical symbols, such as $H_0 : \mu_A = \mu_B$. In this set of symbols, H_0 denotes the null hypothesis, and μ_A and μ_B are the hypothesized parametric means for groups A and B.

Stochastic hypotheses are commonly tested to evaluate stability of a numerical contrast for two (or more) groups. When stability was examined for only a single group in Chapters 7 and 8, the observed data could be rearranged in only a limited manner. When more than one group of data is available, however, diverse rearrangements can be constructed. For those constructions, the stochastic hypotheses are used for assumptions that can be applied both in making the rearrangements and in drawing conclusions afterward.

This chapter is concerned with the strategy of forming hypotheses and making the subsequent decisions. Chapters 12 through 15 describe the specific "tests" that produce the rearrangements and results used for the decisions.

11.2   Basic Strategies in Rearranging Data

The popular statistical procedures used to rearrange data for two groups have such well-known names as *t-test*, *Z-test*, *chi-square test*, and *Fisher exact probability test*. Other procedures, such as the *Pitman-Welch test* and *Wilcoxon test*, are less well known.

Regardless of their fame, the procedures all use the same basic strategy: forming a hypothesis, contemplating a distribution, and reaching a decision. The procedures differ in the method used to form the rearranged distributions; and the tactic chosen for the rearrangement will determine the way in which the hypothesis is stated and evaluated. Regardless of how the procedure is done, however, rejection of the hypothesis leads to the conclusion that the comparison is "statistically significant" and that the contrasted results are stable.

11.2.1   Parametric Sampling

Parametric sampling is the traditional basis of the "rearrangements" used for testing statistical hypotheses and making inferential conclusions. The sequence of events in the parametric method for contrasting two groups has many similarities to what was done in Chapters 7 and 8 for evaluating a single group.

1. Using features of the observed data, parameters are estimated for a parent population.
2. Repetitive samples are theoretically drawn from the parent population, but each "sampling" consists of two groups rather than one.
3. The anticipated results in the array of two theoretical samples are converted to the value of a single group's "test statistic," such as t or Z.
4. The pattern of results for the selected test statistic will have a specific mathematical distribution, from which a P value can be determined.
5. Instead of a P value, a confidence interval can be demarcated, using appropriate theoretical principles, for the location of the parameter.
6. From the P value or confidence interval, a decision is made to reject or not reject the selected hypothesis.

All of these steps occur in parametric tests of inference, whether aimed at a single central index or at a contrast of two central indexes. When two central indexes are compared, however, the procedure has a different goal; the population parameters are estimated in a different way; and a different type of conclusion is drawn. The goal is to determine whether the contrast in the two central indexes is distinctive enough to depart from the hypothesized parameter. The parameters for the theoretical parent populations are usually estimated under a "null hypothesis" that they are the same; and if the null hypothesis is rejected, we conclude that the observed indexes are stochastically different.

The mathematical reasoning is as follows: Suppose $\overline{X}_A$ and $\overline{X}_B$ are observed as the mean values for two groups with sizes n_A and n_B. We assume that each group is a random sample from corresponding parent populations having the parametric means μ_A and μ_B. Using the same respective group sizes, n_A and n_B, we now repeatedly take theoretical random samples from these two populations. Each pair of samples has the mean values $\overline{X}_{A_j}$ and $\overline{X}_{B_j}$ and the increment $\overline{X}_{A_j} - \overline{X}_{B_j}$. As the sampling process continues, the results form a series of increments in two sample means, $\{\overline{X}_{A_j} - \overline{X}_{B_j}\}$. This series of increments can be regarded as coming from the single group of a third parent population, which consists solely of increments formed by each of the items $\overline{X}_{A_j} - \overline{X}_{B_j}$. Applying the null hypothesis, we now assume that $\mu_A = \mu_B$, i.e., that the two groups come from parent populations having the same parametric mean. With the null-hypothesis assumption that $\mu_A - \mu_B = 0$, the parametric mean of the third population will be 0. The observed value of $\overline{X}_A - \overline{X}_B$ is then regarded as a sampling variation among increments of means in samples taken from the third population, whose parametric mean is $\mu = 0$.

For example, suppose the observed results are $\overline{X}_A = 7$ and $\overline{X}_B = 12$, with $\overline{X}_A - \overline{X}_B = -5$. If we drew repeated sets of two samples from a parent population and calculated the difference in means for each set, we might get a series of values such as 2, −1, 7, 4, −8, ... These values would form the sampling distribution for a difference in two means, taken from a theoretical population whose mean difference is assumed to be 0. The theoretical sampling distribution and the result of −5 that was actually observed in the two groups are then appraised for the decision about P values and confidence intervals.

The Z test and t test, which will be discussed in Chapter 13, are the two most common parametric procedures used for this purpose. The popular chi-square test, applied to binary data, will be discussed in Chapter 14.

11.2.2   Empirical Procedures

Although theoretical parametric sampling is the traditional statistical method of forming rearrangements, modern electronic computation has allowed two additional strategies to evaluate stability of a contrast. The new strategies are called *empirical*, because they depend only on the observed data, without invoking any theoretical populations or anticipated parameters. The two types of empirical methods are permutation (or randomization) procedures, which are discussed in the next section, and bootstrap procedures, discussed in Section 11.2.2.2.

11.2.2.1   Permutation Tests — For a permutation test of two groups, the data are first combined into a single larger group, which is pooled under the null hypothesis that the distinguishing factor (such as treatment) has the same effect in both groups. The pooled data are then permuted into all possible arrangements of pairs of samples having the same size as the original two groups. The index of contrast, such as an incremental mean, is determined for each of these paired samples. The distribution of the indexes of contrast is then examined to determine P values under the null hypothesis.

For example, consider the two groups of data $\{1, 2\}$ and $\{3, 4\}$, having the respective means 1.5 and 3.5. If the two groups are pooled into a single "population," $\{1, 2, 3, 4\}$, Table 11.1 shows the six possible permuted arrangements that divide the data into two groups, each with two members. The table also shows the mean and increment in means for each pair of samples. If one pair of samples were randomly selected from these six possibilities, the chances would be 2/6 (= .33) for getting an incremental value of **0**, 1/6 for a value of **+1.0**, 1/6 for **−1.0**, and so on.

TABLE 11.1

Distribution of Incremental Means in Permutation Procedure for Two Groups of Data, $\{1, 2\}$ and $\{3, 4\}$

Sample A	$\overline{X}_A$	Sample B	$\overline{X}_B$	$\overline{X}_B - \overline{X}_A$
1, 2	1.5	3, 4	3.5	2.0
1, 3	2.0	2, 4	3.0	1.0
1, 4	2.5	2, 3	2.5	0
2, 3	2.5	1, 4	2.5	0
2, 4	3.0	1, 3	2.0	−1.0
3, 4	3.5	1, 2	1.5	−2.0

Permutation tests are also called *randomization tests*, for two reasons. First, the subsequent P values denote probabilities for random occurrence of any of the permuted arrangements. Second, large group sizes can produce too many possible permutations for display and examination of the complete tabulation, as illustrated in Table 11.1. For example, about 1.38×10^{11} permuted arrangements can be formed from two groups that each contain 20 members. The appraisal of the full display can be dramatically eased, however, with some of the condensation tactics discussed in Chapter 12.

If those condensations cannot be applied, a different "shortcut" approach is to form permutations as a resampling exercise, by assigning members of the pooled array of data randomly (without replacement) to each of the two compared groups. As each new pair of samples is generated, the corresponding index of contrast is noted and added to the distribution of those indexes. The distribution can then be examined for P values (or other attributes) after a suitable number of pairs of samples has been randomly generated. The total number of pairs of samples can be quite large, ranging from 1000 to 10,000 or more. Nevertheless, for two groups containing 20 members each, the distribution of indexes of contrast will be easier to obtain from 10,000 samplings than from the total of 1.38×10^{11} possible arrangements.

The term *Monte Carlo sampling* can be applied for this approach, which checks a large but truncated series of samples, rather than all possibilities. Monte Carlo sampling relies on applying random choices to an underlying model. In this instance, the underlying model forms a permuted arrangement of the available data, rather than a sampling-with-replacement procedure, which is used for bootstrap tests.

The empirical permutation methods for contrasting two groups have existed for many years, long before modern computation became available; and the methods have many names. They are sometimes called *non-parametric*, because no parameters are estimated, or *distribution-free*, because the resampled results generate their own *ad hoc* distribution, without involving a theoretical mathematical model. The best known empirical procedure is a permutation technique, discussed in Chapter 12, that is eponymically called the *Fisher exact probability test* or *Fisher exact test*. Other reasonably well-known empirical procedures, more commonly called *non-parametric rank tests*, are the *Wilcoxon signed-ranks test* and the *Mann-Whitney U test*; they are discussed in Chapter 15.

11.2.2.2   Bootstrap Tests

11.2.2.2   Bootstrap Tests — In a permutation "resampling," the existing members of data are rearranged to form distinctive combinations. In a bootstrap resampling, the observed data are used as a "parent population," from which random sampling is done, with each individual member being replaced after its random selection. The permutation procedure requires a pooling of two (or more) groups of data, which can then be rearranged appropriately. The bootstrap resampling, however, can be done with a single group of data, as shown earlier in Section 6.4.1.1. Thus, the group of data {1, 6, 9} could form 27 possible resampled groups ranging from {1, 1, 1} to {9, 9, 9}, as shown in Table 6.1.

Bootstrap resampling is seldom used to compare two groups of data, but can be employed in two different ways to construct confidence intervals or P values for the index of contrast.

11.2.2.2.1 Confidence Interval.   For a confidence interval, each group is maintained separately; and a resampling is done, with replacement, within the group. The results of such a resampling for the previous two groups {1, 2} and {3, 4} are shown in Table 11.2.

Each group can produce four bootstrapped samples with corresponding means, shown in the upper part of the table. Each of the four samples for one group can be matched by one of four samples from the second group, and the 16 possible increments in means are shown in the lower half of the table. The distribution of the 16 increments shows values of 1.0 and 3.0 each occurring once, 1.5 and 2.5 each occurring four times, and 2.0 occurring six times. The range spanned from 1.5 to 2.5 would include 14 or 87.5% of the 16 possible values. Thus, the observed increment of 2 would be surrounded by an 87.5% confidence interval that extends from 1.5 to 2.5.

11.2.2.2.2 P Value.   For a P value, the two groups are pooled, and pairs of samples, containing two members each, are formed, with replacement. As 4 possible choices can be made each time, a total of 16 (= 4 $\times$ 4) samples can be obtained for each group, and the increment of means in the two samples

TABLE 11.2

Bootstrap Procedure to Form Confidence Interval for Incremental Means of Two Groups, {1, 2} vs. {3, 4}

Bootstrapped Samples			
Group {1, 2}		Group {3, 4}	
Contents	Mean	Contents	Mean
1, 1	1.0	3, 3	3.0
1, 2	1.5	3, 4	3.5
2, 1	1.5	4, 3	3.5
2, 2	2.0	4, 4	4.0

Incremental Means in 16 Possible Bootstrapped Samples			
Mean in Sample {1, 2}	Mean in Sample {3, 4}		
	3.0	3.5	3.5	4.0
1.0	2.0	2.5	2.5	3.0
1.5	1.5	2.0	2.0	2.5
1.5	1.5	2.0	2.0	2.5
2.0	1.0	1.5	1.5	2.0

can be formed in $16 \times 16 = 256$ ways. The distribution of increments can extend from 0, when the two samples have similar means, to a peak value of 3, when the compared samples are {1, 1} vs. {4, 4}.

Neither of the two bootstrap methods is regularly used for contrasts of two groups, although the methods can often be applied for other stochastic challenges.

11.2.3   Relocation Procedures

A different new strategy, which depends on "relocations" rather than resamplings, is analogous to the jackknife procedure. The jackknife itself is seldom used in "elementary" statistics but is often applied in multivariable statistics, as discussed elsewhere,[1] for getting or checking the values of the estimated parameters. The tactic about to be discussed now is a type of simultaneous jackknife maneuver for two groups. With only one group available in Chapter 7, the jackknife tactic could do no more than remove members from the group. With two groups available, members can be exchanged or otherwise relocated.

11.2.3.1   Unit Fragility Test — The relocations create a series of altered groups, analogous to the altered series produced by the jackknife removals in Section 7.7.3. For these altered groups, the most interesting stochastic approach is to compare the central indexes *descriptively*. Instead of examining distributions to determine P values and confidence intervals, we check to see whether the differences (or other distinctions) in the compared indexes exceed the boundaries selected for *quantitative* zones of significance or insignificance.

For example, suppose the proportions of success are being compared as $p_A - p_B$ for two treatments, where A is expected to be better than B. Suppose the value of $\delta \geq .15$ is set as the boundary for an increment that is quantitatively significant, and that $\zeta \leq .04$ is demarcated as the boundary for quantitatively insignificant increments. With these boundaries, the compared result will be deemed quantitatively significant if $p_A - p_B$ is $\geq .15$, insignificant if $p_A - p_B$ is $\leq .04$, and inconclusive in the intermediate zone where $.04 < (p_A - p_B) < .15$.

To illustrate the relocation process, suppose the results of a clinical trial show $p_A = 10/20 = .500$ and $p_B = 6/18 = .333$. The observed increment of $.500 - .333 = .167$ would be regarded as quantitatively significant because it exceeds $\delta = .15$. If one member of the numerator group in the larger p_A were moved from A to B, however, the result would become $p_A = 9/20 = .450$ and $p_B = 7/18 = .389$. The increment of $.450 - .389 = .061$ would no longer be quantitatively significant. We might therefore decide that the originally observed "significant" result is *not* statistically stable because the boundary of quantitative significance would no longer be exceeded if one person were relocated.

The relocation strategy, called the *unit fragility procedure*, has been proposed[2] for evaluating the change that might occur in two proportions, p_A and p_B, if a single unit is moved from one numerator to the other. Thus, if $p_A = r_A/n_A$ and $p_B = r_B/n_B$, the new proportions might be $p'_A = (r_A + 1)/n_A$ and $p'_B = (r_B - 1)/n_B$. If the move went in the other direction, the new proportions would be $p''_A = (r_A - 1)/n_A$ and $p''_B = (r_B + 1)/n_B$. With the first change, the comparison of $10/20 = .500$ vs. $6/18 = .333$ would become $11/20 = .550$ vs. $5/18 = .278$, an increment of .272. With the second change, the results would become $9/20 = .450$ vs. $7/18 = .389$, an increment of .061.

The changes could be evaluated either intrinsically or against an extrinsic standard, such as $\delta \geq .15$ (or $\zeta \leq .04$). For the intrinsic evaluation, the increment between the two proportions in one instance would rise by .105 [= .272 − .167], and in the other instance, the increment would fall by .106 [= .167 − .061]. The absolute amount of change in the *increment* is the same (except for rounding) in either direction, whether the shifted unit makes the value of r_A become $r_A + 1$ or $r_A - 1$.

The amount of change, called the *unit fragility*, can be expressed with the formula, $f = N/(n_1 n_2)$ where $N = n_1 + n_2$. This result for $10/20$ vs. $6/18$ is $38/(20 \times 18) = .106$. Thus, with the unit fragility procedure, the observed increment of .167 would rise or fall by a value of .106. In reference to change from the intrinsic value of the original increment of .167, the *index of proportionate fragility* is relatively high, at $.106/.167 = .63$. In reference to an extrinsic boundary, the reduction of .106 would make the original increment become .061, which is no longer quantitatively significant. With either type of boundary, we could conclude that the observed contrast of $10/20$ vs. $6/18$ is *not* stable.

Perhaps the most striking feature of the unit fragility procedure is the appraisal of "statistical significance" in a purely descriptive manner, without recourse to probabilities. When *quantitative* boundaries are established for "significant" and "insignificant" differences, the fragility (an inverse of "stability") for the observed result can be determined by whether it crosses those boundaries after a potential unitary change.

11.2.3.2 Application in Mental Screening

11.2.3.2 Application in Mental Screening — The idea of checking stability without resorting to probability is a striking departure from a century of the now traditional paradigms of "statistical inference." Although the new approach has received serious discussion,[2,3] many years will probably elapse before its value becomes recognized by investigators or accepted by statisticians. Regardless of the ultimate fate of the unit fragility tactic, it offers an excellent method for doing a prompt "in-the-head-without-a-calculator" appraisal of the observed results. With this type of "mental screening," the analyst evaluates the data from the counterpart of a simple "physical examination," before doing any calculations as a "laboratory work-up."

This type of screening was done, without being called "unit fragility," when decisions were made earlier in Section 1.1.3 that the comparison of .500 vs. .333 was unstable as 1/2 vs. 1/3 and stable as 150/300 vs. 100/300. In the first instance, a unit fragility shift could reverse the direction of the increment from $.500 - .333 = +.167$ to $(0/2) - (2/3) = -.667$. In the second instance, a one-unit shift would make the altered increment become $(149/300) - (101/300) = +.160$, which hardly changes the original incremental result of .167. For small numbers, such as 1/2 vs. 1/3, the comparison is easily done with mental rearrangements that do not require a calculator.

Exercise 11.1 offers an opportunity to try this type of "mental screening" for a set of dimensional data.

11.3 Formation of Stochastic Hypotheses

The fragility procedure creates a new type of "inference-free" statistics that may not become popular for many years; and the standard, customary inferential procedures will be individually discussed in Chapters 12 through 15. The rest of this chapter is therefore devoted to the traditional inferential reasoning that occurs when statistical hypotheses lead to conventional decisions about stochastic significance. The basic principles used for a contrast of two groups are also applicable to most other types of stochastic contrast.

In the traditional reasoning, hypotheses are established for tests that answer the question, "What if?"; and the answers always depend on stochastic probabilities found in theoretical or empirical random sampling from a distribution. The hypotheses will differ according to the type of question being asked in each test, the type of answer that is desired, and the procedure selected to explore the questions and answers. Nevertheless, certain basic concepts are fundamental to all the procedures, regardless of how they are done.

11.4   Statement of Hypothesis

As the opposite of what we want to prove, the *null* hypothesis is set up for the goal of being rejected, i.e., declared nullified. With the usual aim of confirming that the observed difference is big, important, or "significant," the opposite null hypothesis is customarily set at the value of 0. In parametric procedures, the statement for means would be H_0: $\mu_A - \mu_B = 0$ (which is H_0: $\mu_A = \mu_B$), and for proportions, H_0: $\pi_A = \pi_B$.

In other instances, to be discussed in Section 11.8 and Chapters 23 and 24, the investigator wants to confirm that an observed difference is small, unimportant, or "insignificant." For this purpose, the stochastic hypothesis is set at a nonzero large value, such as δ, with a parametric statement such as H_0: $\mu_A - \mu_B \geq \delta$. In the rest of this chapter (and in Chapters 12 through 15) the null hypotheses are all set essentially at 0, but the distinction in nomenclature should be kept in mind to avoid confusion later. The null hypothesis is called *null* because it is being evaluated for rejection, not because its value is 0.

11.5   Direction of the Counter-Hypothesis

The counter-hypothesis represents the contention to be supported or the conclusion to be drawn when the null hypothesis is rejected. In the usual logic of the mathematical arrangement, the statistical counter-hypothesis represents the investigator's goal in doing the research. Thus, if the aim of a clinical trial is to show that Treatment A is better than Treatment B, the investigator's goal is A > B. When the statistical null hypothesis is stated as A = B, the original goal of A > B becomes the counter-hypothesis.

A prime source of the one-tail vs. two-tail dispute in interpreting probabilities is the *direction* of the counter-hypothesis. Suppose the null hypothesis is stated as A − B = C. If the hypothesis is rejected, the conclusion, which is A − B ≠ C, states an inequality, but not a direction. It does not indicate whether A − B is > C or < C.

For example, if the research shows that $\bar{X}_A - \bar{X}_B = 5$, do we want to support the idea that $\bar{X}_A$ is at least 5 units larger than $\bar{X}_B$? If so, the counter-hypothesis is $\bar{X}_A - \bar{X}_B \geq 5$. Do we also, however, want to support the possibility that $\bar{X}_B$ might have been at least 5 units larger than $\bar{X}_A$? For this bidirectional decision, the counter-hypothesis is $|\bar{X}_A - \bar{X}_B| \geq 5$.

The choice of a uni- or bidirectional counter-hypothesis is a fundamental scientific issue in planning the research and interpreting the results. The issue was briefly discussed in Chapter 6, and will be reconsidered in Section 11.8.

11.6   Focus of Stochastic Decision

The focus of the stochastic decision can be a P value, a confidence interval, or both.

11.6.1 P Values

The customary null hypothesis makes an assumption about "equivalence" for the two compared groups. If searching for a P value, we determine an external probability for the possibility that the observed difference (or an even larger one) would occur by stochastic chance if the hypothesis about equivalence is correct.

11.6.1.1 Parametric Tests — In parametric testing, the concept of *equivalence* refers to parameters. If the two compared groups have mean values $\overline{X}_A$ and $\overline{X}_B$, we assume that the groups are random samples from parent populations having the identical parameters $\mu_A = \mu_B$.

11.6.1.2 Empirical Tests — In empirical procedures, if no parameters are involved or estimated, the hypothesis of equivalence refers to the treatments, risk factors, or whatever distinguishing features are being compared in the groups. To contrast success rates for rearranged groups receiving either Treatment A or Treatment B, we can assume that the two treatments are actually equivalent. The scientific symbols for this stochastic hypothesis are $T_A \backsimeq T_B$.

11.6.2 Confidence Intervals

With either parametric or bootstrap procedures for confidence intervals, we examine the array of possible results that would occur with rearrangements of the observed data. The methods of forming these rearrangements will depend on whether the stochastic hypothesis is set at the null value (of equivalence for the two groups) or at an alternative value, discussed in Section 11.9, which assumes that the two groups are different.

When the rearranged results are examined, the decision about an acceptable boundary can be made according to intrinsic or extrinsic criteria. In one approach, using intrinsic criteria, the main issue is whether the hypothesized parameter is contained *internally* within the confidence interval. Thus, in the conventional parametric approach, with the null hypothesis that $\mu = 0$, the hypothesis is rejected if the value of 0 is *excluded* from the estimated confidence interval. For example, if the observed difference is $\overline{X}_B - \overline{X}_A = 7$, we would check stochastically to see whether the hypothesized parametric value of 0 is contained in the confidence interval constructed around 7.

The second approach depends on an *extrinsic* descriptive boundary that indicates how large (or small) the observed difference might really be. For this type of decision, regardless of whether **0** is included in the confidence interval, we might want to check that the interval excludes a value as large as **20**.

11.6.2.1 Parametric Tests — With parametric testing, a confidence interval is constructed around the observed distinction, which is usually an increment such as $\overline{X}_A - \overline{X}_B$. If the two groups are stochastically different, the null-hypothesis parametric value of $\mu_A - \mu_B = \mu = 0$ will be excluded from this interval. The ultimate decision may therefore rest on four constituents: (1) the selected level of confidence, (2) the magnitude of the zone formed by the confidence interval, (3) inclusion (or exclusion) of the "true" parametric value of 0 in that zone, and (4) inclusion (or exclusion) of any "undesirable" or inappropriate values.

For example, suppose two means have an incremental difference of 175 units, and suppose we find that the 95% confidence interval for this difference is constructed as 175 ± 174, thus extending from 1 to 349 units. Since the parametric value of 0 is not included in this zone, we might reject the null hypothesis and conclude that the two means are stochastically different. On the other hand, because their true difference might be anywhere from 1 to 349 units, we might not feel secure that the observed difference of 175 is a precise or stable value, despite the "95% confidence."

11.6.2.2 Empirical Procedures — With empirical procedures, we inspect results for the indexes of contrast in the series of resamples, as discussed earlier (and later in Chapter 12). A series of permuted samples can be prepared under the "null hypothesis," but a specific confidence interval is not constructed *around the observed difference*. Consequently, the main goal in inspecting the permuted results is to note the range of possible values. This range can be expressed in the counterpart of a zone of percentiles. Thus, if two groups have $\overline{X}_B - \overline{X}_A = 7$ as the difference in means, a permutation procedure might show that 95% of the possible differences extend from **−8** to **+36**. With a bootstrapping procedure, however, the confidence intervals show the array of results that can occur around the observed difference.

11.6.3 Relocation Procedures

Relocation procedures do not use the customary forms of statistical inference. The strategy is stochastic because it answers a question about what might happen, but no mathematical hypotheses are established, and no probability values are determined. The decision depends on potential changes in the *observed* results. For the "unit fragility" procedure discussed in Section 11.2.3.1, these changes were evaluated with a form of reasoning analogous to confidence intervals.

11.7 Focus of Rejection

Because the main goal of stochastic hypothesis testing is to determine whether the hypothesis should be rejected, a focus must be established for the rejection.

11.7.1 P Values

For P values, an α level is chosen in advance as the critical boundary, and the hypothesis is rejected if the test procedure produces $P \le \alpha$ (As noted later in Section 11.12, the value of α is often set at .05.) If $P > \alpha$, the hypothesis is conceded but *not* actually accepted.

The reason for the latter distinction is that rejecting the null hypothesis of equivalence allows the stochastic conclusion that the parameters or treatments are different, but much stronger evidence is needed to accept the null hypothesis and conclude that they are essentially equivalent. The absence of proof of a difference is not the same as proof that a difference is absent. For example, if two treatments have success rates of .25 vs. .40, coming from 1/4 vs. 2/5, we cannot reject the stochastic null hypothesis. Nevertheless, we could not be confident that the two treatments are actually equivalent.

The reasoning for a stochastic hypothesis thus has three possible conclusions: rejected, conceded, and accepted. These three categories are analogous to the verdicts available to Scottish juries: guilty, not proven, and not guilty. Accordingly, we can reject or concede a null hypothesis, but it is not *accepted* without further testing. The stochastic procedures needed to confirm "no difference" will be discussed later in Chapters 23 and 24.

11.7.2 Confidence Intervals

A confidence interval is usually calculated with a selected test statistic, such as the Z_α or $t_{v,\alpha}$ discussed in Section 7.5.4, that establishes a $1 - \alpha$ zone for the boundaries of the interval. This zone can be evaluated for several foci. The first is whether the anticipated (null-hypothesis) parameter lies inside or outside the zone. If the parametric value of μ is *not* contained in the zone of the interval, we can conclude that $P \le \alpha$ and can reject the null hypothesis. This result of this tactic is thus an exact counterpart of the reasoning used for α and P values.

Two more foci of evaluation are the upper and lower boundaries of the interval itself. Do these boundaries include or exclude any critical *descriptive* characteristics of the data? For example, suppose the increment of 175 units in two means has a confidence interval of 175 ± 200 and extends from −25 to 375. Because **0** is included in this interval, we cannot reject the hypothesis that the two groups are parametrically similar. On the other hand, because of the high upper boundary of the confidence interval, we could also not reject an alternative hypothesis that the two groups really differ by as much as 350 units. Conversely, as discussed earlier, if the confidence interval is 175 ± 174, and goes from 1 to 349, it excludes 0. The null hypothesis could be rejected with the conclusion that the two groups are "significantly" different. Nevertheless, the true parametric difference might actually be as little as 1 unit.

This double role of confidence intervals—offering an inferential estimate for both a parameter and descriptive boundaries—has elicited enthusiastic recommendations in recent years that the P value strategy be replaced by confidence intervals. Some of the arguments for and against the abandonment of P values will be discussed later in Section 11.12 and again in Chapter 13.

11.7.3   Relocation Procedures

For P values and confidence intervals, the rejection of the stochastic hypothesis will depend on the magnitudes selected either for α or for the corresponding Z_α or $t_{\nu,\alpha}$. Relocation decisions, however, depend on the descriptive boundaries set quantitatively for the large "significant" δ or the small "insignificant" ζ. The quantitative boundaries, which have received almost no attention during all the stochastic emphases, are crucial for decisions with relocation procedures, but are also needed both to evaluaute the extreme ends of confidence intervals and, as discussed later, to calculate sample sizes or to establish alternative stochastic hypotheses.

11.8   Effect of One- or Two-Tailed Directions

The choice of a one-tailed or two-tailed direction for the counter hypothesis determines how to interpret an observed P value, or how to choose the level of α used in forming a confidence interval.

11.8.1   Construction of One-Tailed Confidence Intervals

Just as a two-tailed P value of .08 becomes .04 in a one-tailed interpretation, the chosen level of α for a $1 - \alpha$ confidence interval really becomes $\alpha/2$, if we examine only one side of the interval. To illustrate this point, suppose Z_α is set at $Z_{.05}$ for a 95% confidence interval calculated as $\bar{X} \pm Z_{.05}(s/\sqrt{n})$. The upper half of the interval includes .475 of the distribution of means that are potentially larger than X, and the lower half of the interval includes the other .475 of the distribution, formed by means that are potentially smaller. If we are interested only in the upper boundary and ignore the lower one, however, the lower half of the interval really includes .50 of the distribution, i.e., *all* of the potentially smaller values. The confidence interval would be larger than the stated level of .95, because it would really cover $.975 = 1 - .025 = 1 - (\alpha/2)$ of the potential values.

In the first example of Section 11.7.2, suppose we wanted the 175 unit increment in two means to be definitely compatible with a parametric value of 350. The lower half of a two-tailed 95% confidence interval would include only a .475 proportion of the values that are potentially smaller than 175. If we are not interested in any of the smaller values, however, and want to know only about the larger ones, we would dismiss all .50, not just .475, of the potential values that are smaller than 175.

Accordingly, if we want a decision level of α for a strictly one-tailed confidence interval, examining only one boundary or the other but not both, the originally chosen α should be 2α, which will become α when halved. Therefore, for a strictly one-tailed confidence interval at the .05 level of α, the calculation would be done with $Z_{.1} = 1.645$, rather than $Z_{.05} = 1.96$.

The $\pm$ sign in the customary calculation can be confusing for the idea of a one-tailed confidence interval. The lower and upper value produced by construction of central index $\pm [Z_\alpha$ (standard error)] will regularly seem strange for a decision that allegedly goes in only one direction. In proper usage, however, a one-tailed confidence interval should be constructed with a $+$ or $-$ sign, but not both. Thus, if we want to reject the null hypothesis for a positive result, such as d, the one-tailed confidence interval is calculated as $d - [Z_\alpha$ (standard error)] and then checked to see if it excludes 0. If we want to consider the alternative possibility that d is really much larger, the one-tailed interval would be $d + [Z_\alpha$ (standard error)], which would be checked to see if it excludes the larger value.

11.8.2   Origin of Two-Tailed Demands

During the early growth of statistical inference in the 20th century, the mathematical hypotheses were almost always bidirectional. The bidirectional approach probably became established in the days when substantial statistical thought, particularly by R. A. Fisher and his disciples, was devoted to agricultural experiments in which two active treatments, A and B, would be compared to determine which was more effective. Since placebos were not used in the agricultural work, it was reasonable to expect that either A or B might be superior; and a bidirectional scientific hypothesis was entirely appropriate.

As statistical methods became increasingly used in medical and psychosocial research, the reviewers and editors began to demand that claims of "significance" be accompanied by P values; and a level of $\alpha = .05$ was set for the boundary of "significance." For the small groups of animals or people who were often studied in the research, the investigators soon discovered that a "nonsignificant" two-tailed P value could sometimes become "significant" if given a one-tailed interpretation. (An example of this event occurred in Exercise 7.4.)

The conversion to one-tailed interpretations could thus salvage results that might otherwise be dismissed as "nonsignificant." For example, an investigator studying the cultural ambiance of different cities and finding a two-tailed P value of .09 for the superiority of Bridgeport over New Haven, could transform the result to a one-tailed $P < .05$. Although the superiority of Bridgeport had not been anticipated when the research began, the investigator might nevertheless claim that the research had produced "significant" stochastic support for the concept.

To avoid this type of retrospective manipulation for research hypotheses that had not been clearly stated in advance and that were developed to fit the observed data, the demand was made that all values of P or α be interpreted in a two-tailed manner. This policy has now become well established at prominent medical journals and at various agencies where research results are evaluated.

11.8.3   Controversy about Directional Choices

In modern medicine, however, many investigations are deliberately aimed in a single direction. In particular, whenever efficacy is compared for an active agent vs. placebo, the goal is almost always to show superiority for the active treatment. If Excellitol is being tested as a new analgesic agent, we want to show that it relieves pain better than placebo. If the observed results show that placebo is better than Excellitol, the next step would *not* be to seek stochastic support for the results. Instead, we would look for a different, more effective active agent.

A reasonable argument might then be offered that Excellitol, although better than placebo in relieving pain, might be worse in producing more adverse side effects such as nausea. If so, however, the data about nausea would be recorded in a variable other than pain. The results for the pain and nausea variables would be tested separately, with each test having its own null hypothesis. Therefore, when we stochastically test the results in variables for pain relief and for occurrence of nausea, each test could be done with the one-tailed hypothesis that results for Excellitol will be larger than those for placebo.

If you accept the latter approach, it leads to a subtle problem. Suppose the patient gives a separate single "global" rating for the *overall* effect of treatment. This rating will incorporate both the good things such as pain relief, and the bad things such as nausea. Should this overall rating be interpreted with a one-tailed or two-tailed hypothesis? Because we may not know in advance whether the nauseous effects of Excellitol are severe enough to overwhelm its anticipated analgesic benefits, we might argue that placebo could turn out to be a better overall agent. Therefore, the hypothesis should be two-tailed. On the other hand, returning to the investigator's original goal, the aim of the research is to show superiority for Excellitol. It will receive no further investigative or public attention if it does not produce a better overall rating. Therefore, the hypothesis should be one-tailed.

The decisions about unidirectional vs. bidirectional hypotheses can become much more complex, particularly when the research is concerned with effects of more than one treatment, with stopping (rather than starting) a treatment in a clinical trial, and with diverse other situations. Because the decision in each situation may involve subtle substantive issues, an easy way to avoid the subtle problems is to insist that all hypotheses be examined in a two-tailed direction. The policy has the advantage of being clear and easy to enforce, but also has some distinct disadvantages. According to the opponents, the policy is too rigid: it substitutes arbitrary mathematical dogma for careful scientific reasoning; and it needlessly raises the expenses (and risks) of research because much larger group sizes are needed to obtain stochastic significance for the same quantitative results.

For example, suppose we anticipate finding that the mean for Treatment A is 4 units better than placebo in a study where the standard deviation of the pooled data is expected to be 15. The formula for sample-size calculations will be discussed later in greater detail, but a simple example can be instructive here. To calculate sample size for two equal-sized groups that would produce a two-tailed P value of .05 for the anticipated distinction, we would choose $Z_{.05} = 1.96$ and solve the equation:

$$1.96 \leq \frac{4}{15/\sqrt{n}}$$

where n is the size of one group. The result would be $(1.96)(15)/4 \leq \sqrt{n}$ and so $n \geq [(1.96)(15)/4]^2$ = 54. If we want only a one-tailed P value of .05, however, $Z_{.1}$ would be 1.645. The required sample size would drop to $n \geq [(1.645)(15)/4]^2 = 38$. The number of patients (and cost) for conducting the trial would be proportionately reduced by 30% [= (54 − 38)/54].

11.8.4 Compromise Guidelines

Different authorities have taken opposing positions on this issue, and the controversy is currently unresolved. In one policy, tests of hypotheses should always be two-tailed; in the other policy, one-tailed tests are allowed in appropriate circumstances.

The following "compromise" guidelines would probably be acceptable to all but the most rigid adherents of the two-tailed policy:

1. Always use a two-tailed procedure if an advance unidirectional hypothesis was *not* stated before the data were examined.
2. A one-tailed test is permissible, however, if the appropriate hypothesis was stated before the data were examined *and* if the direction of the hypothesis can be suitably justified.
3. If the "significance" reported with a one-tailed test would not persist with a two-tailed test, the distinction should be made clear in the text of the report.
4. Because your statistical colleagues will generally be happier with two-tailed tests, use them whenever possible. Thus, if the "significance" achieved with a previously stated one-tailed hypothesis remains when the test is two-tailed, report the two-tailed results.

Regardless of whether you decide to work at levels of α, 2α, or $\alpha/2$, however, another basic and controversial question (although currently less prominent) is whether *any* rigid boundary should be set for the stochastic decisions. This question is discussed in Section 11.12.

To avoid all of the foregoing reasoning and arguments, investigators can report the exact value of the two-tailed P, and then let the reader decide. This approach, which was not possible with the older tabulated "look-up" values that would allow only statements such as P > .05 or P < .05, can now be used when modern computer programs report exact values such as .087 or .043 for the two-tailed P. Receiving this result, the reader is then left to interpret it with whatever authoritative guidelines seem most persuasive. The only problem with the "computerized-P" approach is that (as discussed later) the one-tailed P is not always simply half of the two-tailed P.

11.9 Alternative Hypotheses

As the opposite of the null hypothesis, the counter-hypothesis merely states a direction. It does *not* state a magnitude. Suppose we have observed that $\overline{X}_A = \overline{X}_B + 5$. The null hypothesis for testing this result is $\mu_A - \mu_B = 0$. The subsequently determined P value or confidence interval reflects the probability of observing a difference of≥ 5 if the null hypothesis is correct, but the counter-hypothesis does not specify the magnitude of the difference. The counter-hypothesis is merely $|\mu_A - \mu_B| > 0$ if two-tailed, and $\mu_A - \mu_B > 0$ if one-tailed.

If we are concerned about how large the difference might really be, it becomes specified with an *alternative* hypothesis. For example, if we want to show that $\overline{X}_A - \overline{X}_B$ is not really as large as 12, the alternative hypothesis would be $\mu_A - \mu_B \geq 12$.

An alternative hypothesis is often stipulated when the observed result appears to be "negative," i.e., when the customary null hypothesis is *not* rejected. For example, if $P > .3$ for the stochastic test when $\overline{X}_A - \overline{X}_B = 5$, we can conclude that a "significant" stochastic difference was not demonstrated. We might wonder, however, whether an important quantitative difference was missed. If 12 is chosen as the magnitude of this difference, we could reappraise the data under the alternative hypothesis that $\mu_A - \mu_B \geq 12$. If the latter hypothesis is rejected, we could then conclude that the observed result of $\overline{X}_A - \overline{X}_B = 5$ is not likely to reflect a difference that is at least as large as 12.

For showing that an observed difference is stochastically significant, the level of α indicates the likelihood of a *false positive* conclusion if the ordinary null hypothesis $(\mu_A - \mu_B = 0)$ is rejected when it is correct. If an alternative hypothesis is correct, however, we run the risk of a *false negative* conclusion when the null hypothesis of 0 is conceded. The ideas will be discussed in detail later in Chapter 23, but two main points can be noted now. The first point is that the extremes of the confidence interval are often explored for questions about the possibility of false negative conclusions. For example, an observed increment of .08 in two proportions might be regarded as "nonsignificant" both quantitatively (because it is too small) and stochastically, because $P > .05$ and because the 95% confidence interval, from $-.06$ to $+.22$, includes 0. The possibility of a quantitatively significant difference (e.g., $\geq .15$) cannot be dismissed, however, because the confidence interval extends to .22.

The second point is that although examining the extremes of confidence intervals is an excellent way to "screen" for alternative possibilities, an alternative hypothesis (such as $\pi_A - \pi_A \geq .15$) is often formally tested for showing that an observed difference is "insignificant." An additional stochastic boundary, called β, is usually established for this decision. The level of β indicates the likelihood of a *false negative* conclusion if the alternative hypothesis is rejected when it is correct.

In statistical jargon, the false-positive conclusion is often called a *Type I error*, and the false-negative conclusion, a *Type II error*. The value of $1 - \beta$ is often called the statistical *power* of the study, i.e., its ability to avoid a Type II error. This additional aspect of "statistical significance" introduces a new set of ideas and reasoning that will be further discussed in Chapter 23.

11.10   Multiple Hypotheses

Another important question is what to do about α when a series of comparisons involves multiple hypotheses about the same set of data or multiple tests of the same basic hypothesis. The value established for α indicates only the chance of getting a false positive result in a *single* comparison where the null hypothesis is true. With multiple comparisons, however, the level of α may be misleading. For example, suppose we do 20 randomized trials of a treatment that is really no better than placebo. If we use a two-tailed level of $\alpha = .05$ for each trial, we might expect by chance that one of those trials will produce a "significant" result. If we use a one-tailed level of $\alpha = .1$, two of the trials might produce such results.

11.10.1   Previous Illustration

This same problem occurred earlier in considering whether the dice were "loaded" if two consecutive 7's were tossed. In the multiple events that occur when the two dice are tossed on many occasions, a pair of consecutive 7's can readily appear by chance if the dice are perfectly fair. Because the probability of tossing a 7 is $6/36 = 1/6$, the probability of getting two consecutive 7's is $(1/6)(1/6) = 1/36$. At a dice table where the action is fast, two consecutive 7's could readily appear in the short time interval consumed by 36 tosses.

To determine the chance of getting *at least one* **7** in several consecutive tosses, we can note that the chance of getting it in one toss is 1/6 and the chance of not getting it is 5/6. Therefore, the chance of not getting a **7** is (5/6)(5/6) = .69 for two tosses, $(5/6)^5$ = .40 for five tosses, and $(5/6)^{20}$ = .03 for 20 tosses. Thus, the chances that a **7** will appear at least once are .17 (= 1/6) in one toss, .31 (= 1 − .69) in two tosses, .60 in five tosses, and .97 in twenty tosses. If the null hypothesis is that the tossed dice are "loaded" to avoid a value of **7**, the hypothesis will regularly be rejected by chance alone if tested on multiple occasions.

When you carry your knowledge of statistics into the pragmatic world of gambling casinos, this phenomenon may help you decide when to bet against a shooter who is trying to make a non-7 "point" before tossing a 7.

11.10.2 Mechanism of Adjustment

In the world of medical research, the chance results that can emerge from multiple testing may require an adjustment or precaution, which usually involves a change of the α level for individual decisions. As seen in the previous illustration of tossing dice, the false positive boundary of α for a single stochastic test becomes a true positive probability of $1 - \alpha$. For two tests, the true positive probability is $(1 - \alpha)$ $(1 - \alpha)$, so that the false positive boundary becomes $1 - (1 - \alpha)^2$. For k tests, the false positive boundary becomes $1 - (1 - \alpha)^k$. Consequently with k tests, the α level for a false positive decision is really lowered to $1 - (1 - \alpha)^k$. This formula indicates why, if 1/6 was the chance of a 7 appearing once, its chance of appearing at least once in 20 tosses was $1 - [1 - (1/6)]^{20} = 1 - (5/6)^{20} = 1 - .03 = .97$.

Many proposals have been made for strategies that lower α to an individual value of α' that allows the final overall level of $1 - (1 - \alpha')^k$ to be $\leq \alpha$. The diverse strategies have many eponymic titles (Duncan, Dunnett, Newman-Keuls, Scheffe, Tukey) based on various arrangements of data from an "analysis of variance." The simplest, easiest, and most commonly used approach, however, is named after Bonferroni. In the Bonferroni correction for k comparisons, $\alpha' = \alpha/k$. Thus, for four comparisons, an α of .05 would be lowered to $\alpha' = .05/4 = .0125$ as the level of P required for stochastic significance of each individual comparison. With $\alpha' = .0125$, the "final" level of $\alpha = 1 - (.9875)^4 = 1 - .95 = .05$.

11.10.3 Controversy about Guidelines

Although the Bonferroni correction is often used as a mechanism for *how* to do the adjustment, no agreement exists about *when* to do it.

Suppose an investigator, believing active treatment A is better than active treatment B, does a randomized trial that also includes a placebo group (for showing that both treatments are actually efficacious). Should the α level be lowered to $\alpha/3$ for the three comparisons of A vs. B, A vs. placebo, and B vs. placebo? As another issue, suppose an investigator regularly checks the results of an ongoing trial to see if it should be stopped because a "significant" result has been obtained? If k such checks are done, should each check require an α' level of α/k? Yet another question is what to do about α in "data dredging" or "fishing expeditions" where all kinds of things might be checked in more than 500 comparisons searching for something "significant." If α is lowered from .05 to the draconian level of .0001 for each comparison, even a splendid "fish" may be rejected as "nonsignificant" when caught.

Because the answers to these questions involve more than mathematical principles alone, no firm guidelines (or agreements) have been yet developed for managing the challenges. The issues are further discussed in Chapter 25.

11.11 Rejection of Hypothesis Testing

Regardless of whether the decisions are one-tailed or two-tailed, the most difficult task in all of the stochastic reasoning is to choose a boundary for rejecting null hypotheses or drawing conclusions from confidence intervals.

11.11.1   Complaints about Basic Concepts

Some authors avoid this choice entirely by rejecting the basic ideas of testing stochastic hypotheses and drawing conclusions about "significance." For example, in the encyclopedic four volumes called, *The Advanced Theory of Statistics*, Maurice Kendall and Alan Stuart[4] refuse to use the terms *null hypothesis* and *significance* because they "can be misleading." Reservations about stochastic testing were also stated by two prominent leaders in the American statistical "establishment," William Cochran and Gertrude Cox:[5] "The hard fact is that any statistical inference made from an analysis of the data will apply only to the population (if one exists) of which the experiments are a random sample. If this population is vague and unreal, the analysis is likely to be a waste of time."

In a remarkable book called *The Significance Test Controversy*,[6] published over 30 years ago, investigators mainly from the psychosocial sciences lamented the harm done by "indiscriminate use of significance tests." The editors of the book concluded "that the significance test as typically employed ... is bad statistical inference, and that even good statistical inference ... is typically only a convenient way of sidestepping rather than solving the problem of scientific inference."

Amid the many attacks (and defenses) in the 31 chapters of the book, none of the writers mentioned the idea of evaluating *stability* of the numbers. The main complaints about "significance testing" were that the research could not be statistically generalized because it usually contained "convenience" groups rather than random samples, that errors in the reliability of the basic data were usually ignored by the tests, that *significance* should denote substantive meaning rather than a probabilistic magnitude, and that infatuation with stochastic significance had overwhelmed the priority of attention needed for substantive significance.

In one of the chapters of the book, Joseph Berkson, the leading medical biostatistician of his era, objected to the null hypothesis because "experimentalists [are not] typically engaged in disproving things. They are looking for appropriate evidence for affirmative conclusions. ... The rule of inference on which [tests of significance] are supposed to rest has been misconceived, and this has led to certain fallacious uses."

11.11.2   Bayesian Approaches

The proponents of Bayesian inference are willing to calculate stochastic probabilities, but complain that the classical frequentist approaches are unsatisfactory. Some of the complaints[7,8] are as follows:

1. It is counter-intuitive and may be scientifically improper to draw conclusions about "more extreme values" that were not observed in the actual data.

2. Two groups will seldom if ever be exactly equivalent, as demanded by the null hypothesis.

3. Confused by the contradictory method of forming hypotheses, many readers mistakenly believe that P values represent the probability that the null hypothesis is true.

4. Conventional confidence intervals do not solve the problem, since they merely indicate the potential frequentist results if the same study had unlimited repetitions.

5. Frequentist approaches are "rigidly" dependent on the design of the research, whereas Bayesian methods "flexibly" allow the application of subjective probabilities, derived from all available information.

In the frequentist approach, the stochastic conclusion indicates the probability of the data, given the hypothesis. In the Bayesian approach, the stochastic conclusion is a "posterior" determination of the probability of the hypothesis, given the data. This determination requires that a subjective appraisal (i.e., an enlightened guess) of a value for the prior probability of the hypothesis be multiplied by the value of a likelihood function, which is essentially the probability of the data given the hypothesis. In an oversimplified summary of the distinctions, the Bayesian's conclusive P value is produced when the frequentist's conclusive P value is modified by a subjective prior probability, and denotes the chance that the prior hypothesis is correct.

The controversy recently received an excellent and often comprehensible discussion in a special issue of *Statistics in Medicine*,[9] where the respective "cases" were advocated and later attacked on behalf of either frequentism[10] or Bayesianism[10] in clinical trials.

11.12 Boundaries for Rejection Decisions

Despite the cited reservations and denunciations, stochastic tests of significance have survived, prospered, and prevailed. They are now routinely demanded by editors, reviewers, granting agencies, and regulatory authorities. As an investigator, you usually cannot escape the tests if you want to get your research funded or its publication accepted; and as a reader, you will find results of the tests appearing in most of the papers published in respectable journals. The Bayesian alternatives may have many merits, but they are seldom used.

Regardless of whether the customary tests are good or bad, worthwhile or harmful, they are there; and they will continue to be there for the foreseeable future. Accordingly, like it or not, we have to consider the daunting task of setting boundaries for decisions to reject a stochastic null hypothesis.

In stochastic hypotheses the observed result always has a chance, however tiny, of having occurred under the null hypothesis. The decision to reject the hypothesis will therefore be wrong if it was true on that occasion. The value set for α indicates the frequency with which we are willing to be wrong. Thus, if α is set at .05, we accept the chance of being wrong in one of every twenty times that the null hypothesis is rejected. (The wry comment has been made that "Statisticians are the only members of society who reserve the right to be wrong in 5% of their conclusions.")

Relatively few people would calmly accept the idea that their decisions in daily life would have so high a frequency of error. Physicians practicing medicine (with or without the additional scrutiny of lawyers) might be unable to maintain an unperturbed *aequanimitas* if one clinical decision in 20 was flagrantly wrong. Nevertheless, if statistical inference requires hypothesis testing, a boundary must be set for the rejection zone.

11.12.1   P Values and α

Since probability values are measured in a continuum that extends from 0 to 1 (or from 0% to 100%), choosing a boundary to demarcate a small enough level of α is particularly invidious. The decision is somewhat like answering the question, "How large is *big*?" or "How much is *enough*?" If asked one of those two questions, you would probably answer, "It all depends."

Nevertheless, a specific boundary was suggested many years ago by R. A. Fisher,[11] when he introduced the name *tests of significance* for the rearrangement procedures. As noted earlier, Fisher set α at .05 because about two standard deviations around the mean would span the 95% inner zone of data in a Gaussian distribution. He wrote, "It is convenient to take this point (i.e., α = .05) as a limit in judging whether a deviation is to be considered significant or not. Deviations exceeding twice the standard deviation are thus formally regarded as significant."

In a posthumous biography, Fisher's daughter[12] stated that he later came "to deplore how often his own methods were applied thoughtlessly, as cookbook solutions, when they were inappropriate or, at least, less informative than other methods." In subsequent writings after his initial proposal of .05, Fisher himself did not maintain the 5% boundary. He repeatedly referred to using a "1% level or higher" for stochastic decisions; and eventually he began to discourage the use of *any* fixed boundary. "The calculation is absurdly academic," he wrote in 1959, "for in fact no scientific worker has a fixed level of significance at which from year to year, in all circumstances, he rejects hypotheses; he rather gives his mind to each particular case in light of his evidence and his ideas."[13]

Although many other leaders in the world of statistics have also deplored the fixed boundary of .05, it has become entrenched in medical research. Reviewers and editors may adamantly refuse to publish results in which the P value reached the disastrous heights of .051, while happily accepting other studies that had unequivocal "significance," with P = .049. Like many past medical doctrines that were maintained long after they had been discredited, the "$P \leq 0.5$" boundary will probably continue until it is replaced by something better (or equally doctrinaire).

11.12.2   Confidence Intervals

The problem of choosing a boundary for α is not eliminated by current arguments that P values be replaced by confidence intervals for stochastic decisions. The main contentions in the dispute are whether more information is provided by a P value or a confidence interval; but the choice of a *boundary* is not discussed. Because of the dominant role of α and Z_α (or t_α) in both calculations, a confidence interval is a type of "reciprocal" P value, as shown later in Chapter 13. A boundary of α must be chosen regardless of whether we calculate P to see if $P \leq \alpha$, or choose Z_α (or t_α) and then inspect the contents of the calculated confidence interval. The decision about rejecting the null hypothesis is based on exactly the same data and reasoning, whether the α boundary is examined directly with P or indirectly with the lower (or upper) limit of a confidence interval calculated with Z_α or t_α.

Consequently, the main advantage of a confidence interval is *not* the avoidance of an arbitrary α boundary for stochastic decisions. Instead, the confidence interval shows an "other side" that is not displayed when the null hypothesis is conceded because of a too large P value. For example, the null hypothesis would have to be conceded if an observed difference in means was 175, with 102 as the standard error of the difference. The Z value would be $175/102 = 1.72$, which is below the Z_α of 1.96 required for $2P < .05$; and the 95% confidence interval, calculated as $175 \pm (1.96)(102)$, would extend from -25 to 375, thus including 0. The same stochastic decision of "nonsignificant" would be reached with either approach as long as $\alpha = .05$. The main merit of the confidence interval, however, would be its upper limit of 375, indicating that the "nonsignificant" difference of 175 might be as large as 375.

On the other hand, if α were given a one-tailed interpretation, $Z_1 = 1.645$. The Z value of 1.72 exceeds this boundary, so that P would be $< .05$; and the confidence interval calculated as $175 - (1.645)(102)$ would have a lower limit of 7.2, thus excluding 0. With the one-tailed boundary for α, both methods (the P value and confidence interval) would lead to rejection of the null hypothesis and a stochastic proclamation of "significance."

11.12.3   Descriptive Boundaries

Perhaps the only way to avoid a boundary for stochastic decisions about "significance" is to convert the focus of the decision. Instead of examining *probabilities* for events that might happen when the data are rearranged, we might directly inspect the *descriptive* possibilities.

For example, suppose we set **300** as the lowest value of δ for quantitatively significant increment between two groups. With this boundary, an observed value below δ would not be dismissed if a reasonable rearrangement would bring the results above δ. With this approach, the observed value of 175 in the foregoing example would be regarded as "nonsignificant" if the stochastic α was set at the two-tailed value of .05. On the other hand, with a reasonable rearrangement of the data (in this instance, using a 95% confidence interval), the value of $\delta = 300$ would be included in the zone of -25 to 375. The observed increment, despite its failure to pass the stochastic hurdle of "significance," could *not* be dismissed as insignificant.

If the stochastic α had the one-tailed value of .1, however, the increment of 175 would be regarded as "significant." Nevertheless, if we set **30** as the highest descriptive boundary of ζ for a quantitatively *insignificant* difference, the one-tailed 95% confidence interval that extends from 7.2 to 343 would include the **30** value for ζ (as well as the **300** value for δ). This interval would be too descriptively unstable for a decision in either direction.

To replace stochastic boundaries by descriptive boundaries would make things much more complex than their current state. We would have to choose not only descriptive boundaries for both δ and ζ, but also a method for rearranging the data. The "fragility" technique of unitary removals and relocations offers a method that can avoid hypothesis testing, P values, and choices of α, while producing a result analogous to a confidence interval.

Although an approach based on *descriptive* boundaries seems worthwhile and scientifically desirable, it departs from the established paradigms and involves many acts of judgment about which consensus would not be easily attained. Consequently, the entrenched boundaries of α— which are entrenched only because they got there first — are likely to be retained for many years in the future. You might as well get accustomed to their current hegemony, because you will have to live with it until scientific investigators decide to confront the basic descriptive challenges and create a new paradigm for the evaluations.

References

1. Feinstein, 1996; 2. Feinstein, 1990; 3. Walter, 1991; 4. Kendall, 1951, pg. 171; 5. Cochran, 1950; 6. Morrison, 1970; 7. Berry, 1993; 8. Brophy, 1995; 9. Ashby, 1993; 10. Whitehead, 1993; 11. Fisher, 1925; 12. Box, J.F., 1978; 13. Fisher, 1959.

Exercises

11.1. In a properly designed laboratory experiment, an investigator finds the following results in appropriately measured units:

Group A: 1, 12, 14, 16, 17, 17

Group B: 19, 29, 31, 33, 34, 125

The difference in mean values, $\overline{X}_A = 12.8$ vs. $\overline{X}_B = 45.2$, seems highly impressive, but the investigator is chagrined that the t test (discussed in Chapter 13) is not stochastically significant, presumably because of the particularly high variability in Group B. What relatively *simple* procedure (i.e., no calculations) might the investigator do to get evidence that the distinction in the two groups is stable enough to be persuasive?

11.2. In Section 1.1.3, the quantitative contrast between 8/16 and 6/18 seemed quantitatively impressive because the increment of $.500 - .333 = .167$ seemed reasonably large. How would you interpret the results of a unit fragility test for this comparison?

11.3. In the examples cited in this chapter, when the observed result turned out to be "nonsignificant," the *upper* end of the confidence interval was examined as a possibly "significant" value. In what "nonsignificant" circumstance would you want to examine the *lower* end of the confidence interval as a possibly significant value?

11.4. Although you may not yet have had much pragmatic experience in testing stochastic hypotheses, you have probably had some "gut reactions" to the controversy about using one-tailed or two-tailed criteria for P values. What are those reactions and what policy would you establish if you were appointed supreme czar of stochastic testing?

11.5. These questions refer to the choice of $\alpha = .05$ as the boundary for customary decisions about stochastic significance.

    11.5.1.   Are you content with this boundary? If so, why? If not, why not, and what replacement would you offer?

    11.5.2.   In what kind of circumstance would you want to change the value of α to a more "lenient" boundary, such as .1 or perhaps .2?

    11.5.3.   In what kind of circumstance would you want a more strict boundary, such as .01 or .001?

    11.5.4.   What would be the main pragmatic consequences of either raising or lowering the customary value of α? How would it affect the sample sizes and costs of research? How would it affect the credibility of the results?

11.6. About two decades ago, the editor of a prominent journal of psychology stated that he wanted to improve the scientific quality of the published research. He therefore changed the journal's policy from using $\alpha = .05$ for accepting statistical claims, and said that henceforth no research would be published unless the P values were <.01. How effective do you think this policy would be in achieving the stated goal? What kind of research do you think would be most affected by the new policy?

11.7. Here is an interesting optional exercise if you have time. In Section 11.10.1, we noted that the chance of getting two consecutive **7**'s in two tosses of dice was .03, and that the chance of not getting a **7** in two tosses was .69. These two apparently opposite probabilities do not add up to 1. Why not?

12

Permutation Rearrangements: Fisher Exact and Pitman–Welch Tests

CONTENTS

Of the main methods that rearrange two groups of data for stochastic tests, permutation procedures are particularly easy to understand. Unlike parametric methods, no theoretical assumptions are required about hypothetical populations, parameters, pooled variances, or mathematical model distributions; and unlike jackknife or relocation methods, the process involves no arbitrary removals or displacements. Everything that happens emerges directly from the empirically observed data. Furthermore, for contrasts of two groups, a permutation procedure is not merely statistically "respectable"; it is often the "gold standard" for checking results of other stochastic procedures.

The permutation strategy relies on the idea that when two groups of observed data are compared under the null hypothesis, the data can be pooled into a single larger group. The entire larger group is then permuted into all possible rearrangements that assign the data into batches of two groups of appropriate size. The results in the rearranged groups form a distribution that can be evaluated for P values and, if desired, for a counterpart of confidence intervals.

The best known permutation arrangement procedure, discussed in this chapter, is called the *Fisher exact probability test*. It was first proposed by R. A. Fisher[1] in 1934 and amplified by J. O. Irwin[2] in 1935. The eponym often cited is the *Fisher–Irwin test*, *Fisher exact test*, or *Fisher test*, although the last term may sometimes be ambiguous because Fisher also devised so many other procedures.

12.1 Illustrative Example

Suppose an investigator finds that the success rates in a clinical trial are 75% for new Treatment A and 33% for old Treatment B. The ratio of .75/.33 is 2.27; the direct increment is $.75 - .33 = .42$; the number needed to treat is 2.4; the proportional increment is $(.75 - .33)/.33 = 127\%$; and the odds ratio is $(.75/.33) \times (.67/.25) = 6.1$.

All of these quantitative comparisons are highly impressive and would strongly support the investigator's claim that the distinction is quantitatively significant. On the other hand, if the actual sources of the observed numbers were 3/4 vs. 1/3, the claim might be instantly rejected. With so few people under study, the observed distinction could be merely a "fluke," arising from chance alone, even if the two treatments are identical in the long run. Our quantitative enthusiasm would be overridden by our stochastic skepticism.

If the proportions of .75 and .33 arose from 450/600 vs. 200/600, however, we would have no problem in accepting the idea that the quantitatively significant difference is also stochastically significant. Chance alone could hardly be responsible for the observed increment when the groups are this large. (In fact, as we shall see later, the P value for this distinction is less than one in a million if the two treatments are really equivalent.)

With many other sets of data, however, the result of the stochastic contrast for .75 vs. .33 would not be evident "by eye," and would be more difficult to evaluate. Such contrasts might occur if the numbers were 9/12 vs. 5/15, or 3/4 vs. 100/300, or 150/200 vs. 1/3. In these situations, the indexes of contrast would have the same quantitatively significant values previously noted for the increment, ratio, NNE, proportional increment, and odds ratio. We would not immediately be able to decide, however, whether the distinction is stochastically significant.

The Fisher Exact Test, which is a valuable method for making the stochastic decisions, will be first illustrated for the comparison of 3/4 vs. 1/3. (With larger numbers, an unwieldy amount of tabulation is needed to show all the possibilities.)

12.2 Formation of Null Hypothesis

We begin by assuming that the two treatments are equivalent, i.e., $T_A \backsimeq T_B$. With this assumption, the seven people who were treated in the two groups should have had exactly the same outcome, whether they received Treatment A or B. If we identify those seven people individually with the letters a, b, c, d, e, f, and g, their results can be listed as follows for the 3/4 success rate in Treatment A and 1/3 in Treatment B:

Treatment A		Treatment B	
Person	Outcome	Person	Outcome
a	Sucess	*e*	Sucess
b	Sucess	f	Failure
c	Sucess	g	Failure
d	Failure		

Persons *a*, *b*, *c*, and *e* are shown in italics to indicate that they were the successful members of the groups. The others—d, f, and g—were failures. According to the null hypothesis, each person's outcome would have been the same whether treated with A or B.

12.3 Rearrangements of Observed Population

In the combined data, seven people were originally divided so that four (*a*, *b*, *c*, and d) were in one group and three (*e*, f, and g) were in the other. The seven people could have been divided in many other ways, however, while preserving an arrangement that gives Treatment A to four people and Treatment B to three. With a complete permutation of the data, we can see all of the possible ways in which this arrangement can occur, and we can determine their effects on the observed results. The arrangements are shown in Table 12.1, which you should examine carefully.

The first line of Table 12.1 shows the original observations. The remaining 34 lines show all the other possible arrangements that contain four persons in Group A and three in Group B. Each arrangement is accompanied by the corresponding success rates that would be found in Groups A and B, and by the incremental difference in the two rates.

The results of the 35 arrangements in Table 12.1 are summarized in Table 12.2. Of those 35 arrangements, one would have produced an increment of 100% in favor of A; twelve would have produced an increment of 42% in favor of A; eighteen would have produced an increment of 17% in favor of B; and four would have produced an increment of 75% in favor of B. If we happened to pick one of those 35 arrangements randomly, the chances are .029 (= 1/35) that the increment would be 100%, .343 (= 12/35) that the increment would be 42%, .514 (= 18/35) for an increment of −17%, and .114 (= 4/35) for −75%. The chances of getting an increment as large as the one we observed in favor of A, or even larger, would therefore be .029 + .343 = .372. The chance of getting an increment that is smaller than what was observed (or even negative) would be

TABLE 12.1

Complete Permutation Distribution of Data for Two Groups with Success Rates 3/4 vs. 1/3

Identification of Arrangement	People in Treatment A	People in Treatment B	Success Rates for: A	B	Incremental Difference of A − B
1	a,b,c,d	e,f,g	3/4 (75%)	1/3 (33%)	42%
2	a,b,c,e	d,f,g	4/4 (100%)	0/3 (0%)	100%
3	a,b,c,f	d,e,g	3/4 (75%)	1/3 (33%)	42%
4	a,b,c,g	d,e,f	3/4 (75%)	1/3 (33%)	42%
5	a,b,d,e	c,f,g	3/4 (75%)	1/3 (33%)	42%
6	a,b,d,f	c,e,g	2/4 (50%)	2/3 (67%)	−17%
7	a,b,d,g	c,e,f	2/4 (50%)	2/3 (67%)	−17%
8	a,b,e,f	c,d,g	3/4 (75%)	1/3 (33%)	42%
9	a,b,e,g	c,d,f	3/4 (75%)	1/3 (33%)	42%
10	a,b,f,g	c,d,e	2/4 (50%)	2/3 (67%)	−17%
11	a,c,d,e	b,f,g	3/4 (75%)	1/3 (33%)	42%
12	a,c,d,f	b,e,g	2/4 (50%)	2/3 (67%)	−17%
13	a,c,d,g	b,e,f	2/4 (50%)	2/3 (67%)	−17%
14	a,c,e,f	b,d,g	3/4 (75%)	1/3 (33%)	42%
15	a,c,e,g	b,d,f	3/4 (75%)	1/3 (33%)	42%
16	a,c,f,g	b,d,e	2/4 (50%)	2/3 (67%)	−17%
17	a,d,e,f	b,c,g	2/4 (50%)	2/3 (67%)	−17%
18	a,d,e,g	b,c,f	2/4 (50%)	2/3 (67%)	−17%
19	a,d,f,g	b,c,e	1/4 (25%)	3/3 (100%)	−75%
20	a,e,f,g	b,c,d	2/4 (50%)	2/3 (67%)	−17%
21	b,c,d,e	a,f,g	3/4 (75%)	1/3 (33%)	42%
22	b,c,d,f	a,e,g	2/4 (50%)	2/3 (67%)	−17%
23	b,c,d,g	a,e,f	2/4 (50%)	2/3 (67%)	−17%
24	b,c,e,f	a,d,g	3/4 (75%)	1/3 (33%)	42%
25	b,c,e,g	a,d,f	3/4 (75%)	1/3 (33%)	42%
26	b,c,f,g	a,d,e	2/4 (50%)	2/3 (67%)	−17%
27	b,d,e,f	a,c,g	2/4 (50%)	2/3 (67%)	−17%
28	b,d,e,g	a,c,f	2/4 (50%)	2/3 (67%)	−17%
29	b,d,f,g	a,c,e	1/4 (25%)	3/3 (100%)	−75%
30	b,e,f,g	a,c,d	2/4 (50%)	2/3 (67%)	−17%
31	c,d,e,f	a,b,g	2/4 (50%)	2/3 (67%)	−17%
32	c,d,e,g	a,b,f	2/4 (50%)	2/3 (67%)	−17%
33	c,d,f,g	a,b,e	1/4 (25%)	3/3 (100%)	−75%
34	c,e,f,g	a,b,d	2/4 (50%)	2/3 (67%)	−17%
35	d,e,f,g	a,b,c	1/4 (25%)	3/3 (100%)	−75%

.514 + .114 = .628. For the two-tailed probability of getting an increment of $\geq 42\%$ in either direction, the chance is .029 + .343 + .114 = .486 or 17/35.

TABLE 12.2

Summary of Results in Table 12.1

Success Rates for:		Increment A–B	No. of Arrangements	Identification of Arrangements in Table 12.1
Treatment A	Treatment B			
4/4 (*100%*)	0/3 (*0%*)	100%	1	2
3/4 (*75%*)	1/3 (*33%*)	42%	12	1,3,4,5,8,9,11,14,15,21,24,25
2/4 (*50%*)	2/3 (*67%*)	–17%	18	6,7,10,12,13,16,17,18,20,22, 23,26,27,28,30,31,32,34
1/4 (*25%*)	3/3 (*100%*)	–75%	4	19,29,33,35

12.4 Probability Values

With the concepts and results of the previous two sections, we can set up the following table of relative frequencies or probabilities for each of the possible outcomes.

Distinction in Outcome	Probability
A is 100% better than B	$p_1 = 1/35 = 0.029$
A is 42% better than B	$p_2 = 12/35 = 0.343$
B is 17% better than A	$p_3 = 18/35 = 0.514$
B is 75% better than A	$p_4 = 4/35 = 0.114$
	TOTAL = 1.000

Note that the sum of these four probabilities is 1.000, although sometimes the sums of the total probabilities in a permutation distribution may be slightly different from 1 because of rounding errors. Thus, if we listed the foregoing probabilities in two decimal places rather than three, the sum would be .03 + .34 + .51 + .11 = .99.

For stochastic considerations, we contemplate the full external rather than isolated individual probability of an event. As discussed earlier, the *external probability* consists of the observed individual probability, plus the probability of getting an event that is more extreme. In the foregoing table of events, the first outcome is more extreme than the second in the same direction. Thus, the external probability of having Treatment A exceed Treatment B by at least 42% is the sum of the first and the second probabilities. A capital P is usually used for this purpose, and we could write (for the cited event) $P = p_1 + p_2 = .029 + .343 = .372$.

If we have no preconception that one treatment is better than the other, we would want to know the two-tailed external probability values for chances that either one of the two treatments is superior by an increment as high as 42%. To answer this question, we would include not only the probabilities p_1 and p_2, but also p_4, from the "other side" of the results, where B would be 75% better than A. The two-tailed probability that a difference of 42% (or greater) might arise by chance is thus $2P = \Sigma(p_1 + p_2 + p_4)$ = .029 + .343 + .114 = .486. [The odds in this clinical trial would be about "even money" that if the two treatments are equivalent, one of them will appear to be at least 42% better than the other.]

The interpretation of the P values will depend on the level and direction set for α. In the foregoing comparison of Treatments A and B, the 100% difference of 4/4 vs. 0/3, with its P value of .029, would be stochastically significant if α were set at .05 but not at .02 or .01.

12.5 Simplifying Calculations

Except for arbitrary decisions about the level of α and the unilateral or bilateral directions of P, the foregoing activities were quite straightforward. We were able to determine the exact value of P by considering all the permutation patterns that could have occurred in the actual, observed data. The procedure has one major disadvantage, however: it can be a nuisance to do if all of the possible combinations must be individually prepared, tabulated, analyzed, and counted. Fortunately, the calculations can be greatly simplified by using the numbers of permutations and combinations of a group of objects.

12.5.1 Formulas for Permutations and Combinations

From the earlier discussion in Section 8.4.2.2, you may recall that a total of n objects can be permuted into n! sequential arrangements, where $n! = (n)(n-1)(n-2)(n-3)...(1)$. This "sequential" permutation can then be converted into "consequential" combinations indicating the number of ways in which r items can be selected from n items. The formula is

$$\binom{n}{r} = \frac{n!}{r!(n-r)!}.$$

For a simple example, consider the number of combinations of two letters that could be chosen from the four letters *a*, *b*, *c*, *d*. The first choice could be done in four ways and the second in three, making $4 \times 3 = 12$ possible pairs. Each of those pairs can be permuted in $2 \times 1 = 2$ ways. There are thus $12/2 = 6$ possible combinations. From the formula for combinations, we would find this number as $4!/[(2!)(2!)] = 6$. To verify the process, we can list the six possibilities: *ab*, *ac*, *ad*, *bc*, *bd*, and *cd*.

Note that the formula of $n!/[r!(n-r)!]$ indicates the number of ways in which we can select r items from a group containing n items. If we want to know about the remaining group that contains the "residue" of $n - r$ items, we do not need a second formula, because the contents of that group will always be uniquely determined after the first group is chosen. Thus, if we choose the letters *b*, *c*, *e*, and *g* from a group containing *a*, *b*, *c*, *d*, *e*, *f*, and *g*, the remaining second group will be *a*, *d*, and *f*. Therefore, the formula $n!/[r!(n-r)!]$ will indicate the number of ways in which we can divide n objects into two groups, one containing r members, and the other containing $n - r$ members.

12.5.2 Application to the Fisher Exact Test

The formula for combinations can be used to simplify calculations for the Fisher Exact Probability test. With the two proportions, 3/4 vs. 1/3, we first determine the number of ways of dividing seven people into two groups, containing four people in one group and three in the other. The result is $7!/(4! \times 3!) = 5040/(24 \times 6) = 35$. This is the quick way of determining that 35 arrangements are possible for Table 12.1.

Next, we consider each of the four possible tabular arrangements for success and failure, preserving the "marginal totals" of four successes (S) and three failures (F), with four people in Treatment A and three people in Treatment B. The four possible tables are as follows:

	I		II		III		IV		
	S	F	S	F	S	F	S	F	Total
Treatment A	4	0	3	1	2	2	1	3	4
Treatment B	0	3	1	2	2	1	3	0	3
TOTAL	4	3	4	3	4	3	4	3	7

In each of the four tables just cited, the marginal totals are identical, but the cells differ internally. These are the four tables whose distinctive outcomes were summarized in Sections 12.3 and 12.4.

In each of the foregoing tables, we also have to consider the distribution of the four successful and three unsuccessful patients. Table II contained three successes in one treatment and one success in the other. This arrangement could be done in $4!/(3! \times 1!) = 4$ ways. Simultaneously, the three failure patients would have to be distributed so that two were in one treatment and one in the other. This arrangement could be done in $3!/(2! \times 1!) = 3$ ways. Consequently, Table II could be prepared in $4 \times 3 = 12$ ways.

Analogously, for Table III, the successful patients could be divided in $4!/(2! \times 2!) = 6$ ways and the failures in $3!/(2! \times 1!) = 3$ ways, so that this table could be formed in $6 \times 3 = 18$ ways. For Table IV, the number of possibilities would be $[4!/(3! \times 1!)] \times [3!/(3! \times 0!)] = 4 \times 1 = 4$ ways; and for Table I, the number of possibilities is $[4!/(4! \times 0!)] \times [3!/(3! \times 0!)] = 1 \times 1 = 1$ way. These calculations have produced the same frequencies that were determined previously from the long listing in Table 12.1. The summary of those frequencies in Table 12.2 showed 1, 12, 18, and 4 ways of getting the four respective tables, I, II, III, and IV.

12.6   General Formula for Fisher Exact Test

To develop the general formula for the Fisher Exact Test, suppose a total of N people have been divided so that n_1 are treated with A and n_2 are treated with B. The total number of possible arrangements for those people — preserving n_1 in one group and n_2 in the other — is $N!/[(n_1!) (N-n_1)!] = N!/(n_1!)(n_2!) = N!/(n_1!n_2!)$.

Now suppose that f_1 of the people were post-therapeutic successes and f_2 were failures (where $f_1 + f_2 = N$). The marginal totals of the table will be as follows:

	Success	Failure	Total
Treatment A			n_1
Treatment B			n_2
TOTAL	f_1	f_2	N

Two of the marginal totals — n_1 and n_2 — are fixed by the decision to maintain the original arrangement, which had n_1 members in one group and n_2 in the other. We thus have $N!/(n_1!n_2!)$ ways of achieving the basic arrangement. The other two marginal totals — f_1 and f_2 — are unchangingly fixed by our null hypothesis that the two treatments have identical effects. The remaining room for variation thus occurs among the four cells — a, b, c, d — of the table, which can now be fully shown as follows:

	Success	Failure	Total
Treatment A	a	b	n_1
Treatment B	c	d	n_2
TOTAL	f_1	f_2	N

[Note that a, b, c, d here refer to numbers of people in the four cells of this table. These are *not* the individual people who were labeled for discussion in Section 12.2.] The f_1 people who are successes can be arranged in $f_1!/a!c!$ ways, and the f_2 people who are failures can be arranged as $f_2!/b!d!$. The total number of possible arrangements for successes and failures in this particular table is thus

$$\frac{f_1!}{a!c!} \times \frac{f_2!}{b!d!}.$$

If we want to know the probability of getting this particular table among all the possible tables that could have been obtained, we divide the foregoing number by $N!/n_1!n_2!$. The result is

$$\frac{\dfrac{f_1!}{a!c!} \times \dfrac{f_2!}{b!d!}}{\dfrac{N!}{n_1!n_2!}}$$

Rearranging terms, we get

$$p_i = \frac{f_1!f_2!n_1!n_2!}{a!b!c!d!N!} \qquad [12.1]$$

where the subscript i on p_i denotes the particular table that is being considered. To get the remainder of the probabilities, the remaining tables must be examined in the appropriate directions. Because the marginal totals remain fixed throughout, the term $f_1!\, f_2!\, n_1!\, n_2!/N!$ will be the same for each table. It can be calculated separately for the first table and then used repeatedly thereafter. The pattern of probabilities in the sequence of tables is sometimes called the *hypergeometric distribution*.

12.6.1   Another Example of Calculations

In a clinical trial, Treatment C had a success rate of 1/5 (20%), whereas Treatment D had a success rate of 4/6 (67%). What is the likelihood that the difference arose by chance if the two treatments are actually identical?

To answer this question with the Fisher test, the observed results are first arranged as

	Success	Failure	Total
Treatment C	1	4	5
Treatment D	4	2	6
TOTAL	5	6	11

The "direction" of these results shows an incremental success rate of 47% (= 67% − 20%) in favor of Treatment D. Keeping the marginal totals fixed, we now want to look in two different "directions" to see what other tables can be constructed with an incremental success rate of 47% or higher. Looking in the same "direction," we seek results where the increment of ≥ 7% is in favor of Treatment D. If the observed table is abbreviated as $\begin{Bmatrix} 1 & 4 \\ 4 & 2 \end{Bmatrix}$, the second, third, and fourth tables with similar or more extreme results in the same and in opposite directions are:

$$\begin{Bmatrix} 0 & 5 \\ 5 & 1 \end{Bmatrix} \qquad \begin{Bmatrix} 5 & 0 \\ 0 & 6 \end{Bmatrix} \qquad \begin{Bmatrix} 4 & 1 \\ 1 & 5 \end{Bmatrix}$$

| SAME DIRECTION (0% vs. 83%) | OPPOSITE DIRECTION (100% vs. 0%) | OPPOSITE DIRECTION (80% vs. 17%) |

The p value for the original table is $(5!\ 6!\ 5!\ 6!)/(1!\ 4!\ 4!\ 2!\ 11!) = 1.870129870 \times 10^2/(1!\ 4!\ 4!\ 2!) = 0.162$. If we let $1.870129870 \times 10^2 = k$, the p value for the second table is $k/(0!\ 5!\ 5!\ 1!) = 0.013$. The p value for the third table is $k/(0!\ 5!\ 6!\ 0!) = .002$. The p value for the fourth table is $k/(1!\ 4!\ 5!\ 1!) = 0.065$.

Consequently, the one-tailed P value in the same direction is $0.162 + 0.013 = 0.175$. (It covers the observed result plus another that is more extreme.) The P value on the other side is $.002 + .065 = .067$. The two-tailed P value is $0.175 + .067 = 0.242$.

12.6.2   Additional Considerations

Several other things will be helpful if you do the calculations for a Fisher Exact Test yourself, or if you want to check whether a computer program does them correctly. [Sometimes a "locally constructed" computer program does things wrong by getting the allegedly 2-tailed P value either from only the observed table or from the observed table plus only the others that are more extreme in the same direction].

12.6.2.1   *Total Number of Examined Tables* — The total number of tables that can be examined is one more than the smallest of the four marginal totals. Thus, if f_1 is the smallest number of the marginal values, the total number of tables is $f_1 + 1$.

For example, suppose the original table is $\left\{ \begin{smallmatrix} 4 & 2 \\ 8 & 17 \end{smallmatrix} \right\}$. The marginal totals here are 6, 25, 12, and 19, so that 6 is the smallest marginal value. According to the "formula," we would expect a total of 7 tables. They are as follows:

$$\left\{ \begin{array}{cc} 6 & 0 \\ 6 & 19 \end{array} \right\} \left\{ \begin{array}{cc} 5 & 1 \\ 7 & 18 \end{array} \right\} \left\{ \begin{array}{cc} 4 & 2 \\ 8 & 17 \end{array} \right\} \left\{ \begin{array}{cc} 3 & 3 \\ 9 & 16 \end{array} \right\} \left\{ \begin{array}{cc} 2 & 4 \\ 10 & 15 \end{array} \right\} \left\{ \begin{array}{cc} 1 & 5 \\ 11 & 14 \end{array} \right\} \left\{ \begin{array}{cc} 0 & 6 \\ 12 & 13 \end{array} \right\}$$

The reason for $f_1 + 1$ tables is that we can start with one table having f_1 and 0 in one row; we then form additional f_1 tables until reaching the opposite arrangement (0 and f_1) as the endpoint in that row.

12.6.2.2   *Number of Same-Direction Tables* — If we simply want to determine how many additional tables will give us a more extreme result *in the same direction*, the answer is the smallest number in any of the four cells. The reason is that our quest toward the extreme direction will make this smallest number even smaller and the quest will end when the number reaches 0.

Thus, if we start with the table $\left\{ \begin{smallmatrix} 4 & 2 \\ 8 & 17 \end{smallmatrix} \right\}$, there will be two tables that are more extreme in the same direction. They are $\left\{ \begin{smallmatrix} 5 & 1 \\ 7 & 18 \end{smallmatrix} \right\}$ and $\left\{ \begin{smallmatrix} 6 & 0 \\ 6 & 19 \end{smallmatrix} \right\}$.

12.6.2.3   *Two-Tailed Calculations* — In the procedures described earlier, we had to determine and calculate the tables separately for each "tail" of probability. This process is necessary whenever the two items in each pair of marginal totals are unequal, i.e., $f_1 \neq f_2$ *and* $n_1 \neq n_2$. If either one of these pairs has equal members, i.e., $f_1 = f_2$ or $n_1 = n_2$, the two tails of probability will be symmetrical, and the two-tailed P value can be determined merely by finding the one-tailed value and doubling it.

For example, suppose the table under consideration is

	Success	Failure	Total
Treatment E	10	3	13
Treatment F	5	8	13
TOTAL	15	11	26

The more extreme tables in the same direction are:

$$\left\{ \begin{array}{cc} 13 & 0 \\ 2 & 11 \end{array} \right\} \left\{ \begin{array}{cc} 12 & 1 \\ 3 & 10 \end{array} \right\} \left\{ \begin{array}{cc} 11 & 2 \\ 4 & 9 \end{array} \right\}$$

The analogous tables in the opposite direction are:

$$\left\{ \begin{array}{cc} 2 & 11 \\ 13 & 0 \end{array} \right\} \left\{ \begin{array}{cc} 3 & 10 \\ 12 & 1 \end{array} \right\} \left\{ \begin{array}{cc} 4 & 9 \\ 11 & 2 \end{array} \right\} \left\{ \begin{array}{cc} 5 & 8 \\ 10 & 3 \end{array} \right\}$$

The latter set of tables has the same interior cells as the first four tables and will yield the same individual p_i values.

12.6.2.4   *Two-Tailed Stopping Point* —

If $n_1 \neq n_2$ and $f_1 \neq f_2$, the tables in the opposite direction must be examined separately to find the one for which the absolute difference in proportions begins to be less than what was observed originally.

For example, in Section 12.6.1, the values of 4/6 vs. 1/5 had a difference of 47%. In the opposite direction, a difference of 47% or larger was noted for two sets of results: 1/6 vs. 4/5 and 0/6 vs. 5/5. The latter two tables would be the ones whose individual p_i values would be added to provide the P component for the "tail" on the other side.

An algebraic formula can be developed to establish the particular table where the stopping point occurs on the other side. For the general $\begin{Bmatrix} a & b \\ c & d \end{Bmatrix}$ table shown in Section 12.6, suppose that the two proportions under comparison are a/n_1 and c/n_2. Suppose also that $a/n_1 > c/n_2$, so that $(a/n_1) - (c/n_2) = e$, where e is a positive number. Since $f_1 = a + c$, it can be shown algebraically that $e = (Na - n_1f_1)/n_1n_2$. When we examine the other tail, the corresponding cells will be a′, b′, c′, and d′, and we shall want to have $(c'/n_2) - (a'/n_1) \geq e$. Substituting the previous value of e into the latter equation, substituting $f_1 = a' + c'$, and working out the algebra, we get

$$a' \leq \frac{2n_1f_1}{N} - a$$

To show how this formula works, consider the previous table $\begin{Bmatrix} 4 & 2 \\ 8 & 17 \end{Bmatrix}$. The increment in the original proportions under comparison is $(4/6) - (8/25) = .35$, where $a = 4$, $n_1 = 6$, $c = 8$, $n_2 = 25$, $f_1 = 12$, and $N = 31$. To find the value of a′ on the "other side" of the tables, we calculate $a' \leq [(2)(6)(12)/31] - 4 = 4.65 - 4 = 0.65$. Thus, a′ must be less than 0.65, and its only possible integer value would be 0. To prove this point, the table $\begin{Bmatrix} 0 & 6 \\ 12 & 13 \end{Bmatrix}$ shows an increment of $(0/6) - (12/25) = 0 - .48 = -.48$; and the next table $\begin{Bmatrix} 1 & 5 \\ 11 & 14 \end{Bmatrix}$ shows an increment of $(1/6) - (11/25) = .167 - .44 = -.27$, which is smaller in absolute magnitude than the observed increment of .35. Consequently, the other tail contains only one table to be examined.

12.6.2.5   *Limitation of Hand Calculators* —

With today's electronic hand calculators, the largest number that can be managed is 10×10^{99}, which usually appears as "10 E 99." Consequently, the largest manageable value of n! is $69! = 1.7112 \times 10^{98}$. Because of this limitation, the Fisher Exact Test cannot be done directly on a hand calculator if the total group size is ≥ 70.

There are various ways to trick the machine. For example, suppose $N = 75$ in Formula [12.1], but all other numbers are ≤ 69. You can first get $f_1!$, then divide by a!, then multiply by $f_2!$, then divide by b!, and so on, going "up and down" to keep the result relatively small. When you reach the division by 75!, do not use it directly. Instead, divide by 69!, and then do repeat subsequent individual divisions by 70, 71, 72,..., 75. In the B.E.C. (before electronic computation) era, the entire calculation was done by using the logarithms of n!, which are still available in handbooks of scientific or statistical tables. Today, however, if a Fisher Exact Test is sought for a sample size ≥ 70, the best approach is to go directly to the capacity of a digital computer, rather than trying to use a hand calculator.

Even if $N \leq 69$, however, you may still need to arrange for an oscillating rather than direct computational process to avoid exceeding a value of 10×10^{99}. Instead of multiplying $f_1! \, f_2! \, n_1! \, n_2!$ to get the numerator, and then dividing by each term in the denominator, you can oscillate the calculational sequence as $f_1!/N! \times f_2!/a! \times n_1!/b!$ and so on.

12.7   Application of Fisher Test

The Fisher exact probability test can be applied to any comparison of two proportions. They will form a "fourfold" or 2×2 table whose rearrangements can then be developed. The Fisher test is particularly valuable for tables having "small" numbers in the cells. For tables with "large" numbers, almost identical two-tailed P values will be produced by the chi-square test (discussed in Chapter 14), which is usually preferred because it is easier to calculate.

12.7.1   Small Numbers

The criteria for demarcating "small" and "large" numbers, as noted later in Chapter 14, vary with recommendations from different statistical authorities. Because the Fisher test is the "gold standard," its use in all situations (particularly if a computer is available to do the calculations) will help avoid worries or disputes about what is *small* or *large*. If you think (or suspect) that the numbers in any cell are small, the chi-square test may be unreliable (and its "corrections" are controversial); and so the Fisher test should definitely be used.

12.7.2   One-Tailed Tests

Because the chi-square test produces a two-tailed P value, the Fisher test should also be used if you want a one-tailed P value for data in which you suspect that the two tails are not symmetrical.

12.7.3   Controversy about "Fixed" or "Random" Marginals

Although any 2×2 table can be submitted to a Fisher test, the particular proportions being compared can be constructed in different ways. Consider the fourfold table $\begin{Bmatrix} a & b \\ c & d \end{Bmatrix}$ with the n_1, n_2 row totals and f_1, f_2 column totals shown in Section 12.6. In a randomized trial, we set fixed values of n_1 and n_2, but values of f_1 and f_2 emerge from the trial. In a case-control study, where groups are chosen from the outcome events, we fix the values of f_1 and f_2, but the n_1 and n_2 values emerge from the ascertainment process. In a general community cross-sectional survey, we fix the value of N, but the marginal totals of n_1, n_2, f_1, and f_2 emerge from the results of the survey.

These three different ways of getting "fixed" or "random" values of the marginal totals have led to a statistical dispute about whether all four observed marginal totals are appropriately regarded as "fixed" in the Fisher test and also in the chi-square test. The controversy has been useful for generating graduate-school theses in statistics, but can otherwise be generally ignored. For pragmatic scientific purposes, the four marginal totals can be regarded as fixed; and the Fisher test calculations can be done as previously described.

12.8   "Confidence Intervals" from Fisher Test

In the customary Gaussian construction (discussed in Chapter 13), a confidence interval is placed symmetrically around the observed increment of the two central indexes. In the Fisher test, however, a standard error is not determined to allow use of the Gaussian procedure. Nevertheless, an inner percentile zone that corresponds to a confidence interval can be determined directly from the array of sequential tables in the Fisher Exact Test.

The array of tables indicates the potential spread of data for proportions contrasted under the null hypothesis. The associated p_i value of probability for each table indicates the relative frequency of the corresponding increment in proportions $p_A - p_B$ in the total distribution. Addition of the p_i values in both directions for adjacent tables produces an inner zone of probability. The values of the $p_A - p_B$ increments at the ends of the selected zone will then correspond to the limits of a confidence interval. It will surround the null hypothesis, rather than the observed increment, but it will offer exact boundaries for a demarcated zone of potential increments.

Furthermore, if the analyst wants to know about the occurrence of increments more extreme than the observed value, an exact probability can be found by adding the appropriate p_i's in the Fisher tables. Consequently, the tabular components of the Fisher procedure offer both an empirical and inferential method for stochastic decisions. From the permuted rearrangement of the observed data, the analyst can determine exactly what has happened or might have happened.

For example, consider the stochastic contrast of $18/24 = .75$ vs. $10/15 = .67$. The 2×2 table for this comparison is

$$
\begin{array}{cc|c}
18 & 6 & 24 \\
10 & 5 & 15 \\
\hline
28 & 11 & 39
\end{array}
$$

Because 11 is the smallest marginal total, the Fisher test will involve an examination of 12 tables. The extreme ends are shown in Table 12.3.

TABLE 12.3

Extreme Ends of array of Tables for Fisher Exact Probability Test of $18/24 = .75$ vs. $10/15 = .67$

Table Number	I		II		III		...	VIII		IX		X		XI		XII	
Constituents ⎰	13	11	14	10	15	9	...	20	4	21	3	22	2	23	1	24	0
⎱	15	0	14	1	13	2	...	8	7	7	8	6	9	5	10	4	11
Value of p_A	.542		.583		.625		...	.833		.875		.917		.958		1.0000	
Value of p_B	1.000		.933		.867		...	.533		.467		.400		.333		.267	
Value of $p_A - p_B$	−.458		−.350		−.242		...	.300		.408		.517		.625		.733	
Value of Fisher p_i	.0014		.018		.082		...	.041		.0078		8.2×10^{-4}		4.3×10^{-5}		8.0×10^{-7}	

A reasonably symmetrical 95% confidence interval will extend to the locations where the sums of p_i values exceed .95 for the interior tables or, alternatively, where the probability sums =.025 for the tables in each tail. Because of the discrete values of p_i for each of the constructed tables, the sums may not add up exactly to .025 in each tail. In the array of Table 12.3, the best boundaries occur at Table II, for which $p_2 = .018$, and at Table IX, for which $p_9 = .0078$. The sum of the extreme probabilities is $.0014 + .018 = .0194$ for Tables I and II, and, on the other end, $8.66 \times 10^{-3} = .00866$ for Tables IX through XII. The total external probability is $.0194 + .00866 = .028$. In the two interior tables (III and VIII) that are demarcated within the outer boundaries, the corresponding values of the increments for $p_A - p_B$ are −.242 and .300. Thus, the zone created by the boundaries of −.242 to +.300 occupies 97.2% of the potential increments. (The p_i values for the remaining tables, not shown in Table 12.3, are $p_4 = .200$, $p_5 = .282$, $p_6 = .241$, and $p_7 = .127$. The total spanned by the individual probabilites in Tables III through VIII is .972.)

As a more simple example, the data in the clinical trial of Section 12.6.1 would have the following rearrangements in the Fisher test.

Compared Proportion	Increment	p_i value
0/5 vs. 5/6	−83%	.013
1/5 vs. 4/6	−47%	.162
2/5 vs. 3/6	−10%	.433
3/5 vs. 2/6	27%	.325
4/5 vs. 1/6	63%	.065
5/5 vs. 0/6	100%	.002

The zone from −10% to 27% will cover $.433 + .325 = .758$ or about 75% of the possible increments. If extended from −47% to 63%, the interval will span an additional $.162 + .065 = .227$ of the possibilities, so that the total inner percentile range will cover $.758 + .227 = .985$ of the increments. Thus, an $ipr_{98.5}$ will extend from −47% to 63%.

This approach places the "confidence interval" around the value of the null hypothesis (which here is the equivalence assumption of 0), rather than in the more customary location, discussed later, around the value of the observed increment. Nevertheless, conventional P values are determined from what lies outside the 95% (or other selected) boundary of sampled values, obtained via resamplings or parametric theories, that are centered at the null hypothesis. Because Chapters 13 and 14 discuss the conventional locations of confidence intervals for comparing two central indexes, the last main point to be noted now is that the customary parametric approach for the confidence interval of two contrasted proportions may not always yield one of the realistic values shown in the foregoing tabulation of Fisherian rearrangements. [The disparities will be illustrated in Chapter 14.]

Although the Fisher-table method might offer an elegant solution to the problem of getting confidence intervals for comparisons of two proportions, the method has not been automated and does not appear in the computer programs offered by such "package" systems as BMDP or SAS. If you want to use the method, you will have to work out a suitable approach. The simplest tactic is to start at the "terminal" Fisher tables at each end and then work toward the center, as in Table 12.3.

12.9   Pitman–Welch Permutation Test

A permutation rearrangement can also be applied to dimensional data with results expressed as a difference in two means rather than two proportions. The strategy of stochastically contrasting two means by rearranging the permuted probabilities was described independently by two statisticians[3,4] whose names are joined here for the *Pitman–Welch* commemorative eponym.

Because the data are dimensional rather than binary, the calculations can become much more complex than in a contrast of two proportions, where each individual item of data was either a **0** or a **1**. The binary data allow probabilities to be determined with the simplifying calculations that use permutations and combinations for the **0/1** values. Because each item of dimensional data can have different values, the same type of simplification cannot be used. Nevertheless, with the "short cuts" noted in the following example, the computations can be substantially eased.

12.9.1   Example of a Contrast of Two Means

In four patients who received Treatment A, the measured results were 8, 11, 13, and 21 units, so that the mean was 53/4 = 13.25 units. For Treatment B, the results were 19, 25, 31, and 37 units, with a mean of 112/4 = 28.00 units. Is this difference of 14.75 units stochastically significant?

To answer this question, we could contemplate all the ways of arranging the eight values — 8, 11, 13, 19, 21, 25, 31, and 37 — into two groups, each containing four members. We could calculate the mean for each group in the arrangement, find the difference in means for each pair of groups, and determine how often the difference equals or exceeds 14.75. For the eight values divided into two groups of four each, there would be 8!/(4!)(4!) = 70 arrangements to consider.

Table 12.4 shows 35 of these arrangements. Because the two groups each contain the same number of four members, the second set of 35 arrangements would simply be a mirror image of what is shown in Table 12.4, with all of the Group A results appearing as Group B and vice versa. This type of symmetry occurs in permutation tests whenever the two compared groups have the same number of members. If the numbers are unequal, the entire set of possible arrangements must be considered.

12.9.2   Summary of Distribution

The 35 arrangements in Table 12.4 can be summarized as follows:

Observed Difference in Means	Frequency
15.75	1
14.75	1
10 to 14	3
7 to <10	5
4 to <7	7
0 to <4	7
−4 to <0	7
−7 to <−4	2
−10 to <−7	2
TOTAL	35

TABLE 12.4

Permutation Arrangements in Comparing Means of Two Groups

Data for Treatment A	Group A Mean	Data for Treatment B	Group B Mean	Mean Group B – Group A
8,11,13,19	12.75	21,25,31,37	28.50	15.75
8,11,13,21	13.25	19,25,31,37	28.00	14.75*
8,11,13,25	14.25	19,21,31,37	27.00	12.75
8,11,13,31	15.75	19,21,25,37	25.50	9.75
8,11,13,37	17.25	19,21,25,31	24.00	6.75
8,11,19,21	14.75	13,25,31,37	26.50	11.75
8,11,19,25	15.75	13,21,31,37	25.50	9.75
8,11,19,31	17.25	13,21,25,37	24.00	6.75
8,11,19,37	18.75	13,21,25,31	22.50	3.75
8,11,21,25	16.25	13,19,31,37	25.00	8.75
8,11,21,31	17.75	13,19,25,37	23.50	5.75
8,11,21,37	19.25	13,19,25,31	22.00	2.75
8,11,25,31	18.25	13,19,21,37	23.00	4.75
8,11,25,37	19.75	13,19,21,31	21.50	1.75
8,11,31.37	21.25	13,19,21,25	20.00	−1.25
8,13,19,21	15.25	11,25,31,37	26.00	10.75
8,13,19,25	16.25	11,21,31,37	25.00	8.75
8,13,19,31	17.75	11,21,25,37	23.50	5.75
8,13,19,37	19.25	11,21,25,31	22.00	2.75
8,13,21,25	16.75	11,19,31,37	24.50	7.75
8,13,21,31	18.25	11,19,25,37	23.00	4.75
8,13,21,37	19.75	11,19,25,31	21.50	1.75
8,13,25,31	19.25	11,19,21,37	22.00	2.75
8,13,25,37	20.75	11,19,21,31	20.50	−0.25
8,13,31,37	22.25	11,19,21,25	19.00	−3.25
8,19,21,25	18.25	11,13,31,37	23.00	4.75
8,19,21,31	19.75	11,13,25,37	21.50	1.75
8,19,21,37	21.25	11,13,25,31	20.00	−1.25
8,19,25,31	20.75	11,13,21,37	20.50	−0.25
8,19,25,37	22.25	11,13,21,31	19.00	−3.25
8,19,31,37	23.75	11,13,21,25	17.50	−6.25
8,21,25,31	21.25	11,13,19,37	20.00	−1.25
8,21,25,37	22.75	11,13,19,31	18.50	−4.25
8,21,31,37	24.25	11,13,19,25	17.00	−7.25
8,25,31,37	25.25	11,13,19,21	16.00	−9.25

* = observed result.

We now have the answer to the basic question. An absolute difference of 14.75 units or more occurs twice in these 35 arrangements and would appear four times in the full total of 70 arrangements. The one-tailed P value is 2/70 = .03, and the two-tailed P value is 4/70 = .06.

12.9.3 Simplified Arrangement

To shorten (or avoid) all these calculations, we can note that the observed results for the group receiving Treatment A contain the three members with the lowest values (8, 11, 13) of the total array of values: 8, 11, 13, 19, 21, 25, 31, and 37. The fourth observed value in Treatment A is 21, yielding the mean difference of 14.75 in the two groups. If we look for a difference in mean values that is more extreme, i.e., even larger, than 14.75, the only way to get it is if the fourth member of Group A were 19 rather than 21. For the group of values 8, 11, 13, and 19, the mean would be 12.75. The mean for 21, 25, 31, and 37 would be 28.50; and the difference in means would be 15.75.

Because there are only two ways of getting a mean difference that is at least as large as 14.75, the one-tailed P value will be 2/70 or .03. Because there are 4 members in each treatment group, 35 (or half) of the possible 70 arrangements will be symmetrical. Thus, there will be one arrangement in which the values 19, 25, 31, and 37 appear in Group A, while 8, 11, 13, and 21 appear in B; and another arrangement in which 21, 25, 31, and 37 appear in A, with 8, 11, 13, and 19 in B. Consequently, the probabilities on the "other side" will be distributed in a manner similar to those of the "first side." Thus, the two-tailed P value will be .03 + .03 = .06.

If α is set at .05, the one-tailed but not the two-tailed probability will be "statistically significant."

12.9.4 "Confidence Intervals"

Like the Fisher test, the Pitman–Welch procedure offers P values for the null hypothesis, but does not produce confidence intervals around the observed distinction. Nevertheless, from the probability values associated with each arrangement of the data, a counterpart of confidence intervals can be formed to show extreme limits on either side. For example, the results in Table 12.4 show that 2 of the 35 one-sided arrangements have incremental means that are >13. Among the 35 arrangements on the other side, 2 would have incremental means that are <–13. Consequently a zone from −13 to +13 would cover 66/70 = .94 of the data—an ipr_{94} for the spread of possible increments in means. Because these intervals are not arranged, however, around the observed difference (which is 14.75 in this instance), the Pitman–Welch procedure is seldom used for the stochastic goal of forming a confidence interval around the observed distinction in means. The conventional procedure for the latter goal will be discussed in Chapter 13.

12.9.5 Additional Application

The Pitman–Welch procedure is an excellent way to manage the problem previously stated in Exercise 11.1, where the difference seemed obviously "significant," but where high variability in the data prevented the t-test from giving stochastic confirmation. In Exercise 11.1, a group of 12 items was divided into two groups of 6 each, so that the number of possible arrangements is $12!/[(6!)(6!)] = 924$. Because all of the "low" values were in Group A and all of the "high" ones were in Group B, the observed data are at the extreme ends of the two-group distribution. Any other arrangement will lead to a smaller increment. Because there is a "mirror" extreme table at the other side, the 2-tailed P value is 2/924 = .002 for the observed result.

References

1. Fisher, 1934; 2. Irwin, 1935; 3. Pitman, 1937; 4. Welch, 1937.

Exercises

The assignment is relatively light to allow you to digest all the reading material.

12.1. In Section 12.6.1, the two-tailed P value was determined from only four possible tables of the observed data. How many more such tables are there? Calculate the p value for each such table, and show that the sum of all the p values for all the tables is unity.

12.2. In Section 12.1, we compared the proportions, 9/12 (75%) vs. 5/15 (33%). Perform a Fisher Exact Probability Test for both tails of this stochastic contrast. (Be sure to show your constituent results.)

12.3. In a randomized clinical trial, an investigator finds the following dimensional results: For Treatment X: 2, 8, 11, and 13 units; and for Treatment Y: 1, 3, and 6 units. Perform a Pitman–Welch probability test on the difference in means, in both possible directions.

13

Parametric Sampling: Z and t Tests

CONTENTS

The procedures described in Chapter 12 are simple, direct, relatively easy to understand, and empirical. They use the evidence that was actually observed, and they require no excursions into a hypothetical world of parent populations and parameters. The tests can be used for stochastic contrasts of any two binary proportions, two means, or even, if desired, two medians. (In the last instance, the permuted samples would show the distribution of differences in medians, rather than means.)

Permutation tests, however, are not the customary methods used today for evaluating stochastic hypotheses. Instead, the conventional, traditional approaches rely on parametric procedures that are well known and long established. You may have never heard of the Fisher and Pitman-Welch tests before encountering them in Chapter 12, but your previous adventures in medical literature have surely brought a meeting somewhere with the two-group (or "two-sample") Z and t tests.

They are based on the same principles described in Chapter 7 when the Z and t procedures were used in parametric inference for a single group. In this chapter, the principles for one group are expanded to their most common application: a contrast of two groups.

13.1 Differences in Permutation and Parametric Principles

For the Fisher and Pitman-Welch permutation procedures described in Chapter 12, the central indexes of the two observed groups were converted to a *single* group of increments. The distribution of the rearranged group of increments showed all the potential differences that could occur, for the Fisher test, in the two proportions, and for the Pitman-Welch test, in the two means. Decisions about P values or confidence intervals were then made from what was found in that distribution.

This same type of activity occurs when two groups are contrasted with parametric methods. A single group is formed from the observed results in the two groups; a set of samples is constructed; and decisions are made from the distribution of the samples. The permutation and parametric procedures differ mainly in that the parametrically constructed samples are theoretical, rather than empiric, and that the distribution is examined for a test statistic, rather than for increments of the central indexes. The main advantage of the parametric procedure is that the test statistic theoretically has a specific mathematical distribution, which presumably will always be the same, regardless of what actually occurred in the two observed groups. The mathematical distribution has previously known probabilities for each value of the parametric test statistic, which can thus be promptly used for decisions about P values and confidence intervals.

This advantage is what made the parametric procedures so popular in the days before ubiquitous digital computation. With permutation techniques, the single group of re-arranged increments forms a unique structure that must be calculated *ad hoc* for each pair of contrasted groups. Although easy to understand, the calculations were usually difficult to do. With parametric techniques, the single theoretical distribution of the test statistic can be applied for a contrast of almost any two groups; and the test statistic itself has a formula that makes calculation relatively easy. The hard part, however, is to understand the mathematical reasoning that underlies the theoretical construction.

13.2 Parametric Comparison of Two Means

In common forms of statistical inference, the summary index for contrasting two groups is the direct increment of the two central indexes. For two observed means, $\overline{X}_A$ and $\overline{X}_B$, the increment is $\overline{X}_A - \overline{X}_B$ or $|\overline{X}_A - \overline{X}_B|$; and for two proportions, p_A and p_B, the increment is $p_A - p_B$ or $|p_A - p_B|$. For parametric procedures, these increments are converted to the standardized values of the test statistics Z or t. In the discussion that follows, the conversion process and reasoning will first be described for contrasting two means. The contrast of two proportions will be discussed later in Section 13.8.

As you might expect from Chapter 7, the Z and t procedures for comparing two means are quite similar. With both procedures, we form the same "critical ratio," which is the test statistic called Z or t. With both procedures, the critical ratio consists of the observed increment in means divided by its standard error. With both procedures, the critical ratio can be interpreted with a P value or used to construct a confidence interval. With both procedures, the critical ratio is interpreted in reference to a parametric mathematical model of the "sampling distribution." The only difference between the two procedures is in the mathematical model. For large groups, the model is the Gaussian Z distribution; for small groups, the model is the "Student" t distribution, selected for the appropriate degrees of freedom.

Although the basic operations are similar for the t and Z procedures, and for contrasting two groups rather than examining only one, a new strategy is needed to estimate the parametric standard error for an increment in means. For this strategy, the observed two groups of data are converted into a theoretical sample consisting of *increments in means*, and the standard error is found as the standard deviation in that sample.

The basic principles of that process, discussed in the rest of this section, involve a lot of mathematics, but should not be too difficult to understand. It is worth reading if you want to know about a prime doctrine in the "ethos" of parametric inference. If not, skip to Section 13.3.

13.2.1 Basic Principles

For two observed means, $\overline{X}_A$ and $\overline{X}_B$, in groups having the respective sizes n_A and n_B, with total size $N = n_A + n_B$, the parametric reasoning assumes that Group A is a random sample from a population having μ_A as mean and σ_A as standard deviation, and that Group B analogously has the populational parameters μ_B and σ_B.

We now do a repetitive theoretical sampling process as in Chapter 7, but on each occasion, we draw a pair of samples, not just one. One sample, with n_A members, is taken from population A and has $\overline{X}_{A_j}$ as its mean. The other sample, of size n_B, is taken from population B and has $\overline{X}_{B_j}$ as its mean. We then subtract those two sampled means to form a single item of "new" data, which is the increment in means, $\overline{X}_{A_j} - \overline{X}_{B_j}$.

As the theoretical sampling process is repeated over and over, each time yielding different values of $\overline{X}_{A_j}$ and $\overline{X}_{B_j}$, the increments in those two means form a distribution having its own parametric mean, and its own parametric variance and standard deviation. The next step is to determine what they are.

13.2.2 Variance in Increments of Two Means

To determine the parametric variance of the increments $\{\overline{X}_{A_j} - \overline{X}_{B_j}\}$, we resort to a concept that appeared in Appendix 7.1, with an illustration in Table 7.4. The concept is that the variance of either a sum *or* difference in two variables is equal to the sum of their variances. For the series of means sampled from population A, the parametric variance will be σ_A^2/n_A, which is estimated as s_A^2/n_A.

The corresponding parametric variance for the means in population B will be σ_B^2/n_B, estimated as s_B^2/n_B. The variance of the distribution of increments in means could therefore be estimated as

$$\hat{\sigma}_C^2 = s_C^2 = (s_A^2/n_A) + (s_B^2/n_B) \qquad [13.1]$$

Although this sum offers a satisfactory estimate for σ_C, a problem will arise for the stochastic null hypothesis.

13.2.3 Estimation of Parametric Variance

The appropriate estimate for the parametric variance depends on what we have in mind for the null hypothesis. If the null hypothesis assumes that the two means are equal, i.e., $\mu_A = \mu_B$, we imply that the data forming the increments in the two sample means, $\overline{X}_A$ and $\overline{X}_B$, came from the same single population, having 0 as its parametric mean, i.e., $\mu_C = \mu_A - \mu_B = 0$, with σ as the standard deviation of the data. After making the assumption that $\mu_A = \mu_B$, however, do we also assume that $\sigma_A = \sigma_B = \sigma$? With the latter assumption about variance, we cannot estimate $\hat{\sigma}_C$ directly from s_A^2 and s_B^2, because s_A and s_B may not be equal. If we do not assume that $\sigma_A = \sigma_B$, however, $\hat{\sigma}_C$ can readily be estimated from the sum of $s_A^2/n_A + s_B^2/n_B$ in Formula [13.1].

In most circumstances, the null hypothesis assumes that the two groups are parametrically equal for both the means *and* the variances, i.e., that $\mu_A = \mu_B$ and $\sigma_A = \sigma_B = \sigma$. In other situations discussed in Section 11.9 and later in Chapter 23, however, the stochastic assumption is an *alternative* hypothesis that the two means are different, i.e., $\mu_A \neq \mu_B$. In the latter situations, we do not require that $\sigma_A = \sigma_B$.

If $\sigma_A \neq \sigma_B$, the parametric variance of the increments of means can be correctly estimated with Formula [13.1]; but for most ordinary uses of the two-group Z or t test, the null hypothesis assumes equivalence of both means and variances. Consequently, because the observed s_A^2 will seldom equal s_B^2, we need a new way to estimate σ with the idea that $\sigma_A = \sigma_B$. For this tactic, we estimate σ_A and σ_B as the "average" value of s_A and s_B, found from their *pooled variance*, called s_p^2. The pooling process was shown earlier in Section 10.5.1.1. The group variances, S_{XX_A} in Group A and S_{XX_B} in group B, are added to form $S_{XX_A} + S_{XX_B}$ as the pooled group variance. This sum is then divided by the combined degrees of freedom to form the average pooled variance of the total data as

$$s_p^2 = \frac{S_{XX_A} + S_{XX_B}}{\nu_A + \nu_B} = \frac{S_{XX_A} + S_{XX_B}}{n_A - 1 + n_B - 1} \qquad [13.2]$$

The degrees of freedom are calculated as

$$\nu_c = \nu_A + \nu_B = n_A - 1 + n_B - 1 = N - 2$$

because, as noted in Section 7.5.2, the estimate of μ_c as $\mu_A - \mu_B$ requires estimates for μ_A and μ_B. Therefore, two degrees of freedom are lost from the total group size, N. Because $S_{XX_A} = (n_A - 1)s_A^2$ and $S_{XX_B} = (n_B - 1)s_B^2$, a convenient working formula is

$$s_p^2 = \frac{(n_A - 1)s_A^2 + (n_B - 1)s_B^2}{n_A - 1 + n_B - 1} \qquad [13.3]$$

For example, suppose a group of 8 people have a mean chloride value of 101.25, with s = 4.30. Another group of 15 people have a mean chloride value of 96.15 and s = 4.63. To find the pooled variance, Formula [13.3] would produce

$$s_p^2 = \frac{(7)(4.30)^2 + (14)(4.63)^2}{7 + 14} = \frac{429.55}{21} = 20.45$$

and $s_p = \sqrt{20.45} = 4.52$. This result is what would be anticipated as a "common standard deviation" for the two groups: the value of s_p lies between the two observed values of $s_A = 4.30$ and $s_B = 4.62$; and the pooled value in this instance is closer to s_B, because Group B had a larger size for n_B.

13.2.4   Construction of Standard Error

The value of the parametric variance, σ_C^2, in the theoretical samples of increments of means is the square of the standard deviation, σ_C, in those samples. This standard deviation is the *standard error* needed for the denominator of the critical ratio.

If we were *not* using a pooled standard deviation, s_p, the standard error could promptly be calculated for the cited two groups of chloride values using Formula [13.1] and inserting

$$s_C^2 = \frac{(4.30)^2}{8} + \frac{(4.63)^2}{15} = 2.31 + 1.43 = 3.74$$

so that $s_C = 1.93$.

When a pooled standard deviation is used, however, s_p^2 is substituted for both s_A^2 and s_B^2 in Formula [13.1]. The result is a slightly different estimate, designated as $\hat{\sigma}_{c'}$, and calculated as

$$s_{C'}^2 = \hat{\sigma}_{C'}^2 = \frac{s_p^2}{n_A} + \frac{s_p^2}{n_B} = s_p^2 \left(\frac{1}{n_A} + \frac{1}{n_B} \right) = s_p^2 \left(\frac{n}{n_A n_B} \right)$$

For the example under discussion,

$$s_{C'}^2 = (20.45)\left[\frac{1}{8} + \frac{1}{15}\right] = (20.45)(.1917) = 3.92$$

so that $s_{C'} = 1.98$.

13.2.5   Similarity of the Two Estimates

According to the type of null hypothesis being tested, either s_c or $s_{c'}$ will represent SED, the *standard error of the difference* in two means.

As in various other mathematical niceties — such as when to use t or Z — the distinction between $\hat{\sigma}_C$ and $\hat{\sigma}_{C'}$ (or between s_C and $s_{C'}$) is theoretically important. Pragmatically, however, the distinction often makes little difference, because s_C and $s_{C'}$ are usually quite similar, as in the values of 1.93 and 1.98 for the example here. In fact, with development of the algebra, it can be shown that

$$s_C^2 - s_{C'}^2 = \hat{\sigma}_C^2 - \hat{\sigma}_{C'}^2 = \frac{(N-1)(n_B - n_A)(s_A^2 - s_B^2)}{(N-2)(n_A n_B)} \qquad [13.5]$$

The result shown in Formula [13.5] will be slightly positive or negative according to the relative magnitudes of n_B vs. n_A and s_A vs. s_B. If the original sample sizes or variances are similar, so that $n_B = n_A$ or $s_A = s_B$, the values of s_C^2 and $s_{C'}^2$ will be identical.

Nevertheless, it is useful to know the rules and to "play the game" properly. You would probably do just as well in a "surgical scrub" if you used an ordinary good soap, rather than the special chemical solution that is usually provided. You keep your operating-room colleagues happy, however, by using the special chemical. Analogously, you will keep your statistical colleagues happy by using the pooled standard deviation, s_p, and the pooled standard error, $s_{C'}$, to test a zero null hypothesis, and the unpooled s_C to test the nonzero alternative hypotheses discussed later.

13.2.6   Estimating the Parametric Mean

The last step needed to form the critical ratio for the test statistic is to estimate the parametric mean of the distribution of increments in means, formed as

$$\mu_c = \mu_A - \mu_B$$

In Section 7.3.7.2, we learned that the parametric mean is best estimated, on average, from the value of the observed mean. Therefore, $\hat{\mu}_A$ is best estimated by the observed $\overline{X}_A$, and $\hat{\mu}_B$ by the observed $\overline{X}_B$. Accordingly, the value of μ_C is best estimated as

$$\hat{\mu}_c = \hat{\mu}_A - \hat{\mu}_B = \overline{X}_A - \overline{X}_B$$

13.3   Z or t Tests for Means in Two Groups

With the principles cited throughout Section 13.2, we are now ready to use t or Z for stochastic tests on a difference in two means. The critical ratio will be

$$\frac{\left(\begin{array}{c}\text{Observed}\\\text{Difference}\\\text{in Means}\end{array}\right) - \left(\begin{array}{c}\text{Parametric}\\\text{Difference}\\\text{in Means}\end{array}\right)}{\text{Standard Error of Difference}}$$

Under the parametric null hypothesis that $\mu_A = \mu_B$, the second term in the numerator of this ratio vanishes. The standard error of the difference in means can then be estimated in two ways. For the conventional null hypothesis, the standard error is estimated as $s_{C'}$ from the pooled variance, s_p. The critical ratio becomes

$$t \text{ (or } Z) = \frac{\overline{X}_A - \overline{X}_B}{s_{C'}} \qquad [13.6]$$

When $s_{C'}$ is calculated with Formula [13.4] and s_p with Formula [13.3], the "working" formula becomes

$$t \text{ (or } Z) = \frac{\overline{X}_A - \overline{X}_B}{\sqrt{\dfrac{(n_A - 1)s_A^2 + (n_B - 1)s_B^2}{n_A - 1 + n_B - 1}} \sqrt{\dfrac{1}{n_A} + \dfrac{1}{n_B}}} \qquad [13.7]$$

Formula [13.7] is used for an ordinary "two-sample" Z or t test.

The alternative formula, used for the "alternative hypotheses" discussed later, places s_C rather than $s_{C'}$ in the denominator. With Formula [13.1] for s_C, the critical ratio is

$$t \text{ (or } Z) = \frac{\overline{X}_A - \overline{X}_B}{\sqrt{\dfrac{s_A^2}{n_A} + \dfrac{s_B^2}{n_B}}} \qquad [13.8]$$

The reference distribution for interpreting the test statistic formed in either Formula [13.7] or [13.8] depends on sample size. For larger groups, we use the standard Gaussian Z distribution. For smaller groups, the t distribution is applied, with $v = n_A - 1 + n_B - 1 = N - 2$.

The interpretation can produce either P values or confidence intervals or both. P is found as the appropriate value associated with the calculated critical ratio of Z or t_v. A confidence interval is constructed by first choosing Z_α or $t_{v,\alpha}$ for the selected $1 - \alpha$ level of confidence. The standard error of the difference is then multiplied by Z_α (or $t_{v,\alpha}$), and the interval becomes calculated as

$$(\overline{X}_A - \overline{X}_B) \pm Z_\alpha s_{C'}$$

or as

$$(\overline{X}_A - \overline{X}_B) \pm t_{v,\alpha} s_{C'}$$

13.3.1 Example of Calculations

For the two groups of chloride values that were cited in Section 13.2.3, $\overline{X}_A - \overline{X}_B = 101.25 - 96.15 = 5.1$. The two possible values for SED (calculated in Section 13.2.4) were 1.93 for s_C and 1.98 for $s_{C'}$. The critical ratio (calculated with $s_{C'}$) would be

$$\frac{101.25 - 96.15}{1.98} = \frac{5.1}{1.98} = 2.576$$

For groups having 8 and 15 members, $v = 7 + 14 = 21$. The critical ratio (or "test statistic") would therefore be interpreted from t_{21} in Table 7.3 as a 2-tailed P value for which $.01 < 2P < .025$. At the α rejection level of .05, this result is "significant."

To determine a 95% confidence interval around the observed increment, we first find $t_{21,.05} = 2.080$. After calculation of $(2.080)(1.98) = 4.12$, the interval will be $(\overline{X}_A - \overline{X}_B) \pm 4.12 = 5.1 \pm 4.12$, and extends from .98 to 9.22. Because the null-hypothesis value of 0 is excluded, the result is "significant."

More examples and opportunities for calculation are available in the Exercises at the end of the chapter.

13.3.2 Crude Mental Approximation

A crude mental approximation can sometimes be useful as a "screening" test for a "significant" confidence interval. For the approximation, the two individual standard errors, $s_{\overline{X}_A}$ and $s_{\overline{X}_B}$, are simply added as

$$s_{C''} = \frac{s_A}{\sqrt{n_A}} + \frac{s_B}{\sqrt{n_B}} \qquad [13.9]$$

If the results for each group have been summarized with standard errors (rather than standard deviations), the two standard errors can be added immediately. For the example at the end of Section 13.2.3, however, "standard errors were not listed for each group of chloride values. We therefore use Formula [13.9] to calculate the crude combined standard error as $s_{C''} = (4.30/\sqrt{8}) + (4.63/\sqrt{15}) = 1.520 + 1.195 = 2.715$. It is larger than either $s_C = 1.93$ or $s_{C'} = 1.98$.

The value of $s_{C''}$ will always exceed the value of s_C obtained from Formula [13.1]. (You can prove this statement by squaring formula [13.9] and comparing $s_{C''}^2$ with s_C^2 in Formula [13.1].) Consequently, any confidence intervals calculated with $s_{C''}$ will be larger than those calculated with s_C and almost always larger than those calculated with $s_{C'}$.

The value of the enlarged crude $s_{C''}$ interval can then be used for a quick, mental answer to questions about stochastic significance. The first step is to approximate Z_α or $t_{\nu,\alpha}$ as 2 for a 95% confidence interval and then double the $s_{C''}$ value of 2.715 to produce 5.430. The confidence interval will *not* include 0 whenever the doubled crude value of $s_{C''}$ is *less* than $|\overline{X}_A - \overline{X}_B|$. In this instance $\overline{X}_A - \overline{X}_B$ is 5.1 and the doubled $s_{C''}$ is $> |\overline{X}_A - \overline{X}_B|$. We therefore cannot promptly conclude that "significance" exists. If $2s_{C''}$ were smaller than 5.1, however, we could reach the conclusion of stochastic significance without needing the formal test.

Thus, a working rule for the "in-the-head" approach is:

1. Add the two standard errors.
2. Double the added value.
3. If the doubled value is distinctly smaller than the difference in the two means, the result is stochastically significant at $2P < .05$.
4. Otherwise, do the formal test. (In this instance, as shown in Section 13.3.1, the formal value of 2P turned out to be $<.05$.)

When the two means and their standard errors are cited on a "slide" during an oral presentation, the use of this mental tactic, followed by an appropriate comment, can sometimes make you seem like a wizard. Beware of "false negative" conclusions, however. You will seldom commit a "false positive" error in claiming "significance" if $2s_{C''}$ is $< |\overline{X}_A - \overline{X}_B|$; but if not, the formal test should be done.

13.3.3   Summary of Procedure

Although permuted non-parametric methods (such as the Pitman-Welch test) will probably eventually replace the t test and Z test, the two parametric procedures will remain popular for many years to come. For readers who want a synopsis of "cookbook" directions, two recipes are cited below for the t test. The same recipes are used for Z, when degrees of freedom can be ignored with larger samples (e.g., N > 40).

13.3.3.1   Getting a P Value

1. For each group, A and B, calculate a mean, group variance (or "sum of squares"), and a standard deviation. The respective formulas are $\overline{X} = \Sigma X_i/n$; $S_{XX} = \Sigma X_i^2 - [(\Sigma X_i)^2/n]$; and $s = \sqrt{S_{XX}/(n-1)}$.
2. Add $S_{XX_A} + S_{XX_B}$ or, alternatively, $(n_A - 1) s_A^2 + (n_B - 1)s_B^2$. Divide the sum by $n_A + n_B - 2$. The result is the pooled variance, s_p^2, in the data.
3. Calculate the estimated standard error of the difference in means as $s_p\sqrt{(1/n_A) + (1/n_B)}$. [It is calculated directly as $\sqrt{(s_A/n_A^2) + (s_B/n_B^2)}$ for the "alternative" hypothesis.]
4. Choose a value of α and decide whether the result will be interpreted in a two-tailed or one-tailed direction. For a one-tailed test, t is associated with half the probability value of a

two-tailed test. (All these directional decisions should be made *before* the value of t is calculated, and preferably before any of the statistical analysis begins.)

5. Calculate t as:

$$(\overline{X}_A - \overline{X}_B) / [s_p \sqrt{(1/n_A) + (1/n_B)}]$$

6. Using $n_A + n_B - 2$ degrees of freedom, look up the corresponding P value in Table 7.3 or in a more complete table.

7. Using the preselected value of α, decide whether the P value allows you to reject the null hypothesis and to proclaim stochastic significance.

13.3.3.2 *Getting a Confidence Interval* — If you prefer to use the confidence interval technique for checking stability, the steps are as follows:

1. Carry out the previous steps 1 to 4 to find the estimated standard error of the difference, $s_p \sqrt{(1/n_A) + (1/n_B)}$.

2. Select the $1 - \alpha$ level of confidence and find the value of $t_{v,\alpha}$ that is associated with this value of α, with $v = n_A + n_B - 2$.

3. Multiply the selected t value by $s_p \sqrt{(1/n_A) + (1/n_B)}$.

4. Obtain the $1 - \alpha$ confidence interval by adding and subtracting the result of step 3 to the value of $\overline{X}_A - \overline{X}_B$.

5. Concede or reject the null hypothesis according to whether this confidence interval includes or excludes the value of 0.

After you have finished the procedure, particularly if the conclusion is what you had hoped for, obtain a Guinness product and drink a toast to the memory of William S. Gosset. If you prefer, get a German beer and say "prosit" for Carl F. Gauss.

13.3.4   Electronic Computation

With modern electronic computation, you may never actually have to do the calculations of t or Z. If properly commanded, an appropriate program will do the calculations and promptly give you the results.

You may also never have to use tabular arrays, such as Table 7.3, either to find the associated P values or to guess about interpolated results when the calculated t or Z lies between the values tabulated at P levels of .2, .1, .05, .025, .01, etc. Many "packaged" computer programs today will use the mathematical formulas of standard t and Gaussian distributions to obtain the exact probabilities associated with any value of t and Z. The printout will show you both the t or Z value and a precisely calculated external probability such as P = .063.

The only potential problem in the printouts is that they may not show the actual magnitude of very tiny P values. If P is below .00005, the result may be printed as P = .0000. At even tinier P values, below 1×10^{-16}, the printout may show P = •. Unless you know about these symbolic conventions, the printout may initially be confusing.

The calculational formulas are necessary if you have to do the computations yourself, if you want to check whether an electronic program has done them correctly, or if you occasionally do a mental screening of presented results. You also need to know about the underlying strategy when you decide about 1- or 2-tailed interpretations of P.

13.3.5   Robustness of Z/t Tests

A statistical test is called *robust* if it is "insensitive" to violations of the assumptions on which the test is based. For example, because the means of small-sized groups do not have a Gaussian distribution, the Z procedure is *not* robust and will give inaccurate results at small group sizes. The t distribution is therefore used for small groups when P values are interpreted for the "critical ratio" in Formula [13.7].

For the two-group t or Z procedures, the underlying assumption that is most likely to be violated is the idea that the observed variances, s_A^2 and s_B^2, come from the same parametric population, with variance σ^2, estimated by the pooled variance, s_p^2. If s_A^2 and s_B^2, however, are highly heteroscedastic (which is a splendid word for having dissimilar variances), the invalid assumption might lead to defective values for the critical ratio and its interpretation. To avoid this potential problem, some statisticians will do a "screening" check that the ratio of variances, s_A^2/s_B^2, does not greatly depart from 1. This screening is seldom used, however, because most of the concerns were eliminated after a classical study by Boneau.[1] He did a series of Monte Carlo samplings showing that the t test was "remarkably robust" except in the uncommon situation where *both* the group sizes *and* the variances in the two groups are substantially unequal. In the latter situation, the best approach is to use a Pitman-Welch test.

13.3.6 Similarity of F Test

The published literature sometimes contains a report in which the means of the two groups have been stochastically contrasted with an F test. The F test strategy, which is customarily used in a procedure called *analysis of variance* (discussed later in Chapter 29), was originally developed for contrasting the means of three or more groups, rather than two. For two-group contrasts, however, the calculated value of F is the exact square of the critical ratio used for t, and the squared ratio is interpreted with an F, rather than t, distribution. Nevertheless, the P values that emerge from the F test in a two-group contrast are identical to those obtained with a t test.

The F test is also used when heteroscedasticity is checked for the ratio of the two variances, s_A^2 and s_B^2.

13.4 Components of "Stochastic Significance"

Formula [13.7] indicates that the stochastic calculation of t or Z is a product of several components, which produce the conversion of quantitative into stochastic indexes. One of these components is the standardized increment, which you may recall from Section 10.5.1. The other two components reflect the size and partition of the total group under examination. The diverse components become apparent if we rewrite Formula [13.7] as

$$t \text{ or } Z = \frac{\overline{X}_A - \overline{X}_B}{s_p} \times \frac{1}{\sqrt{(1/n_A) + (1/n_B)}} \qquad [13.10]$$

13.4.1 Role of Standardized Increment

In Chapter 10, the standardized increment was briefly introduced as an index of contrast to describe "effect size" in a comparison of two central indexes. With s_p as a common standard deviation for two groups of dimensional data, having means $\overline{X}_A$ and $\overline{X}_B$, the standardized increment for the contrast is

$$\frac{\overline{X}_A - \overline{X}_B}{s_p}$$

The standardized increment is a descriptive index of contrast because it involves no act of inference (other than the use of degrees of freedom in the calculation of s_p). The s_p factor, however, makes the standardized increment an index of contrast that uniquely provides for variability in the data. This provision is absent in all of the other indexes of contrast discussed in Chapter 10.

The provision for variability gives the standardized increment another vital role (noted earlier) as the bridge that connects descriptive and inferential statistics for a contrast of two groups. The t or Z (and also later the chi-square) test statistics are all constructed when the standardized increment is multiplied by factors indicating the magnitude (and partition) of group sizes. The stochastic statistics of t, Z, and chi-square are thus a product of factors for the standardized increment and group sizes.

13.4.2   Role of Group Sizes

The group sizes are reflected by $1/\sqrt{(1/n_A) + (1/n_B)}$, the other factor in Formula [13.10]. Because $(1/n_A) + (1/n_B) = N/n_A n_B$, division by this factor can be rewritten as the multiplicative entity $\sqrt{n_A n_B/N}$, which is the *group size factor*. Thus,

$$t \text{ (or Z)} = \frac{\text{Standardized}}{\text{Increment}} \times \frac{\text{Group Size}}{\text{Factor}}. \qquad [13.11]$$

The group size factor is decomposed into two parts when the total group, N, is divided into the two groups, n_A and n_B. If we let $k = n_A/N$, then $n_A = kN$ and $n_B = N - n_A = (1 - k)N$, and the group size factor will become $\sqrt{kN(1-k)N/N} = \sqrt{k(1-k)}\sqrt{N}$.

The value of $(k)(1 - k)$ will depend on the partition of n_A and n_B. If the group sizes are equal, $n_A = n_B = N/2$ and $(k)(1 - k) = 1/4$ so that $\sqrt{(k)(1-k)} = .5$. As the partition becomes more unequal, $\sqrt{(k)(1-k)}$ will become smaller. Thus, if $n_A = 20$ and $n_B = 80$, $\sqrt{(.2)(.8)} = .4$. If $n_A = 10$ and $n_B = 190$, $\sqrt{(.05)(.95)} = .22$. If we call $\sqrt{(k)(1-k)}$ the *group partition factor*, the stochastic test result becomes a product of three factors:

$$t \text{ (or Z)} = \frac{\text{Standardized}}{\text{Increment}} \times \frac{\text{Group}}{\text{Partition}} \times \frac{\text{Total}}{\text{Size}}$$
$$\text{Factor} \quad \text{Factor}$$

or

$$t \text{ (or Z)} = \frac{\overline{X}_A - \overline{X}_B}{s_p} \times \sqrt{k(1-k)} \times \sqrt{N} \qquad [13.12]$$

Formula [13.12] offers a striking demonstration of the role of group sizes in achieving stochastic significance. The values of t (or Z) will always increase with larger groups, because $\sqrt{N}$ is a direct multiplicative factor. The values will also increase with equally partitioned groups, because $\sqrt{k(1-k)}$ achieves its maximum value of .5 when $n_A = n_B$. The values get smaller as the proportion for k departs from the meridian of .5 toward values of 1 or 0.

13.4.3   Effects of Total Size

Of the various components of Formula [13.12], the most dramatic is the total group size, N. No matter how small the magnitudes may be for the standardized increment and the group partition factor, a sufficiently large value of $\sqrt{N}$ can multiply their product into a value that exceeds the Z_α (or $t_{\nu,\alpha}$) needed for stochastic significance. Conversely, even if the standardized increment is quantitatively impressive and the group partition factor is a perfect .5, the result for the test statistic will still fail to achieve stochastic significance if $\sqrt{N}$ is too small.

For example, suppose the standardized increment is an extraordinarily low value of .001 and the group partition factor is a greatly unbalanced .04. To exceed the value of $Z_\alpha = 2$ for stochastic significance, all we need is

$$2 \leq 5 \, (.001)(.04) \sqrt{N}$$

and so

$$\sqrt{N} \geq 2/(.001)(.04) = 50,000$$

The necessary value of N will be the square of this value, which is 2.5×10^9 or 2.5 billion. Archimedes is said to have remarked, "If you give me a lever long enough and strong enough, I can move the earth." If the total group size is large enough, *any* observed distinction can be stochastically significant.

Conversely, suppose the standardized increment is an impressively high value of .75 and the group-partition factor is a splendid 0.5. The total product will fail to exceed a value of $Z = 2$ if

$$2 \geq (.75)(.5) \sqrt{N}$$

which occurs when

$$\sqrt{N} \leq 2/[(.75)(.5)] = 3.27$$

This situation would arise with a total group size of $(3.27)^2 = 10.7$ or anything smaller than 10.

13.4.4 Simplified Formulas for Calculation or Interpretation

Formula [13.10] can be converted to

$$t \text{ (or Z)} = \left(\frac{\overline{X}_A - \overline{X}_B}{s_p}\right)\sqrt{n_A n_B/N} \qquad [13.13]$$

In addition to its use in computing the value of t or Z, the formula offers a way of promptly interpreting both quantitative and stochastic significance. The standardized increment, $(\overline{X}_A - \overline{X}_B)/s_p$, can be used as a guide to interpreting quantitative significance. The group size factor, $\sqrt{n_A n_B/N}$, will indicate the role played by the numerical sizes of the groups in converting the standardized increment to stochastic significance.

13.4.4.1 Equal Group Sizes — When the groups have equal sizes, so that $n_A = n_B = n = N/2$, Formula [13.13] can receive two simplifications. The factor $\sqrt{n_A n_B/N}$ will become $\sqrt{(n)(n)/(2n)} = \sqrt{n/2}$. The value of s_p^2 earlier in Formula [13.3] will become

$$[(n - 1) s_A^2 + (n - 1) s_B^2]/[2(n - 1)] = (s_A^2 + s_B^2)/2$$

so that the values of s_C and $s_{C'}$ are identical. Formula [13.13] will then become

$$t \text{ (or Z)} = \frac{\overline{X}_A - \overline{X}_B}{\sqrt{(s_A^2 + s_B^2)/2}}(\sqrt{n/2})$$

which can be further reduced to

$$t \text{ (or Z)} = \frac{\overline{X}_A - \overline{X}_B}{\sqrt{s_A^2 + s_B^2}}(\sqrt{n}) \qquad [13.14]$$

(Remember that *n* here is the size of one group.)

13.4.4.2 Use of Cited Standard Errors — In many instances, the investigators report the results of the two means, the two group sizes, and the two standard errors as SE_A and SE_B. If you want to check the claims for t (or Z), the SE values would have to be converted to standard deviations as $\sqrt{n_A}(SE_A)$ and $\sqrt{n_B}(SE_b)$. To avoid this work, you can use the "alternative-hypothesis" Formula [13.8] and estimate s_C^2 directly as $(SE_A)^2 + (SE_B)^2$. Because the group size factor is incorporated when standard errors are determined, as $(s_A^2/n_A + s_B^2/n_B)$, Formula [13.8] becomes simply

$$t \text{ (or Z)} = (\overline{X}_A - \overline{X}_B)/\sqrt{(SE_A)^2 + (SE_B)^2} \qquad (13.15)$$

This formula will be slightly inaccurate, because the variance was not pooled, but the results are usually close enough for a quick "screening" check of reported values.

If the groups have equal size, Formulas [13.14] and [13.15] produce identical results, because the denominator of [13.15] becomes $\sqrt{(s_A^2 + s_B^2)}/\sqrt{n}$.

13.5 Dissidence and Concordance in Significance

The formulas cited in Sections 13.4.1 through 13.4.4 indicate why separate evaluations are needed for quantitative and stochastic significance, and why the two evaluations may sometimes disagree. Because of small group size, a quantitatively significant difference may fail to achieve stochastic significance. Because of huge group size, a quantitatively trivial difference may become stochastically significant.

The distinctions also help explain some of the problems we encountered in Chapter 10 when trying to choose the magnitude of a quantitatively significant increment. Suppose we decide that we want *concordant* results for *both* stochastic and quantitative significance. Because $Z \geq 2$ (or 1.96) is the minimum boundary for stochastic significance at two-tailed $\alpha = .05$, the magnitude needed for a quantitatively significant increment will vary with the group size. If the total group size is 40, equally divided into two groups of 20, the formula will be

$$2 \leq (S.I.)(.5)\sqrt{40}$$

and so the required standardized increment (S. I.) must exceed $2/[(.5)\sqrt{40}] = .63$. If the sample size is larger, perhaps 100, and still equally divided, stochastic significance will occur when the standardized increment exceeds $2/[(.5)\sqrt{100}] = .40$. With a larger, equally divided total group of 300, the required standardized increment must exceed $2/(.5)(\sqrt{300}) = .23$.

Unless we carefully separate what is quantitatively important from what is stochastically significant, decisions about quantitative importance will be dominated by mathematical calculations of probability. The scientific boundaries set for magnitudes that are quantitatively important will frequently have to change—as noted earlier—according to the clinical, populational, or other biologic implications of the observed results. A much less scientifically acceptable source of varying boundaries, however, is the stochastic caprice caused by changes in group size.

In a particular biologic setting, a standardized increment of .4 either is or is not quantitatively significant; and it may or may not be derived from numbers large enough to be stochastically significant. The decision about *quantitative* significance, however, should depend on its magnitude and connotations in a biologic setting, not on the size of the groups under study. This principle will be further discussed and illustrated with many examples in Chapter 14.

13.6 Controversy about P Values vs. Confidence Intervals

During the past few years, the stochastic dominance of P values has been threatened by advocates of confidence intervals; and a lively dispute has developed between the "confidence couriers" and the "P-value partisans." The advocates of confidence intervals want to supplement or replace P values because the single value of P does not give the scope of information offered by a confidence interval. The defenders want the P value preserved because it indicates the important distance from the stochastic boundary of α. Many highly respected statisticians and statistical epidemiologists have lined up on both sides of the controversy, urging either the use of confidence intervals or the retention of P values.

The confidence couriers seem to be winning the battle in prominent clinical journals. After presenting "tutorial" discussions to educate readers about the use of confidence intervals, the editors proudly announce their enlightened new policies demanding confidence intervals instead of (or in addition to) P values. The enlightened new policies are presumably expected to bring medical literature out of the statistical "dark ages" induced by previous editorial policies that set the demand for P values.

13.6.1 Fundamental Problems in Both Methods

An even-handed reaction to this controversy would be to agree with both sides, since both sets of contentions are correct and both sets of approaches are useful. In fact, as suggested by some of the disputing participants, truly enlightened editors could ask for both types of information: confidence intervals (to show the potential range of results) and P values (to keep authors and readers from being infatuated or deceived by an arbitrarily chosen interval).

Regardless of the opposing viewpoints, however, the argument itself resembles a debate about whether to give an inadequate medication orally or parenterally.[2] The argument ignores the reciprocal similarity of P values and confidence intervals, while also overlooking four fundamental problems: (1) the absence of clearly stated goals for the statistical procedures, (2) the arbitrariness of the α and Z_α boundaries that determine both the interpretation of P values and the magnitude of confidence intervals, (3) the continuing absence of standards for descriptive boundaries of δ for "big" and ζ for "small" distinctions in quantitative significance, and (4) the distraction of both P values and confidence intervals from the challenge of setting *scientific* standards for those quantitative boundaries.

13.6.1.1 Goals of the Statistical Procedures —

What do investigators (and readers) really want in a stochastic test? What questions would they really ask if the answers, somewhat in the format of a game of *Jeopardy*, were not previously supplied by P values and confidence intervals?

Probably the main questions would refer to the stability of the results and their range of potential variation. When two central indexes are contrasted, a first question would ask whether they arise from groups containing enough members to make the contrast stable. Although this question requires a definition or demarcation of *stability*, the idea of stability is not a part of conventional statistical discourse, and no quantitative boundaries have been considered or established. Consequently, the currently unanswerable question about stability is usually transferred to an answerable question about probability. An α boundary is established for the level of probability, and the results are regarded as "statistically significant" when $P \leq \alpha$ or a $1 - \alpha$ confidence interval has suitable borders. The conclusion about statistical significance is then used to infer stability.

If boundaries were directly demarcated for stability, however, questions about a range of potential variation could be referred to those boundaries. For example, an observed distinction that seems to be "big" could be accepted as stable if the potential variations do not make it become "small." A distinction that is "small" could be accepted as stable if it does not potentially become "big." For these key decisions, however, investigators would have to set quantitative boundaries for *big* and *small*. The boundaries might vary for the context of different comparisons but could be established for appropriate circumstances. If these boundaries were given priority of attention, the investigators could then choose a method—fragility relocations, parametric theory, bootstrap resampling, etc.—for determining a range of potential variation.

Probably the greatest appeal of the purely probabilistic approach is that it avoids the scientific challenge of setting *descriptive* boundaries. The stochastic α boundary, which refers to probability, not to substantive magnitudes, becomes the basis for evaluating all quantitative distinctions, regardless of their scientific components and contexts. With a generally accepted α level, such as .05, the stochastic decision can promptly be made from a P value or from a $1 - \alpha$ confidence interval. As noted earlier and later, the .05 boundary may be too inflexible, but it serves the important role of providing a "standard criterion."

When the range of potential variation is examined with confidence intervals, however, the data analyst may sometimes make an *ad hoc* "dealer's choice" for the selected level of α. The extremes of potential variation (denoted by the ends of the constructed confidence intervals) can then be interpreted with individual *ad hoc* judgments about what is big or small. Without established standard criteria for either a stochastic or quantitative boundary, confidence intervals can then be used, as discussed in Section 13.6.1.3, to achieve almost any conclusion that the data analyst would like to support.

These problems will doubtlessly persist until investigators reappraise the current statistical paradigm for appraising probability rather than stability. If the basic question becomes "What do I want to know?" rather than "What can I do with what is available?" the answer will require new forms of inferential methods aimed at quantitative rather than probabilistic boundaries.

13.6.1.2   Reciprocal Similarity of P Values and Confidence Intervals — When α is
used as a stochastic boundary, the reciprocal similarity of P values and confidence intervals can be shown
from the construction and "location" of the concomitant stochastic hypothesis. In ordinary stochastic
tests of a two-group contrast, the "location" of the tested hypothesis can be cited as Δ. For the conventional
null hypothesis, symbolized as H_0, the value assigned to Δ is 0. Thus, in a contrast of two means $\overline{X}_A$
and $\overline{X}_B$, with parameters μ_A and μ_B, the hypothesis is H_0: $\Delta = \mu_A - \mu_B = 0$.

In the conventional 2-group Z test, after a boundary is chosen for α, a "decision interval" for two-
tailed P values is constructed around the null hypothesis value of 0, extending from $-Z_\alpha$ to $+Z_\alpha$. If d_0 is
the observed difference for $\overline{X}_A - \overline{X}_B$, and if SED is its standard error, the critical ratio for the observed
Z_0 is calculated as $Z_0 = d_0/(SED)$. The null hypothesis is conceded if Z_0 falls inside the interval of $0 \pm$
Z_α, and is rejected if Z_0 is outside. Thus, a two-tailed P value will achieve stochastic significance if $|Z_0|$
$> Z_\alpha$.

The *confidence interval* for comparing two groups is constructed not around $\Delta = 0$, but around the
observed value of d_0. After α is chosen and Z_α is determined, the $1 - \alpha$ interval is calculated as $d_0 \pm Z_\alpha$
(SED). The null hypothesis is conceded if its value of 0 falls inside this interval and is rejected if 0 is
outside. Thus, the stochastic requirement for "significance" is $|d_0| - Z_\alpha$ (SED) > 0. When both sides of
the latter expression are divided by SED to express the result in standard error units, the symbolic
formulation becomes $|d_0/SED| - Z_\alpha > 0$, which is $|Z_0| - Z_\alpha > 0$ or $|Z_0| > Z_\alpha$ — the same demand as
previously.

Because the requirement for stochastic significance is exactly the same whether Z_0 is converted to a
confidence interval or to a P value, confidence intervals are essentially a type of "reciprocal" for P values.
For the P value, we calculate $|d_0|/SED = Z_0$ and compare Z_0 directly with Z_α. For the confidence interval,
we calculate $|d_0| - Z_\alpha$ (SED) and compare the result against 0.

13.6.1.3   Scientific Standards for Descriptive Boundaries — When extending from $|d_0| -$
Z_α (SED) to $|d_0| + Z_\alpha$ (SED), the confidence interval demonstrates how large $|d_0|$ might really be. Beyond
their stochastic roles, the two ends of the confidence interval might therefore make an extra contribution
to quantitative decisions about importance or "clinical" significance for the observed results. During
most of the latter half of the 20th century, however, this type of quantitative significance has been
restricted to stochastic rather than substantive decisions. When scientists begin to exhume or reclaim
significance from its mathematical abduction, they will realize, as discussed in Chapter 10, that quantitative decisions depend on purely *descriptive* rather than *inferential* boundaries. Therefore, a descriptive
scientific question cannot be suitably answered when the product of an inferential choice, Z_α, multiplies
an inferential estimate of SED, to form an arbitrary mathematical entity, Z_α (SED). Aside from obvious
problems when the Gaussian Z_α and SED do not adequately represent "eccentric" data, the doubly
inferential product gives no attention to the investigator's *descriptive* concepts and goals.

As crucial scientific boundaries for quantitatively significant and insignificant distinctions, respectively,
δ and ζ must be chosen with criteria of scientific comparison, not mathematical inference. Consequently,
the stochastic intervals constructed with Z_α and SED calculations do not address the fundamental
substantive issues, and attention to the stochastic results may disguise the absence of truly scientific
standards for the quantitative boundaries.

13.6.1.4   Potential Deception of Confidence Intervals — One immediate problem pro-
duced by the absence of standards is that an investigator who wants to advocate a "big" difference may
focus on the upper end of the confidence interval, ignoring the lower end, which might extend below
the null hypothesis level of 0 (or 1, for a ratio). Although the observed distinction would not be
stochastically significant and might be dismissed as too unstable for serious attention, the investigator
may nevertheless claim stochastic support for the "big" difference. This type of abuse evoked a protest
by Fleiss,[3] who said the problem would be prevented if P values were always demanded. If both ends
of the confidence interval are always reported, however, and if the lower end goes beneath the null-
hypothesis boundary, readers of the published results can readily discern the potential deception of a
unilateral focus.

A more substantial deception, against which the reader has no overt protection, occurs when the confidence interval itself has been "rigged" to give the result desired by the investigator. This type of "rigging" is readily achieved if α is abandoned as a stochastic criterion, so that a fixed level of α is no longer demanded for a $1 - \alpha$ confidence interval. If nonspecific "confidence intervals" can be formed arbitrarily, a zealous analyst can choose whatever level of α is needed to make the result as large or small as desired.

To illustrate this point, suppose the observed increment is $d_o = 8.0$, with a standard error of SED = 4.0. To make the confidence interval *exclude* 0, we can choose a relatively large α such as .1. With $Z_{.1} = 1.645$, the component for the two-tailed 90% confidence interval will be $1.645 \times 4.0 = 6.58$, and the interval, constructed as 8.0 ± 6.58, will extend from 1.42 to 14.58, thereby excluding 0. To make the interval include 0, however, we can choose a smaller α, such as .02. With $Z_{.02} = 2.32$, the two-tailed 98% component will be $2.32 \times 4 = 9.28$. Constructed as 8.0 ± 9.28, the confidence interval will include 0 by extending from -1.28 to 17.28. To give the interval an unimpressive upper end, let $\alpha = .5$. The 50% confidence interval constructed with $Z_{.5} = .674$, will now be 8.0 ± 2.7, extending only to 10.7. To give the interval a much higher upper end, let $\alpha = .001$. The 99.9% confidence interval, with $Z_{.001} = 3.29$, will then be 8.0 ± 13.16, and its upper end will exceed 21.

As a customary standard for stochastic decisions, $\alpha = .05$ may have all the invidious features of any arbitrary choice, but it has the laudable virtue of being a generally accepted criterion that cannot be altered whenever, and in whatever direction, the data analyst would like. Unless the proponents of confidence intervals agree on using a fixed (although suitably flexible) boundary for α, stochastic decisions will become an idiosyncratic subjective process, based on the analyst's personal *ad hoc* goals for each occasion.

Until editors and investigators reach a consensus on this matter, you should be wary of any confidence interval that is reported as merely a "confidence interval." If not accompanied by an indication of $1 - \alpha$ (such as 95%, 90%, 50%), the uninformative result may be deceptive. If the $1 - \alpha$ level is reported but departs from the customary 95%, a suitable (and convincing) explanation should be provided for the choice.

13.6.2 Coefficient of Stability

A commonsense approach, which avoids all of the mathematical manipulations, is to make up your own mind by examining the ratio, SED/d_o, which is the two-group counterpart of the coefficient of stability for the central index of one-group. In previous discussions, the coefficient for one group seemed "stable" if its value was $\leq .1$. For the greater variability that might be expected in two groups, this criterion level might be raised to a higher value such as .3, .4, or .5. The criterion can then be used to decide whether the increment (or other distinction) in central indexes for the two compared groups is relatively stable or unstable. As you evaluate the ratio, SED/d_o, for the coefficient of stability in two groups, however, remember that its inverse, d_o/SED, produces the value of Z_o used for determining P values, and that $P < .05$ when $Z_o \geq 2$. If you feel assured by $\alpha = .05$, then "stability" seems likely when SED/d_o is $\leq .5$. If you want a much smaller SED/d_o ratio to persuade you of stability, the corresponding Z_o values will be much larger than 2, and the corresponding P values will become .01 or .001. In the example just described, with $d_o = 8$ and SED = 4, the coefficient of potential variation is .5, which is just at the border of "stochastic significance" or "stability."

To do this type of assessment, however, the SED, and not just the confidence interval, would always have to be cited as a necessary part of truth in reporting.

13.7 Z or t Tests for Paired Groups

Section 7.8.2.2 was concerned with the "paired one-group t test" that can be done when individual members of the two groups are paired, usually in a before-and-after arrangement of data values. Sometimes, however, the data may represent results of a "cross-over" study where each person received treatment A and then treatment B. In yet other situations, two parts of the same person may be paired for comparing therapeutic responses. (Suncream A may be tested on the right arm and Suncream B on the left arm.) In all of these "paired" circumstances, two groups of data are collected, but they can readily be converted to a single group and tested with the one-group (or "one-sample") rather than two-group test.

For this procedure in Section 7.8.1, the pairs of individual data for variable V and variable W were converted to a single group of differences, $d_i = V_i - W_i$, for which we found the mean difference ($\bar{d}$), the group variance (S_{dd}), the standard deviation (s_d), and the standard error ($s_d/\sqrt{n}$). We then calculated and interpreted

$$t \text{ (or Z)} = \frac{\bar{d}}{s_d/\sqrt{n}}$$

13.7.1   Effect of Correlated Values

The main reason for converting the data and doing a one-group rather than two-group t (or Z) test is that the two-group test makes the assumption that the two sets of data are *independent* for each group. In a crossover, before-and-after, or analogous "paired" arrangement, however, each person's second value is not independent; it will usually be correlated with the first value. The explanation for this effect was shown in Appendixes 7.1 and 7.2. For a difference in two paired variables, $\{W_i\}$ and $\{V_i\}$, the group variance is $S_{WW} - 2S_{WV} + S_{VV}$. If the two variables are independent, the covariance term $S_{WV} \sim 0$. If the variables are related, however, S_{WV} has a definite value and its subtraction will produce a substantial reduction in group variance for the paired values.

For example, consider the following before-and-after values for three people:

Person	"Before" Value	"After" Value	Increment
1	160	156	4
2	172	166	6
3	166	161	5

The values of the mean and standard deviation for the Group B ("before") values, will have $\bar{X}_B = (160 + 172 + 166)/3 = 166$ and $s_B = 6$. For the Group A ("after") values, the corresponding results will be $\bar{X}_A = (156 + 166 + 161)/3 = 161$ and $s_A = 5$. The values of group variance would be $S_{bb} = (n_B - 1)s_B^2 = 72$ and $S_{aa} = (n_A - 1)s_A^2 = 50$. The increment in the two means will be $166 - 161 = 5$; the pooled group variance will be $72 + 50 = 122$; and its stochastic average will be $122/[(3-1) + (3-1)] = 30.5$, so that the pooled standard deviation, s_p, is $\sqrt{30.5} = 5.52$. As a separate single group of data, however, the paired increments have the same incremental mean, $\bar{X}_d = (4 + 6 + 5)/3 = 5$, but much lower values for variance: $S_{dd} = 2$ and $s_d = 1$. In this instance $S_{dd} = S_{aa} - 2 S_{ab} + S_{bb}$; and S_{ab} can be calculated as $\Sigma X_{A_i} X_{B_i} - N\bar{X}_A\bar{X}_B = 80238 - 3 (166)(161) = 60$. The value for S_{dd} becomes $50 - 2 (60) + 72 = 2$.

Because s_d becomes much smaller than s_p, the paired t (or Z) test is more likely to achieve stochastic significance than the "unpaired" or two-group test. In the foregoing example, the *paired* calculation for t is $5/(1/\sqrt{3}) = 5/.58 = 8.66$. The *unpaired* or two-group calculation is $t = (5/5.52)(\sqrt{(3)(3)/6}) = 1.11$. The paired result would be stochastically significant at $2P < .05$, but the unpaired two-group result would not.

13.7.2   Paired vs. Two-Group Arrangements

Because the paired one-group test is more likely to produce stochastic significance than the two-group test, you may wonder why investigators seeking the accolade of stochastic "significance" do not always use the paired test. Why bother with the two-group test?

The answer to this question is that most sets of data for two groups cannot be individually paired. In most studies, the members of the two groups were obtained or treated separately, i.e., "independently," and the two group sizes are usually unequal, i.e., $n_A \neq n_B$. A pairing can be done, however, only when the research has been specifically designed for a paired arrangement of data in the individual persons under investigation.

The reduction in variance that allows stochastic significance to be obtained more easily with the paired individual arrangement also allows the use of smaller groups. This distinction is responsible for the avidity with which investigators try to do "crossover studies" whenever possible. Unfortunately, for reasons noted elsewhere,[4] such studies are seldom possible — and even when they are, a formidable scientific problem can arise if the effects of Treatment A are "carried over" when the patient transfers to Treatment B.

13.7.3 Arbitrary Analytical Pairings

The pairing tactic is sometimes applied to check or confirm results noted with a two-group comparison. Using a type of resampling, the analyst randomly selects members of Group A to be paired with randomly selected members of Group B. Results are then calculated for the randomly selected "paired sample," and many such samples can be constructed to see if their results verify what was previously found for the two groups. The procedure, which keeps each group intact, differs from the combination of both groups that precedes a Pitman-Welch type of permutation resampling.

In the days before modern forms of multivariable analysis, a paired arrangement of members of two groups could be used to "match" for other pertinent variables beyond the main variable under analysis. For example, as part of the original research used to indict cigarette smoking as a cause of early mortality, the Surgeon General's Committee[5] asked Cuyler Hammond to reanalyze the original data of his long-term cohort study,[6] and to compare mortality rates for "a 'matched pair' analysis, in which pairs of cigarette smokers and non-smokers were matched on height, education, religion, drinking habits, urban-rural residence and occupational exposure."[5]

13.8 Z Test for Two Proportions

Although commonly used for two means, the Z test can also be applied to evaluate a difference in two proportions, $p_A = r_A/n_A$ and $p_B = r_B/n_B$. Because the variance of a proportion is pq, we can use Formula [13.1] to substitute appropriately and find that the variance of the increment, $p_A - p_B$, will be $(p_A q_A/n_A) + (p_B q_B/n_B)$. Under the null hypothesis that $\pi_A = \pi_B$, we estimate a common value for π as $P = (n_A p_A + n_B p_B)/N = (r_A + r_B)/(n_A + n_B)$. The estimated variance (or squared standard error) of the difference will then be $(PQ/n_A) + (PQ/n_B) = NPQ/n_A n_B$. The test statistic will be calculated as

$$Z = \frac{p_A - p_B}{\sqrt{NPQ/n_A n_B}} = \frac{p_A - p_B}{\sqrt{PQ}} \times \sqrt{\frac{n_A n_B}{N}} \qquad [13.16]$$

You may already have recognized that this formula is an exact counterpart of [13.13] for dimensional data. The standardized increment, which is $(p_A - p_B)/\sqrt{PQ}$, is multiplied by the group-size factor, which is $\sqrt{n_A n_B/N}$.

To illustrate the calculations, consider the contrast of 18/24 (75%) vs. 10/15 (67%). The common value for P would be $(18 + 10)/(24 + 15) = .718$ and $Q = 1 - P = .282$. The standardized increment will be $(.75 - .67)/\sqrt{(.718)(.282)} = .178$. The group size factor will be $\sqrt{(15 \times 24)/39} = 3.04$ and the product for Z will be $(.178)(3.04) = .54$. The result will not be stochastically significant if $\alpha = .05$.

13.8.1 Similarity to Chi-Square Test

As noted later in Chapter 14, the value of Z in Formula [13.16] is the exact square root of the test statistic obtained when the chi-square test is applied to a contrast of two proportions. Accordingly, although the chi-square test is more conventional, the Z test can be used just as effectively for comparing two proportions.

13.8.2   Continuity Correction

You may remember that a continuity correction was recommended back in Section 8.6.1 when the Z procedure is applied to a proportion. Although not all authorities are agreed, this correction can also be applied when two proportions are compared. For the correction, 1/2 is subtracted from the numerator of the larger proportion, and 1/2 is added to the numerator of the smaller proportion. Thus, if $p_A = r_A/n_A$ and $p_B = r_B/n_B$, and if $p_A > p_B$, the correction is

$$Z_C = \frac{[r_A - (1/2)]/n_A - [r_B + (1/2)]/n_B}{\sqrt{NPQ/n_A n_B}}$$

The algebra can be simplified if you recognize that the numerator of this expression becomes $p_A - p_B - [(1/2)(N/n_A n_B)]$. If we let $G = N/n_A n_B$, the expression becomes

$$Z_C = \frac{p_A - p_B - (G/2)}{\sqrt{PQG}}$$

In the foregoing example, $G = 39/(15 \times 24) = .108$, and $G/2 = .054$. The corrected value would be

$$Z_C = \frac{.75 - .67 - .054}{\sqrt{(.718)(.282)(.108)}} = \frac{.0293}{\sqrt{.02187}} = .198$$

The continuity result is identical to what is achieved as the square root of chi-square when the latter is calculated with an analogous continuity correction in Chapter 14. The desirability of the correction will be discussed in that chapter.

13.8.3   Standard Error for Alternative Hypothesis

For the alternative hypothesis, when we assume that $\pi_A \neq \pi_B$, the common value for π is *not* estimated as $P = (n_A p_A + n_B p_B)/N$. In this situation, the standard error is determined as $\sqrt{(p_A q_A/n_A) + (p_B q_B/n_B)}$, not with $\sqrt{NPQ/n_A n_B}$ as in Formula (13.16).

If you work out the algebra, the difference in the two squared standard errors turns out to be minor. Thus, if we let

$$k = \frac{NPQ}{n_A n_B} - \left(\frac{p_A q_A}{n_A} + \frac{p_B q_B}{n_B} \right)$$

the value of k becomes

$$k = \frac{n_A - n_B}{n_A n_B}(p_A q_A - p_B q_B) + \frac{(p_A - p_B)^2}{N} \qquad [13.17]$$

For example, for the comparison of 18/24 vs. 10/15, the conventional standard error is $\sqrt{(39)(.718)(.282)/(24)(15)} = .148$. The standard error for the alternative hypothesis is $\sqrt{[(18)(6)/(24)] + [(10)(5)/(15)]} = .150$. According to Formula [13.17], k turns out to be $-.00069$, which is essentially $(.148)^2 - (.150)^2$.

13.9   Sample Size for a Contrast of Two Means

The last topic discussed in this chapter is the calculation of sample size for a contrast of two means. The calculational challenge occurs most commonly in clinical trials, where the contrast is usually between two proportions, rather than two means; and the clinical-trial calculations often involve the simultaneous consideration of both a null and an alternative hypothesis, as discussed later in Chapter 23. Nevertheless, particularly in laboratory experiments, an investigator may want to know the sample size required to show stochastically that the mean is "significantly" larger for Group A than for Group B.

The process once again involves the type of anticipatory estimates that were discussed in Section 8.8.3, and the conversation between investigator and statistician often evokes the same kind of frustrating guesswork. The decisions require six choices: two estimates, a quantitative distinction, a stochastic boundary, a direction, and a sample partition. The estimates, distinctions, and boundaries are commonly shown with Greek letters to denote that they have been guessed or assigned, rather than actually observed.

One of the estimates is $\hat{\mu}_B$, the mean expected in Group B. The other estimate is $\hat{\sigma}_p$, the common (or pooled) standard deviation of data in the two groups. For example, we might estimate that Group B will have a mean of 32.0, and that the common standard deviation is 12.3. The quantitative distinction is labeled δ, the anticipated magnitude for the impressive or "quantitatively significant" increment in means between Group A and Group B. After δ is chosen, the anticipated mean in Group A is estimated as $\hat{\mu}_A = \hat{\mu}_B + \delta$. If we want the mean in Group A to be at least 25% larger than in Group B, we set δ at 8.0, so that the mean expected for Group A should exceed 40.0.

The next step is to chose a stochastic boundary for α, which can be set at the conventional .05. Because we expect Group A to exceed Group B, a direction has been stated, and the Z_α corresponding to a one-tailed $\alpha = .05$ would be $Z_{.1} = 1.645$. If we wanted to comply with the customary preference for two-tailed tests, however, the anticipated difference would be $|\mu_A - \mu_B| = \delta$ and the $\alpha = .05$ would be bi-directional, so that $Z_{.05} = 1.96$. Finally, for sample partition, we can make the customary choice of equal-size samples, so that $n_A = n_B = n$, and $N = 2n$.

With all of these decisions completed, the rest is easy. The sample size can be calculated by putting all the Greek and other values into the appropriate formula for either a Z test or a confidence interval.

13.9.1 Z-test Formula

For the Z-test sample-size calculation, Formula [13.13] receives appropriate substitutions to become

$$Z_\alpha = [(\hat{\mu}_A - \hat{\mu}_B)/\hat{\sigma}_p]\sqrt{n^2/2n}$$

Squaring both sides and rearranging terms produces

$$(n/2) = \frac{Z_\alpha^2 \hat{\sigma}_p^2}{(\hat{\mu}_A - \hat{\mu}_B)^2} \qquad [13.18]$$

and because $\hat{\mu}_A - \hat{\mu}_B = \delta$ and $\hat{\sigma}_p^2 = s_p^2$, the sample size for one group is

$$n = 2Z_\alpha^2 s_p^2/(\delta)^2 \qquad [13.19]$$

Substituting the foregoing data and using a two-tailed test, we get

$$n = \frac{(2)(1.96)^2(12.3)^2}{(8.0)^2} = 18.2$$

The required sample size will be 19 members in each group. The total sample size will be 38.

13.9.2 Confidence-Interval Formula

With the confidence-interval approach, we want the expected difference, d_o, to exceed 0 at the lower end, so that

$$d_o - Z_\alpha(SED) > 0$$

Because SED is $s_p\sqrt{N/(n_A n_B)}$, we can substitute appropriately and rearrange terms to get

$$\delta > Z_\alpha\, s_p\, \sqrt{2n/n^2}$$

which becomes

$$n > 2Z_\alpha^2 s_p^2 / \delta^2$$

yielding the same result as previously in Formula [13.19].

13.9.3   Adjustment for t Distribution

If we worry that the sample size of 38 is not quite large enough to justify using Z rather than t, the value of $t_{36,.05} = 2.028$ can be substituted for $Z_{.05} = 1.96$ in the foregoing formulas. The result will be

$$n > 2(2.028)^2 \, (12.3)^2/(8.0)^2 = 19.4$$

With a sample size of 20 members in each group, the degrees of freedom will be 38, and $t_{38,.05}$ will be 2.0244. Substituting $(2.0244)^2$ for $(2.028)^2$ in the foregoing calculation produces $n > 19.33$, and so we can keep the sample size as 20 in each group.

13.9.4   One-Tailed Result

Because Z_α^2 (or t_α^2) appears in the numerator of the calculation, the sample size is always larger for two-tailed than one-tailed decisions. For one-tailed calculations, we would use $Z_{.1} = 1.645$ or $t_{38,.1} = 1.686$. The sample size in Formula [13.19] would be reduced to

$$n > 2(1.686)^2 \, (12.3)^2/(8.0)^2 = 13.4$$

and the total sample size would become $2 \times 14 = 28$.

13.9.5   Augmentation for "Insurance"

After all the precise calculations have been completed, with all their exact mathematical stipulations, the results are usually altered by an act of pure judgment. To provide "insurance" against such phenomena as loss of members, "unusable data," or any other potential reduction in the effective size of the research group, a cautious investigator will almost always increase the number that emerged from the mathematical calculations. The amount of augmentation usually exceeds the calculated amount by 10%, 20%, or even more, according to a background "judgment" based on the losses encountered in previous instances of the same type of research. The mathematical calculations may have had splendid quantification, but the ultimate decision depends on augmentations that come from the "hunch" of previous experience.

References

1. Boneau, 1960; 2. Feinstein, 1998a; 3. Fleiss, 1986; 4. Feinstein, 1985; 5. Surgeon General's Advisory Committee on Smoking and Health, 1964; 6. Hammond, 1958; 7. Mohr, 1982.

Exercises

13.1. In Exercise 11.1, you were informed that the t test gave a "nonsignificant" result for the two cited groups of data. Please verify this statement. Why does the t test "fail" to confirm "significance" for these obviously "significant" results?

13.2. In Exercise 12.3, you did a Pitman-Welch test on the mean difference of two groups. For Group A, the data were 2, 8, 11, and 13; for Group B, the data were 1, 3, and 6. Perform a t test on this difference and compare the stochastic conclusions with what you found using the Pitman-Welch test.

13.3. In a randomized clinical trial, one group of babies was fed Formula A from birth to age six months; and the other group was fed Formula B. The two groups can be assumed to have had identical weights at birth. At the end of six months, the weight gains in pounds for members of the two groups were as follows:

Group A: 5, 7, 8, 9, 6, 7, 10, 8, 6

Group B: 9, 10, 8, 6, 7, 9

13.3.1. Considering each group individually, calculate a 95% confidence interval and a 99% confidence interval for the mean. (Show the cogent intermediate steps in your arrangement of calculations.)

13.3.2. Considering each group individually, what is the probability that this group arose from a parent population in which the mean weight gain is 6.7 pounds?

13.3.3. Use two different approaches (t test and confidence interval) to show whether the difference in the means of the two groups is "statistically significant" at the level of $2P < .025$.

13.3.4. Forgetting the differences in the formula feeding, assume that the members of Groups A and B constitute the entire population of babies in which you are interested. What procedure would you use (and show the calculations) to determine whether there is something peculiar about the baby who gained only 5 pounds?

13.4. Here is a chance to let current activities be enlightened by a repetition of past history. In 1908, Gosset reported data showing the comparative effects of two drugs in producing sleep in 10 patients. For each patient, he noted the amount of sleep obtained without medication and the additional hours of sleep gained after treatment (1) with hyoscyamine and (2) with hyoscine. The table below reproduces the data from an original publication, except for a replacement by modern symbols for mean and standard deviation.

Additional hours' sleep gained by the use of two drugs ("Student," 1908)

Patient	Hyoscyamine	Hyoscine	Difference
1	+0.7	+1.9	+1.2
2	−1.6	+0.8	+2.4
3	−0.2	+1.1	+1.3
4	−1.2	+0.1	+1.3
5	−0.1	−0.1	0
6	+3.4	+4.4	+1.0
7	+3.7	+5.5	+1.8
8	+0.8	+1.6	+0.8
9	0	+4.6	+4.6
10	+2.0	+3.4	+1.4
$\overline{X}$	+0.75	+2.33	+1.58
s	1.79	2.00	1.23

The results in this table can be stochastically evaluated with a two-group or one-group test. Do both procedures and compare the results. What is the reason for any differences you observed? Can you demonstrate the source of the differences?

13.5. At a medical meeting you are attending, a renowned professor presents "statistically significant" results showing $\overline{X}_A = 16$, $SE_A = 4$, and $n_A = 81$ for Group A; and $\overline{X}_B = 25$, $SE_B = 6$, and $n_B = 64$ for Group B. Everyone seems to be impressed by the large difference. During the discussion period, however, a member of the audience, who has been sitting placidly taking no notes and doing no apparent calculations, arises to dispute the professor's contention. The commentator says that the difference is *not* "statistically significant" and says, in addition, that the data should *not* have been reported with mean values as summaries of the results.

Everyone is now shocked or outraged by the temerity, skill, or chutzpah of the commentator. The challenged professor responds by saying that he does not understand the mathematics and calls for help from his statistician, who happens to be present in the audience, accompanied by a large volume of computer printout. Intrigued by the dispute, the chairperson declares a brief intermission, while the statistician checks the results. After the intermission, the professor returns to the podium and confesses, somewhat abashedly, that he mistakenly looked at the wrong section of printout in finding the "significant" P value. Furthermore, he says that the statistician has also expressed reservations about using means to summarize the results.

  13.5.1. What do you think the commentator did to decide that the results were not "statistically significant"?
  13.5.2. What is the correct P value for this comparison?
  13.5.3. On what basis do you think the commentator rejected the means as summary indexes?
  13.5.4. What would you recommend as a strategy for an improved alternative summary and analysis?

13.6. In a report in *The Lancet*, the authors did a crossover study in 10 patients with refractory noctural angina.[7] For the control night the bed was placed with the head in a semi-erect position; and for the test night it was put in a feet-down position. The authors wrote that "Results were compared by means of student's t test (non-paired, two-tailed). All numerical results were expressed as mean ± standard error of the mean."

The table below is a copy of what was published as Table II in the report.[7]

Effects of Feet-Down Position on Number of Pain Episodes and Number of Isosorbide Dinitrate Tablets Taken

Patient No.	No. Pain Episodes		No. Tablets	
	Control	Test	Control	Test
1	6	0	6	0
2	2	0	4	0
3	2	0	2	0
4	7	0	10	0
5	3	1	4	1
6	5	0	5	0
7	3	0	5	0
8	2	0	2	0
9	3	1	6	2
10	4	0	4	0
Mean ± SEM	3.7 ± 1.8	0.2 ± 0.4*	4.8 ± 2.3	0.3 ± 0.7*

* $p < 0.001$.

  13.6.1. A value of "$p < 0.001$" is shown for the comparison of "No. pain episodes" in the *Control* and *Test* results. Verify this claim, and show how you verified it.
  13.6.2. Can you think of a simple procedure, which can be done mentally without any calculation, that would promptly give you essentially the same result for the P value in the table? (This is one of those questions where you immediately see how to get the answer—or you don't. If you don't, go on to the next question and don't spend a lot of time deliberating.)

13.7. If you have time, and want to check your understanding of some of the basic principles involved in this and preceding chapters, try answering the following "top ten" questions:

  13.7.1. For a two-group t (or Z) test, why do we subtract the two means? Why not form a ratio of some other index of contrast?
  13.7.2. In the two-group tests, the incremental deviation is calculated as $X_i - \bar{X}$ for the members of each group. Is this the best way to indicate discrepancies between individual values and the central indexes?
  13.7.3. Why are standard deviations calculated by first squaring and summing the individual deviations? Why not use them directly?
  13.7.4. Why is the sum of squared deviations divided by n − 1 rather than n for inferential calculations? What is the justification for getting an "average" value by using one fewer than the number of available members in a group?

13.7.5. What is a *standard error of the mean*? What errors were created during the measurement process, and why don't the investigators find and fix the errors before doing all the statistical analyses?

13.7.6. In the formula for a t (or Z) test, the increment in the numerator is divided by a standard error in the denominator. Why are the two terms divided? Why aren't they added or multiplied?

13.7.7. What is the meaning of *degrees of freedom*? What type of incarceration and subsequent liberation occurred before the data received their "freedom"? And why does it have different "degrees"?

13.7.8. What is a P value? It has immense importance in the uriniferous aspects of human physiology, but what is it statistically? Why does it have so dominant a role in deciding whether research results are "significant" or "nonsignificant"?

13.7.9. What are you confident about in a "confidence interval"? When might your confidence be statistically unjustified? When would the confidence be unjustified for other reasons?

13.7.10. What is the meaning of an α level for "false positive conclusions"? Are they an inevitable consequence of the errors in "standard errors"? Why is α regularly set at .05?

14

Chi-Square Test and Evaluation of Two Proportions

CONTENTS

To do a stochastic contrast (for "statistical significance") of two proportions, the following three methods have already been discussed in Chapters 11–13:

1. *Fragility test*: The unit fragility test (Section 11.2.3.1) is simple, is easy to understand, and uses a commonsense approach that might be applied if investigators were directly appraising stability, without being affected by previous mathematical instruction. The fragility test, however, is new, generally unfamiliar, and currently unaccompanied either by a long track record or by recommendations from what R. A. Fisher once called "heavyweight authorities."

2. *Fisher Exact Test*: Generally regarded as the "gold standard," the Fisher exact test (Chapter 12) should always be used when the constituent numbers are small. It can also be applied if the numbers are large, but usually needs a computer for the calculations. The only disadvantages of the Fisher test are that most current computer programs have not been automated to produce confidence intervals routinely or to do advance calculations of sample size.

3. *Z test*: The Z test (Section 13.8) for the increment in two proportions is easy to do with a hand calculator and requires only that the group sizes be adequately large. Unlike the first two methods, the Z procedure can readily be applied to get conventional confidence intervals or to calculate sample size.

Despite the availability of these three methods, however, two proportions are usually stochastically compared with a fourth procedure to which the rest of this chapter is devoted. Called *chi-square* (rhymes with "eye square"), the procedure is probably the most commonly applied statistical tactic in group-based clinical or epidemiologic research. The chi-square test is popular because it is easy to calculate from the frequency counts of categorical data; and it is versatile enough for many additional applications that will be described later. For two proportions, the chi-square test yields the same result as a Z test; and, when the constituent numbers are large enough, the chi-square (or Z) test produces a stochastic conclusion almost identical to what emerges from a Fisher exact test.

14.1 Basic Principles of Chi-Square Reasoning

The chi-square test relies on a hypothetical "model" for the set of "expected" frequencies in categories of the data. The expected and observed frequencies in each category are then arranged in a ratio as

$$(\text{observed} - \text{expected})^2 / \text{expected}$$

and the sum of these ratios forms the test statistic,

$$X^2 = \Sigma \left[\frac{(\text{observed} - \text{expected})^2}{\text{expected}} \right] \qquad [14.1]$$

The calculated results for X^2 are interpreted with a theoretical sampling distribution from which we find the associated P value and then decide to concede or reject the hypothesis that formed the model being tested.

14.1.1   Two Sources of Models

The model that produces the expected values can come from one of two different assumptions for the null hypothesis. One assumption refers to the apportionment of categories in the simple univariate distribution of a *one-way* table. The proportions may be assumed either to be equal, such as 25% for each of four categories, or to occur in a specific ratio, such as the 9:3:3:1 distribution of *AB*, *Ab*, *aB*, and *ab* in genetic mixtures. The X^2 test for the observed univariate distribution will indicate how well the expectations fit the observed categorical frequencies. Rejection of the null hypothesis leads to the conclusion that the anticipated model fits the data poorly. This type of procedure, illustrated later in Section 14.7.1, is called a *goodness-of-fit chi-square test* and is usually applied to a one-way table of categories, not to the proportions compared in a 2 × 2 table.

The latter comparison is usually done with a different assumption, which is the null hypothesis that the two variables under examination are *independent*, i.e., that one of the variables, such as type of treatment, has no effect on the other variable, such as successful outcome. In the chi-square test of independence, which is commonly applied to two-way tables, the expected values emerge from the observed data, not from a previous belief about apportionment. Subsequent rejection of the null hypothesis leads to the conclusion that the two variables are not independent, i.e., that successful outcome is affected by type of treatment.

14.1.2   Illustration of Test of Independence

In its most frequent and world-renowned application, X^2 (pronounced ex-square) is used to compare two proportions, such as the occurrence of anemia in 6% (6/95) of a group of men and in 13% (14/105) of a group of women. For the stochastic comparison, the proportions are usually "unpacked" to form a 2 × 2 (or fourfold) contingency table, having a structure such as Table 14.1.

TABLE 14.1

2 × 2 Table Showing Contingency Counts for Presence of Anemia in a Group of 200 Men and Women

	Anemic	Not Anemic	Total
Men	6	89	95
Women	14	91	105
Total	20	180	200

Under the null hypothesis of independence, we assume that the two variables, sex and anemia, in Table 14.1 are independent, i.e., unrelated. We therefore expect men and women to be similar in their proportions of anemia and non-anemia. To determine these proportions, we use the *total* results in the data as the best source of the parametric estimates. Thus, from the marginal totals in the table, the "true" proportional parameters would be estimated as 20/200 = .10 for anemia and 180/200 = .90 for non-anemia.

With these parametric estimates, the expected frequency counts in the cells of the table would be .1 × 95 = 9.5 for anemia and .9 × 95 = 85.5 for non-anemia in the 95 men, and .1 × 105 = 10.5 and .9 × 105 = 94.5 correspondingly for the 105 women. For calculating the observed/expected ratios in Formula [14.1], the upper left cell in Table 14.1 would produce $(6 - 9.5)^2/9.5 = (-3.5)^2/9.5$. After the remaining appropriate ratios are formed and added, the value for X^2 would be

$$X^2 = \frac{(-3.5)^2}{9.5} + \frac{(3.5)^2}{85.5} + \frac{(3.5)^2}{10.5} + \frac{(-3.5)^2}{94.5} = \frac{12.25}{9.5} + \frac{12.25}{85.5} + \frac{12.25}{10.5} + \frac{12.25}{94.5} = 2.73$$

When checked as shown shortly, the associated 2P value for this X^2 exceeds .05. Thus, there is a reasonable stochastic chance (i.e., greater than 1 in 20) that men and women — at least in the group under study here — do indeed have similar occurrence rates of anemia.

14.1.3 The χ^2 Distribution

The critical ratio that forms the calculated value of X^2 is an arbitrary stochastic index or "test statistic," which has a mathematical sampling distribution called chi-square, written as χ^2. (This same phenomenon occurred earlier for the "critical ratio" of test statistics that were referred to a t or Gaussian Z distribution. In the previous activities, however, the same names, t or Z, were used for both the test statistics and the corresponding distributions of "continuous" dimensional data. For the "discontinuities" of categorical data, a distinction can be made between X^2, the calculated test statistic, and χ^2, the theoretical continuous distribution.)

The "discovery" of the chi-square distribution is usually ascribed to Karl Pearson, but it is now believed to have been introduced in Germany in 1863 by the physicist, E. Abbe,[1] and publicized in 1876 by another physicist, F. R. Helmert.[2]

The mathematical idea behind the χ^2 distribution (if you are curious to know) involves the sum of squares for a series of individual Gaussian variables, X_j, each with standard deviation, σ_j. When each variable is cited as a standardized deviate, $Z_j = (X_j - \bar{X}_j)/\sigma_j$, the sum of squares for ν such independent deviates is

$$\chi^2_\nu = Z^2_1 + Z^2_2 + \cdots + Z^2_\nu \qquad [14.2]$$

The subscript "ν" denotes that ν independent standard "normal variates" contributed to the sum. The sampling distribution of χ^2_ν would produce a family of curves, analogous to the family we found for the t distribution, with ν being the degrees of freedom for each curve.

Figure 14.1 shows the probability density, analogous to that of a Gaussian curve, for several members of the family of χ^2 curves, each marked with n degrees of freedom. Unlike Z and t curves, the χ^2 curves are not symmetrical. Like the Z and t curves, however, the χ^2 curves are interpreted for the external probability area that remains under the curve beyond a particular value of χ^2.

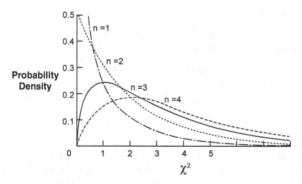

FIGURE 14.1
Probability density of chi-square distribution for different degrees of freedom marked n. (For further details, see text.)

14.1.4 Degrees of Freedom and Interpretation of χ^2

The χ^2 distribution is well suited for interpreting the test statistic, X^2, determined as $\Sigma[(observed - expected)^2/expected]$. The proof of the correspondence between X^2 and χ^2 lies buried somewhere in the annals of mathematical statistics and will not be exhumed here. (Shouts of "hurrah" are permissible, but not encouraged.)

The sampling distribution of χ^2 in its family of curves will have different external P values according to the degrees of freedom in the particular calculated value of X^2. Table 14.2 shows the correspondence of values for χ^2, ν, and P.

To apply Table 14.2 for the X^2 of 2.73 in the data of Table 14.1, we first determine the degrees of freedom in the data. One approach to this decision is to recognize that the increment in two proportions can be converted to a "Z-deviate" using Formula [13.16]. When entered in Formula [14.2], the squared value of Z would be a single member of a χ^2 family and would, therefore, have one degree of freedom.

TABLE 14.2

Correspondence of Two-Tailed External P Values for X^2 Values at Different Degrees of Freedom (marked v)

v	0.90	0.80	0.70	0.60	0.50	0.40	0.30	0.20	0.10	0.050	0.0250	0.010	0.0050	0.0010
1	0.0158	0.0642	0.148	0.275	0.455	0.708	1.074	1.642	2.706	3.841	5.024	6.635	7.879	10.828
2	0.211	0.446	0.713	1.022	1.386	1.833	2.408	3.219	4.605	5.991	7.378	9.210	10.597	13.816
3	0.584	1.005	1.424	1.869	2.366	2.946	3.665	4.642	6.251	7.815	9.348	11.345	12.838	16.266
4	1.064	1.649	2.195	2.753	3.357	4.045	4.878	5.989	7.779	9.488	11.143	13.277	14.860	18.467
5	1.610	2.343	3.000	3.355	4.351	5.132	6.064	7.289	9.236	11.070	12.833	15.086	16.750	20.515
6	2.204	3.070	3.828	4.570	5.348	6.211	7.231	8.558	10.645	12.592	14.449	16.812	18.548	22.458
7	2.833	3.822	4.671	5.493	6.346	7.283	8.383	9.803	12.017	14.067	16.013	18.075	20.278	24.322
8	3.490	4.594	5.527	6.423	7.344	8.351	9.524	11.030	13.362	15.507	17.535	20.090	21.955	26.124
9	4.168	5.380	6.393	7.357	8.343	9.414	10.656	12.242	14.684	16.919	19.023	21.666	23.589	27.877
10	4.865	6.179	7.267	8.295	9.342	10.473	11.781	13.442	15.987	18.307	20.483	23.209	25.188	29.588
11	5.578	6.989	8.148	9.237	10.341	11.530	12.899	14.631	17.275	19.675	21.920	24.725	26.757	31.264
12	6.304	7.807	9.034	10.182	11.340	12.584	14.011	15.812	18.549	21.026	23.337	26.217	28.300	32.909
13	7.042	8.634	9.926	11.129	12.340	13.636	15.119	16.985	19.812	22.362	24.736	27.688	29.819	34.528
14	7.790	9.467	10.821	12.078	13.339	14.685	16.222	18.151	21.064	23.685	26.119	29.141	31.319	36.123
15	8.547	10.307	11.721	13.030	14.339	15.733	17.322	19.311	22.307	24.996	27.488	30.578	32.801	37.697
16	9.312	11.152	12.624	13.983	15.338	16.780	18.418	20.465	23.542	26.296	28.845	32.000	34.267	39.252
17	10.085	12.002	13.531	14.937	16.338	17.824	19.511	21.615	24.769	27.587	30.191	33.409	35.718	40.790
18	10.865	12.857	14.440	15.893	17.338	18.868	20.601	22.760	25.989	28.869	31.526	34.805	37.156	42.312
19	11.651	13.716	15.352	16.850	18.338	19.910	21.689	23.900	27.204	30.144	32.852	36.191	38.582	43.820

Source: This table is derived from Geigy Scientific Tables, Vol. 2, ed. by C. Lentner, 1982 Ciba-Geigy Limited, Basle, Switzerland.

Accordingly, at one degree of freedom in Table 14.2, the top row shows that the calculated X^2 of 2.73 is just higher than the 2.706 value required for $2P = .10$. Therefore, the stochastic conclusion is $.05 < 2P < .10$.

To confirm the relationship of Z^2 and X^2, note that the increment in the numerator of Formula [13.16] for Z is $(14/105) - (6/95) = .070$, and $\sqrt{n_A n_B/N}$ is $\sqrt{(95)(105)/200} = 7.06$. The denominator term for $\sqrt{PQ}$ is calculated as $\sqrt{(20)(180)/200} = .3$. Therefore, $Z = (.070)(7.06)/.3 = 1.65$ and Z^2 is 2.72, which is identical, except for minor rounding, to the value of X^2 calculated with the observed/expected tactic in Section 14.1.2.

Although this approach is satisfactory to show that a 2×2 table has one degree of freedom, a more general strategy is needed for larger two-way tables.

14.1.5   Controversy about d.f. in 2-Way Tables

X^2 tests are most commonly applied to a 2×2 table having four interior cells, but can also be used for two-way tables with larger numbers of cells. With r categories in the rows and c categories in the columns, the table would have $r \times c$ cells.

The decision about degrees of freedom in an $r \times c$ table gave rise, early in the 20th century, to a heated, bitter battle between two statistical titans: Ronald A. Fisher and Karl Pearson. Fisher emerged the victor, but the personal feud between the two men was never resolved, with Fisher thereafter avoiding (or being denied) publication in the then leading journal of statistics (*Biometrika*), which was edited by Pearson. [Fisher, of course, found other places to publish, but the feud was a juicy scandal for many years. Consider the analogous situation in medicine today if William Osler were alive in the U.S. and writing vigorously, but never publishing anything in the *New England Journal of Medicine*.]

In the argument over degrees of freedom, Pearson contended that a two-way table with r rows and c columns would have $r \times c$ cells, and that the degrees of freedom should therefore be $rc - 1$. Fisher demonstrated that the correct value for degrees of freedom was $(r - 1)(c - 1)$.

He began his argument by "dis-entabling" the data and converting the cells into a linear array. It would have $r \times c$ cells, which could be filled with rc degrees of freedom, choosing any desired numbers. Because the cellular totals must add up to N, one degree of freedom is immediately lost, so that $rc - 1$ choices become "freely" available. Reconstructing the $r \times c$ cells into a 2-way table, however, produces some new constraints. The marginal totals must add up to the grand total (N) in the rows and also in the columns. Therefore, only $r - 1$ marginal totals can be freely chosen for the rows, and each of those choices creates an additional constraint in the cellular freedom, so that $r - 1$ degrees of freedom are lost in the basic cellular choices. Analogously, the column totals create another $c - 1$ constraints. Therefore, the degrees of freedom are $rc - 1 - (r - 1) - (c - 1)$, which becomes $(r - 1)(c - 1)$. Thus, a 4×5 table has $(4 - 1)(5 - 1) = (3)(4)$ $= 12$ degrees of freedom, and a 2×2 table has $(2 - 1)(2 - 1) = 1$ degree of freedom.

The idea can be quickly grasped for a 2×2 table if you consider the marginal totals fixed as follows:

		Column	
Row	1	2	Total
1			n_1
2			n_2
Total	f_1	f_2	N

As soon as you enter a number in any one of these four cells, the values of all the remaining cells are determined. Suppose a is chosen to be the value of cell 1,1. Then cell 1,2 is $n_1 - a$; cell 2,1 is $f_1 - a$; and cell 2,2 is either $n_2 - (f_1 - a)$ or $f_2 - (n_1 - a)$. Consequently, the only available freedom in this table is to choose the value for any one of the cells.

14.1.6 "Large" Degrees of Freedom

The formula $(r - 1)(c - 1)$ should be kept in mind when the value of v is determined for $r \times c$ tables that are larger than 2×2. If v becomes very large, however, you may want to reappraise the planned analysis. For example, a table with 4 categories in the rows and 5 categories in the columns will have 12 degrees of freedom, but the results of such a table are usually difficult to understand and interpret. In fact, many experienced, enlightened data analysts say they regularly try to reduce (i.e., compress) everything into a 2×2 table because they understand it best.

Chapter 27 contains a discussion of tables where r and c are each ≥ 3, and also of special tables constructed in a $2 \times c$ (or $r \times 2$) format where only c (or r) is ≥ 3. [For example, we might consider the sequence of survival proportions for four ordinal stages – I, II, III, and IV — in a table that would have $(2 - 1)(4 - 1) = 3$ degrees of freedom.] In general, however, if the degrees of freedom start getting "large" (i.e., ≥ 6), the table is probably unwieldy and should be compressed into smaller numbers of categories. Therefore, opportunities should seldom arise to use the many lines of Table 14.2 for which the degrees of freedom exceed 6.

14.1.7 Yates Continuity Correction

Another major conceptual battle about χ^2 is still being fought today and has not yet been settled. The source of the controversy is the "continuity correction" introduced by Frank Yates[3] in 1934.

The basic argument was discussed in Section 13.8.2. The distribution of a set of categorical frequencies, or of the X^2 value calculated from them, is discontinuous, but χ^2 has a continuous distribution.

Consequently, χ^2 is the "limit" toward which X^2 approaches as the group sizes grow very large. For a suitable "correction" of X^2, Yates proposed that if we take "the half units of deviation from expectation as the group boundaries, we may expect to obtain a much closer approximation to the true distribution."

The net algebraic effect of the Yates correction was to make the basic Formula [14.1] become

$$X_c^2 = \Sigma \frac{(|O - E| - 1/2)^2}{E}$$

where O = observed values, E = expected values, and the c subscript indicates use of the Yates correction. For practical purposes, the Yates correction usually alters the individual observed–expected deviations to make them less extreme. The corrected value of X_c^2 is then used for entering the standard chi-square tables to find the associated value of P.

The Yates correction soon became established as a chic item of statistical fashion in the days before easy computation was available for the Fisher Exact Test. A manuscript reviewer (or editor) who could find nothing else to say about a paper would regularly ask whether the investigators had calculated their X^2 values ignorantly (without the correction) or sagaciously (with it). To know about and use the Yates correction became one of the "in-group" distinctions — somewhat like knowing the difference between *incidence* and *prevalence* — that separated the pro from the neophyte in the analysis of clinical and epidemiologic data.

In recent years, however, a major assault has been launched against the continuity correction and it seems to be going out of fashion. The anti-Yates-correction argument is that the uncorrected X^2 value gives better agreement than the corrected one when an exact probability (rather than an approximate one, via χ^2 tables) is calculated for the data of a 2×2 table. If the "gold standard" Fisher exact probability test, discussed in Chapter 12, eventually replaces the X^2 test altogether, the dispute about the Yates correction will become moot.

14.2 Formulas for Calculation

Because the chi-square procedure is so popular, many tactics have been developed to simplify the arithmetic with methods that incorporate the "expected" values into the calculations, thereby avoiding the cumbersome $\Sigma[(\text{observed} - \text{expected})^2/\text{expected}]$ formula. The alternative formulas are listed here for readers who may want or need to do the calculations themselves without a computer program. [If you like interesting algebraic challenges, you can work out proofs that the cited formulas are correct.]

14.2.1 2 × 2 Tables

For a 2×2 table constructed as

			Total
	a	b	n_1
	c	d	n_2
Total	f_1	f_2	N

the simplified formula is

$$X^2 = [(ad - bc)^2 N]/(n_1 n_2 f_1 f_2)$$ [14.3]

In words, X^2 is the squared difference in the cross product terms, multiplied by N, divided by the product of the four marginal totals. Thus, for the data in Table 14.1,

$$X^2 = \frac{[(6 \times 91) - (89 \times 14)]^2 \times 200}{95 \times 105 \times 20 \times 180} = \frac{(546 - 1246)^2 \times 200}{35910000}$$

$$= \frac{(-700)^2 \times 200}{35910000} = \frac{98000000}{35910000} = 2.73$$

which is the same result obtained earlier.

14.2.2 Yates Correction in 2 × 2 Table

To employ the Yates correction, Formula [14.3] is changed to

$$X_c^2 = \frac{(|ad - bc| - [N/2])^2 N}{(a + b)(c + d)(a + c)(b + d)}$$ [14.4]

If Yates correction were applied, the previous calculation for Table 14.1 would become $X_c^2 = [700 - (200/2)]^2 [200]/35910000 = (600)^2(200)/35910000 = 2.005$.

14.2.3 Formula for "Rate" Calculations

The results of two proportions (or two rates) are commonly expressed in the form $p_1 = t_1/n_1$ and $p_2 = t_2/n_2$, with totals of $P = T/N$, where $T = t_1 + t_2$ and $N = n_1 + n_2$. The "unpacking" of such data can be avoided with the formula

$$X^2 = \left[\frac{t_1^2}{n_1} + \frac{t_2^2}{n_2} - \frac{T^2}{N}\right]\left[\frac{N^2}{(T)(N-T)}\right] \qquad [14.5]$$

This formula may look forbidding, but it can be rapidly carried out on a hand calculator, after only one manual maneuver—the subtraction of T from N.

The formula can be illustrated if the occurrence of anemia in Table 14.1 were presented as 6/95 = .063 for men and 14/105 = .133 for women. Instead of unpacking these proportions into a table, we can promptly determine that $T = 6 + 14 = 20$, $N = 95 + 105 = 200$, and $N - T = 200 - 20 = 180$. With Formula [14.5], we then calculate

$$X^2 = [(6^2/95) + (14^2/105) - (20^2/200)][200^2/\{(20)(180)\}]$$
$$= [.2456][11.11] = 2.73$$

which is the same result as previously.

Another formula that determines X^2 without fully "unpacking" the two proportions is

$$X^2 = \frac{(n_2 t_1 - n_1 t_2)^2 N}{n_1 n_2 T(N-T)} \qquad [14.6]$$

For the data in Table 14.1, this calculation is $[(105)(6) - (95)(14)]^2(200)/[(95)(105)(20)(180)] = 2.73$.

14.2.4 Expected Values

If you, rather than a computer program, are going to calculate X^2 for a two-way table that has more than 2 rows or 2 columns, none of the simplified formulas can be used. The expected values will have to be determined, and a strategy is needed for finding them quickly and accurately.

The process is easiest to show for a 2×2 table, structured as follows:

	Men	Women	Total
Old	a	b	f_1
Young	c	d	f_2
Total	n_1	n_2	N

In this table, the proportion of old people is f_1/N. Under the null hypothesis, we would expect the proportion of old men to be $(f_1/N) \times n_1$ and proportion of old women to be $(f_1/N) \times n_2$. Similarly, the expected values for young men and young women would be, respectively, $(f_2 n_1)/N$ and $(f_2 n_2)/N$. Consequently, the expected values in any cell are the products of the marginal totals for the corresponding row and column, divided by N. Thus, the expected values here are

	Men	Women
Old	$\dfrac{f_1 n_1}{N}$	$\dfrac{f_1 n_2}{N}$
Young	$\dfrac{f_2 n_1}{N}$	$\dfrac{f_2 n_2}{N}$

For a table of larger dimensions, the process can be illustrated as shown in Figure 14.2. In the cell for row 2, column 1, the expected value is $f_2 n_1/N$—which is the product of the marginal totals for row 2 and column 1, divided by N. In row 1, column 3, the expected value is $f_1 n_3/N$. In row 3, column 2, the expected value is $f_3 n_2/N$.

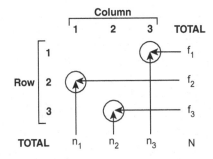

FIGURE 14.2
Diagram showing marginal totals used for calculating expected values in a cell.

14.2.5   Similar Values of $|O - E|$ in Cells of 2 × 2 Table

An important attribute of the observed-minus-expected values in a 2 × 2 table is that their absolute magnitudes are identical in each cell, but the signs oscillate around the table. For example, for Table 14.1, the results in Section 14.1.2. showed that the observed-minus-expected values are

	Anemic	Non-Anemic
Men	−3.5	3.5
Women	3.5	−3.5

A simple formula for the absolute magnitude of the observed-minus-expected value for any cell in a 2 × 2 table is $e = |ad - bc|/N$. For the anemia example, $(ad - bc)/N = [(6 \times 91) - (89 \times 14)]/200 = -700/200 = -3.5$.

With $e = (ad - bc)/N$, the pattern of observed–expected values in the four cells will be:

$$\begin{matrix} -e & e \\ e & -e \end{matrix}$$

The rotating pattern of $+e$ and $-e$ values is useful for checking calculations and for indicating that the four marginal totals (n_1, n_2, f_1, f_2) should be exactly the same in the expected values as in the observed values. Because the (observed −expected)² values of e^2 will be identical in each cell, the main distinctions in X^2 arise from divisions by the expected values. If they are too small, the results may be untrustworthy, as discussed in Section 14.3.1.

14.2.6   Equivalence of Z^2 and X^2

Near the end of Section 14.1.4, we found that Z^2 and X^2 gave identical results for the data of Table 14.1. The equality of Z^2 and X^2 in any 2 × 2 table can be proved by substituting into the previous Formula [13.16] for Z and developing the algebra. The increment of the two binary proportions, $p_1 - p_2$, becomes $(ad -bc)/n_1 n_2$. The common value of P in a 2 × 2 table is $(n_1 p_2 + n_2 p_2)/N = f_1/N$, and $Q = 1 -P$ will be f_2/N. When entered into Formula [13.16], these results lead to

$$Z = \frac{(ad - bc)\sqrt{N}}{\sqrt{n_1 n_2 f_1 f_2}}$$

which is the square root of Formula [14.3] for X^2.

The similarity between Z^2 and X^2 is so striking that in looking for P values you can square Z values if you do not have a Table of χ^2 (at one d.f.) available. For example, in Table 14.2, the X^2 values for

$P = .1, .05,$ and $.01$, respectively, are $2.706, 3.841,$ and 6.635. These are the exact squares of the corresponding Z values in Table 6.3. They produce $(1.645)^2, (1.96)^2$ and $(2.58)^2$.

The equivalence of $Z^2 = X^2$ for a 2×2 table, with 1 degree of freedom, was also shown in the construction of the chi-square distribution in Formula [14.2]. The equivalence helps indicate that for two-group contrasts, the Z procedure is probably the most useful of the three parametric tests: Z, t, and chi-square. Except when group sizes are small enough to be troublesome, the Z test can be used to contrast two means and also two proportions. Perhaps the main reason for noting the similarity of Z and chi-square, however, is that Z is used for calculating confidence intervals and sample sizes, as described in Sections 14.4 and 14.5.

14.2.7   Mental Approximation of Z

A simple mental approximation becomes possible when the Z formula for comparing two proportions is rearranged as

$$\frac{p_1 - p_2}{\sqrt{PQ}} \times \sqrt{(k)(1-k)} \times \sqrt{N} \qquad\qquad [14.7]$$

where $k = n_1/N$ and $1 - k = n_2/N$.

If $\sqrt{(k)(1-k)}$ and $\sqrt{PQ}$ are each about .5 (as is often true), they essentially cancel in the foregoing formula, which becomes

$$Z \cong (p_1 - p_2)\sqrt{N} \qquad\qquad [14.8]$$

To use this formula mentally, without a calculator, begin with the values presented for p_1 and p_2 and for their increment, $p_1 - p_2$. Because Z is "statistically significant" when ≥ 2, this status can be achieved if $|p_1 - p_2|\sqrt{N}$ is strikingly larger than 2. The main job is to see whether $\sqrt{N}$ is large enough to achieve this goal when it multiplies $|p_1 - p_2|$. If denominators are shown for p_1 and p_2, you can quickly add $n_1 + n_2$ to form N and then estimate its square root.

For example, suppose an investigator compares the two proportions $70/159 = .44$ and $300/162 = .19$ as success rates in a trial of Treatment A vs. B. The increment $p_1 - p_2$ is $.44 - .19 = .25$. To exceed 2, this value must be multiplied by something that exceeds 8. Because the total group is bigger than 300, its square root will surely exceed 8. Therefore, your mental screening test can lead to the conclusion that $Z > 2$, and that the result is stochastically significant. The actual calculation would show that $\sqrt{PQ} = .463$, $\sqrt{k(1-k)} = .500$, and $Z = (.440 - .185)\sqrt{321}(.500)/(.463) = 4.93$ for which $2P < 1 \times 10^{-6}$.

Conversely, suppose a speaker compares the proportions $19/40 = .48$ and $12/42 = .29$. The increment of $p_1 - p_2$ seems impressive at $.48 - .29 = .19$, or about $.2$. For the appropriate product to exceed 2, however, the $.2$ value must be multiplied by 10; but the total group size here is below 100, being $40 + 42 = 82$. Because the square root of the group size will not exceed 10, the result cannot be stochastically significant at $2P < .05$ for $Z > 2$. If you want to awe (or offend) the speaker, you can immediately volunteer the warning that the result is not stochastically significant. [The actual calculation would show $\sqrt{PQ} = \sqrt{(.378)(.622)} = .48$, and $\sqrt{(k)(1-k)} = \sqrt{(40/82)(42/82)} = .500$. The value of Z would be $[|.475 - .286|\sqrt{82}](.500)/(.48) = 1.78$. It is close to 2 and will have a one-tailed but not a two-tailed $P < .05$.]

The "mental method" is best for two-tailed rather than one-tailed tests. In the latter, Z need exceed only 1.645 rather than the easy-to-remember "2" of 1.96. In the foregoing example, the closeness of $\sqrt{82}$ to $\sqrt{100}$ might have acted as a cautionary warning that 1.645 could be exceeded in a one-tailed test.

14.3   Problems and Precautions in Use of X^2

The chi-square test became popular because it offered a stochastic contrast for the proportions found in two groups. For a clinical investigator who works with enumeration (counted) data, chi-square was the counterpart of the t test (or Z test) used for contrasting the means in two groups of dimensional laboratory data.

Aside from disputes about how well the X^2 computation fits the χ^2 distribution, many other problems require attention.

14.3.1 Size of Groups

No consistent agreement has been developed for the minimum size of N, or of n_1 and n_2, that will preserve validity in the assumptions about a χ^2 distribution. A compromise solution offered by Cochran[4] is to avoid X^2 and to use the Fisher Exact Probability Test if N < 20, or if 20 < N < 40 *and* the smallest expected value in any cell is less than 5.

14.3.2 Size of Cells

Consistent agreement is also absent about the minimum size of the expected values in the cells. Some authors have said that the X^2 test is not valid if the expected value in any cell is below 5. Others put this minimum expected cell value at 10. Yet others recommend 20.

If you have a suitable computer program, the conflicting recommendations about sizes of groups and cells can be avoided by using the Fisher Exact Test for all 2 × 2 tables.

14.3.3 Fractional Expected Values

The expected values often seem scientifically odd. Given success rates of 8/23 = .35 and 11/16 = .69 for groups of treated and untreated patients, respectively, the observed and expected values for these data are shown in Table 14.3. Just as a "mean of 2.7 children" is one of the reasons for avoiding means and using median values in dealing with discrete integer data, an expected value of "11.8" or "8.2" people seems equally strange in a 2 × 2 frequency table. Nevertheless, these fractions of people are essential for the calculations.

TABLE 14.3

Observed and Expected Values for Data in a 2 × 2 Table

	Observed Values			Expected Values	
	Failure	**Success**	**Total**	**Failure**	**Success**
Untreated	15	8	23	11.8	11.2
Treated	5	11	16	8.2	7.8
Total	20	19	39	20.0	19.0

14.3.4 Is X^2 a Parametric Test?

The X^2 test is sometimes called "non-parametric" because (unlike the usual Z or t test) it does not require dimensional data. Nevertheless, the interpretation of X^2 requires the conventional parametric-type reasoning about sampling from a hypothetical distribution. Besides, as noted earlier, the parametric Z test and X^2 give identical results in the comparison of two proportions.

14.3.5 Controversy about Marginal Totals

As discussed earlier in Section 12.7.3, an academic controversy has developed about the idea of fixing the marginal totals at f_1, f_2, n_1, and n_2 when either X^2 or the Fisher Exact Test is determined for a 2 × 2 table. Because the numbers in the table can be obtained from at least three different methods of "sampling," each method (according to the theorists) can lead to different estimates of parametric values for the observed proportions, and to different strategies for either fixing the margins or letting them vary.

The arguments offer interesting displays of creative statistical reasoning, particularly for estimating sample sizes *before* the research is done. Nevertheless, when the research is completed, the pragmatic reality, acknowledged by many prominent statisticians,[5-7] is that the four marginal totals are f_1, f_2, n_1, and n_2. They are therefore kept intact, i.e., fixed, for the Fisher exact test and for the conventional X^2 test, as well as for the test with Yates correction.

Unless you are planning to write a mathematical thesis on inferential probabilities, the useful pragmatic approach is to follow custom and fix both sets of margins. Besides, as the Fisher test gradually replaces X^2 (or Z) for comparing two proportions, the arguments about estimating the parameters will become historical footnotes.

14.3.6   Reasons for "Success" of Chi-Square

Despite all the cited infelicities, the X^2 test has grown and flourished because it is easy to calculate, reasonably easy to understand, versatile, and robust. Its versatility will be discussed in Section 14.7. Its robustness arises because the results, when converted into probability values, are generally similar to those produced by the "gold standard" Fisher exact probability procedure.

Like the t test, the X^2 test has major intellectual defects and major numerical advantages. The object here is neither to praise nor to condemn the test, but to familiarize you with its usage. Since the X^2 test will probably not be replaced for a long time, it will regularly appear in published literature, and the process of learning about it becomes an act of enlightened self-defense.

Nevertheless, to calculate confidence intervals or to estimate sample size for a contrast of two proportions, the preferred tactic is the Z procedure, not chi-square.

14.4   Confidence Intervals for Contrast of Two Proportions

To use the Z procedure for calculating the confidence interval of a contrast of two proportions, $p_A = t_A/n_A$ and $p_B = t_B/n_B$, the first step is to determine the standard error of the difference.

14.4.1   Standard Error of Difference

An increment of two proportions, like an increment of two means, evokes the same question about "Which standard error?"

14.4.1.1   Customary SED_0 for Null Hypothesis — With the conventional null hypothesis, when we assume that the outcome is unrelated to treatment, the common proportion for the two groups is estimated parametrically as $\pi = (n_A p_A + n_B p_B)/N$. With the observed P used to estimate π, the standard error of the difference, subscripted with 0 to indicate a null hypothesis, will then be

$$\text{SED}_0 = \sqrt{NPQ/n_A n_B} \qquad\qquad [14.9]$$

With Z_α appropriately selected for a $1 - \alpha$ level of confidence, the corresponding confidence interval will be

$$p_A - p_B \pm Z_\alpha \sqrt{NPQ/n_A n_B} \qquad\qquad [14.10]$$

14.4.1.2   Simplified Calculation of SED_0 — The calculation of SED_0 can be simplified by noting that $n_A + n_B = N$ and $t_A + t_B = T$. Then $P = (n_A p_A + n_B p_B)/N = (t_A + t_B)/N = T/N$. The value of $Q = 1 - P$ will be $[N - T]/N$. The product NPQ will then be $T(N - T)/N$, and the calculational formula for [14.9] becomes

$$\text{SED}_0 = \sqrt{[T(N-T)]/[(N)(n_A)(n_B)]} \qquad\qquad [14.11]$$

For example, suppose we want to find the standard error for the difference in two proportions $18/24 = .75$ and $10/15 = .67$. The value of P can be calculated as $(18 + 10)/(24 + 15) = 28/39 = .718$, and Q will be $1 - .718 = .282$. The standard error would become $\sqrt{39(.718)(.282)/(15 \times 24)} = .148$. With the simplified formula, which avoids rounding for values of P and Q, the calculation would be

$$\sqrt{(18 + 10)(6 + 5)/(24 + 15)(24)(15)} = \sqrt{(28)(11)/(39)(24)(15)} = .148$$

14.4.1.3 *Rapid Mental Approximation* — An additional feature of Formula [14.11] allows a particularly rapid "mental" approximation of the standard error of the difference.

This approach is possible because over a reasonable range of values, the ratio of $[(T)(N - T)]/[(n_A)(n_B)]$ will not be too far from 1. (In the cited example, it is $(28)(11)/(24)(15) = .856$.) If the value of $[T(N - T)]/[(n_A)(n_B)]$ is crudely approximated as 1, the standard error of the difference will be approximated as $SED \approx \sqrt{1/N}$.

The $\sqrt{1/N}$ approximation for SED in comparing two proportions is the same $\sqrt{1/N}$ calculation discussed earlier (Section 8.5.1) for the 95% confidence-interval component of a single proportion. In using this "shortcut," remember that the $\sqrt{1/N}$ formula is used for two different approximations: SED for two proportions and 2SE for one proportion. In the example here, $\sqrt{1/39} = .160$ — a value not far from the actual SED of .148.

For the "mental" part of the calculation, you can estimate $\sqrt{1/39}$ as roughly $\sqrt{1/36}$, for which the square root is $1/6 = .167$, which is reasonably close to the actual value of .148. The "mental" feat here is even more impressive because it just happened that way: the numbers in the example were not deliberately "rigged" to produce a close result.

Unlike the results of two means, the results for two proportions are seldom listed with standard errors, which would be $\sqrt{p_A q_A/n_A}$ and $\sqrt{p_B q_B/n_B}$. Therefore, a crude confidence interval component cannot be readily obtained by adding the two standard errors and doubling the result. Applying the "crude" formula of $\sqrt{1/N}$, however, and using the particularly crude value of $\sqrt{1/36} = .167$ in the example here, we could double the approximated SED to get $.167 \times 2 = .234$. Since this value substantially exceeds the observed $p_A - p_B = .083$, we can feel almost sure that the result is *not* stochastically significant at a two-tailed $\alpha = .05$. Essentially the same computational tactic was used for the mental approximation in Section 14.2.7, when $p_A \quad p_B$ was multiplied by $\sqrt{N}$, and the result compared against a value of 2.

14.4.1.4 *SED_H Error for Alternative Hypothesis* — In additional types of stochastic reasoning discussed later in Chapter 23, the assumed alternative hypothesis is that the two "treatments" are different, i.e., the observed values of p_A and p_B are *not* parametrically similar. With this assumption, the appropriate variance of the increment in the two central indexes is calculated, as in Chapter 13, by adding the two observed variances as $(p_A q_A/n_A) + (p_B q_B/n_B)$. Under the alternative hypothesis, the standard error of the difference will be

$$SED_H = \sqrt{(p_A q_A/n_A) + (p_B q_B/n_B)} \qquad [14.12]$$

Thus, if we assumed that one treatment was really different from the other in the foregoing example, the correct standard error would be calculated as

$$\sqrt{[(.75)(.25)/24] + [(.67)(.33)/15]} = .150$$

14.4.1.5 *Simplified Calculation of SED_H* — To avoid problems in rounding, the alternative SED_H is best calculated with the integer values of

$$\sqrt{\{(t_A/n_A)[(n_A - t_A)/n_A]/n_A\} + \{[(t_B/n_B)(n_B - t_B)/n_B]/n_B\}}$$

With hand calculators that can easily do "cubing," a simple computational formula is

$$SED = \sqrt{[(t_A)(n_A - t_A)/n_A^3] + [t_B(n_B - t_B)/n_B^3]}$$ [14.13]

In the foregoing example, the result would be

$$\sqrt{[(18)(6)/24^3] + [(10)(5)/15^3]} = .150$$

14.4.2   Similarity of SEDs

As in a contrast of two means, the two methods of calculation usually produce quite similar results for the standard error of the difference in two proportions. Thus, although Formula [14.9] (or [14.11]) vs. Formula [14.12] (or [14.13]) may produce different results in mathematical theory, the pragmatic values are reasonably close. In the foregoing example that compared $18/24 = .75$ with $10/15 = .67$, the disparity between the SEDs of .148 and .150 is only about 2 parts in 150.

For practical purposes, therefore, the standard error of the difference in proportions can be calculated with either formula, regardless of what assumption is made about the parametric hypothesis. Because the intermediate calculation of P is avoided, the formula of $(p_A q_A/n_A) + (p_B q_B/n_B)$ seems somewhat easier to use on a hand calculator, but $NPQ/n_A n_B$ is usually preferred here because it is also more appropriate for the conventional null hypothesis.

If the result is so borderline that stochastic significance will be lost or gained by choice of the method for calculating SED, the data probably do not warrant any firm conclusions. Besides, both formulas rely on the assumption that increments in the two proportions have a Gaussian distribution. As shown in Chapter 8, however, this assumption does not hold for relatively small group sizes. In such circumstances, the data analyst might want to use the Fisher-test intervals or some other procedure to achieve reality amid the allure of the Gaussian wonderland.

14.4.3   Choice of Z_α Values

After an SED value is determined, the next step in constructing a confidence interval is to choose a value for Z_α. This choice depends on the same questions that have been previously discussed for how much "confidence" we want, and whether it goes in a one- or two-tailed direction.

The questions can be answered with the same reasoning and arguments used previously for dimensional data in Chapter 13, but two distinctions need further consideration for comparisons of binary proportions.

14.4.3.1   Magnitude of α — In most ordinary situations, α is set at a two-tailed level of .05, for which $Z_\alpha = 1.96$. Thus, for the difference in the previously cited comparison of $18/24 = .75$ vs. $10/15 = .67$, with SED = .148, the 95% confidence interval will be

$$(.75 - .67) \pm (1.96)(1.48) = .08 \pm .29$$

and will extend from $-.21$ to $+.37$. Because the interval includes 0, the result is not stochastically significant at $2P \le .05$. On the other hand, we might be reluctant to conclude that the increment of .08 is truly "insignificant" because it might be as large as .21 in favor of "Treatment B" or .37 in favor of "Treatment A" within the extent of the 95% confidence interval.

The magnitude of α becomes particularly important when the stochastic result is "nonsignificant," and the confidence interval is then explored for the possibility that its upper end is impressively high. With a small enough choice of α, e.g., $\alpha = .0001$, Z_α can become large enough to "drag" the interval for any two-proportion increment across whatever descriptive border is set for "high." For example, if the observed increment is .04 and the SED is .03, the customary Z_α will make the confidence interval be $.04 \pm (1.96)(.03)$. It will be "nonsignificant," extending from $-.019$ to $+.099$.

On the other hand, if we set $\alpha = .001$, the Z_α of 3.29 will make the interval become $.04 \pm (3.29)(.03)$. Its upper end will now have the "impressive" value of .14.

14.4.3.2   Focus of Conclusions — In Chapter 10, we saw how an investigator can honestly and legitimately, but somewhat deceptively, make unimpressive results seem impressive. Instead of being cited as unimpressive increments, they can be cited as impressive ratios or proportionate increments. An analogous tactic is available when the investigator chooses Z_α and emphasizes a directional focus for the confidence interval.

If the confidence interval includes the null hypothesis value of 0, the result is not stochastically significant. In this circumstance, many investigators (especially if the group sizes are small) will examine the ends of the interval to see how big $p_A - p_B$ might really be. Such an examination is quite reasonable, but it may sometimes be used zealously by an investigator who is committed to advocating a "significance" that was *not* confirmed stochastically. The investigator may emphasize and focus on only the large potential difference shown at one end of the confidence interval. If Z_α is enlarged, the difference can be made even larger. The other end of the interval, of course, will indicate a reverse possibility—but its existence may then be conveniently ignored. (The prevention of this type of stochastic abuse was one of the reasons cited by Fleiss[8] for insisting on P values.)

In other situations, as discussed earlier in Chapter 13, when the null hypothesis parameter is excluded from the conventional 95% confidence interval, an investigator who is avidly seeking "significance" can ecstatically proclaim its presence. A cautious analyst, however, will examine both the range of the confidence interval and its *smaller* end. If the range is too wide and the smaller end is close to the null-hypothesis value, the relatively unstable result may have "just made it" across the stochastic border. A "fragility shift" of one or two persons might often drastically alter the result and even remove the "significance."

14.4.4   Criteria for "Bulk" of Data

If a confidence interval is being used for descriptive decisions about how big a difference might be, and if Z_α is regularly chosen to be the same value of 1.96 used for a two-tailed $\alpha = .05$, the stochastic tail of the conventional α is allowed to wag the *descriptive* dog of quantitative significance.

Arguing that descriptive significance depends on *bulk* of the data, rather than arbitrary stochastic boundaries, some analysts may prefer to use Z values that reflect differences established by bulk of data, not by stochastic doctrines about level of α. For example, a two-tailed $Z_{.75} = 1.15$ will span 75% of the Gaussian increments, and $Z_{.50} = .6745$ will span 50%. The inner 50% of the data is the interquartile range spanned by a box plot. In the early days of statistical inference, before α was set at .05 by R. A. Fisher's edict, the 50% zone of $.6745 \times$ standard error was regarded as the "probable error of a mean." The investigators were satisfied with the idea that a mean might reasonably vary within this 50% zone, and they did not demand a larger zone that spanned 95% of the possibilities.

If this same idea is used for a *descriptive* possibility regarding the upper boundary of a "nonsignificant" increment, the confidence interval might be better calculated with Z_α set at smaller values of .6745 (or perhaps $Z_{.75} = 1.15$), rather than with the arbitrary 1.96. For example, when the previous contrast of $18/24 = .75$ vs. $10/15 = .67$ failed to achieve stochastic significance, the potential interval ranged from $-.21$ to $+.37$ if calculated with the Gaussian $Z_\alpha = 1.96$. With Z_α set at a descriptive .6745, however, the interval would be $.08 \pm (.6745)(.150)$ and would extend from .02 to .18. We are not concerned about the low end here, but the upper value of .18—which produces an interval spanning 50% of the potential increments—might be a more realistic estimate for the *descriptive* range of the upper boundary in denoting how much larger p_A might be than p_B.

This type of estimate may become attractive when data analysts begin to give serious attention to descriptive rather than inferential decisions about "significance" in statistical comparisons.

14.5   Calculating Sample Size to Contrast Two Proportions

Advance sample sizes are usually calculated, before the research begins, to avoid the frustration of finding quantitatively impressive results in group sizes too small to achieve stochastic significance. The calculation seems to use a relatively simple formula noted later, but the procedure involves decisions, assignments, and directional estimates that have important but often overlooked consequences. In most situations, the investigator expects to observe $d_o = p_A - p_B$ as an increment in two proportions, and also hopes that d_o will exceed δ, which is the lower level of quantitative significance. After choosing an α level of stochastic significance, the investigator wants a sample size whose capacity will produce P < α, or a suitably small $1 - \alpha$ confidence interval.

14.5.1 "Single" vs. "Double" Stochastic Significance

In most trials, the investigators would like to get stochastic significance at the chosen level of α for an observed d_o having a "big" value that is $\geq \delta$. In the past two decades, however, statisticians have worried about a different problem that occurs when the anticipated d_o turns out to be smaller than δ. The stochastic conclusion that such results are nonsignificant may then be a "Type II" or "false negative" error. These conclusions differ from the "Type I" or "false positive" errors that are presumably avoided by a suitably small choice of α. Avoidance of Type II errors involves considerations of statistical "power" that will be discussed in Chapter 23. The main point to be noted now, however, is that an investigator who wants to avoid both false positive and false negative errors will enlarge the sample size substantially by seeking "double stochastic significance" at the level of α and also at a later-discussed level of β.

The rest of the discussion here describes the conventional methods of determining sample sizes that will achieve "single significance" at the chosen level of α. For the customary "single-significance" null-hypothesis contrast of two proportions, sample sizes are calculated with the Z procedure, which yields the same results when used with either a P-value or confidence-interval strategy. The "prospective" calculations are conceptually more difficult than "retrospective" appraisals after the research is completed, however, because no data are available in advance. Everything must be assigned and estimated. In addition to choosing assignments for δ and α, the investigator must estimate both π_B and the common value of π.

14.5.2 Assignments for δ and α

Sample-size decisions begin with two assignments. The first is to set a boundary for δ, the magnitude of the impressive quantitative distinction desired (or expected) between p_A and p_B. As noted earlier (Chapter 10), this choice will depend on the conditions being investigated.

The second assignment sets a level for α. This decision is crucial in both prospective and retrospective stochastic activities because the corresponding level of Z_α is used prospectively to calculate sample size, and retrospectively either to evaluate an observed Z_o for "significance" or to calculate the magnitude of the confidence interval.

As noted in earlier discussions, the choice of α involves decisions for both magnitude and direction. The customary boundary, .05, can be made larger or smaller in special circumstances (such as the multiple-comparison problem mentioned in Chapter 11). The customary direction is two-tailed, so that the Gaussian value of $Z_\alpha = Z_{.05} = 1.96$. If the direction is one-tailed, however, the level of α is doubled, and $Z_{2\alpha} = Z_{.10} = 1.645$.

14.5.3 Estimates of π_A, π_B, and π

The next decisions involve three estimates, for which a plethora of symbols can be applied. We can use p_A to represent an observed value, $\hat{p}_A$ for an estimated value, and π_A for a parametric assumption about p_A or $\hat{p}_A$. To avoid the confusion of probabilities and proportions that can be represented with p or P symbols, we shall here use "hatted Greeks," such as $\hat{\pi}_A$, for estimated values. The main basic estimate is $\hat{\pi}_B$, the value anticipated for $\hat{p}_B$ in the "reference" group, which can be receiving no treatment, placebo, or a compared active agent. After $\hat{\pi}_B$ is chosen, p_A can be immediately estimated as $\hat{\pi}_A = \hat{\pi}_B \pm \delta$. For reasons discussed throughout Section 14.6, however, the choice between $+\delta$ or $-\delta$ is usually avoided, and the increment is usually estimated in a noncommittal two-tailed manner as $|\hat{\pi}_A - \hat{\pi}_B| = \delta$.

As the counterpart of the common proportion, P, the value of π is estimated as

$$\hat{\pi} = (n_A \hat{\pi}_A + n_B \hat{\pi}_B)/N \qquad [14.14]$$

The counterpart of $Q = 1 - P$ cannot be easily written in Greek (which has no symbol for Q), and is therefore expressed as $1 - \hat{\pi}$. The requirements of Formula [14.14] bring in the values of n_A, n_B, and N for which sample size will eventually be calculated.

14.5.4 Decision about Sample Allocation

Although aimed at determining the total sample size, N, the Z formula cannot be applied until the standard error of the difference is estimated. For this estimate, we need to use $\hat{\pi} = (n_A \hat{\pi}_A + n_B \hat{\pi}_B)/N$, but, in addition to not knowing the value of N, we do not know the values of either n_A or n_B.

14.5.4.1 *Equal Sample Sizes* — The approximation of n_A and n_B is usually resolved by assuming that the two groups will have equal size, so that $n_A = n_B = N/2$. We can then use $n = N/2$ for the size of each group. With this decision, the value of $\hat{\pi}$ becomes $(n\hat{\pi}_A + n\hat{\pi}_B)/2n = (\hat{\pi}_A + \hat{\pi}_B)/2$. The value of $N/(n_A n_B)$ becomes $2n/[(n)(n)] = 2/n$. The value of SED_0 is then estimated as

$$\sqrt{2\hat{\pi}(1 - \hat{\pi})/n} \qquad [14.15]$$

(With the alternative-hypothesis formula, the estimated standard error for SED_H would be $\sqrt{[\hat{\pi}_A(1 - \hat{\pi}_A) + \hat{\pi}_B(1 - \hat{\pi}_B)]/n}$.)

14.5.4.2 *Unequal Sample Sizes* — If for some reason the investigator wants unequal sized groups, the process is still relatively easy to manage. In this situation the samples will be divided as $n_A = kN$ and $n_B = (1 - k)N$, where k is a prespecified value for the sample-allocation fraction. For example, if twice as many people are wanted in the treated group as in the control group, and if n_B is the size of the control group, the sample-allocation fraction will be $k = 1/3$, with $1 - k = 2/3$. The value of $\hat{\pi}$ will be $(kN\hat{\pi}_B + (1 - k)N\hat{\pi}_A)/N = k\hat{\pi}_B + (1 - k)\hat{\pi}_A$. The value of $N/n_A n_B$ will be $N/[(kN)(1 - k)N] = 1/[(k)(1 - k)N]$. The standard error would then be estimated from the $NPQ/(n_A n_B)$ formula as $\sqrt{[k\hat{\pi}_B + (1 - k)\hat{\pi}_A]/(k)(1 - k)N]}$. If k is specified as $1/3$, the formula would be $\sqrt{[(\hat{\pi}_B/3) + (2\hat{\pi}_A/3)]/[2N/9]}$, which becomes $\sqrt{[3\hat{\pi}_B + 6\hat{\pi}_A]/2N}$.

In all the estimates discussed here, the samples will be calculated, in the conventional manner, as having equal sizes.

14.5.4.3 *Tactics in Calculation* — With

$$Z_0 = \frac{d_0}{SED} \qquad [14.16]$$

as the customary formula for getting to a P value, we now seem to have everything needed to calculate sample size by suitably substituting into Formula [14.16], where d_0 = observed difference in the two proportions, SED = standard error of the difference, and Z_0 is the value of Z for the observed results. The substituted values will be the anticipated $\delta = |\hat{\pi}_A - \hat{\pi}_B|$ for d_0; and the anticipated SED, for equal sample sizes, will be SED = $\sqrt{2\hat{\pi}(1 - \hat{\pi})/n}$. When these values are substituted, we can solve Expression [14.16] for n (or N if an appropriate formula is used for unequal sample sizes).

The Z value at δ will be calculated as

$$Z_\delta = \frac{\delta}{\sqrt{2\hat{\pi}(1 - \hat{\pi})/n}} \qquad [14.17]$$

For stochastic significance we want Z_δ to exceed the selected level of Z_α. Therefore,

$$\frac{\delta}{\sqrt{2\hat{\pi}(1-\hat{\pi})/n}} \geq Z_\alpha \qquad [14.18]$$

To solve for n, we square both sides and determine that

$$n \geq \frac{2\hat{\pi}(1-\hat{\pi})(Z_\alpha^2)}{\delta^2} \qquad [14.19]$$

14.6 Problems in Choosing $\hat{\pi}$

Formula [14.19] is the standard recommendation for calculating sample size if the goal is to achieve results in which either $P < \alpha$ or the $1-\alpha$ confidence interval has a suitable lower end. The formula relies on the assumption that π will be calculated for equal sized groups as $(\hat{\pi}_A + \hat{\pi}_B)/2$, but the formula does not indicate whether $\hat{\pi}_A$ is expected to be larger or smaller than $\hat{\pi}_B$. If $\hat{\pi}_A = \hat{\pi}_B + \delta$, $\hat{\pi}$ becomes $\hat{\pi}_B + (\delta/2)$. If $\hat{\pi}_A = \hat{\pi}_B - \delta$, $\hat{\pi}$ becomes $\hat{\pi}_B - (\delta/2)$.

14.6.1 Directional Differences in Sample Size

The different directional possibilities for π can substantially affect the variance calculated as $\hat{\pi}(1-\hat{\pi})$ in the numerator of Formula [14.19]. For example, suppose $\delta = .15$ is set as an impressive difference in two proportions and $\hat{\pi}_B = .33$ is estimated for Group B. If Group A has a larger value, $\hat{\pi}_A$ will be $.33 + .15 = .48$, $\hat{\pi}$ will be $(.33 + .48)/2 = .405$, and $\hat{\pi}(1-\hat{\pi})$ will be $(.405)(.595) = .2410$. Conversely, if Group A has a smaller value, $\hat{\pi}_A$ will be $.33 - .15 = .18$, $\hat{\pi}$ will be $(.18 + .33)/2 = .255$, and $\hat{\pi}(1-\hat{\pi})$ will be $(.255)(.745) = .1900$.

With Z_α set at a two-tailed 1.96 for $\alpha = .05$, the insertion of the foregoing values in Formula [14.19] will produce $n \geq [2(.2410)(1.96)^2]/(.15)^2 = 82.3$ for the first estimate, and $n \geq [2(.1900)(1.96)^2]/(.15)^2 = 64.9$ for the second. The first sample size will exceed the second by the ratio of the two variances, which is $.2410/.1900 = 1.27$, a proportionate increase of 27%.

Consequently, the direction of the anticipated increment in proportions does more than just affect the choice of a one- or two-tailed level of α. It extends into the "guts" of calculating SED and, thereby, sample size.

14.6.2 Compromise Choice of $\hat{\pi}$

The different values of n occurred because the value of $\hat{\pi}_A$ was estimated directionally as $\hat{\pi}_B + \delta$ in one instance and as $\hat{\pi}_B - \delta$ in the other. For a noncommittal two-tailed hypothesis, a compromise decision using $\delta/2$, can produce estimates for a different $\hat{\pi}_A'$ and $\hat{\pi}_B'$ instead of $\hat{\pi}_A$ and $\hat{\pi}_B$. With this compromise, the value $\hat{\pi}'(1-\hat{\pi}')$ will always have the same result whether $\hat{\pi}_A$ is larger or smaller than $\hat{\pi}_B$.

Thus, we can estimate $\hat{\pi}_B'$ as $\hat{\pi}_B - (\delta/2)$ and $\hat{\pi}_A' = \hat{\pi}_B + (\delta/2)$. Alternatively, $\hat{\pi}_B'$ can be estimated as $\hat{\pi}_B + (\delta/2)$ and $\hat{\pi}_A'$ will be $\hat{\pi}_B - (\delta/2)$. In both situations, $|\hat{\pi}_A' - \hat{\pi}_B'|$ will be δ; the common proportion $\hat{\pi}'$ will be $(\hat{\pi}_A' + \hat{\pi}_B')/2 = \hat{\pi}_B$; and the "compromise" value of $\hat{\pi}'(1-\hat{\pi}')$ will be $\hat{\pi}_B(1-\hat{\pi}_B)$.

In the foregoing example, with δ set at .15, $\hat{\pi}_A'$ might be $.33 + .075 = .405$ and $\hat{\pi}_B$ would be $.33 - .075 = .255$, with $\hat{\pi}' = (.405 + .255)/2 = .330$, which is the value of $\hat{\pi}_B$. Alternatively, $\hat{\pi}_A'$ could be $.33 - .075 = .255$ and $\hat{\pi}_B'$ would be $.33 + .075 = .405$, yielding the same result for $\hat{\pi}'$.

In giving the same result for the substitute values of $\hat{\pi}'(1-\hat{\pi}')$, regardless of direction, the compromise choice of $\hat{\pi}_B(1-\hat{\pi}_B)$ avoids the two conflicting sample-size estimates created by a directional choice, but the compromise uses $\hat{\pi}_B$ for the single estimated value.

14.6.3   "Compromise" Calculation for Sample Size

With the compromise tactic, the "theoretical" Formula [14.19] becomes the "working" formula

$$n \geq \frac{2\hat{\pi}_B(1 - \hat{\pi}_B)(Z_\alpha^2)}{\delta^2} \qquad [14.20]$$

For the data under discussion, Formula [14.20] will produce $n \geq [(2)(.33)(.67)(1.96)^2]/(.15)^2 = 75.5$. As might have been expected, this value lies between the two previous estimates of 82.3 and 64.9. With the compromise choice, the results should be stochastically significant, at $2P \leq .05$, if the sample size exceeds 76 persons in each group. The total sample size would be 152.

The compromise tactic has two potential hazards. One of them occurs in a really close situation where p_A turns out to be $p_B + \delta$. The compromise sample size—which is smaller than the 166 needed for the larger estimate—may just fail to bring the calculated P value or confidence interval across the desired stochastic border. The second hazard is a scientific problem discussed in the next section.

14.6.4   Implications of Noncommittal (Two-Tailed) Direction

Although statistically comforting and conventional, a noncommittal two-tailed direction has important scientific implications. They suggest that the investigator is disinterested in the direction of the results, does not care which way they go, and is essentially working in a *laissez faire* manner, without a *scientific* hypothesis. The indifference, of course can be statistically proper and valuable if $p_A - p_B$ might acceptably go in either direction, for which a two-tailed null hypothesis is necessary.

The *scientific* idea being tested in the research itself, however, is the counter-hypothesis of the stochastic null hypothesis, which is established as $\hat{\pi}_A - \hat{\pi}_B = 0$, so that it can be rejected. With the rejection, we accept the counter-hypothesis, but it can be either a directional $\hat{\pi}_A - \hat{\pi}_B$, with $\Delta > 0$ or $\Delta < 0$, or a noncommittal $|\hat{\pi}_A - \hat{\pi}_B|$ with $\Delta \neq 0$.

Very few scientific investigators would be willing to invest the time and energy required to do the research, particularly in a full-scale randomized trial, without any idea about what they expect to happen and without caring which way it turns out. Furthermore, if the expectation were actually completely indifferent, very few agencies would be willing to fund the research proposal. A distinct scientific direction, therefore, is almost always desired and expected whenever an active treatment is compared against no treatment or a placebo; and even when two active treatments are compared, the investigator is almost never passively indifferent about an anticipated direction.

Nevertheless, the noncommittal two-tailed approach has been vigorously advocated, commonly employed, and generally accepted by many editors, reviewers, and readers. The one-tailed approach, however, is probably more important when the results are interpreted afterward than when sample size is calculated beforehand.

The reason for the latter statement is that the selection of $\hat{\pi}$ often becomes a moot point after the augmentations discussed in Section 14.6.5, which usually increase the calculated sample size well beyond the largest value that emerges from different choices of $\hat{\pi}$. Thus, the possibility of a one-tailed interpretation is most important after the study is completed, particularly if p_A and p_B have a relatively small increment.

14.6.5   Augmentation of Calculated Sample Size

Regardless of how $\hat{\pi}$ is chosen, cautious investigators will always try to enroll groups whose size is much larger than the calculated value of n.

If everything turns out exactly as estimated, the observed value of $|p_A - p_B| = d_o$ will be just $\geq \delta$, and d_o/SED should produce a value of Z_o that exactly equals or barely exceeds Z_α. The expected result can easily be impaired, however, by various human and quantitative idiosyncrasies. Some or many of the people enrolled in the trial may drop out, leaving inadequate data and a reduced group size. Some of the anticipated success rates may not turn out to be exactly as estimated.

For example, suppose the investigator enrolls 76 persons in each group of the foregoing trial, but data became inadequate or lost for two persons in each group. Suppose the available results came close to what was anticipated for the two groups, but the actual values were $p_A = 36/74 = .486$ and $p_B = 25/74 = .338$. When Z_o is determined for these data, the result is $[(36/74) - (25/74)]/\sqrt{[(61)(87)]/[(148)(74)(74)]} = .1486/.0809 = 1.84$, which falls just below the $Z_\alpha = 1.96$ needed for two-tailed "significance." (With everything already determined and calculated, it is too late for the investigator now to claim a unidirectional hypothesis and to try to salvage "significance" with a one-tailed P.)

For all these reasons, the calculated sample size is always augmented prophylactically. With the augmentation, some of the ambiguities in one/two-tailed directions and decisions for the estimated $\hat{\pi}$ are eliminated, because the sample size usually becomes large enough to manage all the stochastic possibilities. On the other hand, if many of the augmented people really do drop out or produce unusable data, the results may eventually depend on the originally calculated sample size. In such circumstances, the decisions for magnitude and direction of α, and the estimates of $\hat{\pi}$ and SED, can have important effects in either inflating the calculated sample size or reducing the eventual stochastic significance.

14.6.6 "Fighting City Hall"

This long account of problems in calculating sample size for two proportions is relatively unimportant if you are a reader of reported results, rather than a doer of research. As a reader, you will see what was observed and reported, together with the calculated P values and confidence intervals. You need to know the difference between one- and two-tailed decisions in the calculations and contentions, but the original sample-size strategies do not seem important. (They do become important, however, as noted later in Chapter 23, if the observed difference, d_o, was substantially smaller than the anticipated δ and became stochastically significant only because of an inflated sample size.)

As an investigator, however, your ability to carry out the research will directly depend on the estimated sample size. If it is too big, the project may be too costly to be funded, or too unfeasible to be carried out. Accordingly, you will want to get the smallest sample size that can achieve the desired goals of both quantitative and stochastic significance. For this purpose, you would use unidirectional scientific hypotheses, uncompromised choices for π, and one-tailed values of Z_α. You may then need "ammunition" with which to "fight city hall," if your statistical consultants or other authorities disagree.

The customary advice is to calculate sample size in a perfunctory manner by estimating $\hat{\pi}_B$, using the compromise $\delta/2$ strategy for estimating $\hat{\pi}_A{}'$ and $\hat{\pi}_B{}'$ and then employing Formula [14.20]. The value of $\hat{\pi}_A$ is almost never estimated, however, as $\hat{\pi}_B - \delta$. Not fully aware of the numerical consequences of the bidirectional or unidirectional decisions, an investigator may not realize that the subsequent sample sizes can sometimes become much larger than they need to be. Fearing accusations of statistical malfeasance, an enlightened investigator may be reluctant, even when scientifically justified, to insist on declaring a direction, changing from a two-tailed to one-tailed value of Z_α, or estimating $\hat{\pi}_A$, when appropriate, as $\hat{\pi}_B - \delta$ rather than $\hat{\pi}_B \pm \delta/2$.

The great deterrent for most investigators, of course, is the risk of defeating "city hall" in the calculated sample-size battle, but then losing the "war" for statistical approval when the final results are submitted for publication. If the reviewers insist on a two-tailed Z_α, the group sizes that so efficiently yielded a one-tailed P < .05 may not be big enough to succeed in rejecting the *two*-tailed null hypothesis. The results themselves may then be rejected by the reviewers.

In an era of cost–benefit analyses for almost everything, however, some of the exorbitant costs of huge sample sizes for large-scale randomized trials might be substantially reduced if appropriate re-evaluation can be given to the rigid doctrine that always demands nondirectional, noncommittal two-tailed approaches for all research.

14.7 Versatility of X² in Other Applications

Because stochastic contrasts for two proportions can readily be done with the Z or Fisher Exact procedures, chi-square is particularly valuable today for its role in other tasks that are briefly mentioned now to keep you from leaving this chapter thinking that chi-square may soon become obsolete. Except for the following subsection on "goodness of fit," all the other procedures will be discussed in later chapters.

14.7.1 "Goodness of Fit"

The "observed minus expected" tactic is regularly employed (see Section 14.1.1) to determine how well a particular model fits the observed categorical frequencies in a "one-way table," for a single group of univariate data.

For example, in genetic work with certain organisms, we expect the ratios AB:Ab:aB:ab to be 9:3:3:1. A set of real data may not follow these ratios exactly, but their goodness of fit to the expected model can be determined using chi-square. The expected values in each category would correspond to the cited ratios multiplied by the total number of observations. Thus, if a group of genetic observations gave corresponding totals of 317, 94, 109, and 29, we could calculate X^2 for the expected ratios as follows:

GROUP	AB	Ab	aB	ab	TOTAL
Observed Value	317	94	109	29	549
Expected Ratio	9/16	3/16	3/16	1/16	1
Expected Value	308.8	102.9	102.9	34.3	$548.9 \cong 549$
$(0-E)^2/E$	0.22	0.78	0.36	0.82	$2.18 = X^2$

With 4 groups and 3 degrees of freedom, the value of P for $v = 3$ at $X^2 = 2.18$ is $> .05$ and so we cannot reject the idea that the observed data are well fitted to the 9:3:3:1 ratio.

Some statisticians, such as J. V. Bradley,[9] refer to this use of chi-square as a test for "poorness of fit." The name seems appropriate because the stochastic test can "prove" only that the selected "model" fails to fit well, not that it is good or correct. The decision that the model is correct is an act of scientific judgment rather than statistical inference.

An alternative to the chi-square goodness-of-fit test for a one-way table is cited here mainly so you can savor the majestic sonority of its eponymic designation. Called the *Kolmogorov–Smirnov test*,[10,11] it compares the *cumulative* frequencies of the observed distribution against the cumulative frequencies of the expected distribution. (The chi-square test compares the observed and expected frequencies for individual rather than for cumulative categories.)

14.7.2 McNemar Test for "Correlated Proportions"

The X^2 test was adapted by Quinn McNemar, a psychologist, for examining "correlated proportions" in a manner that reduces two sets of results to one set, somewhat like the one-sample Z (or t) procedure for dimensional data. Being often used in medical research to test *agreement* among observers, the McNemar procedure will be discussed among the indexes of concordance in Chapter 20.

14.7.3 Additional Applications

Additional applications of X^2, all to be discussed later, can be listed as follows: getting a Miettinen-type of confidence interval[12] for an odds ratio, testing for stochastic significance in 2-way tables where either the rows or columns (or both) have more than 2 categories, evaluating linear trend for binary proportions in an ordinal array, doing the Mantel–Haenszel test for multiple categories in stratified odds ratios, and preparing the log-rank test calculations to compare two survival curves.

14.8 Problems in Computer Printouts for 2 × 2 Tables

If you do a chi-square test yourself, the formulas cited earlier are easy to use with a hand calculator. If you do not have a printing calculator to show that you entered the correct numbers, always do the calculation twice, preferably with different formulas. If you use a "packaged" computer program for a 2×2 table, always try to get the results of the Fisher Test as well as chi-square.

The main problems in the computer programs are that a confusing printout may appear for the Fisher Test and that a deluge of additional indexes may appear as unsolicited (or requested) options. Because 2×2 tables are so common, their analytic challenges have evoked a plethora of statistical indexes, which can appear in the printouts. Many of the additional expressions are used so rarely today that they are essentially obsolete. Other indexes were developed for tables larger than 2×2, but are available if someone thinks they might be "nice to know about" in the 2×2 situation. Still other indexes represent alternative (but seldom used) approaches to evaluating stochastic significance.

The diverse additional indexes are briefly mentioned here so that you need not be intimidated by their unfamiliarity when deciding to ignore them.

14.8.1   Sources of Confusion

The Fisher Test results can be presented in a confusing manner. In one packaged program (SAS system), the results are called "left," "right," and "2-tail." The sum of the "left" and "right" probability values, however, exceeds 1 because the original (observed) table was included in the calculation for each side. This confusion is avoided in the BMDP system.

The BMDP system, however, offers results for a chi-square test of "row relative symmetry" and "col relative symmetry." The calculation and meaning of these results, however, is not adequately described in the BMDP manual. Communication with the BMDP staff indicates that the test is used to assess results in 2×2 tables that are agreement matrixes (see Chapter 20). For most practical purposes, and even for agreement matrixes, the "symmetry" chi-square tests can be ignored.

14.8.2   Additional Stochastic Indexes

Beyond the results for Fisher exact test and for X^2 with and without the Yates correction, X^2 can be presented with two other variations. One of them, called *Mantel–Haenszel X^2*, is calculated with $N - 1$ replacing N in the customary formula of $[(ad - bc)^2 N]/(n_1 n_2 f_1 f_2)$ for a 2×2 table. The reason for the change, discussed in Chapter 26, is that Mantel and Haenszel calculate variance with a finite-sampling correction.

The other stochastic test, sometimes called the *log likelihood* chi-square, was first proposed by Woolf.[13] It is usually symbolized as G, and calculated as $2\Sigma[o_i \times \ln(o_i/e_i)]$. In this formula, the symbols o_i and e_i refer respectively to the observed and expected values in each of the four cells, and *ln* is the natural logarithm of the cited values. G is interpreted as though it were an X^2 value, which it closely approximates. For a 2×2 table having the conventional format shown in Section 14.2.4, an easy calculational formula is $G = 2[a (\ln a) + b (\ln b) + c (\ln c) + d (\ln d) + N (\ln N) - n_1 (\ln n_1) - n_2 (\ln n_2) - f_1(\ln f_1) - f_2 (\ln f_2)]$. When applied to the data in Table 14.1, this calculation produces $G = 2.81$, whereas the previous X^2 was 2.73.

Although some statistical writers[14,15] believe that G is routinely preferable to X^2, both of the extra approaches just cited for X^2 add little beyond the customary stochastic tests used for 2×2 tables.

14.8.3   Additional Descriptive Indexes

As noted in subsequent chapters, a 2×2 table can also be analyzed with diverse indexes of an *association* between two variables. The indexes are mentioned here as a brief introduction before you meet them, perhaps uninvitedly, in computer printouts. Although sometimes valuable for larger tables (as discussed in Chapter 27), the indexes of association for 2×2 tables usually add nothing beyond confusion to what is already well conveyed by the increments and ratios (see Chapter 10) used as indexes of contrast.

14.8.3.1 ϕ Coefficient of "Correlation" — The ϕ index, calculated as $\sqrt{X^2/N}$, is the "correlation coefficient" for a 2×2 table. ϕ is mentioned later in Chapter 20 as a possible (but unsatisfactory) index of concordance and has a useful role, discussed in Chapter 27, in indexing associations for larger tables.

14.8.3.2 Obsolete Indexes of 2 × 2 Association

— The five additional indexes cited in this section were once fashionable, but almost never appear in medical literature today. The *contingency coefficient, C,* is calculated as $\sqrt{X^2/(N + X^2)}$. *Cramer's V,* which is a transformation of X^2, reduces to ϕ for a 2 × 2 table. In a table having the form $\begin{Bmatrix} a & b \\ c & d \end{Bmatrix}$, *Yule's Q* is $(ad - bc)/(ad + bc)$. Yule also proposed an *index of colligation,* $Y = (\sqrt{ad} - \sqrt{bc})/(\sqrt{ad} + \sqrt{bc})$. The *tetrachoric correlation* is a complex coefficient involving a correlation of two bivariate Gaussian distributions derived from the probabilities noted in the 2 × 2 table.

14.8.3.3 Indexes of Association in Larger Tables

— Several other indexes of association, developed for application in tables larger than 2 × 2, sometimes seek prestige and fame by appearing in computer printouts of analyses for 2 × 2 tables. Those indexes, discussed later in Chapter 27, are *Gamma, Kendall's tau-b, Stuart's tau-c, Somers' D,* and several variations of *lambda* and of an "*uncertainty coefficient.*" The results of all these indexes can safely be disregarded for 2 × 2 tables.

14.8.3.4 Indexes of Concordance

— Tests of concordance, as discussed later in Chapter 20, can be done when each variable in a two-way table offers a measurement of the same entity. The agreement (or disagreement) in these measurements is expressed with indexes such as McNemar symmetry and Kappa. They would pertain only to the special type of "agreement matrix" discussed in Chapter 20, not to an ordinary 2-way table.

References

1. Abbe, 1906; 2. Wallis, 1956, pg. 435; 3. Yates, 1934; 4. Cochran, 1954; 5. Gart, 1971; 6. Yates, 1984; 7. Cormack, 1991; 8. Fleiss, 1986; 9. Bradley, 1968; 10. Kolmogorov, 1941; 11. Smirnov, 1948; 12. Miettinen, 1976; 13. Woolf, 1957; 14. Everitt, 1977; 15. Williams, 1976; 16. Norwegian Multicenter Study Group, 1981; 17. Petersen, 1980; 18. Steering Committee of the Physicians' Health Study Research Group, 1989.

Exercises

14.1. In a randomized clinical trial of timolol vs. placebo in patients surviving acute myocardial infarction,[16] the total deaths at an average of 17 months after treatment were reported as 98/945 in the timolol group and 152/939 in the placebo group. The authors claimed that this difference was both quantitatively and statistically significant. What calculations would you perform to check each of these claims? What are your conclusions?

14.2. Here is the verbatim summary of a clinical report:[17] "Twelve patients with chronic mucocutaneous candidiasis were assigned by random allocation to a 6-month course of treatment with Ketoconazole or placebo in a double-blind trial. All six recipients of Ketoconazole had remission of symptoms and virtually complete regression of mucosal, skin, and nail lesions, whereas only two of the six receiving placebo had even temporary mucosal clearing, and none had improvement of skin or nail disease. The clinical outcome in the Ketoconazole-treated group was significantly more favorable (p $\doteq$ 0.001) than in the placebo-treated group."

What procedure(s) do you think the authors used to arrive at the statistical inference contained in the last sentence of this summary? How would you check your guess?

14.3. In Mendelian genetics theory, the crossing of a tall race of peas with a dwarf race should yield a ratio of 3:1 for tall vs. dwarf peas in the second generation. In his original experiment, J. G. Mendel got 787 tall and 277 dwarf plants in a total of 1064 crosses. Is this result consistent with the 3:1 hypothesis? If so, why? If not, why not?

14.4. In the famous Physicians' Health Study,[18] the investigators reported a "44% reduction in risk" of myocardial infarction for recipients of aspirin vs. placebo. The results had "P < .00001" for 139 myocardial infarctions among 11,037 physicians in the aspirin group, compared with 239 infarctions among 11,034 physicians assigned to placebo. For purposes of this exercise, assume that the "attack rate" in the placebo group was previously estimated to be 2%.

    14.4.1.   What feature of the reported results suggests that the sample size in this trial was much larger than needed?

    14.4.2.   Before the trial, what sample size would have been calculated to prove stochastic significance if the estimated attack rate were reduced by 50% in the aspirin group?

    14.4.3.   The authors report that they enrolled "22,071" physicians, who were then divided almost equally by the randomization. How do you account for the difference between this number and what you calculated in 14.4.2?

14.5. Exercise 10.6 contained the statement that a comparison of two "baseball batting averages, .333 vs. .332, can become stochastically significant if the group sizes are large enough." What should those group sizes be to attain this goal? Do a quick mental estimate and also a formal calculation.

15

Non-Parametric Rank Tests

CONTENTS

Empirical procedures, such as the permutation tests discussed in Chapter 12, can be regarded as *non-parametric* because they do not use the parametric estimates that are required for the t, Z, and chi-square tests. In customary statistical usage, however, the name *non-parametric* is often reserved for a different set of procedures, discussed in this chapter, that use the *ranks* of the observed data rather than the original values. The procedures are often called *non-parametric rank tests* or simply *rank tests*.

15.1 Background Concepts

Rank tests were introduced as a pragmatic analytic procedure because Frank Wilcoxon, a statistician working at Lederle Laboratories, was "fed up with the drudgery of computing one t statistic after another and was looking for something simpler."[1] To get a simpler procedure for two groups, Wilcoxon converted all the dimensional values to ranks, formed an easy-to-calculate sum of ranks for each group, constructed a test statistic from the increment in the two sums, and determined P values from the sampling distribution of the test statistic.

When introduced in 1945, however, Wilcoxon's approach[2] was generally disdained, because it "wasted" information by converting precise dimensional values into ordinal ranks. The approach was labeled "rough-and-ready" or "quick-and-dirty" and was regarded as both inefficient and inferior to the parametric procedures that used Gaussian or other mathematical theories.

The main virtues of the non-parametric procedures, however, came from two advantages that Wilcoxon had not anticipated when he tried to avoid the calculational "drudgery" of t tests for dimensional data. One advantage was that rank tests could be applied directly to ordinal data that were expressed in ranks. Ordinal rating scales, although also sometimes deprecated by classical statisticians, were becoming the best and often the only mechanism for expressing medical phenomena, such as pain, distress, and dysfunction, that could not be measured dimensionally. Ordinal grades became increasingly necessary (and respectable) for such clinical ratings as stage of disease (**I, II, III**), baseline condition (**excellent, good, fair, poor**), and responses to therapy (**much worse, worse, same, better, much better**). Other data for ordinal analysis came from visual analog scales,[3–5] which were commonly applied for rating diverse forms of severity, using dimensional-looking numbers that did not have the equi-interval attributes of measured dimensions.

The ordinal and visual analog ratings could readily be analyzed stochastically today with permutation procedures such as the Pitman-Welch test, but in the precomputer era, the non-parametric rank tests seemed an ideal way to do the job. No one could complain that information was being "lost," because the ordinal data were not converted; they were maintained in their original ratings or quasi-dimensional ranks. The rank tests could also avoid alternative complaints that might arise if the ordinal ratings were regarded as dimensions and managed with t or Z tests.

A second major advantage of rank tests was that they could be applied, without fear of violating mathematical assumptions, to the many sets of dimensional data that had eccentric, non-Gaussian distributions. Furthermore, as noted later, the rank tests could sometimes demonstrate stochastic significance that cannot be achieved in situations where the t and Z tests become "handicapped" by large variance in the eccentric distributions.

15.2 Basic Principles

A rank test uses a hybrid of the empirical and parametric strategies discussed for two-group stochastic tests in Chapters 12 through 14. In both of those strategies, we begin with an index of contrast, which is usually an increment in two means or in two binary proportions, but can also be expressed as a ratio. We next choose a "test statistic" that will be examined stochastically. The test statistic can be either the focal index itself (in empirical tests) or a special stochastic index, such as Z, t, or X^2 (in parametric tests). We then examine the way in which the test statistic would be distributed in a sampling arrangement formed under the null hypothesis. From the possibilities that would occur in that distribution, we determine a P value or a confidence interval for the focal index.

The main difference between the empirical and parametric methods is in forming the rearranged "sampling distribution" of the test statistic. Empirically, the sampling distribution of the index of contrast is constructed from appropriate resamplings or permutations of the observed data, as in the Fisher exact probability or Pitman-Welch test. Parametrically, the test statistic is a special stochastic index — such as Z, t, or X^2 — whose distribution is derived from known mathematical characteristics of the parametric sampling procedure. The non-parametric rank tests are "hybrids," because they also prepare a special stochastic index, which is then rearranged according to empirical permutations.

The purpose of this chapter is to introduce you to the basic operational methods of the "classical" non-parametric rank tests. You need not remember any of the formulas, because you can either look them up when you need them or get a suitable computer program to do all the work.

15.3 Wilcoxon Two-Group Rank-Sum Test

Perhaps the best way to demonstrate the rank-test strategy is with a simple example of the type that led Wilcoxon to devise the procedure.

15.3.1 Illustration of Basic Strategy

Suppose we wanted to compare the dimensional values for {76, 81, 93} in Group A vs. {87, 95, 97} in Group B. To do a t-test for this contrast we would have to calculate values such as S_{xx} for both groups, get the pooled variance, etc. To avoid these calculations, Wilcoxon decided to do a permutation test, somewhat like the Fisher or Pitman-Welch procedure. Instead of permuting the dimensional values of the data, however, he permuted their ranks.

After a null hypothesis is formed, the six items under examination can be combined into a single group and placed in order of magnitude as 76, 81, 87, 93, 95, and 97. The corresponding ranks are 1, 2, 3, 4, 5, 6. (The process yields exactly the same results if the ranks are reversed as 6, 5, 4, 3, 2, 1.) In the observed data, ranks 1, 2, and 4 occurred in Group A and 3, 5, and 6 in Group B.

Because the sum of N consecutive integers is $(N)(N + 1)/2$, the sum of the ranks in these two groups will always be fixed at $21 = (6 \times 7)/2$. Consequently, as the distinctions between the groups increase, the increment in the sum of ranks for each group will enlarge. For example, the widest possible separation for these six items would occur if Group A contains the smallest values 76, 81, and 87, with Group B containing 93, 95, and 97. For this arrangement, the sum of ranks would be $1 + 2 + 3 = 6$ in Group A, and $4 + 5 + 6 = 15$ in Group B. The difference, $15 - 6 = 9$, is the largest obtainable increment in the rank sums for two groups that each contain three members. In our observed data, the sums of ranks are $1 + 2 + 4 = 7$ in Group A and $3 + 5 + 6 = 14$ in Group B. The difference in sums is $14 - 7 = 7$.

15.3.2 Arrangement of Permutations

By examining permutations of the summed ranks, Wilcoxon developed the distribution of the expected increments and could establish probabilities for their occurrence. For the six ranks — 1, 2, 3, 4, 5, 6 — divided into two groups of three members each, a total of $6!/[3! \times 3!] = 20$ combinations are possible.

The arrangement of these combinations for the first ten patterns is shown in Table 15.1. The remaining ten patterns are identical to those shown in Table 15.1, except that the contents are reversed for Groups A and B. The absolute differences in sums of ranks for the 20 possibilities in the total distribution are shown in Table 15.2.

Under the null hypothesis that the two groups are taken from the same underlying population, the observed difference of 7 (or larger) in the sum of ranks would randomly occur with a relative-frequency chance (i.e., P value) of .2. The maximum difference of 9 would have a two-tailed P = .1.

TABLE 15.1

Permutations and Incremental Sum of Ranks for Two Groups
with Three Members Each*

Contents, Group A	Sum of Ranks, Group A	Contents, Group B	Sum of Ranks, Group B	Absolute Difference in Sum of Ranks
1,2,3	6	4,5,6	15	9
1,2,4	7	3,5,6	14	7
1,2,5	8	3,4,6	13	5
1,2,6	9	3,4,5	12	3
1,3,4	8	2,5,6	13	5
1,3,5	8	2,4,6	12	4
1,3,6	9	2,4,5	11	2
1,4,5	9	2,3,6	11	2
1,4,6	11	2,3,5	10	1
1,5,6	12	2,3,4	9	3

* An additional 10 possibilities are produced by reversing the contents of Groups A and B.

TABLE 15.2

Summary of Distribution Illustrated in Table 15.1*

Absolute Difference in Sum of Ranks	Frequency	Relative Frequency	Descending Cumulative Frequency
9	2	.1	.1
7	2	.1	.2
5	4	.2	.4
4	2	.1	.5
3	4	.2	.7
2	4	.2	.9
1	2	.1	1.0
Total	20	1.0	

* Note that Table 15.1 shows half of the total distribution.

15.3.3   Choice of Test Statistic

The strategy just described is used in essentially all of the diverse forms of non-parametric rank tests, which differ mainly in the construction of the index used as a test statistic.

In Wilcoxon's original formulation, he chose the smaller of the two sums of ranks to be the test statistic. Because the total sum of N ranked integers is $(N)(N + 1)/2$, each of the two groups should have half this value, i.e., $(N)(N + 1)/4$, under the null hypothesis of equivalence. Extensive tables of P values can then be constructed for the smaller of the two rank sums under the null hypothesis. The tables are usually condensed to show critical values of the test statistic for conventional α levels such as .05 and .01. Table 15.3 shows such an arrangement for sizes ranging from 2 to 20 in the two groups. (For larger groups, the non-parametric test statistic can receive the parametric conversion discussed in Section 15.4.4.)

15.3.4   Illustration of Procedure

Suppose a written examination for medical licensure has been given to five people from School A and to four from School B. Their scores in the exam are as follows:

School A: 78, 64, 75, 45, 82

School B: 93, 70, 53, 51

TABLE 15.3

Required Value of Smaller of Two Rank Sums to Attain P Values of .05 or .01 in Wilcoxon Two-Group Rank Sum Test, Arranged According to Size of Groups*

N_1	α	\(N_1\) (Smaller Sample)																		
		2	3	4	5	6	7	8	9	10	11	12	13	14	15	16	17	18	19	20
4	.05			10																
	.01																			
5	.05		6	11	17															
	.01				15															
6	.05		7	12	18	26														
	.01			10	16	23														
7	.05		7	13	20	27	36													
	.01			10	16	24	32													
8	.05	3	8	14	21	29	38	49												
	.01			11	17	25	34	43												
9	.05	3	8	14	22	31	40	51	62											
	.01		6	11	18	26	35	45	56											
10	.05	3	9	15	23	32	42	53	65	78										
	.01		6	12	19	27	37	47	58	71										
11	.05	3	9	16	24	34	44	55	68	81	96									
	.01		6	12	20	28	38	49	61	73	87									
12	.05	4	10	17	26	35	46	58	71	84	99	115								
	.01		7	13	21	30	40	51	63	76	90	105								
13	.05	4	10	18	27	37	48	60	73	88	103	119	136							
	.01		7	14	22	31	41	53	65	79	93	109	125							
14	.05	4	11	19	28	38	50	62	76	91	106	123	141	160						
	.01		7	14	22	32	43	54	67	81	96	112	129	147						
15	.05	4	11	20	29	40	52	65	79	94	110	127	145	164	184					
	.01		8	15	23	33	44	56	69	84	99	115	133	151	171					
16	.05	4	12	21	30	42	54	67	82	97	113	131	150	169	190	211				
	.01		8	15	24	34	46	58	72	86	102	119	136	155	175	196				
17	.05	5	12	21	32	43	56	70	84	100	117	135	154	174	195	217	240			
	.01		8	16	25	36	47	60	74	89	105	122	140	159	180	201	223			
18	.05	5	13	22	33	45	58	72	87	103	121	139	158	179	200	222	246	270		
	.01		8	16	26	37	49	62	76	92	108	125	144	163	184	206	228	252		
19	.05	5	13	23	34	46	60	74	90	107	124	143	163	182	205	228	252	277	303	
	.01	3	9	17	27	38	50	64	78	94	111	129	147	168	189	210	234	258	283	
20	.05	5	14	24	35	48	62	77	93	110	128	147	167	188	210	234	258	283	309	337
	.01	3	9	18	28	39	52	66	81	97	114	132	151	172	193	215	239	263	289	315

* This table is derived from Schor, S.S. *Fundamentals of Biostatistics*. New York: Putnam's Sons, 1968.

A data analyst determines that $\overline{X}_A = 68.8$, $s_A = 14.89$, $\overline{X}_B = 66.75$, $s_B = 19.47$; and then claims (after doing a t test) that the results are not stochastically significant. Another analyst might then argue, however, that the t test is improper and that a ranks test is more appropriate, because the examination scores are arbitrary ratings rather than truly dimensional data and, therefore, should not be analyzed with dimensional tactics.

For the Wilcoxon Rank Sum test, we rank the total set of observations, irrespective of group, and then find the sum of ranks in each group. The results are as follows:

Group A		Group B	
Observed Value	Rank	Observed Value	Rank
78	7	93	9
64	4	70	5
75	6	53	3
45	1	51	2
82	8		
Sum of Ranks	$R_A = 26$		$R_B = 19$

[If you do a rank test yourself, rather than with a computer program, always check your calculations by seeing that the total of the two rank sums is equal to the value of $(N)(N+1)/2$. In this instance $26 + 19 = 45 = (9 \times 10)/2$.]

The smaller of the two rank sums here is $R_B = 19$. In Table 15.3, with a smaller group of 4 members and a larger group of 5, the value of R_B would have to be ≤ 11 to attain a 2P value of $\leq .05$. Consequently, the observed result for R_B is too large to be stochastically significant. [The only way stochastic significance could be obtained in the situation here is to get $R_B \leq 11$ with ranks 1, 2, 3, and 4 or ranks 1, 2, 3, and 5 in Group B.]

15.4 Mann-Whitney U Test

To avoid using the somewhat crude sum of ranks, Mann and Whitney[6] developed a different, more subtle indexing strategy, which relies on the sequential placement of ranks. The index reflects the number of times, in the ranked total arrangement, in which a value (or "mark") in one group precedes that of the other group. The sequential placement index, called "U," will have two sets of values: one for the number of times that Group A marks precede those of Group B, and the other, for the number of times that Group B marks precede those of Group A.

Under the null hypothesis, the two U indexes should be about equal. If the two compared groups are different, one of the U indexes should be substantially smaller than the other. The values of U will have a sampling distribution for groups of sizes n_A and n_B; and P values can be found for magnitudes of the smaller value of U in that distribution.

The stochastic results for P turn out to be essentially identical for the Wilcoxon rank-sum approach and for the Mann-Whitney sequential-placement U approach. Nevertheless, the Mann-Whitney approach is usually preferred, perhaps because it has better academic credentials (the paper was published in the *Annals of Mathematical Statistics*), but mainly because its stochastic and descriptive properties have several advantages to be discussed later. In view of the similarity of results, however, the Mann-Whitney U procedure now often receives the eponym of *Wilcoxon-Mann-Whitney*.

15.4.1 Illustration of Procedure

For a Mann-Whitney analysis, the 11 examination grades in the previous example from Schools A and B would be ranked, from lowest to highest, as follows:

45	51	53	64	70	75	78	82	93
A	B	B	A	B	A	A	A	B

The test statistic, U, can be determined as the number of times a B mark precedes an A mark. Thus, the first A mark, 45, is preceded by no B marks. The next A mark, 64, is preceded by two B marks. The next A mark, 75, is preceded by three B marks (51, 53 and 70); and the last two A marks, 78 and 82, are each preceded by the same three B marks. Thus, the value of U is:

$$U = 0 + 2 + 3 + 3 + 3 = 11$$

In the extreme instance, if School A had the five highest scores and School B had the four lowest scores, the results would be:

45	51	53	64	70	75	78	82	93
B	B	B	B	A	A	A	A	A

In this situation, each of the A marks would be preceded by four B marks and the value of U would be:

$$U = 4 + 4 + 4 + 4 + 4 = 20$$

If we had reversed our enumeration technique and counted the occasions on which a B mark is preceded by an A mark, rather than vice versa, we would have obtained, for the first instance:

$$U' = 1 + 1 + 2 + 5 = 9$$

In the second instance, for the extreme example, $U' = 0$.

It can be shown mathematically that $U + U' = n_A n_B$, where n_A and n_B are the respective sizes of the two groups under consideration. Thus, for the examples being discussed, $n_A = 5$ and $n_B = 4$, so that $n_A n_B = 20$. In the first example $U = 11$ and $U' = 9$. In the second example, $U = 20$ and $U' = 0$. In both examples, $U + U' = 20$.

15.4.2   Simplified Procedure

Because the process of determining U (or U') can become a nuisance if the group sizes are large, a simpler method is used. By some algebra that will not be shown here, it can be demonstrated that, if we use the subscripts 1 and 2 for Groups A and B, and if the sums of ranks are R_1 for Group A and R_2 for Group B, then

$$U_1 = R_1 - [n_1 (n_1 + 1)/2] \qquad \text{and} \qquad U_2 = R_2 - [n_2 (n_2 + 1)/2] \qquad [15.1]$$

One of these values will be U and the other will be U'. In the example here, $U_1 = 26 - [5(6)/2] = 11$; and $U_2 = 19 - [4(5)/2] = 9$. These are the same values found earlier with the A-before-B or B-before-A sequential placement procedure.

15.4.3   Use of the U/P Table

Table 15.4 gives the values of P for .025 (one-tail) or .05 (two-tail) decisions, associated with the *smaller* of the two values of U or U'. For the data under discussion, Table 15.4 shows that with $n_2 = 5$ and $n_1 = 4$, U must equal 1 or less for a P value of .05 or lower. Therefore, since $U = 9$, we again conclude that $P > .05$.

15.4.4   Z/U Relationship for Large Groups

When n_1 and n_2 become large (e.g., > 20), the sampling distribution of U approaches that of a Gaussian distribution, having as its mean

$$\hat{\mu}_U = n_1 n_2 / 2 \qquad [15.2]$$

and standard deviation

$$\hat{\sigma}_U = \sqrt{\frac{(n_1)(n_2)(n_1 + n_2 + 1)}{12}} \qquad [15.3]$$

TABLE 15.4

U/P Table for Wilcoxon-Mann-Whitney U Test

(Larger) n₂ (Smaller) n₁	Smallest Permissible Value of U for 2-Tailed P = .05																
	4	5	6	7	8	9	10	11	12	13	14	15	16	17	18	19	20
3		0	1	1	2	2	3	3	4	4	5	5	6	6	7	7	8
4	0	1	2	3	4	4	5	6	7	8	9	10	11	11	12	13	13
5		2	3	5	6	7	8	9	11	12	13	14	15	17	18	19	20
6			5	6	8	10	11	13	14	16	17	19	21	22	24	25	27
7				8	10	12	14	16	18	20	22	24	26	28	30	32	34
8					13	15	17	19	22	24	26	29	31	34	36	38	41
9						17	20	23	26	28	31	34	37	39	42	45	48
10							23	26	29	33	36	39	42	45	48	52	55
11								30	33	37	40	44	47	51	55	58	62
12									37	41	45	49	53	57	61	65	69
13										45	50	54	59	63	67	72	76
14											55	59	64	67	74	78	83
15												64	70	75	80	85	90
16													75	81	86	92	98
17														87	93	99	105
18															99	106	112
19																113	119
20																	127

This table is derived from Smart, J.V., *Elements of Medical Statistics*. Springfield, IL: Charles C Thomas, 1965.

For large group sizes, therefore, Table 15.4 can be avoided. The observed value of U can be converted into a Z test, using the formula:

$$Z = \frac{U - \hat{\mu}_U}{\hat{\sigma}_U} = \frac{U - \frac{n_1 n_2}{2}}{\sqrt{\frac{n_1 n_2 (n_1 + n_2 + 1)}{12}}}$$ [15.4]

This result can then be interpreted using either a table of probabilities associated with Z, or the last row (with $\nu = \infty$) in a t/P arrangement such as Table 7.3.

15.5 Management of Ties

All of these attributes make the Wilcoxon-Mann-Whitney U Test quite easy to use if the data come from dimensions that have been converted to ranks or if the data are expressed in an unlimited-ranks scale. In most medical situations, however, the ordinal data are expressed in a limited number of grades that will produce many ties when the results are ranked. The ties then create problems in choosing scores for the ranking process and also in the analysis of the test statistic.

15.5.1 Illustrative Example

Table 15.5 shows the results of a randomized double-blind trial of active agent A vs. placebo in the treatment of congestive heart failure. Because the outcome was expressed in a 4-category ordinal scale of improvement, the Wilcoxon-Mann-Whitney U procedure is an appropriate stochastic test for the contention that the active agent was better than placebo.

TABLE 15.5

Results of Clinical Trial for Treatment of Congestive Heart Failure

		Ordinal Scale for Improvement of Patients			
Treatment	**Worse**	**No Change**	**Improved**	**Much Improved**	**TOTAL**
Placebo	8	9	19	10	46
Active Agent	2	8	29	19	58
TOTAL	10	17	48	29	104

15.5.2 Assignment of Ranks

To establish the ranks here, we begin at the "low" end of Table 15.5, with 10 patients who were **worse**. Their mean rank will be $(1 + 2 + \cdots + 10)/10 = 5.5$. The next 17 patients had **no change**. They share the ranks 11 to 27, and their mean rank will be $(11 + 12 + 13 + \cdots + 27)/17 = 323/17 = 19$.

An easy method can be used to get a cumbersome sum such as $(11 + 12 + \cdots + 27)/17$. The hard way is to enter all the numbers into a calculator, step by step, pushing the buttons 17 times to get all the numbers entered and added, and then dividing their sum by 17 to get the average value. The easy method relies on remembering that the average value of a sequence of integer numbers — $n_A, n_A + 1, n_A + 2, n_A + 3, \ldots,$ n_B — is simply $(n_A + n_B)/2$. Thus, $(11 + 27)/2 = 38/2 = 19$, which is the same as $323/17$.

The next 48 patients, sharing the ranks 28 through 75, were **improved**. They tie at the average rank of $(28 + 75)/2 = 51.5$. The remaining 29 patients, who were **much improved**, have the average rank of $(76 + 104)/2 = 90$.

To be sure that the assignment of ranks is correct, recall that the sum of ranks for the 104 patients in the trial should be $(104)(105)/2 = 5460$. The sum of ranks for the placebo group is $(8 \times 5.5) + (9 \times 19) + (19 \times 51.5) + (10 \times 90) = 44 + 171 + 978.5 + 900 = 2093.5$. The sum of ranks for the actively treated group is $(2 \times 5.5) + (8 \times 19) + (29 \times 51.5) + (19 \times 90) = 3366.5$. The total is $2093.5 + 3366.5 = 5460$.

15.5.3 Determination of U and Z Values

With the two sums of ranks available, the corresponding U values can be calculated with Formula [15.1] as

$$U_{placebo} = 2093.5 - [(46)(47)/2] = 1012.5$$

and

$$U_{active} = 3366.5 - [(58)(59)/2] = 1655.5$$

[To check accuracy of the calculation, note that $1012.5 + 1655.5 = 2668 = (46)(58)$.] Because $U_{placebo}$ is the smaller value, it will serve as U for the subsequent evaluation.

To do a Z test here, we would use Formulas [15.2] and [15.3] to get $\hat{\mu}_U = (46)(58)/2 = 1334$ and $\hat{\sigma}_U = \sqrt{(46)(58)(105)/12} = \sqrt{23345} = 152.79$. Substituting into Formula [15.4], we then get:

$$Z = \frac{1012.5 - 1334}{152.79} = -2.10$$

The result is stochastically significant, but is not strictly accurate because we have not taken account of ties.

15.5.4 Adjustment for Ties

If t_i is the number of observations tied for a given rank, we can determine

$$T_i = (t_i^3 - t_i)/12 \qquad [15.5]$$

for each rank, and then calculate ΣT_i. In the cited example, for ratings of **worse**, $t_1 = 10$; for **no change**, $t_2 = 17$; for **improved**, $t_3 = 48$; and for **much improved**, $t_4 = 29$. We would have

$$\Sigma T_i = \frac{(10^3 - 10) + (17^3 - 17) + (48^3 - 48) + (29^3 - 29)}{12} = \frac{14790}{12} = 11732.5$$

The value of T_i is used to modify the estimate of the standard deviation of U in Formula [15.3]. The modified formula is:

$$s_U = \sqrt{\left(\frac{n_1 n_2}{N(N-1)}\right)\left(\frac{N^3 - N}{12} - \Sigma T_i\right)} \qquad [15.6]$$

where $N = n_1 + n_2$.

For our observed data,

$$s_U = \sqrt{\left[\frac{(46)(58)}{(104)(103)}\right]\left[\frac{104^3 - 104}{12} - 11732.5\right]}$$

$$= \sqrt{[0.24907][81997.5]} = \sqrt{20423.12} = 142.9$$

This value of s_U can then be used to calculate Z as:

$$Z = \frac{U - \mu_U}{s_U} = \frac{1012.5 - 1334}{142.9} = -2.25$$

With some simple algebra, not shown here, it can be demonstrated that the subtraction of ΣT_i always reduces the variance, so that $s_U \le \sigma_U$. Consequently, the Z value calculated with s_U will always be larger than the Z calculated with $\hat{\sigma}_U$. Thus, the effect of adjusting for ties is to raise the value for Z, thereby increasing the chance of getting stochastic significance.

In the example just cited, the result was stochastically significant without the adjustment, which becomes unnecessary if the directly calculated value of Z yields a P value that is $< \alpha$. If the uncorrected Z yields a P value substantially $> \alpha$, the adjustment probably will not help. Thus, the adjustment is best used when the uncorrected Z is somewhere near but below the border of stochastic significance.

15.6 Wilcoxon Signed-Ranks Test

Wilcoxon also created a one-group or paired rank test, analogous to the corresponding one-group or paired Z and t tests. To show how the Wilcoxon procedure works in this situation, suppose 6 patients have received treatment intended to lower their levels of serum cholesterol. The results of the before (B) and after (A) differences in Table 15.6 show that four of the six cholesterol levels were reduced. The stochastic question to be answered is whether the reduction might be a chance phenomenon if there had been no real effect.

15.6.1 Basic Principle

To do a parametric one-group t test for these data, we would examine all of the B-A differences, find their mean, and contrast its value stochastically against a hypothesized mean difference ($\bar{d}$) of 0. The process is equivalent to adding all the positive increments, subtracting all the negative increments, and noting their mean difference.

In a rank test, we do something quite analogous, but instead of dealing with the direct values, we work with their ranks. After ranking all of the observed increments according to their *absolute* values,

TABLE 15.6

Initial and Subsequent Levels of Serum Cholesterol

Patient Number	(B) Initial Level	(A) Subsequent Level	(B – A) Increment	Rank
1	209	183	26	4
2	276	242	34	5.5
3	223	235	–12	3
4	219	185	34	5.5
5	241	235	6	1
6	236	247	–11	2

i.e., regardless of negative or positive signs, we take the sum of ranks for all the positive increments and compare it stochastically with the sum of ranks for all the negative increments. Under the null hypothesis, we would expect these two sums to be about the same. If their observed difference is an uncommon enough event stochastically, we would reject the null hypothesis.

15.6.2 Finding the Ranks of Increments

The first step is to examine the increments, B – A, in the observed paired values for each patient. (We expect most of these increments to be positive if the treatment is effective in lowering cholesterol.)

The next step is to rank the differences in order of magnitude, *without regard to sign*, from smallest to largest. In Table 15.6, the smallest increment, 6, is ranked as 1. The next largest increment, –11, is ranked as 2 (even though –11 is arithmetically less than 6). The next increment, –12, is ranked 3; and 26 is ranked 4.

A problem arises when two (or more) increments are tied for the same rank. This problem is solved, as discussed in Section 15.5.2, by giving each increment the rank that is the average value of the ranks for the tied set. Thus, in the foregoing table, the incremental values of 34 and 34 are tied for the 5th rank. Since these two numbers would occupy the 5th and 6th ranks, they are each ranked as 5.5. [If three increments were tied for the 5th rank, they would each be ranked as 6, since the average rank of the three would be $(5 + 7)/2 = 6$. Note that the next increment after those three ties would be ranked as 8, not as 6 or 7. If you forget this distinction and rank the 8th increment as 6 or 7, the results will be wrong.]

15.6.3 Finding the Sum of Signed Ranks

The next step is to find the sum of all the ranks associated with negative and positive increments. In Table 15.5, the two negative increments (–11 and –12) have a rank sum of $2 + 3 = 5$. The four positive increments have a rank sum of $1 + 4 + 5.5 + 5.5 = 16$.

We could have determined the value of 16 either by adding the ranks for the four latter increments, or by recalling, from the formula $(n)(n + 1)/2$, that the total sum of ranks should be $(6)(7)/2 = 21$. Thus, if the negative increments have a rank sum of 5, the positive increments must be $21 – 5 = 16$. The smaller value for the sum of the two sets of ranks is a stochastic index designated as T. In this instance, $T = 5$.

15.6.4 Sampling Distribution of T

The values of T have a sampling distribution for different values of n. Under the null hypothesis, anticipating that about half the signed ranks will be positive and half will be negative, we would expect T to be half of $(n)(n + 1)/2$, which in this instance, would be $21/2 = 10.5$. The smaller the value of T, the greater will be its departure from this expectation, and the less likely is its distinction to arise by chance.

15.6.4.1   Total Number of Possible Values for T — As with any other complete resampling distribution, we first need to know the number of possible values that can occur for T. This result will be the denominator for all subsequent determinations of relative frequencies.

In a contrast of two groups, having n_1 and n_2 members, the number of possible arrangements was $N!/(n_1!)(n_2!)$, where $N = n_1 + n_2$. This approach will not work here because the arrangements involve one group, not two, and also because the permuted ranks can be assembled in various groupings. The six "signed" ranks (in the example here) may or may not all have positive values; and the positive values can occur in none, 1, 2, 3, 4, 5, or all 6 of the signed ranks.

When each possibility is considered, there is only one way in which all 6 ranks can be negative and one way in which all 6 are positive. There are 6 ways in which only one of the ranks is positive, and 6 ways in which five of the ranks are negative (i.e., one is positive). There are 15 ways ($= 6 \times 5/2$) in which two ranks are positive, and 15 in which two are negative (i.e., four are positive). Finally, there are 20 ways in which three ranks will be positive, with the other three being negative. (The 20 is calculated as $6!/[(3!)(3!)]$.) Thus, there are $1 + 1 + 6 + 6 + 15 + 15 + 20 = 64$ possible values for the number of positive rank combinations when $n = 6$. A general formula for this process is $\sum_{r=0}^{n} (n!)/[(n - r)!(r)!]$. For $n = 6$,

$$64 = \frac{6!}{6!0!} + \frac{6!}{5!1!} + \frac{6!}{4!2!} + \frac{6!}{3!3!} + \frac{6!}{2!4!} + \frac{6!}{1!5!} + \frac{6!}{0!6!}$$

15.6.4.2   Frequency of Individual Values of T — Under the null hypothesis, for $n = 6$, we expect T to have a value of $21/2 = 10.5$. Therefore, if T is the smaller sum of signed ranks, we need to determine only the ways of getting values of $T \le 10$. Each of the possibilities in Table 15.7 shows the arrangement that will yield the cited value of T for a sum of six ranks. The number of occurrences is then divided by 64 (the total number of possibilities) to show the relative and cumulative frequency for each occurrence.

TABLE 15.7

Values of T for Possible Arrangements of Positive Values of Six Signed Ranks

Value of T	Identity of Positive Ranks That Are Components for This Value of T	Number of Occurrences	Relative Frequency	Cumulative Relative Frequency
0	None	1	1/64 = .016	.016
1	1	1	.016	.031
2	2	1	.016	.047
3	{3}, {1,2}	2	.031	.078
4	{4}, {1,3}	2	.031	.109
5	{5}, {1,4}, {2,3}	3	.046	.156
6	{6}, {1,5}, {2,4}, {1,2,3}	4	.062	.218
7	{1,6}, {2,5}, {3,4}, {1,2,4}	4	.062	.281
8	{2,6}, {3,5}, {1,2,5}, {1,3,4}	4	.062	.343
9	{3,6}, {4,5}, {1,2,6}, {1,3,5}, {2,3,4}	5	.078	.421
10	{4,6}, {1,3,6}, {1,4,5}, {2,3,5} {1,2,3,4}	5	.078	.500
11	{5,6}, {1,4,6}, {2,3,6}, {2,4,5}, {1,2,3,5}	5	.078	.578

Table 15.7 need not ordinarily be extended beyond $T = 10$, because if T becomes 11, we have begun to look at the other, i.e., negative, side of the summed ranks. When the *absolute* values are summed for the negative ranks, their result will be $T = 10$. For example, the 5 groupings that produce $T = 11$ in Table 15.7 each contain the complement ranks omitted from the counterpart groupings when $T = 10$. (The "complement" of {4, 6} is {1, 2, 3, 5}. The "complement" of $T = 0$ is {1, 2, 3, 4, 5, 6}, for which $T = 21$.)

The cumulative relative frequencies in Table 15.7 show the one-tailed P values for any observed positive value of T. These are one-tailed probabilities because a symmetrically similar distribution could be constructed for the negative signed ranks. To interpret the results, if T = 4, P = .109, and if T = 3, P = .078. If we want the one-tailed P to be below .05, T must be ≤ 2. For the two-tailed P to be below .05, T must be 0.

Arrangements such as Table 15.7 can be constructed for any value of n. A summary of the key values found in such constructions is presented here in Table 15.8, which can be used to find the P values associated with T. For example, Table 15.8 shows what we have just found for the circumstance when n = 6: a T of 2 or less is required for two-tailed P to be ≤ .1, and T must be zero for a two-tailed P of ≤ .05.

TABLE 15.8

Critical Values of T for Signed-Ranks Test

	P: two-tailed test			
	.1	**.05**	**.02**	**.01**
n				
6	2	0		
7	3	2	0	
8	5	3	1	0
9	8	5	3	1
10	10	8	5	3
11	13	10	7	5
12	17	13	9	7
13	21	17	12	9
14	25	21	15	12
15	30	25	19	15
16	35	29	23	19
17	41	34	27	23
18	47	40	32	27
19	53	46	37	32
20	60	52	43	37
21	67	58	49	42
22	75	65	55	48
23	83	73	62	54
24	91	81	69	61
25	100	89	76	68

This table is derived from Smart, J.V. *Elements of Medical Statistics.* Springfield, IL: Charles C Thomas, 1965.

15.6.5   Use of T/P Table

To use Table 15.8, a suitable value must be chosen for n. If any of the observed increments in the data are 0, they cannot be counted as either positive or negative when the sums of ranks are formed. Therefore, zero increments should not be ranked, and the value of n should be the original number of pairs minus the number of pairs that had zero increments.

The 6 patients in Table 15.6 have no zero-increment pairs, and so n = 6. (If there were two zero-increment pairs, we would have had to use n − 2 = 4 for entering Table 15.8.) For all values of n in the table, the value of P gets smaller as T gets smaller. Because our calculated T is 5, we can say that P > .05, regardless of whether the result receives a two-tailed interpretation, or the one tail that might be used because treatment was expected to lower cholesterol. We can therefore conclude that a stochastically distinctive (P < .05, one-tailed) lowering of cholesterol has *not* been demonstrated.

With only six patients in the group, Table 15.8 shows that T would have to be 0 for a two-tailed P < .05 or 2 for 2P ≤ .1. If the third patient had an after-treatment value of 211, so that the B − A increment was 223 − 211 = 12, rather than the observed −12, the value of T would have been 2, and the result would have had a one-tailed P value of .05.

15.7 Challenges of Descriptive Interpretation

All of the foregoing discussion of statistical "machinery" describes the operating procedures of non-parametric rank tests. You need not remember the basic strategy or the specific tactics, as the tests today are almost always done with a suitable computer program. Because the program will produce a P value for *stochastic* significance, your main challenge will be to make decisions about *quantitative* significance.

The latter task will be difficult, however, because ordinal data do not have precise central indexes that can be quantitatively contrasted, and the non-parametric rank tests offer P values, but not confidence intervals.

15.7.1 Disadvantages of Customary Approaches

In the absence of a simple, obvious central index for each ordinal group, the contrasts have been done with several approaches, cited in the next three subsections, that are not fully satisfactory.

15.7.1.1 Dichotomous Compression — As noted earlier (see Section 3.5.1.3), ordinal data can be compressed dichotomously and then summarized as a binary proportion. For example, suppose we want to compare groups A and B, which have the following frequency counts in a five-category ordinal scale:

	Much Worse	Worse	Same	Better	Much Better
Group A	6	10	34	27	19
Group B	37	9	4	36	10

The **better** and **much better** results could be combined to form a "central index" for patients who became **at least better**. The result would be $(27 + 19)/(6 + 10 + 34 + 27 + 19) = 46/96 = .48$ for group A and $46/96 = .48$ for group B. Although the two sets of data have quite different distributions, they would have the same binary proportion for the rating of **at least better**.

15.7.1.2 Median Value — The central index of a set of ordinal data could also be cited according to the median value, but this tactic also has the disadvantage of losing distinctions in the rankings. Thus, the foregoing data for Groups A and B have **same** as an identical median value in each group.

15.7.1.3 Dimensional Conversions — If the Wilcoxon approach "loses" data, an opposite approach can gain "pseudo-data" if we convert the ordinal grades to dimensional codes. Thus, if we assign coded digits of **1** = much worse, **2** = worse, **3** = same, **4** = better, and **5** = much better, and if we then use the digits as though they were dimensional values, an arithmetical mean can be calculated for the ordinal ratings. With this type of coding, the means in the foregoing example would be $[(1 \times 6) + (2 \times 10) + (3 \times 34) + (4 \times 27) + (5 \times 19)]/96 = 3.45$ in Group A and $[(1 \times 37) + (2 \times 9) + (3 \times 4) + (4 \times 36) + (5 \times 10)]/96 = 2.72$ in Group B.

The two groups could now be distinguished as different, but only via the somewhat "shady" tactic of giving arbitrary dimensional values to data that are merely ranked categories. Thus, the customary binary proportions, medians, and means may not offer a fully satisfactory approach for identifying desirable contrasts of central indexes in ordinal data.

15.7.2 Additional Approaches

The non-parametric rank tests were originally developed without attention to an index of *descriptive* contrast. Wilcoxon had no need for one because he could immediately compare the observed dimensional means; he used the non-parametric rank test only for its stochastic simplicity in providing P values. When non-parametric rank tests received further development in the academic world of mathematical statistics, the process was aimed solely at a stochastic, not descriptive, contrast.

Accordingly, we need something that is both legitimately ordinal and also applicable as an index of contrast for two ordinal groups. The next few subsections describe the available options.

15.7.3 Comparison of Mean Ranks

From the data presented in Section 15.5.2, we can determine the mean ranks as $2093.5/46 = 45.5$ in the placebo group and $3366.5/58 = 58.0$ in the actively treated group. These two mean values are "legitimately ordinal" because they emerged from the ranks of the data. No arbitrary dimensional values such as 1, 2, 3, ... were assigned to any of the ordinal categories such as **worse, no change**.

Because these ranks have no associated units, we could contrast the two mean rank values as a ratio, $58.0/45.5 = 1.27$. The result would be impressive if you regard the ratio of 1.27 as quantitatively significant. If you are willing to accept the average-rank values of **5.5, 19, 51.5,** and **90** as being analogous to dimensional data, however, we can also calculate a standardized increment. In the placebo group, the group variance will be $8(5.5)^2 + 9(19)^2 + 19(51.5)^2 + 10(90)^2 - [(2093.5)^2/46] = 39606.745$, and the standard deviation is $\sqrt{39606.745/45} = 29.67$. In the actively treated group, the counterpart results are $2(5.5)^2 + 8(19)^2 + 29(51.5)^2 + 19(90)^2 - [(3366.5)^2/58] = 38361.643$ for group variance and $\sqrt{38361.643/57} = 25.94$ for standard deviation. The pooled standard deviation is $\sqrt{(39606.745 + 38361.643)/102} = 27.6$ and the standard increment (or effect size) will be $(58.0 - 45.5)/27.6 = .45$, which could be regarded as modest (according to the criteria in Chapter 10).

15.7.4 Ridit Analysis

The technique of ridit analysis, proposed by Bross[7] in 1958, is analogous to the tactic just described for assigning values to the ranks. A *ridit*, which is an acronym for "relative to an identified distribution," is calculated for each of a set of ordinal categories and represents "the proportion of all subjects from the reference group falling in the lower ranking categories plus half the proportion falling in the given category." The reference group is usually the total population in the study. After the ridits are determined for each category, the mean ridits can be calculated to compare the two groups. The ridit approach is illustrated here so you can see how it works, but you need not remember it, because (for reasons cited later) it is hardly ever used today.

15.7.4.1 *Illustration of Procedure* — For the data in Table 15.5, the **worse** category occupies $10/104 = .096$ of the total group, and will have a ridit of $.096/2 = .048$. For the **no change** category, which has a proportion of $17/104 = .163$ in the data, the ridit will be $(.163/2) + .096 = .178$. For the **improved** category, with proportion $48/104 = .462$, the ridit will be $(.462/2) + .096 + .163 = .490$. Finally, the **much improved** category, with proportion $29/104 = .279$, will have $(.279/2) + .096 + .163 + .462 = .860$. Because the mean ridit in the reference group is always .5, a check that the ridits have been correctly calculated for Table 15.5 shows $(10 \times .048) + (17 \times .178) + (48 \times .490) + (29 \times .860) = 51.97$ as the sum of the ridits and their mean is $51.97/104 = .5$.

Having established the ridit values, we can calculate the mean ridit of the active-agent group as $[(2 \times .048) + (8 \times .178) + (29 \times .490) + (19 \times .860)]/58 = .553$. The corresponding mean ridit in the placebo group is $[(8 \times .048) + (9 \times .178) + (19 \times .490) + (10 \times .860)]/46 = .433$. Their ratio, $.533/.433$, is 1.23. (Recall, from Section 15.7.3, that the corresponding mean ranks were 58.0 and 45.5, with a ratio of 1.27.) Interpreted as probabilities, the ridit results suggest that an actively treated person has a chance of .553 of getting a result that is better than someone in the placebo group.

Standard errors can be calculated for ridits, and the results can be stochastically examined with a Z test. The textbook by Fleiss[8] shows a simple formula for calculating the standard error of the difference in two mean ridits, $\bar{r}_2$ and $\bar{r}_1$. The value of Z is then determined as $(\bar{r}_2 - \bar{r}_1)/\text{SED}$.

15.7.4.2   Similarity to Mean-Rank Procedure — The ridit values are reasonably similar to what would have been found if the mean ranks in each category had been expressed as percentiles. When divided by 104 (the total group size), the mean rank of 5.5 becomes a percentile of .052, 19 becomes .183, 51.5 becomes .495, and 90 becomes .865. The respective ridits that correspond to these percentiles are .048, .178, .490, and .860.

The mean average ranks in the two groups, 45.5 vs. 58.0, could each be divided by 104 to become "percentiles" of .438 vs. .558. The corresponding ridit means are .433 vs. .533. The respective ratios are 1.27 for the mean ranks and 1.23 for the ridits.

15.7.4.3   Current Status of Ridit Analysis — After being initially proposed, ridit analysis was used in investigations of the epidemiology of breast cancer[9], classifications of blood pressure,[10] life stress and psychological well being,[11] economic status and lung cancer,[12] and geographic distinctions in schizophrenia.[13] The ridit method seems to have gone out of favor in recent years, however, perhaps because of a vigorous attack by Mantel[14] in 1979. He complained that the ridit procedure, although intended "for descriptive purposes," was unsatisfactory for both description and inference. Descriptively, the ordinal ridits emerge arbitrarily from frequency counts in the data, not from a biological or logical scheme of scaling; and inferentially, the formulation of variance for ridits has many "improprieties."

Because stochastic decisions for two groups of ordinal data can be done with a Wilcoxon-Mann-Whitney U test and the mean rank for each group produces essentially the same result as the mean ridit, the ridit technique offers no real advantages. It is mentioned here so you will have heard of it in case it is suggested to you or (more unlikely) encountered in a published report.

15.7.5   U Score for Pairs of Comparisons

Another descriptive approach for categorical frequencies in two groups was proposed by Moses et al.[15] For n_A and n_B members in the two groups, each item of data in Group A can be compared with each item in Group B to produce $n_A \times n_B$ pairs of comparisons. Under the null hypotheses, half of these comparisons should favor Group A and half should favor Group B. When we check the comparisons, we count those favoring Group A, those favoring Group B, and the ties. Their sum should be $n_A \times n_B$.

When this tactic is applied to Table 15.5, there are 16 tied pairs (= 8×2) at the rank of **worse**, 72 (= 9×8) tied pairs at **no change**, 551 (= 19×29) at **improved**, and 290 (= 10×29) at **much improved**, yielding a total of 829 tied pairs. The number of pairs in which active agent scored better than placebo is $8(8 + 29 + 19) + 9(29 + 19) + 19(19) = 1241$. The number of pairs in which placebo scored better than active agent is $2(9 + 19 + 10) + 8(19 + 10) + 29(10) = 598$. The total of $(58)(46) = 2668$ pairs can thus be divided into 1241 that favor active agent, 598 that favor placebo and 829 ties. If we credit half the ties to placebo and half to active agent, the scores become $1241 + (829/2) = 1655.5$ for active agent and $598 + (829/2) = 1012.5$ for placebo.

These numbers should look familiar. They are the values of U calculated for the active and placebo groups in Section 15.5.3. Accordingly, we could have avoided all of the foregoing calculations for pairs of ties, etc. by using the relatively simple Mann-Whitney formulas for determining the two values of U. Conceptually, this result also lets us know that the "sequential placement" strategy of counting A-before-B, etc. is the exact counterpart of determining the just-described allocation of paired ratings.

U_A or U_B can be used as a descriptive index for expressing a group's proportion of the total number of compared pairs. Thus, the proportionate score in favor of active treatment is $1655.5/2668 = .62$. According to Moses et al.,[15] this index suggests that .62 is the random chance of getting a better response to active treatment than to placebo in the observed trial. This *descriptive* attribute of the U index may be more valuable than its role as a stochastic index, because the same stochastic results are obtained with the rank sum and U tests, but the rank sum procedure does not provide a descriptive index.

15.7.6   Traditional Dichotomous Index

Although all of the tactics just described are useful, none of them is familiar, and we have no "intuitive feeling" about how to interpret them. Probably the easiest and simplest "intuitive" approach to Table 15.5, therefore, is to dichotomize the outcome variable and report the percentages of **any improvement** as $(29 + 19)/58 = 82.8\%$ for the active group and $(19 + 10)/46 = 63.0\%$ for placebo. The increment of .198 also produces an impressive NNE of 5.

Although dichotomous compression was unsatisfactory for the example in Section 15.7.1.1, the binary "cut point" was not well chosen in that example. If the binary split had been demarcated to separate the ratings of **worse** and **much worse** (rather than the rating of **at least better**), the proportions of patients who were **worse** or **much worse** would have been $16/96 = .17$ for Group A and $46/96 = .48$ for Group B in that example. A clear distinction in the two groups would then be evident.

In general, whenever two groups of ordinal grades have an evident distinction, it can usually be shown quantitatively with a suitable dichotomous split and cited with binary proportions that are easy to understand and interpret.

15.7.7 Indexes of Association

Yet another way of describing the quantitative contrast of two groups of ordinal data is available from indexes of association and trend that will be discussed much later in Chapter 27.

One index, called Kendall's tau, relies on calculations such as U (in Section 15.4.1) that determine and score the sequence of placement for corresponding ranks. A second descriptive index can be the slope of the straight line that is fitted to the ordinal categories by regression-like methods.

A crude, quick descriptive idea of the association, however, can be obtained by forming a ratio between the observed increment in the sums of ranks and the "no expected" (rather than perfect) difference. For example, in Table 15.5, the sum of ranks would be $(104)(105)/2 = 5460$. If the two groups have equal values in ranks, their sums should be $5460/2 = 2730$ in each group. The departure of each group's rank sum from this value is $3366.5 - 2730 = 636.5$ for the active group, and $2093.5 - 2730 = -636.5$ for the placebo group. The value of $|636.5|/2730 = .23$ indicates how greatly the sums proportionately deviate from an equal separation. Because the increment in rank sums is $3366.5 - 2093.5 = 1273$ and $636.5/2730 = (1273/2)/(5460/2)$, the desired ratio can be obtained simply as

$$\text{(increment in rank sums)/(total sum of ranks)}$$

The value of .23 here is not far from the Kendall's tau value obtained for this relationship in Chapter 27.

15.8 Role in Testing Non-Gaussian Distributions

A non-parametric rank test can be particularly valuable for demonstrating stochastic significance in situations where dimensional data do *not* have a Gaussian distribution. Because the t and Z tests are generally believed to be robust, the parametric tests are almost always used for contrasting two groups of dimensional data. Nevertheless, the non-parametric strategy can be a valuable or preferable alternative in non-Gaussian distributions where the group variance is greatly enlarged by outliers. Consider the dimensional values in the following two sets of data:

Group A: 15, 16, 16, 16, 17, 18, 19, 70; $\overline{X}_A = 23.375$; $s_A = 18.88$.

Group B: 21, 23, 25, 27, 29, 32, 33, 37; $\overline{X}_B = 28.375$; $s_B = 5.42$.

The mean in Group B seems substantially higher than the mean in Group A, but the large variance in Group A prevents the t test from being stochastically significant. With $s_p^2 = 7(18.88^2 + 5.42^2)/14 = 192.92$, the calculation of t produces $(28.375 - 23.375)/[\sqrt{192.92}\ \sqrt{(1/7) + (1/7)}] = 5.00/7.42 = .67$, which is too small to be stochastically significant.

On the other hand, the strikingly high variance in Group A suggests that something peculiar is happening. In fact, when we examine the data more closely, all values in Group A, except for the last (outlier) member, are exceeded by the lowest value in Group B. When converted to ranks, the results are as follows:

Ranks for Group A: 1, 3, 3, 3, 5, 6, 7, 16; Sum = 44.

Ranks for Group B: 8, 9, 10, 11, 12, 13, 14, 15; Sum = 92.

With the lower sum serving as the basic component of U, we get $U = 44 - [(8 \times 9)/2] = 8$. For $2P < .05$ at $n_1 = n_2 = 8$ in Table 15.4, U must be ≤ 13. Therefore, the rank test shows the stochastic significance that was not obtained with the parametric t test. (If this situation seems familiar, it should be. An example of analogous data appeared as Exercise 11.1, and the example will surface again here as Exercise 15.3.)

15.9   Additional Comments

Two other important features to be noted about non-parametric rank tests are claims about the reduced "power-efficiency" of the tests, and the availability of other procedures beyond those that have been discussed.

15.9.1   "Power-Efficiency" of Rank Tests

Non-parametric tests were seldom used until Wilcoxon first began writing about them. Because he converted dimensional data to ranks, many complaints arose about the "loss of information," even though — as noted in Section 15.8 — the "loss" can sometimes be highly desirable.

   A different complaint about rank tests was that they had a reduced "power-efficiency." The idea of statistical *power*, which will receive detailed discussion in Chapter 23, refers to the ability of a stochastic test to reject the null hypothesis when a quantitative difference is specified with an alternative hypothesis. Compared with parametric procedures for dimensional data, non-parametric rank procedures were less "efficient," requiring larger sample sizes for this special "power" of "rejection."

   The complaint is true, but is seldom relevant today because the rank tests are almost always used for ordinal data, not for conversions of dimensional data. Besides, all the calculations of "efficiency" and "power" are based on Gaussian distributions. As shown in Section 15.8, however, a rank test can sometimes be more "powerful" than a parametric test in showing stochastic significance when distributions are not Gaussian.

15.9.2   Additional Rank Tests

Many other tests, which rarely appear in medical literature, are also available (if you want or need to use them) for one or two groups of ordinal data. The tests are labeled with a dazzling array of eponyms that include such names as Cramer-von Mises, Jonckheere-Terpstra, Kruskal-Wallis, Kuiper, Kolmogorov-Smirnov, Moses, Savage, Siegel-Tukey, and Van der Waerden. The tests are well described in textbooks by Bradley,[16] Siegel and Castellan,[17] and Sprent.[18]

15.9.3   Confidence Intervals

Because ranked categorical data have discrete values, confidence intervals calculated with the usual mathematical methods are inappropriate because they can produce dimensional results that are realistically impossible. Nevertheless, mathematical formulas have been proposed and are available[19] for calculating the confidence intervals of medians or other quantiles. As computer-intensive statistics begin to replace the traditional mathematical theories, realistic confidence intervals, if desperately desired for ordinal data, can be obtained from a bootstrap procedure or from the array of possibilities that emerge with permutation rearrangements.

15.10   Applications in Medical Literature

A one-group or two-group rank test appears regularly although infrequently in medical literature. For example, the Wilcoxon-Mann-Whitney U tests were recently applied to evaluate ordinal data for "level of alertness" in a study of analgesia for the pain of sickle cell crisis[20] and to compare distributions of blood manganese and magnetic-resonance-imaging pallidal index in patients with liver failure vs. controls.[21] Wilcoxon Rank Sum tests were used to compare numbers of swollen joints in a clinical trial of oral collagen treatment for rheumatoid arthritis[22] and to compare several ordinal-scaled baseline factors among hospitalized patients who did or did not consent to participate in a study of pressure ulcers.[23] When patients with bacteremia or fungemia were compared with a control group,[24] the Wilcoxon rank sum test was used for dimensional variables because they "were not normally distributed." In a trial of topical training therapy for "photoaged skin,"[25] with effects graded in a 5-category ordinal scale ranging from 0 = absent to 4 = severe, the signed-rank test was used for bilateral, paired comparisons of treated forearms, and the U test for "facial efficacy." The signed-rank test was also used to compare differences in serum gastrin levels from one time point to another.[26]

In a study of cancer in the offspring of cancer survivors,[27] the investigators applied an "exact version of the non-parametric rank sum test," and in another instance a bootstrap procedure was used "to correct for loss of power of the Mann-Whitney U test due to the small sample size and tied observations."[28] With increasing availability in "packaged" computer programs, the bootstrap and exact permutation methods may begin to replace both the traditional parametric and the conventional non-parametric rank tests. The key decision for the rank procedures will then be the choice of a particular descriptive index of contrast (such as U or one of the others cited throughout Section 15.7) to be used as a focus of the bootstraps or permutations.

A randomized permutation procedure was also used in an intriguing controversy when data were reanalyzed for a randomized double-blind, placebo-controlled crossover trial that had shown efficacy for a 10^{-12} dilution of *Rhus toxicodendron 6c* as "active" homeopathic treatment for fibrositis.[29] For the crossover, 30 patients "received active treatment and an identical placebo for one month each in random sequence," without an intervening "washout" period. In the original analysis, the mean number of "tender points" after each phase of treatment was 14.1 for placebo and 10.6 for the "active" agent. The associated P value was <0.005 with the Wilcoxon rank sum test. The reanalysis of data[30] was done with "randomization tests," however. "When the original data set was randomized 20,000 – 50,000 times," the results showed much higher, "non-significant" P values. The reanalyst concluded that the trial "provides no firm evidence for the efficacy of homeopathic treatment of fibrositis."

The cogent point of contention, however, was *not* the use of a randomization rather than rank test. Instead, the reanalyst found a "treatment period interaction," which means that the effects of whatever occurred in the first period of treatment had "carried over" into the second. According to conventional wisdom[31] for such circumstances, "the only safe procedure is to restrict attention to the first treatment period only." The impressive P values vanished when the analysis was confined to the first period effects alone.

15.11   Simple Crude Tests

Two other tests mentioned here could have been cited in various previous chapters, but were saved for now because they can be applied to ordinal as well as dimensional data. Called the *sign test* and the *median test*, they are easy to do and easy to understand, although relatively "crude." Nevertheless, they can sometimes promptly answer a stochastic question without resort to more complex work. They are sometimes called "quick and dirty" tests, but the "dirty" epithet is unfair. They are "dirty" only because they compress dimensional and ordinal data into binary scales. If stochastic significance is obtained at the "crude" binary level of compression, however, the more "refined" conventional tests are almost never necessary.

15.11.1   Sign Test

The sign test is a particularly easy way to determine stochastic significance for matched-pair data in which two groups have been reduced to one. The *signs* of the results are compared against the null-hypothesis expected value of equality in the positive and negative values.

For example, in Table 15.6, under the null hypothesis for the six comparisons, we would expect three to be positive and three negative. A P value for the observed results can then be calculated from the binomial expansion of the hypothesis that $\pi = .5$. Thus, if all 6 observations were positive, the one-tailed probability would be $(0.5)^6 = (1/2)^6 = 1/64 = .016$. The probability of getting exactly five positive differences and one negative would be $5(0.5)^5 (0.5) = 5(1/2)^6 = 5/64 = .078$. For getting 5 or more differences in a positive direction, the one-tailed P value would be $.016 + .078 = .094$. As this value already exceeds $P = .05$, the observed result (4 positives and 2 negatives) will probably not be stochastically significant.

The sign test is particularly useful as a rapid mental way of calculating stochastic significance when the paired results go exclusively in one direction. For example, if all results go in the expected direction for five matched pairs, the one-tailed P value will be $(1/2)^5 = 1/32 = .03$. In this circumstance, stochastic significance could be promptly declared without any further calculations. (The tactic was used earlier in the answer to Exercise 13.6.2.)

15.11.2   Median Test

In another simple stochastic procedure, the data are divided at the median value for the two groups. The arrangement forms a 2×2 table, which can then be tested appropriately with either the Fisher test or chi-square.

For example, in the congestive-heart-failure illustration of Table 15.5, the median value of the ratings is **improved**. Partitioned on one side of this median, the data form a 2×2 table as

	Below Improved	Improved or Much Improved	TOTAL
Placebo	17	29	46
Active Agent	10	48	58
TOTAL	27	77	104

The X^2 test for this table produces $[(17 \times 48) - (10 \times 29)]^2 104/[(27)(77)(58)(46)] = 5.2$, with $2P < .025$. Thus, the stochastic significance of this set of data could have been promptly demonstrated with a simple median test, avoiding the more complex Wilcoxon-Mann-Whitney U test.

In the days before easy electronic calculation (and sometimes even today), the median test could also be used for two groups of dimensional data. For example, consider the dimensional results shown for Group B and the eccentrically distributed Group A in Section 15.8. The median for the total of 16 items is at rank 8 1/2, which is between the values of **21** and **23**, at **22**. If the two groups are partitioned at the median, the frequency counts produce the following table:

	Number of Items		
	Below Median	Above Median	TOTAL
Group A	7	1	8
Group B	1	7	8
TOTAL	8	8	16

A crude, uncorrected, and inappropriate chi-square test for these data produces $X^2 = 9.0$, with $2P < .005$. A more appropriate Fisher Test yields $p = .005$ for the observed table and an even smaller value, $p = .00008$, for $\begin{Bmatrix} 8 & 0 \\ 0 & 8 \end{Bmatrix}$. The two-tailed P will be about .01. Thus, stochastic significance for these data could have been promptly shown with the median test, again avoiding the more cumbersome Wilcoxon-Mann-Whitney U test.

References

1. Daniel, 1984; 2. Wilcoxon, 1945; 3. Clarke, 1964; 4. Aitken, 1969; 5. Huskisson, 1974; 6. Mann, 1947; 7. Bross, 1958; 8. Fleiss, 1981; 9. Wynder, 1960; 10. Kantor, 1966; 11. Berkman, 1971; 12. Brown, 1975; 13. Spitzer, 1965; 14. Mantel, 1979; 15. Moses, 1984; 16. Bradley, 1968; 17. Siegel, 1988; 18. Sprent, 1993; 19. Campbell, 1988; 20. Gonzalez, 1991; 21. Krieger, 1995; 22. Trentham, 1993; 23. Allman, 1995; 24. Leibovici, 1995; 25. Weiss, 1988; 26. Klinkenberg-Knol, 1994; 27. Mulvihill, 1987; 28. Avvisati, 1989; 29. Fisher, 1989; 30. Colquhoun, 1990; 31. Armitage, 1982; 32. Keelan, 1965.

Exercises

15.1. In the clinical trial discussed at the end of Section 15.10, the investigators[29] said they were eager to avoid "flaws in the design" of previous trials of homeopathic treatment. They therefore "designed a trial to clarify these results by overcoming the methodological criticisms while retaining a rigorous design." For example, beyond the features described in Section 15.10, the investigators used the following methods: "After entry, there was no further contact between the homeopathic doctor and the patient until the treatment was finished, The clinical metrologist dispensed the treatment and performed the assessments and analyses blind." What aspect of this trial would make you clinically believe that the trial was *not* well designed, and that a "treatment period interaction" was probably inevitable?

15.2. For 10 diabetic adults treated with a special diet, the fasting blood sugar values (in mg./dl.) before and after treatment were as follows:

Person	Before	After
A	340	290
B	335	315
C	220	250
D	285	280
E	320	311
F	230	213
G	190	200
H	210	208
I	295	279
J	270	258

To test whether a significant change occurred after treatment, perform a stochastic contrast in these data using a paired t-test and the signed-rank test. Are the stochastic results similar?

15.3. The data in Exercise 11.1 received a Pitman-Welch test in Section 12.9.5, and a t-test in Exercise 13.1. This chapter gives you the tools with which you can again demonstrate the occasional "inefficiency" of the t test by checking the same data set in three new ways:

15.3.1.   With a Wilcoxon-Mann-Whitney U test;

15.3.2.   With a sign test; and

15.3.3.   With a median test.

Do those tests, showing your intermediate calculations and results. (Because the sign test requires a single group of data or paired data, you will need some moderate ingenuity to apply it here.)

15.4. Random samples of students at two different medical schools were invited to rate their course in Epidemiology using four categories of rating: poor, fair, good, or excellent. At School A, the course is taught in the traditional manner, with a strong orientation toward classical public health concepts and strategies. At School B, the course has been revised, so that it has a strong emphasis on clinical epidemiology. The student ratings at the two schools were as follows:

	Poor	Fair	Good	Excellent	Total
School A	5	18	12	3	38
School B	1	3	20	12	36

A medical educator wants to show that this distinction is quantitatively and stochastically significant.

15.4.1. How would you express the results for quantitative significance?

15.4.2. How would you test for stochastic significance?

15.4.3. If you did a non-parametric rank test in 15.4.2, what is another simpler way to do the contrast?

15.4.4. From what you noted in the *quantitative* comparison, can you think of a simple "in-the-head" test for demonstrating stochastic significance for these data?

15.5. The table below is taken from the first report[32] of the efficacy of propranolol in the treatment of angina pectoris. In a randomized, double-blind, crossover design, the 19 patients who completed the trial received either propranol or placebo for four weeks, followed by the other agent for the next four weeks. Each of the three variables in the table below had values of $P < .05$ for the superiority of propranol over placebo. Looking only at the data for *Severity of Angina*, what *mental* test can you do to persuade yourself that P is indeed <.05?

Case No.	No. of Attacks of Pain		No. of Glyceryl Trinitrate Tablets Taken		Severity of Angina (Grades 1–6)	
	Propranolol	Placebo	Propranolol	Placebo	Propranolol	Placebo
1	37	68	37	68	3	4
2	121	116	61	56	6	6
3	19	47	19	46	2	3
4	14	26	15	25	2	3
5	16	79	16	79	2	4
6	4	6	4	6	2	2
7	24	24	24	24	4	4
8	118	100	0	0	4	4
9	5	4	5	8	2	2
10	10	27	10	14	3	4
11	31	19	6	5	4	4
12	31	46	41	71	2	3
13	59	64	59	64	3	4
14	86	175	119	203	6	6
15	1	8	3	21	2	4
16	4	8	3	4	2	2
17	103	96	115	92	3	3
18	6	44	19	43	2	2
19	38	75	38	75	4	4

15.6. A renowned clinical investigator, who has just moved to your institution, consults you for a statistical problem. He says the *Journal of Prestigious Research* has refused to accept one of his most important studies of rats because he failed to include results of a t test for a crucial finding. "Then do the t test," you tell him. He looks at you scornfully and says, "I did it before the paper was submitted." "Oh," you respond ruefully, "and I suppose it did not quite make 'significance'." "That is right," he says, "I tried to get away without reporting the P value, but the reviewers have insisted on it." "Why not add a few more rats?" you suggest. "I cannot," he replies. "My lab at Almamammy U. was dismantled three months ago before I came here. The technician who did all the work is gone, and there is no way I can set things up to test any more rats now. I felt so sure the results were significant when I first saw them that I did not bother to check the t test at the time. Had I done so, I would have added more rats to the study. Do you have any ideas about what I might do now?" "Let me see your data," you say.

He shows you the following results, expressed in appropriate units of measurement:

$$\text{Group A: } 11, 17, 21, 52; \ \overline{X}_A = 25.25; \ s_A = 18.30$$

$$\text{Group B: } 1, 7, 8, 9; \ \overline{X}_B = 6.25; \ s_B \ 3.59$$

You look at the results for a moment, do a simple calculation at your desk with a paper and pencil, then say to him, "You need not do anything. Your results are significant now at a two-tailed P < .05." After further discussion of what you did and how to report it, the investigator departs with a feeling of awe and wonder at your remarkable genius. The paper is accepted by the *J. Prest. Res.* and, as a grateful statistical "patient," he sends you a bottle of an elegant champagne.

What did you do at your desk?

16

Interpretations and Displays for Two-Group Contrasts

CONTENTS

A two-group contrast is probably the most common statistical comparison in medical research. As noted in Chapters 10 through 15, the comparison involves separate attention to description and inference. The descriptive focus is on quantitative distinctions in the data; the inferential focus is on stochastic appraisal of the quantitative distinctions.

This chapter is devoted to methods of interpreting and displaying the distinctions. The first section shows new graphic ways in which box plots and quantile-quantile plots offer a "visual interpretation" of the quantitative and stochastic decisions. The rest of the chapter discusses principles that can be used to produce effective (and ineffective) displays of the comparisons.

16.1 Visual Integration of Descriptive and Stochastic Decisions

If concepts of *Z tests, t tests, P values,* and *confidence intervals* had not been developed, decisions about significant differences might be made by examining the observed data directly, without any calculated stochastic boundaries.

16.1.1   Comparison of Observed Distributions

In one type of inspection, two groups of dimensional (or ordinal) data can be compared for the distributions shown in their histograms or frequency polygons.

This type of display, shown in Figure 16.1, was used to compare the distribution of urinary excretion of a fixed dose of lithium given to three groups of factory workers demarcated according to tertiles of serum uric acid.[1] Perhaps the greatest advantage of such displays is their demonstration, discussed in Section 16.1.1.2, of the extraordinary amount of overlapping data that can achieve such stochastic accolades as "P < .001."

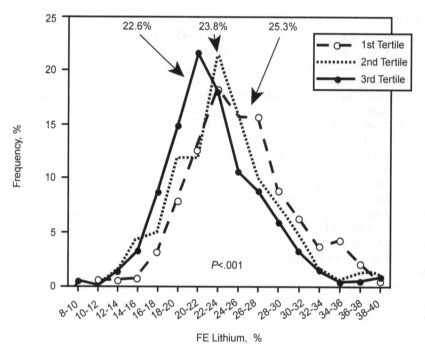

FIGURE 16.1

Frequency distributions of the fractional excretion (FE) of lithium by tertiles of serum uric acid in 568 male factory workers. Statistics by analysis of variance for differences between the means. [Figure and legend taken from Chapter Reference 1.]

16.1.1.1   Back-to-Back Stem-and-Leaf Diagrams — An approach that shows all data points in both groups is a back-to-back arrangement of stem-and-leaf diagrams, suggested by Chambers et al.[2] These diagrams, as shown here in Figure 16.2, offer an excellent way of reviewing the data yourself. The diagrams have the advantages of being easy to construct, compactly showing all the items as well as the shape of the two distributions, while avoiding the problems of multiple points at the same location, overlapping frequency polygons, and also the large vertical extent needed for a range of values that go from 18 to 82 in Figure 16.2.

The main disadvantage of either frequency polygon or stem-and-leaf direct displays, however, is the absence of summary indexes to help in the *quantitative* comparison of results. If the direct graphic displays show little or no overlap, the two groups are clearly different; but because such dramatic separations are rare, a more effective approach is needed for routine usage.

16.1.1.2   Permissiveness of Stochastic Criteria — If you begin examining the actual data—rather than P values, standard errors, and confidence intervals—you will discover the extraordinary amounts of overlapping spread, as shown in Figure 16.1, that can achieve stochastic "significance" in conventional criteria for a contrast in *means*.

```
                98 | 1 |
         443322100 | 2 | 4
     9888877766655 | 2 | 7889
           3221110 | 3 | 001112223334
         999876665 | 3 | 5555667889999
         433332210 | 4 | 0011234
               976 | 4 | 55668999999
      444433322000 | 5 | 001234444
         999987665 | 5 | 5566699
          44331100 | 6 | 00001334
       98888766665 | 6 | 5577789
      4333222110 0 | 7 | 00111122233444444
 99388877666555555 | 7 | 55666667777889
                21 | 8 | 00
```

FIGURE 16.2

Back-to-back stem-and-leaf diagrams of monthly average temperature for Lincoln (left) and Newark (right). [Figure and legend taken from Chapter Reference 2.]

To illustrate what happens, suppose we have two sets of Gaussian data, with different means, $\overline{X}_A$ and $\overline{X}_B$, but with similar group sizes, $n_A = n_B = n$, and equal variances, $s_A^2 = s_B^2$. The two groups will have a common mean, $\overline{X} = (\overline{X}_A + \overline{X}_B)/2$ and a common variance, $s_p = s_A = s_B = s$. As shown in Figure 16.3, the Gaussian distributions in the two groups will overlap on both sides of $\overline{X}$.

The cross-hatching on the right side of X shows the data from Group B that overlap in group A; and the cross-hatching on the left side of X shows the data from Group A that overlap in Group B. These two cross-hatched zones constitute the zone of central overlap. With some algebra not shown here, it can be demonstrated that if each curve has an area of 1, the magnitude of the central overlap is $1 - 2p_c$, where p_c is the one-tailed probability corresponding to $Z_c = |\overline{X}_B - \overline{X}_A| / (2s_p)$, for the proportion of data lying between each mean and the location of $\overline{X}$.

For example, suppose $\overline{X}_A = 146.4$ and $\overline{X}_B = 140.4$, with $s_p = 9.85$. The value of Z_c will be $(146.4 - 140.4) / [2 (9.85)] = .309$, for which the one-tailed $p_c = .121$. The area of central overlap will be $1 - [2 (.121)] = .758$.

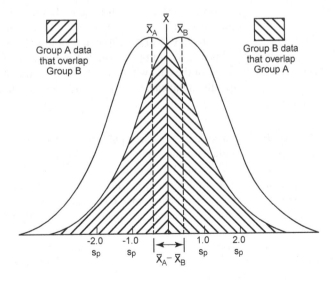

FIGURE 16.3

Patterns of central overlap at $P < .05$ for two Gaussian distributions with equal sample sizes and variances. Central overlap is the sum of the two shaded zones. For further details, see text.

The magnitude of central overlap can be determined from the value of Z_c that produces stochastic significance. Thus, for two means, $\overline{X}_A$ and $\overline{X}_B$, with group sizes n_A and n_B and a pooled common standard deviation s_p, the *stochastic* criterion for "significance" at a two-tailed $\alpha = .05$ is

$$\overline{X}_A - \overline{X}_B \geq 1.96 s_p \sqrt{N/(n_A n_B)}$$

For equal sample sizes, with $n_A = n_B = N/2 = n$, the value of $\sqrt{N/(n_A n_B)}$ becomes $\sqrt{2/n}$, and the foregoing formula becomes $\overline{X}_A - \overline{X}_B \geq (1.96\sqrt{2/n})s_p$, which is $(\overline{X}_A - \overline{X}_B)/s_p \geq 1.96\sqrt{2/n}$. Because $Z_c = (\overline{X}_A - \overline{X}_B)/2s_p$, we can substitute appropriately and promptly determine that

$$Z_c \geq 0.98\sqrt{2/n}$$

for stochastic significance with $\alpha = .05$ in the comparison of two means. Table 16.1 shows the effect of enlarging n on values of $\sqrt{2/n}$, on $Z_c = 0.98\sqrt{2/n}$, on the corresponding one-tailed p_c for Z_c, and on the zone of central overlap, calculated as $1 - 2p_c$. As group sizes enlarge, the value of $\sqrt{2/n}$ becomes smaller, thus making the "significance" criterion easier to satisfy. The value of Z_c also becomes smaller, thus reducing the proportion of the nonoverlapping data and increasing the proportion of the central overlap.

TABLE 16.1

Effect of Increasing Group Size (n) on Proportion of "Central Overlap" for a Stochastically Significant Contrast of Means at $\alpha = .05$

n	$\sqrt{2/n}$	$Z_c = .098\sqrt{2/n}$	p_c = Nonoverlapping Proportion in One Curve	$1 - 2p_c$ = Proportion of Central Overlap
4	.707	.693	.256	.488
5	.632	.620	.232	.536
10	.447	.438	.169	.662
15	.365	.350	.137	.726
20	.316	.309	.121	.758
50	.200	.196	.078	.844
100	.141	.138	.055	.890
200	.100	.098	.039	.922

For example, when $n = 20$, $0.98\sqrt{2/n} = .309$, for which $p_c = .121$ and $1 - 2p_c = .758$. Consequently, despite stochastic significance, the Group A and Group B distributions shown in Figure 16.3 will have a "central overlap" of about 76%. About 38% of the Group A data would overlap the distribution of Group B below the common mean $\overline{X}$, and about 38% of the Group B data would overlap the distribution of Group A above $\overline{X}$. The pattern for this result is further illustrated in Figure 16.4.

For $n = 50$, $0.98\sqrt{2/n} = .196$, and 84.4% of the data will be in a state of central overlap. For $n = 200$, the contrast of means will be stochastically significant at $P = .05$, despite a central overlap for more than 92% of the data.

16.1.1.3 *Illustration of Permissiveness* — For a published illustration of permissiveness in central overlap, Figure 16.5 here is modified (to show only the data points and means) from the original illustration[3] used to compare blood pressure in "100 diabetics and 100 nondiabetics." Do the two sets of data in Figure 16.5 look substantially different to you? Regardless of what your answer may be, Figure 16.6 shows the original illustration, in which a 95% confidence interval extended from 1.1 to 10.9 around the increment of 6.0 in the two means. The interval excludes 0 and therefore denotes stochastic significance at $2P < .05$.

In a related illustration, shown here as Figure 16.7, the presented data had the same pattern and same means as in Figure 16.5, but with only 50 members in each group. The 95% confidence interval is now larger and includes the null value of 0, so that the difference is no longer stochastically significant. Figure 16.7 was originally intended to show the effect of sample size in achieving stochastic significance but might also be used to demonstrate the peculiarity of regarding these two groups as "significantly

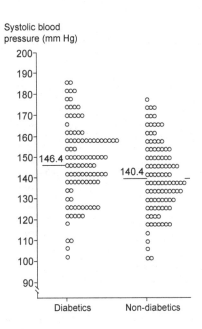

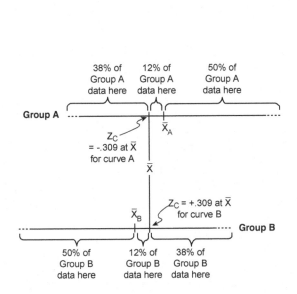

FIGURE 16.4

Overlap of data for two Gaussian groups of 20 members each, with $\overline{X}_A > \overline{X}_B$, similar standard deviations, and P = .05. Beginning at the common mean $\overline{X}$, 38% of the data in Group A overlap the distributions of Group B, and 38% of the data in Group B overlap the distribution of Group A. For further details, see text.

FIGURE 16.5

Systolic blood pressures in 100 diabetics and 100 non-diabetics with mean levels of 146.4 and 140.4 mm Hg, respectively. [Figure and legend taken from Chapter Reference 3.]

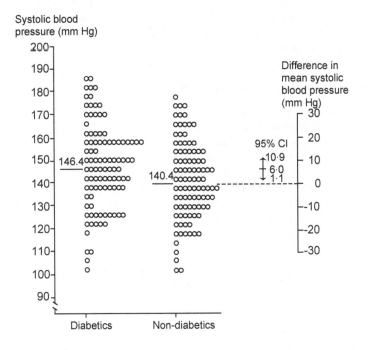

FIGURE 16.6

Systolic blood pressures in 100 diabetics and 100 non-diabetics with mean levels of 146.4 and 140.4 mm Hg, respectively. The difference between the sample means of 6.0 mm Hg is shown to the right together with the 95% confidence interval from 1.1 to 10.9 mm Hg. [Original figure and legend as presented in Chapter Reference 3.]

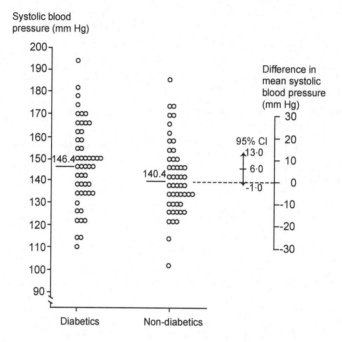

FIGURE 16.7
Same as Figure 16.6, but showing results from two samples of half the size — that is, 50 subjects each. The means and standard deviations are as in Figure 16.6, but the 95% confidence interval is wider, from −1.0 to 13.0 mm Hg, owing to the smaller sample sizes. [Figure and most of legend taken from Chapter Reference 3.]

different" in Figure 16.6, but not in Figure 16.7. If the large overlap of data and small *quantitative* increment (6.0) in the means of Figure 16.7 did not impress you as "significant," why were you impressed with essentially the same pattern of data and *quantitative* distinction in Figure 16.6? (Further discussion of Figures 16.6 and 16.7 is invited in Exercise 16.1.)

16.1.2   Stochastic Comparison of Box Plots

After recognizing the large amount of overlapping data permitted by the conventional criteria for stochastic significance, you may want to consider overlap in bulk of the data, rather than confidence intervals for central indexes, as a stochastic mechanism for deciding that two groups are "significantly" different. A splendid way to inspect overlap is the comparison of "side-by-side" box plots, for which certain types of overlap can be readily "translated" into Gaussian stochastic conclusions.

16.1.2.1   No Overlap of Boxes — Bounded by the interquartile range or H-spread, each box contains 50% of the group's data. If Group A has the higher median, the boxes will not overlap if the lower quartile value for Group A exceeds the upper quartile value for Group B. In symbols, this requirement is $Q_{L_A} > Q_{U_B}$. If the two boxes do not overlap, as shown in Figure 16.8, the two groups can promptly be deemed stochastically different.

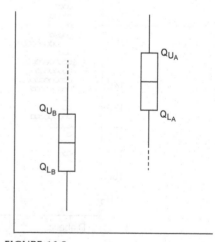

FIGURE 16.8
Non-overlapping box plots for Group A and B, with $Q_{L_A} > Q_{U_B}$. At least 50% of the data in each group have no overlapping values.

When converted into Gaussian principles for contrasting two means, the *descriptive* no-overlap-of-boxes criterion is much stricter than the usual stochastic demands. In a Gaussian distribution, $Z_{.5} = .674$ demarcates a standard-deviation zone containing 50% of the data on either side of the mean. For the spread of Gaussian data, the foregoing relationship would become $(\overline{X}_A - .674s_A) > (\overline{X}_B + .674s_B)$, which requires that $(\overline{X}_A - \overline{X}_B)$ be $> .674(s_A + s_B)$. Assuming that the group sizes are equal and that s_A and s_B are approximately equal at a common values of s_p, this descriptive requirement is $\overline{X}_A - \overline{X}_B > 1.348s_p$.

As noted in Section 16.1.1.2, for a two-tailed P < .05 in a comparison of two means for equal-sized groups, the Gaussian demand for *stochastic* significance is that $(\overline{X}_A - \overline{X}_B)/s_p$ must exceed $1.96\sqrt{2/n}$. As group sizes enlarge, $\sqrt{2/n}$ will become progressively smaller, thus making this demand easier to meet for the same values of $\overline{X}_A - \overline{X}_B$ and s_p. For equal group sizes $1.96\sqrt{2/n}$ need merely be smaller than twice the values of $0.98\sqrt{2/n}$ shown in Table 16.1. The largest of these doubled values, 1.386, will occur when n in each group is as small as 5.

Consequently, a pair of box plots showing no overlapping boxes with group sizes of ≥5 (for essentially Gaussian data) will almost always achieve two-tailed stochastic significance at P < .05.

16.1.2.2   Half-H-Spread Overlap Rule —

A more lenient but still effective stochastic criterion can be called the "Half-H-spread overlap" rule. It is pertinent, as shown in Figure 16.9, if the median for Group A is higher than the upper quartile for B and if the lower quartile of A is higher than the median of B. In symbols, the principle can be expressed as $Q_{L_A} > \tilde{X}_B$ and $Q_{U_B} < \tilde{X}_A$. If the overlap does not extend beyond the cited quartiles, no more than 25% of the data from Group B can be contained in the basic H-spread of Group A, and no more than 25% of the data from Group A can be in the H-spread of Group B.

Although apparently a lenient criterion, the Half-H-spread-overlap rule is still more demanding than the usual Gaussian stochastic standards, because the rule refers to the spread of the actual data, not to the more restricted scope of confidence intervals for an increment of two means. Because the inner 50% of Gaussian data spans a two-tailed $Z_{.5} = .674$, the upper quartile for a Gaussian group B would be at $\overline{X}_B + .674s_B$; and the corresponding lower quartile for Group A would be $\overline{X}_A - .674s_A$. The "Half-H-spread" rule, expressed in Gaussian terms, would demand that

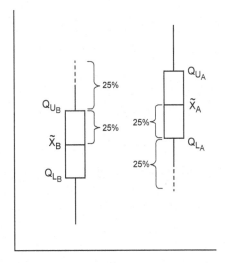

FIGURE 16.9
Less than Half-H-spread overlap in two box plots with $Q_{L_A} > \tilde{X}_B$ and $Q_{U_B} < \tilde{X}_A$.

$$(\overline{X}_B + .674s_B) < \overline{X}_A \quad and \quad (\overline{X}_A - .674s_A) > \overline{X}_B$$

which becomes the simultaneous requirement that

$$(\overline{X}_A - \overline{X}_B) > .674s_A \quad and \quad (\overline{X}_A - \overline{X}_B) > .674s_B$$

Consequently, the requirement is that

$$(\overline{X}_A - \overline{X}_B) > .674(\text{larger value of } s_A \text{ or } s_B)$$

If we let s represent this larger value, $\overline{X}_A - \overline{X}_B$ exceeds .674s when the Half-H-spreads do not overlap. In Table 16.1, the values of $0.98\sqrt{2/n}$, when doubled to produce $1.96\sqrt{2/n}$, show that two-tailed stochastic significance at $\alpha = .05$ will occur here for equal group sizes at all values of n above 20.

Thus, the "physical examination" of overlap in box plots can be used as a quick screening test for stochastic significance of two compared groups. The mathematical values calculated in this section and in Section 16.1.2.1, however, rest on the assumptions that the data are Gaussian, with equal sizes and variances in both groups. Nevertheless, the results will not be too disparate from these calculations if those assumptions do not hold. In general, the contrast will almost always be stochastically significant at 2P < .05 if the two boxes have no overlap at all or if they have no more than a Half-H-spread overlap for group sizes ≥20.

16.1.2.3   Published Examples — Because the box plot is a relatively new form of display, its full potential as a visual aid has not yet been fully exploited for stochastic decisions. For scientists who want descriptive communication and who would prefer to decide about "significance" by directly examining quantitative distinctions in "bulks" of data, a contrast of box plots offers an excellent way to compare the spreads of data and the two bulks demarcated by the interquartile zones. The comparative display of two box plots can thus be used not only to summarize data for the two groups, but also to allow "stochastic significance" to be appraised from inspections of bulk, not merely from the usual P values and confidence intervals. Because box-plot displays have been so uncommon, however, few illustrations are available from published literature.

Figure 16.10 shows such a display, which was presented in a letter to the editor.[4] The spread is completely shown for the data, which are not Gaussian, because the boxes and ranges are not symmetrical around the median (marked with an asterisk rather than a horizontal line). Stochastic significance can promptly be inferred for this contrast because the two boxes are almost completely separated. The only disadvantage of this display (and of the associated text of the letter) is that the group sizes are not mentioned.

Figure 16.11 shows another contrast of box plots, obtained during a previously mentioned (Chapter 10) study, by Burnand et al.,[5] of investigators' decisions regarding quantitative significance for a ratio of two means. The group sizes are indicated; and the medians are drawn with lines (rather than asterisks). The "whiskers" for each group cover an ipr_{95}, rather than the "fence" and "outlier" tactic proposed by Tukey. With almost no overlap in the boxes, the obvious differences in the groups will also be stochastically significant.

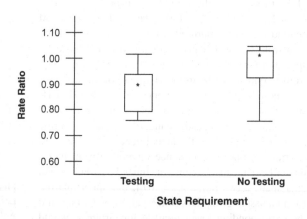

FIGURE 16.10

Box plots of rate ratios for involvement in a fatal crash by licensed drivers 65 years of age or older in 20 states. according to whether the state required vision testing for relicensure. Rate ratios represent the comparison of rates for drivers 65 years of age or older with those for drivers 45 to 64 years of age. Bars indicate the total range, boxes the range from the 25th to the 75th percentile, and asterisks the median value. [Figure and legend taken from Chapter Reference 4.]

In a study of cardiac size on chest films, shown in Figure 16.12, Nickol et al.[6] presented box-plot contrasts for three variables in three ethnic groups. The investigators stated that "every comparison (in these data) differed significantly (p < 0.001)." Using the Half-H-spread exclusion principle, the box plots for the investigated groups show obviously significant differences between Africans and Asians in cardiac diameter, between Africans and Caucasians in cardiothoracic ratio, and between Africans and Caucasians in age.

16.1.2.4   Indications of Group Size — One disadvantage of box plots is that group sizes are not routinely indicated. The sizes can easily be inserted, however, at the top of each "whisker," as shown in Figure 16.11. Some writers have recommended[7] that the width of the boxes be adjusted to reflect the size of each group. Since unequal widths might impair the discernment of lengths in the boxes, the group sizes are probably best specified with a simple indication of N for each group.

16.1.2.5 Notched Box Plots — To make the results more stochastic, the box plot can be marked with a central notched zone that covers the distance $\tilde{X} \pm [(1.57)(\text{ipr}_{50})/\sqrt{n}]$. In these symbols $\tilde{X}$ is the median, ipr_{50} is the interquartile range (between the top and bottom of the box), n is the group size, and 1.57 is analogous to a Z_{α} factor, chosen here to provide a suitably sized counterpart of the confidence interval for a median. The increment in two medians is stochastically significant if the notched interval of one box does not overlap the median of the other.

Figure 16.13 shows notched box plots for CD4 lymphocyte counts in two main groups of men, each divided into three subgroups.[8] The notch-spread criterion for "significance" is analogous to the Half-H-spread-overlap rule, but is easier to fulfill because the potentially overlapping distance is smaller. The Half-H-spread rule is much easier to use, however, and avoids the need for extra measurement of notch length.

16.1.3   Quantile-Quantile Plots

Despite its use as a *descriptive* summary of data, the box-plot contrast discussed throughout Section 16.1.2 was employed for *stochastic* decisions. An elegant way of contrasting the *quantitative* distinctions of two groups, regardless of their sizes, has been devised by Wilk and Granadesikan.[9] They originally proposed "quantile (Q-Q) plots, percent (P-P) plots, and hybrids of these" to compare an observed univariate group with a proposed theoretical distribution for the group, but the tactic can be used to contrast distributions for two different groups. The quantile technique, which relies on quintiles, quartiles, medians, etc., is probably easier to apply than the percent P-P plot, which relies on cumulative percentiles.

The quantile-quantile (Q-Q) graph creates a "pairing," otherwise unattainable with nonpaired data, in which the respective X and Y values at each point are the corresponding quantiles of the compared Groups A and B. The two groups can then be compared descriptively according to the line connecting the Q-Q points. If points lie along the "identity" line X = Y, the two groups have similar results. If the line goes through the origin with slope 1.2, the values in one group are in general 20% higher than in the other.

The method has seldom been used in medical literature, so the illustration here has another source. In Figure 16.14, the ozone concentrations for Stamford vs. Yonkers are plotted with a large array of quantiles, such as 2nd percentile, 5th percentile, 10th percentile, quartile, median, for each group. A much simpler line, however, could be drawn for just three points: the median and the lower and upper quartiles in each group. Four additional points — the lower and upper quadragintile values and the 10- and 90-percentile values might be added for more complete detail.

C.P. Jones[10] has pointed out that the relationship of lines and crossings in the Q-Q plot can be used to demonstrate descriptive differences in location, spread, and shape for the two compared groups of data. Jones has also proposed a simple "projection plot" in which the difference in each pair of quantile values is plotted against their average value. With this arrangement, the identity line passes horizontally through the increment of 0.

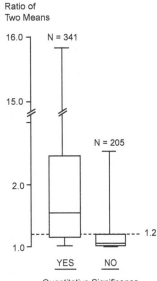

FIGURE 16.11

Box-plot distribution of the ratio of two means according to the investigators' decision about "quantitative significance." 95% of the data is located between the horizontal lines at the ends of the top and bottom "whiskers" (the inner 95-percentile range). The central 50% of the data is located within the top and bottom ends of the box (the inner 50-percentile or interquartile interval). The median transects the box. The best boundary that separates quantitatively significant from non-significant distinctions is a dashed line drawn at a ratio of 1.2. [Figure and legend taken from Chapter Reference 5.]

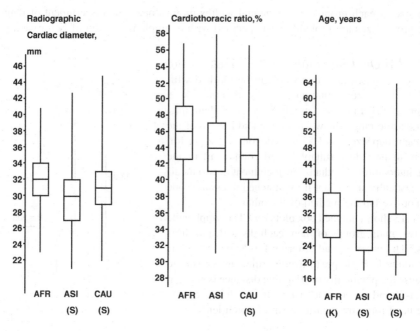

FIGURE 16.12
Box-and-whisker plots of the distribution of the data for radiographic cardiac diameter, cardiothoracic ratio, and age, by ethnic groups; AFR = African, ASI = Asian, CAU = caucasian. The box encloses the interquartile range, and is transected by a heavy bar at the median. The whiskers encompass the 25% of data beyond the interquartile range in each direction (after Tukey, 1977). Skew was statistically significant in 5 groups of data marked (S), $p < 0.05$, but was of very moderate degree in all but the data for Age of caucasian subjects. Age in African subjects showed kurtosis marked (K), $p < 0.05$, of mild degree. [Figure and legend taken from Chapter Reference 6.]

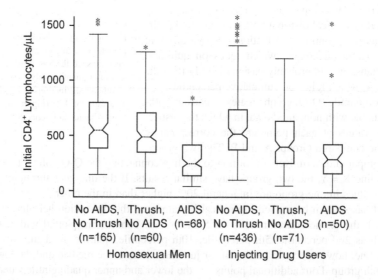

FIGURE 16.13
Distributions of CD4+ lymphocyte counts in injecting drug users and homosexual men, with each cohort divided into individuals who did or did not develop acquired immunodeficiency syndrome (AIDS) or thrush, as described in the text. Boxes indicate median and upper and lower hinges; "waists" around the medians indicate 95% confidence intervals of the medians. The lowermost and uppermost horizontal lines indicate fences, either 1.5 interquartile ranges away from the first and third quartiles or at the limit of the observations, whichever was smaller. Outliers (values beyond the fences) are marked by asterisks. [Figure and legend taken from Chapter Reference 8.]

16.2 Principles of Display for Dimensional Variables

Graphs and other visual displays of dimensional data have usually been prepared in an *ad hoc* arbitrary manner, according to the standards (or whims) of the artist to whom the investigator took the data. This *laissez faire* policy was sharply attacked several years ago in a landmark book by Edward Tufte, *The Visual Display of Quantitative Information*.[11] He offered an invaluable set of principles for both intellectual communication and visual graphics in the display of data. Some of those principles have been used in the discussion here.

Results for a dimensional variable in two groups can usually be effectively compared from suitable summary statements that indicate the central index, spread, and size for each group. If this information is provided in the text or in a table, additional visual displays may be unnecessary. If presented, however, the displays should convey distinctions that are not readily apparent in the summary statements. The main such distinction is the distribution of individual data points. Their portrait can promptly let the reader distinguish spreads and overlaps that are not always clear in the verbal summaries.

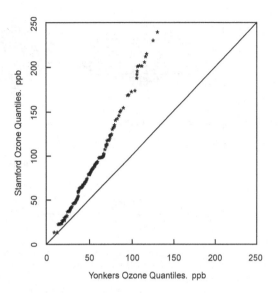

FIGURE 16.14
Empirical quantile-quantile plot for Yonkers and Stamford ozone concentrations. The slope is about 1.6, implying that Stamford levels are about 60% higher than Yonkers level. [Figure taken from Chapter Reference 2.]

16.2.1 General Methods

The main challenges in displaying individual points of dimensional data are choices of symbols, methods of portraying multiple points at the same location, and selection of summary indexes.

16.2.1.1 *Symbols for Points* — In most instances, dimensional values are shown in a vertical array within the arbitrary horizontal width assigned for columns of each compared group. Because each group usually occupies its own column, different symbols are seldom needed for the points of different groups.

A simple, circular, filled-in dot, enlarged just enough to be clearly visible, is preferable to open circles, squares, triangles, crosses, diamonds, and other shapes. The other shapes become useful, however, to distinguish one group from another when two or more groups are contrasted within the *same* vertical column.

16.2.1.2 *Multiple Points at Same Location* — Multiple points at the same vertical location can be spread out in a horizontal cluster as ······, and the arbitrary width of the columns can be adjusted as needed. If the spread becomes too large, the points can be split and placed close together in a double or triple tier. A remarkable "cannonball" spread of points is shown for multiple groups[12] in Figure 16.15.

Instead of appearing individually in a cluster (or "cannonball") arrangement, the multiple points are sometimes combined into a single expanded symbol, such as a large circle, whose *area* must appropriately represent the individual frequencies. The area is easy to identify if the symbol is a square, but is difficult to appraise if it must be calculated for a circle or other non-square symbol. Enlarged symbols can be particularly useful in a two-dimensional graph, whose spacing cannot be arbitrarily altered to fit the

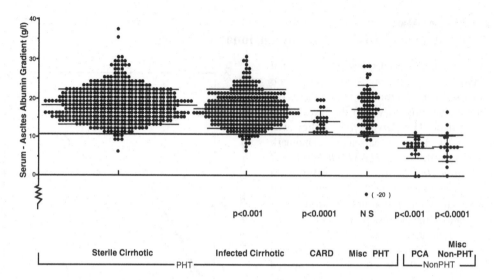

FIGURE 16.15

Serum-ascites albumin gradient in ascites, classified by presence or absence of portal hypertension. Statistical comparisons are to the sterile cirrhotic group by unpaired *t*-test. CARD = cardiac ascites; Misc Non-PHT = miscellaneous-nonportal-hypertension-related; Misc PHT = miscellaneous portal-hypertension-related; NS = not significant; PCA = peritoneal carcinomatosis. Mean ± SD bars are included as well as a horizontal line at 11 g/L, the threshold for portal hypertension. All groups differed significantly (*P* < 0.05) from the sterile cirrhotic samples by analysis of variance with the Dunnette test. [Figure and legend taken from Chapter Reference 12.]

individual cluster. In comparisons of categorical groups, however, the enlarged symbols usually keep the viewer from discerning individual frequency counts.

16.2.1.3   Choice of Summary Symbols

16.2.1.3   Choice of Summary Symbols — The decisions about summary symbols for indexes of central tendency, spread, and size depend on whether the purpose of the display is descriptive communication or stochastic inference. Many displays seem to be aimed at stochastic decisions, showing bars and flanges for means and standard errors but not points of data. Because the summary indexes can readily be presented in verbal text or tables, the display seems wasted if it does not show the individual data points and if the summary does not indicate spread of the data rather than indexes for stability of the mean.

If the visual goal is really stochastic, a separate problem arises from the choice of a standard error. For a stochastic Z (or t) test, or for a confidence interval, the statistical formula uses a standard error calculated from the combined (or "pooled") variance in the two groups. Thus, for purely stochastic displays, each group should have an identical standard error, derived from the combined variance. If the standard errors are shown individually for each group, they might be used for the type of crude mental evaluations described in Section 13.3.2, but the exact sizes of the standard errors are often difficult to discern from the graphical display.

Probably the main value of showing standard errors is to "market" the results by disguising spread of the data. Because the standard deviation is divided by $\sqrt{n}$, the standard error is always smaller than the SD and makes things look much more compact, tidy, and impressive. The SE becomes progressively smaller with enlarging sample sizes, thus allowing two big groups of data with a dismayingly large amount of overlap to appear neatly separated.

If aimed at the appropriate goal of descriptive communication, the display of individual points will often suffice to show the data, because the corresponding summary values will usually appear in text or tables. An appropriate choice of summaries, however, can be valuable for descriptive (and even stochastic) evaluations of "bulk," as discussed earlier. The summaries are also necessary for large data sets having too many points to be shown individually. The comparison of two box plots is the best current method of showing these summaries. With suitable artistic ingenuity, the individual points might even be shown inside each box, and they could replace (or be shown alongside) the "whiskers" beyond the box.

Some good and bad examples of two-group dimensional displays are shown in the sections that follow. Because some of the displays will be adversely criticized, the sources of publication are not identified, and the names of some of the original variables have been changed.

16.2.2   Conventional Displays of Individual Data Points

This subsection contains displays of various conventional arrangements of the points of data for two comparisons.

Figures 16.16 and 16.17 show the points of data directly, without any indexes of spread. In Figure 16.17, the location of the means would probably be easier to identify if they were shown with lines rather than asterisks, if the legend called them *means* rather than *averages*, and if the vertical scale on the far left had more "tick marks."

In Figure 16.18, a solid line has been added to show the mean, and dashed lines to show SE in each direction. As noted earlier, the main value of displaying SE alone is that a difference in means cannot be stochastically significant if the SE values overlap. If they do *not* overlap, however, a t value or confidence interval for the difference must still be calculated to demonstrate stochastic significance. For a very wide gap between the ranges of the two SE zones, the mental calculation described earlier (Section 13.3.2) is easier to do from the stated summary indexes than from trying to measure the size of the gap in a graph.

In Figure 16.19, a desirable line has been drawn near the bottom of each group to separate all the data points having values of 0. The arrangement allows each of those points to be seen without the crowding that occurs in the points above the line in the left column.

Figure 16.20 makes a laudable effort to show all the data points, but communication is impeded by the overlapping circles and by the many diverse symbols, which are generally used only once or twice. The display probably would have been much easier to read and interpret if each person were shown with a dot, group means with lines, and special individuals identified with a label on the graph and an arrow pointing to the dot.

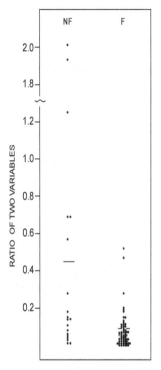

FIGURE 16.16
Graph shows ratio of two variables in nonfailing (NF) and failing (F) conditions.

In Figure 16.21, a logarithmic scale is used to cover the wide range of values for data points shown in a single vertical array for three groups, with different symbols. The three groups are so clearly separated that no summary expressions are needed to emphasize the distinctions. In Figure 16.22, data points are also shown for three groups, together with indications of mean and SEM for each group. In the original report, no stochastic calculations were presented for the textual claim that the special amine was "consistently raised in uraemia," but the separation of the data points indicates that no such calculations were needed. The display of SEM values thus seems redundant, particularly as no claims were made for stochastic distinctions between the "blind-loop" and "control" groups.

Figure 16.23 is remarkable for displaying the summary results with medians and an inner 80-percentile zone rather than with Gaussian indexes. The authors[13] say they wanted to avoid Gaussian assumptions and that "this type of presentation is easily understood by most people." The research was used, however, to establish a zone of normal values in 704 "healthy asymptomatic aircrewmen." The 10th and 90th percentile boundary points were chosen "arbitrarily … [as] conservative reference values for the response of healthy men to treadmill exercise" and also "to exclude individuals having subclinical conditions." Despite the excellent clarity of the visual display, many clinicians will have doubts about establishing a "range of normal" by arbitrarily excluding 20% of apparently healthy persons.

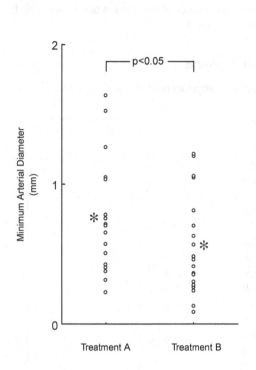

FIGURE 16.17
Minimum arterial diameter for subjects receiving treatments A or B.

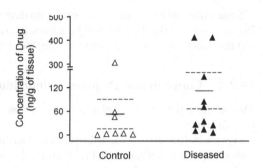

FIGURE 16.18
Means and standard errors for two groups.

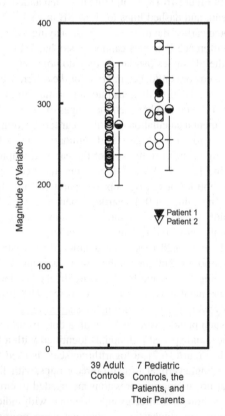

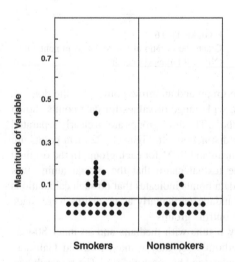

FIGURE 16.19
Segregation of clusters of data points at value of 0.

FIGURE 16.20
Magnitude of measured variable in (at left) 39 normal adults and (at right) the 7 children with other neurologic diseases who were used as controls (open circles), including 2 following a ketogenic diet (circles framed by squares); Patient 1; his parents (solid circles); Patient 2; and her mother (circle with slash). Half-filled circles to the right of each group represent means, and the vertical scales are marked in increments of 1 SD from the mean, with the results for Patients 1 and 2 excluded. The level of the variable for Patients 1 and 2 was more than 3 SD below the mean for either group of control subjects.

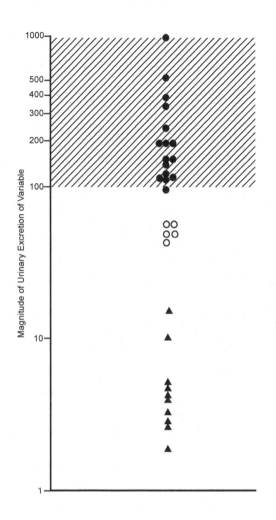

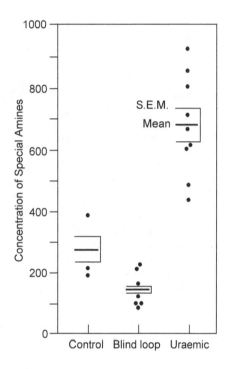

FIGURE 16.21
Urinary excretion of cited variable during water-deprivation tests in 10 children with histiocytosis and diabetes insipidus (triangles) and 21 children with histiocytosis but no symptoms of diabetes insipidus (circles). The hatched area represents the range in healthy children.

FIGURE 16.22
Special amine concentrations in control, blind-loop, and uremic subjects.

16.2.3 Bar Graphs

For large groups, which may have too many individual data points to be easily displayed, the results are often shown with bar graphs. The lengths of the bars show the means, and flanges are added to show dispersion (usually SE). Figure 16.24 gives an example of this tactic for comparing results, in two groups of about 48 animals marked with cross-hatched or black bars, at different times after special administration of insulin. The symbols "N.S." and "p < 0.05" are added to show the absence or presence of stochastic significance at each time point of comparison. This type of graph offers little that cannot be discerned from the data summaries for each contrast, but a visual display may be valuable for showing the trend of results over time.

A particularly complex bar chart, which probably tries to do too many things, is shown in Figure 16.25. The lengths of the bars indicate the means, but the quartile and median values are appended, together with a special symbol (Δ) for demarcating the increment in means. This same information could probably have been communicated, with greater artistic ease and visual effectiveness, in two contrasted box plots.

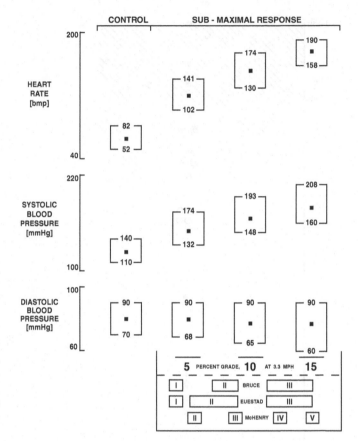

FIGURE 16.23

Control and submaximal treadmill exercise measurement data are shown as median (■) with 10th and 90th percentiles. Submaximal data are presented for the 5, 10 and 15 percent grade within the Balke-Ware treadmill protocol; the relationship between these three grades and other treadmill protocol stages is depicted at the bottom of the figure. The numbers of subjects with complete data for each of the measurements are 698 for control; 699, 700, and 503, respectively, for three submaximal responses. [Figure and legend taken from Chapter Reference 13.]

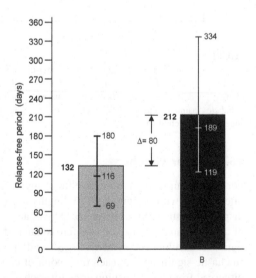

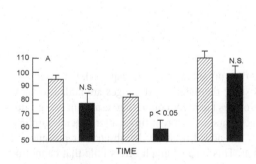

FIGURE 16.24

Blood-glucose in diabetic animals treated with special insulin.

FIGURE 16.25

Average relapse-free period after treatment in groups A and B, shown in the height of columns with corresponding median values, and 1st and 3rd quartiles in 2,045 patients.

Note that the half-H-spreads do not overlap, consistent with a statement in the text that the 73-day difference in medians is "highly significant with non-parametric tests."

16.2.4 Undesirable Procedures

The next set of illustrations shows some particularly unattractive or undesirable procedures. In Figure 16.26, information that could readily have been understood with simple, direct summaries has been displayed in bar graphs. Beyond the basic redundancy, the graphs do not indicate the group sizes or the identity of the top flanges as either SD or SEM. The artist has also "volumized" the bars with an unnecessary third dimension. As a final undesirable touch, the legend erroneously states that the bar graphs are histograms.

Figure 16.27 is another volumized bar graph, which also omits showing group sizes. The unidentified "SED" at the far right of the graph is presumably standard error of the difference, explained in the text only as having been obtained "from the error mean squared of the respective ANOVA (analysis of variance) table." Aside from the flaws in display, however, the data themselves may not have been appropriately analyzed. According to the text of the report, all the results were obtained in two sets of crossover studies of 6 patients. In one crossover, the patients went from a supine to a tilted position, and in each position they were untreated or received a particular treatment. The research was thus aimed mainly at contrasting the two sets of changes in a single group, but the results are presented as though four groups were being compared.

Figure 16.28 shows two of several similar structures displaying blood pressure and heart rate in response to five different treatments given to 14 patients. The original legend listed only the abbreviations used for the treatments and had no other identifying information. What at first seems to be an incomplete box plot for the blood pressure values could eventually, by careful reading of the text, be discerned as bars having mean systolic pressure on the top of each "box" and diastolic pressure on the bottom. The flanges represent standard deviations. In the lower display for heart rate, the circles are presumably central indexes, whose actual value is effectively obscured by the circles, and whose identity — as means or medians — is not listed in either the original legend or the original text.

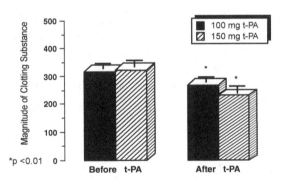

FIGURE 16.26
Histograms of plasma levels of clotting substance before and after (4.2 ± 0.3 hours) tissue-type plasminogen activator (t-PA) at the two doses. Levels were significantly lower after treatment with the two doses (p < 0.01) but similar for each.

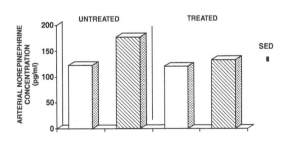

FIGURE 16.27
Bar graphs showing changes in arterial plasma norepinephrine concentration during 30° head-up tilting before and after treatment. Data are shown for patients in the supine position (open bars) and after 30° head-up tilting (shaded bars).

Figure 16.29 is a counterpart, in two groups, of the useless display of complementary proportions shown earlier in Figure 9.1 for one group. The information for both groups could have been communicated more simply and directly with a straightforward comparison of the constituent numbers.

Figure 16.30 has been nominated for an "Oscar" in malcommunication. The only virtue of the figure—its display of data points—is negated by ineffective or inadequate marks and labels. The upper and lower bars for each box show only the range for each group. Two different measurement scales are distinguished by ∗ and ∗∗ symbols, which are confusing because they are normally used to signify magnitude of P values rather than scales of measurement. The unidentified dashed horizontal lines must be discerned, from the text, as means. Sample sizes are not identified and must be either counted from the dots or searched in the text.

Figure 16.31 at first seems to have many merits. It shows box plots and cites actual values for pertinent boundaries on each plot. The legend, however, is confusing in describing an "NL" (presumably "normal") hatched bar for "blood urea nitrogen," although the graph refers to "serum creatinine." Furthermore, the meaning of the hatched NL bar is not clear. Does the "NL" symbol indicate a range of normal, or does its hatched bar represent a box plot analogous to the others on that graph? A more cogent statistical problem, however, is that the data in this crossover study have been displayed as though two groups were involved. A more effective portrait would have shown the results of *change* for individual patients.

Figure 16.32 asks the reader to compare histograms for the distribution of atypical lobules per breast in two groups. Despite the merit of showing the actual distributions, the portrait has no value in helping summarize the data for interpretation. The associated table of data, copied here from the original publication, makes relatively little contribution beyond listing a relatively useless "average" (presumably mean) value for the eccentric distributions. The original discussion of the statistical analysis and your invitation to improve things are contained in Exercise 16.2.

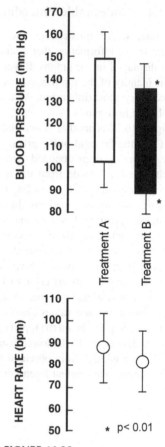

FIGURE 16.28
Blood pressure and heart rate during each treatment regimen.

16.3 Displaying Binary Variables

The frequency counts for a binary variable in two groups form a 2×2 table, and each group's results are easily summarized as a binary proportion. The main visual decision is how to orient the rows and columns of the table itself.

16.3.1   Orientation of 2 × 2 Table

If the research has the cause–effect architectural structure of a randomized trial, observational cohort, or etiologic case-control study, the most scientific arrangement places the alleged causal agents in the rows and the outcomes in the columns. This format is used because readers are accustomed to looking at horizontal scientific symbols for the sequence of cause → effect. Table 16.2 is organized in this "longitudinal" direction of observation and reasoning. In longitudinal studies, the rows indicate the

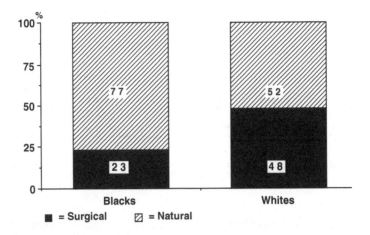

FIGURE 16.29
Percentages of black women and white women by type of menopause.

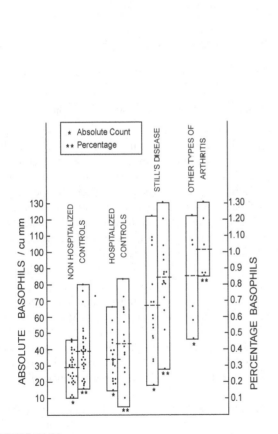

FIGURE 16.30
Absolute number and percentage of basophils in controls and in children with arthritic conditions.

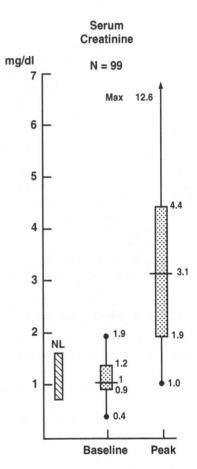

FIGURE 16.31
Changes in renal function induced by treatment in patients receiving immunotherapy for advanced cancer. The arrow indicates that the maximum level for serum creatinine was greater than 7 mg/dL. Hatched bar shows blood urea nitrogen.

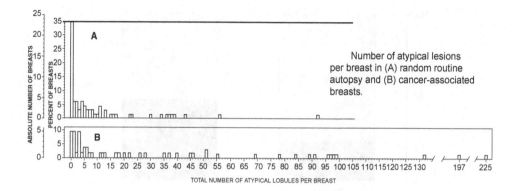

Number of atypical lesions per breast in (A) random routine autopsy and (B) cancer-associated breasts.

Comparison of 119 autopsy and cancer-associated breasts.

Item	Autopsy	Cancer-associated
Number of breasts	67	52
Average age (years)	63.47	60.80
Age range (years)	25-96	28-89
Average number of AL per breast	9.96	37.40
Range in number of AL per breast	0-92	0-225

FIGURE 16.32
Reproduction of histograms and tabular data for a comparison of "atypical lobules per breast" in two groups.

denominator groups, n_1 and n_2, that have been exposed or nonexposed to the alleged "cause"; and the columns show frequencies for the outcome fates, f_1 and f_2, for the forward direction of observation.

In an etiologic case-control study, however, the groups are chosen according to presence or absence of the outcome event. They are then "followed backward" to determine previous exposure to the alleged "cause." To keep a scientific format, the table can still have the same horizontal orientation with "causes" in the rows; but the n_1 and n_2 totals for the "sampling" are now listed in the columns for the selected outcome groups that are the appropriate denominators. The arrangement is shown in Table 16.3.

16.3.2   Individual Summaries

Because of structural differences in the research, the n_1 and n_2 denominators for longitudinal and case-control studies have different locations in the tables and must be expressed with different binary proportions.

For the longitudinal data of Table 16.2, n_1 and n_2 are marginal totals for the rows. The proportions of success, which would be $p_1 = a/n_1$ and $p_2 = c/n_2$, could then be compared as an increment $p_1 - p_2$ or as a "risk" ratio, p_1/p_2. (If "risk of success" seems like an inappropriate phrase, it can be replaced by the risk ratio for failure, expressed as q_2/q_1.)

For the case-control study shown in Table 16.3, the analogous calculation of a/f_1 and c/f_2 in the rows is forbidden, as noted earlier (in Section 10.7.3), because patients were not chosen according to their exposure or nonexposure. If two proportions in this table are to be compared directly, they would have to refer to antecedent exposure, as $e_1 = a/n_1$ and $e_2 = b/n_2$. Because these proportions have relatively little intuitive meaning and cannot be used to express risk, they are seldom given much attention. Instead, the odds ratio, ad/bc, is usually cited as a single index of contrast, with the hope that it will adequately approximate the risk ratio. (The topic, mentioned in Chapter 10, is further discussed in Chapter 17.)

TABLE 16.2

Architectural Structure of a Longitudinal "Cause–Effect" 2 × 2 Table

| | Alleged Outcome | | |
	Present (Success)	Absent (Failure)	Total
Present (Active Treatment)	a	b	n_1
Absent (Comparative Treatment)	c	d	n_2
Total	f_1	f_2	N

TABLE 16.3

Architectural Structure of Etiologic Case-Control Study

| | Alleged Outcome | | |
Alleged Cause	Present (Diseased Case)	Absent (Nondiseased Control)	Total
Present (Exposed)	a	b	f_1
Absent (Non-exposed)	c	d	f_2
Total	n_1	n_2	N

16.3.3 Graphic Displays

If graphic displays have any merit at all for a 2 × 2 table, their main role would be to show the direction of observation and to compare magnitudes for the appropriate proportions.

Figures 16.33 and 16.34 show the "tabular box-graphs" that have been proposed[14] for this purpose. In both instances, the 2 × 2 table contains the data $\begin{bmatrix} 20 & 10 \\ 15 & 46 \end{bmatrix}$, and both box-graphs are drawn as "unitary squares." The dividing lines, however, are arranged to show the different directions and interpretations of the research architecture. The proportions for the selected denominators of the two main groups are shown by the placement of thick horizontal or vertical lines, and the thinner perpendicular vertical or horizontal lines are then placed to show the appropriate proportions in each group of either success for the cohort study or exposure for the case-control study.

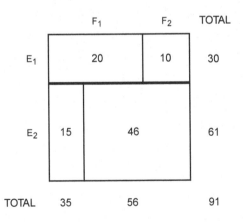

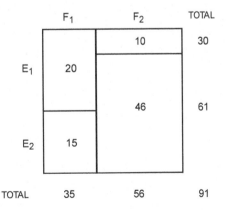

FIGURE 16.33
Tabular box-graph for a cohort study. The horizontal line is drawn at a distance of 0.33 (=30/91) in the unitary square. The two vertical lines are drawn at distances of 0.67 (=20/30) and 0.25 (=15/61).

FIGURE 16.34
Tabular box-graph for a case-control study. The vertical line is drawn at a distance of 0.38 (=35/91). The two horizontal lines are drawn at distances of 0.57 (=20/35) and 0.18 (=10/56).

To display each constituent of an odds ratio, Figure 16.35 has a "quadrant-hub" arrangement of four contiguous squares, whose magnitudes for each side are $\sqrt{a}$, $\sqrt{b}$, $\sqrt{c}$, and $\sqrt{d}$ for the four cells of the 2×2 table. The substantial differences in magnitude of the ad vs. bc squares in Figure 16.35 is consistent with the odds ratio of 6.1 $[= (20 \times 46)/(10 \times 15)]$.

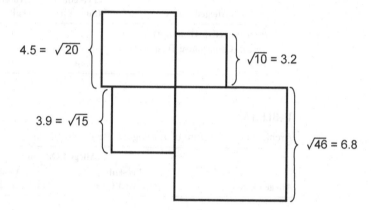

FIGURE 16.35
Contiguous squares showing cell sizes in a 2×2 table. [Figure and legend taken from Chapter Reference 14.]

The graphical displays in the squares of Figures 16.33 through 16.35 do not communicate much beyond what is readily discerned from direct inspection of the corresponding table, but they can be used if you want tables to receive an artistic emphasis that might help compensate for the enormous visual attention given to dimensional graphs in statistical illustrations.

A visually esthetic but intellectually unattractive arrangement shows the spinning-top shapes of Figure 16.36. The implications of the shapes themselves are difficult enough to understand; but the legend — which is reproduced here exactly as published — is inscrutable.

16.4 Displaying Ordinal Data

Because of the problems of getting adequate summary indexes (discussed throughout Section 15.7), there is no single ideal method for visual display of ordinal categories. The available methods of arrangement will inevitably differ according to the goal of the display. Is it intended to compare the *overall distribution* of categories in the two groups, or to do a *category-by-category* comparison? Bar charts can be used for either purpose, but the organization of the bars will differ.

FIGURE 16.36
Change with age of numbers of people at risk by virtue of having bone masses below an arbitrary threshold. Pendular shapes represent normal distribution of bone mass in two populations with different fracture risks (equivalent to cases and controls) at two different ages. For each population mean bone mass has been reduced between the two ages by 1.5 standard deviations of the distribution (--------), an amount fully in accord with that implied by cross-sectional studies as occurring between age 50 and 85. Risk threshold intersects distributions at (from left to right) 2.5, 1.0, 1.0, −0.5 standard deviations from means, resulting in stated ratios of numbers at risk in the two populations (shaded areas).

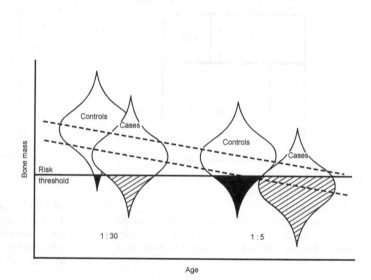

16.4.1 Overall Comparisons

The "divided bar-chart," also called a "component bar-chart," has been a standard method of showing the distribution of constituent categories for two groups. Figure 16.37 is a schematic drawing of the arrangement, with the ordinal categories arrayed in vertical tiers that obscure both the shape of the distribution, and the comparison of individual categories.

A preferable way of displaying this same information is the divided dot chart proposed by Cleveland and McGill.[15] Figure 16.38, which shows their dot chart for the same information that appears in Figure 16.37, allows magnitude to be clearly identified for each category, while also displaying shape of the overall distributions.

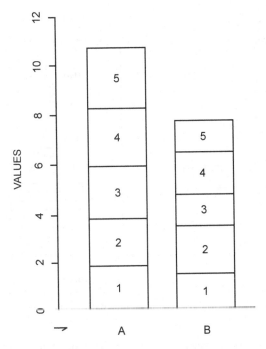

FIGURE 16.37
Divided (or "component") bar chart for ordinal categories in two groups. [Figure and legend taken from Chapter Reference 15.]

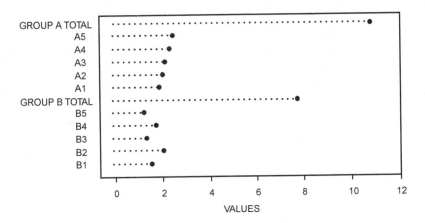

FIGURE 16.38
Divided dot chart for data of Figure 16.37. [Figure taken from Chapter Reference 15.]

16.4.2 Category-by-Category (Side-by-Side) Comparisons

Perhaps the most effective way to show category-by-category comparisons, however, is to place the bars opposite one another on a single vertical stalk.[16] If just a few categories are included, this type of arrangement resembles a traffic signpost, as in Figure 16.39. If the ordinal data have many categories that are shown without spaces, as in Figure 16.40, the portrait may look like the layers of the "Michelin man." The latter tactic has often been used to construct a "population pyramid," which compares demographic components for two regions. The tactic can also be used to construct a type of back-to-back histogram, shown in Figure 16.41 for the distributions of CD-4 counts in two groups of men.[17]

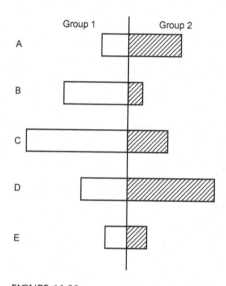

FIGURE 16.39
"Traffic signpost" arrangement. [Figure and legend taken from chapter Reference 16.]

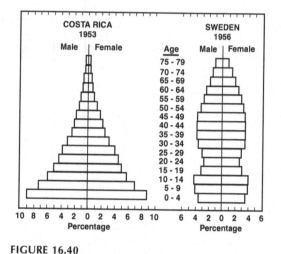

FIGURE 16.40
"Michelin-man" arrangement, showing "population pyramid" often used in demographic comparisons.

If the layered categorical-bar arrangements of Figure 16.39 are converted to dot charts, as shown in Figure 16.42, the results produce a "Christmas tree" effect.[16]

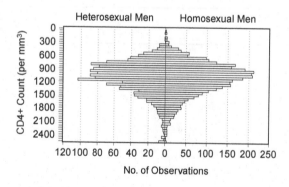

FIGURE 16.41
Distribution of CD4+ counts in HIV-negative heterosexual and homosexual men in San Francisco. [Figure and legend taken from Chapter Reference 17.]

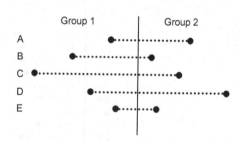

FIGURE 16.42
"Christmas tree" dot chart for the 5-category, 2-group data of Figure 16.39. [Figure taken from Chapter Reference 16.]

16.5 Nominal Data

For two groups of nominal data, no visual structure improves the comparison that can be obtained with a well-organized table showing the frequency counts (or relative frequencies) for each of the nominal categories in each group. If visual adornment is desired, a side-by-side category dot chart is probably the best approach.

16.6 "Bonus" Displays

As a reward for your completing this chapter, here are two "bonuses" of interesting features in data display.

16.6.1 New Haven–New York Timetable

In Edward Tufte's second book, *Envisioning Information*,[18] he denounces the visual display used for the schedule of Metro North trains from New York to New Haven. His critique is replicated in Figure 16.43.

In Figure 16.44, however, Tufte shows a revised improved schedule, done as a student project at Yale University in 1983. Whatever be the merits of the criticism and the new design, travelers on this railroad route will recognize that the old format is still being used almost 20 years later. (Tufte does not mention whether the improved version was ever brought to the attention of railroad officials.)

NEW YORK TO NEW HAVEN

Bold sans serif capitals weak in distinguishing between two directions:
NEW HAVEN TO NEW YORK   NEW YORK TO NEW HAVEN

MONDAY TO FRIDAY, EXCEPT HOLIDAYS

Column headings repeated 3 times and 24 AM's and PM's shown due to folded sequence of times. The eye must trace a serpentine path in tracking the day's schedule; and another serpentine for weekends:

Leave	Arrive	Leave	Arrive	Leave	Arrive
New York	New Haven	New York	New Haven	New York	New Haven
AM	AM	PM	PM	PM	PM
12:35	2:18	2:05	3:45	T 6:25	8:10
5:40	7:44	3:05	4:45	T 7:05	8:56
7:05	8:45	T 4:01	5:45	T 8:05	9:45
8:05	9:45	4:41	6:25	T 9:05	10:50
9:05	10:45	T 4:59	6:53	10:05	11:45
10:05	11:45	XT 5:02E	6:33	11:20	1:05
11:05	12:45	XT 5:20	7:08	12:35	2:18
12:05	1:45	X 5:42	7:26	.....	.....
1:05	2:45	XT 6:07E	7:46	.....	.....
PM	PM	PM	PM	PM	PM

Poor column break, leaving last peak-hour train as a widow in this column.

Too much separation between leave/arrive times for the same train.

Too little separation between these unrelated columns.

Most frequently used part of schedule (showing rush-hour trains) is the most cluttered part, with a murky screen tint and heavy-handed symbols.

SATURDAY, SUNDAY & HOLIDAYS

AM	AM	PM	PM	PM	PM
12:35	2:18	2:05	3:45	7:05	8:45
5:40	7:37	S 3:05	S 4:45	H 8:05	H 9:45
8:05	9:45	4:05	5:45	9:05	10:45
10:05	11:47	5:05	6:48	11:20	1:00
12:05	1:45	6:05	7:48	12:35	2:18
PM	PM	PM	PM	AM	AM

Rules segregate what should be together; a total of 41 inches (104 cm) of rules are drawn for this small table.

The service shown herein is operated by Metro-North Commuter R.R.

Wasted space in headings cramps the times (over-tight leading, in particular). Well-designed schedules use a visually less-active dot between hours and minutes rather than a colon.

REFERENCE NOTES
Economy off-peak tickets are not valid on trains in shaded areas.
Check displays in G.C.T. for departure tracks.
E-Express
X-Does not stop at 125th Street.
S-Saturdays and Washington's Birthday only.
H-Sundays and Holidays only.
T-Snack and Beverage Service.
HOLIDAYS-New Year's Day, Washington's Birthday, Memorial Day, Independence Day, Labor Day, Thanksgiving and Christmas.

Ambiguity in coding; both x and E suggest an express train, or even E for Economy.

FIGURE 16.43
Edward R. Tufte's critique[18] of the Metro North Railroad schedule of trains from New York to New Haven.

NEW YORK → NEW HAVEN
Grand Central Station

Monday to Friday, except holidays		Saturday, Sunday, and holidays	
Leaves New York	Arrives New Haven	Leaves New York	Arrives New Haven
12.35 am	2.18	12.35 am	2.18
5.40 am	7.44 am	5.40 am	7.37 am
7.05	8.45		
8.05	9.45	8.05	9.45
9.05	10.45		
10.05	11.45	10.05	11.47
11.05	12.45 pm		
12.05 pm	1.45	12.05 pm	1.45 pm
1.05	2.45		
2.05	3.45	2.05	3.45
3.05	4.45	3.05 Saturdays only 4.45	
4.01	5.45	4.05	5.45
4.41	6.25		
4.59	6.53		
X 5.02 ● 6.33		5.05	6.48
5.20 ● 7.08			
5.42 ● 7.26			
X 6.07 ● 7.46		6.05	7.42
6.25	8.19		
7.05	8.56	7.05	8.45
8.05	9.45	8.05 Sundays only 9.45	
9.05	10.50	9.05	10.45
10.05	11.45		
11.20	1.05 am	11.20	1.00 am
12.35 am	2.18	12.35 am	2.18

(Boxed area labeled: Economy off-peak tickets are not valid on trains in boxed areas.)

X   Express
●   Does not stop at 125th Street

Holidays: New Year's Day, Washington's Birthday, Memorial Day. Independence Day, Labor Day, Thanksgiving and Christmas.

NEW YORK → NEW HAVEN
Grand Central Station

Monday to Friday, except holidays		Saturday, Sunday, and holidays	
Leaves New York	Arrives New Haven	Leaves New York	Arrives New Haven
12.35 am	2.18	12.35 am	2.18
5.40 am	7.44 am	5.40 am	7.37 am
7.05	8.45		
8.05	9.45	8.05	9.45
9.05	10.45		
10.05	11.45	10.05	11.47
11.05	12.45 pm		
12.05 pm	1.45	12.05 pm	1.45 pm
1.05	2.45		
2.05	3.45	2.05	3.45
3.05	4.45	3.05 Saturdays only 4.45	
4.01	5.45	4.05	5.45
4.41	6.25		
4.59	6.53		
X 5.02 ● 6.33		5.05	6.48
5.20 ● 7.08			
5.42 ● 7.26			
X 6.07 ● 7.46		6.05	7.42
6.25	8.19		
7.05	8.56	7.05	8.45
8.05	9.45	8.05 Sundays only 9.45	
9.05	10.50	9.05	10.45
10.05	11.45		
11.20	1.05 am	11.20	1.00 am
12.35 am	2.18	12.35 am	2.18

(Boxed area labeled: Economy off-peak tickets are not valid on trains in boxed areas.)

X   Express
●   Does not stop at 125th Street

Holidays: New Year's Day, Washington's Birthday, Memorial Day. Independence Day, Labor Day, Thanksgiving and Christmas.

FIGURE 16.44
Proposed improvement for schedule shown in Figure 16.43. [Figure taken from Chapter Reference 18.]

16.6.2   Sexist Pies

Several years ago the New Yorker magazine[19] published a cartoon, shown here as Figure 16.45, in which pie graphs depicted the alleged distribution of male and female thoughts. You can make your own decision about whether the data are worth converting to a dot chart.

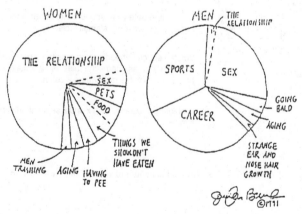

FIGURE 16.45
Proposed distribution of gender-related cognitive foci. [Figure taken from Chapter Reference 19.]

References

1. Cappuccio, 1993; 2. Chambers, 1983, pg. 60; 3. Gardner, 1986; 4. Nelson, 1992; 5. Burnand, 1990; 6. Nickol, 1982; 7. McGill, 1978; 8. Margolick, 1994; 9. Wilk, 1968; 10. Jones, 1997; 11. Tufte, 1983; 12. Runyon, 1992; 13. Wolthius, 1977; 14. Feinstein, 1988b; 15. Cleveland, 1984; 16. Singer, 1993; 17. Sheppard, 1993; 18. Tufte, 1990; 19. New Yorker Magazine, 1991; 20. Baer, 1992.

Exercises

16.1. (Note: To answer the following questions, you should not have to do *any* counting or locating of individual points on the graphs.)

    16.1.1. Using the data shown in Figure 16.6, determine a coefficient of potential variation, i.e., stability, for the mean difference in the two groups. Are you impressed with the stability? Why or why not?

    16.1.2. Determine a coefficient of variation for the data in each group. Are you impressed that the means are suitable representatives of the data? Why or why not?

    16.1.3. The authors state (see legend of Figure 16.7) that the groups in Figure 16.6 have the same standard deviations as in Figure 16.7. Verify this statement.

    16.1.4. Although you might think that the two groups in Figure 16.7 were randomly chosen as half of the groups in Figure 16.6, the points on the graphs contain contradictory evidence. What is that evidence? How do you think the data were really obtained for the two figures?

16.2. The text that follows appeared in a leading journal of American research and contains the only quantitative information — together with what appeared in Figure 16.32— of a published report on preneoplastic lesions in the human breast:

> The *t*-test was used to examine the hypothesis that the means of the populations of the two samples (routine autopsy and cancer-associated) are equal when the sigmas are equal but unknown. If the two samples are drawn from the same population they must necessarily have the same sigma and mean. If the *t*-test rejects the hypothesis that the means are equal while the sigmas are equal but unknown, then the populations are different within the confidence interval that is drawn from the *t*-test. In this instance the *t*-test indicates that the two samples are not drawn from the same population, with less than 1 percent chance for error. All *P* values were less than 0.1. These results show a positive correlation between AL and cancer-associated breasts in the human.

    16.2.1. If this manuscript were submitted now and you were asked to review the statistical analysis, what comments would you make?

    16.2.2. Using the available information cited here and in Figure 16.32, prepare and show an alternative (improved) graphic presentation for the results.

16.3. Figure E.16.3 appeared in the report of a study[20] that compared two new technologies — gradient echo magnetic resonance imaging (MRI) and ^{99m}Tc methoxyisobutyl-isonitrile single-photon emission computed tomography (MIBI-SPECT) — for their ability to define myocardial scars. The abbreviation DWT in the vertical ordinate refers to diastolic wall thickness, whose magnitudes on MRI were compared with the MIBI-SPECT designation of scar or no scar.

By visual inspection and mental computation only, without using a calculator, how could you determine whether the ± 1 and ± 2 citations on the graph are standard deviations or standard errors?

16.4. Figure E.16.4 shows the data points and geometric means for two groups.

    16.4.1. What alternative expression would you propose as an index of central tendency for these groups?

    16.4.2. What problem would occur if you tried to do a t (or Z) test on the data shown in the graph?

    16.4.3. What alternative simple strategy can you use to demonstrate stochastic significance for this contrast?

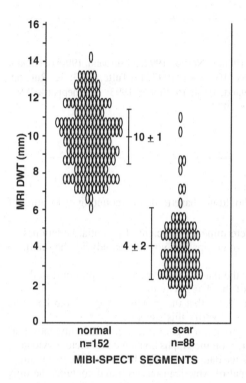

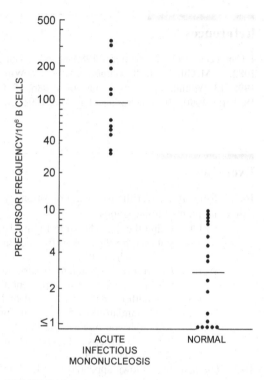

FIGURE E.16.3

Comparison of MIBI-SPECT and MRI assessed DWT. Distribution of DWT obtained from segments graded normal and scar by MIBI-SPECT. DWT was significantly ($p < 0.001$) higher in normal segments than in segments graded as scar. [Figure and legend taken from Chapter Reference 20.

FIGURE E.16.4

Frequency and geometric mean of spontaneous B-cell outgrowth in the peripheral blood of patients with acute Epstein-Barr-virus-induced infectious mononucleosis and of normal persons seropositive for Epstein-Barr virus. The geometric mean is indicated by the horizontal bar.

16.5. In the displays in Figure 16.12, each box shows a lower quartile, median, and upper quartile for the group. [The whiskers show the full range of data, i.e., from the 0th to the 100th percentile.] The actual values for the three quartile points of data can be estimated from the ordinates on the graph. Using this information for each group, prepare a quantile-quantile graph for the comparison of age in Africans and Caucasians.

16.6. Here is another "find-and-fix" set of exercises. From any published literature at your disposal, find an unsatisfactory graph, chart, or other visual display for two groups of data. (If you cannot find a drawing, a badly organized table can be substituted.) For each unsatisfactory display, indicate what is wrong and how you would improve it, sketching the improved arrangement. If possible, find such suboptimal displays for 2-group data that are

      16.6.1. Binary

      16.6.2. Dimensional

      16.6.3. Ordinal

    If you cannot find any "juicy" bad displays for these data, and are desperate, a particularly "good" display can be substituted.

16.7. In a scientifically famous legal case, called *Daubert v. Merrell Dow Pharmaceuticals, Inc.* (in which Bendectin was accused of causing birth defects), the U.S. Supreme Court reviewed a previous legal doctrine, called the Frye rule. The rule had been used by judges in lower courts to make decisions about admissible evidence in "toxic tort" cases involving the adverse effects of pharmaceutical substances or other products accused of "risk." According to the Frye rule, the only admissible courtroom evidence should have been published in peer-reviewed journals; and any positive contentions about "risk" should have been accompanied by "statistically significant" evidence. The opponents of the Frye rule — who were the plaintiffs in the Daubert case — wanted a more lenient approach. It would allow "expert witnesses" to introduce unpublished data and also, when P values were not "statistically significant," the potential magnitude of risks could be estimated from the upper ends of confidence intervals. *Amicus curiae* briefs were filed on both sides by a prominent array of institutions and individuals. The Frye rule was defended by the American College of Physicians, AMA, *New England Journal of Medicine*, a consortium of Nobel laureate scientists, and other persons (such as ARF) who argued that the dropping of standards would fill courtrooms with "junk science." The Frye rule was opposed by some prominent scientists, statistical epidemiologists, and legal groups (mainly attorneys for plaintiffs) who argued that P values were too rigid a standard and that peer-reviewed publication was neither a guarantee of, nor a requirement for, good scientific work.

Briefly discuss what position you would take in this dispute. What position do you think was taken by the Supreme Court?

17

Special Arrangements for Rates and Proportions

CONTENTS

Several prominent ambiguities have already been noted when central indexes are chosen and contrasted for binary data. The central index itself is ambiguous, because information coded as 0, 0, 0, ..., 1, 1, 1 can be cited with either of two complementary proportions, p or q. Thus, the same group might have a success rate of 29% or a failure rate of 71%. Another problem occurs for reporting changes. Choosing one central index rather than the other would not affect results when standard deviations are calculated as $\sqrt{pq}$ or when two-group increments are formed as $|p_1 - p_2| = |q_1 - q_2|$. The results can differ dramatically, however, if proportionate incremental changes are cited with either p or q in the denominator. Thus, a drop in the death rate from .09 to .07 could be cited proportionately as either a 22% decline in mortality $[= (.07 - .09)/.09]$ or an equally correct 2% rise in survival $[= (.93 - .91)/.91]$.

Beyond these ambiguities, however, the complexities of binary proportions create several profound scientific and statistical problems that are discussed in this chapter. The problems arise from the custom of calling the proportions "rates," from their different sources of numerators and denominators, from their static or dynamic temporal constructions, from the uniqueness of the odds ratio as a statistical index of contrast, and from the special epidemiological jargon used for comparisons of rates.

17.1 Ambiguous Concepts of a Rate

Like *probability*, the idea of a *rate* is a fundamental concept in statistics; and like *probability*, *rate* is difficult to define. As noted in Chapter 6, probabilities can be subjective or objective, isolated or cumulative, empirical or theoretical, frequentist or Bayesian. Rates have many more sources of diversity, inconsistency, and confusion.

17.1.1 Non-Biostatistical Rates

In nonmedical branches of science and daily life, a *rate* is often constructed as a quotient of different components, cited in the different units of measurement. Velocity (or speed) is a rate in which distance traveled, divided by duration of time, is listed in expressions such as **km per hr**. This usage suggests that a *rate* reflects something occurring over a period of time. The rate of an automobile's gasoline consumption, however, is cited without reference to time, in such terms as **miles per gallon**.

Although the foregoing examples suggest that a *rate* is a quotient of two different constituents, such quotients also receive other names. When a quantity of calcium is divided by a quantity of fluid, the quotient is called a *concentration*, expressed in such units as **mg/dl**. A quantity of red blood cells divided by a quantity of fluid, however, is not called a *concentration*. It is called a *count* if the cells are enumerated and a *hematocrit* if their packed volume is measured. If the units of measurement are similar, but the measured entities are different, yet another word may be used. The quotient formed when a concentration of serum albumin is divided by a concentration of serum globulin is called a *ratio* and is unit-free. Many unit-free quotients, however, are not called ratios. They are called *rates*. Thus, a quotient of two quantities of money, such as the amount of interest for the principal of a bank loan, is called an *interest rate*. It is expressed as a unit-free proportion (or percentage). Although many proportions are called *percentages* as well as *rates*, other names are sometimes used. A baseball player's proportion of number of hits per number of times at bat is called an *average*.

In maintaining the inconsistencies just noted for the world beyond, the rates examined in biostatistics may or may not be proportions; the proportions may or may not be rates; and the ratios may be either or neither.

17.1.2 Complexity in Biostatistical Rates

Valiant attempts[1] are sometimes made to define a *rate* as "a measure of change in one quantity (y) per unit of another quantity x … [which] is usually time." Although a desirable standard, this definition is constantly ignored in the literature of medicine and public health. For practical purposes, a *rate* is almost anything that the user of the term wants it to be and that editors are willing to publish.

Any rate can readily be described (rather than defined) as a quotient of two quantities, a/n, in which a numerator, *a*, is divided by a denominator, *n*. In biostatistics, these quantities are usually frequency counts rather than measured dimensions. The quantities come from enumerations of either groups of people or events that occur for people, not from dimensional amounts of such entities as distance, gasoline, calcium, or fluid. The inconsistencies and ambiguities of biostatistical rates (and non-rates) arise from differences in what goes into the denominator, what goes into the numerator, and even what goes into the virgule, which is the "/" mark between denominator and numerator.

Regardless of what the a/n quotient is called, it is always a *proportion* if the number counted in the numerator is a specific subset of the entity identified and counted in the denominator. If a denominator group of 60 people contains 20 men and 40 women, the proportion, not the rate, of men in the group is .33 = 20/60. If the numerator for those people, however, represents an event — such as death, success, or occurrence of a disease — the analogous proportion is often called a *rate*. Thus, if 20 of the group of 60 people die, have successful outcomes after treatment, or develop streptococcal infections, the enumerated 20 people are still a subset of the denominator of 60, and the quotient of .33 = 20/60 is still a proportion; but it will often be called, respectively, a *death* (or *mortality*) *rate*, a *success rate*, or an *attack rate*.

The next two main sections discuss the complexities produced by the different components and nomenclature used when rates express probabilities of risk, and when they denote different directions and durations of time. The main problems in these complexities are scientific: the diverse terms may be difficult to understand or remember, and the enumerations may have dubious accuracy.

17.2 Components of Probabilities for Risk

The rate with which a particular event occurs in a group of people is often called a *probability* or *risk* for occurrence of the event. This structure, which uses the quotient of two frequency counts to form a rate of risk, is unique in medical biostatistics. The weatherman may say there is an 18% chance or "risk" of rain, but does not derive the forecast from enumerations. In biostatistics, however, if 10 members of a group of 2000 people die in the next year, the proportion, .005 (= 10/2000), is often called a *mortality rate* and is further cited

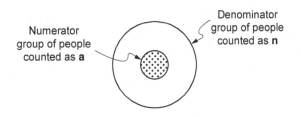

Proportion − a/n = "rate" of an event

FIGURE 17.1
Set and subset for a proportion.

as the probability or *risk* of death for that group. This rate or risk, like all frequentist probabilities, is constructed as a proportion. The denominator contains the enumerated people who are candidates for the risk of death; the numerator contains the count of those who died; and the rate is the proportion or relative frequency of death. The subset structure of a proportion is shown in Figure 17.1.

The basic idea is familiar and easy to understand, but clinicians and public-health epidemiologists produce confusion by using the same name — *mortality rate* — for death rates calculated from substantially different components in the numerators and denominators. Furthermore, when the necessary components are not specifically counted, the calculations may produce quasi-proportions and quasi-risks that are statistically reasonable, but scientifically inaccurate.

17.2.1 Sources of Denominators

The basic source of different rates is the group of people who constitute the denominator. In public-health statistics, this group is the general population of a community or region. At any particular point in time, some of the people in that region are sick, but most are healthy. In clinical work, however, the denominator group is usually a collection or "case series" of patients with a particular clinical ailment. The different proportions of subsequent death in these two different denominator groups, however, are often given the same name: *mortality rate*.

Suppose a community contains 4000 people of whom 80 are known to have lung cancer, and suppose 20 of those patients die in the ensuing year. The rate of death for lung cancer in that year will often be expressed as a *mortality rate* of .005 (= 20/4000) in public-health reports and as a *mortality rate* of .25 (= 20/80) in clinical reports. The distinctive sources that produce these disparate mortality rates for the same disease in the same year are shown in Figure 17.2. With more precise citation, the result for the public-health denominator is often called an *annual cause-specific mortality rate*, whereas the result for the clinical denominator may be called a *one-year mortality rate*.

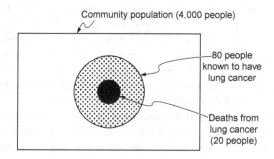

FIGURE 17.2
Sources of numerators and denominators for 20/4000 = .005 as "cause-specific annual mortality rate" for lung cancer, and for 20/80 = .25 as "one-year mortality rate" for lung cancer.

To avoid the ambiguity of using *mortality rate* for both types of denominators, the term *case-fatality rate* has been proposed as a substitute name for the clinical citation. Clinicians do not like to give up *mortality rate*, however, because they often refer to its complementary proportion, *survival rate*. Thus, the one-year survival rate for lung cancer in the foregoing group would be expressed as .75 = 60/80. This term creates no conflict in public-health statistics, which seldom refer to a survival rate.

The public-health data sometimes contain demographic calculations for rates that reflect survival, but the results are called "longevity" or "life expectancy," not "survival." Accordingly, the idea of a death rate is regularly expressed by public-health investigators as *mortality rate* for a regional denominator, and by clinical investigators as the complementary proportion, *survival rate*, for a clinical denominator. The two citations of death rates, however, are not at all complementary. In the foregoing example, the public-health mortality rate is .005, but the clinical survival rate is .75. Confusion often occurs when clinical investigators ignore the distinctions and refer to their clinical results as a mortality rate of .25.

17.2.2   Quasi-Proportions

A different type of problem arises when the public-health rates are regarded as proportions and used to express probabilities or risks. Because of inevitable difficulties in getting the data, these rates are really quasi-proportions; and their accuracy may sometimes be uncertain or dubious.

The challenge of finding and counting everyone to enumerate the entire human denominator of a large region or community is a daunting task. When this task is done every ten years, the census bureau is highly gratified if the enumeration seems reasonably complete. Aside from the problem of being completely counted, however, the denominator in a highly mobile society is constantly changing as various people move into or out of the region and other people die or are born. Because of depletions by deaths and out-migration and augmentations by births and in-migration, the denominators for inter-censal years (such as 1991, 1992, ..., 1999) depend on estimates derived from the counts obtained at the most recent census year (such as 1990). For inter-censal years, the basic decennial census results are altered according to counts of intervening annual births and deaths in the region, and then modified from educated guesses about annual out-migration and in-migration.

These estimates, without which no denominators would be available, make the regional mortality rates become quasi-proportions, rather than true proportions. The proportions are "quasi" because the counts of deaths, cancers, or other events in the numerators are *not* specific subsets of the people who were individually identified and counted in the denominators. The rates appear to be relative frequencies for a set and subset, but they are really a quotient of frequencies from two different sources, for groups counted in two different ways. The numerators come from an actual count of death certificates submitted to a regional agency, such as a state health department. These numerator counts can be accepted as complete, because a dead body cannot legally be disposed until a death certificate is prepared. The denominators for each of the nine inter-censal years, however, are not actual counts. They come from whatever formulas were used to estimate the augmentations and depletions that occurred after the actual counts in the census year.

Because two different groups of people are sources of the counted and estimated numbers, the regional rates of death are sometimes called *heterodemic*. In contrast, the rates of death in clinical groups are usually a *homodemic* true proportion: Everyone in the clinical denominator is suitably enumerated at the beginning of the observation period and is suitably accounted for afterward; and the numerator is a true subset of the denominator.

17.2.2.1 Problems of In- and Out-Migration —

Under-enumeration of a region is a striking problem, whose magnitude is difficult to determine. For various social, cultural, or other reasons, the census takers can seldom count everyone who lives in the region.[2] The counted regional population in Figure 17.3 is therefore shown as a smaller subset of the actual regional population.

With geographic migration both into and out of a region, some or many of the people originally enumerated in the denominators may later move elsewhere. The rectangle counted as the regional population in Figure 17.3 can be later depleted by a non-counted number of out-migrants while being simultaneously augmented by a non-counted number of in-migrants. If the two migrating groups are similar in both numbers and composition (such as age-sex distribution), the counted denominator will be essentially

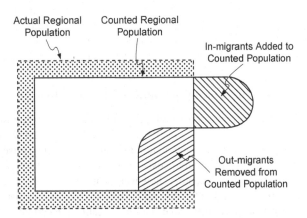

FIGURE 17.3
Sources of denominators in regional rates.

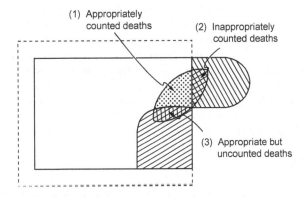

FIGURE 17.4
Sources of appropriate deaths, counted and uncounted, and of deaths inappropriately counted in the regional population of Figure 17.3. For further details, see Figure 17.3 and text.

unchanged. Otherwise, the actual denominator will be different from the estimated denominator.

For the numerators, all of the deaths are usually counted completely in industrially developed countries. As shown in Figure 17.4, however, the deaths may not always be associated with the denominators from which they emerged. The originally enumerated people who remain and die in the region will be suitably managed. The out-migrants who die elsewhere, however, may be counted in the denominator of Region A but in the numerator of Region B. The in-migrants who die in Region A may be counted in its numerator, while appearing in the denominator of Region B.

17.2.2.2 Problems of Under-Enumeration —

With suitable monitoring, data, and adjustments, the migratory phenomena may not produce major inaccuracies in the results. The main problem will then be the basic errors caused by census under-enumeration. For example, in many regions of the United States, the African-American or Hispanic population is regularly undercounted. The community leaders may then complain that the falsely low count has deprived their group of suitable political representation. A fascinating legal battle may then occur as the regional district, supported by an array of prominent statisticians, sues the government, supported by a different array of prominent statisticians, asking that the census be adjusted for the undercount.[3,4]

During the legal and political skirmishes, however, an unrecognized biostatistical problem is that the falsely low denominators, when divided into the accurate numerators obtained from death certificates, will also lead to falsely elevated mortality rates. Thus, if 500 correctly counted deaths occur among 100,000 people erroneously counted as 90,000, the true death rate is .005, or 5 per thousand; but it will proportionately increase by 12% when reported as 5.6 per thousand.

17.2.3   Inaccurate Numerators for Specific Diseases

If the numerators consist of *all* deaths and the appropriate denominators are suitably counted or estimated, the regional death rates may be reasonably accurate. Life insurance companies have managed to develop and maintain a profitable enterprise by using *total* death rates to anticipate longevity and set suitable costs for the premiums charged in policies.

For more than a century, however, death certificates have been used for much more than counts of total mortality. From the different diagnoses that may be listed on each death certificate, a single disease has been selected as the sole "cause of death"; the counts of these "causes" are then used as numerators for calculations called *cause-specific mortality rates*. These rates have been used to represent the frequency of occurrence, or "incidence rates," of those diseases.

The errors produced by this peculiar custom have received thorough discussion elsewhere[5,6] and are too extensive for more than a brief outline of all their lamentable consequences. The rates of "incidence" are fundamentally erroneous because they reflect death, not occurrence of disease; the rates are inevitably too low because only one of the patient's many identified diseases is counted; the numerators contain counts of diagnoses rather than diseases and will vary with changes in diagnostic concepts and technology; the reported diagnoses may depend on inconsistent idiosyncrasies in the physicians who fill out the death certificates; and when one of the cited diseases is chosen as *the* cause of death, the selection criteria will vary both from one decade to the next and with inconsistent application during the coding process at official agencies, such as a Bureau of Vital Statistics or (in the U.S.) the National Center for Health Statistics.

17.2.4   Quasi-Risks

Aside from the problem of accurate counts for numerators and denominators, the regional rates are seldom accurate as probability estimates of risk. The problem here arises from the concept of risk itself. Individual persons are "at risk" for a particular event if they are suitably susceptible to that event *and* if it has not yet occurred. Risk of death is easy to identify because any living person has that risk. If the numerator event, however, is a "causal disease," such as cancer of the uterus or gallbladder, rather than death itself, any woman who has had a hysterectomy, or anyone with a previous cholecystectomy, is not at risk. Furthermore, someone in whom the numerator event has already occurred is also not at risk of developing it. Thus, a woman who is now pregnant is not at risk for becoming pregnant, and the development of coronary heart disease is not a risk for someone who already has angina pectoris.

When a regional population is entered into a denominator for calculating a rate that will represent a risk, however, the counted group will include not only the people who are truly at risk, but also those who are not at risk either because they are not susceptible to the numerator event or because they already have it. To identify the three separate categories of people — the at-risk, no-risk, and already affected groups — is seldom possible or feasible, however, in large communities. Consequently, because the denominator will almost inevitably be too large, the "risks" calculated for the community or region will be too small. The magnitude of error in these quasi-risks will depend on the relative proportions of the three types of constituent groups in the denominator. For some diseases — such as the cancers, infarctions, and other chronic diseases often found unexpectedly at necropsy after having been clinically "silent" and unsuspected or undiagnosed during life[7,8] — the errors can be substantial.

17.2.5 Bilateral Units of Observation

A distinctly clinical problem in identifying constituents of the denominator arises when therapy is aimed at preventing or treating conjunctivitis, glaucoma, otitis media, diabetic neuropathy, or any other potentially bilateral disease for which a person may have two anatomic candidates, rather than one. In this circumstance, the main issue is whether to count persons or anatomic entities. If we study 24 persons, do we count the denominator group as 24 persons or as 48 eyes and/or ears?

The answer to this question may vary from one study to another and will often depend on whether the therapy is prophylactic or remedial. With prophylactic therapy, we probably want to count susceptible people who may develop the outcome event on one anatomic side or the other (or both). For remedial therapy, however, we may want to determine what happens to each treated entity. Sometimes a patient with similar involvement on both sides might even be used as a "self-control" for comparing two treatments.

17.2.6 Proportionate Mortality Rates

Another potentially confusing entity is the *proportionate mortality rate*, symbolized as PMR. This proportion is almost never used in clinical work, but often appears in public-health or occupational epidemiology. The denominator for the PMR proportions is the collection of all deaths in a group or region during a particular time interval. The numerators are the counts of deaths ascribed to individual diseases. Thus, at the end of a year in a region with a total of 400 deaths, of which 50 are attributed to coronary heart disease, the PMR for coronary disease will be $50/400 = .125$.

These calculations avoid the problem of erroneous counts in the denominator population, but magnify all the difficulty of getting accurate classifications and numbers for the "cause of death" cited in the numerators. Furthermore, the PMR values, although true proportions, cannot be used as probabilities for risk. They describe constituents in the univariate nominal spectrum of deaths, not the risk in living people.

The PMR has often been used in occupational epidemiology to examine death rates for workers in different industries. Getting the true death rate for an industry would involve the arduous task of identifying all the "exposed" employees in the denominator and following them as a cohort thereafter to discern the numerator fatalities. Instead, the deaths alone can be determined relatively easily (often from claims filed for "benefits"); and sometimes occupation is also listed on the death certificate. With either approach for relating deaths and occupation, a PMR can be constructed from death data alone, without the need for cohort studies.

Beyond the scientific difficulties of the PMR tactic, however, an additional mathematical problem is produced because the total of all proportionate mortality rates must add up to 1 (or 100%). Therefore, if the death rate declines for one disease but remains stable for a second disease, the PMR may rise for the second disease. Thus, if infectious diseases are substantially eliminated or reduced as causes of death, the PMR results can increase for chronic diseases, such as arteriosclerosis and cancer, even though the latter diseases may be occurring with unchanged lethality or even less often than before.

17.3 Temporal Distinctions

All of the problems just cited arise from counting the numerators and denominators in a rate such as a/n. A quite different problem is due to time. For each person enumerated in the denominator, the numerator event may have been counted at the same time, at a later time, or more than once. This distinction gives the virgule ("/") a special temporal role beyond merely denoting division of a numerator by a denominator to form a/n. The virgule can imply a direction, duration, or repetition of events for an interval of time.

17.3.1   Cross-Sectional or Longitudinal Directions

The group of people in the denominator can be observed in either a static or forward direction. In static or *cross-sectional* observation, the condition counted in the numerator is observed at essentially the same time as the denominator condition. Thus, if we can simultaneously count the population of a region and the corresponding number of people with AIDS, we can calculate a "point prevalence" for AIDS in that region. In clinical work, group A streptococcal infection has a cross-sectional prevalence of 15% if we find 30 such infections in a survey examination of 200 schoolchildren.

In *longitudinal* observation, the numerator condition (or event) occurs afterward, at a serial time later than the original denominator condition. (The word *longitudinal* is itself a peculiar title. The name has no more of a *forward* connotation than *latitudinal*, but probably became popular because of its resemblance to "longevity," which implies a forward direction of follow-up.)

A major distinction between cross-sectional and longitudinal data is the number of examinations required for each person. In a cross-sectional study, all the information can be obtained in essentially a single examination, which identifies the person's age, sex, clinical state, or other descriptions of the condition counted in the denominator. The same examination can also identify the existence of a streptococcal infection, dietary habit, or previous exposure to a risk factor that may be counted in the numerator. To note the incidence of a longitudinal event, however, each person under observation must be examined on at least two occasions. If the 200 school children are examined repeatedly or at least one more time during the next year, and if 50 of them are found to have developed new streptococcal infections, the *attack rate* or *incidence rate* per person is 25% (= 50/200).

17.3.1.1   Incidence vs. Prevalence

17.3.1.1   Incidence vs. Prevalence — The difference between *incidence* and *prevalence* is a key distinction in epidemiologic nomenclature. *Prevalence* refers to what is there now; *incidence* refers to what happens later. Deaths are always an incidence event, but the occurrence of a disease may represent prevalence or incidence, according to when and how the occurrence was discovered. If a woman is suitably examined today and found to be free of breast cancer, its discovery two years from now is an incidence event. If she received no previous examinations the breast cancer discovered two years from now is usually called *incidence* because it seems to be "new," but it may also be a revealed *prevalence* that would have been discovered had she been suitably examined today.

Clinicians constantly misuse the word *incidence* in referring to such *prevalence* events as the proportions of women, antecedent myocardial infarction, or college graduates observed in a counted group of people. The distinction is particularly important for the case-control studies discussed in Section 17.5.2, where all of the retrospective phenomena represent prevalence, not incidence. [If you accept the idea that rates involve a change over time, *incidence rate* is a satisfactory term, but *prevalence rate* is not, because prevalence does not involve a change over time.]

17.3.1.2   Spectral Proportions — Clinicians also often misuse the idea of incidence when reporting proportions for the univariate age or sex spectrum of a disease. For example, suppose the spectrum of a clinical group of patients with omphalosis contains 70% men, and also 5% children, 20% young adults, 50% middle-aged adults, and 25% elderly adults. These results will regularly be reported with the comment that omphalosis has a higher "incidence" in men than in women, and has its highest "incidence" in middle-aged adults. Because the denominator of these univariate proportions is the number of patients with omphalosis, the results represent neither incidence nor prevalence in a group at risk. They show proportions in the univariate spectrum of distribution for each variable in the group of patients collected at whatever medical setting was the source of the research.

17.3.2   Durations

Because all incidence events involve observation during a duration of time, a temporal period becomes the third component of an incidence rate. As a longitudinal quotient, a/n has two components, but in strict symbolism, it is $a/n/t$, where t is the interval of time. The extra symbol for t is commonly omitted, however, because the results are usually cited in such phrases as *annual mortality rate* or *3-year survival rate.* The time duration becomes more evident when a streptococcal infection incidence rate of .60 over 3 years becomes reported as an average annual incidence of .20. [This type of simple average can be erroneous for mortality rates. If .60 of a cohort dies over 3 years, and if the annual mortality rate is said to be .20, the survival rate each year will be .80. At the end of 3 years, the proportion of people still alive will be $.80 \times .80 \times .80 = .51$. The 3-year mortality rate will be .49, not .60.]

Time durations also become an evident and integral part of the computation process when actuarial or other methods, discussed in Chapter 22, are used to adjust incidence rates for numerator losses.

17.3.3 Repetitions

In many incidence rates, the numerator condition is a "failure event" — such as death, occurrence of myocardial infarction, or unwanted pregnancy — that ends each person's period of observation. Sometimes, however, the numerator is a streptococcal or urinary tract infection that can occur repeatedly.

The repeated-occurrence events produce two types of problems in deciding how to express the attack rates. The first problem is whether to count the number of events or the number of persons in whom events occurred. For example, suppose 45 urinary tract infections are noted when 300 women are followed for an interval of time. Does the "45" represent 45 infections in different women, or perhaps 10 infections in one woman, 5 infections in each of 3 women, 2 infections in each of 8 women, and 4 women who had 1 infection each. Either approach can be used, but if the numerator refers to infected women rather than number of infections in this group, the attack rate is 16/300 rather than 45/300.

A second problem involves a decision about how to express unequal durations for people who have been followed for different lengths of time. If the numerator is a single "failure" event, unequal durations of observation can be managed with the actuarial methods of "survival" adjustment described in Chapter 22. Because these adjustments cannot easily be used for repeated events, the customary procedure is to convert the denominator from a count of persons to a sum of person-durations. Thus, if 20 women have been followed for 0.5 years, 30 for 1 year, 50 for 1.5 years, 60 for 2 years, 90 for 2.5 years, and 50 for 3 years, the denominator would contain 610 person-years of follow-up, calculated as $(20 \times .5) + (30 \times 1) + (50 \times 1.5) + (60 \times 2) + (90 \times 2.5) + (50 \times 3)$. If 45 urinary tract infections occurred in that group during that duration, the attack rate would be $45/610 = 7.4\%$ per patient-year.

17.4 Issues in Eligibility

When the problem of quasi-risks was discussed in Section 17.2.4, persons were regarded as ineligible for the denominator if they could not possibly develop the numerator event, or if it had already occurred.

17.4.1 Exclusions for New Development

The previous existence of the event seems an appropriate reason for exclusion if the study is concerned with conditions such as cancer, coronary disease, cerebrovascular disease, or pregnancy, whose new development is the main focus of the research. If no attempt is made to remove the ineligible persons, the denominator will be wrong, and the subsequent incidence rates will be inaccurate.

For example, suppose we institute a program to prevent a relatively common ailment, such as coronary disease, in a community of 100,000 people. If 2000 people have coronary disease that is already present (but perhaps unrecognized), the eligible denominator should be 98,000. At the end of the program, suppose coronary disease has become identified in 1500 of the 2000 people who already had it, and in 1000 new cases. The correct incidence rate would be $1000/98,000 = .0102$. The incidence rate may be incorrectly cited, however, as $2500/100,000 = .025$.

17.4.2 Inclusions for Repetitions

A different type of problem arises if the numerator event can occur repeatedly, because persons who have had it once may get it again. Clinical examples of such events are recurrent episodes (often called "attacks") of streptococcal infection, rheumatic fever, asthma, acute pulmonary edema, epileptic seizure, migraine headache, urinary tract infection, transient ischemic attack, syncope, severe depression, pregnancy, or dysmenorrhea. In these circumstances, persons who have already had the event once are not merely eligible for inclusion in the denominator; they may sometimes be the main focus of the research.

For example, continuous prophylactic medication would seldom be given to prevent rheumatic fever, epilepsy, asthma, migraine, or urinary tract infection in someone who has never had an episode, but might be used for persons whose susceptibility to *recurrence* has been demonstrated by an initial attack. On the other hand, continuous prophylactic medication to lower blood sugar, blood pressure, or blood lipids might be used in persons who may or may not have already manifested a "vascular complication."

In the absence of a standard set of guidelines, the decisions about eligibility for repetition are arbitrary. Regardless of what is chosen, however, the criteria should always be clearly stated in the published report, and the results should always be analyzed separately for persons with and without previous episodes of the numerator event.

17.5   The Odds Ratio

The odds ratio is a unique statistical index of risk. Calculated as (p_A/p_B) (q_B/q_A), it is applicable only to a contrast of two proportions (p_A vs. p_B) and, in the world of medicine, is used almost exclusively for epidemiologic statistics.

As discussed earlier throughout Section 10.7, the odds ratio in a fourfold table is constructed as ad/bc. It is a contrast not of the actual proportions, but of the numbers in the four cells that are components of the proportions. The two denominators for the proportions themselves would be constructed either with (a + b) and (c + d) or with (a + c) and (b + d). Thus, a simple ratio that contrasts the two proportions might be [a/(a + b)]/[c/(c + d)]. Because the denominators are ignored or "ablated," the odds ratio has an appeal that makes it sometimes regarded as the best single index for summarizing results of a 2×2 table.

In the world of epidemiology, however, the main attraction of the odds ratio is that it makes etiologic research easy to do. In suitable circumstances, the odds ratio obtained from a quick, inexpensive case-control study can approximate the risk ratio obtained from a protracted, expensive cohort study. A specific numerical example of this accomplishment was not cited earlier and is offered now.

17.5.1   Illustration of Numbers in a Cohort Study

Suppose omphalosis usually occurs in about one person per thousand, and suppose we suspect that tea drinking helps cause omphalosis, raising its rate of occurrence to about five per thousand. To get supportive evidence for this etiologic suspicion, we might assemble a cohort of 10,000 people, of whom 2000 are tea drinkers and 8000 are non-tea drinkers. After following these people for the next 20 years, we might find that omphalosis had developed as shown in Table 17.1.

TABLE 17.1

Occurrence of Omphalosis in a Hypothetical Cohort Study

	Omphalosis	No Omphalosis	Total
Tea Drinkers	10	1990	2000
Non-Tea Drinkers	8	7992	8000
TOTAL	18	9982	10,000

For the people in Table 17.1, the risk (i.e., the rate of occurrence) of omphalosis is 10/2000 = .005 in tea drinkers and 8/8000 = .001 in non-tea drinkers. These two risks can be contrasted in a single index, the direct *risk ratio*, which is .005/.001 = 5.

Alternatively, we can calculate an odds ratio from these data by determing the odds for tea drinking in omphalotic patients (= 10/8 = 1.25) and in non-omphalotic patients (= 1990/7992 = .249). The odds ratio will be 1.25/.249 = 5.02 and (in this instance) will be quite similar to the risk ratio.

To do the cohort study, however, would require assembling 10,000 people — tea drinkers and non-tea drinkers — and following them for the next 20 years to determine which persons develop omphalosis. This type of huge, long-term project does not attract many potential investigators, even if ample funds were available to collect the 10,000 people and maintain them under observation for the next 20 years. As a substitute research structure, the "retrospective" *case-control study* offers an alternative simpler strategy for exploring the etiologic question.

17.5.2 Illustration of Numbers in a Case-Control Study

Instead of starting at the beginning of the causal pathway, with "exposed" tea drinkers and "non-exposed" non-tea drinkers, the investigator starts at the end, assembling a group of people who have already developed omphalosis. A comparative group, called *controls*, is chosen from persons without omphalosis.

After being selected, members of the case and control groups are asked about their antecedent intake of tea. From this interview, each person might be classified as a tea-drinker or non-tea drinker, and a fourfold table is created. If no distortions (or biases) have occurred in the itinerary between tea-drinking (or non-tea-drinking) and the subsequent occurrence (or nonoccurrence) of omphalosis, the proportion of tea drinkers noted in the cases and controls will be the same as what would have been found in the larger, longer, forward-directed cohort study of 10,000 people.

For example, suppose the investigator assembles 90 cases of patients with omphalosis, and 90 controls who lack omphalosis. In the omphalosis group, the odds for tea drinking should be 10/8, and so 10 of every 18 cases should be tea drinkers. Of 90 cases, 50 would be tea drinkers. In the non-omphalosis group, the odds for tea drinking should be 1990/7992. For only 90 controls, the appropriate number would be about 18 tea drinkers. The investigator's fourfold table would produce the results shown in Table 17.2.

TABLE 17.2

Case-Control Study of the Same Topic Presented in Table 17.1

	Cases	Controls	Total
Tea Drinkers	50	18	68
Non-Tea Drinkers	40	72	112
TOTAL	90	90	180

The results in Table 17.2 do not allow a risk or incidence rate to be determined because the patients were not assembled as tea drinkers or non-tea drinkers. If the "risk" of omphalosis were calculated in the tea drinkers of this table, the result would yield the unbelievably high 50/68 = .74, instead of the correct rate of .005 found in Table 17.1. Similarly, the "risk" of omphalosis in non-tea drinkers would be 40/112 = .36, which is about 360 times higher than the true risk of .001. Furthermore, if a "risk ratio" were calculated from these two "risks," the result would be .74/.36 = 2.06, which is substantially lower than the true risk ratio of 5.

On the other hand, if the odds ratio for this table is calculated as (50/40)/(18/72) or (50 × 72)/(40 × 18), the result is 5 and is identical to the true risk ratio. [The algebra that accounts for this similarity was shown earlier in Section 10.7.4.1 and in Appendix A.10.1 of Chapter 10.]

17.5.3 Ambiguities in Construction

Just as odds can always be stated for or against a particular occurrence, the odds ratio is always ambiguous because it can always be constructed in two ways. In a table that has $\begin{Bmatrix} a & b \\ c & d \end{Bmatrix}$ as its four cells, the columns could equally well have been reversed, so that the same four numbers would be $\begin{Bmatrix} b & a \\ d & c \end{Bmatrix}$. The rows might also have been reversed to make the table either $\begin{Bmatrix} d & c \\ a & b \end{Bmatrix}$ or $\begin{Bmatrix} c & d \\ b & a \end{Bmatrix}$. The first and fourth of these four arrangements will produce ad/bc as the odds ratio. The second and third will produce the reciprocal value, bc/ad.

The choice of arrangements and expressions depends on what point is being communicated. If we think that exposure helps promote a disease, the odds ratio is usually constructed with the *exposed-and-diseased* cell in the upper left corner. The ad/bc odds ratio will then exceed 1. If exposure protects against disease (as in tests of vaccines), this arrangement will produce an odds ratio below 1.

On the other hand, if exposure is believed to protect against disease, we may want to cite the risk ratio for the unexposed group. In the latter instance, the cell for the *unexposed-and-diseased* group is placed in the upper left corner, and the ad/bc odds ratio will exceed 1. Thus, an odds ratio that indicates a reduced or "protective" risk of 0.23 in the exposed group also indicates an increased or "promoted" risk of 1/.23 = 4.35 in the unexposed group.

17.5.4   Incalculable Results

The word *incalculable* is often used to denote something too large to be precisely quantified. For odds ratios, however, this word literally means "cannot be calculated"— an event that happens whenever any one of the four cells has a value of 0. Because we must be able to determine both ad/bc and bc/ad, a zero cell would produce an unacceptable division by 0.

Reluctant to give up the cherished odds ratio, biostatisticians have proposed that 0.5 be added to each cell when this problem arises. Consider the controversial case-control study[9] that associated clear-cell adenocarcinoma of the vagina or cervix (CCVC) with intrauterine gestational exposure to diethylstilbestrol (DES). The results were as follows:

Antecedent Exposure to DES	Cases of CCVC	Control Group
Exposed	7	0
Non-Exposed	1	32

With the "add 0.5 to each cell" tactic, the odds ratio in these data would be calculated as $(7 + .5)(32 + .5)/[(0 + 0.5)(1 + .5)] = 325$.

17.5.5   Stochastic Appraisals

Like any other index of contrast, the odds ratio can be appraised stochastically with a P value or confidence interval.

17.5.5.1   P Values — As in any 2×2 table, a P value for the results of an odds ratio can be obtained with a Fisher exact test or a chi-square test. In many epidemiologic studies, the numbers are small enough to warrant the Fisher test.

17.5.5.2   Confidence Intervals — Determining a confidence interval for the odds ratio is tricky because it does not have a symmetrical span of values, and because it is constructed from two quotients, not one.

If the odds ratio exceeds 1, its value can range in the interval from 1 to almost infinity. If the ratio is <1, however, the values can range only in the relatively small interval between 1 and 0. To avoid this inappropriate asymmetry, confidence intervals are usually calculated for the natural logarithm ("ln") of the odds ratio. Because ln 1 = 0, these intervals will be spread symmetrically around zero. Thus, if the odds ratio is 4, ln 4 = 1.39; if the ratio is 0.25 (= 1/4), ln .25 = −1.39. When the symmetric logarithmic calculation is converted to ordinary numbers, however, the interval will then be asymmetrical.

Because the confidence interval involves two quotients that can often have small numerical constituents, the calculation has evoked several mathematical strategies. They are mentioned here mainly so you will have heard of them and be able to recognize that the different results do not always agree. You need not try to learn (or even understand) the formulas. The three most prominent methods are eponymically named for Woolf,[10] Cornfield,[11] and Miettinen.[12] Generically, they are sometimes called respectively the simple, exact, and test-based methods. In several mathematical comparisons,[13,14] Cornfield's exact method was the preferred approach, particularly for small sample sizes.

17.5.5.2.1 Woolf Simple Method. Using o as the symbol for odds ratio, a standard error can be calculated for ln o in a relatively simple method proposed by Woolf.[10] The method relies on calculating standard error of ln o with the formula

$$SE = \sqrt{(1/a) + (1/b) + (1/c) + (1/d)} \qquad [17.1]$$

The a, b, c, d symbols are the frequency counts in each cell after 0.5 has been added to the cell. After the confidence interval is prepared in the usual manner as ln $o \pm Z_\alpha$ (SE), the limits of the interval are converted to customary units by taking the antilogarithm, i.e., $e^{\ln(o)}$, for the lower and upper values.

For example, in Table 17.2, SE $= \sqrt{(1/50.5) + (1/18.5) + (1/40.5) + (1/72.5)} = \sqrt{.112} = .335$. The logarithmic 95% confidence interval will be ln $5 \pm (1.96) (.335) = 1.609 \pm .657$. This confidence interval will extend from .953 to 2.266. Because $e^{.953} = 2.59$ and $e^{2.266} = 9.64$, the boundaries for the 95% confidence interval around the odds ratio of 5 will be 2.59 and 9.64. For the table in Section 17.5.4, SE $= \sqrt{(1/7.5) + (1/0.5) + (1/1.5) + (1/32.5)} = \sqrt{2.83} = 1.68$; and ln $325 \pm (1.96) (1.68) = 5.784 \pm 3.298$. Suitable calculations and conversions will then show that the 95% confidence interval for this odds ratio extends from 12 to 8794.

Breslow and Day[15] are willing to construct confidence intervals this way, but Gart and Thomas[16] say the limits will generally be too narrow, especially for small-sized groups. Fleiss[17] recommends using Formula [17.1] to gauge "precision" for the odds ratio but not to calculate the actual confidence interval.

17.5.5.2.2 Cornfield Exact Method. In a tactic originally suggested by Fisher[18] and reminiscent of the array of tables used for the Fisher exact test, Cornfield[11] developed an exact method for getting an odds ratio's confidence interval. The calculations are complex and computer-intensive because iterative numerical solutions are required for quartic equations. Because of the calculational complexity, Cornfield's method is seldom used. If you do a lot of this work, however, you might want to get and use the appropriate computer program. [The Cornfield method is *not* available in standard SAS, BMDP, or other packages, but can be found in the EPIINFO Version 5 available from the Centers for Disease Control.[19]]

17.5.5.2.3 Miettinen Test-Based Method. Probably the most common approach today is Miettinen's "test-based" method,[12] which uses the X^2 test statistic calculated for the 2×2 table, preferably[15] without Yates correction. The confidence interval will be

$$\ln o \pm o(Z_\alpha/X) \qquad [17.2]$$

where X is the square root of the X^2 statistic, and where Z_α would be 1.96 for a two-tailed $\alpha = .05$. Because the formula can be rewritten as ln o $[1 \pm (Z_\alpha/X)]$, the confidence limits could be expressed in a power of o as

$$o^{[1 \pm (Z_\alpha/X)]} \qquad [17.3]$$

For example, for the values of $\begin{Bmatrix} 50 & 18 \\ 40 & 72 \end{Bmatrix}$ in Table 17.2, $o = 5.0$; $X^2 = 24.2$; and X $= 4.92$, so that $1.96/4.92 = .398$ and $1 \pm .398$ yields .602 and 1.398. The value of $5.0^{.602}$ is 2.63 and $5.0^{1.398}$ is 9.49. (With Woolf's method, the corresponding values were 2.59 and 9.64.) For the table $\begin{Bmatrix} 7 & 0 \\ 1 & 32 \end{Bmatrix}$ in Section 17.5.4, the uncorrected X^2 is 33.94 and X $= 5.83$, so that $1.96/5.83 = .336$. With $1 - .336$ becoming .664, the lower confidence limit is $325^{.664} = 46.33$; and the upper limit is $325^{1.336} = 2269.22$. (With Woolf's method, the corresponding limits were 12 and 8794.) Thus, in both of the two cited examples, the Miettinen method produced narrower intervals than the Woolf method.

17.5.5.3 Tests of Fragility — A rapid crude (or "commonsense") method to appraise stability for an odds ratio is to do a unit fragility test. For this test, relocate one unit of the data while keeping the marginal values constant, and then recalculate the odds ratio. For example, the table in Section 17.5.4 is already at a maximum value in one direction. The unit relocation can move things only in the other direction toward $\begin{Bmatrix} 6 & 1 \\ 2 & 31 \end{Bmatrix}$. The odds ratio for the latter table is $(6 \times 31)/(2) = 93$, which is a drop of 71% $[= (325 - 93)/325]$ from the original value. This demonstration of substantial descriptive "instability" can be compared against the stochastic result of the Fisher test, which would produce $P = 4.0 \times 10^{-7}$ for the extreme data in the observed original table.

For $\begin{Bmatrix} 50 & 18 \\ 40 & 72 \end{Bmatrix}$ in Table 17.2, however, the odds ratio of 5 has much less fragility. A shift of one unit produces $\begin{Bmatrix} 49 & 19 \\ 41 & 71 \end{Bmatrix}$ in one direction and $\begin{Bmatrix} 51 & 17 \\ 39 & 73 \end{Bmatrix}$ in the other. The corresponding odds ratio would become 4.47 or 5.62. The proportionate fragility would be a drop of $.53/5 = 11\%$ or a rise of $.62/5 = 12\%$. The result is still not impressively stable, but with $X^2 = 4.92$, the 2P value is $<.05$.

17.5.6 Quantitative Appraisal of Odds Ratio

When boundaries of "quantitative significance" were discussed in Chapter 10, the odds ratio received relatively little discussion among the other indexes of contrast. The quantitative importance of an odds ratio is particularly difficult to evaluate because the appraisal strongly depends on the context, rather than the magnitude itself. Furthermore, the magnitude may be directly distorted by the context.

17.5.6.1 "Inflation" of "High" Rates — Consider the "high" rates (usually $\geq .1$) that are found in many clinical studies, such as a randomized trial in which the compared success rates are $p_A = .5$ and $p_B = .3$. The simple ratio of $p_A/p_B = .5/.3 = 1.67$ would indicate the higher "risk" of success with treatment A. The simple ratio of $q_B/q_A = .7/.5 = 1.4$ would indicate the higher risk of failure with treatment B. The odds ratio, however, multiplies these two "risks" to produce $(p_A/p_B)(q_B/q_A) = (.5/.3)(.7/.5) = 2.33$, which substantially inflates the value for either simple ratio.

The inflation is the mathematical reason why the odds ratio should *not* be used if the smaller of the two rates is not small enough. If not close to 1, the value of $q_B = 1 - p_B$ will be divided by a smaller q_A, and the product will inflate the value of p_A/p_B. Scientifically, of course, there is no reason to use the odds ratio when the actual values of p_A and p_B have been determined in a clinical trial or cohort study. In the latter two situations, the desired "risk" ratio can be expressed directly either as p_A/p_B or as q_B/q_A, but not as their product.

17.5.6.2 No Effect on "Low" Rates — In most public health studies of etiologic "risk factors," the odds ratio will not produce substantial inflation because the compared rates of disease occurrence are relatively small, i.e., $< .01$. For example, in Table 17.1, $p_B = .001$ and $p_A = .005$, and $q_B/q_A = .999/.995 = 1.004$. The odds ratio of 5.02 would be hardly changed from the simple risk ratio of 5. If the risk ratio were still 5, but obtained from $p_A = .05$ and $p_B = .01$, the value of q_B/q_A would be $.99/.95 = 1.04$ and the odds ratio would become 5.2, which is moderately but not substantially inflated above 5. If the risk ratio of 5 came from $p_A = .5$ and $p_B = .1$, however, q_B/q_A would be $.9/.5 = 1.8$, and the odds ratio would increase to 9.

17.5.6.3 Criteria for Quantitative Significance — For the reasons just cited, odds ratios are particularly difficult to interpret out of context. In clinical studies of therapy, the odds ratio usually is mathematically undesirable because of potential inflation and is also unnecessary because the compared results can be effectively (and better) evaluated with more conventional indexes of contrast, such as the direct increment or number needed to treat. When etiology is investigated with an epidemiologic case-control study, however, the "sampling method" usually precludes the calculation of direct increments or ratios. The odds ratio then becomes the only index of contrast available for evaluation.

Although the evaluation is highly judgmental, various authorities[20,21] have stated that odds ratios <3 represent "weak associations" that often may not warrant serious attention because the small elevations above 1 hardly exceed the "noise" that can be expected from ordinary sources of inaccuracy and bias in the raw data. In a study of quantitative conclusions for published odds ratios, Burnand et al.[22] found that 2.2 seemed to be an average minimum level for quantitative significance.

Because odds ratios are so difficult to interpret, they are not well understood by workers in the health-care field, and they can be seriously misleading or deceptive if presented to laymen when investigators seek either to obtain "informed consent" or to advocate a particular belief. A much more effective and "honest" approach is to determine or estimate an incidence rate for the control-group "risk," use the odds ratio to calculate the corresponding rate for the "exposed" or "treated" group, and convert the increment in incidence rates to an NNE for the number needed for one event. An opportunity to do this conversion appears in Exercise 17.6 at the end of the chapter.

17.5.6.4   Lod Scores — Odds have received an entirely new use in molecular genetics, to quantify the strength of linkage for an observed association between two traits in families. The odds are determined as a ratio of posterior and prior probabilities. The numerator is the posterior probability of observing the distributional pattern of the two traits' frequency of re-combination under the hypothesis of linkage. The denominator is the analogous prior probability, assumed to be 0.5, under the null hypothesis of no linkage. The decimal logarithm of this ratio is called a *lod score*; and a lod value of 3, i.e., odds of 1000 to 1, is required to assert that linkage exists.[23,24]

17.5.7   Combination of Stratified Odds Ratios

A simple 2×2 table is sometimes stratified, according to an additional variable, into a series of 2×2 tables. For example, Table 17.1 might be divided into separate 2×2 tables for men and women, or for different durations of tea drinking. The table in Section 17.5.4 might be partitioned according to whether the women did or did not have pregnancy problems such as cramping, bleeding, or spotting. The separate odds ratios calculated for each stratum can then be appropriately combined to form an odds ratio that has been "adjusted" for imbalances in the strata. The adjustment method, called the *Mantel–Haenszel procedure*, is discussed in Chapter 26.

17.5.8   Scientific Hazards of Odds Ratios

Despite all the mathematical cavils, the main hazard of the odds ratio is scientific, not statistical. It is regularly used for a cause–effect inference about an etiologic agent or "risk factor," but the research structure itself may contain few or sometimes *no* scientific precautions against biased or inaccurate results.

Randomized trials were developed to provide these precautions in cause–effect reasoning about the action of therapeutic agents; and the precautions are equally pertinent in cause–effect reasoning for etiologic agents. Although the precautions could be applied in case-control studies, suitable efforts are seldom made. Consequently, case-control studies become an easy prey for the susceptibility bias, performance bias, detection bias, and transfer bias — discussed elsewhere[6] — that can occur innately in any form of cause–effect relationship. Beyond the innate biases, the investigator has the opportunity to introduce two additional biases — exclusion bias and ascertainment bias — when the groups of cases and controls are chosen and interviewed.

Thus, in exchange for the ease of doing etiologic research with the mathematical splendor of the odds ratio, case-control studies create formidable scientific problems in deciding whether the result is valid or credible.

17.6   Specialized Terms for Contrasting Risks

As noted in Chapter 10, two central indexes are most commonly contrasted as an increment or ratio. Exactly those same ideas occur in a contrast of two epidemiologic rates. Because the rates are regarded as risks, however, an elaborate specialized jargon has been developed for the citations. Emanating from the world of public health, which emphasizes preventing disease by reducing risk factors, the jargon uses terms such as *attributable risk* and *etiologic fraction*, which indicate "editorial" conclusions about the data rather than scientific descriptions of "news."

An additional complication in the nomenclature is that the risks—which usually refer to the rate of death or the incidence rate for a particular disease—can be considered and compared for three sets of people, rather than two. The three sets are: a regional community population, a group of persons exposed to a particular etiologic agent or risk factor, and a group of persons who are unexposed. The risks are then contrasted in ways that imply the quantitative consequences of exposure or non-exposure. To avoid the threat of clarity amid all the other complexity, the same ideas have received many different names, and occasionally the same name is given to different ideas.

Card-carrying epidemiologists themselves often have difficulty remembering all the terms and distinctions, which are listed here mainly so you will have met them and know roughly what they mean when they appear in published literature. The "glossary" that follows is intended merely to cite the nomenclature and quantitative constituents, not to justify, praise, question, or condemn the associated assumptions and reasoning about cause–effect relationships. Whenever the literary exposure becomes too risky to your intellectual tranquillity, advance promptly to Section 17.7.

17.6.1 Glossary of Symbols and Terms

The three rates under discussion as risks can be represented with the following symbols:

p_E = rate of event (e.g., occurrence of disease or death) in an exposed group of people

p_U = rate in an unexposed group of people

p_C = rate in a community (regional) population

The proportion of the community exposed to a risk factor is e, and the proportion of unexposed people will be $1 - e$. The rate of the event in the community will be

$$p_C = ep_E + (1 - e)p_U$$

17.6.2 Increments

The increment in risk represents the alleged excess of the disease that is caused by exposure. The increment can be expressed in two ways. *Attributable risk* is used for the increment $p_E - p_U$. It is also called the *rate difference* or *risk difference*. *Attributable community risk* is used for the increment $p_E - p_C$. It is also called the *attributable population risk*. Substituting $p_C = ep_E + (1 - e)p_U$ and working out the algebra produces $(1 - e)(p_E - p_U)$. The *attributable community risk* is thus the *attributable risk* multiplied by the proportion of unexposed people.

17.6.3 Ratios

A single simple ratio expresses the contrast of rates for exposed/un-exposed risk as $r = p_E/p_U$. To compensate for the simplicity, this ratio has an exuberance of names. It has been called *risk ratio*, *relative risk*, *rate ratio*, *incidence rate ratio*, and *relative rate*. All of these statistical names refer to essentially the same entity. The term that will be used here is *risk ratio*.

17.6.3.1 *Nonstatistical Sources of Confusion in Nomenclature* — The reason that odds ratios are so attractive in epidemiology is that under the suitable conditions discussed earlier for a retrospective case-control study, the odds ratio, *o*, can be used to approximate the risk ratio, *r*, that might be obtained in a cohort study. (In fact, many case-control investigators improperly use the term *risk ratio* or *relative risk* when reporting results of an *odds ratio*.)

In the customary use of pertinent words, however, the term *cases* refers to persons with the focal disease, and *controls* refers to persons who do not have it. The case-control structure is thus used for diagnostic marker studies (see Chapter 21) and for other cross-sectional clinical investigations[6] in which a disease and a focal entity are associated in a concurrent, forward, or uncertain direction of timing, rather than in the retrospective direction of etiologic research. To separate the backward from the other directions of inquiry, the term *trohoc* (which is *cohort* spelled backward) was proposed[25] for retrospective case-control studies. The term has been "deprecated"[26] or actively resented, however, by many public-health epidemiologists, who insist that *case-control* is a satisfactory name, despite the directional ambiguity.

At least six alternative names have been proposed for retrospective case-control studies, not to clarify the problem of direction, but to remove the confusion produced when "control" is used for an outcome event rather than for the customary scientific designation of a comparative agent.[6] Four additional terms are *case-comparison study*, *case-compeer study*, *case-history study*, and *case-referent study*. Another alternative, *case-base study*, can indicate the choice of controls from the regional "base" population rather than from the available other clinical conditions that are often used as "controls." A sixth term, *case-exposure* study, has been proposed[27] when "the controls who are obtained concurrently with cases are representative of the exposure experience of the population from which the cases are drawn."

The last term can add to the confusion produced when *case-control* is also used (erroneously) for a cohort study in which the exposed persons are called "cases," and the non-exposed are called "controls." Despite all the peer-reviewing and editing, this flagrant error occasionally appears in prestigious medical journals.[28,29]

17.6.3.2 Confidence Interval for Risk Ratio —

When a cohort study has actually been done, with the outcome events found in a/n_E exposed people and in c/n_U unexposed people, the risk ratio is $r = (a/n_E)/(c/n_U)$. A confidence interval can be obtained[30] for the logarithmic transformation of r by calculating

$$SE(\ln\ r) = \sqrt{(1/a) - (1/n_E) + (1/c) - (1/n_U)}$$

This result is then managed like the standard error of the logarithm of the odds ratio, and the final confidence limits are the exponentiated values of $\ln r \pm Z_\alpha [SE (\ln r)]$.

17.6.4 Cumulative Incidence and Incidence Density

Another source of confusing jargon about rates is that the term *incidence rate* can be applied to two different mathematical phenomena. One of them is the conventional, standard scientific idea: the proportion of people in a specified population who have developed the cited event during the course of specified time period. Mathematicians call this the *cumulative incidence rate*. The second usage refers to the proportionate number of new cases during a very small or "instantaneous" time period. This idea has different names: *incidence density, instantaneous incidence rate*, and *hazard rate*. The two approaches are used later in Chapter 22 when interval mortality rates indicate the hazards from which the cumulative incidence, or *survival rate*, is then calculated.

Most epidemiologic case-control studies claim to use "incidence-density" arrangements, in which exposure histories are compared for "incident cases" and for control "noncases who are still at risk of becoming cases." In a "cumulative-density" arrangement, however, the control group is "no longer at risk of becoming cases." The latter situation is pertinent for investigating reproductive outcomes such as congenital deformities or vaccine efficacy during an epidemic. Hogue et al.[31] have pointed out that the case-control odds ratio can suitably approximate the risk ratio in incidence-density studies, but must receive special checks and modification in cumulative-incidence studies.

17.6.5 Proportionate Increments

Proportionate increments are particularly popular because, as discussed in Chapter 10, they make the results seem more impressive than ratios alone, and also because they allow additional editorial claims about etiology and prevention. The calculations and titles will depend on what is chosen for comparison in the reference group or denominator.

When the attributable risk is divided by the risk in the non-exposed group, the proportionate increment is formed as $(p_E - p_U)/p_U = r - 1$. This *excess relative risk* is also called the *relative effect.*

Prevented fraction reports the same comparison as the excess relative risk, but the exposure is expected to prevent rather than promote the disease. Since p_U should exceed p_E, the proportionate increment is expressed as $(p_U - p_E)/p_U = 1 - r$. With exposure having a protective effect, r will be < 1, and the value of $1 - r$ will range from 0 to 1. This term, often used for evaluating vaccines, is also called *protective efficacy.*

For *etiologic fraction* (for *exposed group*), the attributable risk, $p_E - p_U$, is divided by the risk in the exposed group to form $(p_E - p_U)/p_E = 1 - (1/r) = (r - 1)/r$. It is also called the *attributable proportion* or *attributable risk percent*. It indicates the proportion of disease that would presumably be removed from the exposed group if everyone became unexposed.

Etiologic fraction (for *community*) uses a different increment, formed by the excess of the community rate beyond the unexposed rate. This increment is then divided by the community rate to produce $(p_C - p_U)/p_C$. Substituting $p_C = ep_E + (1 - e)p_U$, and carrying out the rest of the algebra, this expression reduces to $[e(r - 1)]/e(r - 1) + 1$. The result, which is also called the *population attributable risk percent*, is regarded as the proportion of community cases attributable to the exposure. The implication is that these cases would be prevented if the exposure were eliminated.

The calculations can be illustrated with data presented by Cole and McMahon[32] for a case-control study of smoking and bladder cancer in men. The data were as follows:

	Cases	Controls
Smokers	284	261
Nonsmokers	59	114
TOTAL	354	375

Because bladder cancer is a relatively rare disease, the odds ratio, calculated as $(284 \times 114)/(261 \times 59) = 2.10$, can be used as a surrogate for the risk ratio. The proportion of exposure in the general population can be estimated from the control group as $e = 261/375 = .696$. Inserting this information into the foregoing formula, the community etiologic fraction is found to be $(.696) (1.10)/[(.696) (1.10) + 1] = .43$. Thus, if the underlying reasoning and data are correct, the men of a smoke-free society should achieve an apparently impressive 43% reduction in the former incidence rate of bladder cancer. Because the former rate is not stated, however, the actual magnitude of the reduction is unknown.

17.7 Advantages of Risk Ratios and Odds Ratios

If you have survived the tour through all the foregoing formulas, you may have noted a fascinating thing about r, the risk ratio: it avoids the need for knowing any of the basic values for p_E, p_U, or p_C. Except for the direct increments cited in Section 17.6.2, all the other formulas do not require getting any scientific evidence or doing any specific research to find the actual occurrence rates for the disease (or death) in the exposed, unexposed, or community populations. Everything is taken care of by the mathematical arrangements. Such impressive information as "excess relative risk," "etiologic fractions," and "prevented fractions" can all be determined from a single item of information, r, which is the risk ratio for p_E/p_U. (In one instance, we also need an estimate for e.)

Consequently, an easy, inexpensive, retrospective case-control study can avoid the laborious cohort research necessary to find p_E, p_U, or p_C. With the risk ratio approximated by the ad/bc odds ratio of the 2×2 table and with the value of e estimated from results in the "control" group [e.g., as $b/(b + d)$], we can produce a gigantic mathematical buffet that extends from risk ratios to etiologic fractions. As noted earlier in the text, Francis Galton once wrote[33] that the ancient Greeks, had they but known it, would have worshipped the Gaussian curve as a god. The retrospective case-control study and odds ratio, if available, might have received the same deification from ancient Greek epidemiologists.

17.8 Adjustments for Numerators, Denominators, and Transfers

A quite different statistical strategy for epidemiologic rates is to "adjust" them mathematically for additional major problems, not hitherto cited, in either the numerator or denominator constituents.

The incidence data in a longitudinal study must often be adjusted for "numerator losses." The "lost" people were counted when they entered the denominator, and their status was known at some subsequent time of observation; but they then became "lost to follow-up" and their ultimate status is unknown for counting the outcome event in the numerator as **dead/alive, success/failure,** etc. To adjust the ongoing depletion of the cohort, the denominators are successively decremented over time, using either conventional actuarial or the currently popular Kaplan-Meier "life-table" methods. The methods of adjustment, often called *survival analysis*, are discussed in Chapter 22.

A different type of adjustment, used in both longitudinal and cross-sectional studies, is done for "denominator imbalances." This problem arises when we want to compare incidence rates or prevalence in two groups, but we know that the composition of the groups is biased by a "confounding" factor that affects the rates. For example, the comparison of birth rates in two groups of people would be unfair if one group contained mainly men and postmenopausal women, whereas the other group contained mainly women aged 18 to 45. An adjustment called "standardization" is often done to help "equalize" the disproportionate denominator components that would distort the comparison of the unadjusted "crude" rates. This process, discussed in Chapter 26, leads to the "age–sex adjustments," "stratum-specific rates," and other adaptations for which epidemiologic data are famous (or infamous).

A third type of problem, which is difficult to adjust, occurs when epidemiologic cohorts are assembled from volunteers, or from the people who are still available many years after the initial serial time at which the cohort observations began. The problem, a scientific issue in assembly of groups, is beyond the scope of a mainly statistical discussion.

17.9 Interdisciplinary Problems in Rates

As might be expected when the same ideas and names are used for rates in substantially different groups, major interdisciplinary problems have occurred about the propriety of the activities. Public-health researchers may contend that clinicians should not apply the name *cohort* or talk about *rates* if the denominator refers to clinical groups, rather than regional populations. Clinicians may respond that the public-health cohorts are studied mathematically, rather than with direct examinations, and that the population-based rates of "disease" are too inaccurate to warrant scientific credibility, particularly when results in different regions or eras are used for major decisions in public policy.

Because the problems are currently unresolved (with few attempts having been made to achieve resolution), both the public-health and the clinical investigators continue their unchanged use (or abuse) of the process. Although public-health mortality rates are regularly adjusted or "standardized" for unbalanced demographic composition of denominators, clinical mortality rates are seldom adjusted for corresponding imbalances caused by differences in severity of the denominator conditions. Although extensive variations in accuracy and consistency of diagnostic citation[5,6] make death-certificate data untrustworthy, a single selected "cause of death" continues to be used for public-health tabulations of the incidence of different diseases.

A striking example of scientific defects in both the clinical and public-health approaches is the use of *infant mortality rates* as indicators of national or regional quality of health care. The denominator of these rates consists of infants who were born alive. The numerator consists of live-births who died in the next year. What is ignored in both denominators and numerators are the fates of the products of conception. No adjustments are made for spontaneous or induced abortions; and in particular, no adjustments are made for stillbirths or for infants born in a precarious state of life.

If left alone, the precarious infants may promptly die, be recorded as stillbirths, and appear in neither numerators nor denominators of the infant mortality rates. If given vigorous resuscitation and excellent care, however, many of the precarious births will survive, but those who do not will augment the numerator of deaths. In this way, excellent care in the delivery room and in special neonatal nurseries can help salvage life for many babies who formerly would have been "stillbirths." The result, however, can also lead to a paradoxical *increase* in the infant mortality rates.

Despite these problems, few attempts have been made to adjust the infant mortality rates for "precarious" states (which include very low birth weights) or for the local clinical customs used to identify a precarious baby who is resuscitated but who dies soon afterward.[34] The rates of infant mortality can rise or fall according to whether the clinician decides to list such babies either as *stillbirths* (thereby filling out one official certificate) or as *live births* followed by *deaths* (thereby having to fill out two official certificates).

References

1. Elandt-Johnson, 1975; 2. Freedman, 1991; 3. Ericksen, 1985; 4. Hamilton, 1990; 5. Gittlesohn, 1982; 6. Feinstein, 1985; 7. McFarlane, 1987; 8. Burnand, 1992; 9. Herbst, 1972; 10. Woolf, 1955; 11. Cornfield, 1956; 12. Miettinen, 1976; 13. Gart, 1982; 14. Brown, 1981; 15. Breslow, 1980; 16. Gart, 1972; 17. Fleiss, 1981, pg. 64; 18. Fisher, 1934; 19. Dean, 1990; 20. Wynder, 1987; 21. Cornfield, 1987; 22. Burnand, 1990; 23. Bale, 1989; 24. Risch, 1992; 25. Feinstein, 1973; 26. Last, 1988; 27. Hogue, 1981; 28. Koivisto, 1984; 29. Eagles, 1990; 30. Katz, 1978; 31. Hogue, 1983; 32. Cole, 1971; 33. Galton, 1889; 34. Howell, 1994; 35. Greenwald, 1971; 36. Labarthe, 1978; 37. McFarlane, 1986.

Exercises

17.1. A major controversy has occurred about apparent contradictions in biostatistical data as researchers try to convince Congress to allocate more funds for intramural and extramural investigations supported by the NIH. Citing improved survival rates for conditions such as cervical cancer, breast cancer, and leukemia, clinicians claim we are "winning the war" against cancer. Citing increased incidence rates for these (and other cancers), with minimal change in mortality rates, public-health experts claim that the "war" has made little progress, and we should focus on prevention rather than cure.

      17.1.1.   What explanation would you offer to suggest that the rising incidence of cancer is a statistical consequence of "winning" rather than "losing" the battle?

      17.1.2.   What explanation would you offer to reconcile the contradictory trends for survival and mortality rates, and to suggest that both sets of results are correct?

      17.1.3.   What focus of intervention would you choose for efforts to *prevent* breast cancer, cervical cancer, or leukemia?

17.2. Practicing pediatricians constantly make use of "growth charts" to show the range of normal growth for children. The charts are constructed in the general format shown for weight in Figure E.17.2.

    The data for these charts are obtained as follows. A collection of "normal" children is assembled, measured, and divided into groups according to age. For each age group, the distribution of weight is noted and converted into percentiles. The percentile points are then entered on the graph for each age group and the points are joined to form the lines.

    Pediatricians use these graphs to follow their cohorts of well children and to determine whether the children are growing in a normal manner.

      17.2.1.   Were the data on the graph obtained from cohort research? If not, what designation would you give to the data structures?

      17.2.2.   Do you perceive any clinical biostatistical problems arising from any disparity you have noted?

17.3. The drawing shown in Figure E.17.3 gives a diagrammatic representation of the occurrence and course of instances of a particular disease in six members of a group of 300 persons. The other 294 persons remained free of the disease. For this group of 300 persons, calculate

17.3.1. Point prevalence on July 1, 1993.
17.3.2. Incidence rate, July 1, 1993 to June 30, 1994.
17.3.3. Period prevalence, July 1, 1993 to June 30, 1994.

[Epidemiologists use the term *period prevalence* for the sum (i.e., point prevalence plus incidence) of all encountered instances of disease.]

17.4. In patients receiving radiotherapy for lung cancer, the 6-month survival rate is found to be 32% at the West Haven VA Hospital, and 54% at Yale-New Haven Hospital. A newspaper reporter discovers this difference and has prepared an article about the incompetent physicians working at the VA. The managing editor, after a few inquiries, discovers that the same physicians design and supervise radiotherapy at both institutions. The newspaper reporter then plans a major "exposure" of the unsatisfactory radiotherapy equipment purchased by the Veterans Administration, but the managing editor discourages the work after learning that the VA patients are transported by shuttle bus and usually receive their radiotherapy at Yale-New Haven Hospital. The reporter, who has been told to subside by the irritated managing editor, now alerts and urges the district congressman to conduct public hearings about the fatal fumes or other lethal ambiance of the shuttle bus. A day before the public hearings are due to begin, the congressman's assistant, at a cocktail party, meets a quantitative clinical epidemiologist. The QCE person, when told about the impending excitement, makes a few statistically oriented remarks that persuade the congressman to call off the investigation immediately and to abandon further pursuit of the subject. What do you think might have been said?

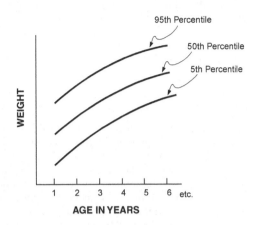

FIGURE E.17.2
Format of pediatric growth curves.

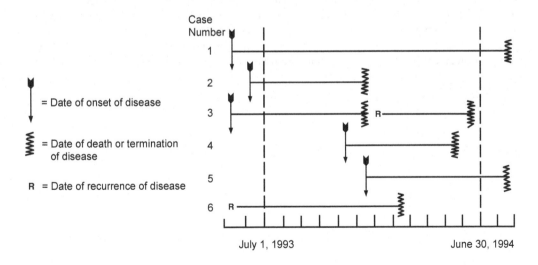

FIGURE E.17.3
Occurrence patterns of disease in 6 cases.

17.5. After the original report[9] of the case-control study mentioned in Section 17.5.4, a second case-control study[35] was published with the following results:

Antecedent In-Utero Exposure to DES	Cases of Clear-Cell Vaginal Cancer	Control Group
Exposed	5	0
Non-Exposed	0	8

   17.5.1. What is the odds ratio for this table?
   17.5.2. Although DES is now almost universally regarded as a transplacental carcinogen, and although millions of women who were exposed to DES *in utero* now live in cancerophobic terror waiting for the clear cells to strike, the two cited case-control studies are the only "controlled" epidemiologic evidence that supports the carcinogenic belief. In a subsequent large cohort study (the "DESAD" project[36]), *no* clear-cell cancers were found after about 25 years since birth in any of about 2000 adult women exposed in utero to DES or in a corresponding number of women in the non-exposed matched group, born at the same time as the exposed cohort.
             Several cantankerous clinical epidemiologists[37] (from New Haven) have disputed the "established wisdom," contending that the case-control studies were poorly conducted and that a cause–effect relationship has not been proved. What do you think were some of the main arguments offered by the "heretics"?
   17.5.3. Assuming that the DES/CCVC relationship is real, causal, and has odds ratios as large as those you have noted and/or calculated, why do you think no cases of clear-cell cancer were found in the exposed DESAD cohort?

17.6. In a case-control study, the odds ratio for development of endometrial cancer was found to be 4.3 for postmenopausal women taking replacement estrogen therapy. (The results have been disputed because of a problem in "detection bias," but can be accepted as correct for this exercise.) To inform a patient of the risk of this cancer if she decides to take replacement therapy, you want to convert the odds ratio to a value of NNE. You can assume that the customary incidence of endometrial cancer is .001. What calculations would you do, and what result do you get for NNE?

17.7. In an immaculately conducted case-control study, the investigators found an odds ratio of 6 for the development of an adverse event after exposure to Agent X. You have been invited, as an expert consultant, to comment about establishing public policy for management of the problem revealed by this research. Assuming that the study was indeed "immaculate" (so that research architecture need not be further evaluated), you have been allowed to ask no more than four individual questions before you reach your judgment. What sequence of four questions would you choose, and why?

Part III

Evaluating Associations

All of the statistical strategies discussed so far were intended to evaluate one group or to compare two groups of data. When we now begin "comparing" two variables rather than two groups, the bad news is that the different types of variables will require diverse new arrangements and many new *descriptive* indexes for the results. The good news, however, is that only a few indexes are needed for most of the common descriptive activities; the additional arrangements involve no new forms of statistical *inference*, which is used with the same basic principles as before.

The arrangements of two variables are generally called *associations*, but the associations can have many different goals and structures. The aim might be to discern *trend* in the relationship of two different variables or to note *concordance* for two variables that describe the same entity. The trends can be an interdependent *correlation* or a dependent *regression*; the concordances can refer to *conformity* or to *agreement*.

The diverse associations that can be formed between *two* variables are discussed in the next few chapters. In more advanced activities, when the associations become multivariate, the statistical strategies are more complicated, but they should not be too hard to grasp if you clearly understand what happens for only two variables.

18

Principles of Associations

CONTENTS

Suppose we have measured weight and serum cholesterol in each member of Group A and Group B. The results could be summarized with the univariate and the two-group contrast indexes discussed in Parts I and II of the text. Indexes of location and dispersion could express the univariate values of weight and cholesterol separately in each group. Indexes of contrast could compare the weights and the cholesterol values in Group A vs. Group B. If we wanted to know, however, whether cholesterol tends to rise or fall with increasing levels of weight, we currently do not have a suitable method of expression. To summarize the trend in two variables, we need a new approach, using indexes of association.

Association is a heavy-duty word in statistics. Except for univariate results in a single group of data, *all* statistical arrangements can be regarded as associations of either two variables or more than two.

18.1 Two-Group Contrasts

Although not so designated, the two-group contrasts in Chapters 10 through 17 were really associations of two variables. One of them had a binary scale, identifying the two contrasted groups as A or B, exposed or nonexposed, treated or untreated. The second variable, which was the analytic focus for the two-group comparison, was a dimension (such as age), a binary attribute (such as success/failure or alive/dead), an ordinal grade, or a nominal category. When the results of the second variable were summarized with means, medians, standard deviations, or proportions, the group identity, cited in the first variable, became a subscript (such as A and B, or 1 and 2) in the symbolic expressions $\overline{X}_A$ and $\overline{X}_B$, or p_1 and p_2. The use of two variables is readily apparent if we consider the way the original data would have been coded. An X variable would have identified group membership as A or B (or in some other binary code), and a Y variable would have identified the "result," which would then be summarized for two means as $\overline{Y}_A$ and $\overline{Y}_B$.

The arrangement of data is illustrated in the following layout for four variables that can each receive a two-group contrast. The first column identifies each person; the second column is the X variable, identifying group membership as A or B; and the remaining four columns show Y variables that can be binary, dimensional, ordinal, or nominal.

Person	X Variable	Y Variable			
		Success	Age	Urine Sugar	Color of Eyes
1	B	0	28	Trace	Brown
2	A	1	34	1+	Blue
3	A	0	19	3+	Hazel
4	B	1	42	None	Brown
⋮	⋮	⋮	⋮	⋮	⋮

The two-group contrasts could compare Group A vs. Group B for proportions of success, mean (or median) age, or distributions of urine sugar or color of eyes.

In most instances, however, the idea of *association* is used for situations in which the X variable is dimensional, ordinal, or nominal rather than binary. According to the scale of the corresponding Y variable, the bivariate arrangement will then have a bi-dimensional, bi-ordinal, multi-group, or other format that cannot be summarized with a relatively simple index of *contrast*, and will require new statistical indexes.

18.2 Distinguishing Features of Associations

The indexes that describe associations are prepared for different goals, orientations, and patterns. The goals can be to evaluate trends or concordances; the orientation of variables can be dependent or nondependent; and the patterns can have the diverse formats produced when each variable is expressed in four possible types of scale. These basic distinctions are discussed in the next few sections before we turn to the corresponding statistical principles.

18.2.1 Goals of Evaluation

All of the associations to be discussed here and in the next three chapters refer to a relationship between two variables, but the bivariate relationships can be examined for diverse goals and cited in diverse indexes that reflect the types of variables under examination.

The goals can be aimed at describing *concordances* for the agreement between two similar variables or *trends* for gradients of change, contrast, or correlation between two different variables.

18.2.1.1 Concordances — The distinguishing feature of a *concordance* is that the two associated variables describe exactly the same substantive entity and are cited in exactly the same (i.e., "commensurate") scales. Despite the similarity of scales and measurements, however, the two variables come from different sources, such as different observers, different systems of observation, or two sets of measurements by the same observer. The goal of the analyses is to summarize the *agreement* (or *disagreement*) between the two sets of measurements.

For example, we might check for *inter-observer variability* when two pathologists each give diagnostic "readings" to the same set of slides, for *intra-observer variability* when the same pathologist reads the slides on a second occasion, for *sensitivity* and *specificity* when diagnostic marker tests are checked against the "gold standard" diagnoses, or for *quality control* when the same set of chemical specimens is measured at two different laboratories.

18.2.1.2   Trends — In an evaluation of trend, the two associated variables describe different entities, such as body weight and serum cholesterol. If each variable is ranked in a dimensional or ordinal scale, the goal is to determine the corresponding "movement" for the two sets of rankings. As one variable changes, the trend is shown by the gradient that occurs as the second variable rises, falls, or stays the same. Does serum cholesterol get lower as people get thinner? Does income go up as educational level increases? Is severity of pain related to the amount of fever? All of these questions are answered by examining trends in ranked variables that have dimensional or ordinal scales.

Unless each variable can be ranked, however, the trend cannot always be assessed as a pattern of movement. Because binary and nominal scales do not have successive ups or downs, the idea of *rising* or *falling* cannot be used to express trend in bivariate relationships between religion and occupation, height and choice of hospital, or level of pain and a nominal set of therapeutic agents A, B, C, and D. Nevertheless, even for non-ranked variables, gradients can often be identified in a second variable when changes occur in the first. These gradients will be further discussed in Section 18.2.2.3.

18.2.2   Orientation of Relationship

The two associated variables can be oriented in a dependent or nondependent direction. In a dependent relationship, one variable is believed to affect or influence the other. Thus, we may think that body weight affects serum cholesterol or that treatment produces a successful outcome. These orientations go in one direction because we are not likely to believe that a successful outcome influences the *preceding* treatment or (in most instances) that serum cholesterol influences weight.

A somewhat confusing jargon has been developed for describing the directional distinction. The variable that does the influencing can be called *independent*, *predictive*, or *explanatory*. The affected variable can be called the *dependent*, *target*, or *outcome* variable. In the usual graphic arrangement, shown in Figure 18.1, the independent variable is marked X, and labeled as the *abscissa* in a horizontal direction. The dependent variable is called Y, labeled as the *ordinate*, and placed in a vertical direction. (If you have trouble remembering which is which, a good mnemonic is that alphabetically X precedes Y; and abscissa precedes ordinate.)

Figure 18.2 shows the collection of data points for a dependent relationship of the dimensional variables, serum cholesterol and body weight.

Figure 18.3 shows an analogous set of data points for the dependent relationship of two binary variables, success and treatment. In this instance, success is coded as **0** if absent, and **1** if present; and Treatment is coded **0** for A and **1** for B. The clusters of points at the graph locations of (0, 0), (0, 1), (1, 0) and (l, 1) correspond to the frequency counts that would appear in a 2 × 2 contingency table.

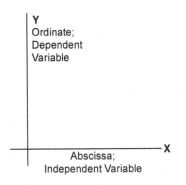

FIGURE 18.1
Graphic outline for data of an independent and dependent variable.

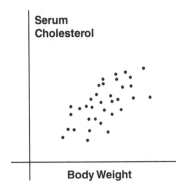

FIGURE 18.2
Relationship of *serum cholesterol* vs. *body weight* as dimensional variables.

As discussed earlier (Section 9.3.1), the axis of contingency tables is usually shifted and rotated, so that the *independent* variable appears in the rows and the *dependent* (or outcome) variable is in the columns. Table 18.1 shows the customary tabular arrangement that would express the data in Figure 18.3.

TABLE 18.1

Tabular Arrangement of Data in Figure 18.3

Treatment	Outcome		TOTAL
	Success	Failure	
A	9	11	20
B	20	6	26
TOTAL	29	17	46

In a *nondependent* relationship, we simply see how the two variables go together, without necessarily implying that one of them is independent and the other dependent. A nondependent association might be examined for the relationship of hematocrit and hemoglobin, or for serum cholesterol and white blood count. Nondependent relationships are sometimes called *interdependent* if the two variables seem distinctly associated — such as hemoglobin and hematocrit — without having a specific dependent orientation.

In evaluations of concordance, the relationship is dependent if one of the variables is regarded as the "gold standard"; and the analysis is concerned with *accuracy* or *conformity* rather than mere *agreement*. Thus, indexes of *sensitivity, specificity,* and *predictive accuracy* all have a directional orientation, whereas other indexes of concordance, such as *proportional agreement*, do not.

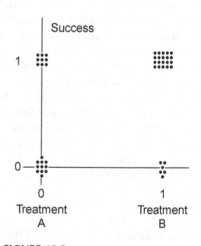

FIGURE 18.3

Relationship of *outcome* (success/failure) vs. *treatment* (A/B) as binary variables.

18.2.2.1 Trends in Ranked Variables — If both
variables can be ranked, trends can easily be examined either nondependently or in a specific directional orientation.

18.2.2.2 Trends for Binary Variables — Although
binary variables do not seem to have ranks, their **0/1** characteristics can readily be used for expressing trends. The two categories of an *independent* binary variable delineate two groups, such as **A** and **B** for *treatment* or **men** and **women** for *sex*. The binary, dimensional, or ordinal results of the *dependent* variable will then indicate the "trend" as the independent variable "moves" from one binary category to the other. These "trends" are the *contrasts* that were discussed throughout Chapters 10 to 17 when the independent variable identified Groups A and B, and the results were compared for such outcomes as the success rates, p_A vs. p_B, for a binary dependent variable, and as the means, $\bar{X}_A$ vs. $\bar{X}_B$, for a dimensional variable, such as *blood sugar*.

For an independent ordinal variable, the results of a binary or dimensional *dependent* variable can be summarized and compared according to changes in rank of the independent variable. For example, suppose the dependent variable is the outcome state of being alive or dead at a particular point in time. Figure 18.4 shows this state for 5 people at four time intervals after zero time. Figure 18.5 is a "survival curve" that summarizes the results for these five people, showing binary proportions of survival at different ranked points in time.

If the ranks refer to severity of illness rather than time, the binary proportions of survival can be shown in a table called a *prognostic stratification* for the *clinical staging system*. Table 18.2 displays results for this type of arrangement.

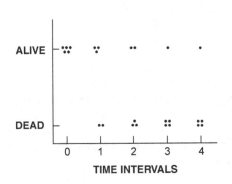

FIGURE 18.4
Data for survival in a group of 5 persons.

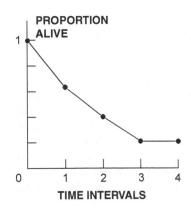

FIGURE 18.5
"Survival Curve" (survival proportions over time) for data in Figure 18.4

TABLE 18.2

Prognostic Stratification Showing Relationship of 5-Year Survival to Clinical Stage of Disease

Variable X (Clinical Stage of Disease)	Variable Y (5-Year Survival Proportions)
I	16/20 (80%)
II	23/50 (46%)
III	21/70 (30%)
IV	6/60 (10%)
TOTAL	66/200(33%)

18.2.2.3 *Special Arrangements for Nominal Variables*

— Because ordinal and dimensional variables can be ranked and binary variables can acquire magnitudes when summarized as proportions, the main problems in describing trend occur for nominal variables. A set of unranked categories, A, B, C, D,…, cannot be put into an ordered arrangement for discerning a specific trend.

If used as the dependent outcome event, a nominal variable is sometimes compressed into a binary variable, and the trend is shown with binary proportions. For example, consider a set of diseases—in heart, lungs, brain, liver, etc.—that can be the outcome associated with such independent variables as a binary *sex*, an ordinal *social class*, a dimensional *age*, or a nominal *ethnic group*. If the nominal dependent variable is dichotomized as **cardiovascular disease** vs. **other**, the binary proportions of cardiovascular disease could promptly be examined in relation to each of the independent variables.

If the *independent* variable is nominal, a similar type of compressed dichotomization would allow simple comparisons. For example, suppose the independent variable, *religion*, contains the four categories **Christian, Hindu, Jewish,** and **Moslem**. The dependent variables might be the dimensional *weight*, the ordinal *stage of clinical severity*, or the binary *college graduate*. The results of the dependent variables could be contrasted in simple arrangements such as **Christian** vs. **All Others** or in pairs of categories such as **Jewish** vs. **Moslem**.

Sometimes, however, the independent nominal variable is kept intact, and the results of the dependent variable are examined simultaneously in all three (or more) of the nominal categories. The indexes for this type of multicategorical arrangement are discussed in Chapter 27.

18.2.3 Patterns Formed by Constituent Variables

The main statistical complexity of bivariate associations is produced by the diverse patterns formed with different scales for the constituent variables. Because each of the two variables can be cited in four possible scales — binary, dimensional, ordinal, or nominal — indexes of descriptive association will be needed for 16 (= 4 × 4) possible patterns. Additional possibilities will occur when the relationships are concordant, or nondependent and dependent trends. The rest of this section, which provides an outlined inventory of the diverse formats, is intended only to let you know about the many different indexes. Fortunately, only a few of them regularly appear in medical research.

The diagram in Figure 18.6 shows 16 possible patterns for co-relationships in scales of an independent and dependent variable. The bi-dimensional pattern in the heavily stippled central zone is the classical and most frequent arrangement; it will be discussed throughout Sections 18.3 and 18.4, and again in Chapter 19. In the three lightly stippled central zones, both variables can be ranked. In seven of the outer zones, around the top and left side of the diagram, at least one of the variables is binary; and in the remaining five zones, at least one of the variables is nominal. These 16 possible patterns will not all occur, however, for concordances or for nondependent trends.

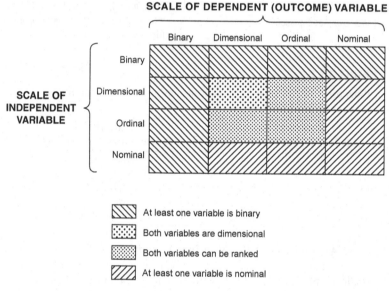

FIGURE 18.6

Possible patterns of co-relationship for two variables, each expressed in four possible scales.

18.2.3.1   Concordance — Because concordance can be measured only when both variables are commensurate — i.e., expressed in exactly the same scales — only four patterns are possible. They arise when the two examined variables are expressed in the same binary-binary, dimensional-dimensional, ordinal-ordinal, or nominal-nominal scales for the same entities. The possible arrangements are shown in Table 18.3. The indexes of concordance for these four patterns of data will be discussed in Chapter 20.

TABLE 18.3

Four Patterns of Variables for Assessing Concordance

		Scale of Variable A			
		Binary	**Dimensional**	**Ordinal**	**Nominal**
Scale of Variable B for Same Entity	Binary	•			
	Dimensional		•		
	Ordinal			•	
	Nominal				•

18.2.3.2 Nondependent Trend — The trend in nondependent correlations can be expressed for four patterns in which the scales for the two variables are binary-binary, ..., or nominal-nominal. For example, the dimensional scales for hematocrit and hemoglobin, although different in magnitude, would form a dimensional-dimensional pair. Six additional patterns can occur, however, when the two associated variables have different types of scales. The additional pairs of scales can be binary-dimensional, binary-ordinal, binary-nominal, dimensional-ordinal, dimensional-nominal and ordinal-nominal as shown in Table 18.4. The names of some of the indexes, as cited in the footnote to Table 18.4, will be discussed either in Chapter 19, or later in Chapter 27.

TABLE 18.4

Patterns of Variables and Statistical Indexes for a Nondependent Correlation*

		Scale of Variable A			
		Binary	**Dimensional**	**Ordinal**	**Nominal**
Scale of Variable B for	Binary	A			
Different Entity	Dimensional	B	C		
	Ordinal	D	E	F	
	Nominal	G	H	I	J

* Examples of correlation indexes, discussed in either Chapter 19 or later in Chapter 27, for these bivariate scales are:
A: ϕ; B: Biserial coefficient; C: Pearson's r; D: Pearson's r or same as F; E: Jasper's multiserial coefficient; F: Spearman's rho, Kendall's tau, gamma, or Somers D; G: ϕ; H: Eta; I: Lambda or Freeman's theta; J: ϕ.

Because the two variables are associated without a direction, the correlations for each pair will be symmetrical, whether the variables are listed directionally in a dimensional-ordinal or ordinal-dimensional orientation. For example, the correlation between the dimensional *height* and the ordinal *social class* or between the nominal *religion* and the binary *sex* would be the same regardless of how the variables are arranged.

18.2.3.3 Dependent Trend — For dependent associations, however, all 16 patterns can occur asymmetrically, as shown in Figure 18.6.

18.2.3.3.1 Binary Constituents. The upper row and left-hand column of Figure 18.6 contain seven patterns in which the independent and/or dependent variable is binary. If independent, the binary variable forms the two groups whose contrasts were previously discussed. If the dependent variable for the two groups is also binary, the contrast (or association) can be shown in a 2 × 2 table, with the results expressed as an index of association or comparison for two proportions. In the other illustrations throughout Chapters 10 to 17, the dependent variables were dimensional values of *blood sugar* (summarized as means) or ordinal values of *improvement*. An independent binary variable could be associated with a nominal dependent variable if we compared *choice of occupation* (**doctor, lawyer, homemaker**, etc.) in *women* and *men*.

A binary dependent variable was associated with a dimensional (or ordinal) independent variable for the "survival curve" constructed in Figure 18.5. Each point on the curve showed the proportion of people who were alive (or dead) at various times after the onset of observation. The binary proportion of survivors could also be associated with an independent variable that is ordinal (e.g., *severity of clinical stage*) or nominal (e.g., different categories of *diagnosis*). In the latter two situations, the results will usually be shown with tables (such as Table 18.2) rather than graphs.

18.2.3.3.2 Nominal Constituents. The lower row and right-hand column of Figure 18.6 contain five patterns in which at least one constituent variable is nominal. These associations will require special arrangements, some of which were mentioned earlier.

18.2.3.3.3 Both Constituents Rankable. For the associations shown in the central four stippled zones of Figure 18.6, both variables can be ranked, being either dimensional or ordinal. This type of jointly ranked relationship is what most people have in mind when thinking about "associations." In particular, the dimensional-dimensional (or "bi-dimensional") pairing is the pattern that gave rise to the well-known ideas of *regression* and *correlation*.

18.3   Basic Mathematical Strategies for Associations

In any form of statistical analysis, the most pertinent basic question is, "What do I really want to know?" The answer to this question indicates the basic *goal* of the analysis. The next question might be, "What statistical strategy is used for this purpose?" The answer indicates the basic *operational principle* used for achieving the goal. The third question is, "What particular index, procedure, or test is used to carry out the strategy?" The answer indicates the particular statistical *method* applied to execute the basic operational principle.

For example, in Part I of the text, one of the goals was to select a single value that would represent a group of dimensional data. The main operational principle for achieving this goal was to choose an item that was "central" in the group. The mode, median, (arithmetic) mean, and geometric mean were methods available to carry out the principle. The choice of the method depended on what we wanted to use as a "central" index.

In Parts I and II of the text, we discovered that the investigator's goals and the operational principles of statistical analysis do not always coincide. For example, if the goal is to evaluate numerical stability for a contrast of two groups, the prime statistical strategy is often *not* aimed directly at stability. Instead, various arrangements of mathematical probability are used to find a P value or a $1 - \alpha$ confidence interval for the summary indexes of the observed contrast. The parametric sampling and the permutation or resampling methods are individual procedures for getting the desired P values or confidence intervals.

Analogous types of disparity between goals and operational principles can arise in the statistical methods developed for indexes of association. These indexes have achieved the general status of established tradition, widespread acceptance, and ubiquitous usage. Nevertheless, if common sense has not been obliterated during all the mathematical explanations and computations, you may sometimes note that what you get is not necessarily what you want.

18.3.1   Basic Mathematical Principles

To summarize a single group of data, the operational principles use a central index and an index of dispersion. To summarize a contrast of two groups, the main principles rely on increments and ratios. For associations, the mathematical principles employ *estimations* and *covariations*. With estimations, one variable is used to estimate (or predict) the value of the other. With covariations, an index of magnitude or strength is determined for the relationship between the two variables.

18.3.1.1   Estimations — For the univariate dimensional data, $\{Y_i\}$, shown on the left of Figure 18.7, suppose we had to guess the value of any individual Y_i that might be chosen from this set. If G is the chosen guess, the individual error will be $Y_i - G$.

From what was learned in univariate statistics (Section 4.6.2), we know that the average absolute error, $|Y_i - G|$, will be smallest if G is chosen to be the median of the data set, and that the average squared error, $(Y_i - G)^2$, will be smallest if G is the mean. Accordingly, the best guess would be either the mean or the median of the Y_i values.

Now suppose that values of an associated variable, X_i, are available for each Y_i, as shown on the right side of Figure 18.7. The pattern of points suggests that the estimates of Y_i could be substantially improved if we made use of the X_i values. For this purpose, we can fit the points with an algebraic model* that

---

* Many types of "models" — including clusters of categories, algorithmic flow charts, and other mathematical or quasi-mathematical structures — can be used in statistical analysis. Models arranged in the form of an equation will be called *algebraic*, a term that seems preferable to *equational*.

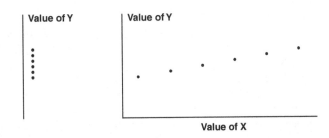

FIGURE 18.7
Display of values, on left, for $\{Y_i\}$ alone, and,
on right, for $\{Y_i\}$ with corresponding $\{X_i\}$.

expresses Y as a "function" of X. The model used most commonly (for reasons discussed later) is the straight line:

$$\hat{Y}_i = a + bX_i. \tag{18.1}$$

In this expression, the "^" symbol over $\hat{Y}_i$ indicates that it is estimated from the corresponding observed value of X_i. The value of a is the *intercept* of the equation, representing the value of $\hat{Y}_i$ when $X_i = 0$. The value of b is the *slope* of the line indicating the number of units of change in $\hat{Y}_i$ for each unitary change of X_i. (The calculation of a and b is discussed in Chapter 19.)

18.3.1.2   *Errors in Estimation* — For each $\hat{Y}_i$ estimated with X_i, the absolute error of the estimate will be $|\hat{Y}_i - Y_i|$ and the squared error will be $(\hat{Y}_i - Y_i)^2$. We can express the accomplishment of the algebraic model by comparing the total errors made when we used only the univariate "guesses" from values of Y alone, versus errors in the bivariate estimates of $\hat{Y}$, using values of X. The expression for proportionate reduction in error would be calculated as

$$\frac{\text{Errors with Y alone} - \text{Errors using X}}{\text{Errors with Y alone}} \tag{18.2}$$

If the expression used the sums of squared errors, the "guesstimates" made from the mean of Y alone would be $S_{yy} = \Sigma(Y_i - \overline{Y})^2$. With S_r as the symbol, the corresponding sum of squared errors for estimates with $\hat{Y}_i$ would be $S_r = \Sigma(Y_i - \hat{Y}_i)^2$. The formula for proportionate reduction in errors would be

$$\frac{S_{yy} - S_r}{S_{yy}} \tag{18.3}$$

The idea of reducing error or improving accuracy is a fundamental principle in constructing indexes of association, and the proportionate reduction in errors is commonly used as an index of the association.

Errors in estimation can also be reduced for associations that are not dimensional. For example, suppose Y is a binary variable showing that the 5-year survival rate is 33% (= 66/200) for a particular disease. If we had to make individual predictions for each patient from the univariate information alone, the best guess would be to predict that everyone will be dead at 5 years. The prediction will be wrong in 66 patients and right in 134.

Now suppose that the patients were classified, as in Table 18.2, into four ordinal stages of disease, expressed as Variable X. Using results of the additional variable, we can form another set of predictions. For the 80% survival rate in Stage I, the prediction of **alive** would be correct in 16 patients and wrong in 4. For Stages II, III, and IV, where the survival rates are below the meridian of 50%, we would predict **death** for everyone. The prediction would be correct, respectively, for 27, 49, and 54 patients and wrong in 23, 21, and 6 patients of those three stages. The total number of predictive errors in the 200 patients would become $4 + 23 + 21 + 6 = 54$; and the proportionate reduction in errors would be calculated, from the 66 with Y alone and the 54 using X, as

$$\frac{66 - 54}{66} = 18\%$$

18.3.1.3   Covariations — The other main principle for indexing an association is to cite the magnitude (or "strength") of covariation in the relationship between the two variables. As X increases, how vigorously does the gradient rise or fall in Y? For example, in Table 18.2, the survival rate drops from 80% to 10% during three "steps" from Stage I to Stage IV, so that the "average" decrease is 70%/3 = 23% for each change of stage.

The gradient of change is easy to discern when results are expressed in the ordinal-binary arrangement of Table 18.2, but a more general approach is needed to show *covariance* when both variables are dimensional. The index should denote the simultaneous change of the two variables in a set of paired points, $\{X_i, Y_i\}$, for each person, i.

Considering each variable alone, the "changes" within X can be cited as the amount by which each item, X_i, deviates from a reference point, which is most commonly chosen to be the arithmetical mean, $\overline{X}$. The deviation, $X_i - \overline{X}$, will then indicate the amount by which any individual value, X_i, has changed from the mean. Similarly, for the other variable Y, the deviation of $Y_i - \overline{Y}$ would indicate the corresponding change in Y_i.

This principle was used to calculate *variance* and *standard deviation* as indexes of univariate dispersion. For n items in variable X, the individual deviations from the mean are squared and added to form the group variance, $S_{xx} = \Sigma(X_i - \overline{X})^2$, which is then divided by n − 1 (or n) to form the variance. A similar process would produce $S_{yy} = \Sigma(Y_i - \overline{Y})^2$ as the group variance in variable Y. The square roots of the two variances would be the corresponding standard deviations.

The two individual deviations for the pair of X_i and Y_i values at point i will have a *bivariate* role if they are multiplied. The product, $(X_i - \overline{X})(Y_i - \overline{Y})$, is the *codeviation* that indicates the simultaneous change as the two variables "move" from their respective means to reach point i. The codeviation product will be positive if both deviations are positive, so that X_i becomes greater than $\overline{X}$, and Y_i greater than $\overline{Y}$. The product will also be positive if both deviations are negative, with X_i and Y_i each becoming less than their corresponding means. If the deviations for $X_i - \overline{X}$ and $Y_i - \overline{Y}$ have opposite signs, the codeviation product will be negative, indicating that the two variables have moved in opposite directions. The greater the absolute magnitude of each codeviation, the greater the amount of movement in a jointly positive or negative direction.

For "movement" within an *individual* variable, the univariate deviations were squared and added to form $S_{xx} = \Sigma(X_i - \overline{X})(X_i - \overline{X})$ and $S_{yy} = \Sigma(Y_i - \overline{Y})(Y_i - \overline{Y})$. For the two variables "moving" together, the individual codeviations are added to form a sum of products that can be called the *group covariance*, symbolized as

$$S_{xy} = \Sigma(X_i - \overline{X})(Y_i - \overline{Y})$$ [18.4]

The average value, obtained when S_{xy} is divided by n (or by n − 1 for inferential purposes) is called the *covariance*. As a quantitative index of co-relationship between two variables, covariance will have a high positive score if the variables generally move together in the same direction, a high negative score if they generally move oppositely, and a score near 0 for no distinct pattern.

18.3.1.3.1   Illustration of Calculations.   To demonstrate the way that covariance indicates co-relationship, consider the illustrative set of data for X_i and Y_i of eight persons in Table 18.5. In addition to the basic values of $\{X_i\}$ and $\{Y_i\}$, the table shows values for $\overline{X}$, $\overline{Y}$, $X_i - \overline{X}$, $Y_i - \overline{Y}$, $(X_i - \overline{X})^2$, $(Y_i - \overline{Y})^2$, and $(X_i - \overline{X})(Y_i - \overline{Y})$. Figure 18.8 is a "scattergraph" for the eight points listed in Table 18.5. In Figure 18.9, the scattergraph has been redrawn, with the axes of origin placed at the mean values of X and Y, forming four quadrants that locate each point according to the deviation units for each variable.

18.3.1.3.2   Pattern and Quantification of Covariance.   The X and Y deviations at each point are both positive in Quadrant I of Figure 18.9 and both negative in Quadrant III. In both of these quadrants the co-deviation product will be positive. Conversely, in Quadrants II and IV, the X and Y deviations go in opposite directions, one being positive and the other negative; and the product of co-deviations in these quadrants will be negative. This distinction is also shown by the values of $(X_i - \overline{X})(Y_i - \overline{Y})$ in

TABLE 18.5

Deviations, Squared Deviations, and Codeviations for an Illustrative Set of Data

| Person | Variables | | $X_i - \bar{X}$ | $(X_i - \bar{X})^2$ | $Y_i - \bar{Y}$ | $(Y_i - \bar{Y})^2$ | $(X_i - \bar{X})(Y_i - \bar{Y})$ |
	X	Y					
A	1	39	−3.88	1 5.05	−27.13	736.04	+105.25
B	2	90	−2.88	8.29	+23.87	569.78	−68.75
C	3	50	−1.88	3.53	−16.13	260.18	+30.32
D	4	82	−.88	.77	+15.87	251.86	−13.97
E	6	43	+1.12	1.25	−23.13	535.00	−25.91
F	7	95	+2.12	4.49	+28.87	833.48	+61.20
G	8	51	+3.12	9.73	−15.13	228.92	−47.21
H	8	79	+3.12	9.73	+12.87	165.64	+40.15
Sum	39	529	0	52.88	0	3580.88	+81.13
Mean	$\bar{X} = 4.88$	$\bar{Y} = 66.13$	0	6.61	0	447.61	10.14

Note: Divisor for all mean values = 8.

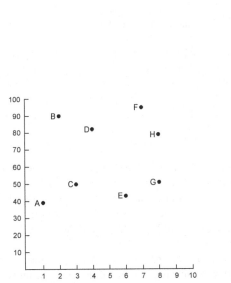

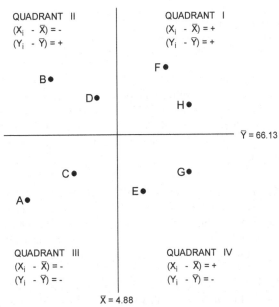

FIGURE 18.8
"Scattergraph" of data in Table 18.5.

FIGURE 18.9
Mean values of X and Y used as axes for scattergraph of data in Table 18.5 and Figure 18.8.

Table 18.5. For persons A, C, F, and H, whose points lie in Quadrants I or III, each co-deviation is positive. For persons B, D, E, and G, whose points lie in Quadrants II or IV, the products are negative.

To show the general impact of co-deviations, arbitrary collections of illustrative points (not the ones shown in Figure 18.8 and 18.9) have been placed in the appropriate quadrants of Figures 18.10 and 18.11. In Figure 18.10, where all the codeviate points lie in the first and third quadrants, the swarm of points shows a distinct positive relationship between X and Y. In Figure 18.11, where all of the points lie in the second and fourth quadrants, the pattern shows a distinct negative or inverse relationship. (An important feature of terminology for co-relationships is that *negative* means something going in a direction distinctively opposite to *positive*. In many medical uses, the word *negative* refers to "none" or "normal"; but in the absence of a distinct co-relation, the correct word is *none*, not *negative*. To avoid possible confusion, however, a negative co-relationship is often called *inverse*.)

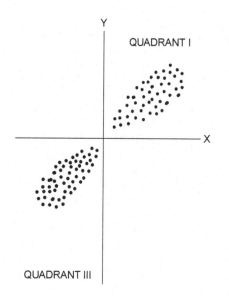

FIGURE 18.10
Positive correlation effect evident from "swarm" of co-deviate points in Quadrants I and III of a scattergraph.

FIGURE 18.11
Negative correlation effect evident from "swarm" of co-deviate points in Quadrants II and IV of scattergraph.

As the average value of $\Sigma(X_i - \overline{X})(Y_i - \overline{Y})$, the covariance could quantitatively indicate the positive or negative strength of the relationship. For example, the group of eight points in Figure 18.8 do not show a strong relationship in either direction. Their average codeviance (as shown in Table 18.5) is 10.14. On the other hand, if we consider only the contributions of points A, C, F, and H (in Quadrants I and III), their average co-deviance is +236.93/4 = +59.23; and for just the points B, D, E, and H, the average co-deviance is –155.83/4 = –38.96.

18.3.1.4   *Correlation Coefficient* — Although helping quantify a co-relationship, the average magnitude of S_{xy} depends completely on the arbitrary units in which X and Y are expressed. If each value of Y in Table 18.5 were ten times larger (e.g., 390, 900, 500,...rather than 39, 90, 50,...) the values of Y would be ten times larger for the mean and deviations, and the values of S_{xy} and S_{xy} /n would also be ten times larger. Nevertheless, the basic relationship between X and Y would remain the same.

18.3.1.4.1   Product of Standardized Deviates.   To eliminate this problem, each variable can be expressed in the Z-scores that form standardized deviates, thereby making S_{xy} free of dimensional units. Thus, if s_x is the standard deviation of the X values, the entity $(X_i - \overline{X})/s_x$ is dimension-free, cited in standard-deviation units above or below the mean of X. The counterpart entity, $(Y_i - \overline{Y})/s_y$, has a similar structure for values of Y. Each product of the standard deviation scores would be

$$\left(\frac{X_i - \overline{X}}{s_x}\right)\left(\frac{Y_i - \overline{Y}}{s_y}\right)$$

and the sum of these standardized codeviations would be $\Sigma[(X_i - \overline{X})(Y_i - \overline{Y})]/s_x s_y$, which is $S_{xy}/[(s_x)(s_y)]$. The mean value of this sum (using n as the divisor) would be $(S_{xy}/n)/[(s_x)(s_y)]$. Because $s_x = \sqrt{S_{xx}/n}$ and $s_y = \sqrt{S_{yy}/n}$, some further algebra will show that the new index would be

$$r = \frac{S_{xy}}{\sqrt{S_{xx}S_{yy}}} \qquad\qquad [18.5]$$

(The same result would emerge if each divisor were n – 1 rather than n.)

This index is customarily symbolized as *r* and called the *correlation coefficient*. It is also sometimes called *Pearson's r*, to commemorate Karl Pearson, who helped popularize its use for expressing correlation. In older statistical language, values of $X_i - \overline{X}$ and $Y_i - \overline{Y}$ were called the "first moment around the mean." For this reason, the correlation coefficient is sometimes called the *product-moment coefficient*.

Some additional algebra, shown in Chapter 19, will demonstrate that r has a maximum positive value of +1 and a maximum negative value of −1. Thus, when the "standardized" dimension-free r has values close to +1 or −1, the two variables have a strong relationship. When r is close to 0, they have little or no relationship.

18.3.1.4.2 Example of Calculations. The sums of appropriate columns in Table 18.5 show that $S_{xx} = 52.88$, $S_{yy} = 3580.88$, and $S_{xy} = 81.13$. Substituting these values in Formula [18.5], the correlation coefficient for the data is

$$r = \frac{81.13}{\sqrt{52.88 \times 3580.88}} = \frac{81.13}{435.15} = 0.186$$

which indicates the weak positive relationship evident in Figure 18.8. If you do these calculations yourself, some computing formulas can greatly ease the job. Just as $\Sigma(X_i - \overline{X})^2 = \Sigma X_i^2 - n\overline{X}^2$ was best calculated as $S_{xx} = \Sigma X_i^2 - [(\Sigma X_i)^2/n]$, the best "hand-calculator" formula for the group covariance is

$$S_{xy} = \Sigma X_i Y_i - [(\Sigma X_i)(\Sigma Y_i)/n] \qquad [18.6]$$

For example, as shown in the Sum row of Table 18.5, $\Sigma X_i = 39$ and $\Sigma Y_i = 529$. The additional items needed for the quick calculations are $\Sigma X_i^2 = 243$, $\Sigma Y_i^2 = 38561$, and $\Sigma X_i Y_i = 2660$. These items would lead to $S_{xx} = 243 - [(39)^2/8] = 52.88$ and $S_{yy} = 38561 - [(529)^2/8] = 3580.88$. The group covariance, $S_{xy} = \Sigma(X_i - \overline{X})(Y_i - \overline{Y})$, was originally calculated in Table 18.5 by directly adding each codeviation to get +81.13. The quick-calculation Formula [18.6] would produce $2660 - [(39)(529)/8] = 81.13$.

18.3.2 Choice of Principles

According to the goals, orientation, and patterns of data, indexes of association will be formed with principles of estimation or principles of covariation, and sometimes with both. For example, to demonstrate closeness of agreement in appraising concordance or to make specific predictions, the emphasis is on principles of estimation. To appraise trend in the two variables, the focus is on covariation.

The two indexes of expression — for estimation and covariation — will indicate different attributes of the association. A weak relationship can produce highly accurate estimations, and a strong relationship may have many errors. For example, in Figure 18.7, Y seems to have a weak relationship to X: the values of Y go up only slightly as X increases. Yet the estimates of Y made from X might have perfect accuracy because a straight line would fit the data so well. Conversely, in Table 18.2, the two variables have a strong (although inverse) relationship, but the error rate in predictions is proportionately reduced only 18%.

18.4 Concept and Strategy of Regression

Regression has become the well established name for a process that fits a mathematical "model" to data of a dependent variable. The same term is also regularly used in calling the result a *regression line*.

18.4.1 Historical Background

Fitting a mathematical model was *not* the idea, however, when the term *regression* was originally proposed in 1885 by Francis Galton, who is often regarded (at least in English-speaking countries) as the founder of biometry. While studying familial manifestations of genetics, Galton compared the height of parents and the corresponding height of their children. Fitting a straight line to the plot of points presented here in Figure 18.12, Galton[1] noted a phenomenon that he initially called *reversion* but later

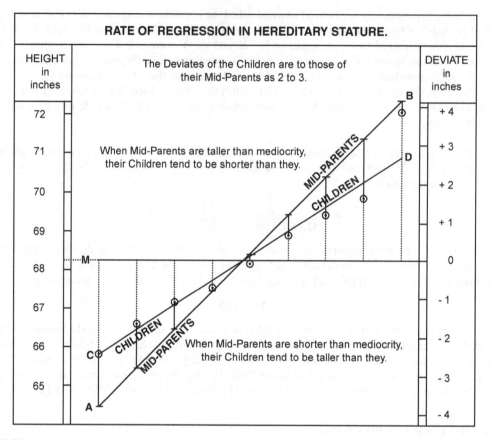

FIGURE 18.12
Format of graph displayed by Francis Galton to demonstrate "regression toward mediocrity." [Figure derived from Chapter Reference 1.]

termed *regression toward mediocrity*. The tallest parents tended to have children who were shorter than themselves; and the shortest parents tended to have correspondingly taller children. The extreme values of tall or short height for the parents were associated, in the children, with heights that were closer to the mean for each variable.

18.4.2   Regression to the Mean

The phenomenon Galton noted as reversion to mediocrity is today called *regression to the mean* and is still regularly encountered, but not in Galton's format. In subsequent repeated measurements of people who initially have the highest (or lowest) values of blood pressure or serum cholesterol in a group, the originally extreme values often tend to regress toward the mean of the group. The data analyst then has to decide whether the change was due to treatment or whether values that were higher because of random variation had later regressed to the mean.[2,3] [An analogous event, occurring in professional sports, is sometimes called the "outstanding rookie's second-year slump." The person who may have randomly been the best player among the first-year rookies may regress to the mean in the next year, and is thought to have "slumped."]

   Galton used the term *regression* for the straight line that he drew through the bivariate dimensional points for heights of parents and children in Figure 18.12, but the mathematical strategy that fit the line to the data had nothing to do with either the biologic idea of regression to the mean, or the statistical idea that with random variations in measurement, the extreme values on one occasion subsequently become closer to the mean. Nevertheless, the term *regression* became rapidly accepted and thoroughly entrenched for a totally different idea: the mathematical procedure of fitting a line to a set of bivariate dimensional data.

18.4.3 Straight-Line Models and Slopes

Although many kinds of curved lines can be fitted to a bi-dimensional set of points, the standard approach uses a rectilinear, i.e., straight-line, model, $Y = a + bX$, which is mathematically arranged to do its best job in fitting the data. The fit may be good or poor, but the slope of the straight line indicates a trend that is constant throughout all zones of the data. Consequently, no matter how well the line fits, the single value of its slope will be misleading if the data have different gradients in different zones. Thus, if we want to know the *general* trend of the data, the single slope may be a quite satisfactory average, but if we want to know about the trends in different zones, the single slope may produce serious distortions of what is happening.

The problem is illustrated for bi-dimensional data by the three sets of points shown in Figure 18.13. Figure 18.14 shows the results of applying a best-fitting straight-line model to each set of points. As expected from the pattern of points, the left-hand set of data is excellently fit by the straight line. The middle set of data is relatively well fit by the straight line, which will be given credit for a good achievement, according to the customary indexes of fit (discussed in Chapter 19). Nevertheless, the slope of the line will fail to show the three different gradients present in the three zones of data: small gradients at the low and high ends of the X variable and a large gradient in the middle.

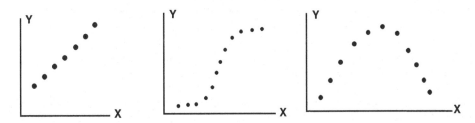

FIGURE 18.13
Patterns for three sets of bi-dimensional points.

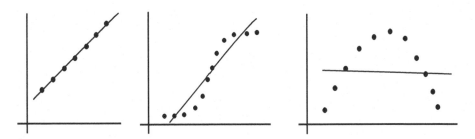

FIGURE 18.14
Best-fitting straight lines for the patterns shown in Figure 18.13.

For the right-hand set of data in Figures 18.13 and 18.14, the straight line will have a slope close to 0, indicating no relationship between X and Y. Nevertheless, X and Y have the strong relationship that is evident from visual inspection of the pattern. The straight line will completely distort this pattern, by failing to capture the large gradient, at the beginning of the X variable, that later reversed into another large gradient going in the opposite direction.

18.4.4   Reasons for Straight-Line Models

Looking at the obvious curves in the middle and right side of Figures 18.13 and 18.14, you may wonder why the data were fitted with a straight line. With alternative algebraic formats, a curve could have been created to fit each set of data almost perfectly. For example, the middle set of data could be fit exactly with a curve such as $\ln[Y/(1 - Y)] = a + bX$. The right-hand set of data could be fit exactly with a curve such as $Y = a -(X-b)^2$. Why not use curves rather than straight lines?

The five main reasons for routine use of straight-line models are: (1) the curvilinear models are usually difficult to choose; (2) the straight-line model is standard and easy to interpret; (3) it produces indexes for both estimation and co-relation; (4) in bivariate data, the straight-line model can be used for both the dependent relationship of *regression* and the interdependent relationship of *correlation*; and (5) in bivariate data, the correlation coefficient is the standardized regression coefficient. These distinctions are discussed in the next five subsections.

18.4.4.1   *Problems in Choosing Curves* — The curvilinear patterns in the data of Figures 18.13 and 18.14 were reasonably obvious. If you are familiar with the shape of different curves, you would have promptly recognized the S-shaped "logistic" pattern of the middle set of data and the inverted-U parabola of the right-hand set.

In many instances, however, the corresponding correct shape is not immediately apparent. For example, consider the pattern of points in Figure 18.15. This set of points could be fit by many different curves. The pattern could be part of a descending exponential curve having the form $Y = e^{a-bX}$, but could also be part of a polynomial expression such as $Y = a + bX + cX^2 + dX^3 + fX^4$, or a segment of a giant oscillating curve, such as a sine or cosine wave. From the limitless number of curves that might be fitted to these data, an appropriately programmed computer could readily find one that fits excellently, but we would not know whether the selected curve is correct for the true relationship between X and Y. The excellent fit might be an artifact in which the "best" fit may not be the right fit.

A more substantial problem arises when the pattern of points does not have an obvious shape. Consider the set of data shown in Figure 18.16. This pattern looks more like the customary results of medical research than any of the illustrations in Figures 18.14 or 18.15. The data set of Figure 18.16 does not have an obvious rectilinear or curvilinear pattern. Because these data could be assigned to almost any selected pattern, the straight-line format has the advantage of being "standard." It avoids the arbitrary choice of a candidate from one of the many possible curves.

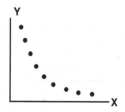

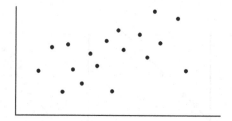

FIGURE 18.15
Pattern of points for which the appropriate curve has many possibilities

.FIGURE 18.16
Patterns of points for which no linear pattern seems immediately apparent.

18.4.4.2   *Problems in Interpreting Curvilinear Results* — If the goal is to evaluate trend, the result of a straight line is easy to interpret: the trend is the slope. With the line expressed as $Y = a + bX$, its slope, b, is called the *regression coefficient*. It indicates that Y changes by the amount of b units for every unitary change in X. With curvilinear models, however, trends are much more difficult and sometimes impossible to determine. Suppose the curve is expressed as $Y = a + bX - cX^2 - dX^3 + eX^4$. The trend, i.e., the change in Y as X changes, could eventually be determined from this curve, but the process would not be easy. The trends would differ in different sectors of the X values, and a great deal of computation would be needed to determine the locations of the sectors and the magnitude of the trends.

Consequently, a straight-line model has a second major advantage: The single regression coefficient for slope is easy to interpet as an index of trend for the co-relationship.

18.4.4.3   The "Two-Fer" Bonus — All regression models, whether straight lines or curves, are mathematically constructed (as noted in Chapter 19) to produce a "best fit" for the estimated values of Y. While producing this estimate, however, the straight-line model has the "two-fer" advantage of offering a bonus: the regression coefficient, b, is an easy-to-interpret index of the co-relationship between Y and X.

18.4.4.4   Indexes for Both Correlation and Regression — For any two variables, X and Y, we can assume either that Y depends on X or that X depends on Y. For the first assumption, the regression line takes the form

$$Y = a + bX$$

For the second assumption, the regression line has different coefficients expressed as

$$X = a' + b'Y$$

As noted later in Chapter 19, these two lines are seldom identical. They will usually have different values for a and a′ and for b and b′; and the trend that is manifested by the regression coefficient will differ if we regress Y on X or X on Y. As both regression lines are legitimate, what do we do if interested not in regression, but in correlation? Suppose we want to know the interdependent trend between the two variables, rather than the slope of Y on X or the slope of X on Y?

The answer to this question involves another act of mathematical elegance that will be demonstrated in Chapter 19. The correlation coefficient, r, which indicates interdependent trend, is obtained like a geometric mean, as the square root of the product of the two slopes, b and b′. In other words,

$$r = \sqrt{(b)(b')}$$

Thus, the fourth advantage of the straight-line model is that the bivariate correlation coefficient is the geometric mean of the two possible regression coefficients.

18.4.4.5   Correlation and Standardized Regression — The advantage just mentioned may not immediately seem impressive. To get the correlation coefficient symmetrically, as the square root of bb′, is a neat mathematical feat, but why should anyone be excited about it? The answer to this question, as demonstrated later in Chapter 19, is that the ordinary regression coefficient is affected by the units of measurement. In quantifying the dependent trend between Y and X, the regression coefficient will be larger or smaller according to whether X is measured in days, weeks, or years and Y in pounds or kilograms. In bivariate data, however, the correlation coefficient, as discussed throughout Section 18.3.1.4, is analogous to a standardized Z-score that is unaffected by units of measurement. The correlation coefficient, r, is a standardized regression coefficient, having exactly the same value whether Y is regressed on X or X is regressed on Y.

The fifth advantage of the bivariate straight-line model, therefore, is that the correlation coefficient can be used in a standardized way to compare the strengths of different co-relationships, regardless of the units in which the variables were measured.

18.4.5   Disadvantages of Straight-Line Models

In exchange for these many advantages, straight-line models have the flaws that have already been cited. The actual pattern of the data may be distorted by its transmogrification into a linear pattern, and the single, constant index of trend, although correct on average, may be wrong in many zones of the data.

The problem is not altered by using the correlation coefficient, r, rather than the regression coefficient, b, as an index of trend. Because the correlation coefficient seems to have been constructed as a product of standardized deviates for X and Y, without invoking a linear model such as Y = a + bX, we might expect the correlation coefficient to be unaffected by linearity in the data. That expectation is wrong, because the "linear" deviates of $X_i - \overline{X}$ and $Y_i - \overline{Y}$ were used to form the products calculated as covariance. These products can give a distorted account of the co-relationship if X and Y do not have a rectilinear pattern. Besides, as noted later in Chapter 19, r will have the same flaws as b because it can be calculated simply as a "standardized" transformation of b.

The distortion of non-rectilinear dimensional patterns was shown earlier in Figures 18.13 and 18.14. The distortion of zones can be seen in the previous results of Table 18.2, where the survival proportions were 80% in **Stage I**, 46% in **Stage II**, 30% in **Stage III**, and 10% in **Stage IV**. Without any special mathematical concepts, the trend of this relationship is easily shown by the incremental gradient in survival rates from one stage (or zone) to the next. The overall survival gradient is 70% (= 80 −10) between Stages I and IV, but the intermediate zonal gradients are distinctly unequal. They have a drop of 34% between Stages I and II, 16% between Stages II and III, and 20% from III to IV. These inequalities show that the trend is not the same in different zones of data, although the *average* gradient for the three increments would be about 70%/3 ≃ 23%. With certain techniques discussed later, a straight line could be fitted to these data. The slope of that line would show the average decline in survival proportions between Stages I and IV. The constant value of the slope, however, would not indicate the distinct differences in component gradients for the zones. The question about overall trend in the data would get a reasonable, respectable answer, but the answer would not reveal the striking differences in the inter-zonal trends.

A crucial basic issue for the investigator, therefore, is: What kind of trend do we want to know about? Is it the average overall trend or the distinctive differences that can occur in the constituent zones of the data? The answer to this question is pertinent not only when bivariate data are fitted with straight-line models but particularly in multivariable analysis, where everything may depend on the results achieved with "linear models." According to what we really want to know, these models can be entirely correct statistically, while producing gross distortions scientifically.

18.5   Alternative Categorical Strategies

Despite the possible problems and distortions, the straight-line mathematical models have generally been quite successful. In fact, this approach was used (without being deliberately identified) when two central indexes were contrasted in Chapter 10. If we code X = 0 for all members of Group A and X = 1 for all members of Group B, the pattern of points for dimensional data is as shown in Figure 18.17. The means for these two groups could be expressed as $\overline{Y}_A$ for Group A and $\overline{Y}_B$ for Group B. The increment of $\overline{Y}_B - \overline{Y}_A$ is really the slope of the line joining the mean values of Y as X moves from **0** (for Group A) to **1** (for Group B).

This process is easy to conceive and illustrate because we could arbitrarily set the values of X at **0** and **1** for the two groups. If X has its own dimensional values, however, the data might have the bi-dimensional pattern shown in Figure 18.16. Despite the many cited virtues of the straight-line model, the pattern of data in Figure 18.16 does not intuitively suggest that a straight line (or any other linear shape) should be fitted. What can be done instead?

The main alternative strategy is to abandon the idea of fitting the data with straight lines or any other arbitrary mathematical shape. Instead, the data are divided into categories (or zones), and the results are examined directly within those zones. Diverse mathematical tactics can be used during the examinations — but no attempt is made to fit the data into the overall "shape" of a mathematical model.

18.5.1   Double Dichotomous Partitions

In one approach, the bi-dimensional data of Figure 18.16 are converted into two groups. A dichotomous partition at the median value of X will produce two groups of equal size, as shown in Figure 18.18. The mean values of Y can then be determined in each group and compared as an increment.

In another possible approach, the data of Figure 18.16 become a "double dichotomy" when another partition is added at the *median* of the *total* set of Y values. This partition would divide Figure 18.18 into the four categories shown in Figure 18.19. The values above and below the median could then be called

high and **low**, and binary proportions could be compared for the occurrence of high values in the two groups. With the median arbitrarily assigned here to the higher group, the data in Figure 18.19 would form the following 2×2 table.

| | Value of Y | | | Proportion of |
Value of X	<Median	≥Median	Total	"High" Values of Y
<Median	6	3	9	.33
≥Median	3	6	9	.67

These results immediately show that Group B (with X values ≥ median) has a larger proportion of high values of Y than Group A.

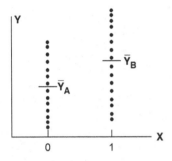

FIGURE 18.17
Pattern of points and means for two-group contrast where X = 0 for Group A and X = 1 for Group B.

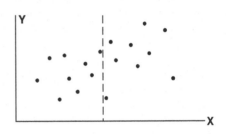

FIGURE 18.18
Median drawn through X variable to divide data of Figure 18.16 into two groups.

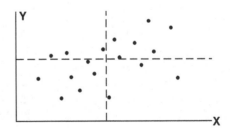

FIGURE 18.19
Medians drawn through X and Y variables to divide data of Figure 18.16 into four groups.

18.5.2 Ordinal Strategies

The main objection to a dichotomous split for the X variable is that the result shows a contrast rather than a distinctive trend. Whenever only two groups are compared, one set of values will almost always (on average) be *higher* or *lower* than the other, but the contrast does not convey a *rising* or *falling* sense of movement.

The trend in movement of the data can be explored, however, if the X variable is partitioned into more than two categories. For dimensional values of X, this partition can produce a set of three, four, five, or more ordinal categories. The trend can then be examined for summaries of the Y variable as a mean, median, or proportion in each of those categories.

To produce a definite central category, the X variable is often split into an odd number of zones. To avoid invidious choices of boundaries and to distribute the data into relatively equal-sized groups, the split is usually done with quantiles of X. The simplest partition divides X at its tertiles. As shown in

Figure 18.20, a tertile split for the X variable of Figure 18.16 produces two boundaries and divides the abscissa into three categorical zones. The proportions of "high" Y values in those three categories of X are .33 (2/6), .50 (3/6), and .67 (4/6). Although the group sizes are small, the equal gradients are compatible with a "linear" relationship.

If relatively abundant, the data are often partitioned at the quintiles, which will divide X into five equal-sized ordinal groups. The trend can readily be discerned from the summary value of Y in each group as X "moves" from the lowest to highest category.

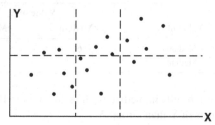

18.5.3   Choosing Summaries for Y

In choosing a summary value to show the trend of Y in each category, we could use a mean or median, but neither of these values would immediately indicate the stability of the data. With dimensional summaries, a second index, such as a standard deviation or ipr_{95},

FIGURE 18.20
Tertile partition for X and median partition for Y in the data of Figure 18.16.

would be needed to help denote stability. Consequently, although many data analysts will check the trend in Y by examining medians or means, many other analysts prefer to inspect the binary proportions in each zone, expressed as p = t/n, where t is the count in the "high" or other category demarcated for the binary split of n members. The single value of p immediately shows the magnitude of the binary proportion, and the constituent elements, t/n, will immediately indicate the stability. With the latter approach, the Y variable would be split at its median *for the total data* (as shown in Figure 18.20), and each of the X groups would be summarized, as in Section 18.5.2, for the proportion of values that lie either above or below the median.

18.5.4   Comparison of Linear-Model and Categorical Strategies

For another set of bi-dimensional data, shown in Figure 18.21, a straight line could be fitted (by methods to be discussed in Chapter 19) as $\hat{Y}_i = 6.39 + 0.118X_i$. An alternative categorical approach, with quintile partitions for X and a binary split for Y, is shown in Figure 18.22. Using **I, II, ..., V** for the five zones of X, the binary proportions for high values of and Y in each zone are **I**: .20(1/5); **II**: .33(2/6); **III**: .50(3/6); **IV**: .60(3/5); and **V**: .80(4/5). The numbers are small, and all of the proportions are unstable. Nevertheless, the upward trend in the data seems quite clear.

The overall gradient across the five quintiles is .80 − .20 = .60, which produces an average gradient of .60/4 = .15 for each of the four changes in the 5 categories of X. Because X ranges from 0 to 50, the average span in each zone is 10 units. The average gradient in each zone is thus .15/10 = .015. When Y changes from low to high values, the mean of the 14 low (i.e., ≤10) values of Y is 6.07, and the mean

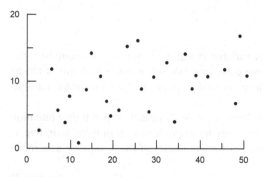

FIGURE 18.21
Set of bi-dimensional data.

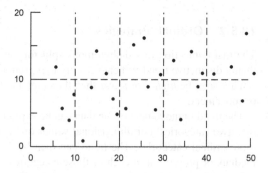

FIGURE 18.22
Quintile partition for X and median partition for Y in data of Figure 18.21.

of the 13 high values is 12.92. Thus, the average change from a low to high value is 6.85 units (= 12.92 – 6.07) in Y. Accordingly, the average change in Y is (6.85)(.015) = .103 per unit change in X. This average value, obtained with only a crude binary-quintile split, is reasonably close to the coefficient of 0.118 obtained when the average slope was calculated with the regression-model equation.

18.5.5 Role of Categorical Examination

You can decide for yourself whether you prefer to use a line or a series of central indexes to discern the trend of data in such Figures as 18.16 or 18.21. In this instance, both approaches lead to essentially the same conclusion: a generally rising trend. (The denominators are too small in each of the five zones to draw any firm conclusions about major changes in trend *between* adjacent zones.)

The alternative categorical strategies often play a role analogous to that of a history and physical examination in clinical practice, but they can also be the "gold standard" for showing exactly what is happening. They allow you to inspect the data directly, without being constrained by whatever emerges from application of a straight-line or other arbitrary algebraic model. The alternative categorical strategy may sometimes be just as arbitrary as a straight line, but the arbitrariness is chosen by you rather than by mathematical doctrines. One of the magnificent intellectual contributions of modern electronic computation is *not* the capacity for complex calculation, but the ability to let you easily explore your own data. With these explorations, you can do commonsense "clinical" evaluations that might otherwise be lost amid the mathematical elegance and computational splendor.

This type of exploration can promptly reveal the distortions that may occur in relatively simple bivariate analyses. For example, if you did not plot a graph of points for the collections of data in the middle and right sides of Figure 18.13, you would not know about the curving patterns. If you then examined only the value of b for the slope of the regression lines, you would totally miss the changing trends in different zones. A categorical examination of trends in tertile or quintile splits of the X variables, however, would promptly indicate the distinctions that were missed by the straight-line model.

A further advantage of categorical evaluations occurs, as discussed elsewhere,[4] in multivariable analyses. The algebraic models rely on a series of mathematical assumptions about straight-line or other shapes for the data, but the basic assumptions are often difficult to check or confirm. If you really want to know about trends in different zones of the data, the exploration of categorical groups becomes the "gold standard" for determining whether a mathematical model has distorted the results.

References

1. Galton, 1885; 2. Davis, 1976; 3. Healy, 1978; 4. Feinstein, 1996.

Exercises

Because this chapter is intended mainly to describe background strategy and ideas, the exercises do not involve many statistical operations or calculations.

18.1. Here are two opportunities to improve your skill in the "physical examination" of graphs.

> 18.1.1. Figure E.18.1.1 shows a straight line drawn for the points of two variables. Without knowing how the line was determined and without trying to verify its coefficients, what is one simple thing you can do mentally, without any formal calculations or specific manipulations, to determine that the line is drawn *correctly* on the graph?

> 18.1.2. The intercept seems to be wrong for the straight line in Fig. E.18.1.2; because the line does not meet the Y-axis at a value of –0.91. What feature of the graph suggests that the cited value is correct? How could you check it? Does the slope seem correct? Does the line seem to fit properly?

18.2. In any published literature at your disposal, find a paper where the authors used a straight-line pattern to summarize the trend in a set of bivariate dimensional data. The points of data should have been shown in a graph, together with an equation for the corresponding line. Although you do not yet know how that line was formulated, submit a replicate copy of the graph (indicating its publication source) and describe your comfort or discomfort in accepting the line as a "summary" of the bivariate relationship.

After describing your response, make "guesstimates" or other arrangements of the data points to prepare an alternative analysis that might help confirm or refute your reaction. You get extra credit if you find a graph that left you uncomfortable, give good reasons for the discomfort, and prove your point with the alternative analysis.

18.3. The most common associations that appear in medical literature involve either bi-dimensional data or the doubly dichotomous "contrast" shown in a 2×2 table. Examining the tables or graphs of any published papers that are conveniently available, find two examples of associations that are *not* either bi-dimensional or "double dichotomies." Show and label the skeleton structure of categories and/or dimensions (not the actual data) in the table or graph that connects the two variables.

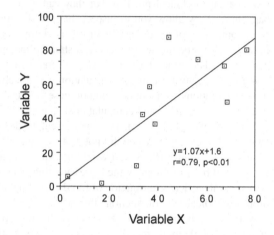

FIGURE E.18.1.1
Relationship between Variable Y and Variable X in 11 persons.. A significant correlation was found ($y = 1.07x + 0.02$, $r = 0.79$, $2P < 0.01$).

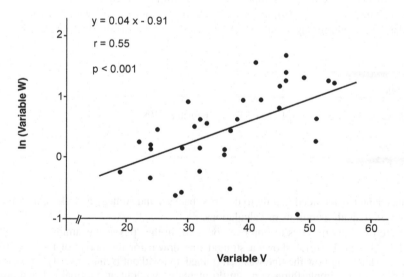

FIGURE E.18.1.2
Data and regression analysis for relationship of Variable W vs. Variable V. Variable W was appraised as a logarithm because of an "uneven distribution."

19

Evaluating Trends

CONTENTS

Like any set of strategic principles, the estimations and covariations discussed in Chapter 18 need operational methods to obtain specific results and to evaluate the accomplishments. This chapter is devoted to the most commonly used "classical" methods that produce regression and correlation analyses for bi-dimensional data.

The first four main sections of the chapter contain many statistical concepts and indexes that "set the stage" before the pragmatic "show" of applications and abuses arrives in Sections 5 and 6. The lengthy discourse is justified because everything previously discussed in the text (for one and two groups) and almost everything that follows (for more complex statistical activities later and even for multivariable analyses) can be regarded as extensions of the basic principles used for correlation and regression.

19.1   Linear Model of Regression

Anyone who has seen straight-line graphs for expressing the data of physics or chemistry will be immediately familiar with using the *slope* of the line as an index of a targeted relationship. If Y depends on X, and if the straight line is expressed as $Y = a + bX$, the slope of the line is b. If Y tends to rise as X rises, the line will slope upward and b will be positive; if Y tends to fall as X rises, the line will slope downward and b will be negative. The steeper the slope, the greater will be the absolute magnitude of b, and the stronger the relationship. If the line is essentially horizontal, showing no substantially upward or downward slope, b will be close to zero, suggesting that Y has little or no relationship to X.

When this same principle is used in bivariate analyses, we first make the assumption that X and Y have a rectilinear relationship, and we then find the slope of the straight line that best fits the data. There will actually be two possible lines: one in which Y depends on X, and the other in which X depends on Y.

19.1.1   Regression Coefficient

If Y depends on X, the line expressed as

$$\hat{Y}_i = a + bX_i$$

represents the *regression* of Y on X. The $\hat{Y}_i$ estimates the value of Y that lies on the line for each observed value of X_i. The Y_i symbol, without the hat, represents the corresponding observed value in the data.

As shown later (in Appendix A.19.2) the value of the intercept, *a*, is calculated as $\overline{Y} - b\overline{X}$. Accordingly, the line is regularly written in the form of deviations as

$$\hat{Y}_i - \overline{Y} = b(X_i - \overline{X}) \qquad [19.1]$$

When $X_i = \overline{X}$, $\hat{Y}_i = \overline{Y}$. Therefore, the line always passes through the mean of the two variables. When $X_i = 0$, $\hat{Y}_i = \overline{Y} - b\overline{X} = a$, and so the line intersects the y-axis at the *intercept* value of a. The slope of the line, b, is called the *regression coefficient*.

19.1.1.1   Method of Calculation — Of the various approaches that might be used for determining the appropriate values of *a* and *b* for the data, the traditional and still most popular strategy is the "principle of least squares." According to this principle, b is chosen to give the smallest possible (i.e., the "least") value to the quantity $\Sigma(Y_i - \hat{Y}_i)^2$. Each $Y_i - \hat{Y}_i$ value represents the residual deviation between the observed Y_i and the estimated $\hat{Y}_i$; and the goal is to minimize the sum of squares for the residual deviations. With the symbol r (for regression or residual), this sum is $S_r = \Sigma(Y_i - \hat{Y}_i)^2$.

The desired minimization of squared deviations in S_r occurs when

$$b = \frac{S_{xy}}{S_{xx}} \qquad [19.2]$$

A proof of this assertion is given in Appendix 19.1; and the proof in Appendix 19.2 shows that as soon as we know *b*, we can determine

$$a = \overline{Y} - b\overline{X} \qquad [19.3]$$

Consequently, for the data in Table 18.5, where $S_{xy} = 81.13$ and $S_{xx} = 52.88$, we can calculate b = 81.13/52.88 = 1.53; and with $\overline{Y} = 66.13$ and $\overline{X} = 4.88$, we find that a = 66.13 – (1.53) (4.88) = 58.64.

The regression coefficient, b, has an intuitively appealing construction. As the covariance of the XY values, S_{xy}/n shows the way that the two variables change simultaneously. As the variance of the X values, S_{xx}/n shows the changes that occur in X alone. When S_{xy}/n is divided by S_{xx}/n to form S_{xy}/S_{xx}, we would expect to index the changes that occur in Y as changes occur in X. This index is exactly what is calculated as the slope of the line. (The same S_{xy}/S_{xx} value would emerge if each divisor for the group values were n − 1 rather than n.)

19.1.1.2 *Expression and Graph of Regression Line*

— As soon as b and a are found, we can immediately draw the regression line on a graph. Equation [19.1] shows that the line passes through the point $(\overline{X}, \overline{Y})$; and when $X_i = 0$, the line goes through (0, a). To draw the line, these two points are located and connected on the graph.

Thus, the regression line for Y on X in the data of Table 18.5 would be $\hat{Y}_i = 58.64 + 1.53X_i$. The line could promptly be drawn in Figure 19.1 by connecting the points (0, 58.64) and the bivariate mean, (4.88, 66.13). The regression coefficient indicates that Y rises by a factor of 1.53 for each unit of rise in X.

19.1.1.3 *Calculating Estimates of* $\hat{Y}_i$

— After the equation is established for $\hat{Y}_i = 58.64 + 1.53 X_i$, each estimate of $\hat{Y}_i$ can be determined for the corresponding X_i, as shown in Table 19.1. The deviations of each Y_i value from the regression line can also be determined (if desired) as $Y_i - \hat{Y}_i$.

19.1.2 The "Other" Regression Line

The foregoing calculations were based on the assumption that Y depended on X. The other assumption, i.e., that X depends on Y, would produce an analogous set of calculations for the line

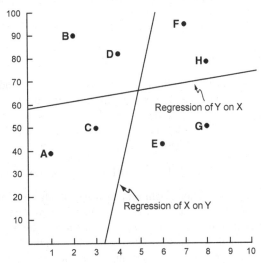

FIGURE 19.1
The two possible regression lines for the data points in Table 18.5.

$$\hat{X}_i = a' + b'Y_i$$

It would have suitably different values for b′, which is the regression coefficient of X on Y, and for a′, which is the X-intercept when $Y_i = 0$. The "other" straight line would be expressed as $(\hat{X}_i - \overline{X}) = b'(Y_i - \overline{Y})$ and the best-fitting line would occur when $b' = S_{xy}/S_{yy}$, with $a' = (\overline{X} - b'\overline{Y})$.

TABLE 19.1

Estimated Values of $\hat{Y}_i$ and Deviations around the Regression Line for Data in Table 18.5

Person	X_i	Y_i	$\hat{Y}_i$	$Y_i - \hat{Y}_i$
A	1	39	60.17	−21.17
B	2	90	61.70	28.30
C	3	50	63.23	−13.23
D	4	82	64.76	17.24
E	5	43	67.82	−24.82
F	7	95	69.35	25.65
G	8	51	70.88	−19.88
H	8	79	70.88	8.12

For the data of Table 18.5, the calculations would produce $b' = S_{xy}/S_{yy} = 81.13/3580.88 = .0227$ and $a' = 4.88 - (.0227)(66.13) = 3.38$. The "other" line for the regression of X on Y would be expressed as $\hat{X}_i = 3.38 + .0227Y_i$; it passes through the points (3.38, 0) and (4.88, 66.13), as shown in Figure 19.1.

19.1.3   Correlation and Standardized Regression

The formulas for the two regression coefficients, b and b′, demonstrate the remarkable property of the correlation coefficient noted in Section 18.3.1.4. To be suitably nondependent or interdependent, the correlation coefficient must get to a value that lies between the two "dependent" regression coefficients. It does so by becoming a "geometric mean," taking the square root of their product.

Thus,

$$r = \frac{S_{xy}}{\sqrt{S_{xx}S_{yy}}} = \sqrt{\frac{(S_{xy})(S_{xy})}{(S_{xx})(S_{yy})}} = \sqrt{bb'} \qquad [19.4]$$

This attribute of the correlation coefficient also indicates an important feature of its structure. When the co-deviations were standardized to form the correlation coefficient, the idea of a straight line was not invoked or even mentioned. Nevertheless, as shown in Formula [19.4], the correlation coefficient involves straight-line reasoning, because it represents the geometric mean of slopes for the two straight lines that would best fit the bivariate relationship. For the data in Table 18.5,

$$r = \sqrt{bb'} = \sqrt{[(81.13)/(52.88)][(81.13)/(3580)]} = \sqrt{(1.53)(.0227)} = .186$$

The correlation coefficient also has another important attribute. Like the covariance, a regression coefficient relies on the raw values in which the data were expressed. Thus, if *time* is cited in days rather than months, or *temperature* in Fahrenheit rather than Celsius scales, the corresponding regression coefficient will be substantially altered, even though the basic relationship remains unchanged. For this reason, a regression coefficient is best interpreted when expressed in a standardized form that is dimension-free. The *standardized* regression coefficient can be obtained by working with the Z-score standardized values of Y and X. The algebraic activity to demonstrate this process is shown in Appendix 19.3, and the result is pleasing. Regardless of whether Y is regressed on X, or vice versa, the standardized regression coefficient is the same: it is r.

In other words, r is not just the correlation coefficient; it is also the "standardized" regression coefficient when either of the two regression lines is expressed in standard-deviation units.

19.1.4   Alternative Approaches

The "least squares" method for getting the values of a and b for the regression line is traditional, well known, straightforward, and easy to understand. It has several potential problems, however, that can become important in diverse circumstances, and particularly when an analogous linear model and method are later used in multiple regression for more than one independent variable. These problems can arise because (1) the linear model of regression is aimed at best fit, not best trend; (2) the least squares method may not always yield the best fit; and (3) the mean may not be the best central index for expressing deviations.

For example, a better fit might sometimes be obtained by minimizing the sum of absolute deviations. The median might sometimes be a better central index than the mean for either the squared or absolute deviations. A method called *maximum likelihood*, which is discussed elsewhere,[1] might sometimes be a better way to find the coefficients, regardless of what is chosen for a central index and expression of deviations. Furthermore, when deviations are minimized with the goal of getting a best fit for the estimates, the trend expressed by b is merely a secondary by-product of the calculations. Different approaches, using resampling or other tactics requiring a computer, might be aimed primarily at finding a best coefficient of trend, letting the estimate of fit become a secondary product.

The focus on best fit rather than best trend is entirely reasonable. The observed Y_i values are available as "gold standard" references for determining the accuracy of estimates made by $\hat{Y}_i$, but no analogous reference slope is available to appraise accuracy for different selections of b. Consequently, the b that emerges from the least-square minimization of $\Sigma(Y_i - \hat{Y}_i)^2$ rests on five important assumptions: (1) the data for $\{X_i, Y_i\}$ are suitably fit by a straight line; (2) we minimize the sum of squared deviations, $\Sigma(Y_i - \hat{Y}_i)^2$, rather than other entities, such as the sum of absolute deviations, $\Sigma|Y_i - \hat{Y}|$; (3) the deviations are all measured from the means, rather than some other central index, such as the median; (4) we use the least-squares rather than other potential methods for determining the best-fitting coefficients; and (5) the entire process is aimed mainly at getting a best accomplishment for the estimated fit rather than the identified trend. In diverse circumstances, particularly for nonlinear patterns of data and in multivariable regression, some or all of these assumptions may not be valid or optimal.

Despite these limitations, the linear, least-squares mathematical model for simple regression of two variables is relatively "robust" and has been used with great success for many years. The limitations are important to remember, however, when "linear" conclusions are drawn from the results, whether in simple bivariate or later in multivariable regression. Investigators using the regression process, particularly in clinical epidemiology or public health, are often much more interested in the impact (i.e., trend) of the individual independent variables, than in estimating values for the dependent $\hat{Y}_i$. The quantified results for trend can sometimes be deceptive when emerging from a rectilinear model, relying on squared deviations from means, that was aimed at estimates, not trends.

Assuming that the least-squares regression method is satisfactory, however, we can proceed to evaluate its accomplishments.

19.2 Accomplishments in Estimation

The descriptive *accomplishments* of the regression model are expressed with statistical indexes that reflect the goals of making estimates and assessing trends. Appraisal of the estimates, discussed in this section, will let us know how good a job the model has done in fitting the data. Appraisal of trend, considered in Section 19.3, will indicate the impact of the independent variable.

19.2.1 Components of Estimations

As noted earlier (Section 18.3.1.2), improvements in estimation are expressed as a proportion,

$$\frac{\text{Errors with Y Alone } - \text{ Errors Using X}}{\text{Errors with Y Alone}}$$

This expression is simple to use if each estimate can be marked **right** or **wrong** for categorical data. For dimensional data, however, the "errors" are deviations in each $Y_i - \hat{Y}_i$. To determine "errors," these deviations are converted to sums of squares and partitioned into several forms of "group variance." The partition process is discussed here in detail because the principles are used not only in simple bi-dimensional regression, but also later in other types of regression and in the procedure called *analysis of variance*. The partitions also appear in computer printouts of results for any type of regression analysis.

19.2.1.1 Partition of Deviations

When $\hat{Y}_i$ is estimated from X_i, the original deviation, $Y_i - \overline{Y}$, is decomposed into two parts:

$$Y_i - \overline{Y} = (Y_i - \hat{Y}_i) + (\hat{Y}_i - \overline{Y}) \qquad [19.5]$$

Each of these deviations has a name:

- $Y_i - \overline{Y}$ is the original or basic deviation.
- $Y_i - \hat{Y}_i$ is the residual or "error" deviation from the regression model.
- $\hat{Y}_i - \overline{Y}$ is the "model" deviation, representing the increment between estimates from the regression model and from the original basic "model," which was the mean.

For example, for person A in Tables 18.5 and 19.1, the deviations are −27.13 for $Y_i - \overline{Y}$, −21.17 for $Y_i - \hat{Y}_i$, and −5.96 for $\hat{Y}_i - \overline{Y}_i$. The last value could have been obtained by direct substitution as $60.17 - 66.13 = -5.96$, or by subtracting the other two deviations to get $-27.13 - (-21.17) = -5.96$.

19.2.1.2 Partition of Variance

The three component deviations for each person in the group can be squared and added to form a group variance (or "sum of squares"), which can be divided by the appropriate degrees of freedom to produce a mean variance.

The jargon that describes the activities is sometimes confusing because the term *variance* is regularly used for the sum of squares of a group variance, rather than for its mean value. Thus, in discussing "reductions in variance," the speaker (or writer) will often refer to variance as a group value, such as $\Sigma(Y_i - \overline{Y})^2$, not to a mean value, such as $\Sigma(Y_i - \overline{Y})^2/(n-1)$. This "abusage" of *variance* is too common and convenient to be avoided here, so beware of the distinctions.

19.2.1.2.1 Basic Group Variance.

The basic group variance available to be "improved" is

$$S_{yy} = \Sigma(Y_i - \overline{Y})^2$$

Representing the "indigenous errors" that will be reduced by the subsequent algebraic model, S_{yy} is often called the *sum of squares* or *corrected sum of squares*, particularly in computer printouts.

Because Y_i can be chosen from n values, and $\overline{Y}$ represents one estimated parameter, the degrees of freedom in $Y_i - \overline{Y}$ are $n - 1$. Thus, the mean value of the original group variance is

$$\Sigma(Y_i - \overline{Y})^2/(n-1)$$

The square root of this value is the standard deviation for the $\{Y_i\}$ data.

19.2.1.2.2 Residual ("Error") Variance.

The group variance for $Y_i - \hat{Y}_i$, symbolized as $S_r = \Sigma(Y_i - \hat{Y}_i)^2$, is often called (with the word "group" omitted) *residual variance* or *error variance*. In Table 19.1, the sum of squared values of $Y_i - \hat{Y}_i$ is $S_r = \Sigma(Y_i + \hat{Y}_i)^2 = 3456.41$.

As shown in Formula [A.19.1] of Appendix 19.1, S_r can also be expressed in values of S_{xx}, S_{yy}, and S_{xy} (as well as b). The expression is

$$S_r = S_{yy} - 2bS_{xy} + b^2S_{xx} \qquad [19.6]$$

This formula is conceptually useful for showing that S_r consists of a weighted sum of the two group variances, S_{xx} and S_{yy}, minus the weighted covariance, S_{xy}. The way that S_r reduces variance is via the subtracted covariance. Because the "weight" for b is calculated as S_{yy}/S_{xx}, the expression in [19.6] becomes

$$S_r = S_{yy} - (S_{xy}^2 / S_{xx})$$ [19.7]

which shows that S_r will always be smaller than S_{yy} except when $S_{xy} = 0$. Thus, fitting a regression line should almost always reduce the original "basic" group variance.

Formula [19.7] also shows a "shortcut" method for determining the value of $S_r = \Sigma(Y_i - \hat{Y}_i)^2$. We could painstakingly square and add each of the $Y_i - \hat{Y}_i$ values in Table 19.1 to get $S_r = 3456.41$. With the shortcut, we substitute in Formula [19.7] to get $S_r = 3580.88 - [(81.13)^2 / 52.88] = 3456.41$.

19.2.1.2.3 Mean Square Error. To calculate a mean for S_r, the value for degrees of freedom is $n - 2$. It represents the n degrees of freedom in Y_i minus the 2 that are used when two parameters are estimated for $\hat{Y}_i$ in the bivariate regression. (A further discussion of this idea appears in Appendix A.19.4.) The residual mean variance when S_r is divided by $n - 2$ is symbolized as $s_{y.x}^2$ and often called the "mean square error" or "MSE" in computer printouts. The y.x symbol indicates the regression of Y on X. The calculation is

$$s_{y.x}^2 = S_r/(n-2)$$ [19.8]

The smaller the value of "mean square error," the better is the fit of the regression line. For the 8 items of data in Table 19.1, the "mean square error" is $3456.41/6 = 576.0$.

Although seldom used to express goodness of fit, the mean square error appears later (Section 19.4.2.2) for determining, if desired, a confidence interval for the estimated values, $\hat{Y}_i$. The concept becomes particularly important in multivariable analysis, when fit is compared for different regression models.

19.2.1.2.4 Model Variance. The group variance for the model deviation is usually called *model variance* and symbolized as

$$S_M = \Sigma(\hat{Y}_i - \overline{Y})^2$$ [19.9]

The value of S_M can be found algebraically by substituting $\hat{Y}_i = \overline{Y} + b(X_i - \overline{X})$ for $\hat{Y}_i$ in Expression [19.9]. It becomes $S_M = \Sigma[b(X_i - \overline{X})]^2 = b^2 S_{xx}$; and because $b = S_{xy}/S_{xx}$,

$$S_M = S_{xy}^2/S_{xx}$$ [19.10]

Substitution of Formula [19.10] into Expression [19.7] produces

$$S_r = S_{yy} - S_M$$ [19.11]

which shows that the model variance is the amount by which S_{yy} is reduced to form the residual variance. If we happen to know the values of S_r and S_{yy}, we can always find the model variance as

$$S_M = S_{yy} - S_r$$ [19.12]

From Table 18.5, we know that $S_{yy} = 3580.88$, and from Table 19.1, we could determine that $S_r = \Sigma(Y_i - \hat{Y}_i)^2 = 3456.41$. With this long approach, $S_M = 3580.88 - 3456.41 = 124.47$. Alternatively, we could substitute the known values of S_{xy} and S_{xx} in Formula [19.10] to get $S_M = (81.13)^2/52.88 = 124.47$.

The *mean* of the model variance is used for various complex statistical activities discussed later in the text. In the simple bivariate analysis under discussion now, S_M has only one degree of freedom, calculated from the 2 degrees of freedom in $\hat{Y}_i$ minus the 1 degree of freedom in $\overline{Y}$. Thus, the mean value of S_M in bivariate analysis is $S_M/1 = S_M$.

19.2.2 Sum of Partitioned Variance

Another way of rewriting Formulas [19.11] and [19.12] is

$$S_{yy} = S_r + S_M$$ [19.13]

This expression demonstrates an extraordinary feature of the partition of sums of squares in the basic group variance: the results are arranged in a manner identical to the partition of deviations in Formula [19.5], where

original deviation = residual deviation + model deviation

For the group variances in Formula [19.13],

original variance = residual variance + model variance

This remarkable attribute of the partition of variance gave rise to the statistical domain called *analysis of variance*, and is also constantly used in multivariable analysis. In the simple regression of two variables, the attribute is interesting but not especially important. It is responsible, however, for the "analysis-of-variance table" in which results are usually displayed in computer printouts.

19.2.3 r^2 and Proportionate Reduction of Variance

With all of the necessary concepts and symbols now available, we can return to the main focus of the agenda: expressing the proportionate reduction of group variance as (Errors with Y alone – Errors using X)/(Errors with Y alone). Because S_{yy} represents the "errors" in estimates with Y alone, and S_r represents the "errors" in estimates using X, the expression becomes

$$\text{Proportionate reduction}_{\text{in group variance}} = \frac{S_{yy} - S_r}{S_{yy}} \qquad [19.14]$$

Because $S_{yy} - S_r = S_M$ (Formula [19.12]), the proportionate reduction in group variance is S_M/S_{yy}. Because $S_M = S_{xy}^2/S_{xx}$ in Formula [19.10], the desired index of proportionate reduction is

$$r^2 = \frac{S_{xy}^2}{S_{xx}S_{yy}} \qquad [19.15]$$

which is the square of the correlation coefficient, r.

Sometimes called the *coefficient of determination*, r^2 indicates the proportion of basic group variance that has been reduced or statistically "explained" by the X variable. Consequently, if we really want to know about the error reduction accomplished by a bivariate regression line, or by a correlation of two variables, the best index to examine to indicate the accomplishment is r^2 rather than r.

Formula [19.15] also indicates that for a quicker, simpler (or kinder, gentler) calculation of proportionate reduction in group variance, we need not go through the process of finding all the $Y_i - \hat{Y}_i$ values to get $S_r = \Sigma(Y_i - \hat{Y}_i)^2$. Instead, we can directly substitute appropriate values in the formula for r^2.

In the data for Table 18.5, $S_{xy} = 81.13$, $S_{xx} = 52.88$, and $S_{yy} = 3580.88$. With Formula [19.15], we can promptly calculate $r^2 = (81.13)^2/[(52.88)(3580.88)] = .0348$. With the longer approach, using values of S_{yy} and S_r, the calculated r^2 would be $(3580.88 - 3456.41)/3580.88 = 124.47/3580.88 = .0348$.

If we knew the value of r^2 and S_{yy} but did not know S_r, it could easily be found by expressing Formula [19.14] as $S_{yy} - S_r = r^2 S_{yy}$, and so

$$S_r = (1 - r^2)S_{yy} \qquad [19.16]$$

In this instance, $S_r = (1 - .0348)(3580.88) = 3456.27$, which is the same value as before, except for minor differences due to rounding.

19.2.4 Interpretation of r^2

Formula [19.14] shows that r^2 has a maximum value of 1 when $S_r = 0$, i.e., when the regression line fits perfectly, so that $\Sigma(Y_i - \hat{Y}_i)^2 = 0$. Conversely, r^2 has a minimum value of 0 when $S_{yy} = S_r$. As noted in Formula [19.6], the minimum of 0 occurs when $b = 0$, implying that the data are fitted with a line parallel to the X axis. This line, of course, will be at the level of the mean, $\overline{Y}$.

Many people are surprised to discover that r^2 is always *smaller* than r (except in the rare situations where r is either 0 or 1). If a number's absolute magnitude lies between 0 and 1, the number becomes smaller when squared. Thus, if $r = .6$, $r^2 = .36$; and if $r = .2$, $r^2 = .04$. Because $0 \le r^2 \le 1$, values of r that sometimes seem moderately impressive may lose their quantitative stature when considered for their job in reducing variance. An apparently large, respectable correlation coefficient, such as .5, has reduced only 25% of the variance, and a coefficient of .3 has reduced only 9%.

For the data in Table 18.5, the r^2 value of .0348 shows the poor relationship expected from an inspection of points in Figure 18.8.

19.2.5 F Ratio of Mean Variances

As noted in Section 19.2.3, the r^2 value for proportionate reduction in group variance is S_M/S_{yy}. A different way of expressing the accomplishments, however, is to form a ratio not from group variances, but from the *mean* of the group variances, S_M and S_r.

The result is the F ratio that is famous in the analysis of variance and in multivariable analyses, but hardly needed in simple linear regression for two variables. The reason is that in simple regression S_M has only one degree of freedom, so its mean is $S_M/1 = S_M$; and S_r has $n - 2$ degrees of freedom, so its mean is $S_r/(n - 2)$. Because $S_r = (1 - r^2)S_{yy}$, according to Formula [19.16], the ratio of mean variances will be

$$F = S_M/[S_r/(n-2)] = \frac{S_M(n-2)}{S_{yy}(1-r^2)}$$

and because $r^2 = S_M/S_{yy}$,

$$F = \frac{r^2(n-2)}{1-r^2} \qquad [19.17]$$

As noted later (Section 19.4), this value of F is identical to the square of the ratio formed when the customary value of t or Z is calculated to test stochastic significance for r or r^2. Unlike r^2, which is easily interpreted because it always has a "standard" range from 0 to 1, F can have an extensive spread of values. F will approach 0 as r^2 approaches 0, but will approach infinity as r^2 approaches 1. Therefore, F can be (and is) used as a *stochastic* index, but it has little or no value as a *descriptive* index of accomplishment.

19.3 Indications of Trend

The co-relations of the two variables are expressed with two descriptive indexes: the regression coefficient, b, for dependent trend, and the correlation coefficient, r, for interdependent trend.

19.3.1 Magnitude of b

As an index of dependent trend, the magnitude of b demonstrates the direct impact or effect of variable X on variable Y. Despite the adequacy of this result in a specific research project, the values of b are difficult to interpret because (as noted earlier in Section 19.1.3) they will vary with different units of measurement for X and Y. Consequently, b is best evaluated as a dimensionless, standardized value.

19.3.2 Standardized Regression Coefficient

The value of r has a double role in simple linear regression. In addition to being the interdependent correlation coefficient, r is the standardized value of the slope, whether the regression coefficient refers to the line regressing Y on X or X on Y.

If you know the values of b, s_x, and s_y, but do not know r, it can be obtained as

$$r = bs_x/s_y \qquad [19.18]$$

If you know b′ for the regression of X on Y,

$$r = b's_y/s_x \qquad [19.19]$$

Because $s_x = \sqrt{S_{xx}/(n-1)}$ and $s_y = \sqrt{S_{yy}/(n-1)}$, the value of s_x / s_y is $\sqrt{S_{xx}/S_{yy}}$. Thus, without calculating s_x and s_y, we could determine r for the data in Table 18.5 by using the known values of b = 1.53, S_{xx} = 52.88, and S_{yy} = 3580.88. The result will be r = 1.53 $\sqrt{52.88/3580.88}$ = .186. This result is the same as what was obtained in Section 19.1.3 when r was calculated as $\sqrt{bb'}$. It is also essentially identical to what would occur as the square root of r^2 = .0348 in Section 19.2.3, yielding $\sqrt{.0348}$ = .1865.

19.3.3 "Quantitative Significance" for r

Almost 50 years ago, J.P. Guilford[2] recommended the following arbitrary standards for interpreting r:

<.20:	slight, almost negligible relationship
.20–.40:	low correlation; definite but small relationship
.40–.70:	moderate correlation; substantial relationship
.70–.90:	high correlation; marked relationship
>.90:	very high correlation; very dependable relationship

A much more lenient set of standards was proposed by another statistical psychologist, J. Cohen.[3] After asserting that "the state of development of much of behavioral science is such that not very much variance in the dependent variable is predictable," Cohen set the standards for r at the following relatively low levels:

≥.10:	small effect
≥.30:	medium effect
≥.50:	large effect

Cohen stated that most investigators in his field would regard values of r = .50 as being "about as high as they come."

Investigators elsewhere, however, may not be persuaded by Cohen's "affirmative action" criteria for psychologic correlations. Although no formal boundaries have been established for "quantitative significance" in the magnitude of r^2, most investigators and data analysts agree that a bivariate relationship is particularly unimpressive if the X variable fails to "explain" (i.e., proportionately reduce) at least 10% of the basic group variance in Y. Accordingly, $r^2 \geq .10$ is often used (but not applied rigidly) as a boundary for quantitative significance. If $r^2 = .10$ is about as low as one might accept for a substantial proportionate reduction in group variance, the corresponding minimum value for a quantitatively significant r becomes $\sqrt{.10} = .32$. The latter level is recommended by Fleiss,[4] and is essentially the same as the value of 0.30-0.32 found by Burnand et al.[5] in their study of minimum boundaries used for quantitative significance in medical-literature publications. [For quantitative effects, Burnand et al. also regarded $r \geq .45$ (reducing 20% of variance) as "substantially significant" and $r \geq .60$ as "highly significant."]

The selected criteria should always be used flexibly, however, because each result must be interpreted in context. For example, as noted later in Chapter 20, a correlation coefficient of .94, although strikingly impressive, may not indicate good agreement for two different methods of measuring the same substance. Conversely, in such fields as psychology and sociology, where correlation coefficients are often .06, .04, or lower, a value of r as "high" as .1 (which represents only a 1% reduction of variance) may sometimes be regarded as indicating a significant relationship.

The important point to bear in mind is not the choice of criteria, but the importance of evaluating the quantitative magnitude of correlation (r) or "explained variance" (r^2) from the descriptive coefficients, *not* from the associated P values.

19.4 Stochastic Procedures

In bi-dimensional analysis, the three main descriptive indexes — r^2, b, and r — are evaluated stochastically with parametric procedures. Empirical rearrangements of data could be used but are seldom applied.

For the parametric reasoning, the observed set of n points, $\{X_i, Y_i\}$, and the regression line, $\hat{Y}_i = a + bX_i$, are regarded as a random sample from a larger parametric population whose true regression line is $Y = \alpha + \beta X$. The estimate is done with $n - 2$ degrees of freedom, for reasons discussed in Appendix A.19.4. The parametric null hypothesis is that $\beta = 0$ (indicating no relationship between X and Y). The P value reflects the external probability that the observed or an even larger value of b or r would have occurred by chance under the null hypothesis.

The parametric reasoning and strategy, presented in Appendixes 19.5 and 19.6, show that r^2, b, and r can all be stochastically tested with exactly the same critical ratio, which is

$$t \text{ (or } Z) = \frac{r\sqrt{n-2}}{\sqrt{1-r^2}} \qquad [19.20]$$

19.4.1 P Values

The critical ratio in Formula [19.20] is converted to a P value, using Z for large groups, or t, with $n - 2$ degrees of freedom, for small groups. (Because the squared ratio is the same as F in Formula [19.17], the Z or t test gives the same result as a stochastic test on F.)

For the data in Table 18.5, t would be calculated from Formula [19.20] as

$$.186(\sqrt{8-2})/\sqrt{1-.0348} = .464.$$

At six degrees of freedom in Table 7.3, P is between .404 and .553, and is not stochastically significant. We could therefore decide stochastically that X is essentially unrelated to Y, although the quantitative decision of "unrelated" was already made much earlier when we noted the small descriptive values for r^2 and r.

19.4.2 Confidence Intervals

Confidence intervals can be calculated, if desired, for each of the diverse statistical components under discussion: a, b, r, and even two forms of $\hat{Y}_i$. For most practical purposes, the "confidence" analysis seldom extends beyond r (or b). Becasue most analyses in medical literature do not go even that far, the rest of this section is optional reading. It is here if you ever need or want it, or if you have become exhilarated by the ideas and are ecstatically awaiting more mathematics. If you are surfeited by all of this stage setting, however, the pragmatic "show" begins in Section 19.5.

19.4.2.1   Confidence Intervals for r and b — The stochastic focus in simple regression is almost always a P value; and confidence intervals are seldom constructed for r or b. A confidence interval around r (or b), however, could help support a conclusion that the relationship is *not* significant.

If the P value exceeds the α boundary (usually set at .05), a *stochastically* significant relationship has *not* been shown. The investigators may then improperly conclude that X and Y are not related, but the "no-relationship" conclusion requires evidence that a quantitatively significant value was *excluded* from the appropriate 95% confidence interval. To get a confidence interval, the easiest approach (See Appendix 19.7) is to calculate the "standard error" of r as

$$SE_r = \sqrt{1 - r^2}/\sqrt{n - 2} \qquad [19.21]$$

The confidence interval around r is then constructed, using t, as

$$r \pm t_{v,\alpha}\sqrt{(1 - r^2)/(n - 2)} \qquad [19.22]$$

For the data in Table 18.5, the standard error of r is $\sqrt{1 - .0348}/\sqrt{6} = .401$ and $t_{.05,6} = 2.447$. The confidence interval will be $.186 \pm (2.447)(.401) = .186 \pm .981$; it extends from $-.795$ to the (impossibly) high value of 1.167. Although stochastic significance was not demonstrated, we cannot exclude the possibility that a quantitatively significant relationship might be present in the "universe" represented by this small data set.

To convert the confidence interval to an expression that surrounds the slope b = 1.53, use Formula [A.19.7] in the Appendix. The previous confidence interval for r is multiplied by s_y/s_x, which is $\sqrt{S_{yy}/S_{xx}} = \sqrt{3580.88/52.88} = 8.229$. The interval would become $8.229[.186 \pm .981] = 1.53 \pm 8.07$; and it would go from -6.54 to 9.60. Note that the 1.53 in this calculation coincides with the value of b in these data.

19.4.2.2   Confidence Interval for Estimated Values of $\hat{Y}_i$ — In published graphs, the estimates made by the regression line are sometimes accompanied by a "confidence band," which consists of two lines showing upper and lower confidence limits along the range of potential variation for the line of estimated points, $\hat{Y}_i$. The drawing always looks peculiar because the lines that form the confidence band are not straight. They are convex curves on either side of the regression line, as shown in Figure 19.2.

The reason for this peculiarity is that at an individual location of $\hat{X}_i$, the $\hat{Y}_i$ value of the regression line is actually estimating the mean value, $\overline{Y}_i$, of all the Y_i points that may be present at that location. Thus, for a series of individuals Y_i at location X_i, the mean of the series will be $\overline{Y}_i$, and

$$\hat{Y}_i - Y_i = (\hat{Y}_i - \overline{Y}_i) + (\overline{Y}_i - Y_i)$$

The customary concave "confidence bands" are shown for estimates of the $\overline{Y}_i$ mean values at each X_i. For this calculation, mathematical tactics not shown here produce the formula

$$s_{\hat{Y}_i}^2 = s_{y \cdot x}^2 \left[\frac{1}{n} + \frac{(X_i - \overline{X})^2}{S_{xx}} \right] \qquad [19.23]$$

With a suitably chosen $t_{v,\alpha}$, the confidence interval around each estimated value on the line becomes

$$\hat{Y}_i \pm t_{v,\alpha}(s_{\hat{Y}_i})$$

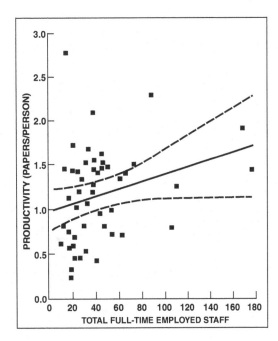

FIGURE 19.2

Curved confidence-interval lines for regression line showing academic productivity (i.e., papers published per person) in relation to total full-time employed staff at British universities. [The figure is taken from Chapter Reference 6.]

In Formula [19.23], $s^2_{y \cdot x}$, $1/n$, and S_{xx} are all constant, but $X_i - \overline{X}$ enlarges as X_i gets farther from the mean in either direction. The enlarging $(X_i - \overline{X})^2$ term produces the symmetrically concave curves, which are closest to the regression line at the bivariate mean, $(\overline{X}, \overline{Y})$.

19.4.2.3   Additional Evaluations — Four additional evaluation procedures, relegated to the Appendix, are confidence intervals for individual points and for the intercept, comparisons of two regression lines, and transformations of r.

19.5   Pragmatic Applications and Problems

Regression and correlation coefficients are among the most frequently used indexes in statistics and are probably the most commonly abused. This section is concerned with the valuable applications. Section 19.6 discusses the abuses.

19.5.1   "Screening" Tests for Trend

Correlation and regression coefficients are commonly used in medical literature as a "screening" (or sometimes definitive) test for *whether* two variables are related and for the average magnitude of the trend. If the variables seem to be distinctly related, the investigator can then speculate or do additional research about reasons for the relationship.

19.5.1.1   "Physical Examination" for "Abnormalities" — Before any statistical conclusions are formed from r, b, or P values, the graphical portrait of points should always receive a "physical examination." The goal is to find "abnormalities," such as distinctly curved patterns or major reversals in trend, that may make a straight-line inappropriate for the data. If the points are diffusely spread with no obvious pattern as in Figures 18.8 and 18.16, the rectilinear analysis is satisfactory for identifying an average trend. In such situations, a poor fitting line may be useless for accurate estimates, but can be valuable for denoting the average trend in the data, particularly if the analyst does not compare results in the zones, as suggested in Chapter 18. If the graph shows an obvious curving pattern, however, as in Figures 18.13 and 18.14, a rectilinear analysis may yield distorted results.

Figure 19.3 gives an excellent example of a published "screening process," which was especially easy to do in this instance[7] because the graph has points on both the X and Y sides of a (0,0) central axis. The points do not show an obviously curved pattern; and the straight line seems appropriate, with about equal numbers of points above it and below it throughout the graph.

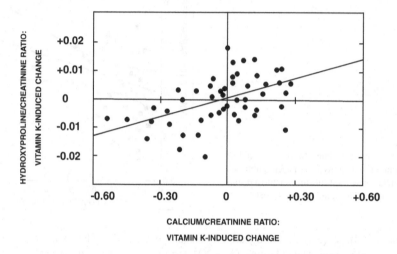

CALCIUM/CREATININE RATIO:

VITAMIN K-INDUCED CHANGE

FIGURE 19.3
Correlation between the vitamin K-induced changes in Ca^{2+} and hydroxyproline excretion. The straight line was fitted with a computer program equipped for linear regression calculations and the r value was +0.437. [Figure and legend taken from Chapter Reference 7.]

After checking that a straight-line is suitable, the analyst can easily determine trend from the calculated value of r, which is readily obtained from computer programs. Many investigators prefer to cite b as the main quantitative index of the dependent relationship, but r has the advantage of being standardized, relatively unaffected by arbitrary units of measurement, and easy to interpret.

19.5.1.2 *"Physical Diagnoses" of b or Wrong Lines* — Skillful physical examiners can sometimes make good visual guesses of b without any calculations. One approach is to locate (and determine the slope of) a line that will have about equal numbers of points above and below it, consistent with a least squares sum for $\Sigma(Y_i - \hat{Y}_i)^2$. The visual approach may be tricky, however, if the X or Y axes have unequal-sized increments produced by logarithmic or other transformations, or if the axes have been truncated or changed in mid-course. Such axes, however, also provide opportunities for the artist to place graphic lines improperly and for the error to be diagnosed with simple physical examination.

For example, visual inspection would suggest that the solid line for Group A has been calculated or drawn incorrectly in Figure 19.4, which shows results of a clinical trial[8] intended to find the effects of recombitant human erythropoietin on the packed cell volume (PCV) and serum erythropoietin (s-EPO) in patients donating blood before elective surgery. The solid squares are distributed so that about 32 of them are above the corresponding solid line and only about 11 are below that line.

Furthermore, the corresponding regression line seems to have a wrong intercept. In the line, which is reported to be $\log(s\text{-EPO}) = -.04(PCV) + 2.72$, the customary Y-intercept cannot be checked because neither axis reaches zero, but the graph shows the X-intercept, where log s-EPO appears to be 0 when PCV is about 42.5. Inserting the latter value into the stated regression equation produces the disagreeing result that for PCV = 42.5, log s–EPO = (−.04)(42.5) + 2.72 = 1.02, which is about 1. Therefore, something must be wrong. (The problem may arise from the artist's forgetting that the Y axis has a break between 0 and 1.)

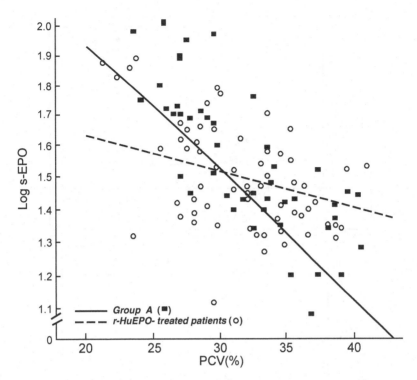

FIGURE 19.4

Relation between log s-EPO and PCV after surgery. Regression line equations: group A (■), log s-EPO = $-0.04 \times$ PCV (%) + 2.72 (r = -0.76. p = 0.01); all r-HuEPO-treated patients (○), log s-EPO = $-0.01 \times$ PCV (%) + 1.82 (r = -0.38. p = 0.01). [Figure and legend taken from Chapter Reference 8.]

A quick, crude way to check the value of b is to determine the range of X and Y dimensions as $(X_{max} - X_{min})$ and $(Y_{max} - Y_{min})$ and then to estimate b as the ratio of (range of Y)/(range of X). For example, the solid squares in Figure 19.4 have a Y range from about 1.1 to 2, and an X-range from about 24 to 40. The crude slope would be $-0.9/16 = -.06$, which is not far from the stated value of $-.04$.

19.5.1.3 Taxonomy of Visual Patterns for r — Even with advanced skill in physical diagnosis of graphs, most examiners have difficulty anticipating the values of r or r^2. The difficulty arises from having to guess not just b, but also variances in the X and Y axes. Values of r near 0 or 1 are relatively easy to anticipate if the points have mainly a horizontal spread or a pattern that clearly looks like a straight line, but visual "diagnosis" is difficult for the intermediate zones between r = .2 and r = .8.

A collection of 10 graphs, excerpted from published medical literature, has been assembled here in Figures 19.5, 19.6, and 19.7, producing a taxonomy of visual patterns for r values ranging from near 0 to near 1. Visual guesses for r seem relatively easy for the extreme values near 0 and 1, but the zones between .2 and .8 do not have any obvious quantitative "diagnostic" signs.

Perhaps the main take-home message here is to be wary of any specifically quantitative claims based on regression and correlation coefficients. If r is big enough and stable, it supports the idea that the two variables are related on average. If the investigator claims they are closely or linearly related, however, and if the coefficient for b is offered as a confident *prediction* of future values, beware of the often contradictory graphical evidence.

19.5.2 Predictive Equations

Although developed to allow Y_i to be estimated from X_i, the equation $\hat{Y}_i = a + bX_i$ rarely has a close enough fit to be used for *individual* predictive estimates in most medical research. Such estimates might

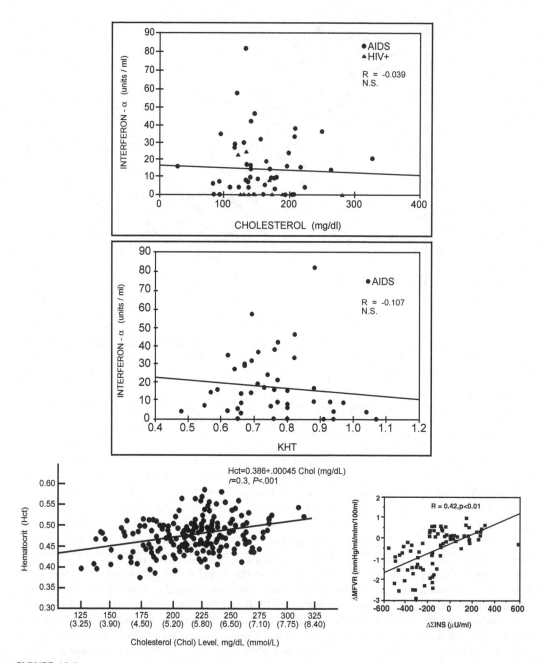

FIGURE 19.5
Four graphs showing r values from .04 to .42.

be attempted when r ≥ .9, but few analysts would be willing to make specific predictions from the extensive variability shown, despite "r = .94," in the lower right graph of Figure 19.7.

Predictive equations are regularly used for exact estimates, however, when diverse (usually chemical) substances are measured with laboratory technology. The magnitude of the measured substance (such as a concentration of serum calcium) is usually converted into the magnitude of another entity (such as the voltage on a spectrophotometer), and a "calibration curve" is constructed, as shown in Figure 19.8, for the voltage values at known magnitudes of the substance. If the calibration points produce a closely

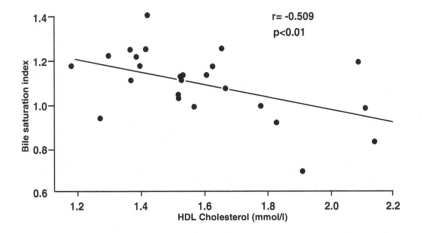

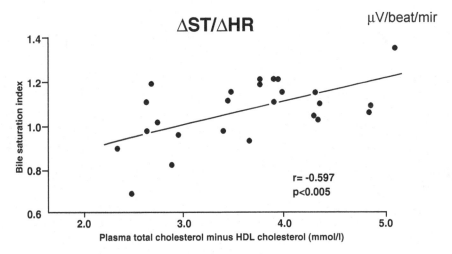

FIGURE 19.6
Two graphs showing r values from .51 to .60.

fitting straight line, the equation is then used to estimate the values of future "unknown" substances. For pragmatic application, the equation has a reverse biologic orientation. Biologically, the voltage readings depend on the concentrations in the serum, but pragmatically, future concentrations will be estimated from the voltage readings. Accordingly, the voltages are plotted as the X variable and concentrations as Y.

Equations of this type are invaluable in modern laboratories, but are misapplied if the goal is to compare measurements of the *same* substance, such as serum calcium, by two different methods, such as flame photometry vs. spectrophotometry. If the analytic aim is to determine agreement rather than trend, the best approach is a concordance method described in Chapter 20.

19.5.3 Other Applications

Although screening for trend and making predictive estimates are the most common applications, regression/correlation procedures can be applied for some of the other goals noted in the next few subsections.

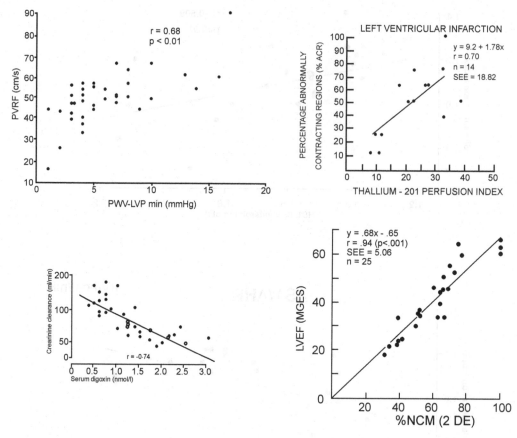

FIGURE 19.7
Four graphs showing r values from .68 to .94.

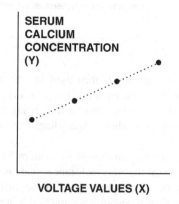

SERUM
CALCIUM
CONCENTRATION
(Y)

VOLTAGE VALUES (X)

FIGURE 19.8
Relationship of serum calcium concentration and voltage values in a chemical measurement system. The four points are the known "calibration" values of calcium specimens. The dotted line represents the "relationship" used to estimate future values of Y from observed values of X in unknown specimens.

19.5.3.1 *Summarizing Individual Time Trends* — Each person's individual data (in a group of people) may be a series of measurements over a period of time. For example, the response to cholesterol-lowering treatment may comprise serum cholesterol measurements at baseline and at four time intervals thereafter. To summarize individual results, a regression equation can be fitted for each person's trend over time; and the individual regression coefficients can represent the main "outcome" variable.

19.5.3.2 "Smoothing" Vital Statistics Rates — The annual rates of incidence (or prevalence) in vital statistics phenomena (such as birth, death, or occurrence of disease) often show oscillations from one year to the next. To avoid these oscillations, the analysts may try to "smooth the curve" by using a "running average," in which each year's value is calculated as a mean of values for the current, preceding, and following year. Thus, the incidence rate for 1992 might be an average of the rates for 1991, 1992, and 1993. In an alternative approach, a lengthy (or the entire) sequence of time points is "smoothed" by conversion to a regression line.

19.5.3.3 Curvilinear and Quadratic Regression — If the plot of points is obviously curved, the data analyst can try to preserve a "linear" format by transforming the X (or Y) variable into expressions such as log X or 1/X. The regression line is then constructed as $\hat{Y}_i = a + b \log X_i$ or $\hat{Y}_i = a + b(1/X_i)$.

In other situations, however, X may be retained without transformation, but expressed in a frankly curvilinear polynomial such as

$$\hat{Y}_i = a + bX + cX^2 + dX^3 + ...$$

The most common polynomial format, called *quadratic regression*, adds only one extra quadratic term, X^2, as $\hat{Y}_i = a + bX + cX^2$.

A quick screening "diagnosis" for the shape of the relationship can be shown by the ratio of the standard deviation (or its square) to the mean of the subset of Y_i values in equally spaced intervals of X_i. The regression model is linear if this ratio remains about constant, and log linear (i.e., $\log Y = a + bX$) if the ratio progressively increases. If the square of the standard deviation increases in proportion to the mean, the regression model is quadratic (i.e., $Y = a + bX + cX^2$).

19.5.3.4 Time Series and Financial Applications — Some bivariate analyses are intended to show the "secular" changes during calendar time of a dependent variable, such as the population or economic status of a geographic region. The statistical goal might be satisfied with a best-fitting straight line for population size as Y variable and for time as the X variable. The patterns of data, however, may form a curve with wavy or irregular shapes that are not well fitted with a straight line; or the data analyst may want to make particularly accurate predictions for the future, based on what was noted in the past.

The association may therefore be described not with a crude straight-line model, but with a polynomial or other complicated algebraic expression called a *time series*. The relationship is still bivariate, but the complex expression (with t for time) may be something like $\hat{Y}_i = a + bt + ct^2 + dt^3 + ...$ Time-series relationships are commonly used in economics to help predict stock-market prices or in meteorology to forecast weather. Having seldom been usefully employed in clinical or epidemiologic activities, time-series analysis will not be further discussed here.

In financial enclaves, an ordinary linear regression model, $Y = a + bX$, is sometimes used to express the performance of individual stocks during a period of time, such as a month or year. In this model, Y represents daily prices of the stock and X represents the corresponding values of a market index, such as the Dow-Jones average. The b coefficient, called *beta*, indicates the stock's movement in relation to the market (or "how much the market drives the stock"), but the a intercept, called *alpha*, indicates unique attributes of the stock itself. According to the theory, alpha should equal zero on average, but stocks with a high positive alpha are believed to have a high likelihood of going up rapidly in price. (The standard deviation of the Y values is sometimes used as an index of "volatility.")

19.6 Common Abuses

The four most common types of abuse for correlation and/or regression procedures are: (1) drawing "significant" conclusions from stochastic P values, while ignoring the actual quantitative significance of the relationship; (2) failure to check whether a straight-line model is suitable for the actual shape of the relationship; (3) ignoring the potential influence of outliers; and (4) concluding that a causal relationship has been shown when high values of correlation indicate a strong association.

19.6.1   Stochastic Distortions

Formula [19.20] for the stochastic t value can be re-written as

$$t = \left(\frac{r}{\sqrt{1-r^2}} \right) \sqrt{n-2} \qquad [19.24]$$

In this formula, the $r/\sqrt{1-r^2}$ ratio is analogous to a standardized increment. Its changing value for different values of r is shown in Table 19.2. On the left side of the table, with small values of r (below .4), the value of $1-r^2$ and the enlarged $\sqrt{1-r^2}$ will be close to 1, and so the ratio of $r/(\sqrt{1-r^2})$ will be essentially r. On the right side of the table, as r enlarges above .5, the ratio becomes strikingly larger than r.

TABLE 19.2

Values of r, $1-r^2$, and $r/\sqrt{1-r^2}$

r	$1-r^2$	$r/\sqrt{1-r^2}$	r	$1-r^2$	$r/\sqrt{1-r^2}$
.05	.9975	.05	.5	.75	.58
.1	.99	.10	.6	.64	.75
.15	.9975	.15	.7	.51	.98
.2	.96	.20	.8	.36	1.3
.25	.9375	.26	.85	.2775	1.6
.3	.91	.31	.9	.19	2.1
.4	.9165	.44	.95	.0975	3.0

To get across the stochastic boundary for "significance" at $P \leq .05$, t must be at least 2. (The requirement is somewhat higher with small group sizes.) Because the ratio exceeds 2 when $r \geq .9$, this magnitude of r will almost always be stochastically significant. At levels of $r \geq .5$, relatively small values of n will make the product high enough when the ratio of $r/\sqrt{1-r^2}$ is multiplied by $\sqrt{n-2}$. The most striking effect occurs at small values of r, however, where sufficiently large group sizes for n will always produce a t value that exceeds 2. The most trivial value of r can thus become stochastically significant if n is big enough.

For example, with a negligibly small r value of .01, the P value will be < .05 if the sample size is huge, such as 40,000, because the value of t calculated with the foregoing formula will be

$$t = \frac{.01\sqrt{39,998}}{\sqrt{1-.0001}} = 2.00$$

When suitably converted, Formula [19.24] shows that

$$n = \left[t^2(1-r^2)/r^2 \right] + 2 \qquad [19.25]$$

Formula [19.25] can promptly show the group sizes that will transform r values into stochastic significance. Using $t = 2$ as a rough guide, the required value will be $n = [4(1-r^2)/r^2] + 2$. Table 19.3 shows the values of n needed to get $t \geq 2$ for different values of r. For example, a correlation coefficient of .7, which has reduced less than half of the original group variance ($r^2 = .49$), will be stochastically significant if obtained with as few as 7 people. (One more person will actually be required here because t must exceed 2 as group sizes become very small. In this instance, t would have to be about 2.37, rather than 2; and Formula [19.25] would produce $n = 7.85$ rather than 7.) An r value of .2, which has reduced only 4% of the original variance, will be stochastically significant if the group size exceeds 98.

For this reason, the associated P value is the *worst* way to determine whether a correlation coefficient is quantitatively significant. Nevertheless, either to avoid making a scientific judgment about the magnitude of r or to escape the distressing implications of low values for r (or r^2), many investigators use

TABLE 19.3

Values of n Required for Stochastic Significance (P ≤ .05) at Cited Value of r

r	.03	.05	.1	.2	.3	.4	.5	.6	.7
r^2	.0009	.0025	.01	.04	.09	.16	.25	.36	.49
n	4443	1598	398	98	43	23	14	10	7

only a stochastic calculation of P to claim that an association is "significant." This pernicious abuse of statistics is abetted by reviewers and editors who allow the authors to "get away with it."

In 1978, Eugene A. Stead, a medical academician well known[9] for maintaining "common sense" in the midst of technologic onslaughts, was reproached, as the contemporary editor of *Circulation*, by the authors[10] of a paper in which "information regarding statistical significance of certain [r correlation coefficients] ... was deleted." Stead defended[11] the editorial deletion by saying that "the P value is frequently misleading [and that] ... when the number of observations is large ... a relationship between two variables at the mathematical level does not necessarily translate into a useful relationship at the patient care level."

This type of intellectual vigor seems to be disappearing among editors today. For example, in Figure 19.9, which is reproduced exactly as published,[12] the investigators showed "three data points" for each of "63 men ... who had stable angina pectoris ... and a positive exercise test with ST-segment changes indicative of ischemia." Without citing a value of r or r^2, the authors concluded that "For this range of carboxyhemoglobin values, there was a decrease of approximately 3.9 percent in the length of time to the ST end point for every 1 percent increase in the carboxyhemoglobin level."

You can decide for yourself whether the claimed precision of the linear relationship is really supported by the points in Figure 19.9. The decision can be helped by checking in a table of t/P values to find that the highly impressive "P ≤ 0.0001" requires a value of t ≥ 4. Inserting n = 3 ×63 = 169 into Formula [19.25] produces 169 = [16(1 − r^2)/r^2] + 2, which can be solved to show that $11.44r^2 = 1$. Consequently, an r^2 value as small as 1/11.44, or about .09, could be associated with the "impressive" findings and subsequent quantitative precision of the relationship claimed by the investigators.

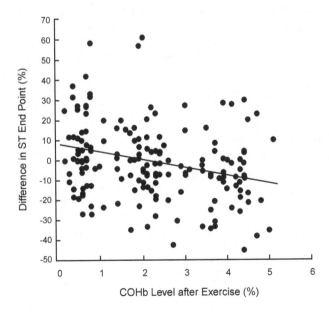

FIGURE 19.9

Dose-Response Relation between the Percentage Change in the Length of Time of the Threshold Ischemic ST-Segment Change (ST End Point) and the Carboxyhemoglobin (COHb) Level after Exercise. Each subject is represented by three data points. The regression shown represents the mean slope of the individual regressions for each subject when y = 3.9 (percentage of COHb) + 8.0 (P ≤ 0.0001). [Figure and legend taken from Chapter Reference 12.]

The abuse of P values is now so thoroughly entrenched that many published reports do not even show values of r, b, or the regression equation. They are replaced entirely by P values. The P values themselves are also sometimes replaced by "stars" (usually asterisks) in which * represents < .05, ** is < .01, and *** is < .001. The starry results, showing neither descriptive values nor the actual P values, may then appear in a celestial table that is bereft of any scientific evidence of quantitative effect. [The use of stars to indicate P values seems to have been introduced,* in a textbook discussion of regression methods, by the distinguished statisticians, G.W. Snedecor and W.G. Cochran.[13]]

Because P values are so affected by group size, they should never alone be trusted for decisions about "significance." A sole reliance on P values may also substantially distort decisions about "nonsignificance." If the P value is >.05 because only four patients were studied, a strong correlation coefficient, as high as .8, might be dismissed as "nonsignificant" (without confirmation by a confidence interval).

19.6.2   Checks for Linear Nonconformity of Quantified Trends

When b and r are determined, the bivariate pattern is fitted with a straight line whose slope is constant and unchanging throughout all zones of the data. Nevertheless, as shown in Chapter 18, some data sets will not be suitably analyzed with a straight line. For other data sets, as in the right side of Figure 18.13, a straight line is obviously the wrong model. It will produce a fallacious result, with r and b near 0, suggesting no relationship, although the two variables actually have a close parabolic relationship. In yet other situations, as in the middle of Figure 18.13, a straight line will produce a reasonably good fit, but the slope of the line will be misleading. It will be too high in the lower and upper ends of the data and too low in the center. (In other situations, such as Figure 19.9, the appropriate regression line may not be curved, but may fit so poorly that any claims for a *precise* relationship must be doubted.)

19.6.2.1   Quantitative Impact of "Risk Factors" — Checking the fit of the line becomes important when a quantified trend in "risk factors" is claimed on the basis of coefficients obtained with various forms of regression analyses. The customary statement is something like "You gain 3.4 years of life for every fall of 5.6 units in substance X." Because the claims usually come from data in which the outcome event is a **0/1** binary variable for life or death, the regression lines (or "surfaces" in multivariable analysis) cannot be expected to have the close fit that might be anticipated for dimensional measurements of biochemical or physiologic variables.

Therefore, before any quantitative contentions, the analyst should first determine whether the data have curved patterns and whether a rectilinear regression model is appropriate. As noted by Concato et al.,[14] however, many published quantitative claims have not been checked for linear conformity between the regression model and the data.

19.6.2.2   Plots of Residual Values vs. X_i — A conventional mathematical method of doing this check is to examine the plot of the residual values, $Y_i - \hat{Y}_i$, against X_i. If a straight line gives a proper fit, the plot of residuals should show points that vary randomly around 0 as X goes from its lowest to highest values. If the residuals show a pattern — i.e., contiguous zones where all of the values are > 0 or < 0 — the data have a curved shape, and the straight line is an inappropriate model that produces a misfit.

This method of checking residuals is commonly used in multivariable analysis. In simple bivariate analysis, however, a much simpler and easier option is to inspect the graph of the original points for Y_i vs. X_i. This simple graph is always easy to plot, and a computer will do it, if asked. If the points show a clear non-rectilinear pattern — as in the middle and right side of Figure 18.13 — the straight line is a poor or potentially unsatisfactory model. If the points show a diverse scatter with no evident pattern, as in Figure 18.16, and if all you want to know is the *average* trend in their relationship, a straight line can be satisfactory.

---

* The introduction probably came in the 5th edition in 1956, as the tactic is not mentioned in the 1st edition (written by Snedecor alone) in 1937, or in the 4th edition in 1946.

The bivariate graph of points should always be drawn and inspected, and it should preferably be displayed in the published report. For drawing conclusions about a bi-dimensional relationship, a single graphic picture can be worth more than 1000 "words" of statistical calculations.

19.6.2.3   Anscombe's "Quartet" — F. J. Anscombe (Professor Emeritus of Statistics at Yale University) constructed[15] an ingenious illustration of the problems inherent in doing regressions and interpreting coefficients without carefully examining the graph of the data. He prepared four different sets of bivariate data that all had the same summary values. For each set of data, $n = 11$, $\overline{X} = 9.0$, $\overline{Y} = 7.5$, $S_{xx} = 110.0$, $S_{yy} = 41.25$, and $S_{xy} = 55.01$. Each set of data also had the same $S_r = 13.75$, $S_M = 27.50$, $r^2 = .667$, and the same regression line: $\hat{Y}_i = 3 + 0.5X_i$. From this striking similarity in all pertinent features of the univariate and bivariate statistical summaries, the graphs for the four sets of data could be expected to look quite similar. Nevertheless, the four data sets had the disparate patterns shown in Figure 19.10. Whenever you think that a statistical summary has told you everything, and that you need not bother looking at the graphical portrait, remember the cacophonous music of "Anscombe's quartet"!

19.6.3   Potential Influence of Outliers

In univariate analysis, outlier points could distort the effectiveness with which a mean and standard deviation represented the associated data. In the conventional ("parametric") form of bivariate analysis under discussion here, the adverse effects can be particularly pernicious. The outlier can greatly alter the covariance as well as the variances used in the calculations.

For example, consider the eleven points of the D graph in "Anscombe's Quartet" (Figure 19.10). The first ten points all lie on a vertical straight line that shows no relationship between X and Y. The eleventh point, however, is an outlier. It may represent an error in measurement, a person who does not belong in the group, or someone who is there quite properly. Regardless of the substantive propriety of the outlier, however, it will have the profound statistical impact shown in the summary coefficients and the linear graph.

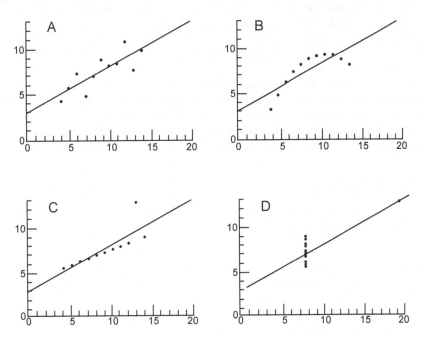

FIGURE 19.10
The four performers in "Anscombe's Quartet." (For details, see text.) [Figure and legend taken from Chapter Reference 15.]

19.6.3.1 Published Illustration of

Problem — If you believe
that Anscombe's imagination was too wild,
and that this type of configuration occurs too
rarely to be regarded as a serious problem,
consider Figure 19.11, which achieved publication in a prominent medical journal.[16] The
investigators did not succeed in exactly repli-
cating Anscombe's D pattern, but they certainly came close.

The best way to avoid such problems is to
look at the data. If you see a pattern such as D
in Figure 19.10 or the graph in Figure 19.11, do
not try to summarize the results with conventional regression and correlation coefficients.

19.6.3.2 Another Published

Illustration — A particularly
dramatic example of the outlier problem
appeared earlier in Figure 19.2. The data in
the graph (and in the study itself) had been
used to conclude that "large science departments ... are more productive than small ones"
in British universities. With that premise, government agencies were thinking about closing

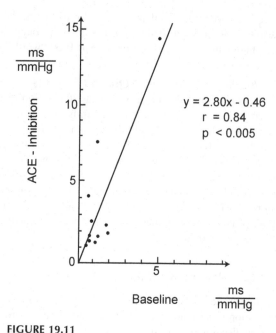

FIGURE 19.11

Relation of the baroreflex sensitivity during ACE inhibition
(*vertical axis*) to the baseline sensitivity (*horizontal axis*). [Fig-
ure and legend taken from Chapter Reference 16.]

small science departments. Two physicists at Sussex University, however, pointed out[6] that the main
effect in Figure 19.2 is produced by the two outlier points on the far right of the graph. These two
points happen to be Oxford and Cambridge Universities, which have other atypical attributes. If the
Oxford and Cambridge points are removed from the data, the effect of department size on productivity
vanishes. Outraged about decisions based on this type of "spurious correlation," one of the physicists
said, "Who's going to have a policy where you start closing university departments on the basis of a
graph that's really fuzzy ... [and] easily destroyed by a very simple commonsense thing [i.e., removing
the two outlier points]."

In ordinary bivariate regression, the effects of outliers can be reduced by transferring from a dimensional to an ordinal analysis, as discussed in Chapter 27, using the ranks of the data rather than absolute
values. (In multivariable analysis, the effect of outliers can be examined with various "influence functions." Some of them use the jackknife method of removing one member at a time, recalculating the
regression coefficients, and seeing how extensively they vary.)

19.6.4 Causal Implications

Scientifically oriented readers probably need no reminder of the old statistical cliché that correlation
does not imply causation. No matter how stochastically and quantitatively significant a correlation
coefficient may be, its magnitude does not imply that the association is a causal relationship.

Most thoughtful scientists today are aware of this distinction, but it is still often disregarded during
some of the etiologically infatuated reasoning that may occur during analyses of alleged causes of chronic
disease. The attendant biases, which are beyond the scope of the discussion here, can distort the true
value of correlation coefficients and lead to erroneous conclusions about etiology.

An important point to bear in mind, however, is that diverse types of strong associations can be found
during various types of "dredging" from the computerized databases that are now widely available. If
you cannot dredge the abundant data to find evidence associating anything that you want to incriminate
and any effect that it allegedly produces, either you or your computer programmer is not very talented.
For example, the annual rise in incidence rates for AIDS in the U.S. can be strongly correlated with

increases in the annual sales of video cassette recorders. Yet no one has proposed — as of now — that the two events are causally related. A few years ago, however, a distinct association was found[17] (in a case-control study) between AIDS and antecedent usage of amyl nitrite "poppers." A chemical etiology was strongly proposed for AIDS before the causal virus was demonstrated, and before the role of amyl nitrite "poppers" was found to be correlated with the sexual activity that transmitted the virus.[18]

A well-known example of the fallacy that correlation implies causation is shown in Figure 19.12, where the population of Oldenburg during the years 1930–36 was plotted against the number of storks observed flying in the city each year.[19] What better evidence could one want to prove that storks bring babies?

19.6.5   Additional "Sins"

Beyond all the problems just cited, many other opportunities are available to abuse the correlation/regression process. Of the many candidate "sins," only five more will be listed here.

19.6.5.1   Retroactive Demarcations — In certain studies the regression line shows a "dose–response" or "exposure–response" relationship when different levels of response are plotted against increasing magnitudes of a pharmaceutical agent or a "risk factor." If the regression line is not impressively "significant," however, the investigator may demarcate the dose–exposure variable into zones and then search for "significance" in pairwise (or other) comparisons of results in the demarcated zones.

If the demarcation is announced beforehand or if it depends on quantiles that are determined inherently by the data, the procedure is scientifically "legitimate." On the other hand, if the investigator makes arbitrary choices after inspecting the pattern of the data, the retroactive demarcations have dubious scientific credibility. They can sometimes be found, however, in studies where a binary variable for "exposure" is neither defined before the analysis nor stated in the text of the published report. Instead, after doing regression analysis for results of different levels of exposure, the investigators may present an odds ratio for response to a yes/no binary demarcation of "exposure." Distressing examples of these retroactive demarcations have been noted[20] in reports of the alleged relationship between endometrial cancer and postmenopausal use of estrogen.

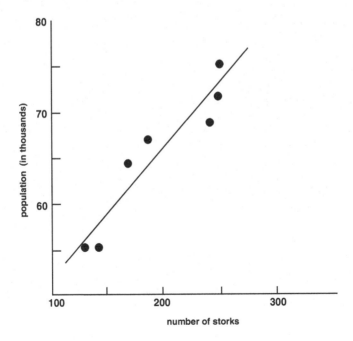

FIGURE 19.12
A plot of the population of Oldenburg at the end of each year against the number of storks observed in that year, 1930–1936. [Figure and legend taken from Chapter Reference 19.]

19.6.5.2 *Comparing Subsequent vs. Baseline Values* —

If variable X represents a person's baseline value at time 1 and if another value of X is obtained for each person at a later time 2, the investigator may plot a graph showing the subsequent values as Y and the baseline values as X. If d is each person's change in values, the graph is really a plot of (X + d) vs. X, and a strong correlation with the baseline values of X is inevitable.

Back in Chapter 7, this type of correlation was the reason for examining change in a single incremental group of (**after – before**) values, rather than comparing two groups of values. In addition to the previously cited impropriety of the graphical line, this problem occurred in the data reported in Figure 19.11. The investigators checked at least nine other variables (plasma renin, noradrenaline, vasopressin, etc.) that might affect baroreflex sensitivity in the displayed group, but concluded that "the only significant correlation (p < 0.005) was found between baroreflex sensitivity before and during ACE inhibition."

A separate biologic correlation is often present, of course, between the amount of *change* in a variable and the initial level. An example of such a relationship is shown with the decreasing exponential curves that depict survival rates in a cohort or levels of radioactive decay over time. The relationship between change and initial levels is called the "Law of the initial value" and its appropriate analytic management is often an improperly managed challenge in biomedical data.[21]

19.6.5.3 *Extrapolation beyond Observed Range* —

Any regression line — whether rectilinear or curved—is constructed to fit the observed values of points, and the estimates are valid only within that range. For example, in most systems of laboratory measurement, voltages can be *rectilinearly* related to chemical concentrations only within a limited range of values. If the concentration becomes too high or too low, the laboratory will transfer to a different system of measurement (and a different linear relationship with voltage).

The problem of beyond-range extrapolation is particularly likely to occur when the X-variable is time, and when a future status is predicted from extrapolations beyond the most recent date in the regression line. The annals of errors in the biomedical or social sciences contain many wrong predictions about populations, economic events, global temperatures, etc. — all derived from beyond-range extrapolation of a regression equation.

19.6.5.4 *Inappropriate Combinations* —

Data from different studies are regularly aggregated for analysis as a single group during meta-analyses or other forms of analytic "pooling." One requirement for pooling is that the individual results be reasonably homogeneous. Testing for "homogeneity" is often neglected, however, because its definition may be inconsistent for statistical components or nonexistent for biologic distinctions.

Figure 19.13 displays a dramatic example of the error that can occur when the directions of individual group regressions are ignored during a combined analysis of the groups. Each of the individual groups shows a distinct negative association, but the aggregate shows a strong trend in the opposite (positive) direction.

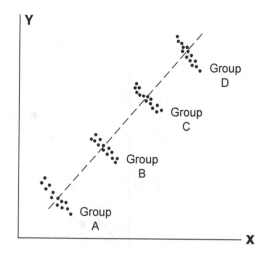

FIGURE 19.13
Misleading aggregate regression line for individual results in four groups.

19.6.5.5 *Inappropriate Fits* —

Almost any collection of data can be fitted with a polynomial or "time series" regression line expressed by

$Y_i = a + bX + cX^2 + dX^3 + \ldots$. Even if the data have no resemblance to a linear structure, the computer can find coefficients for a line that offers "best fit" for the collection of scattered points. Such an accomplishment appears in Figure 19.14, which shows total results for repeated measurements of a cohort of 74 patients receiving antiretroviral therapy after acute or recent HIV–1 seroconversion. The authors concluded that the line in Figure 19.14 "shows the rapid decrease in plasma levels of HIV–1 RNA over time" and that "after 117 days after infection, an inflection point was reached at which HIV-1 levels stopped decreasing and gradually increased." You can decide for yourself whether this interpretation is justified for the data fitted by the line.

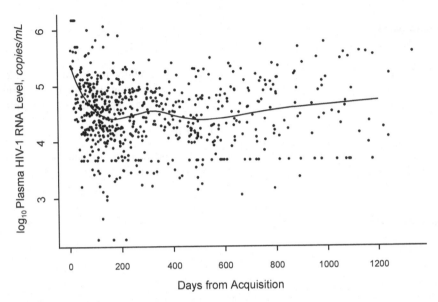

FIGURE 19.14
Scatterplot of plasma HIV-1 RNA levels ($\times 10^3$/mL) and median plasma HIV-1 RNA levels in the cohort from the time of seroconversion. [Figure and legend taken from Chapter Reference 22.]

19.7 Other Trends

Despite substantial length, the discussion in this chapter has covered only the bivariate estimates and trends for two variables that are each dimensional. As noted in Chapter 18, however, many more statistical indexes are needed for trends in relationships that are not bi-dimensional. After this long bolus of reading, you will be pleased to know that most of the additional indexes seldom appear in medical literature, and that their discussion, deferred until Chapter 27, will emphasize only a few that you may be likely to encounter. The topics omitted now and included in Chapter 27 are the following: bi-ordinal coefficients, such as Spearman's rho and Kendall's tau; the expression of linear trend in an ordinal array of proportions; binary and nominal coefficients, such as ϕ; and other indexes of trend in $r \times 2$ or $r \times c$ two-way tables (where $r \geq 3$ and $c \geq 3$).

References

1. Feinstein, 1996; 2. Guilford, 1956, pg. 145; 3. Cohen, 1977, pgs. 78-81; 4. Fleiss, 1981; 5. Burnand, 1990; 6. Cherfas, 1990; 7. Knapen, 1989; 8. Tasaki, 1992; 9. Wagner, 1978; 10. Blankenhorn, 1978; 11. Stead, 1978; 12. Allred, 1989; 13. Snedecor, 1956, pg.126; 14. Concato, 1993; 15. Anscombe, 1973; 16. Osterziel, 1990; 17. Mormor, 1982; 18. Vandenbroucke, 1989; 19. Box, 1978; 20. Horwitz, 1986; 21. Bierman, 1976; 22. Schacker, 1998; 23. Altman, 1988; 24. Sechi, 1998; 25. Saad, 1991; 26. Wintemute, 1988; 27. Reaven, 1988; 28. Beckmann, 1988; 29. Kahaleh, 1989; 30. Godfrey, 1985; 31. Dines, 1974.

Appendix

Additional Formulas and Proofs for Assertions

A.19.1 $S_r = \Sigma(Y_i - \hat{Y}_i)^2$ is a minimum when $b = S_{xy}/S_{xx}$

From Equation [19.1], $\hat{Y}_i - \bar{Y} = b(X_i - \bar{X})$. Transposing $\bar{Y}$ and subtracting Y_i from both sides, we get $\hat{Y}_i - Y_i = \bar{Y} - Y_i - b(\bar{X}_i - X)$. Because $S_r = \Sigma(Y_i - \hat{Y}_i)^2$, the squaring and summing produces $S_r = \Sigma(Y_i - \bar{Y})^2 - 2b\Sigma(X_i - \bar{X})(Y_i - \bar{Y}) + b^2\Sigma(X_i - \bar{X})^2$. Substituting the appropriate symbols, this becomes

$$S_r = S_{yy} - 2bS_{xy} + b^2S_{xx} \qquad\qquad [A.19.1]$$

where S_{yy}, S_{xy}, and S_{xx} are constant for any individual group of data. To find the minimum value, differentiate S_r with respect to b, set the result to 0, and solve. Thus, $\delta S_r / \delta b = -2S_{xy} + 2bS_{xx} = 0$, and so $b = S_{xy}/S_{xx}$.

A.19.2 $a = \bar{Y} - b\bar{X}$

Starting with $\hat{Y}_i = a + bX_i$, subtract Y_i from both sides, then square both sides, and take the sums to produce $\Sigma(\hat{Y}_i - Y_i)^2 = S_r = na^2 + b^2n\bar{X} + nY_i^2 + 2abn\bar{X} - 2an\bar{Y} - 2b\Sigma X_iY_i$. When differentiated with respect to a, all terms will vanish that do not include a. Differentiating and setting the result to 0 produces $\delta S_r/\delta a = 2an + 2bn\bar{X} - 2n\bar{Y} = 0$; and so $a = \bar{Y} - b\bar{X}$.

A.19.3   Standardized Regression Equation is $(Y_i - \bar{Y})/s_y = r(X_i - \bar{X})/s_x$

Divide both sides of equation [19.1] by $s_x s_y$ to produce $(\hat{Y}_i - \bar{Y})/s_x s_y = b(X_i - \bar{X})/s_x s_y$. Transpose and rearrange terms to produce $(\hat{Y}_i - \bar{Y})/s_y = (bs_x/s_y)(X_i - \bar{X})/s_x$. Because $s_y = \sqrt{S_{yy}/(n-1)}$ and $s_x = \sqrt{S_{xx}/(n-1)}$, $s_x/s_y = \sqrt{S_{xx}/S_{yy}}$. Because $b = S_{xy}/S_{xx}$, the factor bs_x/s_y becomes $(S_{xy}/S_{xx})(\sqrt{S_{xx}/S_{yy}})$, which is $S_{xy}/(\sqrt{S_{yy}S_{xx}}) = r$. [With a similar algebraic process, the same result emerges if we start with $\hat{X}_i - \bar{X} = b'(Y_i - Y)$, where $b' = S_{xy}/S_{yy}$. The result is $(\hat{X}_i - \bar{X})/s_x = r(Y_i - \bar{Y})/s_y$.]

A.19.4   Degrees of Freedom for $\hat{Y}_i$

For parametric inference, the observed values of $\{X_i, Y_i\}$ are regarded as a sample from the "true" regression equation, which is cited (using Greek letters for the parameters) as $Y = \alpha + \beta X$. In the calculated equation for $\hat{Y}_i = a + bX_i$, a and b are estimates for the two parameters, α and β. Thus, two degrees of freedom are lost from the n degrees available for choosing $\hat{Y}_i$. An alternative explanation is that a and b are calculated after the parametric means are estimated as $\mu_X = \bar{X}$ and $\mu_Y = \bar{Y}$. Two degrees of freedom are lost for those two parameters.

A.19.5   Parametric Variances of Regression Line

We need to estimate two variances. One of them is $\sigma_{y.x}$, which represents the average parametric variance of the observed Y_i values for the $\hat{Y}_i$ calculated from X_i. The other is the sampling variance or "standard error" of the slope, β. Anything else that is needed can be derived from these two estimates.

A.19.5.1 Variance of $\sigma_{y \cdot x}$ for $Y_i - \hat{Y}_i$

From Formula [19.8] the "mean square error" is estimated as

$$\hat{\sigma}^2_{y.x} \ = \ s^2_{y.x} \ = \ S_r/(n-2) \qquad\qquad \text{[A.19.2]}$$

A.19.5.2 Variance of the Slope β

To determine variance of the slope, the formula $b = S_{xy}/S_{xx}$ is rewritten as $b = \Sigma(X_i - \overline{X})(Y_i - \overline{Y})/S_{xx}$, which becomes

$$b = \frac{\Sigma(X_i - \overline{X})Y_i - \overline{Y}\Sigma(X_i - \overline{X})}{S_{xx}}$$

The second term in the numerator vanishes because $\overline{Y}$ is constant and $\Sigma(X_i - \overline{X}) = 0$ by definition. The rest of the expression is now expanded to form

$$b = \frac{(X_1 - \overline{X})Y_1}{S_{xx}} + \frac{(X_2 - \overline{X})Y_2}{S_{xx}} + \cdots + \frac{(X_n - \overline{X})Y_n}{S_{xx}}$$

If each of the $(X_i - \overline{X})/S_{xx}$ components is expressed as a constant, k_i, we can write

$$b = k_1 Y_1 + k_2 Y_2 + \cdots + k_n Y_n$$

Using "Var ( )" as the symbol for variance, we first determine the effects of a constant in variance. Thus, if $\text{Var}(X) = \Sigma(X_i - \overline{X})^2$, $\text{Var}(kX) = \Sigma(kX_i - k\overline{X})^2 = k^2\Sigma(X_i - \overline{X})^2 = k^2\text{Var}(X)$.

In Appendix A.7.1, we found that the variance of a sum is the sum of the variances. Thus, $\text{Var}(X + Y + W + ...) = \text{Var}(X) + \text{Var}(Y) + \text{Var}(W) + ...$ Consequently, in the foregoing expression of b,

$$\text{Var}(b) = k_1^2 \, \text{Var}(Y_1) + k_2^2 \, \text{Var}(Y_2) + \cdots + k_n^2 \, \text{Var}(Y_n)$$

The average variance of each Y_i value around the regression line was previously shown to be $s^2_{y.x}$. On average, therefore,

$$\text{Var}(b) = s^2_{y.x} \, (k_1^2 + k_2^2 + \cdots + k_n^2)$$

Because $k_i = (X_i - \overline{X})/S_{xx}$ and $k_i^2 = (X_i - \overline{X})^2/S^2_{xx}$, the sum is

$$\Sigma k_i^2 = \Sigma(X_i - \overline{X})^2/S^2_{xx} = S_{xx}/S^2_{xx} = 1/S_{xx}$$

Therefore the variance of the slope is

$$s^2_b = \text{Var}(b) = s^2_{y.x}/S_{xx} \qquad\qquad \text{[A.19.3]}$$

___

A.19.6 Critical Ratio for t or Z Test on b or r

The critical ratio for a t or Z test on the slope will be

$$t \text{ or } Z = \frac{b - \beta}{s_b} \qquad\qquad \text{[A.19.4]}$$

which becomes b/s_b when β is set to 0 under the null hypothesis. From Formula [A.19.2], $s^2_{y \cdot x} = S_r/(n-2)$ and from Formula [19.16], $S_r = (1 - r^2)S_{yy}$. Therefore, $s^2_{y.x} = (1 - r^2)S_{yy}/(n-2)$. Substituting in Formula [A.19.3], we get $s^2_b = (1 - r^2)S_{yy}/[S_{xx}(n-2)]$. When the square root of this result and $b = S_{xy}/S_{xx}$ are substituted, and when terms are suitably rearranged, the critical ratio becomes

$$t \text{ (or } Z) = \frac{r\sqrt{n-2}}{\sqrt{1-r^2}} \qquad\qquad \text{[A.19.5]}$$

The critical ratio for testing b is thus expressed in values of r. Exactly the same calculation is used for a t or Z test on r when the parametric correlation coefficient, ρ, is set to 0 under the null hypothesis.

A.19.7   Confidence Intervals for r and b

In the critical ratio of Formula [A.19.5], $\sqrt{(1-r^2)/(n-2)}$ corresponds to the standard error for the observed value of r. Therefore, a confidence interval for the estimated parameter ρ can be placed around r as

$$\rho = r \pm t_{v,\alpha}\sqrt{(1-r^2)/(n-2)} \qquad\qquad [\text{A.19.6}]$$

If you want a more formal demonstration of the "standard error" approach here, recall from Formula [A.19.4], that a confidence interval for β can be estimated (using t) as

$$\hat{\beta} = b \pm t_{v,\alpha}s_b$$

This becomes

$$\hat{\beta} = \frac{S_{xy}}{S_{xx}} \pm t_{v,\alpha}\sqrt{[(1-r^2)S_{yy}]/[S_{xx}(n-2)]}$$

and then

$$\hat{\beta} = \frac{S_{xy}}{S_{xx}} \pm t_{v,\alpha}\sqrt{\frac{1-r^2}{n-2}}\sqrt{\frac{S_{yy}}{S_{xx}}}$$

Because $\sqrt{S_{yy}/S_{xx}} = s_y/s_x$ and $b = S_{xy}/S_{xx} = rs_y/s_x$, the confidence interval becomes

$$\hat{\beta} = (s_y/s_x)\left[r \pm t_{v,\alpha}\sqrt{(1-r^2)/(n-2)}\right] \qquad\qquad [\text{A.19.7}]$$

The term in the square root sign is the "standard error" for r.

A.19.8   Confidence Interval for Individual Points

If the goal is to estimate an actual point, Y_i, rather than using $\hat{Y}_i$ as the mean value of $\bar{Y}_i$ at X_i, the confidence interval is wider, to encompass the variations in $\bar{Y}_i - Y_i$. The standard error of an estimated point becomes

$$s_{y.x}^2[1 + (1/n) + \{(X_i - \bar{X})^2/S_{xx}\}] \qquad\qquad [\text{A.19.8}]$$

Because the value of 1 in Formula [A.19.8] is so much larger than (1/n) or $(X_i - \bar{X})^2/S_{xx}$, the result is not greatly affected by changes in $X_i - \bar{X}$, and the subsequent wide confidence bands will seem to be relatively straight rather than concave lines.

A.19.9   Confidence Interval for Intercept

Because the intercept is calculated when $X_i = 0$, the corresponding confidence interval can be determined from Formula [19.23], with X_i set to zero.

A.19.10   Comparison of Two Regression Lines

Because most ordinary regression lines in medical research do not give close fits, two lines are seldom compared stochastically. (Two *survival curves* may be compared, as discussed later in Chapter 22, but the stochastic strategy does not use regression principles.)

If a stochastic contrast is desired, however, two regression lines can be compared either for the different slopes or, if the lines seem parallel, for the interlinear vertical distances. The latter evaluation is essentially a comparison of the two intercepts.

If you need to do any of these comparisons, they are clearly discussed, with a worked example, in an excellent paper by Altman and Gardner.[23]

A.19.11   Transformations of r

If X and Y have a joint bivariate Gaussian distribution (which would look like a Gaussian hill), r can be transformed to

$$Z_r = \left(\frac{1}{2}\right) \ln \left(\frac{1+r}{1-r}\right)$$

The distribution of Z_r is approximately Gaussian and its standard error is $1/\sqrt{n-3}$. For the $1-\alpha$ confidence interval we calculate $Z_r \pm (t_{v,\alpha}/\sqrt{n-3})$, and then transform the results with suitable exponentiation. A good worked example of the procedure is also shown by Altman and Gardner.[23]

The data of Table 18.5 obviously do not have a suitable distribution, but can be used for a crude illustration here. In those data, $r = .186$ and $n = 8$; and so $Z_r = (1/2) [\ln(1.186/.814)] = .188$. The value of $\sqrt{n-3}$ is 2.236, and $t_{6,.05} = 2.447$, so that $.188 \pm 2.447 = -2.259$ to 2.635, is the range for Z_r. Because

$$2Z_r = \ln \frac{1+r}{1-r}$$

we exponentiate to get $[(1+r)/(1-r)] = e^{2Z_r}$, which leads to $r = (e^{2Z_r} - 1)/(e^{2Z_r} + 1)$. For $Z_r = -2.259$, this result becomes $r = -.989/1.0109 = -.978$; and for $Z_r = 2.635$, the corresponding result is $r = 193.42/195.42 = .990$. The 95% confidence interval for the observed $r = .188$ would thus extend throughout the wide range from $-.978$ to $.990$ — a result consistent with the diffuse spread in the small data set. Because neither boundary exceeds $|1|$, this range seems more numerically "acceptable" than the range of $-.795$ to 1.167 previously calculated in Section 19.4.2.1 with Formula [19.22].

Exercises

To give you time for all the reading, the exercises that follow are mainly challenges in "physical diagnosis," containing almost no requirements for calculation. (Besides, most regression calculations today are relegated to a computer program.) Nevertheless, because your education would be incomplete if you failed to do at least one set of regression computations yourself, a delightful opportunity is presented in Exercise 19.1.

19.1. A clinical investigator who believes that serum omphalase is closely related to immunoglobulin zeta is disappointed by the nonlinear pattern seen in a graph of the following data:

Immunoglobulin Zeta Level	Serum Omphalase Level
1	35
3	10
5	40
7	30
9	15
10	45
11	80
13	75
15	50
17	60
19	50

The investigator consults a statistician who also happens to be board-certified in diagnostic graphology. The statistician looks at the graph, and promptly announces, "The relationship here is strong and probably stochastically significant."

19.1.1. After plotting the graph on any kind of paper you want to use, try to guess (and explain your guess about) the reasons for the statistician's statement.

19.1.2. Please carry out the computations necessary to determine the regression line, the value of r, and the test of stochastic significance; also draw the line on your graph. Please show all the intermediate computations, so that pathogenesis can be probed if you get a wrong result.

19.2. The data in the scattergraph shown in Figure E.19.2 were recently used to support the claim that "serum lipoprotein(a) levels are elevated in patients with early impairment of renal function" and that the "inverse correlation between serum lipoprotein(a) level and creatinine clearance" points to "decreased renal catabolism as a probable mechanism of lipoprotein(a) elevation in patients with early renal failure." The study was done in 417 patients, referred consecutively to a hypertension clinic in Italy, who were tested one week after antihypertensive drugs were withdrawn. An abnormal creatinine clearance, defined as < 90 mL/min per 1.73 m² was found in 160 of the 417 patients.

Do you agree with the stated claim? Please justify your reasons.

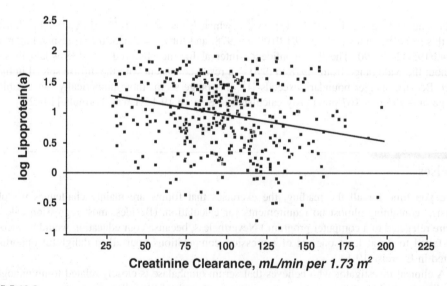

FIGURE E.19.2

Relation between creatinine clearance and log lipoprotein(a). A significant inverse correlation ($r = 0.243$; $P < 0.0001$) was seen. [Figure and legend taken from Chapter Reference 24.]

19.3. The text of Chapter 19 contained no comments about one-tailed or two-tailed interpretations for the P values associated with b or r; and most statistical writers and texts do not discuss the subject. Nevertheless, investigators regularly do research with the anticipation that the slope will definitely go up (or down), and that the correlation will be definitely positive (or an inverse negative). Do *you* believe that one-tailed interpretations should be allowed when a distinct direction has been specified in advance for the slope or correlation coefficient?

19.4. Here is another opportunity to draw conclusions from the physical examination of graphs. Figure E.19.4 is an exact reproduction of what appeared in a publication[25] on "racial differences in the relation between blood pressure and insulin resistance." The investigators studied "116 Pima Indians, 53 whites, and 42 blacks who were normotensive and did not have diabetes." The Pima Indians "were recruited from subjects participating in a longitudinal study on the development of non-insulin dependent diabetes. The whites and blacks were recruited by advertising in the local community." The white and black participants were required to have parents and grandparents who were correspondingly white or black. "Afro-Caribbean and blacks from countries other than the United States were excluded." The selected groups were shown to be similar in mean age and blood pressure. From the results in Figure E.19.4, however, the authors drew the following conclusions: (1) "the Pima Indians had higher fasting plasma insulin concentrations than the whites or blacks"; and (2) in whites, but not in Pima Indians or blacks, "mean blood pressure ... was significantly correlated with fasting plasma insulin concentration (r = 42) and [with] the rate of glucose disposal during the low dose (r = −0.41) and high-dose (r = −0.49) insulin infusions." The authors concluded further that "a common mechanism, genetic or acquired, such as enhanced adrenergic tone, or a cellular or structural defect may constitute the link between insulin resistance and blood pressure in whites but not in other racial groups."

Considering only the graphic evidence, and avoiding discussion of the proposed biologic or physiologic mechanisms, do you think the investigators' conclusions are justified?

19.5. The four figures marked E.19.5.1 through E.19.5.4 are taken directly from published medical reports. In each instance, the author(s) claimed that a significant relationship had been demonstrated. Except for methodologic details describing the measurements and groups, the text offered no statistical information about these relationships, beyond what is shown in the figures. (In one instance, r values reported in the text have been added to the figures.)

For Exercises 19.5.1 through 19.5.4, comment on each of these four analyses, figures, and conclusions. Do you think the authors are justified or unjustified? If you do not like what they did, what would you offer as an alternative?

19.6. Figure E.19.6 shows a scatter-plot of residuals in which the values of $Y_i - \hat{Y}_i$ have been plotted against the values of $\hat{Y}_i$ for a group of 12 bivariate points. What conclusion would you draw from this pattern? If you are unhappy with the problem, what solution would you propose?

19.7. Figure E.19.7 shows the published points and corresponding regression lines for a plot of serum copper vs. pleural fluid copper in three diagnostic categories of patients.

19.7.1. In the text, the authors stated that for the 120 patients with malignant disease the value of r = 0.19 was statistically significant at P < 0.05. Are you convinced that this significance is biologically important? If so, why? If not, why not?

19.7.2. A regression line has been drawn for each of the three cited equations. How can you quickly (by eye test alone) get supporting evidence that these lines correctly depict the stated equation?

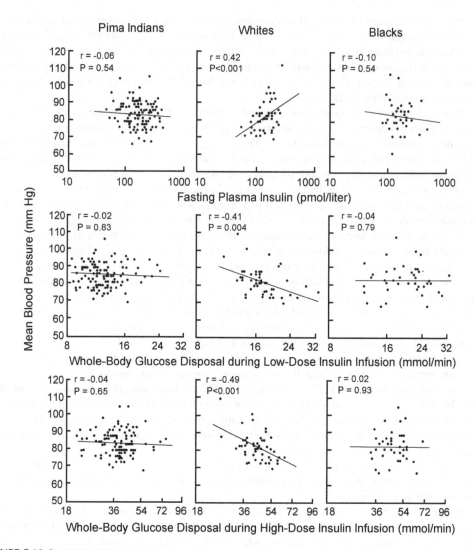

FIGURE E.19.4

Relation between Mean Blood Pressure and Fasting Plasma Insulin Concentration (Top Panel) and Insulin-Mediated Glucose Disposal during Low-Dose (Middle Panel) and High-Dose (Bottom Panel) Insulin Infusions in Pima Indians, Whites, and Blacks, after Adjustment for Age, Sex, Body Weight, and Percentage of Body Fat. The differences among the three groups in the slopes of the regression lines between mean blood pressure and the fasting plasma insulin concentration and insulin-mediated glucose disposal during low-dose and high-dose insulin infusions were statistically significant (P = 0.001, 0.017, and 0.025 for Pima Indians, whites, and blacks, respectively). [Figure and legend taken from Chapter Reference 25.]

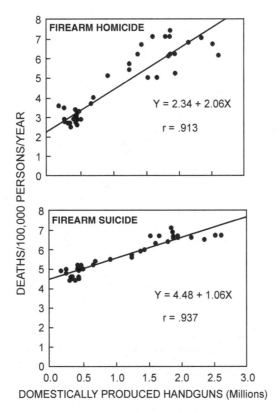

FIGURE E.19.5.1
Handgun availability and firearm mortality: United States, 1946–85. [Figure and legend taken from Chapter Reference 26.]

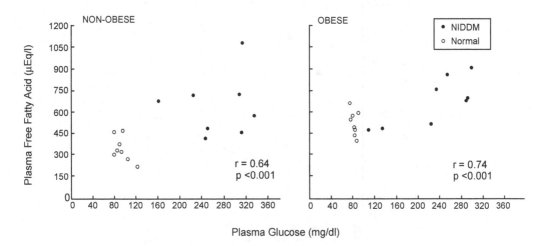

FIGURE E.19.5.2
Relationship between fasting plasma glucose and FFA concentrations in nonobese and obese persons with normal glucose tolerance (open circles) or NIDDM (solid circles). [Figure and legend taken from Chapter Reference 27.]

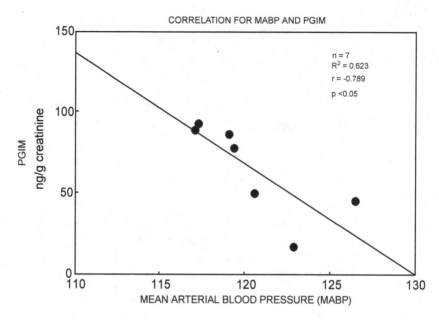

FIGURE E.19.5.3

Correlation of mean arterial blood pressure (MABP) and measured PGI_2 metabolite excretion (PGIM) in seven essential hypertensive patients receiving no medications. Each patient underwent three separate determinations for MABP and PGIM (during control periods 1 and 2 and during the placebo period) for a total of seven independent observations. Regression analysis was performed with the Statistical Analysis System using analysis of variance. [Figure and legend taken from Chapter Reference 28.]

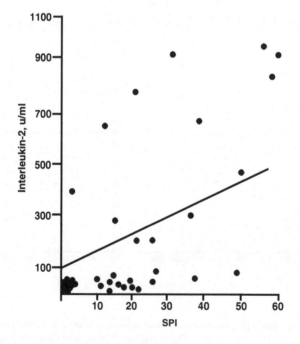

FIGURE E.19.5.4

Interleukin-2 serum level as measured by enzyme-linked immunosorbent assay in 81 sera samples. Data represent the mean of quadruplicate values. [Figure and legend derived from Chapter Reference 29.]

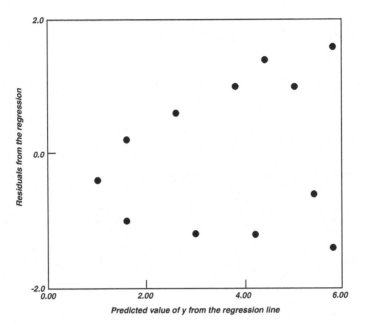

FIGURE E.19.6
[Figure and legend taken from Chapter Reference 30.]

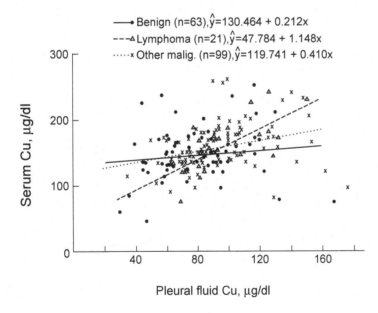

FIGURE E.19.7
Positive relationship between pleural fluid copper and serum copper in the group with malignant disease. [Figure and legend taken from Chapter Reference 31.]

20

Evaluating Concordances

CONTENTS

A striking feature of modern medical statistics has been the relative absence of attention to the scientific quality of raw data. Despite the many methods developed for sampling, receiving, and analyzing data, and for drawing conclusions about importance or "significance," the scientific suitability, accuracy, and reproducibility of the basic information has not been a major focus of concern.

The contemporary statistical emphasis on inference rather than evidence is particularly ironic because problems of "observer variability" were the stimulus about 150 years ago that made C. F. Gauss develop his "theory of errors" in describing the "normal" distribution of deviations from the "correct" value (i.e., the mean) of a measurement. Analogous challenges in "quality control" for chemical variations in beer at the Guinness brewery were the stimulus almost 100 years ago for W. S. Gosset's activities that are now famous as the *Student t test*. After Gaussian and Gossetian theory were established, however, statistical creativity became devoted more to quantity in mathematical variance than to quality in measurement variability.

Until about two decades ago, W. Edwards Deming, a statistician who gave imaginative attention to industrial methods of achieving "quality control," was generally little known or heralded in English-speaking academic enclaves. Nevertheless, Deming's methods are particularly famous in Japan, where they were adopted after World War II and became a keystone of Japanese success in developing high quality products with modern industrial technology.

Because variability in scientific measurement[1] is still distressingly alive, well, and flourishing, the statistical methods of describing the problems have often come from investigators working directly in the pertinent scientific domain. Examining observer variability among radiologists,[2] J. Yerushalmy, an epidemiologist, devised the indexes of *sensitivity* and *specificity* now commonly used in the literature of diagnostic tests. Indexes of biased observation,[3] a special chi-square test for observer variability,[4] and the commonly used *kappa* coefficient of concordance[5] were contributed by two psychologists, Quinn McNemar and Jacob Cohen. Statistical methods for describing accuracy and reproducibility in laboratory data have also been developed mainly by workers in that field,[6] although R. A. Fisher's *intraclass correlation coefficient* has sometimes been applied for laboratory measurements. [Fisher originally proposed[7] the intraclass coefficient, however, to compare results in pairs of brothers, not to analyze diverse measurements of the *same* entity.]

Lacking the mathematical "clout" of statistical theory, the pragmatic challenges of measurement variability are omitted from many textbooks of medical, biologic, and epidemiologic statistics. In many textbook discussions of "association," in fact, trends in measurements of different variables are not distinguished from concordances in different measurements of the same entity.

This chapter is intended to outline some of the main distinctions and challenges in statistical appraisals of concordance and to discuss the diverse indexes of concordance that appear in medical literature.

20.1 Distinguishing Trends from Concordances

The idea of interchangeability is what separates concordance from trend. Trends are assessed to determine whether two different variables are co-related, i.e., whether they "go along together." For concordances, however, the goal is to see whether Variable A can be interchangeably substituted for Variable B. An index of trend may have a high correlation value when derived from the proportionate reduction in group variance for sums of squared errors, but the estimates of $\hat{Y}_i$ may not be good enough to be used as direct substitutes for Y_i.

To illustrate the problem, consider the four data sets in the table below. The values of X are the same in each set, but the corresponding values of Y — in the columns marked $Y_A, Y_B, Y_C,$ and Y_D — represent different methods of measuring X.

X	Y_A	Y_B	Y_C	Y_D
3	3	7	6	4
4	4	8	8	3
5	5	9	10	6
6	6	10	12	5
7	7	11	14	8
8	8	12	16	7
9	9	13	18	10
10	10	14	20	9

The graphs of the four sets of points and the corresponding fitted lines are shown in Figure 20.1.

If assessed for trend, the regression line fits the points perfectly for each of groups Y_A, Y_B, and Y_C, and the line for Group Y_D also fits very well. The r values are 1 for the first three lines, and close to 1 for the fourth. Despite the almost identical high marks for trend, however, only the Y_A line has close agreement; and in the three other lines, the corresponding Y values never agree with those of X. In Y_B, the values are always 4 units higher; in Y_C, they are doubled; and in Y_D, they are alternatingly one unit higher or lower.

None of these disagreements is shown, however, by indexes of trend. The intercepts are different for lines Y_B and Y_C, but similar for lines Y_A and Y_D; the slopes are identical in lines Y_B and Y_D; and the correlation coefficients are extremely high in all three of the disagreeing lines for Y_B, Y_C, and Y_D. Because the customary statistical indexes of trend are not satisfactory, agreement must be described with a different set of indexes, aimed at appraising concordance.

20.2 Conformity vs. Agreement

Although the orientation is either dependent or non-dependent for assessing trend, the orientation of a concordance is aimed at either conformity or agreement. In conformity, the goal is to see how closely the observed measurement conforms to a "correct result," which is available as the "reference," "criterion," or "gold standard" value for each measurement. This concept is usually regarded as *accuracy*, but is best called *conformity*. The idea of *accuracy* is pertinent for technologic measurements, but cannot be readily applied to assess other types of discrepancy, such as whether a clinician's decisions comply with the criteria established by an audit committee. *Conformity* is also preferable because the "gold standard" may sometimes change. Thus, the "correct" answer to the question in a certifying examination ten years ago may no longer be correct today.

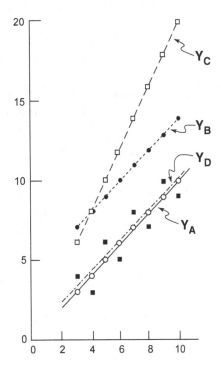

FIGURE 20.1
Graph of the four sets of data in Section 20.1.

Agreement, however, is assessed without a "gold-standard" criterion. We determine how closely two observations agree, but not whether they are correct. For example, suppose two radiologists independently decide whether pulmonary embolism is present or absent in each of a series of chest films. If no information is available about the patients' true conditions, we can assess only the radiologists' agreement. If additional data indicate whether each patient did or did not actually have pulmonary embolism, we can determine each radiologist's accuracy (i.e., conformity with the correct diagnosis) as well as the agreement between them.

When pathologists provide "readings" of histologic specimens, we can assess only the agreement of the observers, unless one of the pathologists is accorded the deified status of always being correct. Two pathologists' readings of cytologic specimens (such as pap smears) would usually be assessed for agreement, but accuracy could also be checked if an appropriate *histologic* decision were available for each smear.

Although studies of observer variability will indicate disagreements among "equal" observers, studies of conformity are done with a "gold standard." For laboratory measurements, the gold standard is provided by a selected reference laboratory or a national Bureau of Standards. For the categorical measurements used in certifying examinations or audits of health care, the "gold standard" is provided by an individual expert or consensus of designated experts.

In a particularly common type of conformity research, the gold standard for a diagnostic marker test is the definitive diagnosis of the selected disease. Diagnostic marker tests and other aspects of conformity are appraised in so many different ways that the topic will receive a separate discussion in Chapter 21. The rest of this chapter is devoted to evaluating agreement.

In the specialized jargon developed for describing the ideas, the results of a study of agreement are sometimes called *reproducibility, repeatability, reliability,* or *consistency.* The first two terms are inadequate if each rater has given only a single rating, and the third term is unsatisfactory because *reliability* is an idea that generally connotes "trustworthiness" beyond mere agreement alone. To describe the general concept, *consistency* is probably the best of the four terms, but fortunately, the assessment of individual (rather than group) agreements is usually called *agreement* (or *concordance*). Indexes of agreement or disagreement will be needed for the individual results and total group patterns that can occur in the four main types of rating scales.

20.3   Challenges in Appraising Agreement

Appraising agreement involves a new set of statistical challenges that arise uniquely when discrepancies are noted and summarized for measurements of the same entities.

20.3.1   Goals of the Research

An important consideration *before* the work is done is to establish the goals of the research. Is it intended to expose and quantify the state of disagreement among the raters, or is the main goal to improve the state of the observational art? In most published studies of concordance, the work seems aimed merely at quantifying disagreement. The investigator does the research, presents the report, and departs in an air of sagacious revelation — but nothing happens thereafter. The disagreement itself becomes exposed, but whatever was causing it is neither discovered nor repaired.

The distinction between "diagnostic" demonstration and "therapeutic" improvement is shown in the names commonly used for the research. When disagreement is investigated for laboratory measurements, the work is usually called *quality control.* The revealed disagreements are confronted and carefully explored; the methods of measurement are checked and improved; and the eventual improvements elevate the quality of the measurement process. In most investigations of disagreement among clinicians, radiologists, and pathologists, however, the work is usually called *observer variability.* Little or no effort is made afterward to remove the defects that have been revealed.

This apparent complacency is probably due to the difficulty of arranging suitable analytic confrontations. In laboratory measurements, the procedures can usually be clearly delineated, so that sources of variation can easily be sought among the component steps of the observational process. For clinicians, radiologists, and pathologists, however, the component steps of the procedure are not clearly discerned when the result is merely stated as a rating — such as **systolic murmur, 1+ enlargement,** or **poorly differentiated adenocarcinoma** — that emerges from a complex act of observation and decision. To determine component steps and criteria for the observational decisions, the observers must meet together, confront the disagreements, and identify the constituent steps of the process. These analytic confrontations may be difficult to arrange because of problems in getting the observers assembled, and also because many observers may dislike the confrontational process and its possible departures from "diplomacy."

If the goal is to improve rather than merely document the problems of observer variability, however, the investigator may have to plan for much more than just getting and comparing the stated ratings. If the observers cannot be assembled for direct confrontation, the solicited information should include attention not only to the "final" ratings, but particularly to the intricate components and criteria of the observational process.

20.3.2   Process, Rater, and Observer

If the *entity* being "measured" is a white blood count, serum calcium, chest film, liver biopsy, answer to an examination question, or clinical decision, the person or apparatus that produces the actual measurement can be called the *rater*. The term *rater* has two advantages over *observer*. First, many decisions are expressed as ratings in a scale of categories, such as **adenocarcinoma** or **1+ cardiac enlargement**, rather than as purely descriptive statements, such as "roseating clusters of multi-nucleated cells" or "outward bulge of apex." Second, when the observed entity requires technologic preparation — such as a radiographic film — variations can arise from the way the technologic apparatus was used in positioning the patient or in taking and developing the film. Since "variability" can arise from both the technologic process that produces an entity and the person who interprets it, the term *rater* indicates the latter source.

The term *observer variability* can then include the combination of variations that can arise from both the process and the rater. In certain technologic measurements where a numerical value is produced without the intercession of a human rater, the variability is usually called *process*, because human variations can still arise when the results are transcribed or transmitted.

20.3.3 Number of Raters

Any comparison requires at least a pair of ratings for each entity, but the pair can come from one rater or two, and sometimes the same entity can receive more than two ratings.

20.3.3.1 *Single Rater* — If the same rater provides both ratings, the comparison can have several formats. In a common arrangement, *intra-rater concordance* is assessed when the rating is repeated by the same observer (such as a radiologist or pathologist) after enough time has elapsed for the first rating to have been forgotten.

In other circumstances, which might be called *intraclass concordance*, two (or more) ratings are available almost simultaneously. This situation can occur when the same laboratory measures aliquots of the same specimen to check repeatability of the process. In another situation, individual ratings are available for somewhat similar entities, such as a pair of twins or brothers. In the latter situations, the ratings cannot be assigned to a specific source, such as Method A vs. Method B, or Sibling A vs. Sibling B, because either one of the ratings can go in the first position. The management of these "unassigned" pairs was the stimulus for development of the intraclass correlation coefficient, discussed later.

20.3.3.2 *Two or More Raters* — The most common test of agreement is the *inter-rater concordance* between two ratings for the same entity, offered by Rater A vs. Rater B. Even when the same entity receives more than two ratings, many investigators prefer to check pairwise concordances for rater A vs. B, A vs. C, B vs. C, etc. rather than calculate a relatively nonspecific single index that covers all the raters simultaneously.

If measurements of the same entities come from three or more raters, concordance can be described for the pertinent pairs of two raters, or for the overall results among the group of raters. Because the mathematical activities become particularly complex for more than two sets of ratings, the challenge of indexing multiple observers will be saved for the end of the chapter in Section 20.9. The main discussion throughout the chapter will emphasize pairwise comparisons for two raters.

20.3.4 Types of Scale

Concordance can be checked only if each entity is rated in commensurate scales, having the same values available for citation in each scale. Statistical indexes will be needed for patterns in which the scales for *both* variables are: *dimensional*, e.g., laboratory measurements; *binary*, e.g., diagnostic marker tests; *ordinal*, e.g., ratings for staging systems or grades of clinical severity; or *nominal*, e.g., histopathologic categories.

20.3.5 Individual and Total Discrepancies

Each of the four patterns of data needs arrangements and indexes to cite individual discrepancies between each pair of ratings and to summarize the total pattern of discrepancies.

20.3.5.1   Categorical Data — For categorical data, the results are arranged in a two-way contingency table that is often called an *agreement matrix*. It shows the frequency counts in each cell formed by the rows and columns for each observer's ratings. Individual pairs of ratings will have different degrees of disagreement according to whether the scales are binary, ordinal, or nominal. Perfect agreements occur in the appropriate diagonal cells; and all other cells show different degrees of partial disagreement that are managed as discussed later.

The frequency counts for perfect or partial agreements in the cells can be added and then divided by the total to show proportions of different types of agreement.

20.3.5.2   Dimensional Data — An ordinary graph of dimensional data can show rater A's results as $\{X_i\}$, and rater B's corresponding measurements as $\{Y_i\}$. Figure 20.2 is an example of such a graph, for agreement between plasma and salivary measurements of caffeine.

The individual discrepancies can be expressed as $d_i = X_i - Y_i$ at each point, i, of the data. The sum of the discrepancies can be converted to a central index, such as a median, or a mean, which will be $\Sigma d_i/N$ for N points of data.

To get a better idea of magnitudes, the individual increments can be squared, added, divided by N, and then reconverted by taking the square root. The value of $\sqrt{\Sigma d_i^2/N}$ is called the *quadratic mean* or *root mean square* (mentioned in Section 3.8.1) of the increments. The smaller the square root value, the better is the agreement. This procedure is analogous to what was done in Section 7.8.1 for deviations in data for two paired groups or for before-and-after results in the same group. The increments here refer to deviations in pairs of measurements for the same N entities.

Other challenges in evaluating agreement for dimensional pairs of data will be discussed later in Section 20.7.

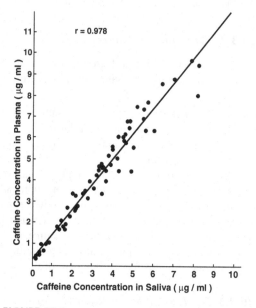

FIGURE 20.2

Correlation between caffeine concentrations in plasma (ordinate) and saliva (abscissa) in 12 subjects after single oral dose over 16 hr.

20.3.6   Indexes of Directional Disparity

Expressions of agreement do not indicate the directional effect of the discrepancies. For example, two raters can generally disagree in an apparently random manner, or one rater may be consistently higher or lower than the other. In addition, the discrepancies may have about the same magnitude in all zones of the data or may get larger or smaller in different zones. The bias in directional disparities will be expressed differently according to the four types of data, and also according to whether the bias refers to raters or to zones of data.

20.3.7   "Adjustment" for Chance Agreement

Another distinctive challenge in studies of concordance is that agreements can arise by chance alone. For example, suppose you know nothing about the substantive content of a certifying examination containing five choices of a single correct answer for each question. With random guesses alone, you should correctly answer 20% of the questions. Analogously, if two radiologists regularly rate 90% of chest films as being *normal*, we could expect their *normal* ratings to agree randomly on 81% (= .90 × .90) of the occasions.

In multiple-choice examinations, "guesses" are penalized when points are subtracted for wrong answers but not for "blanks" where no answer is offered. In studies of concordance, an analogous type of penalty can be used to make adjustment for the number of agreements that might have occurred by chance alone. If the raters are not given a well-chosen challenge, however, the adjustment process can produce an excessive penalty. For example, suppose two radiologists are tested for agreement on the chest films of a university freshman class, for whom about 95% (or more) of the films will be normal. Even if the radiologists achieve almost perfect agreement, they may be harshly penalized because so large a proportion of the agreement ($.90 = .95 \times .95$) might be ascribed to chance alone. Consequently, the distribution in the challenge group becomes particularly important if agreement is adjusted for chance.

Adjustments for chance in categorical data are cited with the Kappa index discussed later, but are seldom (if ever) applied to dimensional scales, for which the same two values have only a remote chance of being chosen randomly from the limitless (or at least large) number of dimensional choices for each variable.

20.3.8 Stability and Stochastic Tests

For tests of stability in small groups, the descriptive index of concordance is usually converted to a stochastic index that is checked with either a Z or chi-square procedure. Fortunately, the modern emphasis on stochastic tests has not extended to the evaluation of concordance. The descriptive indexes are usually reported directly and are seldom replaced by P values or confidence intervals. In fact, stochastic tests are often left unexamined or unreported, because the focus is on descriptive agreement and because the group sizes are usually large enough for the descriptive indexes to be regarded as stable.

Stochastic tests for concordance are discussed in Section 20.8.

20.4 Agreement in Binary Data

If *Yes* and *No* are used to represent the two categories of binary data, four possible results can occur for each pair of ratings. They form the 2×2 agreement matrix of frequency counts shown in Table 20.1.

TABLE 20.1

Agreement Matrix for Binary Data

		Rater A		
		Yes	**No**	**Total**
RATER B	Yes	a	b	f_1
	No	c	d	f_2
	TOTAL	n_1	n_2	N

The two raters **agree** in the *a* and *d* cells, and **disagree** in the *b* and *c* cells, but the results have directional distinctions as follows:

Rater A	Rater B	Result	Location of Cell in Table 20.1
Yes	Yes	Agree	a
No	Yes	Disagree	b
Yes	No	Disagree	c
No	No	Agree	d

If one of the raters is the "gold standard," the other's ratings are correct in the *a* and *d* cells and incorrect in the *b* and *c* cells. Without a gold standard, however, we need a way to summarize agreement rather than conformity.

20.4.1   Proportion (Percentage) of Agreement

Among many statistical proposals for summarizing index for agreement in binary data, only a few expressions are generally popular or valuable.

The most obvious, straightforward, and easiest-to-understand index is the proportion (or percentage) of agreement. It resembles a "batting average" in which the perfect agreements are "hits" and anything else is an "out." In the symbols of Table 20.1, the proportion of agreement is

$$p_o = \frac{a + d}{N} \qquad\qquad [20.1]$$

In the example shown in Table 20.2, the two examiners agreed on 40 candidates, whom both passed, and on 20 others, whom both failed. The proportion or percentage agreement is $(40 + 20)/80 = 60/80 = 75\%$.

TABLE 20.2

Agreement Matrix of Ratings on a Specialty Board
Certification Examination

Ratings by Examiner B	Ratings by Examiner A		
	Pass	Fail	Total
Pass	40	2	42
Fail	18	20	38
TOTAL	58	22	80

The simplicity of the index of percentage agreement is accompanied by three disadvantages. First, it does not indicate how the agreements and disagreements are distributed. Thus, the same value of 75% agreement would be obtained for the two raters in Table 20.2 if the 2×2 agreement matrix for 80 ratings had any of the following arrangements:

$$\begin{Bmatrix} 20 & 18 \\ 2 & 40 \end{Bmatrix} \quad \begin{Bmatrix} 30 & 10 \\ 10 & 30 \end{Bmatrix} \quad \begin{Bmatrix} 60 & 10 \\ 10 & 0 \end{Bmatrix} \quad \begin{Bmatrix} 0 & 10 \\ 10 & 60 \end{Bmatrix}$$

A second disadvantage is that the index does not show whether agreement is better directionally when the examiners decide to pass a candidate than when they decide to fail. A third disadvantage is that the expression of percentage agreement makes no provision for the concordance that might occur by chance alone.

20.4.2 ϕ Coefficient

The ϕ coefficient is an index of association (or correlation) for the data in a 2×2 table. The descriptive index, which is further discussed in Chapter 27, is calculated from the (uncorrected) X^2 statistic as $\phi^2 = X^2/N$, where N =total number of frequency counts. Thus,

$$\phi = \sqrt{X^2/N} = (ad - bc)/\sqrt{f_1 f_2 n_1 n_2} \qquad\qquad [20.2]$$

for the data in Table 20.1. Because X^2 for a 2×2 table is calculated with values that are expected by chance, the ϕ coefficient seems to offer a method of adjusting for chance-expected results in a 2×2 agreement matrix. With Formula [20.2], the value of ϕ in Table 20.2 would be $[(40)(20) - (2)(18)]/\sqrt{(58)(22)(42)(38)} = .535$.

However, ϕ has several disadvantages. First, it is aimed at assessing the trend in two independent variables, rather than concordance between two closely related variables. Suppose the ratings in Table 20.2 were transposed to show the following results:

	Examiner A		
Examiner B	**Pass**	**Fail**	**Total**
Pass	2	40	42
Fail	20	18	38
Total	22	58	80

The percentage of agreement would drop precipitously to only 25% [= (2 +18)/80] but ϕ would have the same absolute value, although in a negative direction, as $-.535$.

Because ϕ can take positive and negative signs, it might indicate whether the agreement is better or worse than might be expected by chance. The construction of ϕ, however, depends on examining the observed-minus-expected values in all four cells of the table. The value of ϕ thus contains individual discrepancies from cells showing agreements *and* disagreements; and it really tells us more than we want to know if the goal is to look at agreement alone or at disagreement alone.

Furthermore, the usual calculation of X^2 refers to N different members, each "rated" for a different variable. In an agreement matrix, however, each member has been rated twice for the same variable. There are really 2N ratings under consideration, not N. Thus, if we rearrange Table 20.2 to show total ratings rather than an agreement matrix for two observers, we would get the 160 ratings that appear in Table 20.3. The two arrangements for the same set of data are often called *matched* (in Table 20.2) and *unmatched* (in Table 20.3). The differences become important later (in Chapter 26) when we consider appropriate tabular structures for appraising results of exposed and non-exposed persons in a matched-pair case-control study.

TABLE 20.3

Total Ratings in Table 20.2

	Rating		
Examiner	**Pass**	**Fail**	**Total**
A	58	22	80
B	42	38	80
TOTAL	100	60	160

Despite these apparent disadvantages, the results of ϕ are usually reasonably close to those of the chance-adjusted kappa discussed in the next section. In fact, it can be shown algebraically that when the marginal totals of Table 20.1 are equal, i.e., $n_1 = n_2$ and $f_1 = f_2$, the values of ϕ and kappa are identical. The ϕ coefficient was recently used, without apparent complaint by editors or reviewers, to adjust for chance in reporting agreement among observers' opinions about whether antihistamine treatment had been used prophylactically during anesthesia.[8]

20.4.3 Kappa

Kappa is now regarded as the best single index to adjust for chance agreement in a 2×2 table of concordance. Specifically designed for this purpose by the clinical psychologist, Jacob Cohen,[5] and medically popularized by J. L. Fleiss,[9] kappa forms a ratio that adjusts the observed proportion of agreement for what might be expected from chance alone.

To illustrate the strategy, consider the situation in Table 20.2. Because Examiner A passes the proportion, p_A, of candidates and Examiner B passes the proportion, p_B, we would expect the two examiners to agree by chance in the proportion $p_A \times p_B$. Similarly, the two examiners would be expected to agree by chance in failing the proportion $q_A \times q_B$. For the data in Table 20.2, $p_A = 58/80 = .725$; $p_B = 42/80 = .525$; $q_A = 22/80 = .275$; and $q_B = 38/80 = .475$. The sum of $(.725)(.525) + (.275)(.475) = .381 + .131 = .512$ would therefore be expected as the chance proportion of agreement for the 80 candidates being rated. Because the observed proportion of agreement was 60/80 = .75, the observed agreement exceeded the chance expectation by .750 −.512 =.238. If the observed agreement were perfect, p_o would be 1 and the result would have exceeded chance by $1 - .512 = .488$. The ratio of the observed superiority to perfect superiority is .238/.488 =.488, which is the value of kappa.

Expressed in symbols, using p_o for observed proportion of agreement and p_c for the agreement expected by chance, kappa is

$$\kappa = \frac{p_o - p_c}{1 - p_c} \qquad\qquad [20.3]$$

20.4.3.1   *Computation of Kappa* — To convert expression [20.3] into a calculational formula, we can use the symbols of the 2×2 agreement matrix. The agreement expected by chance is

$$p_c = p_A p_B + q_A q_B = \left(\frac{f_1}{N} \times \frac{n_1}{N}\right) + \left(\frac{f_2}{N} \times \frac{n_2}{N}\right) = (f_1 n_1 + f_2 n_2)/N^2$$

Because the observed agreement is $(a +d)/N$, the observed minus expected values will be $[(a + d)/N] - (f_1 n_1 + f_2 n_2)/N^2 = [N(a +d) - (f_1 n_1 + f_2 n_2)]/N^2$. The value of $1 - p_c$ will be $[N^2 - (f_1 n_1 + f_2 n_2)]/N^2$, and so the calculational formula for kappa will be

$$\kappa = \frac{N(a + d) - (f_1 n_1 + f_2 n_2)}{N^2 - (f_1 n_1 + f_2 n_2)} \qquad\qquad [20.4]$$

An alternative calculational formula, whose derivation is left as an algebraic exercise for the reader, is

$$\kappa = \frac{2(ad - bc)}{(b + c)N + 2(ad - bd)} \qquad\qquad [20.5]$$

Formula [20.4] is probably most rapid to execute on a hand calculator if the row and column totals are available and if the calculations are suitably organized.

For the two medical-board examiners in Table 20.2,

$$\kappa = \frac{2(40 \times 20 - 2 \times 18)}{(2 + 18)(80) + 2(40 \times 20 - 2 \times 18)} = \frac{1528}{1600 + 1528} = 0.49$$

using Formula [20.5], or

$$\kappa = \frac{80(40 + 20) - (58 \times 42 + 22 \times 38)}{80^2 - (58 \times 42 + 22 \times 38)} = \frac{1528}{3128} = 0.49$$

using Formula [20.4].

20.4.3.2   *Interpretation of Kappa* — Kappa has a range of values from −1 to +1. When the observed agreement is perfect, i.e., $p_o = 1$, kappa will be +1. If the observed agreement equals the chance-expected agreement, so that $p_o = p_c$, kappa will be 0. If the observed agreement is less than the chance expected agreement, i.e., $p_o < p_c$, kappa will become negative. In the special case when both raters choose each of the categories half the time, p_c will be $[(N/2)(N/2) + (N/2)(N/2)]/N^2 = 1/2$. In this case, if the raters also happen to have no agreement at all, so that $a = d = 0$, then p_o will equal 0, and kappa will take on its minimum value of −1, i.e., $[0 - (1/2)]/[1 - (1/2)]$.

Kappa is ordinarily used to measure concordance between two variables, i.e., two raters. If more than two raters (or processes) are under comparison, kappa indexes can be calculated for each separate pairwise agreement, i.e., for A vs. B, for B vs. C, for A vs. C, etc. A summary "group value" could be obtained as the median or other average of the individual kappa indexes. Alternatively, Fleiss[9] has developed a mathematically complicated method that allows calculation of a single generalized kappa for three or more observers.

20.4.3.3 Quantitative Standards

20.4.3.3   Quantitative Standards — Although stochastic P values can be calculated, the quantitative significance of kappa, i.e., its descriptive magnitude, is more important than the associated P value. Thus, P < .05 might be necessary to show that the results are stable, but the P values are otherwise useless for denoting meaningful degrees of observer agreement.

Kappa thus holds the distinction of being one of the few descriptive indexes that has received serious statistical efforts to develop standards for *quantitative* significance. For increments and correlation coefficients, quantitative standards have been proposed by clinical psychologists[10] and clinical epidemiologists.[11] As guidelines for the quantitative strength of agreement denoted by kappa, however, two sets of criteria have been proposed by statisticians: Landis and Koch[12] and Fleiss.[9] The proposals are shown in Figure 20.3. The Fleiss guidelines seem "tougher" than the Landis–Koch guidelines. Fleiss demands values of ≥.75 for **excellent** agreement, whereas Landis and Koch regard .61 − .80 as **substantial** and .81 − 1.00 as **almost perfect**. Fleiss deems everything < .40 as **poor**, a designation that does not occur for Landis and Koch until kappa gets below 0.

Despite the disagreement in criteria for agreement, however, both sets of guidelines can be applauded for their pioneering attempts to demarcate descriptive zones of quantitative significance.

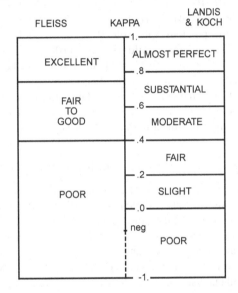

FIGURE 20.3

Scales for strength of agreement for Kappa, as proposed by Fleiss[9] and by Landis and Koch.[12]

20.4.3.4 Problems in Distribution of Challenge

20.4.3.4   Problems in Distribution of Challenge — Values of kappa have important problems, however, that were not considered in the proposals for quantitative guidelines. The problems, first noted by Helena Kraemer,[13] arise when the challenge contained in the research is maldistributed. The chance-expected penalty of kappa may then become unfair to raters who have excellent observational agreement but who are victims of unsatisfactory research architecture.

To illustrate this situation, consider the agreement matrix in Table 20.4. The two radiologists have 97% agreement [= (102 +3)/108] in designating the chest films of first-year university students as normal or abnormal. The expected chance agreement, however, is [(103)(104) +(5)(4)]/108² = .92. Using the formula $(p_o - p_c)/(1 - p_c)$, kappa would be (.97 − .92)/(1 − .92) = .05/.08 =.625. The value of .625 for kappa still indicates an agreement that is "substantial" (according to Landis–Koch) or "fair to good" (according to Fleiss), but the result is much less impressive than the former 97% agreement. Because this problem

TABLE 20.4

Ratings of Chest Films for 108 First-Year University Students

Radiologist B	Radiologist A		
	Normal	Abnormal	Total
Normal	102	2	104
Abnormal	1	3	4
TOTAL	103	5	108

arises from a maldistribution of the challenge group, the two radiologists would need a different research design to allow the remorseless kappa to produce a more impressive value for their excellent agreement.

With expected agreement calculated as $(f_1n_1 + f_2n_2)/N^2$, the penalty factor is substantially increased when $f_1n_1 + f_2n_2$ has relatively high values in relation to N^2. In a special analysis,[14] the penalty factor was shown to have its minimum values when the challenge group is distributed equally so that $f_1 = f_2 = N/2$ and $n_1 = n_2 = N/2$. Accordingly, the two radiologists would receive a better challenge if the test population contained roughly equal numbers of abnormal and normal films, rather than a predominantly normal group.

For example, suppose the 108 challenge cases were distributed as shown in Table 20.5. In this situation, the proportional agreement would still be 105/108 =97%, but the value of $f_1n_1 + f_2n_2$ would be $(54)(55) +(54)(53) = 5832$, in contrast to the previous value of $(103)(104) +(5)(4) = 10732$. Kappa would rise to $[(108)(105) - (5832)]/[(108)^2 - 5832] = .94$, and would indicate much better agreement than before.

TABLE 20.5

Ratings of Chest Films for 108 Selected Patients

| | Radiologist A | | |
Radiologist B	Normal	Abnormal	Total
Normal	53	2	55
Abnormal	1	52	53
TOTAL	54	54	108

If the challenge was not suitably arranged before the research was done, the problem can still be managed, but the management requires replacing the single "omnibus" value of kappa by indexes of specific agreement in different zones.

20.4.4   Directional Problems of an "Omnibus" Index

Regardless of whether kappa or either of the two other indexes is used, a single "omnibus" index cannot answer two sets of directional questions that regularly arise about agreement in zones and bias in raters. In dimensional data, the agreements may get better or worse with changes in the dimensional magnitudes for different zones of the data. For binary data, only two zones occur, but the proportions of agreement may differ in those zones.

This issue is neglected in any "omnibus" index that gives a single value for binary concordance, without distinguishing the two types of agreement for positive and negative ratings. In many evaluations of concordance, however, the goal is to answer two questions about agreement, not just one. Instead of a single summary statement, we may want special indexes to show how closely the raters agree separately on positive decisions and on negative decisions. This problem is particularly prominent, as noted later in Chapter 21, in citing accuracy for diagnostic tests. Omnibus indexes of diagnostic agreement have generally been avoided because they do not separate sensitivity and specificity, or accuracy for positive and negative tests.

20.4.4.1   Indexes of Specific Agreement — Several approaches have been proposed for determining indexes of specific agreement. The most useful for binary data is the specific proportionate agreement for positive and for negative ratings, denoted as p_{pos} and p_{neg}.

If f_1 and n_1 are each observer's total of positive decisions, the expected positive agreement can be estimated as $(f_1 + n_1)/2$. Because positive agreement occurs with a frequency of a, its proportion will be

$$p_{pos} = a/[(f_1 + n_1)/2] = 2a/(f_1 + n_1) \qquad [20.6]$$

The expected negative agreement will be $(f_2 + n_2)/2$ and its proportion will be

$$p_{neg} = d/[(f_2 + n_2)/2] = 2d/(f_2 + n_2) \qquad [20.7]$$

For the two previous sets of challenges to radiologists, the value of p_{pos} will be $(2)(102)/(104 + 103) = .985$ in Table 20.4 and $(2)(53)/(55 +54) = .97$ in Table 20.5. The value of p_{neg} will be $(2)(3)/(4 + 5) = .67$ in Table 20.4 and $(2)(52)/(53 +54) = .97$ in Table 20.5.

For these reasons, when concordance is evaluated in a 2×2 agreement matrix, kappa is probably the best index to use if you are using only one; but the results should always be accompanied by values of

p_{pos} and p_{neg} to indicate what is really happening. The special indexes for the two types of agreement can be obtained easily without any need for adjustments due to chance, because the "expected" value is used for each calculation.

20.4.4.2 McNemar Index of Bias for Binary Data

20.4.4.2 McNemar Index of Bias for Binary Data — Proposing a simple index for biased disagreements in a 2×2 concordance matrix, such as Table 20.1, Quinn McNemar[3] used the following reasoning: If the disagreements occur randomly, the total of $b + c$ in the b and c cells of Table 20.1 should be split about equally between b and c. If the *Yes/No* disagreements occur much more often than *No/Yes* disagreements, or vice versa, the b and c values will be unequal.

The inequality is expressed proportionately in McNemar's index

$$\frac{\mid b - c \mid}{(b + c)} \qquad [20.8]$$

The lowest possible value for this index is 0. It occurs when $b = c$, i.e., when the number of *Yes/No* paired ratings is the same as the number of *No/Yes* ratings. The highest possible absolute value, $\mid 1 \mid$, occurs either when $b = 0$, so that the index is $(-c)/(+c) = -1$, or when $c = 0$, so that the index is $b/b = +1$. When either $b = 0$ or $c = 0$, all the disagreement is in one direction.

Thus, the closer McNemar's index is to zero, the more likely are the two observers to be "unbiased" in their ratings. As the index approaches $\mid 1 \mid$, the observers have increasingly substantial differences in the way they disagree. If one of the observers is regarded as the "gold standard," the McNemar index will be an index of inaccuracy rather than merely bias in directional disagreement.

In Table 20.2, the two observers disagree on $18 + 2 = 20$ occasions. The pattern is Fail/Pass in 18 and Pass/Fail in 2. The McNemar index will be $(2 - 18)/(18 + 2) = -16/20 = -.8$. This relatively high magnitude suggests a substantial difference among the examiners. (The McNemar index is stochastically evaluated with a special chi-square test in Section 20.8.1.) If Examiner A were regarded as the gold standard in evaluating candidates, the McNemar index would show whether Examiner B has biased inaccuracy. In the current situation, however, Examiner B merely seems "tougher" than A, failing more candidates than might be expected if the disagreements went equally in both directions.

The McNemar index was used[15] to denote bias in the diagnosis of toxic shock syndrome when clinicians reviewed scenarios for a series of cases that were identical in history, physical findings, and laboratory tests, but different in sex, and in presence/absence of menstruation or use of tampons. The proportion of biased diagnoses for toxic shock syndrome rose progressively when the same clinical scenarios respectively included a woman rather than a man, a statement about menstruation rather than no statement, and specific mention of a tampon rather than no mention.

The disadvantage of the McNemar index is that the emphasis on disagreements eliminates attention to the rest of the results. For example, the two observers in Table 20.2 would have the same McNemar index of $-.8$ if they seldom agreed, so that the 2×2 matrix was $\begin{Bmatrix} 3 & 2 \\ 18 & 4 \end{Bmatrix}$, or if the disagreements were an uncommon event among all the other concordances in an agreement matrix such as $\begin{Bmatrix} 190 & 2 \\ 8 & 175 \end{Bmatrix}$.

20.5 Agreement in Ordinal Data

For the three or more rows and columns of ordinal data, the paired ratings can have different degrees of "partial" agreement.

20.5.1 Individual Discrepancies

With g ordinal grades, the frequency counts for the two raters will form a $g \times g$ agreement matrix. A straightforward index of proportional agreement can be formed from the sum of frequencies for perfect agreement in cells of the downward left-to-right diagonal. For example, Table 20.6 shows concordance of intraoperative Doppler flow imaging vs. pre-operative biplane ventriculography in rating the severity of

TABLE 20.6

Severity of Mitral Regurgitation as Graded by Ventriculography and by
Transesophageal Doppler Color Flow (TDCF) Imaging (Data from
Chapter Reference 16)

Severity	Severity in Ventriculography					
in TDCF	0	1	2	3	4	Total
0	91	28	11	1	0	131
1	33	20	11	3	2	69
2	6	3	4	1	0	14
3	2	1	5	10	2	20
4	0	0	2	1	9	12
TOTAL	132	52	33	16	13	246

mitral regurgitation in 246 patients.[16] Perfect agreements occur in (91 +20 +4 +10 +9) =134 of the 246 cases, a proportion of 54%.

The disagreements in all the other cells can be managed in two ways. In one approach, they are counted merely as disagreements. In a better approach, however, they are weighted according to the degree of partial disagreement. For example, paired ratings of **0–1** in Table 20.6 would have less disagreement than the pair **0–2**, which in turn would have less disagreement than **0–3**.

20.5.2   Weighting of Disagreements

At least three tactics can be used to create weights for partial disagreements.

20.5.2.1   Categorical-Distance Method — The most simple and commonly used procedure assigns a point for each unit of categorical distance from the diagonal cells of perfect agreement. The subsequent calculations are easier if the weights increase for increasing degrees of agreement, rather than disagreement, as shown in Table 20.7. With g ordinal categories, ranked as **1, 2, 3,..., g**, the maximum disparity is in cells rated as **(1,g)** or **(g,1)**. These cells are given weights of **0**. The next worst disparities will be in cells rated as **(2,g)**, **(g,2)**, **(1,g–1)**, or **(g–1,1)**. These cells are given weights of 1. The grading process continues until the maximum possible weight, **g–1**, is given for perfect agreement in the diagonal cells **(1,1)**, **(2,2)**, **(3,3)**,..., **(g,g)**.

TABLE 20.7

Scheme of Weights for One-Point Units of Agreement in Ordinal Categories

Ordinal	Ordinal Rating by A						
Rating by B	1	2	3	4	...	g–1	g
I	g–1	g–2	g–3	g–4	...	1	0
2	g–2	g–1	g–2	g–3	...	2	1
3	g–3	g–2	g–1	g–2	...	3	2
4	g–4	g–3	g–2	g–1	...	4	3
...	...	...	...	...	⋱	...	...
g–1	1	2	3	4	...	g–1	g–2
g	0	1	2	3	...	g–2	g–1

20.5.2.2   "Squared-Deviation" Method — In an alternative method,[17] partial disagreements are weighted according to "the square of the deviation of the pair of observations from exact agreement." With the previous method of categorical-distance scoring, the partial *agreements* in a 5-category scale might be weighted as **4, 3, 2, 1**, and **0**. With the "squared-deviation" method, the corresponding partial *disagreements* would be rated as **0, 1, 4, 9**, and **16**. The disagreement ratings can be converted to a "unitary scale" when divided by the maximum rating. Thus, if the maximum is 9, the foregoing ratings would be **0**, **.11**, **.44**, and **1**. If the maximum is **16**, the ratings would be **0**, **.0625**, **.25**, **.5625**, and **1**.

The argument offered[17] in favor of the "squared-deviation" proposal is that it is "an intuitively appealing standard usage," with the advantage that "weighted kappa calculated with these weights approximately equals the product-moment correlation coefficient." Since indexes of concordance were developed to avoid possibly misleading results from ordinary correlation coefficients, the "advantage" claimed for the "squared-deviation" method may not be "intuitively appealing" to all potential users.

20.5.2.3 *"Substantive-Impact" Method* — Both the categorical-distance and the "squared-deviation" methods of weighting are chosen according to arbitrary statistical strategies. In a third scheme, the weights are assigned according to the substantive impact of the disparities. For example, if the neoplastic suspiciousness of cervical pap smears is rated as **0**, **1**, **2**, **3**, **4**, a one-category disagreement between **3** and **4** will have fewer consequences than a disagreement between **0** and **1**. With either a **3** or **4** rating, the patient will receive a further "workup" that probably includes colposcopy and cervical biopsy. A disagreement between **0** and **1**, however, can lead to the clinical difference between simple reassurance vs. invasive further testing. Accordingly, a discrepancy between **0** and **1** may be given a much greater "penalty" than any of the other one-category disagreements.

This type of problem is particularly likely to occur when the ordinal rating scale begins with a *null*, *negative*, or *absent* category, followed by categories that have different degrees of a "positive" rating. These null-based scales — such as **0**, **1**, **2**, **3**, **4** for pain or for pap smears — differ from other ordinal scales, such as I, II, III for TNM stage of cancer, where something "positive" is always present. In TNM stages, however, a discrepancy between **I** and **II**, i.e., between a localized state and regional spread, might be regarded as more (or less) serious than the regional vs. distant metastases implied by a discrepancy between **II** and **III**.

Cicchetti[18] has developed a formal procedure for assigning substantive weights for disagreements in what he calls *dichotomous-ordinal* scales, where the extreme rating at one end has a special connotation (usually "normal" vs. a set of "abnormal" ratings). In *continuous-ordinal* scales, the disagreements in adjacent increments have equal connotations. As long as the weights are established before the statistics are computed, the assigned weights seem scientifically reasonable and offer increased flexibility in the evaluation procedure.

A substantive-impact weighting procedure can also be used for appraising concordance in various other situations. For example, substantive weights can be assigned (as noted later in Section 20.6.2) for disagreements among *nominal* categories. When errors are assessed in diagnostic marker tests (see Chapter 21), a false positive rating may sometimes be given a greater (or lesser) "penalty" than a false negative rating.

20.5.2.4 *Other Weightings* — Cicchetti[18] has proposed another weighting scheme that assigns weights as proportions between 0 and 1, and Fleiss[9] mentions two other arrangements beyond those already cited.

20.5.3 Proportion of Weighted Agreement

To form a summary score, the weighted indexes for individual agreements or disagreements are multiplied by frequency counts; the products are added and then converted to suitable proportions.

In the categorical-distance method, suppose f_i is the frequency count in each cell and w_i is the corresponding weight of agreement. The total agreement score for the table will be $\Sigma f_i w_i$. For perfect agreement, all of the N pairs of ratings would be in the diagonal cells getting weights of $g - 1$; and so the perfect score would be $N(g - 1)$. Thus, the weighted proportion of agreement would be

$$p_w = \frac{\Sigma f_i w_i}{N(g - 1)} \qquad [20.9]$$

To illustrate this procedure in the five ordinal ranks of Table 20.6, the perfect-agreement cells all receive weights of **4** for the 134 (= 91 +20 +4 +10 +9) frequencies in those locations. For the remaining cells, disparities of one category occur in the locations of (0,1), (1,0), (1,2), (2,1), (2,3), (3,2), (3,4), and (4,3). Each disparity receives a weight of **3** for the 84 (= 28 +33 +11 +3 +1 +5 +2 +1) frequencies in those locations. Two-category disparities, receiving weights of **2**, occur in the (0,2), (2,0), (1,3), (3,1), and (4,2) locations, which contain 23 (= 11 +6 +3 +1 +2) frequencies. Three-category disparities, with weights of **1**, occur with 5 (= 1 +2 +2) frequencies in the (0,3), (3,0), and (1,4) locations. The maximum possible 4-category disparity, which would receive a weight of **0**, did not occur in the (0,4) or (4,0) cells of the table. Consequently, the total weighted agreement score is $(134 \times 4) + (84 \times 3) + (23 \times 2) + (5 \times 1) = 839$. Because a perfect score would have been $246 \times 4 = 984$, the proportion of weighted agreement for Table 20.6 is $839/984 = 85\%$. (Without weighting, the ordinary proportion of agreement would have been $134/246 = 54\%$.)

With the squared-deviation method, the weighted score for each categorical disagreement would be q_i; the frequency of scores would be f_i; the score for maximum disagreement in N ratings would be $N(g-1)^2$; and the score for proportion of weighted agreement would be

$$p_w = 1 - \{\Sigma f_i q_i / [N(g-1)^2]\} \qquad [20.10]$$

To illustrate this process in the data of Table 20.6, the total score for disagreement would be $(134 \times 0) + (84 \times 1) + (23 \times 4) + (5 \times 9) + (0 \times 16) = 221$. The score for perfect disagreement would be $246 \times 16 = 3936$. The proportion of weighted agreement would be $1 - (221/3936) = .94$. (With the "categorical distance" method, the corresponding value was .85.)

As another example of the weighted scoring process, suppose two clinical pharmacologists, A and B, have independently appraised 30 cases of suspected adverse drug reaction,[19] rating each case as **definite**, **probable**, **possible**, or **unlikely**. The results are shown in Table 20.8.

TABLE 20.8

Agreement Matrix of Two Clinical Pharmacologists, A and B, in Rating the Likelihood of Adverse Drug Reactions in 30 Suspected Cases [Data from Chapter Reference 19]

	Rater A				
Rater B	**Definite**	**Probable**	**Possible**	**Unlikely**	**Total**
Definite	1	2	0	0	3
Probable	1	5	3	1	10
Possible	1	4	5	2	12
Unlikely	1	1	1	2	5
Total	4	12	9	5	30

The index of percentage agreement for the appropriate diagonal cells is

$$\frac{1 + 5 + 5 + 2}{30}(100) = 43.3\%$$

For the *index of weighted percentage agreement* with categorical-distance scoring, a weight of **3** is given for perfect agreement among the four ordinal categories. A one-category disagreement is given a weight of **2**; a two-category disagreement is weighted as **1**; and the maximum disagreement (of three categories) is weighted as **0**. Using Formula [20.9], the index of weighted percentage agreement is calculated as:

$$\frac{(1 + 5 + 5 + 2)(3) + (2 + 3 + 2 + 1 + 4 + 1)(2) + (0 + 1 + 1 + 1)(1) + (0 + 1)(0)}{(30)(3)} = 75.6\%$$

This value is considerably higher than the 43.3% unweighted index of percentage agreement. With the squared-deviation scoring method, using Formula [20.10], the value of $\Sigma f_i q_i$ is $(1 + 5 + 5 + 2)0 + (2 + 3 + 2 + 1 + 4 + 1)1 + (0 + 1 + 1 + 1)4 + (0 + 1)9 = 13 + 12 + 9 = 34$. The score for $N(g-1)^2$ is $30 \times 9 = 270$. The value of p_w is $1 - (34/270) = .874$, which is again higher than the .756 calulated with the categorical-distance method.

20.5.4 Demarcation of Ordinal Categories

In all of the foregoing methods, the analyst began with an array of ordinal categories, and then chose statistical weights for the different degrees of partial agreement or disagreement. A more fundamental scientific challenge can arise, however, in demarcating the array of categories before all the statistical work begins.

Getting commensurate scales is a common problem in observer variability because the raters may use different expressions for their routine activities. Thus, one rater may refer to cardiac size in four categories as **normal, slightly enlarged, moderately enlarged**, or **substantially enlarged**, whereas another rater may use six categories, which include the previous four plus **borderline** (after **normal**) and **massively enlarged** (after **substantially enlarged**). The problem is magnified when the raters use additional categories formed by qualifying expressions such as **compatible with normal** or **consistent with slightly enlarged**.

The investigator's work will be eased if the raters can be persuaded to agree on a common scale of standard categories before the research begins, but the raters may then protest that the standardized scale is an artifact and that the results will not accurately reflect what happens in routine clinical practice. Because every research study creates artificial conditions, this problem cannot be avoided if observer variability is to be investigated at all. Recognizing that perfection may be impossible, the investigator can simply try to use a maximum of clinical "common sense" to achieve a best possible consensus from the participating observers. Sometimes, when several options are available for demarcating or consolidating categories, the investigator can analyze results for each option separately. If the results differ substantially, each set can be reported separately.

For example, in a study of observer variability in mammography,[20] the original scale of four diagnostic categories was **normal; abnormal, benign; abnormal, indeterminate** (i.e., uncertain whether benign or probably malignant); and **abnormal, suspicious of cancer.** For one set of analyses using three ordinal categories, the investigators consolidated the middle two categories into a single **benign/indeterminate** rating. Because some of the mammographers believed that the **indeterminate** group would receive essentially the same subsequent "workup" as the **suspicious-of-cancer group**, another set of three-category analyses was done with the latter two groups collapsed into a single category. Finally, in yet another analysis, all four of the original categories were retained.

20.5.5 Artifactual Arrangements

A different set of problems arises if the observers are accustomed to certain operating conditions that are altered for the research. For example, pathologists and radiologists regularly see accounts of a patient's history before they examine the pertinent slides or films. If the history, suspected as a source of biased interpretation,[21] is not supplied, the observers may then complain that the research process did not conform to reality.

As another example, when the initial interpretation is equivocal, a final conclusion may not be reached until pathologists have ordered and examined additional slides or stains, or until radiologists have checked additional views or other films. If the research arrangement forces the observers to reach a final conclusion without access to the additional options, the investigative process may again be deemed unfair.

This problem is also seldom avoidable within the pragmatic constraints of realities for both ordinary practice and concordance research. The practitioners who volunteer to participate in studies of observer variability may themselves be an unrepresentative sample; and the investigator must hope to come as close as possible to the "average" conditions of clinical practice, while acknowledging that individual idiosyncrasies may have been suppressed and that no investigation can be done without certain artifacts. The Heisenberg principle (which states that the act of observation may change the observed object) pertains not only for the relatively simple phenomena of the world of physics, but particularly for the more complex phenomena of observer variability. Sometimes, however, the artifacts can be effectively used for testing certain hypotheses. Thus, to determine whether the patient's history is indeed a source of bias, the observers may be given and asked to report on selected specimens that have been submitted on two occasions with and without an accompanying history.[21] In one study of radiographic interpretations of change in a sequence of chest films,[22] the radiologists on one occasion reviewed films of the same patients arranged in the chronologic succession and, on another occasion, in a random chronology.

20.5.6   Weighted Kappa

Regardless of the selected categories and weighting scheme, however, the index of weighted percentage agreement does not make provision for the agreement that might be expected by chance. If a correction factor is introduced for chance agreement, the best index for concordance in ordinal data is weighted kappa, κ_w. It is derived from κ after weights are assigned for the magnitude of observed disagreements. κ_w is easier to calculate when based on q, the proportion of disagreements, rather than p, the proportion of agreements. Since $q = 1 - p$,

$$\kappa_w = 1 - \frac{q_o'}{q_c'} \qquad\qquad [20.11]$$

where q_o' = observed proportion of weighted disagreements and q_c' = chance-expected proportion of weighted disagreements. (The "primes" are added to each q to indicate that the quantities are weighted.)

The most commonly used strategy of indexing disagreements for weighted kappa is a reverse counterpart of the categorical-distance method. The varying degrees of disagreement are given "reverse" weights as follows: **0** =perfect agreement (e.g., A and B both report "moderate" pain); **1** =one-category disagreement (e.g., "severe" vs. "moderate"); **2**=two-category disagreement (e.g., "mild" vs. "severe"), and so on up to a maximum weight of **g − 1**, where g is the number of categories in the ordinal scale. (With the other two methods of weighting, the corresponding sequence would be **0, 1, 4, 9,**... for the "squared deviation" method or whatever weights are assigned for the "substantive-impact" method).

In Table 20.9, Table 20.8 has been modified to include the chance-expected cell frequencies (f_c) and assigned cell weights (w_i) of "categorical distance" that would be used in addition to the observed cell frequencies (f_i) in the calculation of κ_w. As in the case of unweighted kappa, f_c is calculated by multiplying the appropriate marginals, i.e., row total by column total, and then dividing by N. Proportions of weighted disagreements are computed by multiplying cell frequencies (f_i or f_c) by the disagreement weight (w_i) assigned to that cell, summing these values over all cells, and then dividing by N.

For the calculation of weighted kappa in Table 20.9,

$$q_o' = \frac{\Sigma w_i f_i}{N}$$

$$= \frac{(0)(1+5+5+2) + (1)(1+4+1+2+3+2) + (2)(1+1+0+1) + (3)(1+0)}{30}$$

$$= \frac{22}{30} = .733$$

and

$$q_c' = \frac{\Sigma w_i f_c}{N}$$

$$= \frac{(0)(0.4+4.0+3.6+0.8) + (1)(1.3+4.8+1.5+1.2+3.0+2.0)}{30}$$

$$+ \frac{(2)(1.6+2.0+0.9+1.7) + (3)(0.7+0.5)}{30} = \frac{29.8}{30} = .933 \; ; \; \text{and}$$

$$\kappa_w = 1 - \frac{.733}{.993} = +.262.$$

TABLE 20.9

Agreement Matrix Containing Observed and Expected Frequencies and
Assigned Weights for Ratings of Adverse Drug Reactions in Table 20.8.
[From Chapter Reference 19]

Rater B	Rater A				
	Definite	**Probable**	**Possible**	**Unlikely**	
Definite	$1(0.4)^{\backslash 0}$	$2(1.2)^{\backslash 1}$	$0(0.9)^{\backslash 2}$	$0(0.5)^{\backslash 3}$	$3 = r_1$
Probable	$1(1.3)^{\backslash 1}$	$5(4.0)^{\backslash 0}$	$3(3.0)^{\backslash 1}$	$1(1.7)^{\backslash 2}$	$10 = r_2$
Possible	$1(1.6)^{\backslash 2}$	$4(4.8)^{\backslash 1}$	$5(3.6)^{\backslash 0}$	$2(2.0)^{\backslash 1}$	$12 = r_3$
Unlikely	$1(0.7)^{\backslash 3}$	$1(2.0)^{\backslash 2}$	$1(1.5)^{\backslash 1}$	$2(0.8)^{\backslash 0}$	$5 = r_4$
	$4 = c_1$	$12 = c_2$	$9 = c_3$	$5 = c_4$	$30 = N$

Note: Numbers in cells represent observed frequencies, (f_a); numbers in parentheses
indicate chance-expected cell frequencies (f_a); numbers in upper right corner
are the assigned weights (w_i) for disagreements.

The quantitative magnitude of κ_w is interpreted in the same way as the magnitude of unweighted
kappa. The values range from -1 to $+1$, with 0 representing chance-expected weighted agreement.

20.5.7 Correlation Indexes

Analogous to the use of ϕ for describing trends between two dichotomous categorical variables, non-
parametric correlation indexes such as r_s (Spearman's rho) and τ (Kendall's tau) — which are discussed
later in Chapter 27 — have sometimes been applied for analyzing concordance in ordinal data. Denoting
trend rather than agreement, however, these indexes refer to *correlation* or general relatedness, not
concordance.

In particular, the correlation indexes ignore systematic bias. If Observer B consistently assigns higher
rankings than Observer A, while using the same order of rankings, the correlation will be excellent
although agreement is poor. On a four-category pain scale, for example, if B reports "mild" pain whenever
A reports "none," "moderate" whenever A reports "mild," and "severe" whenever A reports "moderate"
or "severe," the *correlation* will be quite high, despite only a modest degree of *concordance*.

20.6 Agreement in Nominal Data

Agreement has seldom been assessed for circumstances in which the observer chooses one of a series
of ≥ 3 nominal categories. In one example, citation of four possible body sites of melanoma was compared,
with ordinary (non-weighted) indexes of agreement, for the locations listed in physicians' office records
and in a hospital cancer registry.[23] The usual situation that evokes a choice among nominal categories,
however, is a test of conformity between a series of diagnostic estimates and the "gold standard" results.
The same statistical index is used for expressing either concordance or conformity in nominal data.
Table 20.10 shows the agreement matrix for a hypothetical series of clinical diagnoses of liver disease
and the "gold standard" results of liver biopsy.

Because nominal data cannot be ranked, the only straightforward index for Table 20.10 is the proportional agreement, which would be expressed as $(10 + 20 + 13 + 35)/114 = 78/114 = 68\%$.

20.6.1 Substantively Weighted Disagreements

Although the individual values cannot be ranked, certain pairs of nominal disagreements may be weighted
substantively as "better" or "worse" than others. For example, suppose we were estimating a person's
birthplace in the nominal category of **Alabama, Alaska, Arizona,..., Wyoming**, for one of the 50 United
States. For these predictions, a set of discrepancies might be weighted on the basis of geographic

TABLE 20.10

Nominal Diagnoses by Clinician and by Liver Biopsy in Hypothetical Data Set

Clinical Diagnosis	Results of Liver Biopsy				
	Hepatitis	**Cirrhosis**	**Cancer in Liver**	**Other**	**Total**
Hepatitis	10	3	2	6	21
Cirrhosis	4	20	3	2	29
Cancer in Liver	3	5	13	4	25
Other	2	1	1	35	39
TOTAL	19	29	19	47	114

proximity. Thus, if someone were born in New Hampshire, the estimate of Vermont would be much closer than the estimate of California.

An arbitrary scheme of substantive weights might also be established for disagreements in the diagnoses of Table 20.10. Thus, a disagreement with the diagnosis of *cancer* might be rated as a much worse discrepancy than disagreements for any other pair of diagnoses. In a study[24] of variability in ratings of cell types for the histopathology of lung cancer, a disagreement of **well-differentiated epidermoid** vs. **well-differentiated adenocarcinoma** was weighted more heavily than a disagreement of **poorly-differentiated adenocarcinoma** vs. **large cell anaplastic**.

Unless such substantive *ad hoc* weights are established, the only descriptive index for nominal data is the simple proportion of agreement. Because such studies are uncommon, the results are usually reported without any adjustments for chance. If desired, however, kappa statistics can be calculated by converting the nominal scales into a series of dichotomous scales such as diagnosis A vs. all others, B vs. all others, or C vs. all others. Values of proportional agreement and kappa could then be determined for each of the 2×2 tables created by the dichotomous scales. The final result would be the medians (or means) of the series of values for proportional agreement and kappa.

20.6.2 Choice of Categories

If the observers are accustomed to a free range of expressions, the choice of rating-scale categories can be even more difficult for nominal than for ordinal challenges in observer variability. For example, when interpreting the cell types of a series of histologic specimens of lung cancer, some of the pathologists[24] used sparse numbers of categories such as **epidermoid carcinoma, adenocarcinoma,…**, whereas others used many more categories with additional qualifying details such as **well-differentiated, moderately well-differentiated**, and **poorly differentiated** for the **epidermoid** group and yet other details (**acinar, papillary, bronchiolar**) for the adenocarcinomas.

In such situations, special analytic arrangements may be needed beyond the usual indexes for expressing agreement. In the study just cited, a special set of "spectral numbers" was calculated for the different designations the same slide might have received in both the intra-observer and inter-observer interpretations.

20.6.3 Conversion to Other Indexes

In some nominal-rating circumstances, the results are converted into binary or summated expressions. For example, the nominal-category coding of ethnicity was expressed in binary indexes for each category vs. all others in a study of agreement between birth and death certificates.[25] In another study,[26] ten categories of possible differences were established between the ante-mortem clinical diagnoses and the post-mortem diagnostic decisions. The results of each category were given a point for agreement, no points for disagreement, and a blank for not pertinent. The points were then added to form a type of "batting average" called a concordance score.

A different type of summary score was used when Loewenson et al.,[27] examining the consistency of pathologists' assessments of cerebrovascular atherosclerosis, gave one point for each occlusion noted in the mounted specimens of a set of transversally cut pieces of cerebral arteries. The participating pathologists were then checked for agreement in their total point scores.

20.6.4   Biased Agreement in Polytomous Data

Indexes of bias in direction and magnitude are seldom sought for agreement matrixes expressed in polytomous (i.e., ≥ 3) categories of ordinal or nominal data. When desired, however, a modified McNemar index can be calculated from the rows and columns arranged appropriately around the main diagonal, which contains the cells of perfect agreement. The cells of disagreement are divided into an upper group, above the agreement diagonal, and a lower group below the diagonal. The sum of frequency counts in the upper disagreement cells is U and the corresponding sum in the lower cells is L.

For nominal data, the modified McNemar index is then $|U - L|/(U + L)$. For example, in Table 20.10, the sum of the upper disagreement cells is $U = 3 + 2 + 6 + 3 + 2 + 4 = 20$. The corresponding lower sum is $L = 4 + 3 + 5 + 2 + 1 + 1 = 16$. The index of disagreement would be $(20 - 16)/(20 + 16) = 4/36 = 11\%$. For calculating U and L in ordinal data, the distances from the diagonal, i.e., weighted disagreements, can be taken into account in a manner resembling the tactics used in Section 20.5.2.

20.7   Agreement in Dimensional Data

Expressing agreement for pairs of dimensional data would at first seem to be a relatively simple procedure. We want to know the individual discrepancies, their summary, an indication of inter-rater bias (whether one rater is regularly higher than the other), and an indication of directional bias (whether the discrepancies change with magnitude of the ratings). If the ratings from Raters A and B are cited respectively as X_i and Y_i, these goals can readily be achieved from examining and appropriately analyzing the increments, $d_i = X_i - Y_i$.

This simple approach has been ignored for many years, however. Instead, the paired data are usually analyzed with various types of correlation analysis that are unsatisfactory, as discussed in Section 20.1, because they express trends rather than agreements. Furthermore, at least two different types of correlation analysis have been used — the ordinary least-squares regression procedure discussed in Chapter 19, and an intraclass correlation that makes a brief debut in this chapter, with further discussion in Chapter 29.

20.7.1   Analysis of Increments

The increments noted as $d_i = X_i - Y_i$ can be evaluated directly to offer a summary of results and to provide indications of bias in raters and directions.

20.7.1.1   Direct Increments — Consider the data shown in Table 20.11 comparing two methods, A and B, for measuring serum sodium. A quick look at the data suggests that the methods yield reasonably close results, but a more careful inspection of the individual increments shows that they are respectively -5, -3, -3, -2, -5, -7, -2, -6, -2, and -5 for the values of Method A $-$ Method B in subjects 1 through 10. This examination immediately shows that Method B, in this group of data, always has higher values than Method A. For the 10 increments, $\Sigma d_i = -40$ and $\bar{d} = -4.0$.

To get an idea of relative magnitude for this disparity, we can calculate its relationship to the actual measurements. The mean of the values is 140.0 in Method A and 144.0 in Method B, with an overall mean of 142.0. The ratio of the average disparity to the average measured value will be $-4.0/142.0 = -.028$, which is about a 3% difference.

20.7.1.2   Absolute and Squared Increments — The main problem in examining the means of direct increments is that negative and positive values may cancel one another in situations less

TABLE 20.11

Comparison of Two Methods (A and B) for Determining Serum
Sodium Concentration (in mEq/l) in 10 Subjects

Subject No.	Method A	Method B	Subject Means
1	136	141	138.5
2	142	145	143.5
3	129	132	130.5
4	148	150	149.0
5	140	145	142.5
6	152	159	155.5
7	142	144	143.0
8	134	140	137.0
9	139	141	140.0
10	138	143	140.5
Method means	140.0	144.0	Overall mean: 142.0

extreme than that of Table 20.11. For example, suppose the compared rating systems produce the following values for three persons:

Person	Rating by X	Rating by Y	Deviation: X − Y
1	100	80	20
2	85	95	−10
3	63	73	−10

If we merely added the three deviations, as $\Sigma d_i = \Sigma(X_i - Y_i)$, the result would be 0, which falsely suggests perfect agreement. To eliminate this effect, we can examine either the absolute increments or the squared increments. For absolute increments here, $\Sigma|d_i| = 40$ and their mean would be $40/3 = 13.3$. For squared deviations, the sum would be $\Sigma d_i^2 = 600$. The root mean square, expressed as $\sqrt{\Sigma d_i^2/N}$, would be $\sqrt{600/3} = 14.1$.

Because the mean of the six measured values is 82.7, the ratio of (mean discrepancy)/(mean measured value) would be either $13.3/82.7 = .16$ or $14.1/82.7 = .17$. For the data in Table 20.11, the mean absolute deviation is the same as the mean of direct deviations (because they all have the same sign). The root mean squared deviation is $\sqrt{190/10} = 4.36$, which is close to the direct value of 4.0.

20.7.1.3   Bias in Raters — The bias in raters in Table 20.11 was shown by the mean deviation of −4.0. To indicate the stability of this result, we can put a 95% inner percentile range around it. Bland and Altman[29] have suggested the name "limits of agreement" for this interval. If the data are Gaussian, the interval will extend ±1.96 s.d. above and below the mean discrepancy. In Table 20.11, the standard deviation of the discrepancies is 1.83 and so the "limits of agreement" will be −4.0 ±(1.96) (1.83), a zone that goes from −7.59 to −.41.

The foregoing "limits" were descriptive, being obtained with the standard deviation, not the standard error. For stochastic confirmation of the bias, the standard error of the increments would be $1.83/\sqrt{10} = .579$. A 95% confidence interval would denote stochastic significance by excluding 0 in the extent of −4.0 ± (1.96) (.579), which goes from −2.87 to −5.13.

20.7.1.4   Bias in Zones of Data — An important directional problem arises from the magnitude of discrepancies in different zones of the data. For example, a difference of 10 units seems relatively small if the two measurements are **821** and **831**, but not if the two measurements are **21** and **31**. To deal with this problem, each discrepancy can be indexed as a proportion of the "correct" value (if a "gold standard" exists). In the absence of a gold standard, the mean of the two values, i.e., $(X_i + Y_i)/2$, can be the reference point.

The increments of $X_i - Y_i$ can then be plotted as a dependent variable in a graph where $(X_i + Y_i)/2$ is the independent variable. If unbiased, the incremental values should vary randomly around zero from the smallest to largest values of $(X_i + Y_i)/2$. If a set of the increments becomes all positive or all negative in a particular zone, the measurements are biased in that zone.

Another potential problem in direction, however, is that the incremental values, although balanced around 0, may become much larger (or smaller) with increasing (or decreasing) magnitudes of $(X_i + Y_i)/2$. The enlarging-discrepancy effect would suggest that the measurement process itself — rather than one of the raters — is biased, getting excessive disparities at the extreme values of measurement. A transfer to logarithmic values may sometimes help eliminate the problem.

For the data in Table 20.11, the plot of each d_i vs. the corresponding $(X_i + Y_i)/2$ is shown in Figure 20.4. As expected, all of the increments have negative values, but our main concern here is whether their magnitudes are affected by the size of the corresponding mean values for $(X_i + Y_i)/2$. An eye scan of the graph suggests very little relationship. The points above and below the mean increment of –4 are all within the Gaussian "limits-of-agreement" zone (from –7.59 to –.41) as $(X_i + Y_i)/2$ increases.

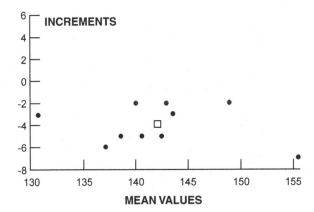

FIGURE 20.4
Plot of increments vs. mean values of X_i and Y_i for data in Table 20.11. □ = Overall mean.

20.7.2 Analysis of Correlation

The analysis of increments can indicate everything we want to know about pairs of dimensional data, but it has often been avoided in favor of correlation analysis. In the latter procedure, the sets of points for $\{X_i, Y_i\}$ are plotted on a graph similar to Figure 20.2, and then receive a set of regression-correlation calculations. Readers can then be impressed with the relatively close fit of the line and with the high values of r (such as .978 in Figure 20.2).

The regression approach can yield a reasonably satisfactory index of agreement provided that the line has a slope of 1 (indicating a 45° angle) and an intercept at the origin. If either of these values significantly deviates from the goal, agreement may be poor, although trend is excellent. Besides, the regressioin/cor-relation approach does not indicate the relative magnitude of individual discrepancies or direction in bias.

Although the superiority of incremental analysis is sometimes regarded as a "modern" discovery, the procedure was used as early as over 60 years ago. When the distinguished Indian statistician, P. C. Mahalanobis[30] was examining the "question of correlation between errors of observation ... in physician measurements," he considered the increment and standard error of the means in the pairs of observation. (Mahalanobis also noted the phenomenon that biased observations occurred more often "than one would expect from the normal theory.")

20.7.3   Analysis of Intraclass Correlation

When R. A. Fisher proposed[7] the intraclass correlation coefficient, he was interested in single measurements of paired entities (such as two brothers) rather than paired measurement of single entities (such as serum sodium). Because the paired entities did not have an assigned position (with Method A as the X_i values and Method B as the Y_i values), either entity could be regarded as X_i or Y_i. Fisher's approach to this situation was to list the entities both ways. He assembled N pairs of an $\{X_i, Y_i\}$ arrangement and then reversed their order to form N interchanged pairs with each Y_i in the X_i position and vice versa. He gave the name *intraclass correlation coefficient* (ICC) to the ordinary correlation coefficient calculated for the 2N pairs of data. The procedure is lucidly described and well illustrated by Robinson.[31] For example, for the three persons whose ratings were reported in Section 20.7.1.2., Fisher's set of analyzed values are shown in the accompanying list at the right.

X	Y
100	80
85	95
63	73
80	100
95	85
73	63

The ICC procedure became popular among statisticians because it used Fisher's analysis-of-variance approach (further discussed in Chapter 29). The "unassigned locations" of the X and Y values were also appealing for psychometric assessments of "reliability" in repeated tests.

20.7.3.1   Sources of Variations — For the intraclass analysis, the results are partitioned according to two main sources of variation: the inter-individual variations among the individuals being rated and the intra-individual variations among the raters. These variations are expressed as means of the pertinent group variances; and appropriate ratios of those mean variances form the interclass correlation coefficient, R_I. The process resembles the partitioning of group variance for linear regression in Chapter 19, but the R_I is calculated from the means of the group variances.

20.7.3.2   Example of Calculation — For the data in Table 20.11, the inter-individual group variance is $S_{XX_A} + S_{XX_B}$. For n members, each group has $n - 1$ degrees of freedom, so the total for degrees of freedom is $2n - 2$. The mean of the group variance will be $(394 + 442)/(20 - 2) = 46.44$. For the intra-individual group variance, $S_{dd} = \Sigma(d_i - \bar{d})^2 = 30$, and there are $n - 1 = 9$ degrees of freedom. The mean will be $30/9 = 3.33$.

If s_I^2 represents the inter-individual variance, and s_o^2 represents the intra-individual variance, the intraclass correlation coefficient is

$$R_I = s_I^2/(s_I^2 + s_o^2).$$
[20.12]

In this instance, $R_I = 46.44/(46.44 + 3.33) = .93$. Because R_I will vary from 0 to 1, the value of .93 seems impressively high (as the ordinary correlation coefficient would be).

20.7.3.3   Problems and Complexities in R_I — An immediately evident problem in R_I is that the high value just noted for the data in Table 20.11 does not indicate the discrepancies — with method B always being higher than method A — that are promptly shown in direct examination of the increments.

A second problem is the way that the s_I^2 term dominates the value of R_I calculated with Formula [20.12]. With large variations in the group of people under study, s_I^2 will have a large value, and R_I will be relatively high regardless of how well or badly the raters perform in producing s_o^2. This distinction gives R_I problems analogous to those of kappa in being greatly affected by the distribution of data in the study group.[32]

For multiple raters rather than two, R_I becomes much more complex, because it is constructed in different ways for different analyses. The complexities, which involve components of the analysis of variance, will be discussed in Chapter 29.

Perhaps the greatest deterrent to using R_I is the difficulty of understanding its construction and interpretation. Many authors have written about R_I, using different formulations, symbols, and interpretations, even for the simple set of two-observer data in Table 20.11. If you intend to use this approach, or want to understand the results, get help from an appropriately knowledgeable and communicative statistician.

Perhaps the last main point to be noted before we leave R_I is that it would seem to be most pertinent pragmatically in quality control studies of laboratory measurements. Nevertheless, R_I seldom appears in the literature of laboratory medicine. Perhaps the investigators have already discovered that R_I does not offer an optimum approach to the challenges.

20.8 Stochastic Procedures

As noted earlier, the *descriptive* indexes are almost universally acknowledged as the main entity to be considered in evaluating concordance. Consequently, P values and/or confidence intervals seldom appear unless the group sizes are particularly small. Nevertheless, various chi-square procedures have been applied for stochastic tests, and the McNemar test is particularly well known. The other procedures, which lead to Z tests for kappa and weighted kappa, are briefly mentioned so you will have heard of them.

The *McNemar chi-square test* warrants special attention because it is regularly used for 2×2 tables that express change as well as agreement. To get a stochastic index for the agreement matrix in Table 20.1, McNemar used the following reasoning: Under the null hypothesis, the b and c cells can be expected to have equal values, which would be $(b + c)/2$. A goodness-of-fit chi-square test between the observed and expected values can be calculated as

$$X_M^2 = \frac{\left(b - \frac{b+c}{2}\right)^2}{\frac{b+c}{2}} + \frac{\left(c - \frac{b+c}{2}\right)^2}{\frac{b+c}{2}}$$

With suitable algebraic expansion and collection of terms, this expression becomes

$$X_M^2 = \frac{(b-c)^2}{b+c} \qquad [20.13]$$

which can be interpreted in a chi-square table with 1 degree of freedom. A continuity correction can be incorporated to make the working formula become

$$X_{M_C}^2 = \frac{(|b-c|-1)^2}{b+c} \qquad [20.14]$$

McNemar recommended that the continuity correction be used when $(b + c) < 10$.

The McNemar index and stochastic test, which will reappear later in Chapter 26 when "matched" arrangements are discussed for case-control studies, have been used[33] to compare rates of agreement between patients and surrogates about preferences for different forms of life-sustaining therapy.

The *conventional X^2 test* can be applied whenever the descriptive results are expressed either in ordinary (unweighted) proportions of agreement or with the ϕ coefficient. In a 2×2 agreement table, however, the McNemar test is often preferred.

Agreement in polytomous matrixes can be tested stochastically with an extension of the McNemar test, called the *Bowker X^2 test* for off-diagonal symmetry. The test is well described, with a worked example, in the textbook by Sprent.[34]

The stochastic procedure for kappa uses its standard error to form either a confidence interval or a Z statistic from which a P value is determined. The formula for calculating the *standard error of kappa* is shown with an illustrative example in Fleiss.[9]

Fleiss[9] also shows the calculation of a *standard error for weighted kappa*. The standard error is used for a confidence interval or a Z statistic.

The *paired t test* can be used for pairs of dimensional data.

20.9 Multiple Observers

The last topic in this long chapter is the problem of analyzing results from multiple observers. In the many indexes and strategies just discussed, *two* (paired) ratings are compared for each entity. Sometimes, however, more than two ratings may be available. For example, in studying observer variability in mammography, Elmore et al.[20] appraised the diverse readings offered by 10 radiologists for each of 150 sets of mammograms.

The strategy that seems most scientifically sensible and easy to understand is to arrange the multiple ratings into pairs of raters, to calculate indexes of concordance for each pair of raters, and then to determine an average result. Thus, for four raters, we might determine kappa indexes for rater A vs. B, A vs. C, A vs. D, B vs. C, B vs. D, and C vs. D. An overall result, if desired, could be the average (as a median or mean) of the six kappa indexes.

20.9.1 Categorical Data

Because the statistical challenge is irresistible, various proposals have been offered to determine an overall generalized index for m raters, each offering n ratings for a set of categorical data. The methods are discussed and demonstrated by Fleiss.[9] Kendall's coefficient W for associating m sets of rankings is presented and illustrated by Sprent[34] and also by Siegel and Castellan.[35]

20.9.2 Dimensional Data

For dimensional data, each of the m raters is regarded as a "class," and the m dimensional values for each of the n rated entities receive a "repeated measures analysis of variance" that leads to the *intraclass correlation coefficient* R_I. The analysis-of-variance strategy used for R_I will be discussed in Chapter 29.

References

1. Elmore, 1992; 2. Yerushalmy, 1969; 3. McNemar, 1955; 4. McNemar, 1947; 5. Cohen, 1960; 6. Barnett, 1979; 7. Fisher, 1941, pg. 213; 8. Lorenz, 1994; 9. Fleiss, 1981; 10. Cohen, 1977; 11. Burnand, 1990; 12. Landis, 1977; 13. Kraemer, 1979; 14. Feinstein, 1990c; 15. Harvey, 1984; 16. Sheikh, 1991; 17. Maclure, 1987; 18. Cicchetti, 1976; 19. Kramer, 1981; 20. Elmore, 1994b; 21. Elmore, 1997; 22. Reger, 1974; 23. Hourani, 1992; 24. Feinstein, 1970; 25. Fendrich, 1992; 26. Friederici, 1984; 27. Loewenson, 1972; 28. Dyer, 1994; 29. Bland, 1986; 30. Mahalanobis, 1940; 31. Robinson, 1957; 32. Bland, 1990; 33. Sulmasy, 1994; 34. Sprent, 1993; 35. Siegel, 1988; 36. Edmunds, 1988; 37. Saunders, 1980.

Exercises

20.1. Table E.20.1 reports two respiratory measurements with each of two flow meters on 17 subjects. The investigator's goal was to see whether the more complex Wright flow meter could be replaced with a simpler-and-easier-to use mini flow meter. [Data and figures taken from Chapter Reference 29.]

TABLE E.20.1

PEFR Measured with Wright Peak Flow and Mini Wright Peak Flow Meter

| Subject | Wright peak flow meter | | Mini Wright Peak Flow Meter | |
	First PEFR (1/min)	Second PEFR (1/min)	First PEFR (1/min)	Second PEFR (1/min)
1	494	490	512	525
2	395	397	430	415
3	516	512	520	508
4	434	401	428	444
5	476	470	500	500
6	557	611	600	625
7	413	415	364	460
8	442	431	380	390
9	650	638	658	642
10	433	429	445	432
11	417	420	432	420
12	656	633	626	605
13	267	275	260	227
14	478	492	477	467
15	178	165	259	268
16	423	372	350	370
17	427	421	451	443

20.1.1.   What would you check to see whether each flow meter yields essentially the same results (i.e., "intra-observer variability") in its two measurements for each subject? Which flow meter seems inherently more "variable"?

20.1.2.   Suppose the investigator, using only the first measurement for each subject, compares the results as shown in Figure E.20.1. For these data, r = .94 with P < .001. [For the questions that follow, use only the first "PEFR" for each method of measurement.]

(a)   From visual inspection of the graph, would you be impressed that the high r value shows excellent agreement? If not, why not?

(b)   What could you do quantitatively to check the excellence of the agreement?

(c)   What would you check to see whether the two measuring systems are biased with respect to one another or to the magnitudes of PEFR? If your check involves calculations, show the results and your conclusions.

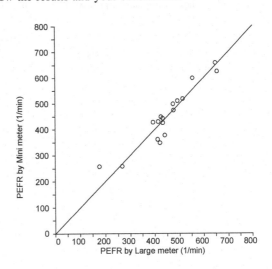

FIGURE E.20.1

PEFR measured with large Wright peak flow meter and mini Wright peak flow meter, with line of equality.

20.2. Table E.20.2 shows dodeciles of "sucrose intake" as reported in two questionnaires repeated at a one-year interval.[17]

20.2.1.   Form a 2 × 2 table by dividing the original 12 × 12 table between the 6th and 7th dodeciles. What are the values of proportional agreement and kappa in the 2 × 2 table?

20.2.2.   What are the values of p_{pos} and p_{neg} in the 2 × 2 table? Do these results convince or dissuade you for the belief that kappa is a good index of concordance here?

20.2.3.   Form a 3 × 3 table by dividing between the 4th and 5th and 8th and 9th deciles. What happens to proportional agreement? Using the categorical-distance method, what is the value of weighted proportionate agreement?

20.2.4.   A compassionate instructor saves you from having to slog through the calculations and tells you that weighted kappa (with the categorical-distance method) is 0.46 for the 3 × 3 table. How does this compare with the value previously obtained for the unweighted (2 × 2) kappa? How do you account for the difference?

TABLE E.20.2

Cross-Classification of Subjects by Dodeciles of Sucrose Intake Measured by a Food Frequency Questionnaire Administered Twice, One Year Apart, to 173 Boston-Area Female Registered Nurses Aged 34–59 Years in 1980–1981 [Taken from Chapter Reference 17.]

Second Questionnaire Dodeciles	First Questionnaire Dodeciles											
	1	2	3	4	5	6	7	8	9	10	11	12
1	7	4	0	1	1	0	1	0	0	0	0	0
2	3	3	4	0	3	0	0	0	0	0	1	0
3	1	0	2	2	2	3	1	2	1	0	1	0
4	1	3	2	3	3	0	1	1	1	0	0	0
5	0	2	1	2	1	5	0	1	2	0	0	0
6	0	1	0	3	1	3	3	3	0	0	1	0
7	1	0	1	0	1	2	3	0	3	1	1	1
8	0	0	2	1	2	1	0	1	2	5	0	1
9	1	1	2	0	0	0	1	2	2	1	3	1
10	0	0	0	1	0	0	4	2	3	1	1	3
11	0	1	0	0	0	1	0	1	0	5	1	5
12	0	0	0	1	0	0	0	1	1	2	5	4

Comment: In the exercises that follow, you are not expected to do any sophisticated calculations such as kappa. Your conclusions should come mainly from visual inspection and "clinical judgment," although you should feel free to check minor arithmetical details, such as sums.

20.3. In a paper on open-heart surgery for aortic valve and/or coronary disease in 100 consecutive octogenarians,[36] the authors concluded that "operation may be an effective option for...selected octogenarians with unmanageable cardiac symptoms." Symptoms were classified and tabulated as shown in Figure E.20.3A.

20.3.1   The authors say that 90 patients were in Class IV for either the NYHA or CCS classifications. What is the source of this number and do you agree with it?

20.3.2.   Are you satisfied that the patients in Class IV (with either rating scale) have been suitably classified? If not, why not?

20.3.3.   In Figure E.20.3B, the authors report the "current functional and ischemic status of the 54 patients who still remain alive" in follow-up durations that are at least one year for all patients and as long as six years for a few. Are you satified with the classifications and results offered in Figure E.20.3B? Is there anything else you might like to know to determine which patients were most benefited by the operation, and whether the authors' claim is justified that the operation is beneficial for "octogenarians with unmanageable cardiac symptoms?"

N.Y.H.A.
Classification

	I	II	III	IV	total
I	-	-	3	28	31
II	-	-	2	8	10
C.C.S. Classification of Angina — III	2	1	2	4	9
IV	30	6	3	11	50
total	32	7	10	51	100

FIGURE E.20.3A

Matrix of Symptoms in All 100 Patients Who Underwent Open-Heart Surgery. Each patient was classified according to both the New York Heart Association (N.Y.H.A.) classifications of functional disability and the Canadian Cardiovascular Society (C.C.S.) classifications of severity of effort angina. Patients who did not have angina were included in C.C.S. Class I, since none of them could exercise strenuously. [Taken from Chapter Reference 36.]

N. Y. H. A.
Classification

	I	II	III	TOTAL
I	33	12	1	46
C. C. S. Classification of Angina — II	3	5		8
TOTAL	36	17	1	54

FIGURE E.20.3B

Functional and Anginal Classification of the 54 Living Patients. [Taken from Chapter Reference 36.]

20.4. Figure E.20.4 shows results of a simpler, speedier electrophoresis method than the standard ("modified K-L columns") method for measuring glycosylated hemoglobin (HbA_1). The authors said the new method was "accurate," but offered no comparative information except what appears in Figure E.20.4 and its legend.

    20.4.1.   What is the meaning of "$S^2y \cdot x = 1.04$" on the graph?

    20.4.2.   Do you agree with the authors' claim that the new method is "accurate"? If not, why not?

20.5. In a study of therapeutic outcome as rated by patients and their psychotherapists, the following frequency counts were reported for 37 patients:

	Rating by Therapist		
Rating by Patient	**Satisfactory**	**Unsatisfactory**	**Total**
Satisfactory	19	1	20
Unsatisfactory	5	12	17
Total	24	13	37

The authors listed the stochastic analytic results exactly as follows:

	X² Value	P Value
Agreement	17.345	< .005
Change	2.667	NS

    20.5.1.   How do you think this stochastic analysis was conducted? Do you agree with it? If not, what would you propose instead?

    20.5.2.   What would you do to check whether the therapists were more optimistic than the patients?

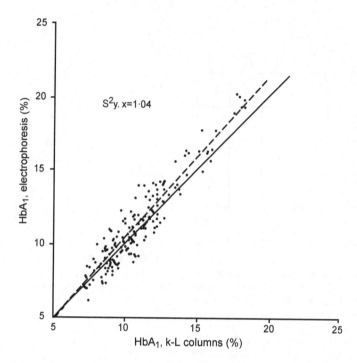

FIGURE E.20.4

Relation between HbA_1 concentrations measured by electrophoresis endosmosis and our own modified Kynoch-Lehmann (K-L) columns (n = 192). HbA_1 by electrophoresis 1.10 HbA_1 by K-L–0.64(—— Line of identity, - - - Regression line). [Taken from Chapter Reference 37.]

21

Evaluating "Conformity" and Marker Tests

CONTENTS

As medical technology began to burgeon after World War II, the diagnostic accuracy of new procedures and tests required quantitative evaluation. As new *therapeutic* technology was developed, however, patient care began to offer many scientific challenges beyond diagnostic decisions alone. The additional decisions demanded that clinicians use the technologic information to estimate prognosis, choose and evaluate therapy, and appraise diverse conditions and changes. Nevertheless, most statistical methods for assessing technology have been devoted to the accuracy of diagnostic tests.

After a brief discussion of nomenclature, most of this chapter is devoted to the diagnostic statistical methods. Some of the additional nondiagnostic challenges in clinical care are noted afterward.

21.1 Concepts of *Accuracy* and *Conformity*

When the same entity is measured in two ways, the agreement in results can be called *accuracy* if one result is accepted as the *correct* entity, which is often called the *reference, criterion*, or *gold standard*. For chemical (and other laboratory) measurements, the criterion result may come from the National Bureau of Standards or from a particular laboratory designated as *the* reference standard. In the usual assessment of accuracy, a tested laboratory's results for a measurement such as serum calcium are compared against the corresponding values obtained in the reference laboratory.

Many *diagnostic* activities, however, do not compare two measurements of exactly the same substance. Instead, the results of one variable, such as serum calcium, are used as a marker test to identify (or "predict") the diagnosis of a disease, such as hypoparathyroidism, that is verified with other methods in the second, or "gold standard," variable. In other activities, a marker test may be evaluated for *efficacy* rather than *accuracy*, because the gold-standard criterion may rely not on a single idea of "correctness," but on a composite combination of costs, convenience, and consequences for right and wrong answers. The idea of *accuracy* may itself sometimes be uncertain, because the gold-standard criterion may not have enduring permanence. For example, the radiologic imaging procedure that is today's "gold standard" might be replaced by a better technique tomorrow.

For all these reasons, the term *conformity* is often better than *accuracy* for assessing agreement between an evaluated entity and the accepted criterion. Nevertheless, *accuracy* is usually applied for tests of diagnostic markers. As a label for the reference criterion, *gold standard* has also become popular and conventional, despite occasional objections that the fluctuating value of gold is undesirable for an allegedly constant criterion.

This chapter is devoted mainly to quantitative methods of expressing conformity. Although diagnostic marker tests are the main topic, conformity can also be appraised for spectral marker tests, which are used for diverse clinical conditions rather than diseases, and for many clinical decisions beyond diagnosis alone. The mathematical methods often appear in medical literature, but they are beset by important, often overlooked, and currently unresolved scientific problems that are discussed in Sections 21.8 and 21.9.

21.2 Statistical Indexes of Diagnostic Efficacy

The idea of diagnostic efficacy was introduced when scientific and statistical problems arose during "screening" for disease in apparently healthy people. After World War II, searches for tuberculosis were done with photofluorography, a simple, quick procedure that produced much smaller films than the customary "gold standard" chest X-ray. In 1947, observer variability and accuracy in the use of photofluorography were reported[1] by a group of physicians working with Jacob Yerushalmy, an epidemiologist. Later that year, Yerushalmy[2] introduced the terms *sensitivity* and *specificity*, which have subsequently become the "established" statistical indexes for appraising diagnostic performance.

21.2.1 Structure of a Decision Matrix

The results of diagnostic tests are usually expressed in a 2×2 table, sometimes called[3] a decision matrix, showing frequency counts for the binary results of **yes/no** for presence of the disease, and **positive/negative** for the marker test. Table 21.1 resembles all other 2×2 tables, but the results are commonly expressed with two statistical indexes aimed at diagnostic efficacy. Two of the indexes, as christened by Yerushalmy, were sensitivity and specificity. *Sensitivity*, which is $v = a/(a + c) = a/n_1$ in Table 21.1, is the proportion of "true positive" results in diseased cases; and *specificity*, which is $f = d/(b + d) = d/n_2$, is the proportion of "true negative" results in the nondiseased controls. Another common index, called *prevalence*, is the proportion of diseased cases in the total group under study, expressed as $P = n_1/N$.

TABLE 21.1

Components of Decision Matrix for Diagnostic Marker Tests

Diagnosis Made from Marker Test	Correct ("Gold Standard") Diagnosis of Disease		Total
	Present	**Absent**	
Positive	a (true positive)	b (false positive)	m_1
Negative	c (false negative)	d (true negative)	m_2
TOTAL	n_1	n_2	N

Note: "Sensitivity" $= a/(a + c) = a/n_1$; "Specificity" $= d/(b + d) = d/n_2$; "Positive predictive accuracy" $= a/(a + b) = a/m_1$; "Negative predictive accuracy" $= d/(c + d) = d/m_2$.

These three indexes — sensitivity, specificity, and prevalence — are commonly used in statistical discussions, and are calculated "vertically" from the columns in the table. In making decisions for individual patients, however, clinicians usually want to know the rates of diagnostic accuracy that are shown "horizontally" in the rows of the table. These different directions of interpretation are the source of the major problems to be discussed shortly.

21.2.2 Omnibus Indexes

The direction of interpretation can be avoided with an "omnibus" index, which offers a single summary for a result that otherwise requires two or more separate citations, such as *sensitivity* and *specificity*.

For a diagnostic marker test, one omnibus expression, called *index of validity*, is essentially the same as *percentage agreement*. In the symbols of Table 21.1,

$$\text{Index of validity} = (a + d)/N$$

Another omnibus index, called *Youden's J*, was suggested as a compensation for error in the "vertical" indexes. The false positive rate in nondiseased people, i.e., $b/(b + d)$, is subtracted from the true positive rate in diseased people, i.e., $a/(a + c)$. When the algebra is developed, Youden's J turns out to be $v - (1 - f) = v + f - 1$, which is simply the sum of sensitivity + specificity $- 1$.

The omnibus simplification that combines these two indexes is also a prime defect. It obscures what is needed for two separate clinical decisions: the accuracy of the marker test in diseased and in nondiseased persons. Furthermore, when the test is applied to an "unknown" group, the clinician will want to know "predictive" accuracy separately for positive and negative results. The omnibus indexes are hardly ever used today because the single combined result does not provide the desired information.

21.2.3 Problems in Expressing Rates of Accuracy

The terms *sensitivity* and *specificity* were quite appropriate when the original research, designed in a case-control manner, contained groups of cases, who were known to have the disease, and controls, who did not. In the case-control design, these two groups served as denominators of the original statistical indexes, which were a/n_1 for sensitivity and d/n_2 for specificity.

21.2.3.1 Problems in Nomenclature

21.2.3.1 Problems in Nomenclature — The case-control approach, however, led to major conceptual problems that have never been easily resolved. One problem is in nomenclature. Since the opposite of a *true positive* is a *false positive*, the latter title might be expected for the additive reciprocal of the "true positive" index of sensitivity. The value of $1 - (a/n_1) = (n_1 - a)/n_1 = c/n_1$, however, refers to false *negative*, not false positive, diagnoses for the diseased cases. Similarly, the additive reciprocal of the *true negative* result for specificity, i.e., $1 - (d/n_2)$, is b/n_2, which refers to *false positive* diagnoses for controls, rather than the intuitively expected idea of false *negatives*.

To avoid confusion, Henrik Wulff[4] proposed using the more precise terms *nosologic sensitivity* and *nosologic specificity* for the "vertical" statistical indexes that are calculated nosologically, from cases and controls whose true state of disease is already known. The precise adjectives have generally been omitted, however, and *sensitivity* and *specificity* are seldom cited with their nosologic prefixes.

21.2.3.2 Problems in Clinical Direction

21.2.3.2 Problems in Clinical Direction — A second problem is in the direction of clinical application. The terms *sensitivity* and *specificity*, although perhaps satisfactory for a case-control structure, do not indicate what a clinician does with a diagnostic marker test. For persons with unknown diagnoses (in clinical practice), the clinician wants statistical indexes to show the marker test's rates of accuracy when results are positive or negative. In Table 21.1, these rates would be determined, respectively, as a/m_1 and d/m_2, not as a/n_1 and d/n_2.

If the statistical nomenclature were concerned with scientific clinical precision, the "predictive" rates might have been called, respectively, *diagnostic sensitivity* and *diagnostic specificity*. An alternative, but longer, pair of designations would have been *diagnostic true positive rate* and *diagnostic true negative rate*. The reciprocal values for these diagnostic rates would have been intuitively easy to understand, because each positive or negative rate would have true and false reciprocal components.

Instead, however, bowing to the established case-control definitions and improperly using the term *predictive* for estimating a concomitant rather than future event, investigators designated the desired clinical rates as *positive predictive accuracy* (for a/m_1) and *negative predictive accuracy* (for d/m_2). Massive ambiguity and confusion can then occur when writers talk about a "false positive rate" or a "false negative rate," without indicating which denominator is used for the rates.

21.2.3.3 Problems of Prevalence

21.2.3.3 Problems of Prevalence — A third and more profound statistical problem was soon recognized. Because comparative differences are often best demonstrated in contrasts for equal numbers of members, the case and control groups chosen for most diagnostic marker research had roughly similar sizes, i.e., $n_1 \simeq n_2$. With this partitioning, the disease had a prevalence of about 50%, i.e., $n_1/N \simeq .5$, in the case-control research. At that level of prevalence, high values of nosologic sensitivity and specificity would be converted into correspondingly high values of predictive diagnostic accuracy.

For example, consider a marker test that has 92% sensitivity and 96% specificity in a group of 50 diseased cases and 50 nondiseased controls. The numerical results, shown in Table 21.2, have relatively high values of .96 for positive and .92 for negative predictive accuracy. The prevalence of the disease in this carefully selected test group, however, is .50 — a situation that seldom occurs in real life, even in tertiary-care hospitals. When the diagnostic marker test is used for screening purposes in the community, the prevalence of disease is substantially lower — at rates of .1, .05, or .001.

Table 21.3 shows the performance of this same diagnostic test when applied to 1,000 persons in a community where prevalence of the disease is .05. The sensitivity and specificity of the test remain the same: .92 in the 50 diseased persons, and .96 in the 950 who do not have the disease. The negative predictive accuracy is even better than before, with a rate of .996 (= 912/916). The positive predictive accuracy, however, falls drastically to a value of .55 (= 46/84), indicating that about one of every two positive results will be a false positive.

The two omnibus indexes of Section 21.2.2 would not be able to detect this problem. The index of validity will be $(46 + 48)/100 = .94$ in Table 21.2 and $(46 + 912)/1000 = .958$ in Table 21.3. The high

TABLE 21.2

Performance of Diagnostic Indexes in a Setting of "High" Prevalence

Marker-Test Result	Diseased Cases	Nondiseased Controls	TOTAL
Positive	46	2	48
Negative	4	48	52
TOTAL	50	50	100

Note: "Sensitivity" = 46/50 = .92; "Specificity" = 48/50 = .96; "Positive predictive accuracy" = 46/48 = .958; "Negative predictive accuracy" = 48/52 = .923.

TABLE 21.3

Performance of Same Test Shown in Table 21.2 in a Setting of "Low" Prevalence

Marker-Test Result	Diseased Cases	Nondiseased Controls	TOTAL
Positive	46	38	84
Negative	4	912	916
TOTAL	50	950	1000

Note: "Sensitivity" = 46/50 = .92; "Specificity" = 912/950 = .96; "Positive predictive accuracy" = 46/84 = .548; "Negative predictive accuracy" = 912/916 = .996.

value of the latter result would completely hide the predictive "lesion" in that table. The lesion will also be missed by Youden's J, which is independent of prevalence, relying only on nosologic sensitivity and specificity. In Tables 21.2 and 21.3, Youden's J will have identical results of $.92 + .96 - 1 = .88$.

21.2.4 Mathematical Conversions for Clinical Usage

Because the indexes of nosologic sensitivity and specificity are unsatisfactory for clinical usage, some other approach was needed. If the original diagnostic marker research had been done in cohort populations and expressed directly in the clinically desired "predictive" indexes, the results (and main problems) of clinical accuracy would have been immediately apparent. Case-control studies, however, were much easier to do than cohort research, and besides, sensitivity and specificity seemed to be inherent, invariant properties of the diagnostic marker test. They presumably reflected the test's performance for the selected disease, regardless of what its prevalence might be.

With this assumption, investigators sought a mathematical method that could easily, without any further work, convert the two nosologic indexes into the desired diagnostic indexes.

21.2.4.1 *Ordinary Algebra* — The conversion can easily be done with simple algebraic symbols, letting $v = a/n_1$ represent sensitivity, $f = d/n_2$ represent specificity, and $P = n_1/N$ represent prevalence. These three symbols can then be algebraically transformed into predictive diagnostic indexes for any group containing N people.

For positive predictive accuracy, we first determine appropriate substitutes for $a/(a + b)$ in Table 21.1. Because $a = vn_1$, and $n_1 = PN$, we can express a as vPN. Because $b = n_2 - d$, with $n_2 = (1 - P)N$ and $d = fn_2$, the value of b becomes $(1 - f)(1 - P)N$. Thus, positive predictive accuracy, abbreviated as *ppa*, becomes $a/(a + b) = vPN/[vPN + (1 - f)(1 - P)N]$, which is

$$ppa = vP/[vP + (1 - f)(1 - P)] \qquad [21.1]$$

When applied to Table 21.3, this formula produces $ppa = (.92)(.05)/[(.92)(.05) + (.04)(.95)] = .04/[.046 + .038] = .046/.084 = .55$, which is the same result obtained previously.

For negative predictive accuracy, we substitute for $d/(c + d)$. The value of d becomes $fn_2 = f(1 - P)N$; and $c = (1 - v)n_1 = (1 - v)PN$. Consequently, with suitable algebraic arrangements, the negative predictive accuracy (*npa*) for $d/(c + d)$ is calculated as

$$npa = [f(1 - P)]/[f(1 - P) + (1 - v)P] \qquad [21.2]$$

For Table 21.3, the calculation would be $(.96)(.95)/[(.96)(.95) + (.08)(.05)] = .912/(.912 + .004) = .912/.916 = .996$, which is also the same result obtained previously.

Formulas [21.1] and [21.2] can easily show why misleading clinical results are produced by case-control studies in which P is about .5. When $P = .5$, $1 - P = .5$, and so ppa becomes $v/[v + (1 - f)]$, i.e., sensitivity/ [sensitivity + (1 − specificity)], and npa becomes $f/[f + (1 - v)]$, i.e., specificity/[specificity + (1 − sensitivity)]. In this situation of high prevalence, if nosologic sensitivity and specificity have essentially similar high values, their counterparts in diagnostic sensitivity and specificity will also have similar high values.

In Table 21.3, however, where prevalence is .05, ppa will be $.05v/[.05v + .95 (1 - f)]$. The result will be strongly affected (and reduced) by the relatively large value of .95 (1 − f) in the denominator. Conversely, npa will be $.95f/[.95f + .05 (1 - v)]$. The result will usually be close to 1, because the .05 (1 − v) term in the denominator, being relatively small, will have little effect.

21.2.4.2   Bayes Theorem — A mathematically "elegant" way of achieving the simple algebraic conversions just described is to use the complex ideas and symbols of Bayes Theorem. Its basis is illustrated with the Venn diagrams of Figure 21.1, which shows the Boolean relationship in a population where one group, D, has the focal disease, and the other group, T, has a positive marker test for that disease. The complementary symbol, $\overline{D}$, represents persons who do not have the disease, and $\overline{T}$, those who have a negative (i.e., nonpositive) result in the marker test. In the combined diagram, the doubly cross-hatched group in the upper left corner represents $D \cap T$, i.e., the "true positive" persons who have both a positive result and the disease. The group of people shown without shading in the lower right corner of Figure 21.1 represent $\overline{D} \cap \overline{T}$, i.e., the true negative group.

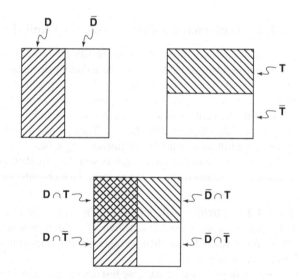

FIGURE 21.1

Rectangular Venn diagrams showing groups in-volved in Bayes Theorem. The left side of the upper section shows the tested "population" di-vided into D, persons who have the disease under study, and not D. The division on the right side shows T, persons with a positive marker test for that disease, and those without. The overlap in the lower section shows the four groups in the customary 2 × 2 table. Persons with $\overline{D} \cap \overline{T}$, who have neither the disease nor a positive test, are represented in the lower right corner.

If the symbol "N( )" is used to represent the number of persons in a particular group, the number of persons with disease D is N(D), and the prevalence of disease D in the total group of N persons is N(D)/N, which is also called the probability of the disease, P(D). Analogously, the prevalence (or probability) of persons with a positive test is $P(T) = N(T)/N$. The prevalence (or probability) of persons with a true positive result is $P(D \cap T) = N(D \cap T)/N$. All of these probabilities represent proportionate occurrence of the cited entities in the total population under investigation.

The other pertinent entities in Bayes Theorem are called *conditional probabilities.* They represent the proportional occurrence of a subgroup within a particular group. Thus, the symbol $P(T|D)$ represents the proportion of positive test results in diseased persons. The expression is pronounced "probability of T, given D"; and the symbol is a vertical "|" mark, not the diagonal "/" mark often used for division.

The proportion of diseased persons among those with a positive test is P(D |T). Figure 21.1 demonstrates the relationships that can be expressed or defined as

$$P(T|D) = P(D \cap T)/P(D) \qquad\qquad [21.3]$$

and

$$P(D|T) = P(D \cap T)/P(T) \qquad\qquad [21.4]$$

Solving these two equations for P(D ∩ T) and then setting the results equal to each other, we get

$$P(D|T) [P(T)] = P(T|D) [P(D)] \qquad\qquad [21.5]$$

Some additional thought about these symbols will reveal that P(D |T) represents positive predictive accuracy; P(T) represents the prevalence of a positive test result; P(T |D) represents the nosologic sensitivity of the marker test; and P(D) represents the prevalence of the disease. In the jargon developed for statistical communication, P(D) is also called the *prior* or *pretest* probability of the disease, and P(D |T) is called its *posterior* or *posttest* probability.

Because we want to know P(D|T), we can solve Equation [21.5] to get

$$P(D|T) = \frac{P(T|D)P(D)}{P(T)} \qquad\qquad [21.6]$$

which is one of the simpler ways of expressing Bayes Theorem for diagnostic marker tests. The more complex expressions are derived by suitable substitutions of "known" values for those that are not known. To get the value of P(T) in Formula [21.6], we note from Figure 21.1 that P(T) = [N(T ∩ D) + N(T ∩ $\overline{D}$)]/N which becomes

$$P(T) = [P(T|D) P(D)] + [P(T|\overline{D}) P(\overline{D})].$$

The cited value for specificity is P($\overline{D}$ ∩ $\overline{T}$)/P($\overline{D}$), which is P($\overline{T}$ |$\overline{D}$). The reciprocal value, 1 – P($\overline{T}$ |$\overline{D}$), will be P(T |$\overline{D}$). The reciprocal value of P(D) is P($\overline{D}$) = 1 – P(D). When the cited value of P(T) is substituted into Equation [21.6], we can use the expressions of conditional probability, and the values for sensitivity, specificity, and prevalence of disease, to write

$$P(D|T) = \frac{P(T|D)P(D)}{[P(T|D)P(D)] + [1 - P(\overline{T}|\overline{D})][1 - P(D)]} \qquad\qquad [21.7]$$

This complex expression for positive predictive accuracy, cited in terms of conditional probabilities, says exactly the same thing as the much simpler algebraic expression in Formula [21.1].

The application of Bayes Theorem can be illustrated with exactly the same data used earlier to show the change in positive predictive accuracy from Table 21.2 to Table 21.3. To apply Formula [21.7], we know that sensitivity, i.e., P(T |D), is .92 and that specificity, i.e., P($\overline{T}$ |$\overline{D}$), is .96. In Table 21.3, prevalence, i.e., P(D), is 50/1000 = .05. To determine positive predictive accuracy, i.e., P(D |T), we now substitute into Formula [21.7] to get (.92)(.05)/[(.92)(.05) + (1 − .96)(1 −.05)] = .55, which is the same result obtained previously.

An analogous expression can be developed for the Bayesian citation of P($\overline{D}$ |$\overline{T}$), which indicates negative predictive accuracy. You can work out the details for yourself or find them cited in pertinent publications elsewhere.

An important (and perhaps comforting) feature of Bayes Theorem is that it is simply a manipulation of the algebraic truism recorded in Expressions [21.3], [21.4], and [21.5]. For most purposes of analyzing diagnostic marker tests, nothing more need be known about Bayes Theorem itself.

21.2.4.3   *Likelihood Ratio* — A more sophisticated manipulation of the Bayesian algebra produces an entity called the *likelihood ratio*. It is used later for other types of diagnostic calculations, but it has become an important intellectual contributor to a new form of stochastic reasoning, called Bayesian inference.

To demonstrate the use of the likelihood ratio, we first note that results in Figure 21.1 for the "false positive" group, $P(\bar{D} \cap T)$, can be included in two expressions as

$$P(T \mid \bar{D}) = P(\bar{D} \cap T)/P(\bar{D}) \qquad [21.8]$$

and

$$P(\bar{D} \mid T) = P(\bar{D} \cap T)/P(T) \qquad [21.9]$$

Solving [21.8] and [21.9] for $P(\bar{D} \cap T)$ and equating the two results, we get

$$P(T \mid \bar{D}) \, P(\bar{D}) = P(\bar{D} \mid T) \, P(T) \qquad [21.10]$$

If Equation [21.10] is solved for $P(T)$, and if the result is substituted for $P(T)$ in Equation [21.6], we get

$$\frac{P(D \mid T)}{P(\bar{D} \mid T)} = \frac{P(T \mid D) \times P(D)}{P(T \mid \bar{D}) \times P(\bar{D})} \qquad [21.11]$$

In Equation [21.11], the far right entity, $P(D)/P(\bar{D})$, is simply the odds for prevalence. It is $(n_1/N)/(n_2/N) = n_1/n_2$, and is also called the *prior odds* of the disease. The value of $P(D \mid T)/P(\bar{D} \mid T)$ on the left side of the equation is the odds for a true positive among positive results. It is $(a/m_1)/(b/m_1) = a/b$, and is also called the *posterior odds* for a positive marker test.

The value of $P(T \mid D)/P(T \mid \bar{D})$ is called the *likelihood ratio*. It converts the prior odds into the posterior odds according to the formula

$$\text{posterior odds} = \text{likelihood ratio} \times \text{prior odds} \qquad [21.12]$$

or

$$\text{likelihood ratio} = \frac{\text{posterior odds}}{\text{prior odds}} \qquad [21.13]$$

Because $P(T \mid D) = \text{sensitivity} = a/n_1$, and $P(T \mid \bar{D}) = 1 - \text{specificity} = 1 - (d/n_2)$, we can express the test's accomplishment for a positive result in the 2×2 decision matrix as

$$\text{positive likelihood ratio} = \frac{\text{sensitivity}}{1 - \text{specificity}} \qquad [21.14]$$

For a negative diagnostic marker result, the prior odds are n_2/n_1 and the posterior odds are d/c. When appropriately arranged, the negative likelihood ratio for a 2×2 table becomes $(d/n_2)/(c/n_1)$, which is

$$\text{negative likelihood ratio} = \frac{\text{specificity}}{1 - \text{sensitivity}} \qquad [21.15]$$

This reasoning becomes pertinent later when likelihood ratios are used to express levels of diagnostic marker results.

21.2.4.4   *Illustration of Likelihood-Ratio Calculations* — To illustrate the numerical activities, the positive likelihood ratio in Table 21.2 is $[46/50]/[2/50] = 23$. The negative likelihood ratio is $[48/50]/[4/50] = 12$. The same results are obtained respectively in Table 21.3, where $[46/50]/[38/950] = 23$, and $[912/950]/[4/50] = 12$. This similarity would be expected because sensitivity and specificity are the same in both tables.

The main difference in the two tables is the prior odds, which is $50/50 = 1$ in Table 21.2, and $50/950 = .0526$ in Table 21.3. Consequently, the two tables have different values for posterior odds, calculated as likelihood ratio × prior odds. The posterior odds for a positive result are $23 \times 1 = 23$ in Table 21.2, and $23 \times .0526 = 1.21$ in Table 21.3. An even simpler way of getting these results for the first row in each table is to note that $46/2 = 23$ in Table 21.2 and $46/38 = 1.21$ in Table 21.3.

After being calculated, the posterior odds must be converted to the probabilities that express diagnostic accuracy. The conversion uses the mathematical "construction" that probability = odds/(odds + 1). Thus, the positive predictive accuracy is $23/(23 + 1) = .958$ in Table 21.1 and $1.21/(1.21 + 1) = .548$ in Table 21.2. Various nomograms[5-7] have been proposed to produce these transformations directly from values for the likelihood ratios and prior probability.

21.2.5 Bayesian Inference

The logic of Formula [21.12] is especially cogent for the statistical reasoning called *Bayesian inference*, which differs from the frequentist methods that underlie all the stochastic strategies discussed in this text. Bayesian inference relies on the likelihood-ratio relationship between prior and posterior odds.

The Bayesian inferential methods are becoming fashionable today, especially for advanced graduate courses and doctoral dissertations in academic departments of statistics. Nevertheless, the value of Bayesian inference is highly controversial,[8,9] and its ultimate role is currently uncertain. A fundamental problem in the dispute is that subjective choices are often used for the values of prior odds. Clinicians who have received decades of exhortation to avoid anecdotal evidence and to get precise documentation for any quantitative statements are often surprised and ruefully chagrined to discover a new brand of mathematical reasoning that allows completely subjective guesses to be made about prior odds.

The main point to be noted now, however, is that Bayes Theorem, in contrast to the complexities of Bayesian inference, is a relatively simple mathematical mechanism for converting the case-control ("nosologic") values of sensitivity and specificity, and the anticipated or observed prevalence of disease, into the desired "predictive" indexes of diagnostic accuracy. This mechanism is what has made Bayes Theorem so famous (or infamous) in the statistical analysis of diagnostic marker tests.

21.2.6 Direct Clinical Reasoning

If all the foregoing mathematical methods had not been developed and subsequently advocated by academic investigators, a simple direct procedure might have been used. When diagnostic-marker tests are applied in cohorts of patients, the results can be promptly expressed in rates of diagnostic accuracy. For the symbols in Table 21.1, these rates would be the "horizontal" values of a/m_1 and d/m_2 that are respectively called *positive* and *negative predictive accuracy*.

In a recent survey of practicing clinicians in diverse specialties, Reid et al.[10] found that the formal mathematical strategies were almost never used. Instead, the clinicians — although often believing that they evaluated the vertical indexes of "sensitivity" and "specificity" — usually examined the *horizontal* results in their own groups of patients. The results were commonly expressed in the reciprocal values of false positive and false negative rates, which would be b/m_1 and c/m_2. With these direct expressions, clinicians could promptly appraise the accuracy of the tests without having to rely on special mathematical calculations, transformations, or nomograms.

The direct, "sensible" clinical cohort approach may eventually replace the indirect case-control mathematical transformations. Because the indirect methods remain popular, however, they create the additional challenges (and problems) discussed in the next few sections.

21.3 Demarcations for Ranked Results

Regardless of whether Bayesian, likelihood-ratio, or direct expressions were used, all of the components discussed so far were dichotomous: the disease was either present or absent, and the diagnostic marker test was either positive or negative. The splendid mathematical tactics applied to these double dichotomies require binary citations for both the disease and the marker test.

Many diagnostic marker (or even gold-standard) tests, however, are expressed in ranked values. They might be dimensional scales for blood glucose, serum calcium, or enzyme tests, or ordinal scales, such as the **none, trace, 1+, 2+, ...** ratings for various urinary tests. Furthermore, many "gold standard" diagnoses are expressed in a three-category scale, containing an equivocal **maybe** or **uncertain**, in addition to the 2-category unequivocal **yes** or **no**.

These problems can be managed with three approaches: (1) converting all gold standards into binary categories, (2) choosing a binary demarcation for ranked results of the marker test, and (3) establishing ordinal zones for the marker test and using a *likelihood ratio*, for efficacy in each zone.

21.3.1   Binary "Gold Standards"

The ranked results of *marker tests* can easily be converted into binary (or ordinal) arrangements that will be discussed shortly. These arrangements, however, will not take care of a *gold-standard* criterion that is not binary. Accordingly, diagnostic marker evaluations are almost always confined to situations in which the gold-standard disease criterion is cited as an unequivocal binary **yes** or **no**. For example, the dimensional scale of a glucose tolerance test for diabetes mellitus or a urinary culture for bacteriuria might be given a **yes/no** binary demarcation such as ≥ 500 for the sum of four glucose levels or $\geq 5 \times 10^3$ for a colony count of bacteria.

The custom of using a binary gold standard can easily be justified when the demarcation comes from dimensional scales such as those used for bacterial counts or the sum of glucose values. If the boundary is disputed, the accuracy of the marker test can be re-calculated at different boundaries. For example, if $\geq 10^5$ colony forming units (CFU) is chosen as the gold-standard threshold for bacterial infection in a urinary culture, and if a different threshold is preferred, the efficacy of the marker test can be determined for alternative boundaries, such as 10^3, 10^4, or 10^6.

Insistence on a binary gold standard, however, creates major difficulties for a three-category scale if the group with an **uncertain** diagnosis is omitted from the clinical reality of diseases that are usually diagnosed in the trichotomous categories[11] of **yes, uncertain,** or **no**. For example, a biopsy specimen may be inadequate for making a definitive diagnostic decision; or the collection of data for a patient with chest pain may lead to the conclusion of possible, but not definite, myocardial infarction.

If the gold-standard results contain only the two groups of unequivocally diseased cases and nondiseased controls, the results for efficacy, although mathematically attractive, may seriously distort what really happens in clinical practice. This potential distortion is constantly ignored, however, for the statistical activities of both published literature and the discussion that follows. Consequently, the pertinent statistical evaluations may be deceptive when published results of marker-test accuracy for binary gold standards are applied in the nonbinary scientific realities of clinical practice.

21.3.2   Receiver-Operating-Characteristic (ROC) Curves

To get the double dichotomy needed for Bayes Theorem, the gold-standard nosologic groups are divided into diseased cases and nondiseased controls, and the ranked results of marker tests are also given a binary demarcation. Without this double binary split, the marker test cannot be indexed for sensitivity and specificity, and cannot be applied thereafter in Bayesian diagnostic analyses. Choosing the best binary split for ranked marker-test values thus became a new statistical challenge. It was approached with a method, developed in engineering, that analyzes a *receiver-operating-characteristic* curve.[12] The popularity of these curves in published reports soon made ROC become a fashionable abbreviation in the mathematics of diagnostic analysis.[3]

21.3.2.1   Inverse Relationship of Sensitivity and Specificity — Table 21.4 shows the relationship of results for a ranked marker (S-T depression in an exercise stress test) and the definitive nosologic state of 150 cases of coronary disease and 150 controls. The 7 ordinal categories used for the marker can be split dichotomously at six locations, marked A, B, ..., E, F in Table 21.4. Each split would produce a different fourfold table, yielding different indexes for sensitivity and specificity. For example, with split C, the fourfold table becomes $\begin{Bmatrix} 73 & 7 \\ 77 & 143 \end{Bmatrix}$, having a sensitivity of $73/150 = .49$ and specificity of $143/150 = .95$. With split D, which produces $\begin{Bmatrix} 103 & 15 \\ 47 & 135 \end{Bmatrix}$, the corresponding indexes are $103/150 = .69$ and $135/150 = .90$.

TABLE 21.4

Results in Diagnostic Marker Study of Coronary Artery Disease and Level of S-T Depression in Exercise Stress Test

	Definitive State of Disease	
Patients with S-T Segment Depression of	Cases of Coronary Disease	Controls Without Coronary Disease
≥ 3.0 mm.	31	0
A _____		
≥ 2.5 mm. but < 3.0 mm.	15	0
B _____		
≥ 2.0 mm. but < 2.5 mm.	27	7
C _____		
≥1.5 mm. but < 2.0 mm.	30	8
D _____		
≥1.0 mm. but <1.5 mm.	32	39
E _____		
≥ 0.5 mm. but < 1.0 mm.	12	43
F _____		
< 0.5 mm.	3	53
TOTAL	150	150

The results of the different demarcations for Table 21.4 are summarized in Table 21.5, which shows that sensitivity and specificity have an inverse relationship: as sensitivity increases, specificity decreases, and vice versa. This relationship is easy to prove algebraically, but can be understood intuitively if you recognize that the denominators for calculating sensitivity and specificity are the same, regardless of the level of demarcation. As the level goes downward, however, the numerator values increase for the sensitivity index and decrease for specificity.

TABLE 21.5

Summary of Nosologic Sensitivity and Specificity Calculated for Demarcations of Table 21.4

Demarcation	Location of Boundary for Abnormal	Number of Cases Included	Sensitivity	Number of Controls Included	Specificity	1 – Specificity
A	≥ 3.0 mm.	31	0.21	0	1	0
B	≥ 2.5 mm.	46	0.31	0	1	0
C	≥ 2.0 mm.	73	0.49	7	0.95	0.05
D	≥ 1.5 mm.	103	0.69	15	0.90	0.10
E	≥ 1.0 mm.	135	0.90	54	0.64	0.36
F	≥ 0.5 mm.	147	0.98	97	0.35	0.65
	TOTAL	150	—	150	—	—

21.3.2.2 Construction of ROC Curves —

If sensitivity is plotted against specificity at each level of the possible split, the shape of the curve will go downward to the right. To make the curve go upward, it is constructed as a plot of sensitivity vs. 1 – specificity. The two pairs of values then rise monotonically.

The ROC curve for the data of Tables 21.4 and 21.5 is shown in Figure 21.2. The curve here has .21 and .31 as the lowest values of sensitivity when 1 – specificity = 0, and .98 as the highest value when 1 – specificity = .65.

In a *useless* marker test, the cases and controls will have similar distributions, and the corresponding values of sensitivity and 1 – specificity will be essentially equal in each row. The ROC curve will be a straight line at a 45° angle.

In a *perfect* marker test, all of the cases will be included in rows that have no controls, and all the controls will appear in rows that begin below the level of the last case. The values of sensitivity will ascend toward a maximum of 1 while 1 − specificity = 0, and will maintain the value of 1 while 1 − specificity gradually rises. The curve will resemble a capital Greek gamma, Γ.

The useless, perfect, and ordinary possibilities for the ROC curves are shown in Figure 21.3. An inverted wedge is formed as the upper and left outer lines of the Γ-shaped perfect test join the diagonal line of the useless test. The results for most ordinary tests fit into that wedge. The closer they approach the Γ shape, the better is the test's performance.

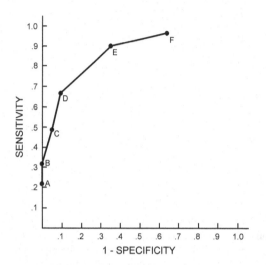

FIGURE 21.2
Receiver-operating-characteristic (ROC) curve for data in Tables 21.4 and 21.5.

FIGURE 21.3
Perfect, useless, and ordinary possibilities for ROC curves of diagnostic marker tests.

21.3.2.3   Choice of Optimal Dichotomous Boundary — The main reason for constructing ROC curves is to choose an optimal dichotomous boundary for the diagnostic marker results. For a perfect test, the choice is easy: it will be the level at which sensitivity = 1, and 1 − specificity = 0. Because perfect tests almost never occur in clinical reality, however, a practical strategy is needed for the decisions. The strategy can be purely mathematical or can involve additional ideas about costs and benefits.

21.3.2.3.1 Mathematical Strategy.   A simple method of choosing an optimal cut-point is to minimize the sum of false positive and false negative test results.[13] Mathematical calculus will show that this point occurs when the slope of the ROC curve is at $(N − T)/T$, where T is the total number of cases and $N − T$ is the number of controls. Because $N ≥ T$, the formula becomes $(N/T) − 1$, and this slope is always positive.

To avoid calculations of slope, the cut-point can be found as the location where the number of accruing false positive values begins to exceed the number of accruing false negatives. Thus, for the data in Table 21.5, the accruing totals for each cut-point are as follows:

Cut-Point	Accruing Totals for:		Total Number of False Results
	Number of False-Negatives	Number of False-Positives	
A	119	0	119
B	104	0	104
C	77	7	84
D	47	15	62
E	15	54	69
F	3	97	100

In downward descent of these boundaries, the false negatives exceed the false positives at cut-point D, but not at point E. The total number of false results is also minimized at cut-point D. Therefore D would be the best choice of demarcation for these data. This point occurs in Figure 21.2 just before the curve begins to flatten its sharp upward slope.

With another mathematical strategy,[13] the chosen cut-point will maximize the predictive accuracy of the test for its *diagnostic* sensitivity and specificity. Yet another mathematical tactic relies on "information content"[3,12,14] of the test, determined from logarithmic calculations of sensitivity, specificity, and prevalence.

21.3.2.3.2 Cost-Benefit Strategies. Each false-positive, true-positive, false-negative, and true-negative diagnostic result can be multiplied by an arbitrary monetary (or other quantitative) value that gives a "weight" to costs and benefits of that result. The score that is calculated for the different possibilities can then be used to find an optimal cut-off boundary in the ROC curve.[3,13]

Despite the mathematical ingenuity, this strategy has had little value beyond its contributions to academic scholarship. The basic problem is making pragmatically realistic choices of quantitative values for the costs and benefits.

21.3.2.3.3 Area under the ROC Curve. Because the ROC curve gets "better" as it approaches the Γ shape, the area under the curve can be used as an index of accomplishment. In the square formed by the coordinates of the graph, a perfect curve will have an area of 1, and a useless curve will cover an area of .5. The areas under most curves will thus range from .5 to 1.

This distinction may not help choose the best cut-point for an individual curve, but can be useful in evaluating the accomplishments of different marker tests. For example, the areas under the corresponding ROC curves could be compared to decide whether S-T segment depressions or CPK enzyme results are the better diagnostic markers for coronary disease.

One problem in using areas under the curve is that a useless test will have a value of .5, which may seem impressive in other contexts, such as correlation coefficients. If the kappa coefficient in Chapter 20 is intended to adjust indexes of agreement for results that might occur by chance, the area-under-the-curve index should be similarly adjusted to reflect its superiority over a useless result. Thus, with an area of only $1 - .5 = .5$ available for showing "superiority," a .8 area under the curve has produced an improvement of only $.8 - .5 = .3$, which is a proportion of $.3/.5 = 60\%$ of what could be accomplished.

The main mathematical flaw in the area-under-the-curve strategy, however, is that the points on the curve may often come from small proportions that are numerically unstable. The problem of stability is discussed in Section 21.4.

21.3.2.4 ROC Curves as Indexes of Prediction — The area under the ROC curve has been proposed as an index for evaluating staging systems or other multivariable mechanisms that produce prognostic predictions rather than diagnostic separations.[15] Aside from the problem of instability in the constituent numbers, the ROC method ignores the principle that staging systems are used for much more than individual forecasts. In the design or evaluation of therapeutic research, a prognostic staging system is most valuable for the way it distributes the patients and provides significant gradients between the stages.[16] Neither of these desiderata is considered in ROC curves that are aimed only at the individual accuracy of each estimate.

21.3.3 Likelihood-Ratio Strategy

To avoid choosing a single binary cut-point, the marker test results can be appraised with likelihood ratios for ordinal zones.[5] The reasoning is as follows: Suppose the numerical results in any row (or zone) of the table are t_i for the cases and s_i for the controls, with $m_i = t_i + s_i$ as the total in that row. The grand total will be T cases and S controls, with $T + S = N$. In any marker test, the *prior* odds of a positive result from the total of cases and controls, will be T/S. In any row (or zone), such as those in Table 21.4, the *posterior* odds for a positive result will be t_i/s_i. As shown earlier in Formula [21.13],

$$\text{likelihood ratio} = \frac{\text{posterior odds}}{\text{prior odds}}$$

Accordingly, the positive likelihood ratio in any zone will be

$$LR_{pos} = (t_i/s)/(T/S)$$

Analogously, the likelihood ratio for a negative result will be

$$LR_{neg} = (s_i/t_j)/(S/T)$$

The major advantage of likelihood ratios is the removal of the grand total denominator, N, so that prevalence does not affect the results. The values of LR_{pos} and LR_{neg} can therefore be calculated directly from the counts in each zone and from the individual columnar totals for cases and controls. In contrast to the separate binary values of sensitivity for cases and specificity for controls, the likelihood ratios offer "stratified" indexes of efficacy for each selected zone of ordinal categories in the cases and controls of the diagnostic marker research.

21.3.3.1   *Example of Calculations* — In Table 21.4, the value for prior odds is T/S = 150/150 = 1. Consequently, the posterior-odds values in each zone will provide the positive and negative likelihood ratios. For positive results, the posterior odds will be $31/0 = \infty$ in the first zone, $30/8 = 3.75$ in the fourth zone, and $12/43 = .28$ in the sixth zone. The posterior odds for the corresponding negative results will be 0, .27, and 3.58. If the value of T/S were .5 rather than 1, however, each of these positive likelihood ratios would be doubled, and each negative ratio would be halved.

21.3.3.2   *Disadvantage of Likelihood Ratios* — Although the conversion to odds gives the likelihood ratio the advantage of avoiding the effects of prevalence, the tactic becomes a disadvantage when the result is actually applied clinically. As noted earlier, the probability value needed for a clinical decision requires special calculations or nomograms to convert the odds values and likelihood ratio for the estimated prevalence of disease in the clinical situation under scrutiny.

The likelihood ratios also have all of the problems of stability (see Section 21.4) that occur for any collection of binary proportions, and the inevitable difficulties (see Section 21.8.3.1) of any index that erroneously relies on having constant values in the varied spectrum of a disease.

21.3.4   Additional Expressions of Efficacy

Eisenberg et al.[17] have proposed two additional ways of expressing diagnostic efficacy. In one method, which can be used only for binary markers, the prior and posterior probability values are subtracted as $P(D|T) - P(D)$, and the incremental change in probability becomes the index of accomplishment. In the second method, the indexes of accomplishment are cited as logarithms (rather than actual values) of odds in the likelihood ratio. The logarithms are preferred, for reasons noted earlier (see Section 17.5.5.2), because of asymmetrical constraints in the range of odds ratios below and above 1. If LR > 1, the values can extend up to infinity; but if LR < 1, the values can range only between 0 and 1. Besides, if LR = 1, i.e., a useless result, log LR will be zero.

21.3.5   Trichotomous Clinical Strategy

From an esthetic mathematical viewpoint, the Bayesian, ROC, and likelihood-ratio approaches offer appealing solutions for the challenges of either dichotomously demarcating or examining ordinal zones of ranked marker-test categories. Nevertheless, a different approach, which uses *no* specific mathematical strategy, may often best represent the way in which many clinicians would interpret the data in Table 21.4.

Clinicians usually want to separate three diagnostic zones for a marker test.[11] In one extreme zone, the disease should almost always be present and, at the other extreme, the disease should almost always be absent. In the middle zone, the marker-test result will be too uncertain, and additional data (or tests) will be needed for diagnostic confidence. For this type of trichotomous clinical partition, the data of Table 21.4 would be divided as shown in Table 21.6. Coronary disease is particularly likely to be present for S-T segment depressions in the upper zone of Table 21.6, and absent in the lower zone. In the middle zone, the results are too "iffy" for diagnostic decisions, and a more confident diagnosis would require further information.

TABLE 21.6

Trichotomous Clinical Summary of Results in Table 21.4

ST Segment Depression	Number of Cases	Controls	Diagnostic Probability of Disease	Positive Likelihood Ratio	Negative Likelihood Ratio
≥ 2.5 mm.	46	0	1.00	∞	0
≥ 0.5 mm. but < 2.5 mm.	101	97	.51	1.04	.96
< 0.5 mm.	3	53	.054	.057	17.5
TOTAL	150	150	.5	1	1

The simple trichotomous approach is particularly easy, effective, and commonly used by clinicians. The approach requires almost no mathematical adjuncts or calculations. Its main disadvantage is that clinical "common sense" may not be cherished or useful for obtaining grants and writing publishable papers.

21.4 Stability of Indexes

Regardless of whether the diagnostic indexes come from direct, Bayesian, ROC, likelihood-ratio, or even "clinical judgment" methods, the indexes can be quantitatively unstable if derived from small numerical components. Their stability can be appraised with the same confidence-interval methods used for proportions and for ratios. If a sensitivity or specificity value is derived from a proportion such as $p = r/n$, a 95% confidence interval can be determined from an appropriately chosen binominal distribution or from the Gaussian calculation of $p \pm 1.96 \sqrt{pq/n}$, where $q = 1 - p$.

Being derived as a ratio of two proportions, likelihood ratios require more complex methods. In any selected zone, the 95% confidence interval for the likelihood ratio can be calculated, according to Simel et al.[18], as

$$\exp[\ln(p_1/p_2) \pm 1.96 \sqrt{(q_1/p_1 n_1) + (q_2/p_2 n_2)}]. \qquad [21.16]$$

The "exp" symbol in this formula is a typographically easy way of writing "e to the power of"; for example, exp (w) is e^w. The value of p_1 is the analog of sensitivity, formed in a particular row by the proportion of (positive results in cases)/(total no. of cases), with $q_1 = 1 - p_1$; and p_2 is the analog of $1 -$ specificity formed by the proportion of (positive results in controls)/(total no. of controls), with $q_2 = 1 - p_2$. According to the symbols developed at the beginning of Section 21.3.3, each $p_1 = t_i/T$ and each $p_2 = s_i/S$.

Confidence intervals are useful not only for indicating the possible "range" of the sensitivity/specificity and likelihood-ratio indexes, but also for considering weak numerical strength as an explanation for situations in which a marker test did not yield the expected high values of efficacy.

A recent proposal[19] that chance corrections be applied to indexes of diagnostic efficacy, analogous to the kappa coefficient used for indexes of agreement, does not yet seem to have evoked suitable evaluations.

21.5 Combinatory and Multivariable Methods

In all the discussion so far, the marker result came from a single diagnostic test. Sometimes, however, the marker can come from a combination of multiple tests or variables.

21.5.1   Simultaneous Tests

Because a single marker test may not be adequate, several marker tests can be combined simultaneously or ordered in a sequence that is prompted by results of previous tests. For example, a composite "dipstick" marker for urinary tract infection may contain two tests, not one. The efficacy of the dipstick marker can then be evaluated for positive results either in both component tests or in only one of the two.

21.5.2   Sequential Tests

A "battery" of tests is often ordered all at once to save time in hospitalized patients. In ambulatory situations, however, the same (or a smaller) set of marker tests may be ordered sequentially in an ad hoc manner. The sequential contribution of each test can be assessed from incremental changes in the likelihood ratios, posterior probabilities, or other indexes of diagnostic efficacy that existed before the additional results were obtained.

Despite the apparent efficacy when used alone, a particular individual test may have unimpressive incremental efficacy when added to other tests. For example, in a discussion of ECG-Tc 99m exercise tests after myocardial infarction, Staniloff et al.[20] and later Ladenheim et al.[21] decried "the incremental information boondoggle: when a test seems powerful but isn't." In analogous comments about the merit of electrophysiologic testing after myocardial infarction, Goldman[22] lamented the absence of proof for a "significant, incremental prognostic value."

21.5.3   Multivariable Analyses

The results of diverse accompanying variables (for demographic, clinical, co-morbid and other pertinent features) can be entered along with the results of the marker test in a multivariable analysis that develops a statistical model for estimating the probability of a particular disease in a particular person. This tactic eliminates all of the "bivariate" statistics devoted to sensitivity, specificity, ROC curves, and likelihood ratios.

Diverse mathematical methods can be used. The multiple variables can be combined with logistic regression,[23] with discriminant function analysis,[24] in a simple point score system formed from regression coefficients,[25] or in an algorithmic succession of categories.[26] The analytic methods can also incorporate[27] a "cost" or "regret" matrix that gives suitable weights to "partial" agreements or disagreements. Although the multivariable approaches have been enthusiastically advocated, their advantages have not yet been well documented.

21.6   Conformity in Laboratory Measurements

The conformity of tests in modern laboratories is commonly assessed with activities called *quality control*. Aimed at mensurational accuracy rather than diagnostic efficacy, the assessments are intended to find and repair disagreements when the same specimen is tested repeatedly in the same laboratory and when the laboratory's results are compared with those of a reference laboratory. For these appraisals of dimensional data, the results can be cited either for variability in agreement or for accuracy in comparison with a reference standard.

In a graphic plot of values for pairs of measurements, a rectilinear regression coefficient of 1 and an intercept of 0 (denoting a straight line slope of 45°, passing through the origin of the graph), would indicate that the two methods on average produce the same result. This apparently excellent index can often be achieved, however, despite considerable disagreement in the individual pairs of measurements. An example was shown earlier in the appraisal of concordance for data set D in Figure 20.1. For this and other reasons noted in Chapter 20, regression coefficients or the Pearson correlation coefficient are *not* a good way to express agreement, but they still continue to be used.[28]

The best alternative index has not yet received a unanimous consensus, but the most commonly recommended method today is the examination of pairwise increments, as discussed in Section 20.7.1. Other procedures regarded as less desirable are checking the standard deviation of the residual error around the regression line[29] or calculating the intra-class correlation coefficient (ICC).

21.7 Spectral Markers

In contrast to a diagnostic marker, which separates a particular disease from all other medical entities of health or illness, a spectral marker usually indicates the status of persons within the spectrum of a particular disease or condition. Thus, a diagnostic marker would denote that a patient has (or does not have) cancer of the colon. A spectral marker would denote that the cancer is in Stage I (or some other stage). The distinction is shown in Figure 21.4.

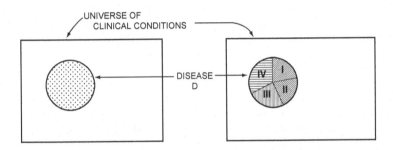

FIGURE 21.4
Diagnostic and spectral markers. In the figure on the left, a *diagnostic marker test* is intended to discriminate between disease D and all other conditions in the clinical universe. In the figure on the right, a *spectral marker test* is intended to discriminate among different portions (such as stages I, II, III, and IV) of the spectrum of disease D.

A spectral marker can be used for many clinical decisions — such as etiology, prognosis, choice of therapy, changes of therapy, or reassurance — other than diagnosis alone. For example, the estrogen receptor test has been used as a spectral marker in estimating prognosis and choosing therapy for patients with breast cancer. The carcinoembryonic antigen (CEA) test, which was introduced as a diagnostic marker for colon cancer, has now been relegated to being a spectral marker, denoting whether metastasis has occurred. In the "staging" role, a spectral marker can sometimes be used in post-therapeutic monitoring to denote transitions in clinical condition. Thus, after removal of a colon cancer, the CEA test may be repeatedly checked to determine whether the cancer has recurred.

In addition to roles in prognosis, therapeutic choices, and post-therapeutic monitoring for a particular disease, spectral markers can denote the "severity" of either a disease or a nonspecific clinical condition. For example, the APACHE index[30] contains a combination of laboratory tests used to indicate the severity of acute illness for patients in an emergency or intensive-care setting.

21.7.1 Use of Spectral Marker without "Gold Standard"

Just as a "gold standard" is used to evaluate the accuracy of a diagnostic marker, an analogous reference criterion can be used for a spectral marker. For example, if a CEA result indicates metastasis, the gold standard is anatomic evidence of the presence (or absence) of metastasis, obtained via imaging, biopsy, surgical inspection, or autopsy. If a laboratory test shows that a bacterium is sensitive to a particular antibiotic, the "gold standard" is (probably) the patient's post-therapeutic response to that antibiotic.

In many instances, however, a direct "gold standard" does not exist; and the spectral marker result becomes the main data used for a decision that must be evaluated some other way. This situation commonly arises when the results of a monitoring test (such as level of serum lithium or intra-ocular pressure) are used to change or adjust therapy; when a scan of the brain in a patient with stroke is used to assure the patient, family, or physician that a surgically remediable lesion is absent; or when indexes of "severity" are proposed for diverse purposes.

21.7.2   Pre-Spective vs. Post-Spective Expressions

A common statistical problem in expressing results of spectral markers (and other variables) is the use of "backward" summaries for results that have "forward" implications. Suppose serum bilirubin levels on admission to the hospital are examined as possible predictors of hepatic encephalopathy. Using a case-control approach, the investigators assemble a case group, whose members have developed encephalopathy, and a control group, whose members have not. The bilirubin levels in the two groups are then summarized, perhaps as means and standard deviations, and then compared. If the results show a significantly higher average level in the encephalopathy group, the investigators may conclude that an elevated bilirubin predisposes to encephalopathy. This conclusion may be correct, but is useless for future application, because it offers no "predictive" information about levels of risk. The results were cited "post-spectively" as baseline values per outcome events, rather than "pre-spectively" as outcome events per baseline values. In a pre-spective citation, the billirubin values would be demarcated into levels such as 0–1.9, 2.0 – 3.9, and ≥ 4.0. A rate of occurrence for encephalopathy might then be cited for each level, with expressions such as 0/100, 1/35, and 4/15.

Investigators may be reluctant to use these citations mainly because they require establishing levels of demarcation—a more difficult task than simply calculating the "post-spective" means and standard deviations. An additional problem is that the rates of occurrence, being obtained from case-control rather than cohort data, do not represent correct values of risk. Nevertheless, such demarcations are regularly used to obtain "dose-response" patterns in case-control data; and odds ratios can be used to avoid the connotation of risks.

The main point is that a "post-spective" citation of summaries for baseline data in the outcome groups does not allow the results to be used in predicting outcomes. For such predictions, the data must be cited "pre-spectively" as outcomes per level of baseline data, not in the reverse manner. This abuse of temporal direction frequently occurs, however.

21.7.3   Problems in Evaluation

The evaluation of spectral markers is a complex challenge that has not yet been fully mastered. The main problem is the delineation of what is being "marked" by the spectral marker. If the CEA test denotes the presence or extensiveness of metastases, its efficacy can be directly checked for that role. If results of upper gastrointestinal endoscopy are used as a marker that affects therapeutic rather than purely diagnostic decisions, the results can be evaluated[31] for the changes they produce in previous plans of treatment. If a clinical staging system is used for prognostic predictions, the results can be checked for the associated gradient in outcomes such as survival rates.

If the test is a marker of severity, however, the results cannot be evaluated without a clear definition of what is meant by *severity*. Does it refer to the amount of medical and nursing care needed for an acute illness, to the anticipated length of stay in an intensive care unit, to the patient's functional limitations, to the costs of care, or to other "gold standards" such as anticipated length of life, "activity" of an inflammatory disease, size of the heart, or size of a myocardial infarction?

Because clinicians have not yet clearly demarcated both the phenomena to be evaluated and the methods of evaluation, the appraisal of spectral markers is currently in a primordial state, awaiting better research ideas and strategies. The clinical inertia in developing strategy for the evaluation process has often led to methods that lack clinical sophistication. For example, many clinicians do not like the APACHE index of acute severity because it seems to be an arbitrary mathematical pastiche of multiple laboratory variables, having no clearly defined pathophysiologic connotations and excluding the subtle effects of co-morbid conditions. Yet these clinicians have not constructed or offered anything better. The DRG (diagnosis-related-group) system of demarcating categories of illness is perhaps the best illustration of the hazards that occur when clinical investigators avoid the scientific challenge of evaluations that can improve efficiency and reduce costs. Few clinicians would approve the way that the DRG "marker" system was constructed[32,33] — but it has become widely disseminated because of the principle of *faute de mieux* (lack of anything better), and because of its sponsorship by third-party payers of health care.

21.8 Scientific Problems in Diagnostic Statistics

Despite all the statistical attention, the evaluation of diagnostic marker tests is beset with five major scientific problems that have often made the diagnostic statistics unsatisfactory either for individual patient-care decisions or for policy evaluations of informational technology. The problems are briefly summarized here because the scientific details and illustrations, which can be found in the cited references, are beyond the scope of a mainly statistical text.

21.8.1 Surrogate vs. Other Diagnostic Roles

In the main evaluations thus far, the result of the marker test was used directly to identify the disease as present or absent. The strategies used for these evaluations will seldom be applicable when a test has other diagnostic roles. The result of the test may act as a definitive gold standard (e.g., liver biopsy or glucose tolerance test), as multidiagnostic information pertinent for many diagnoses (e.g., chest X-ray, abdominal ultrasound), as a prerequisite diagnostic demand (e.g., demonstration of Group A streptococcal infection for rheumatic fever[34]), or as contributory evidence in which a diagnosis is made only when the test's result is combined with other types of data (e.g., enzymes plus ECG plus clinical history for acute myocardial infarction). A test's performance in each of these different roles will require indexes different from those that have been developed for surrogate efficacy alone.

21.8.2 Diagnostic Performance

Not all tests are ordered for the same type of diagnostic performance. A discovery test, used to "screen" persons with no symptoms or overt manifestations of disease,[35] has a job different from that of an exclusion (or "rule-out") test, which, when negative, assures that the disease is absent. Conversely, a confirmation (or "rule-in") test is used to give assurance that the disease is present. Examples of these three distinctions are urinary glucose in screening for diabetes mellitus, a negative echocardiogram to exclude significant cardiac tamponade, and urinary red blood casts to confirm nephronal inflammation. The demands for efficacy will differ with these different functions. A confirmation test needs high specificity, regardless of sensitivity; an exclusion test needs high sensitivity, regardless of specificity; and a discovery test needs both high sensitivity and high specificity to avoid too many false positive and false negative results.

Because of the horizontal-vertical converse reasoning, the nomenclature for these different performances often seems counter-intuitive. A *rule-in* test for the disease should have high specificity in the *nondiseased* group, and a *rule-out* test should have high sensitivity in the *diseased* group. Beyond these paradoxes in nomenclature, however, the different goals of diagnostic marker tests lead to several statistical paradoxes in evaluating performance.

Being usually invoked when suitable suspicion has been aroused by other evidence, the "rule-in" and "rule-out" procedures need not be splendid in both sensitivity and specificity. A discovery test, however — which may be frequently used because of its convenience — is desirable only if it is excellent in both attributes. If too insensitive, it will fail to discover enough cases, and if too nonspecific, it will yield too many false positives. Thus, the simple discovery test used for "general" screening should preferably have a better performance record than the exclusion and confirmation tests used in more "specialized" clinical circumstances.

Another problem in evaluating a test's performance is the choice of a *suitable* "gold standard." Should a fecal occult blood test be evaluated for its ability to detect blood or to detect colorectal cancer? The test may be excellent for identifying blood as an immediate target, but relatively poor for identifying cancer as an anatomic source. Similarly, a urine test for protein may be splendid for identifying protein, but less effective at demonstrating renal disease.

Finally, clinicians may create problems by failing to distinguish between the existence of a disease and its causal role in producing a particular manifestation. Because many diseases can exist "silently," without provoking symptoms or other manifestations,[35] the demonstration of a particular diagnosis may identify the disease without supplying an appropriate pathophysiologic explanation for the patient's overt clinical problems. For example, a patient's angiogram may show major coronary disease despite a history that is negative for angina pectoris and positive for postprandial pain relieved by antacid. In this instance, the existence of the coronary disease does not offer a pathophysiologic explanation for the pain.

When clinicians do not distinguish between existence and explanation, certain diagnostic tests may lead to unnecessary therapy. For example, because the classical symptoms of functional bowel distress are not explained if "silent" gallstones are found on an abdominal ultrasound examination, the removal of the stones would not be expected to offer enduring relief for the symptoms.

21.8.3   Spectral Composition

The fundamental but often unrecognized problem in all of the case-control statistical indexes and mathematical transformations is that they rest on an erroneous assumption of constancy.[36] They assume that sensitivity and specificity, or likelihood ratios, remain the same for any cases of disease and for any control group without disease. This assumption has turned out to be wrong, because the values of the indexes will differ according to demographic, clinical, and/or co-morbid distinctions in the spectrums of patients who constitute the cases and controls.[36–40]

Consequently, the indexes calculated for diagnostic accuracy will vary not just with prevalence but with the spectral composition of the subgroups of patients who receive the test. This unfortunate fact of clinical reality essentially vitiates all of the splendid mathematical theory that has been developed for diagnostic marker analyses. The best approach, as practicing clinicians have already discovered,[10] is to determine diagnostic accuracy for the pertinent collection of patients seen in a particular clinical practice.

The magnitude of this problem in a fixed index of efficacy was quantified by Lachs et al.[39] for a composite dipstick marker test used to diagnose urinary tract infection. Among patients with a "high" prior probability of infection — i.e., those with pertinent suspicious symptoms or other clinical manifestations — the dipstick test had sensitivity 0.92 and specificity 0.42. Among patients with a "low" prior probability — i.e., those who lacked the cited clinical manifestations — the sensitivity and specificity varied directly with the degree of pyuria. For three ordinal groups having 0, 1–5, and >5 leukocytes per microscopic field of spun urine, sensitivity rose progressively from 0.50 to 0.68 to 1.00 and specificity declined progressively from 0.90 to 0.68 to 0.22.

21.8.4   Bias in Data and Groups

Regardless of whether the appraisals are done "vertically" or "horizontally," the results can be biased by problems in the raw data or in the composition of groups. Because the marker test and the gold standard procedure occur in a sequence, the raw data for the results will not be objective if the interpreter of whichever procedure came second is aware of what was found previously. To avoid this type of review bias, the second procedure should always be examined blindly, without the reviewer knowing the previous results.

In composition of groups, the patients chosen to receive the gold-standard test may not equally represent the spectral composition of all possible candidates. The results of *spectrum bias* in these choices may then produce indexes distorted by group imbalances that are diversely called[36,39–42] *work-up, verification,* or *referral bias.*

In ordinary clinical practice, the definitive test may not be ordered for everyone if it seems too costly or possibly hazardous. Accordingly, when diagnostic markers are evaluated from tests done in ordinary clinical circumstances, a definitive result may not be available for many patients, particularly those who had a negative marker test. In this situation, the best way to avoid "workup" (or "spectrum") bias is to get surrogate information for the patient's definitive status. For example, a definitive diagnostic biopsy is almost always done for patients with a "positive" mammogram, but not for those with a "negative" result. Therefore, in a study of mammographic diagnoses, Elmore et al.[43] restricted the eligible "negative" patients to those who had had at least three years of follow-up without evidence of cancer and who had another negative mammogram three years later. A simple long-term follow-up showing absence of the suspected disease may sometimes suffice as a suitable "reference standard,"[44] without repeating the original marker test.

Yet another problem is the *incorporation bias* that arises when the result of a marker test is incorporated into the evidence used for the definitive diagnostic conclusion.[36] For example, if a serum amylase result is used to make definitive diagnostic decisions about acute pancreatitis, the amylase test is no longer merely a marker. It becomes part of prerequisite evidence and should not be checked for sensitivity and specificity.

21.8.5 Reproducibility

A separate but often overlooked problem refers to issues in reproducibility rather than accuracy. Variability can occur whenever the result or interpretation of a test requires human observation and communication. Nevertheless, checks of intra-personal and inter-personal variability are seldom done for the obviously subjective work of radiologists, histopathologists, and cytopathologists, and also for the less obviously subjective laboratory observations used for such examinations as flocculation, dark fields, and white blood cell differential counts.[45]

Unless basic reproducibility has been demonstrated, all the subsequent calculations may sometimes resemble an exercise in futility. The indexes of efficacy will have been determined for data whose fundamental reliability is uncertain.

21.9 Additional Challenges

Many additional major challenges, not yet discussed, are prominently available for thoughtful research in an era of proliferating technology, escalating costs, and increasing complaints about "dehumanized" clinical care.

21.9.1 Diagnostic Evaluations and Guidelines

Despite various recommendations for the contents and phases of evaluation, most diagnostic marker tests still come into widespread clinical usage before they have been adequately evaluated. Reid et al.[46] have recently shown that the proportion of satisfactory evaluations is rising with time but is still not good. Of 34 marker-test appraisals reported in four leading general medical journals during 1990–1993, more than 50% failed to meet at least 3 of 6 methodologic standards and only 6% complied with all 6 standards.

In view of these basic scientific defects, many clinicians are surprised or appalled[47,48] when "guidelines" for using the tests[49–52] are issued by prominent clinical organizations. The organizations may hope to do a "preemptive strike," offering better guidelines than what might otherwise be promulgated by governmental or corporate agencies, but a more fundamental approach would be to convince the public and policy makers that suitable guidelines cannot be constructed because the necessary fundamental research is absent. Arrangements can then be made to carry out the appropriate research.

21.9.2 Non-Diagnostic Roles

As noted earlier, many technologic tests have a critically important role in non-diagnostic decisions, such as estimating prognosis or choosing or monitoring therapy. For example, laboratory tests of an infectious organism's "sensitivity" are done to select appropriate antibiotics, and tests of blood (or sometimes urine) levels may be used to monitor treatment with psychotropic or other chemical agents. An MRI scan of lumbar vertebrae may be intended not to diagnose a herniated disc, but to decide therapeutically whether more than one disc must be treated. The availability of various imagings for neoplastic involvement of abdominal (and other) lymph nodes has replaced the surgical explorations that were formerly done as "staging" for choosing treatment of Hodgkin's or other lymphomatous disease.

These often invaluable clinical contributions of technologic information are neglected in statistical indexes aimed at only diagnostic performance. Consequently, to offer satisfactory appraisal for the total merit of a technologic procedure, new statistical indexes must be developed to account for *all* of a test's contributions to diverse clinical decisions, not just diagnosis alone.

21.9.3 Appraising Reassurance

An important but often neglected merit of technologic tests is the reassurance they bring to clinicians, patients, and patients' families. For example, in most patients with a classical "cerebrovascular accident," the CT or magnetic resonance imaging (MRI) scan of the head seldom alters the main diagnosis, the estimated prognosis, or the therapeutic plans that would have been made without the scan. Nevertheless, by demonstrating that the patient does not have a surgically remediable lesion — such as a meningioma or subdural hematoma — the imaging provides a relatively risk-free form of important reassurance. In the era before the new images, this reassurance required the horrors of pneumoencephalography or the hazards of carotid arteriography.

Many older clinicians would have given the CT scan a Nobel prize for its role merely in providing risk-free reassurance that a stroke is a stroke. Yet the immense human importance of this reassurance is not currently appraised, or even "valued" enough to be regarded as warranting appraisal.

21.9.4 Automated Observations

The automated observation of images has been successfully applied for diagnosing a single state in an electrocardiogram, and is now being used for differential leukocyte counts[53] and for ocular perimetry.[54] Efforts[55] are now in progress to develop automated image analysis in mammography, lung cancer, cervical cytology, and fine needle aspirates of the breast.

Some of the main statistical challenges in the automated-observation process are to choose both a suitable gold standard for the validation and suitable methods of identifying the image. For example, who is the person to be used as "gold standard" for interpreting a leukocyte differential smear or a mammogram? Should the recognition process be aimed at a direct recapitulation of the image or at a transformed attribute? Thus, in differentiating leukocytes, the automated entity is a histogram of light intensities in a grid that covers each cell, not a direct visual "portrait" of the cell.

21.9.5 "DNA" Diagnostic Markers

In the era of molecular biology, many genetic, oncologic, and other diagnoses are explored with markers that use DNA probes or polymorphism analysis.[56-58] Bogardus et al.[59] have recently discussed the striking methodologic flaws in many of these studies, including absence of objectivity, failure to check for test reproducibility, and an unsuitable spectrum of case and/or control groups. Better methods might be demanded sooner rather than later to avoid the devastating human and scientific effects of false positive results for genetic "risk" and of erroneous directions in genetic research.

21.9.6 Neural Networks

A technique still in its infancy does multivariable diagnostic analysis with the special pattern recognition methods of a neural network, rather than with mathematical procedures such as logistic regression. An impressive set of results has been reported[60] for efficacy of neural-network analysis in diagnosing myocardial infarction among adults presenting to a hospital emergency department; and further work is now in progress. To be scientifically acceptable, however, the neural-network results will require careful validation in "external" challenge groups. Most of the work reported thus far has been validated only "internally," in the same group from which the neural-network model was constructed. The credibility of these analytic models will depend on how well they perform when exposed to the challenge of new "unknown" groups, and how well they can identify the most cogent variables.

21.9.7 Constructing "Silver Standards"

When not available or possible, a "gold standard" diagnosis can be obtained by noting the patient's eventual outcome or by using an authoritative diagnosis made *without* the marker result. In the absence of these methods for getting a "gold standard," a new statistical strategy has been proposed[61] to determine efficacy from repeated observations of the marker test. Because "gold standard" results will inevitably be absent for many test procedures, the construction of a suitable alternative "silver standard" (to substitute for the "gold") is an intriguing challenge.

References

1. Birkelo, 1947; 2. Yerushalmy, 1947; 3. McNeil, 1975; 4. Wulff, 1981; 5. Sackett, 1991; 6. Moller-Petersen, 1985; 7. Jaeschke, 1994; 8. Finney, 1993; 9. Kempthorne, 1975; 10. Reid, 1998; 11. Feinstein, 1990a; 12. Metz, 1973; 13. Weinstein, 1980; 14. Diamond, 1981; 15. Steen, 1993; 16. Feinstein, 1996; 17. Eisenberg, 1984; 18. Simel, 1993; 19. Brenner, 1994; 20. Staniloff, 1982; 21. Ladenheim, 1987; 22. Goldman, 1991; 23. Coughlin, 1992; 24. Lachin, 1973; 25. Mann, 1983; 26. Brand, 1982; 27. Kodlin, 1971; 28. Barnett, 1979; 29. Cornbleet, 1978; 30. Knaus, 1991; 31. Lichtenstein, 1980; 32. Thompson, 1975; 33. Fetter, 1980; 34. Special Writing Group, 1993; 35. Feinstein, 1967a; 36. Ransohoff, 1978; 37. Rozanski, 1983; 38. Hlatky, 1984; 39. Lachs, 1992; 40. Feinstein, 1985; 41. Begg, 1991; 42. Knottnerus, 1992; 43. Elmore, 1994b; 44. Hull, 1983; 45. Elmore, 1992; 46. Reid, 1995; 47. Jenkins, 1991; 48. Brook, 1989; 49. Griner, 1981; 50. Sox, 1987; 51. Eddy, 1990; 52. Hospital Association of New York State, 1989; 53. Rosvoll, 1979; 54. Katz, 1988; 55. Cancer Letters, 1994; 56. Wiggs, 1988; 57. Malkin, 1990; 58. Lemna, 1990; 59. Bogardus, 1999; 60. Baxt, 1991; 61. Schulzer, 1991.

Exercises

21.1. About 4% of school-aged children in Megalopolis are believed to be physically abused by their parents. The schools in the city might be able to screen all children for evidence of abuse (e.g., scars, cuts, bruises, and burns), with the intent of follow-up by contacting the suspected parents. School and health officials must be very confident of their suspicions before approaching the parents, however, because a great deal of potential harm can be done either by letting an abused child go undetected or by erroneously suspecting an innocent parent. According to school health officials, the physical examination they use is very reliable: it gives positive results in 96% of abused children, and false positive results in only 8% of nonabused children.

    a.   What is the nosologic sensitivity of the physical examination?

    b.   What is the nosologic specificity of the physical examination?

    c.   If the screening program is implemented in Megalopolis schools, what will be the physical examination's diagnostic sensitivity, i.e., positive predictive accuracy?

21.2. Your hospital has recently acquired a new non-invasive radiologic test to detect deep venous thrombi (DVT). The manufacturer reports impressive test performance data: nosologic sensitivity, 96%; and nosologic specificity, 98%. To evaluate the accuracy of the new test in your hospital, the radiology department invites the first 100 patients suspected of having DVT and evaluated by the new test to receive additional "gold-standard" testing with a lower extremity venogram. This evaluation yields a nosologic sensitivity of 52%, and a specificity of 65%. Cite and briefly discuss at least four possible reasons for the reduction in test performance.

21.3. A new diagnostic test for omphalosis has +LR 10.0, with 95% CI 5.0–20.0. You are seeing a patient whom you suspect of having omphalosis, with a pretest probability ranging from 2 to 20%. Using the nomogram and cited probabilities in Figure E.21.3, indicate the appropriate posttest probabilities. Do you regard this test as diagnostically useful? Please give brief reasons for whatever answer you choose.

21.4. A new outpatient test for rapid detection of group A beta-hemolytic strepococci has a reported nosologic sensitivity of 88%. The fine print accompanying the test instructions, however, has the following statement: "95% CI 76–100%." Given this information, how many patients do you think were initially tested by the manufacturer?

21.5. One stated advantage of calculating likelihood ratios, as opposed to predictive accuracies, is that likelihood ratios do not depend on group prevalence. Explain why this advantage occurs.

21.6. Many prominent textbooks and publications have urged that diagnostic evaluations be done with likelihood ratios and/or the conditional probability methods that use sensitivity, specificity, and prevalence to determine rates of "predictive accuracy." Do you use this approach? If so, please cite and briefly discuss at least three advantages that you have found with it. If you do not use this approach, what are at least three disadvantages that you have noted? What alternative approach do you use or advocate?

21.7. From your clinical background or experience, give an example of a diagnostic marker (not previously cited in the text) that is used mainly as a "rule-in" test and another used as a "rule-out" test. Briefly discuss the reasons that justify the use of each test for the cited purpose.

21.8. From the literature at your disposal, select a study of a diagnostic marker test, and in one or two sentences, outline its basic arrangement. Comment on the selection of case and control groups. If you do not fully approve of the selections, what alternatives would you suggest? Make any other critical comments or architectural suggestions that occur during your review of the study.

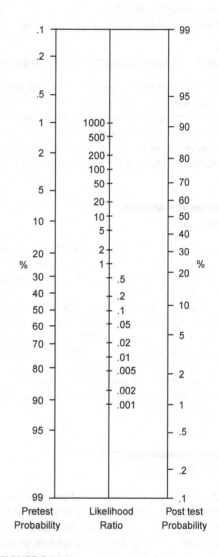

FIGURE E.21.3
Nomogram showing relationship of pretest probability and likelihood ratio to form posttest probability. [Taken from Chapter Reference 57.]

21.9. Find a set of diagnostic criteria for any disease in which you are interested. If the criteria were tested for their diagnostic efficacy, comment on how well the test was done. If the criteria have not been tested, outline the procedure you would suggest for this purpose.

21.10. What ideas do you have about how to evaluate (and quantify) reassurance?

22

Survival and Longitudinal Analysis

CONTENTS

When free-living people are members of a cohort under long-term observation, a baseline "zero-time" status can be identified for each person, but special problems and challenges can arise thereafter. The final outcome may be unknown for members of the cohort who "drop out" or become "lost to follow-up." The intermediate events may be unknown or difficult to interpret for persons who continue to participate in the study, but who make unauthorized changes in the assigned plans or fail to appear for scheduled examinations.

For events that are either unknown or occur under inappropriate circumstances or timing, the statistical analyses cannot be suitably managed with a regression equation that merely has outcome as one variable and time as the other. In other situations, where the follow-up period is aimed not at a single "survival" event, such as death, but at a series of events or changes, the analysis of repeated or multiple outcomes is also not amenable to any of the statistical structures discussed thus far in the text.

This chapter is devoted to methods of serial analysis that have been developed to cope with these challenges. The chapter begins and is mainly concerned with a method called *survival analysis*, which is also known as *life-table* or *actuarial analysis*. Used when each person is followed until the occurrence of a single "failure event," such as death, which concludes the person's period of observation "at risk," the analysis produces the survival curves that commonly illustrate clinical trials and cohort studies. The main discussion of survival analysis is followed by brief accounts of two additional applications: measuring *life expectancy* and evaluating certain *age-period cohort* effects in a general population. The chapter concludes with an outline of another cohort procedure, called *longitudinal analysis*, that is devoted to repeatedly measured serial outcomes, which can be either recurrences of a binary event, such as episodes of streptococcal infection, asthma, or epilepsy, or changes in dimensional variables, such as blood pressure, serum cholesterol, or pulmonary function tests.

22.1 Differences between *Survival* and *Longitudinal Analysis*

Any form of cohort analysis can be regarded as "longitudinal," but the particular methods called *survival analysis* and *longitudinal analysis* collect and analyze the information with different approaches. In a conventional *survival analysis*, each person's outcome data contain a *single* pair of bivariate values: the duration of serial time until the person's exit date and the concomitant binary "exit state," which might be **dead** or **alive**. In a *longitudinal analysis*, each patient's basic outcome data contain *multiple* pairs of bivariate values for the timing and concomitant value of each measurement.

Both the survival and the longitudinal procedures use bivariate temporal data for each cohort, but the bivariate relationship can become trivariate when an additional variable allows results to be compared for two or more cohort groups, such as recipients of Treatment A or B or patients in Stages I, II, and III of a particular disease. The analytic methods can become multivariate when data for additional conditions, such as age and baseline clinical severity, are used to "adjust" the bivariate or trivariate results.

[Note to readers: This long chapter covers the extensive scope of the topic, but the main parts to learn are survival analysis (in Sections 22.2 through 22.5) and life expectancy (Section 22.6). If you are tired by the time you reach Section 22.7, you can go through the rest of the chapter quickly, and need not struggle with the details. — ARF]

22.2 Construction of Survival Summaries

Survival analysis is concerned with an event that concludes the person's period of time "at risk." In the following discussion, the "event" will be a "failure," i.e., death, but the analytic methods are equally pertinent and applicable for other types of concluding events, such as development of a myocardial infarction, stroke, unwanted pregnancy, or even a desired pregnancy.

If time to death were known for each person, the cohort's results could easily be summarized as a mean survival time. When most studies are ended, however, some members of the cohort may still be alive. Their unknown duration of survival will preclude calculation of an accurate mean for the group. (If the unknown durations are omitted for still-alive persons, the mean survival time for the group will be too low.)

This problem can often be avoided, as noted earlier in Section 3.6.4, by summarizing results with a median survival time. It has the double advantage of being easily determined in most groups despite unknown durations for the still-alive persons, while also avoiding distortions of the mean by outlier members with particularly short or long survivals. In fact, as noted later, the median survival time is probably the best *simple* descriptive index for the results.

Nevertheless, neither the mean nor the median would show dynamic features of the survival curve, and neither index would permit effective predictions. If the median survival is 2.3 years, we can predict that 50% of the cohort will be alive at 2.3 years, but we would not know what the survival rates might be at serial times such as 6 months, 1 year, 3 years, or 5 years.

If survival time were known for everyone except those still alive at the end of the study, a summary survival curve could easily be constructed, as shown earlier in Figure 18.5 for the data in Figure 18.4, to depict the proportion of persons alive at each successive time interval. The choice of a suitable "parametric" algebraic expression for these curves has enriched statistical literature with the names of mathematical models called *gamma*, *lognormal*, *Weibull*, *Rayleigh*, and *Pareto* distributions.

A simpler algebraic model is possible, however, if the survival-curve pattern resembles the type of exponential decay that occurs for radioactivity. In this frequent situation, the data can often be fitted with a descending exponential expression, $Y = e^{-ct}$, in which t = time, Y = the corresponding survival proportion (which is 1 at $t = 0$), and c is a constant appropriate for each curve. This expression can promptly be logarithmically transformed into a straight-line model, $\ln Y = -ct$.

The summary expression for Y at each time point, however, is a proportion constructed as $(n - d)/n$, where n is the number of pertinent people at risk and d is the number of persons who have died at or before the cited time. Because the original denominator, n, is always known, this proportion could easily be determined if the numerator status were also known as dead or alive at each time point for each person. Unfortunately, in the realities of human follow-up studies, this status may not always be known; and even if known, the person's condition may not always be easily classified in the simple dichotomy of dead/alive. This difficulty creates the problem of numerator losses — the prime challenge in survival analysis for medical phenomena.

22.2.1 Sources of Numerator Losses

Everyone is known to be alive when the cohort is assembled at each person's zero-state baseline. The cohort is then followed thereafter until a selected "closing" duration, T, which might be five years of serial follow-up for each patient. If a relevant death occurs before time T, the status of the patient is always known for each time point thereafter. If a relevant death has not occurred before time T, however, problems are created by patients who have not been followed for as long as T. Such patients are called *censored*; and the censoring can arise from three (or four) mechanisms.

22.2.1.1 *Insufficient Duration* — In most cohort studies and clinical trials, the group is assembled by accrual during a period of calendar time, rather than being collected and entered into the study all at once on the same day. The research will therefore take much longer in calendar time than the shorter duration, T, that is usually chosen for the maximum length of each patient's serial observation.

For example, suppose a particular study began on January 1, 1993 and ended on December 31, 1999. If T was set at 5 years, everyone who entered the study before January 1, 1995 had a chance to be followed for five years when the study ended; but someone who entered on July 1, 1997 was followed for only 2 1/2 years. If still alive on December 31, 1999, the latter person would have been censored at a follow-up duration of 30 months. In this type of "terminal censoring," the ultimate status of the patient, who is still alive and under observation when the study closes, might easily be determined if the calendar time of the study were extended.

22.2.1.2 *Intermediate Lost-to-Follow-Up* — A more substantial problem is created by intermediate rather than terminal censoring. Intermediate censoring occurs when patients are last seen or

known to be alive at a serial time before T, but are then "lost" or "dropped out" with nothing known of their status thereafter. Such intermediate lost-to-follow-up patients are censored (and called "withdrawn alive") as of the last date on which they were known to be alive.

22.2.1.3   Withdrawn by "Competing Risk" — If any kind of death is the failure event, the problem of a "relevant" death need not be considered. In many cohort studies, however, the failure event is death due to a specific disease. For example, in the follow-up of patients treated for cancer of the breast, the relevant deaths under analysis are usually those ascribed to cancer of the breast. If someone dies of an apparently unrelated myocardial infarction or automobile accident, the death is regarded as part of the "competing risk" of an incidental, non-relevant event. Such patients are censored at the date of death and are also regarded as "withdrawn alive."

22.2.1.4   Altered Therapy — A formidable problem in many randomized clinical trials is what to do about patients who abandon the originally assigned treatment, who may continue it in a poorly maintained schedule, or who may even transfer to the competing opposite therapy. For example, in a trial of medical vs. surgical treatment, some of the patients originally assigned to the medical therapy may later decide to have surgery. In a trial of an active vs. placebo pharmaceutical agent, some of the patients assigned to the active drug may comply so ineffectively that they essentially become an untreated counterpart of the placebo group. A further problem in any trial is the unauthorized use of additional treatment that may affect or obscure the actions of the main assigned agent(s). For example, if antibiotics A and B are being compared for their prophylactic ability to prevent a particular infection, the results may be distorted by patients who also take antibiotic C incidentally for some other reason.

The solution to the altered-therapy problem is controversial. In one popular statistical approach, called "intent-to-treat" (ITT) analysis, any therapeutic changes or supplements are ignored, and everyone is counted as though he or she had received the initially assigned treatment, in the exact regimen or schedule in which it was assigned. The main argument for this approach is that it is statistically "unbiased": the original therapeutic classification is not affected by anything that happened after the initial "sanctifying" randomization. Consequently, the ITT approach makes no adjustments for altered therapy.

The counter-argument is that the ITT approach, although perhaps statistically unbiased, is scientifically improper. With scientific common sense, someone would not be counted as having received surgical treatment if the surgery was not done, nor would patients be counted as having received only medical therapy, if they later had the operation.

Because the ITT controversy has not yet been resolved, a possibly acceptable compromise is to withdraw the patient as censored when the major therapeutic alteration began. This type of withdrawal, if used, becomes a fourth mechanism for censoring.

22.2.2   Adjustment of Denominators

Although patients who have died can be "followed" thereafter for any selected duration of time, the original size of the cohort is progressively reduced when patients are withdrawn as censored. Therefore, the calculated summary expressions at each time point should reflect the smaller numbers of people for whom suitable data are available. This problem — the need to change denominators sequentially after censored losses in the numerators — cannot be readily managed by parametric algebraic models. Accordingly, survival summaries are usually constructed with "non-parametric" methods that do not have an algebraic format and that fit the data in an ad hoc manner. For the post-censoring adjustments, the denominators of the remaining cohort can be decremented by two main mechanisms: a direct or an interval method; and the intervals can have a fixed or varying duration.

22.2.2.1   Arrangement of Data — In the ordinary arrangement of data, each person will have a calendar date for the time of randomization or some other event (such as date of diagnosis or admission) that acts as the zero time for calculating serial duration until the calendar date of exit. The exit state will be listed as the failure event (such as death) or one of the diverse sources of censoring. After the

serial durations are determined, the persons can be listed in ranked order according to the durations. An excerpt of such a list might show the following:

Rank	Duration (mos.)	Exit State
27	17	Dead
28	18	Censored (alive; lost to follow-up)
29	18	Dead
30	19	Dead
31	23	Censored (died in automobile accident)
32	24	Censored (alive; end of observation period)
33	25	Dead

Such a list is used in the two "interval" methods of calculation. For the "direct" type of calculation, however, another entry is needed to denote the maximum duration for which dead patients might have been followed during the calendar time of the study. For example, the patient ranked 29 in the foregoing list died at 18 months, but potentially might have been followed for 48 months, whereas patient 30, who died at 19 months, may have entered the study only two years before its end, so that the maximum survival duration would have been only 24 months.

22.2.2.2   *Direct Method* —

In the direct method of adjustment, the denominator should contain only those persons who could have been followed for the appropriate length of time. Thus, one-year survival rates are calculated only for those persons who could have been followed for at least a year; two-year rates are calculated only for persons who could have been followed for at least two years; and so on.

Persons who died are counted as dead in the interval when they died, and in all subsequent *eligible* intervals thereafter. For example, someone who entered the cohort 18 months ago and who died at 5.4 months of serial time would be eligible for being counted as dead in the 6-month and 1-year but not in the 2-year survival rates. Persons who were censored are counted in the denominators of only the pertinent eligible durations. Thus, someone who was censored at 6.3 months would not be counted in the denominator for the 1-year or 2-year survival rates, but could appear in a 6-month survival denominator. Persons who entered the study 12 months before it ends can be counted in all 6-month or 1-year survival rates, but are not eligible for inclusion in a rate for any subsequent duration, even if they died soon after admission.

If pertinent eligibility for being counted is ignored, substantial biases can be introduced. For example, the direct 2-year survival rates might include the dead but not the still-living members of a group eligible for only 1 year of follow-up.

Table 22.1 shows the way the data of a direct analysis might be summarized for 150 persons who entered a study that lasted for three years, with 50 persons accrued at the beginning of each annual interval. The first row shows the annual occurrence of deaths and losses in the 50 persons who could have been followed for three years. The next two rows show analogous results for persons who could have been followed for only two years or for only one. The third line shows 43 patients remaining and terminally censored in the one-year group after 3 deaths and 4 intermediate losses. The second line shows 39 patients remaining in the second-year group after a total of 5 deaths and 6 intermediate losses during the two-year period.

Table 22.2 shows the direct arrangement of survival for the 150 persons cited in Table 22.1. All 150 persons were potentially eligible for 1-year survival calculations, but the 6 persons lost to follow-up during that year are removed from the denominator. The mortality rate at one year is thus calculated as $9/144 = .0625$. Only 100 persons are potentially eligible for inclusion in 2-year survival rates, but 13 of them have become lost to follow-up (2 in the first year and 11 in the second). With 12 deaths ($= 3 + 3 + 4 + 2$) having occurred in the two-year period, the 2-year mortality is $12/87 = .1379$. Finally, among the 50 persons potentially eligible for 3-year survival calculations, 10 ($= 1 + 6 + 3$) have been lost and 9 ($= 3 + 4 + 2$) have died. The 3-year total mortality rate would be $9/40 = .2250$. The corresponding total survival rates at 1, 2, and 3 years respectively are thus .9375, .8621, and .7750. These results are reasonably close to those noted later with the interval methods.

TABLE 22.1

Summary of Data that Precede a Direct Survival Analysis for 150 Persons

Maximum Duration of Observation for Group	Size of Group	Number of Persons of This Group Who Died in:			Number of Persons Lost to Follow-up in:			Persons Censored at End of Maximum Observation
		1st year	2nd year	3rd year	1st year	2nd year	3rd year	
3 yrs.	50	3	4	2	1	6	3	31
2 yrs.	50	3	2	—	1	5	—	39
1 yr.	50	3	—	—	4	—	—	43

TABLE 22.2

Direct Arrangement of Survival Data for 150 Persons in Table 22.1

Maximum Duration	Number Potentially Eligible	Number of Potentially Eligibles Lost	Number Eligible	Total Deaths in Eligible Group	Mortality Rate	Survival Rate
1 yr.	150	6	144	9	.0625	.9375
2 yrs.	100	13	87	12	.1379	.8621
3 yrs.	50	10	40	9	.2250	.7750

An important point to bear in mind is that if the direct method is used without suitable attention to the "eligible death" group, the mortality rates will become excessively high after the first interval. For example, the group eligible for only 1 year in Table 22.1 had 3 deaths. If those 3 deaths are carried into the 2nd year calculation in Table 22.2, the mortality numerator becomes $12 + 3 = 15$ and the denominator would be $87 + 3 = 90$, so that the total mortality rate at 2 years would be raised to $15/90 = .1666$. The group eligible for only 2 years in Table 22.1 had 5 deaths in those two years. If those 5 deaths plus the other 3 deaths from the only 1-year eligible group were included for the 3rd-year calculation in Table 22.2, the total mortality numerator would be $9 + 8 = 17$ and the denominator would be $40 + 8 = 48$. The total mortality rate would rise to $17/48 = .3542$ and the corresponding survival rate, .6458, would be substantially lower than the correct value of .7750.

When properly calculated, the direct method is simple and obvious, and it has the scientific advantage of being straightforward and promptly understood. The survival rate at each time point indicates the exact number of persons who were eligible to be counted and classified at that point. The direct method, however, does not acknowledge the survival contributions of censored people to the interval in which they were censored. For example, persons who are censored at 23 months make no contribution to the 2-year survival rate, although they survived for 23/24ths of that period.

The direct results thus offer easy comprehension, but an underestimation of the dynamic survival rates. The latter problem could be substantially reduced by calculating the rates at frequent intervals, such as monthly rather than yearly, but a slight underestimate would still remain. Another disadvantage of the direct method is a paradox that can occur when the survival rate is relatively high in the few persons who have (or could have) been followed for the longest durations of time. In such situations, the direct 5-year survival rate may be higher than the corresponding rates at earlier time points.

Perhaps the main disadvantage that makes the direct method seldom used, however, is mathematical. Being calculated directly at each time point, the total survival rates lack the mathematical appeal of a series of interval survival rates, discussed in the next few sections, that are multiplied to form each total survival rate as a cumulative product.

22.2.2.3   *Actuarial (Fixed-Interval) Method* — Long before the outcome of clinical cohorts became a challenge in biostatistics, the actuaries of life insurance companies had developed a method,

called *life tables*, to manage survival analyses. The actuaries particularly wanted to know about life expectancy, so that their companies could set appropriately profitable "premiums" for the cost of policies sold to the public. The derivation of life expectancy from a life-table survival analysis is discussed later in Section 22.6. The analyses themselves, however, rely on constructing a cumulative product of fixed-interval survival rates.

In the latter process, the total observation period for the group is divided into a series of follow-up intervals, such as 0–1 year, 1–2 year, 2–3 year, etc. At the end of each interval, the numbers are catalogued according to persons who were "at risk" when the interval began. They then died or were censored during the interval, or they were alive and under follow-up when it ended. An interval mortality rate is calculated as the number who died divided by an appropriate denominator of those at risk during the interval. The interval mortality rate, which is called the *hazard* for the interval, is then converted to an *interval survival rate*. The final result, called the *cumulative survival rate*, is the product of all the component interval survival rates.

For example, suppose p_t represents the survival proportion for each interval. When the observations begin, everyone is alive and $p_0 = 1$. If p_1 is the interval survival at the end of the first interval, the cumulative survival is $S_1 = 1 \times p_1 = p_1$. At the end of the second interval, with p_2 as its survival proportion, the cumulative survival is $S_2 = S_1 \times p_2$. At the end of the fifth interval, $S_5 = S_4 \times p_5 = p_1 \times p_2 \times p_3 \times p_4 \times p_5$. This construction should be intuitively evident, but can be illustrated as follows:

In a cohort of 100 persons for whom the outcome is always known to be either alive or dead, suppose 10 die in the first interval, 13 in the second, and 24 in the third. The interval survival rates will be $(100 - 10)/100 = .900$ for the first interval, $(90 - 13)/90 = .856$ for the second interval, and $(77 - 24)/77 = .688$ for the third. The cumulative survival rate at the end of the third interval is the product of these three interval rates: $.900 \times .856 \times .688 = .530$. [The direct method of calculation yields the same result: 47 persons have died at the end of the third interval, and so total survival rate at that time is $(100 - 47)/100 = .530$.]

The tricky statistical decision in this approach is the choice of an appropriate denominator for those at risk during each interval. Everyone who died in an interval or who lived through it was at risk throughout the interval, but those who were intermediately censored were not at risk for the entire time. According to an arbitrary but customary convention, half the censored persons are assumed to have been at risk for the interval. (Alternatively phrased, if the interval is one-year long, each intermediately censored person is assumed to have been at risk for half a year. Thus, if 4 persons are censored respectively at 2, 5, 7, and 10 months after the one-year interval began, their total duration of observation in that interval is 24 months, which yields an average of 6 months, or 1/2 year, for each of the 4 persons).

With the actuarial approach for fixed-interval survival rates, the data in Tables 22.1 and 22.2 can be rearranged as shown in Table 22.3. The first line in Table 22.3 begins with all 150 patients, of whom 6 (= 4 + 1 + 1) were intermediately censored during the interval and 9 died. The denominator is adjusted only for the 6 lost patients, and it becomes $150 - (6/2) = 147$. The interval mortality rate is $9/147 = .0612$ and the corresponding survival rate is .9388. Because 43 patients of the "1-yr.-only" group were withdrawn at the end of the first interval, the second-year interval is begun by 92 persons (= $150 - 6 - 9 - 43$), of whom 11 are lost, and 6 die. The adjusted denominator is $92 - (11/2) = 86.5$; the interval mortality and survival rates are respectively $6/86.5 = .0694$ and .9306. The cumulative survival rate at the end of the second year is $.9388 \times .9306 = .8737$.

TABLE 22.3

Fixed-Interval Actuarial Arrangement of Survival Data for 150 Patients in Table 22.2

Interval	At Risk at Beginning of Interval	Lost or "Censored" During Interval	Withdrawn Alive at End of Interval	Died During Interval	Adjusted Denominator for Interval	Mortality Rate for Interval	Survival Rate for Interval	Cumulative Survival Rate
0–1 yr.	150	6	43	9	147.0	.0612	.9388	.9388
1–2 yr.	92	11	39	6	86.5	.0694	.9306	.8737
2–3 yr.	36	3	31	2	34.5	.0580	.9420	.8230

After the 39 remaining persons in the 2-year-only group are censored at the end of that interval, the third-year interval begins with 36 persons at risk, of whom 3 are intermediately censored and 2 die. The interval mortality rate is $2/[36 - (3/2)] = .0580$; and the interval survival rate of .9420 leads to a three-year cumulative survival rate of $.8737 \times .9420 = .8230$. Note that the cumulative survival rates with the actuarial method are only slightly higher than with the direct method for the same data. The differences in the two methods can sometimes be more substantial, however, as shown in Exercise 22.1.

In the actuarial method, each interval usually has the same duration, but sometimes the lengths can vary so that a few intervals might be one year, and others, 6 months long. Regardless of equality in durations, however, the temporal location of the intervals is usually fixed in advance, before the analysis begins. In medical activities, the fixed-interval approach is sometimes called the *Berkson-Gage method*,[1] commemorating the Mayo Clinic statisticians who introduced the actuarial or "life table" method into medical research. The Berkson-Gage eponym also serves to differentiate the fixed-interval method from the *Kaplan-Meier method*, discussed in Section 22.2.2.5, which uses intervals of varying length for the actuarial life-table procedure.

22.2.2.4   Hazard Functions

— Actuaries and demographers who specialize in analyzing the "forces of mortality" in a cohort use the term *hazard* for the interval mortality rates. For example, if a particular population has an annual mortality rate of .007, the hazard of death is .007 for that year.

For interval analyses, the hazard is the proportionate change in cumulative survival rate between any two intervals. Thus, if the cumulative survival rate is S_4 at interval 4 and S_3 at interval 3, the change is $(S_3 - S_4)/S_3$. Because $S_4 = p_4 S_3$, the hazard is $(S_3 - p_4 S_3)/S_3 = S_3(1 - p_4)/S_3 = 1 - p_4$, which is the interval mortality rate. Consequently, if n_3 people are followed for the third interval, and if d_3 persons die during that interval, the hazard is d_3/n_3.

In radioactive decay, the rate of decay at any moment is constantly proportional to the amount of radioactivity, Y, at that moment. The expression for the rate of radioactive decay over time is $dy/Y = -c$, which (if you remember the calculus) becomes converted to $\ln Y = -ct$, and $Y = e^{-ct}$. The value of c in this expression is the constant hazard, or the logarithmic rate of decay, over time.

With your consent to some more mathematics, we can note that if successive temporal values of the cumulative survival curve are denoted as S_t, the general formula for the type of change just discussed is $(S_t - S_{t-1})/S_{t-1}$. This expression (again recalling the calculus) is the time derivative of the natural logarithm of S_t. Thus, if S_t has an exponential format, $\ln S_t = -ct$. To make the latter expression positive, we can examine $-\ln S_t = ct$. If we then take the time derivative, we get $d(-\ln S_t) = c$, which is the value of the hazard.

In the realities of medical events, the survival curve seldom has a perfect exponential shape and the hazard is seldom fixed at a constant value. In customary nomenclature, however, S_t is called the *cumulative survival function*, $-\ln S_t$ is called the *cumulative hazard function*, and $d(-\ln S_t)$ is called the *hazard function*. The values of the *hazard function* at different time points are usually approximated by the interval mortality rate, $q_t = 1 - p_t$.

These ideas about hazards are not particularly important or necessary for the simple life tables under discussion in this chapter, but the concept becomes important in more advanced statistics, when a multivariable procedure, called *proportional hazards analysis* (or "Cox regression"), is used to evaluate the effect of different baseline covariate factors — such as age, stage, anemia — on survival curves. The concept of a hazard is also used in Section 22.4.5 to designate an index called the *hazard ratio*.

22.2.2.5   Variable-Interval Method

— The variable-interval life-table method was created as a result of some "matchmaking" by John Tukey.[2] Knowing about a common interest in time-to-failure events, he brought together workers in two different fields. The workers were Edward L. Kaplan, then at Bell Laboratories, who was studying the "survival" time of vacuum tubes, and Paul Meier, then a biostatistician at Johns Hopkins Medical School, who was interested in analyzing post-therapeutic human survival.

Kaplan and Meier were troubled by the arbitrary fixed-duration intervals and adjustments of the Berkson-Gage method and were especially worried about the effects in small samples. The alternative

Kaplan-Meier strategy[3] was to let the intervals be defined by the observed events: a new interval would be demarcated every time someone died. Anyone who was censored during one of those death-defined intervals would be simply eliminated from the denominator of that interval, as in the direct method of calculation discussed in Section 22.2.2.2. (Because no adjustments are made for a contribution to the interval, the contribution may not be missed if the deaths occur at small enough intervals. Problems can arise, however, when patients are censored during the long intervals that often appear near the right end of many survival curves.)

Because the events must be exactly timed in the Kaplan-Meier method, they cannot be grouped for fixed intervals as in Tables 22.2 or 22.3. Instead, the serial durations and corresponding exit states must be individually examined for each person. To illustrate these entities for the cohort of 150 people under scrutiny in Table 22.3, suppose the nine deaths in the first year occurred at 0.2, 0.3, 0.4, 0.4, 0.5, 0.5, 0.6, 0.7, and 0.9 years, and the six intermediate censorings at 0.3, 0.4, 0.6, 0.6, 0.7, and 0.9 years. To avoid analytic ambiguity, deaths and censorings cannot take place at exactly the same time. Accordingly, when a death and censoring seem to occur identically (as in many time points in this example), the death is assumed to have happened just before the censoring. The death thus terminates the interval, and the censoring is ascribed to the next interval. For example, for the death and censoring that both occurred at 0.3 yr, the death is counted in that interval; the censored person is removed from the denominator of the next interval.

For the remaining persons in Table 22.3, the deaths occurred at 1.1, 1.4, 1.5, 1.5, 1.6, 1.9, 2.3, and 2.8 years; and the intermediate censorings at 1.1, 1.1, 1.4, 1.4, 1.5, 1.5, 1.5, 1.9, 1.9, 1.9, 1.9, 2.3, 2.8, and 2.8 years. In addition, 43 persons of the 1-year-only group were terminally censored at 1.0 year, and 39 persons of the 2-year-only group were terminally censored at 2.0 years.

Table 22.4 shows an appropriate Kaplan-Meier life-table arrangement for the foregoing data. The first interval in Table 22.4 begins with a cumulative survival rate of 1.000 and ends with the death at 0.2 year. The death drops the interval survival rate to 149/150 = .9933; and so the second interval begins with a cumulative survival rate of $1.000 \times 0.9933 = 0.9933$. After the death that ends the second interval at 0.3 yr, the interval survival rate is 148/149 = .9933. The third interval thus begins with a cumulative survival rate of $.9933 \times .9933 = .9866$, and the denominator is reduced to 147 when decremented for the 1 censoring at 0.3 yr. With 2 deaths at 0.4 yr, the interval survival rate for the third interval is 145/147 = .9864, which makes the cumulative survival $.9866 \times .9864 = .9732$.

TABLE 22.4

Variable-Interval (Kaplan-Meier) Arrangement of Data in Table 22.3*

Number of Interval	Cumulative Survival Rate before Death(s)	Time of Death(s) That End(s) Interval	Number Alive before Death(s)	Number of Deaths	Number of Survivors	Interval Survival Rate	Censored before Next Death
1	1.000	0.2	150	1	149	.9933	0
2	.9933	0.3	149	1	148	.9933	1
3	.9866	0.4	147	2	145	.9864	1
4	.9732	0.5	144	2	142	.9861	0
5	.9597	0.6	142	1	141	.9930	2
6	.9529	0.7	139	1	138	.9928	1
7	.9461	0.9	137	1	136	.9927	44(= 1 + 43)
8	.9392	1.1	92	1	91	.9891	2
9	.9290	1.4	89	1	88	.9888	2
10	.9185	1.5	86	2	84	.9767	3
11	.8972	1.6	81	1	80	.9877	0
12	.8861	1.9	80	1	79	.9875	43(= 4 + 39)
13	.8750	2.3	36	1	35	.9722	1
14	.8507	2.8	34	1	33	.9706	2
15	.8257	—	31	—	—	—	—

* Additional data regarding timing are provided in Section 22.2.2.5 of text

The procedure then continues step by step, so that the seventh interval begins with a cumulative survival of .9461 and 137 persons at risk. The interval ends with a death at 0.9 yr. The one person censored at 0.9 yr and the 43 people followed for only 1 year are removed from the denominator of the eighth interval, which ends with a death at 1.1 yr. As the process continues, the thirteenth interval begins with a cumulative survival rate of .8750 and with a "risk group" (number alive) that has been reduced to 36, after removal of all the previous deaths, intermediate censorings, and terminal censorings. The fourteenth interval begins with a cumulative survival of .8507 and with 34 people who are alive and being followed. The interval survival rate of .9706 would make the 15th interval begin with a cumulative survival rate of .8257 and with 33 persons at risk, but no further deaths have occurred, so the table ends here. Note that the sum of deaths (17) plus censorings (102) plus final number at risk (31) in Table 22.4 equals the 150 persons who began. Note also that the Kaplan-Meier cumulative survival rates of .9392, .8750, and .8257 correspond to the respective Berkson-Gage results of .9388, .8737, and .8230 in Table 22.3.

The Kaplan-Meier approach is sometimes called a *product-limit method*, because the cumulative survival is a product of all the component interval survival rates. Because the multiplicative tactic is also used in the Berkson-Gage method, *variable-interval* is a better generic title to distinguish the Kaplan-Meier procedure. The term *actuarial* or *life-table* analysis can be applied to either method, but is usually reserved for the fixed-interval technique.

22.2.3   Display of Results

Graphs for the fixed-interval and variable-interval survival summary curves of Tables 22.3 and 22.4 are shown in Figure 22.1. The fixed interval points are usually connected directly with straight lines; if the intervals are close enough, the lines may resemble a relatively smooth curve. The variable-interval results are usually shown as the flat lines of a "step function." With a drop occurring for the death(s) at each step in the irregular intervals, the curve looks like a staircase with uneven steps. In a strict mathematical portrait, however, the Kaplan-Meier curve would be the horizontal lines of a "step function," without connecting vertical lines. The vertical lines are usually added for visual esthetics, to avoid a ghostly staircase.

The fixed-interval and variable-interval methods usually produce relatively similar results, as in Figure 22.1, but disparities can sometimes occur.

22.2.4   Choice of Methods

As in many other issues in statistical communication, the choice of a survival-arrangement method often depends on the background and viewpoint of the data analyst and reader. Because the denominators are reasonably well decremented for censored patients in all three methods, any one of the three offers a reasonably satisfactory approach. Contemporary biostatisticians (perhaps in deference to Meier) usually recommend the variable-interval method.

To provide prompt and easy-to-understand scientific communication, the direct method is most desirable because it shows the exact constituents of each survival rate, rather than a multiplicative product whose components are not displayed. The survival rates in the direct method are slightly underestimated because the censored patients do not contribute to the interval in which they are censored, but this same disadvantage occurs with the variable-interval method. The variable-interval method gets its advantage only if deaths occur at frequent intervals so that a small duration is available for each censored loss. This same advantage can be gained for either the direct or the fixed-interval method if the rates are determined at arbitrarily frequent intervals. Because the frequency of intervals in the Kaplan-Meier method is data-dependent and cannot be altered, this method can have substantial disadvantages for long intervals that have no deaths but many censorings.

Regardless of which method is used, a problem occurs at the right end of the curve, when the cited proportions of survival may depend on small numbers of observed patients. Although the constituent numbers should always be shown, they are frequently omitted when artists (or computers) prepare the displayed curves. Consequently, a reader may mistakenly believe that a five-year survival rate of 30%

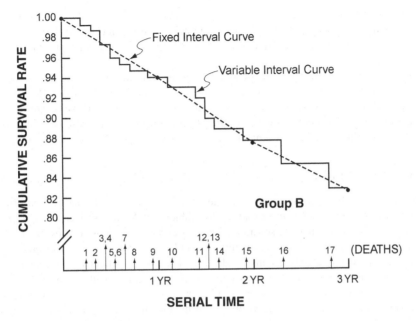

FIGURE 22.1
Survival curves for the data in Tables 22.3 and 22.4. The points and dashed lines show the results obtained with the fixed-interval technique of actuarial analysis. The solid line "staircase" shows the results obtained with the Kaplan-Meier method. The vertical arrows on the abscissa show the timing of the 17 deaths used to demarcate the Kaplan-Meier intervals. In this instance, the fixed-interval and variable-interval methods give similar results at 1, 2, and 3 years.

refers to all 219 members of the initial cohort, when in fact only 10 persons in the entire group may have been followed as long as five years. This deception can be avoided only if editors and reviewers insist on showing the pertinent constituent denominators for each interval of follow-up. In an alternative approach, standard errors and confidence intervals can be calculated (see Section 22.5) and cited for each cumulative rate, but the simplest and best strategy is to let the reader see directly what is happening.

22.3 Scientific Problems and Adjustments

The main scientific problems in constructing survival curves arise from "informative censoring," decisions about competing risks and competing outcomes, "left censoring," and the adjustments that occur with sensitivity and relative survival analyses.

22.3.1 Informative Censoring

In any of the three cited methods for constructing survival curves, the censored patients are regarded as essentially similar to those who continue under observation. The particular reasons that may have led to the censoring are ignored and are not used to modify the post-censoring results. This *laissez-faire* approach can lead to substantial distortions if the censorings were biased, i.e., caused by the effects of treatment or by anything other than random events. The term *informative* is a delicate name for this type of potentially biased censoring.

For example, in a clinical trial of treatment for chronic pain, suppose the failure event is the development (or persistence) of pain severe enough to warrant vigorous supplemental therapy. If Treatment A is particularly effective, many of its recipients may drop out of the study early, without further treatment, because their pain has been "cured." The remaining cohort for Treatment A will then contain only those patients who did not respond promptly. An analysis that does not acknowledge the successful censored patients will misrepresent the true effects of Treatment A. Conversely, many censored patients for Treatment B may have dropped out because of an adverse side effect or other untoward event that is not counted as a "failure." The remaining uncensored cohort will then misrepresent the true effects of Treatment B.

For these reasons, in a scientifically well-conducted study, vigorous efforts are made to determine the reasons why patients dropped out so that they are not listed merely as "lost-to-follow-up." The data might then be analyzed separately according to the reasons why the "informative censoring" took place. In the foregoing example, a separate success (rather than failure) rate might also be calculated (to show the advantages of Treatment A), and a separate adverse-event rate (to show the flaws of Treatment B).

22.3.2   Competing Risks

The competing-risk problem is a variation in the general theme of informative censoring. Special mathematical efforts[4] have been made to adjust life tables for deaths ascribed to "competing" non-relevant causes, and even to calculate separate rates of occurrence for those causes, but relatively little attention has been given to the scientific difficulty of deciding when a cause is truly "non-relevant." For example, suicide would appear to be an unrelated cause of death in a patient with cancer, but sometimes the suicide is brought on by cancer-induced depression. In a patient with a particularly difficult-to-maintain therapy, suicide may have been evoked by the discomforts of the therapy. The problem of competing risks is heightened if the untrustworthy information on death certificates is used to determine the "cause of death."

Because of these difficulties, an unequivocal decision is not always possible about the unrelatedness of death attributed to a competing risk. Many cautious analysts therefore reject any disease-specific attributions and insist on using death itself, i.e., total deaths in the cohort, as the only unequivocal outcome event.

22.3.3   Competing Outcomes

The problem of *competing outcomes* arises when several "hierarchical" entities can be regarded as the failure event, and when occurrence of one of the entities precludes the occurrence of another. For example, suppose the failure event is occurrence of either a stroke or death. If the patient survives a stroke, death can always occur later, but someone who dies cannot have a subsequent stroke. The same type of competitive problem arises if the failure event can be the development of either myocardial infarction or of angina pectoris, which is often ended by myocardial infarction.

Kernan et al.[5] have discussed the misleading results that can occur if the competing outcomes are examined in only a single life-table analysis. The proposed solution for the problem is to do a series of analyses with appropriately chosen categories and combinations of categories for the outcome phenomena.

22.3.4   Left Censoring

In any life-table analysis, an appropriate zero time must be chosen for the start of each person's serial follow-up. In randomized clinical trials, the date of randomization is an easy, obvious choice, and so the zero-time challenge is generally ignored when discussions of survival analysis are limited to randomized trials. In other forms of clinical epidemiologic research, however, a zero-time problem commonly arises when nonrandomized cohorts are assembled to evaluate therapy or to identify either prognostic factors for outcome of disease or risk factors for etiology of disease.

In many situations, the problem is easily resolved by assembling an *inception cohort*, which fulfills all of three requirements. The first requirement is that the cohort consist of persons whose zero time was the date of the first therapy aimed at the disease (or the date of the decision not to treat). The second and third requirements refer to the zero-time event: It should have occurred both during a bounded secular (calendar) interval, such as 1991–1996, and at the institution(s) whose results are under study. The rationale for these criteria is discussed elsewhere.[6]

If a presumably effective therapy is not available, however, as in certain chronic diseases such as multiple sclerosis, zero time may be chosen as the date of first diagnosis. Consequently, the assembled group of patients at a particular specialty center may contain many who have had the disease for 5, 10, 20 years or longer before they appeared for follow-up at that center. Such patients are the residue of cohorts elsewhere whose follow-up began at least 5, 10, or 20 years earlier, but the numbers and fates of the other cohort members are unknown. If patients in the specialty-center cohort are counted as though their zero time was the date of *diagnosis*, the follow-up results for the total group can be substantially distorted.

This problem can be avoided with a tactic called *left censoring*. (The term refers to the period *before* the cohort observations began, rather than to the customary *right* censoring, which occurs afterward.) With left censoring, patients who have already had 10 years of post-diagnostic observation are "admitted" to the cohort at the 10-year interval point of serial time; they are then followed thereafter from the 10-year point onward. The process of left censoring thus leads to *increases* in the post-zero serial denominator, rather than the usual decrements produced by right censoring. The two processes have been engagingly compared by John Kurtzke[7] in "a tale of two censors."

22.3.5 Sensitivity Analysis for Lost-to-Follow-Up Problems

No bias occurs when persons who were still alive at the end of the observation period are terminally censored because of insufficient duration. A possible bias can arise, however, from imbalances in the unknown reasons for "informative censoring" among persons who have become intermediate losses-to-follow-up.

The best way of managing the problem of "unknown reasons" for intermediate losses is to avoid it. Instead of relying on mathematical adjustments for the lost patients, an investigator can improve the scientific quality of the work by getting suitable follow-up information for all patients, even those who may have moved away from the research site. In an excellent early discussion of this problem, Harold Dorn[8] said, "The only correct method of handling persons lost to follow-up is not to have any." Demonstrating the flaws of each proposed method of "adjustment," Dorn concluded that "even a small percentage lost to follow-up, less than five percent of the total number under observation … may seriously bias [the results] … if this group has a relatively large proportion of persons withdrawing due to the condition being studied."

A sensitivity analysis is one mathematical method of approaching the problem of unknown-reason intermediate losses. For this analysis, a final cumulative survival rate is determined *by the direct method* for everyone whose final status was known as **dead** or **alive** for the full period of observation. This rate is then recalculated twice: once with the assumption that all of the intermediate withdrawals were dead in their exit status, and again with the assumption that they are all alive at the end of the full observation period.

The range between the high and low "sensitivity-adjusted" survival rates will usually give a better scientific idea of potential variability in the results than the purely statistical calculation (see Section 22.5) of standard errors or confidence intervals.

22.3.6 Relative Survival Rates

To avoid invidious diagnostic decisions about the cause of competing-risk deaths, *any* type of death can be used as the failure event. Many investigators prefer this total-death approach because it avoids possibly biased or wrong decisions about what is a "relevant" death, and because (in clinical trials) a treatment is not really successful if it reduces relevant but not total deaths. The approach also allows a straight-forward analysis of results without further adjustment for "competing risks."

If uncomfortable about the absence of such adjustments, however, the data analyst can calculate a *relative survival rate*.[9] In the first step of this calculation, a general demographic survival rate is determined from census and general mortality data for a cohort having the same age-sex composition as the group under observation. In this general-census cohort, the expected survival rate, S_E, would presumably reflect all the deaths — relevant and non-relevant — that would occur in ordinary circumstances. The actual survival rate, S_G, for the observed group under study, is then expressed as a relative proportion of the demographically expected general survival rate, S_E. For example, suppose the observed life-table survival rate is 0.62 at the end of five years in a cohort for whom the demographically expected general 5-year survival rate would have been 0.83. The relative survival rate at that time would be 0.62/0.83 = .75.

Despite the advantage of avoiding decisions about deaths due to competing risks, the relative survival rate has two major disadvantages: (1) it can sometimes be paradoxically higher at a later follow-up date than at an earlier date; and (2) if an unusually healthy cohort is being observed or treated, the general population may not be a pertinent comparison group and the relative survival rates may exceed 1.

Relative survival rates are now used much less often than in the past, probably because newer multivariable statistical methods are readily applied to "adjust" the survival results for baseline features, such as age and co-morbidity, that can affect competing risks.

22.4 Quantitative Descriptions

An unfortunate omission in contemporary statistics is the absence of a standard quantitative index to *describe* either a single survival curve or the contrast of two curves.

The slope or standardized slope of a regression line through the data might offer such an index, but it has seldom been applied to survival curves, probably because the denominators vary at different times and the time relationship may not be rectilinear. The area under the survival curve could also be used as a quantitative index, but no routine methods have been developed for calculating area. Besides, the calculated areas might be misleading if two survival curves with relatively similar areas have striking differences in shape (and in the corresponding clinical implications). Figure 22.2 shows two curves with a crossing that can produce many complexities in the analysis and interpretation.

In the absence of a quantitative descriptive index for each curve, survival curves are almost never compared directly. Instead, the usual comparisons are stochastic rather than descriptive, using the tests discussed in Section 22.5. Because the stochastic results depend so strongly on size of the groups, the survival curves themselves should always be inspected and evaluated judgmentally to decide whether the distinctions are quantitatively (rather than just stochastically) impressive.

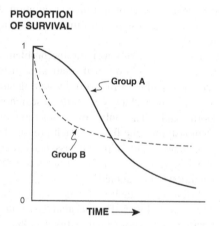

FIGURE 22.2

"Crossing" of survival curves. Sharply different survival curve patterns, but similar areas under the curve, produced by "crossing" of survival in Groups A and B.

Beyond the "physical examination" of the curve itself, however, the median and several other indexes can be used for quantitative summaries of a single curve, and a "hazard ratio" can be used to contrast two curves.

22.4.1 Median Survival Time

The most obvious and readily available statistical index for quantitative description is the median survival time. Although it does not reflect a dynamic pattern, it has the major advantage of being simple and easy to interpret.

The median can always be calculated if all of the censorings are terminal and do not occupy more than half the cohort. If intermediate censorings, with an unknown survival duration, do not have an obvious chronologic pattern and are not common, they might be ignored. If worst comes to worst, the median survival can be determined from the survival curve itself, using the time at which the cumulative survival rate reaches 50%. If the 50% survival mark is a flat "step" line, the median can be estimated at half the duration occupied by the step.

The examination of median survivals was denounced, however, in a frequently cited treatise on the analysis of clinical trials. According to Peto et al.,[10] the median survival is one of the thirteen "bad methods of analysis" that are "either [*sic*] inefficient, misleading, or actually wrong." The main complaint is that the median can be "very unreliable unless the death rate around the time of median survival is still high." Peto et al. therefore urged that median survival times be "treated with great caution, except for diseases in which nearly everyone dies, the data are extensive, and the life table falls rapidly through the whole region between 70% and 30% alive (the region in which the life table is used to estimate the median)."

After delivering this indictment, however, Peto et al. later in the same paper used the "bad method" of median survival to denote quantitative clinical importance for a prognostic distinction in comparing two groups. The authors wrote, "The difference between the relative death rates of 1.3 and 0.4 ... represents a difference between about 18 months and 5 years in median survival time, and is thus of considerable medical significance" (p. 27).

22.4.2   Comparative Box Plots

The absence of satisfactory descriptions for survival curves was lamented by Gentleman and Crowley[11] who said, "In more standard settings, no analysis would be considered complete without a detailed graphical examination of the data." After pointing out the difficulty of trying "to visually decode" the differences in plots of survival curves, the authors recommended several alternative graphic methods. Perhaps the simplest and potentially most useful method is a comparison of "censored-data box plots." Each box is formed by the median, upper quartile, and lower quartile of the successive survival durations in the group. If data have been censored, the pertinent quantile values can be determined from the survival curve itself.

Figure 22.3 shows comparative censored box plots of survival distributions for two treatments. The box plots are called *truncated* because some of the data are missing. (With "severe censoring," the upper quartile point may not be observed, and the truncated box may not have a top.) The median survival, at close to 600 days in Figure 22.3, was distinctly higher for "Treatment One" than the 200-day median for "Treatment Two." The quantitatively significant difference was also stochastically significant, according to the "half-H-spread overlap" rule discussed in Section 16.1.2.2. (A personal communication from Dr. Gentleman has explained

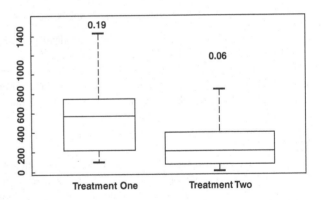

FIGURE 22.3

"Truncated box-plots" comparing data in two survival curves. [Figure derived from Chapter Reference 11.]

a potentially confusing feature of Figure 22.3. The numbers "0.19" and "0.06" represent the survival rate just before the last observed failure in each group.)

22.4.3   Quantile-Quantile Plots

A quantile-quantile plot, another visual approach, allows the two curves to be compared in a dynamic manner. If not readily available from the raw data, the appropriate quantiles of survival for each group can be taken from the life-table graphs. If the quantile-quantile plot is a straight line, its location above or below the "identity" line will promptly indicate the ratio of magnitude by which the quantiles of one curve are larger or smaller for one curve than the other. Although proposed by Waller and Turnbull[12] for checking goodness-of-fit between a model and the censored data, quantile-quantile plots should be readily applicable for comparing two survival curves.

22.4.4   Linear Trend in Direct-Method Survival Rates

If the survival proportions at each interval are calculated with the direct method, rather than with the cumulative products of an interval method, a counted numerator and denominator will be available at each time point. Although the array of binary proportions will not be "independent" (because the same patients may appear repetitively), the points can be fit with a suitably selected regression line.

The simplest model would be an ordinary rectilinear expression, $Y = 1 - bt$, where Y is the survival proportion at each time duration, t. The slope, $-b$, would then be a descriptive quantitative index. If the survival curve seems to have an exponential-decay pattern, however, the slope might best be expressed with the model $\ln Y = -ct$ (see Section 22.2). The value of $-c$ would then be an alternative quantitative index.

22.4.5   Hazard Ratio

The *hazard ratio* is a descriptive index that contrasts the survival rates in two groups at a single selected point in time. Machin and Gardner[13] have described the calculation of this index, together with a formula for its confidence interval.

At any time point in the life table, the hazard ratio for two groups, A and B, compares the total number of observed deaths, symbolized as O_A and O_B, and the number of deaths that might have been expected for the number of persons at risk in each group during that interval. If the number of persons at risk in a particular interval is N_A and N_B, the total number of deaths would be expected to have the same ratio as N_A and N_B. After all the algebra is worked out, the hazard ratio is calculated essentially as

$$R = (O_A/N_A)/(O_B/N_B)$$

In an ordinary 2×2 table for the alive and dead persons of two groups, with $q_A (= 1 - p_A)$ and $q_B (= 1 - p_B)$ representing rates of *mortality*, the hazard ratio is simply the ordinary risk ratio, q_A/q_B. Its main advantage is applicability to the decremented denominators of a life-table arrangement. Unfortunately, even when calculated at the last temporal interval after all observed deaths have occurred, the hazard ratio pertains to only one time point, not to the dynamic pattern in two compared curves.

22.4.6   Hazard Plots

The cumulative survival rates are useful for making predictions and giving an overall view of what is happening to a group, but do not indicate whether the interval "force" or "hazard" of mortality is changing over time. For example, the progressive declines in the cumulative survival curves in Figure 22.1 do not indicate that the annual interval mortality rates (in Table 22.3) are relatively constant around values of .06. Because the latter rates correspond to the annual hazard (see Section 22.2.2.4), data analysts[14] have suggested that important descriptive information can be obtained by inspecting the hazard function, which is essentially a plot of the interval mortality rates over time. The hazard pattern is easier to visualize when the graph has distinctive fixed intervals rather than the erratic oscillations that can occur with particularly small intervals and numbers in the Kaplan-Meier table.

The left side of Figure 22.4 shows the customary cumulative survival rates and the right side shows the annual percentage dying in a study of mortality and possible "curability" for a cohort of patients with breast cancer. Because the hazard function levels off at similar values for the long-term survivors in Stages I–III, the analysts concluded that stage becomes relatively unimportant after 5-year survival. This distinction could be inferred from the relatively parallel cumulative survival curves on the left side of Figure 22.4, but is shown more clearly and distinctly on the right side.

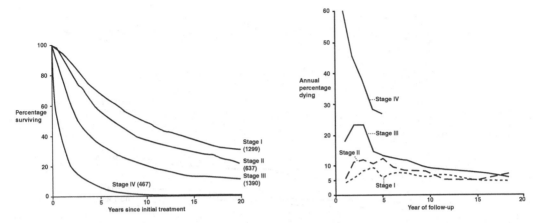

FIGURE 22.4

Cumulative survival (left side) and hazard function (right side) plots for a cohort with breast cancer. In Stage IV, the hazard plot is discontinued because too few patients were alive after 5 years. [Figure taken from Figures 1 and 2 in Chapter Reference 14.]

Plots of hazard functions are also used to check the assumption of "constant hazards" when survival is checked in multivariable analysis with the Cox regression procedure.

22.4.7   Customary Visual Displays

Most life tables are drawn, rather than tabulated, and are depicted in one of the two types of curves in Figure 22.1, emphasizing rates for avoiding the "failure event." The graphs can also go in an inverted direction, however, to show cumulative rates for the "failure" event itself. With suitable artistry, as shown in Figure 22.5, both types of plots for several types of events can be shown in the same graph.

22.5   Stochastic Evaluations

Standard errors and confidence intervals can be calculated at each time point of an individual survival curve; and two curves can be stochastically compared with various adaptions of conventional inferential tests.

22.5.1   Standard Errors

If the cumulative *direct-method* survival rate is S_T at time T, the standard error is determined with the customary calculation for any proportion. The formula will be $\sqrt{S_T(1 - S_T)/n_T}$ where n_T is the number of survivors at time T.

With the intervals of the actuarial methods, the cumulative survival rate is a product of the individual proportions, $p_t = 1 - (d_t/n_t)$, where d_t is the number of persons who died during the preceding interval and n_t is the number of persons at risk in that interval. After the last interval, T, the value of $S_T = p_1 \times p_2 \times p_3 \times \cdots \times p_t \times \cdots \times p_T$. The standard error of S_T is calculated by Major Greenwood's formula[16] as

$$SE_T = S_T\sqrt{\Sigma[(1 - p_t)/(n_t p_t)]}$$

The summation in this formula includes the individual values, from the first to the last interval, of $[(1 - p_1)/(n_1 p_1)] + [(1 - p_2)/(n_2 p_2)] + \cdots + [(1 - p_T)/(n_T p_T)]$. As time progresses, the values of n_t will get smaller, and the magnitude of the standard error will usually be dominated by the relatively large quantities produced by small numbers in the last few terms.

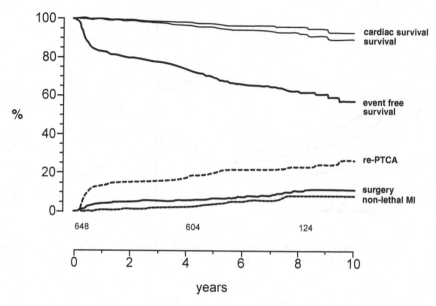

FIGURE 22.5

Long-term prognosis after immediately successful PTCA (percutaneous transluminal coronary angioplasty) in 648 patients. Event-free survival is defined as absence of repeat PTCA, bypass surgery, myocardial infarction, and death. *MI,* Myocardial infarction. [Figure and legend taken from Chapter Reference 15]

22.5.2 Confidence Intervals

With the usual Gaussian assumptions and choices of Z_α, confidence intervals can be calculated for any point on a single curve using Z_α times the standard error. If two curves are being compared, however, standard errors are seldom determined for the differences in successive survival rates. Because the differences are seldom cited with confidence intervals, the stochastic comparison is usually done with methods discussed in the next section.

22.5.3 Comparative Tests

The stochastic comparison of two (or more) survival curves has evoked many statistical tests, most of which can be catalogued as variations of the Wilcoxon rank or chi-square procedures. The most important thing to remember (or beware) about all these tests is that, like all stochastic procedures, they depend on group sizes. No matter how impressive the P value may be, the curves themselves should always be inspected to determine whether their difference is really quantitatively significant.

22.5.3.1 *Wilcoxon-Based Tests* — The Wilcoxon test for comparing ranks in two groups was generalized and applied by Gehan[17] to contrast two or more survival curves. After the Gehan tactic came under criticism,[18] Peto and Peto[19] developed an alternative log rank test that is currently preferred. According to Matthews and Farewell,[20] the Wilcoxon tests attach "more importance" to early deaths, whereas "the log-rank test gives equal weight to all others."

22.5.3.2 *Log-Rank and Chi-Square Procedures* — Several chi-square procedures have been used to form a stochastic index from stratified arrangements of the ranked survival data. Almost all the procedures are derived from a rank test originally devised in 1956 by Richard Savage.[21] The subsequent contributions, from many prominent statisticians, have been succinctly summarized by Breslow.[22]

The most commonly used type of chi-square procedure today is the log rank test, christened by Peto and Peto,[19] who offered that name although the test overtly employs neither logs nor ranks. (According to Gehan,[23] "the log rank statistic is the same as the statistic U(O)" previously proposed by Cox.[24]) The log rank test relies on calculating the observed and expected deaths for each group, using the principle discussed for the hazard ratio in Section 22.4.5. At a particular time interval, if $O_T = O_A + O_B$ for the total and component deaths in groups A and B, and if $N = N_A + N_B$ is the corresponding number of persons at risk of death, the expected number of deaths in each group is $E_A = (N_A/N)O_T$ and $E_B = (N_B/N)O_T$. These entities then receive a conventional chi-square expression for each interval, and the sum of the interval values for each group is calculated as

$$X^2 = \Sigma\{[(O_A - E_A)^2/E_A] + [(O_B - E_B)^2/E_B]\}$$

This result is then interpreted with 1 degree of freedom (when two groups are compared) in a chi-square distribution. Clear worked examples of the procedure have been shown by Peto et al.[10] and also by Tibshirani.[25] Coldman and Elwood[26] offer a worked example that shows calculation of both the Wilcoxon and the log-rank statistics.

To help preserve ambiguity, the log rank procedure is also sometimes called the *Mantel–Haenszel test*, or the *Cox–Mantel* test. According to Haybittle and Freedman,[27] however, the procedures have different operational mechanisms, and a test attributed to Mantel alone[28] is recommended "if a substantial proportion of deaths in one group occur after the other group has been entirely removed from risk" or if the comparison is done with prognostically adjusted groups.

22.5.3.3 ***Permutation Resampling*** — Of various other proposals for stochastically contrasting two survival curves, perhaps the most interesting was Forsythe and Frey's suggestion,[29] almost 25 years ago, that the tests be done with a "permutation technique" of rearrangement. The suggestion appears to have been ignored during the many subsequent proposals of diverse stochastic methods. Now that permutation and diverse resampling methods are becoming well known and regularly employed, the Forsythe-Frey proposal may warrant appropriate "resurrection" and reconsideration.

22.5.4   Sample-Size and Other Calculations

For additional stochastic activities, Freedman[30] has prepared a set of tables showing required sample sizes with the log rank test; and Borenstein[31] has described the challenges (and an appropriate computer program) of planning for "precision" in hazard ratios, attrition rates, and confidence intervals, as well as the "power" discussed in Chapter 23.

22.6   Estimating Life Expectancy

One of the main reasons life insurance companies developed actuarial methods was to estimate life expectancy, not to plot survival curves. The estimates are derived from what is called an *age-cohort analysis*, using the "cross-sectional" or "current" demographic mortality rates available for the age and sex groups of a regional population.

22.6.1   Customary Actuarial Technique

Suppose the annual mortality rates for a general population at a particular calendar period are .00960 at age 55–56, .01054 at age 56–57, and .01156 at age 57–58. If a cohort contains 89,000 persons who are alive at age 55, we would expect that $.00960 \times 89000 = 854$ of them will die in the next year, leaving 88146 (= 89000 − 854) still alive at age 56. If the 854 deaths are evenly distributed throughout the year, the dead persons will have each lived about a half year. The total number of years lived by the cohort during that year will have been 88146 + (0.5)(854) = 88573. During the next year, beginning at age 56, deaths would occur in $88146 \times .01054 = 929$ persons, leaving 87217 alive at age 57. The total years lived by the cohort in the 56–57 year interval will be 87217 + (0.5)(929) = 87682. The number who die in the interval from age 57 to 58 will be $87217 \times .01156 = 1008$, leaving 86209 alive, and a total of $86209 + (0.5)(1008) = 86713$ years lived.

The cumulative total of years lived by the cohort for the three-year period will be $88573 + 87682 + 86713 = 262,968$. The foregoing calculations can be iterated, using the appropriate mortality rates for each successive year of age, to obtain the annual deaths, survivors, and annual years lived at each year of age until almost everyone in the cohort has died.

The annual depletions and additions of the cumulative years-lived data can then be used to determine life expectancy. In the most common procedure, the analysis begins with a "stationary" cohort of 100,000 newborn persons who are then successively depleted by deaths at annual intervals until the cohort size becomes negligible at perhaps age 110. After the deaths and years lived are determined for each annual interval of the cohort, a "future cumulative" total of years lived is also calculated for each year. The future cumulative total consists of the total number of years lived by the cohort at that age, plus the annual total of years lived in all subsequent years. For example, in a stationary cohort of 100,000 persons who start at birth in the U.S., the future cumulative total might be 7,247,519 years. The average life expectancy at birth would then be $7,247,519/100,000 = 72.48$ years.

With the stationary-cohort tactic, life expectancy can be determined for anyone at any age. Suppose 87,217 persons in the stationary cohort are alive at age 57. The future cumulative total number of years lived in that year and in all subsequent years might be 1,895,992. If so, the average remaining life expectancy at age 57 would be $1,895,992/87,217 = 21.74$ years.

22.6.2   Additional Procedures

In the strategy just discussed, the death rates and life expectancies were determined for a general population. The results can be made more demographically specific if the calculations use death rates for annual ages of different sex or ethnic groups.

In addition, extra refinements are sometimes used to determine what would happen to general life expectancy if diseases such as cancer were eliminated. Assuming accuracy of information, the annual death rates for cancer are subtracted from the corresponding total death rate to produce a cancer-free death rate at each year of age. The annual life-table events are then appropriately recalculated, and the new value of life expectancy denotes the arithmetical consequences of eliminating cancer. The increment between this result and ordinary life expectancy (without the conquest of cancer) is usually disappointingly small[32,33] — only about a 2 to 3 year increase in average longevity.

A new life-table "disaggregation technique" was recently used[34] to explore reasons why African-American life expectancy declined, while Caucasian life expectancy rose, during 1984–89 in the United States. The authors concluded that for African-Americans the prime contributions came from HIV infection in both sexes, as well as from homicide in men and cancer in women. The diverse calculations were done, however, without attention to the massive problems caused by census underenumeration of African-Americans, as noted in Chapter 17.

22.7   Dynamic (Age-Period) Cohort Analysis

In the methods just discussed for estimating life expectancy, all of the mortality rates for each age group were cross-sectional. They came from demographic mortality data at a single period in secular time, which would usually be the latest available data for the general population. For example, the estimate of life expectancy for someone in 1993 would rely on the death rates noted for each age group in 1992, or in the closest calendar date (such as 1990) for which trustworthy information is available for census counts, numbers of deaths, and the corresponding age-specific mortality rates. This approach seems quite reasonable for an insurance company, which would want to estimate life expectancy for someone today according to the death rates that pertain today.

In various other circumstances, however, the investigators may take a more "historical" approach, aimed at determining the social or secular effects of changes in calendar time. For example, because of reductions in infant and other annual mortality rates, a cohort of persons born in 1905 might have life expectancies, at each successive age in each successive calendar interval, that differ substantially from a cohort of persons born in 1950. These two cohorts would be unfairly compared, however, if cross-sectional mortality rates were chosen from 1905 for all members of the first cohort, and from 1950 for the second. When persons born in 1905 became 20 years old, they were affected by the annual mortality rate for age 20 that existed in 1925, not in 1905. At age 40, they would be subject to the corresponding mortality rate in 1945. Similarly, the members of the 1950 birth cohort would be expected to die at age 20 according to the corresponding rate for 1970, and at age 40 according to the corresponding rate for 1990.

Analyzing the changing age-specific rates for each calendar period, rather than the "cross-sectional" rates existing at a single calendar year, produces a dynamic approach that has received various names. *Age-period cohort* analysis is the most popular term today, but the approach has also been called a *generation* or *fluent* analysis.

22.7.1　Methods of Construction and Display

Although applicable to general demographic explorations, age-period-cohort analyses have medically appeared most often in epidemiologic research on changes in mortality rates for a particular disease. In an early demonstration in 1947, Margaret Merrell[35] constructed the appropriate analytic grid, shown in Figure 22.6, using age-specific death rates for tuberculosis in Massachusetts men at 10 year intervals from 1880 to 1940. The columns show the "cross-sectional" secular calendar rates and the rows show the pertinent age groups. The demarcated diagonal segment shows the "cohort experience" as persons born in 1880 went through the changing age and secular rates at each period.

Age	1880	1890	1900	1910	1920	1930	1940
0 - 4	760	578	309	209	109	41	11
5 - 9	43	49	31	21	24	11	2
10 - 19	126	115	90	63	49	21	4
20 - 29	444	361	288	207	149	81	35
30 - 39	378	368	396	353	164	115	51
40 - 49	364	336	253	253	175	118	86
50 - 59	366	325	267	252	171	127	92
60 - 69	475	346	304	246	172	95	109
70 +	672	396	343	163	127	95	79

FIGURE 22.6
Age-specific death rates per 100,000 from tuberculosis for Massachusetts males, 1880 to 1940. Rates for the birth cohort of 1880 are indicated in the outlined diagonal strip. [Taken from Chapter Reference 35]

The data are usually plotted with age on the abscissa and age-specific death rates on the ordinate for each "birth cohort." The graphs can become quite complex because the investigators often show both the cross-sectional and the diagonal rates for each cohort. Such an arrangement appears in Figure 22.7, which presents both sets of results for lung cancer in cohorts of U.S. men.[36] The solid lines show the cross-sectional secular rates of age-specific deaths from lung cancer during calendar intervals ranging from 1931–35 to 1971–75. The dashed lines show the "diagonal" rates for the life experience of different birth cohorts, born in approximately 1876, 1881, 1886, 1891, 1896, and 1901.

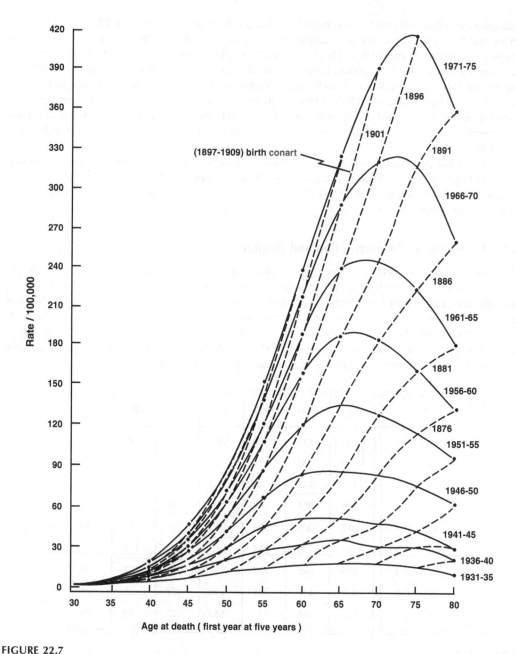

FIGURE 22.7

U.S. white male ling cancer mortality rates per 100,000 by age at death, period of death, and birth cohort. Solid lines show rates of death for the age groups cross-sectionally at each calendar period. Dashed lines show the corresponding rates of death as each birth cohort (marked 1901, 1896, 1891, etc.) goes through its ageing. To avoid too much overlapping, birth cohorts are labelled only for 5-year increments in the midpoints of 9 year intervals, such as "1901" for the interval 1897–1905. [Taken from Chapter Reference 36]

22.7.2   Uncertainties and Problems

Because age-period-cohort analysis seems to be an attractive method of examining the "natural history" of general and disease-specific mortality, various statistical models have been proposed for the procedure. The proposals have been disputed, however, with authorities such as Holford[37,38] favoring and Kupper et al.[36] doubting, the value of "currently available" models. The mathematical disputes refer to the choice of an appropriate statistical model for estimating parameters, and to the "identifiability" problem that arises because the age, period, and cohort effects are interrelated rather than independent.

Regardless of the way this mathematical controversy is resolved, however, the age-period-cohort analytic method has the profound scientific problem of using disease-specific rates of death. The analyses might be much more persuasive if aimed at the credible data of total mortality. As noted in Chapter 17, cause-specific rates of disease can seldom be scientifically accepted as trustworthy data,[4,39,40] regardless of whether the rates come from the idiosyncratic inconsistencies of coded death certificates or from the technologic detection bias that affects results assembed at tumor registries.

22.8 Longitudinal Analysis

In *longitudinal analysis*, the members of a cohort are followed to delineate the results of repeated measurements over time.

22.8.1 Confusion with Longitudinal Cross-Sections

The age-period-cohort procedure is seldom mistaken for a truly longitudinal analysis because the information comes from general mortality data for a population; i.e., individual members of a cohort are not examined or followed. A procedure that is sometimes confused with longitudinal analysis, however, is constantly used by practicing pediatricians to track the location of a child's annual height and weight on a graph showing appropriate percentiles in a reference "growing" population. The data for apparent growth in the reference population, however, come from cross-sections of children at the different ages, not from a longitudinally followed cohort. These analytic structures are often called *longitudinal cross-sections*.

The use of longitudinal cross-sections rather than cohort studies can create complex problems and controversies. The tactic seems to work well for the growth of normal children (as shown in Exercise 17.2), but can produce major distortions in studies of the course of older adults, where various noxious influences, eliminating vulnerable persons at relatively early ages, can lead to deceptive results in the cross-sections of "survivors." The topic is further discussed in Section 22.8.2.5.

22.8.2 Applications of Longitudinal Analysis

Longitudinal analyses for the individual members of a followed cohort have become a prominent statistical challenge only in recent years,[41-43] as pertinent data were made available from long-term clinical trials and epidemiologic cohort studies that were seldom conducted until the past few decades. The analyses have been done to appraise recurrent events, to explore dynamic impacts, to develop longitudinal correlations, to "track" changes, and to validate longitudinal cross-sections.

22.8.2.1 Recurrent Events — Longitudinal analyses become needed when a "failure event" — such as a streptococcal or urinary tract infection, episode of diarrhea, asthmatic attack, or epileptic seizure — can appear recurrently, thus precluding the conventional life-table procedure. Formal longitudinal analyses can be attempted, and proposals have been made[44] to extend the life table to repeated and changing events, but the most commonly used approach for recurrent events is to convert the denominator to person-durations of observation, rather than individual persons.

The results for the group are then cited, for example, as the number of events per patient-year. If certain persons are particularly susceptible to recurrent events, the results can also be cited as number of "eventful" persons per patient-year. Thus, if the recurrent events are streptococcal infections, the "attack rates" can be cited per patient-year either for number of infections or for number of infected persons. The process was discussed earlier in Section 17.3.3.

22.8.2.2   Dynamic Impacts — Longitudinal studies can also be used to investigate two types of dynamic impact. In one situation, the investigators determine the way that subsequent changes in baseline factors can affect (or predict) a single outcome event. In the other situation, individual events or factors are checked for their impact on a dynamic outcome — such as weight, blood pressure, or psychic status — that can change over time.

The first situation is illustrated by the famous Framingham study,[45] in which persons without known heart disease were followed for more than 20 years to study the original values and changes in baseline variables regarded as "risk factors" for the subsequent development of coronary heart disease. The members of the cohort were re-examined in sequential "panels" every few years to check the pertinent variables and to determine whether coronary disease had occurred.

In other studies of dynamic factors, a predictive impact has been noted from declines in pulmonary function[46] and sometimes from a patient's immediate or short-term early response to treatment.[47] Although "time-dependent covariate" and "time series" strategies have been developed for these analyses, an easier and more effective approach may be to record the successive values of pertinent clinical variables and then repeat the prognostic estimation at each new "zero-time" status, after a pertinent short-term interval.

The second type of dynamic longitudinal study, with moving values for the outcomes, has been done to check the impact of naturally occurring events in cohorts of women. For example, pregnancy was appraised for subsequent effects on adiposity,[48] and menopause for impact on depression.[49]

22.8.2.3   Longitudinal Correlations — In another pattern of longitudinal analysis, the changes that occur over time can be correlated with one another. For example, the results of repeated pulmonary function tests may be correlated with concomitant respiratory symptoms, smoking status, and age.[50] Changes in endogeneous testosterone over time may be correlated with age and with changes in triglycerides and high density lipoprotein cholesterol.[51] Serial values of ambient air pollutants, adjusted for temperature, humidity, and time of week or season, did not affect serial peak expiratory flow rates in asthmatic children.[52] The longitudinal correlations may also be used prognostically if data are obtained for a specific target outcome.[53,54]

22.8.2.4   Tracking — The term *tracking* is commonly used for the process of following a patient's course (or "trajectory") in successive values of certain factors, such as blood pressure or serum cholesterol. The analysis will often check whether a person's initial rating or rank persists as time progresses. For example, do children who are in the lower (or upper) percentiles of height and weight at age 2 remain in those percentiles at age 9 or age 19? Does asthma or acute rheumatic fever tend to have the same kinds of manifestations in recurrent episodes as in the initial attack? In a longitudinal follow-up study, when compared with children of parents with coronary artery disease (CAD), the offspring of those with CAD were found to have progressively higher development of cardiovascular "risk factors."[55]

22.8.2.5   Validation of Longitudinal Cross-Sections — A major advantage of longitudinal analysis is the opportunity to resolve disputes about the value of research with longitudinal cross-sections. The effort and expense of long-term follow-up could be avoided if cross-sections of appropriately aged persons yielded the same results that might emerge from following a large single group of persons as they grew older. For example, Margolis et al.[56] contended that short-term follow-up of a suitably analyzed cross-section gave essentially many of the same results obtained in the long-term Framingham cohort. In four contradictory examples, however, longitudinal analyses were used to show the "noncomparability of longitudinally and cross-sectionally determined annual change in spirometry,"[57] to demonstrate the error of previous cross-sectional studies claiming an increase of stillbirth in women who postpone childbearing until their "late twenties,"[58] to refute the wrong results of cross-sectional data for assessing "generational changes in the lifetime risk of depression or other psychiatric disorders,"[59] and to note that cross-sectional estimates of change in urinary symptom severity may underestimate the true effect of aging on prostatism.[60]

22.8.3 Statistical and Scientific Problems

Longitudinal analytic studies have all the difficulties cited earlier for follow-up in any type of cohort research, but the problems are much more complex, occurring from persons, times, and data.

An obvious scientific difficulty is what to do about persons who are "intermediate drop-outs," with subsequent longitudinal measurements that are unknown. Should they be excluded from the analysis, or conversely, with the intention-to-treat principle, should they be listed as though they had been followed to the end, receiving the originally assigned regimen? If the latter, should their most recent set of results be "carried over" and listed as the final data? In timing, the problems involve what to do with repeated measurements that are obtained irregularly when members of the cohort do not comply with the scheduled arrangements. (The problem of irregular long-term measurements seldom occurs when "acute" conditions — such as congestive heart failure, gastrointestinal bleeding, acute myocardial infarction, extremely low birth weight, or non-traumatic coma — have a short-term outcome.) An additional challenge refers to the timing of asymptomatic events (such as major changes that can be shown only in laboratory tests). Chappell and Branch[61] have described the "Goldilocks dilemma" of arranging for follow-up intervals that are neither too short nor too long, but just right.

In data, a major question is what to do about missing subsequent values. Should they be imputed from other members of the cohort or "guesstimated" from a statistical regression of previous values for the individual person? Another set of problems involves the management of both missing data for intermediate tests and wrong timing of tests.

As might be expected, many mathematical models have been proposed[62–65] for analyzing the scientific and statistical complexity. In a particularly clear account, Matthews et al.[66] classified two types of challenges presented by the patterns (peaks or growth) of longitudinal data, indicated the specific questions associated with each challenge, and proposed methods of answering each question. The authors strongly urged that the analyses be constructed from pertinent summaries of each patient's data, rather than with the more customary approach, which uses summaries of the group at different points in time. For example, instead of fitting a regression line through the group's mean values as serial time progresses, we might fit a suitable regression line through each person's data and then try to summarize the set of regression lines.

The choice of optimum analytic methods will doubtlessly be expanded and clarified as more experience is acquired with longitudinal studies.

References

1. Berkson, 1950; 2. Kaplan, 1983; 3. Kaplan, 1958; 4. Chiang, 1961; 5. Kernan, 1991; 6. Feinstein, 1985; 7. Kurtzke, 1989; 8. Dorn, 1950; 9. Ederer, 1961; 10. Peto, 1977; 11. Gentleman, 1991; 12. Waller, 1992; 13. Machin, 1988; 14. Pocock, 1982; 15. Kadel, 1992; 16. Greenwood, 1926; 17. Gehan, 1965; 18. Prentice, 1979; 19. Peto, 1972; 20. Matthews, 1988; 21. Savage, 1956; 22. Breslow, 1984; 23. Gehan, 1972; 24. Cox, 1972; 25. Tibshirani, 1982; 26. Coldman, 1979; 27. Haybittle, 1979; 28. Mantel, 1966; 29. Forsythe, 1970; 30. Freedman, 1982; 31. Borenstein, 1994; 32. Manton, 1980; 33. Tsai, 1982; 34. Kochanek, 1994; 35. Merrell, 1947; 36. Kupper, 1985; 37. Holford, 1983; 38. Holford, 1985; 39. Gittleschn, 1982; 40. Feinstein, 1987c; 41. Plewis, 1985; 42. Dwyer, 1992; 43. Diggle, 1994; 44. Hoover, 1996; 45. Kahn, 1966; 46. Rodriguez, 1994; 47. Esdaile, 1992; 48. Smith, 1994; 49. Avis, 1994; 50. Sherrill, 1993; 51. Zmuda, 1997; 52. Agocs, 1997; 53. Lieberman, 1983; 54. Capdevila, 1994; 55. Bao, 1997; 56. Margolis, 1974; 57. Glindmeyer, 1982; 58. Resseguie, 1976; 59. Simon, 1992; 60. Jacobsen, 1995; 61. Chappell, 1993; 62. Zeger, 1992; 63. Stukel, 1993; 64. Twisk, 1994; 65. Zerbe, 1994; 66. Matthews, 1990.

Exercises

22.1. Here is the "skeleton table" of a set of data for subsequent survival of a group of patients with a particular disease:

(1) Years after Diagnosis	(2) Alive at Beginning	(3) Died during Interval	(4) Lost to Follow-up	(5) Withdrawn Alive	(6) Adjusted Denominator	(7) Mortality Rate	(8) Survival Rate	(9) Cummulative Survival Rate
0–1	126	47	4	15				
1–2		5	6	11				
2–3		2	0	15				
3–4		2	2	7				
4–5		0	0	6				

22.1.1. Using a fixed-interval method of analysis and calculating all rates to at least three decimal places (to avoid errors due to rounding), complete the table.

22.1.2. Using the direct method of decrementing denominators, calculate the cumulative (or "total") survival rates at each of the cited intervals in the table.

22.1.3. Comment on the different results obtained for 5-year cumulative survival rates with the two methods of calculation. Which method would you prefer to use as a clinician evaluating treatment and making decisions in patient care?

22.2. For the data shown in Exercise 22.1, assume that the investigators checked each patient's status every 6 months. The deaths and censored events listed in the data were noted at the following times:

	During Interval		
	Lost to Follow-Up	**"Withdrawn Alive"**	**Deaths at End of Interval**
0–6 mos.	3	5	32
6–12 mos.	1	10	15
12–18 mos.	3	7	3
18–24 mos.	3	4	2
24–30 mos.	0	8	2
30–36 mos.	0	7	0
36–42 mos.	1	3	0
42–48 mos.	1	4	2
48–54 mos.	0	5	0
54–60 mos.	0	1	0

Prepare a Kaplan-Meier analysis for these data.

22.3. Prepare a graph showing the results of the fixed-interval and Kaplan-Meier analyses of these data. (You need not recalculate the previous data of Exercise 22.1.)

22.4. Like the direct method, the variable-interval method does not augment the interval denominators to include contributions from people censored during an interval. In Exercises 22.1 and 22.2, are the results of the variable-interval method more like those of the direct method or those of the fixed-interval method? What is your explanation for the observed distinction?

22.5. The graph in Figure E.22.5 is an exact reproduction from a recent report in a respectable medical journal. If you were reviewing this manuscript for publication, what suggestions would you offer about how to improve the graph?

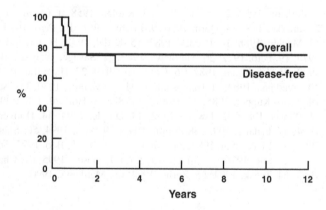

FIGURE E.22.5

Overall and disease-free survival for entire group of 16 study patients.

Part IV

Additional Activities

This last part of the text is devoted to two sets of additional topics in making stochastic decisions and in describing categorical contrasts and associations.

The new stochastic decisions arise when the goals differ from those of previously discussed stochastic tests, almost all of which were aimed at confirming something "big." The new descriptive strategies are used to "adjust" for "confounding variables" and to provide indexes of association for arrangements that cannot be suitably managed with the methods discussed earlier in Part III.

In the stochastic tests discussed thus far, the main goal was to show "stability" and proclaim "significance" for an observed distinction, d_o, that was regarded as quantitatively impressive. Regardless of the index (increment, ratio, etc.) used to describe the impressive quantitative magnitude of d_o, its stochastic confirmation was sought from a P value or confidence interval calculated under the null hypothesis of "no difference." After this calculation, the investigator would conclude that the results were stochastically either "significant" if the null hypothesis was rejected or "nonsignificant" if the hypothesis was conceded.

Beyond confirming a single quantitatively impressive value of d_o, however, stochastic tests can also have many purposes. Sometimes, if d_o is smaller than expected, the goal is to see how large it really might be. This type of exploration can be done with confidence intervals, but can also involve the ideas of capacity, alternative hypothesis, type II errors, power, and doubly significant sample sizes that are discussed in Chapter 23. In other situations, the investigator may want to find and confirm a small rather than large distinction. With this goal, discussed in Chapter 24, the stochastic procedures become re-oriented for testing "equivalence." Another important issue in that chapter is the interpretation of disparities between the investigator's goals and the statistical results. In still other situations, discussed in Chapter 25, the stochastic testing is done on multiple occasions rather than just once. The multiple testing may occur for different hypotheses (called "multiple comparisons") within the same set of data, for repeated sequential tests of the same hypothesis in an accumulating set of data, or for a meta-analytic aggregation of data pooled from a series of individual studies, each of which has already been stochastically tested.

The additional approaches to association occupy the last four chapters. With new descriptive indexes, discussed in Chapter 26, the two-group contrasts discussed in part II can receive special approaches to deal with the problems of "confounding." The approaches involve such tactics as "adjustment," "standardization," and "matching." A different descriptive challenge requires new indexes of association, discussed in Chapter 27, for categorical relationships that are not suitably managed with the strategies previously considered in Part III.

The last two chapters, which contain no Exercises at the end, are intended mainly to familiarize you with two sets of procedures that you may meet in medical literature. For reasons noted in those chapters, you may not do (or want to do) any of these procedures yourself, but they regularly appear in published papers. The non-targeted analyses in Chapter 28 contain methods for reducing multiple variables (or categories) into a smaller set of variables (or categories) without aiming at a specific target variable. The analysis of variance, in Chapter 29, aims at a target variable that is associated with more than two "independent" categories.

The additional stochastic and descriptive topics are not part of the common daily events in medical statistics, but they occur often enough to warrant inclusion among the principles needed by thoughtful readers or users.

Part IV

Additional Activities

23

Alternative Hypotheses and Statistical "Power"

Type II errors are a common event in stochastic testing. They occur when the investigator concedes the null hypothesis and concludes that the observed results are "not significant," although the true distinction is really impressive. These errors are the reverse counterpart of the Type I errors, emphasized in all the stochastic discussions so far, that occur when the null hypothesis is rejected although it is actually true.

In conventional statistical discussions, the stochastic conclusion is often regarded as the fundamental decision in the research. The stochastic strategy is then aimed mainly at either confirming the "correct" decisions or preventing the errors of "false-positive" and "false-negative" conclusions. The research may reach a wrong conclusion, however, for scientific rather than stochastic reasons. In the first part of this chapter, devoted to the diverse sources of wrong conclusions, the scientific problems are discussed first. A knowledge of those problems can often help either to avoid the use of an unsuitable stochastic test or to keep the investigator (and reader) from being deceived by results of an appropriate test.

23.1 Sources of Wrong Conclusions

Assuming that the raw data are themselves correct, a wrong conclusion can be produced by several types of scientific and statistical problems.

23.1.1 Scientific Problems

The main scientific sources of error are biased groups, erroneous hypotheses, and erroneous interpretations.

23.1.1.1 *Biased Groups* — Whether "significant" or "nonsignificant," a statistical result can deviate from truth because the particular group(s) under study did not suitably represent the pertinent population or events. This problem was the source of a particularly famous error in political poll-taking. Before the U.S. presidential election of 1936, a sample of more than 1,000,000 people was assembled by a respectable magazine, *Literary Digest*, from the mailed-in "ballots" of readers and from randomly placed telephone calls. The opinions expressed in this huge sample led to a highly confident prediction that the Republican candidate, Alfred Landon, would win the election overwhelmingly. On Election Day, however, the incumbent Democrat, Franklin Roosevelt, won by a "landslide." A "post-mortem examination" showed that the sampling process had a major bias, which you are invited to diagnose in Exercise 23.1.

In the example just cited, the composition of a single group (potential voters) was biased. When two groups are contrasted for conclusions about cause–effect etiologic or therapeutic relationships, biased comparisons can arise from diverse problems in susceptibility, detection, and other nonstatistical sources of distortion. If the problems are recognized and if appropriate data are available, statistical efforts can be made to adjust for the bias. The best approach, however, is scientific, not statistical. The research should be designed in ways that can avoid or substantially reduce the bias.

23.1.1.2 *Erroneous Scientific Hypotheses* — As discussed in Chapter 11, most research comparisons involve two types of hypotheses. One of them, seldom emphasized in statistical discussions, is the *scientific* hypothesis. It denotes what the investigator expects (or wants) to find in the research. Always cited descriptively, the scientific hypothesis may be stated in phrases such as: "Treatment A is better than Treatment B," or "Agent E causes or promotes development of Disease D." The scientific hypothesis will be wrong if the proposed maneuvers do not, in fact, have the action anticipated by the investigator.

Medical history contains many accounts of erroneous etiologic and therapeutic hypotheses that were scientifically popular in different eras until truth (or suitable corrections) eventually emerged. The scientific sources of these errors were usually wrong qualitative concepts. For many centuries, disease was thought to be caused by imbalances in the four "humors" of the body. The imbalances were then "cured" by such treatments as blood-letting, blistering, purging, and puking. During the 19th century, many contagious diseases were ascribed to miasmal vapors. In the mid-20th century, thousands of premature babies were blinded during an iatrogenic epidemic of retrolental fibroplasia,[1] caused by excessive oxygen therapy given as prophylaxis in the belief that its potential pulmonary benefits could not be accompanied by adverse effects elsewhere in the body.

23.1.1.3 Erroneous Interpretations — When the hypotheses emerge from the data, a correct set of information may be erroneously interpreted.

A major blunder in confusing association with causation was committed by William Farr (the respected "founder" of Vital Statistics) who concluded, from statistical correlations, that cholera was caused by high atmospheric pressure.[2] In the early 20th century, pellagra was erroneously regarded as infectious after it was commonly found in members of a family and in their neighbors.[3]

23.1.2 Statistical Problems

Common statistical sources of error have been the failure to set quantitative boundaries, to appraise stochastic variation, and to understand dissident results.

23.1.2.1 Boundaries for Quantitative Distinctions — As the use of statistical data became popular in the 20th century, a subtle source of error was incorrect beliefs about magnitude. If Treatment A was believed "better" than B, but turned out "worse," the scientific hypothesis itself was wrong. If A was only slightly or trivially better, however, the scientific hypothesis was still correct, but the anticipated magnitude of difference was wrong.

To be examined statistically, such concepts as *better, worse,* or *trivially better* must be converted to quantitative expressions. The scientific difficulty of choosing these expressions was discussed in Chapter 10. Qualitatively, a particular phenomenon (death, "success," relief of symptoms, etc.) must be chosen as the focus of attention; and a particular statistical index (increment, direct ratio, proportionate increment, etc.) must be chosen to cite the quantitative distinction, d_o, observed in the compared treatments. The next statistical step is to demarcate a magnitude that will make this distinction be regarded as "big" or "small."

The choice of these boundaries is often difficult, but they must nevertheless be established to allow statistical procedures to be used, before the research, for calculating a suitable sample size, and afterward, to decide whether the observed distinctions are impressive or unimpressive enough to warrant stochastic "tests of significance."

23.1.2.1.1 Demarcations of "Big" and "Small". Suppose the symbol δ is used for the *lower* boundary of a *big* or quantitatively impressive distinction. If Treatment A is expected to be substantially better than Treatment B, the scientific hypothesis might be cited symbolically as

$$A - B \geq \delta$$

If Treatments A and B are expected to be essentially equivalent, the difference in results will seldom be exactly zero. Consequently, an upper limit, expressed with the symbol ζ, can be established as the *maximum* magnitude of a *small* or quantitatively insignificant distinction. The scientific hypothesis of equivalence, or a tiny difference, could then be quantitatively cited as

$$A - B \leq \zeta$$

23.1.2.1.2 Effects of Quantitative Boundaries. The quantitative boundaries for δ and ζ are arbitrary, but no more arbitrary than the level of .05 usually set for the boundary of α in stochastic tests. With two sets of boundaries available for quantitative and stochastic decisions, however, a gallery of statistical errors becomes possible. Most of this chapter is concerned with possible errors in stochastic decisions when the investigator wanted to find a "big" distinction, i.e., $d_o \geq \delta$. The stochastic examination of "small" distinctions, i.e., the confirmation of "equivalence," is discussed in Chapter 24.

23.1.2.2   *Stochastic Variations* — *Stochastic variation* refers to phenomena that can occur during the action of random chance. Wrong conclusions can occur if these variations are not recognized and suitably accounted for. For example, someone who wins the main prize in a lottery might become rich, but would not immediately be regarded as a talented selector of random numbers. In fact, if the same person wins again and particularly a third time, we might believe something is wrong with the lottery process. On the other hand, if a **12** is tossed with two dice, the chance probability of the occurrence is $(1/6)(1/6) = 1/36 = .028$, but we would not immediately reject the idea that the dice are "fair." The event would regularly happen among a large series of consecutive tosses at a gambling casino's dice table.

23.1.2.2.1 "False Positive" Conclusions.   The customary "tests of statistical significance" are done to avoid erroneous "false positive" conclusions that might arise merely from stochastic variation; and α is set at the level of acceptable errors. Thus, an impressively large incremental success rate could readily arise by stochastic variation alone if two treatments, A and B, are actually equivalent, but produced $p_A = 8/13 = .615$ and $p_B = 4/12 = .333$, with $d_o = .282$, in a study done with small groups.

For these small numbers, the stochastic test of the null hypothesis is best done with the Fisher exact procedure, which would produce $2P = .238$. The mathematical principles, however, are easier to illustrate with the Z test. The standard error of the difference is first calculated with Formula [14.11] as

$$SED = \sqrt{[(8+4)(5+8)]/[(13+12)(13)(12)]} = 0.2$$

The observed value of Z, designated as Z_o, is then calculated as $.282/.2 = 1.41$, for which $2P_o = 0.159$. Although this P value is smaller than the result of the Fisher test, neither procedure would lead to rejection of the null hypothesis with α set at .05.

23.1.2.2.2 "False Negative" Conclusions.   Stochastic variation, however, might also lead to an erroneous "false negative" conclusion. For example, suppose two treatments in a clinical trial really differ substantially (i.e., by at least $\delta = .15$), and suppose at least 25 patients had been entered into each group. If the subsequent results then show that $p_A = 14/29 = .483$ and $p_B = 12/28 = .429$, the value of $d_o = .483 - .429 = .054$ is less than $\delta = .15$. This result is *not* quantitatively significant and is also not stochastically significant with a test in which we first calculate

$$SED = \sqrt{[(14+12)(15+16)]/[(57)(29)(28)]} = .132$$

The value of Z_o is then $.054/.132 = .409$, for which $2P_o = .68$.

To avoid a false negative conclusion, however, we can first check to see whether the observed small value of d_o is a stochastic variation, which differs by chance from the true value of $\delta \geq .15$. An obvious way to check for the latter possibility was discussed in Sections 11.7.2 and 11.9. We determine whether $\delta = .15$ is included in the upper boundary of an appropriate confidence interval around $d_o = .054$. With .132 as the value of SED, the 95% confidence interval is $.054 \pm (1.96)(.132) = .054 \pm .258$. It extends from $-.205$ to $.313$. The result is not stochastically significant because the value of 0 is included, but the confidence interval also includes the value of $.15$. The result might therefore be a stochastic variation from a true difference, between treatments A and B, that is actually as large as $\delta = .15$.

Because the confidence interval component, $Z_\alpha \times SED$, is $.258$ here, the value of $\delta = .15$ would be *included* in the upper part of the confidence interval for all positive values of d_o. The interval would fail to exceed δ only if $d_o < \delta - Z_\alpha(SED)$, which would occur when d_o has a negative value of at least $.150 - .258 = -.108$.

23.1.2.2.3 Clinical Claims of "No Difference".   The situation just described constantly occurs in medical literature when the investigator gets the observed data, finds that the customary P value exceeds the α level of "significance," and then concludes that the study had "nonsignificant" results.

If a confidence interval was not published to show how large the "nonsignificant" difference might have been (or sometimes even if the confidence interval was shown), irate readers will regularly send letters to the editor complaining about the omission. The readers usually contend that the group sizes were too small to prove the claim. The original authors may then respond by citing the confidence intervals (which may often include a "big" result), but offering various justifications for the claim of nonsignificance.

Such arguments have occurred after publication of clinical trials claiming that early discharge from hospital was relatively safe after acute myocardial infarction,[4] that glucagon injections did not improve accuracy of a double-contrast barium enema,[5] that exchanging unsaturated fats did not affect plasma lipoproteins[6], that thoracic radiotherapy did not prolong survival in patients with carcinoma of the lung,[7] and that ritodrine (a beta-adrenergic agonist) was not effective in treating preterm labor.[8] If a big difference is included, the upper boundary of the confidence interval can readily be used to justify the contention that such a difference might exist.

23.1.2.3 *Statistical Dissidence* — The quantitative and stochastic decisions agree if the observed distinction seems quantitatively significant, and if the stochastic test confirms the significance. *Statistical dissidence* occurs when the two sets of results do not agree, so that significance is found quantitatively but not stochastically, or stochastically but not quantitatively. The conclusion will be wrong if a correct quantitative distinction is ignored in favor of the contradictory stochastic result.

The quantitative-yes–stochastic-no type of dissidence was frequently noted in scientific literature as stochastic tests became increasingly used to prevent erroneous conclusions from small groups. The dissidence occurs when the group size is too small to allow stochastic confirmation for a big quantitative distinction. Without the stochastic test, an investigator might claim significance when a quantitatively impressive increment of 15% in success rates of 25% vs. 40% came from numbers as small as 1/4 vs. 2/5. "Tests of significance" were introduced and intended to prevent this problem. The opposite type of quantitative-no–stochastic-yes dissidence, which has become increasingly common when stochastic tests are used as the main or only basis for *scientific* conclusions, is the stochastic proclamation of significance for a small, unimpressive quantitative distinction.

23.1.2.3.1 *"Boundless Significance" and Oversized Groups.* The enormous impact of size in tested groups was shown in earlier discussions of the Z, t, and chi-square tests. If the groups are too small, an impressive quantitative distinction may not be stochastically confirmed; but if the groups are too big, an unimpressive distinction may become stochastically significant.

The latter type of statistical dissidence can occur because the customary calculation of stochastic significance is "boundless." The quantitative boundary of δ is neither used nor needed for determining a conventional P value from $Z_o = d_o/(\text{SED})$ or a confidence interval constructed as $d_o \pm Z_\alpha$ (SED). If the calculated Z_o exceeds Z_α, or if the confidence interval excludes 0, the stochastic result can be proclaimed "significant," regardless of the actual magnitude of d_o. For example, in a study that contains more than 2200 persons in each group, the rates of "success" may be $750/2207 = .34$ in Group A and $819/2213 = .37$ in Group B. The increment of .03 in the two groups may seem small and unimpressive, but it is stochastically significant at $P < .05$, because the big groups lead to a suitably large value of 2.1 for Z_o.

There is no statistical method to prevent erroneous conclusions in this situation. They can be avoided (or "cured") only if investigators (and readers) preserve their scientific judgment and examine the actual magnitude of the observed distinction. If it is not big enough to be impressive, it is not "significant" even if the P value is infinitesimal.

23.1.2.3.2 *Problems of Undersized Groups.* The stochastic dissidence caused when undersized groups are too small to allow rejection of the null hypothesis was illustrated in Section 23.1.2.2.1. In a well-conducted clinical trial that produced $p_A = 8/13 = .615$ vs. $p_B = 4/12 = .333$, the investigator could not get stochastic confirmation for the impressively large quantitative increment of $d_o = .282$.

This problem, although regularly regarded as a defect in "power" of the trial, is actually due to a simpler defect in what might be called *capacity*. As noted later, *power* refers to the ability to reject an alternative hypothesis that the quantitative distinction is large although the observed result may be small. *Capacity*, however, refers to the ability to reject the original null hypothesis when the observed distinction is large.

23.2 Calculation of Capacity

The statistical dissidence just described occurred because the group sizes were too small. If the investigator had really expected to find an increment as large as .282 between the two treatments, the necessary sample size for stochastic significance at a two-tailed P < .05 could have been calculated with the earlier Formula [14.20], using π_B = .333, to get

$$n \geq (2)(.333)(.667)(1.96)^2/(.282)^2 = 21.5$$

At least 22 patients would have been required in each group. With Formula [14.19], for which π would be estimated as (.615 + .333)/2 = .474, the sample size needed for each group would have been

$$n \geq (2)(.474)(.526)(1.96)^2/(.282)^2 = 24.1$$

or at least 25. With either calculation, the actual group sizes of 13 and 12 would lack the capacity to achieve a stochastic 2P < .05.

If δ = .15 had been originally chosen as a boundary for quantitative significance, the sample size required by Formula [14.19] would have been

$$n \geq 2(.4065)(.5935)(1.96)^2/(.15)^2 = 82.4$$

With at least 83 persons in each group, the quantitatively impressive d_o = .282 would easily have yielded 2P < .05.

The cited stochastic defect in capacity can easily be quantified numerically. The foregoing calculations (where d_o = .282 and π was estimated as .474) showed that about 25 persons were required for each group, making a total required size of N_R = 50. Because the actual group, N_o, contained 13 + 12 = 25 people, the capacity was approximately N_o/N_R = 25/50 = 50% of what was needed.

The main point to be noted, however, is that the trial under discussion was defective in its basic *capacity*, not in its *power* to reject an alternative hypothesis, as discussed shortly.

23.3 Disparities in Desired and Observed Results

In a study that begins with the goal of finding a big difference, $d_o \geq \delta$, three possible outcomes can occur. In the first two, the result is "positive," with $d_o \geq \delta$. This "positive" result is then either confirmed stochastically, with $P_o \leq \alpha$, or not confirmed, with $P_o > \alpha$. In the third situation, the result of the trial is "negative," with $d_o < \delta$. In this situation, the investigator hopes that the small d_o is stochastically consistent with a big δ.

23.3.1 General Conclusions

An observed "positive" big distinction, i.e., $d_o \geq \delta$ would be stochastically confirmed if the group size had full capacity, but would not be confirmed, with P > α, if the group size was too small. If the result was "negative," i.e., $d_o < \delta$, the small d_o might be rendered stochastically significant if the group size was huge; but in most reasonable situations, the associated P_o would exceed α, and the distinction would be nonsignificant, both quantitatively and stochastically.

In the last situation, however, an investigator who wanted to find $d_o > \delta$ would be delighted if δ were included in the upper end of the confidence interval for d_o. After savoring the delight, however, a cautious investigator might have a nagging doubt. Suppose the *scientific* hypothesis is wrong, so that d_o is really small, rather than being merely a stochastic variation from δ. Worried about this possibility, the investigator may now want some further stochastic reassurance that can prove or confirm "no difference." Thus, the investigator would ask, "How can I be sure I have not been deluded by random fate? What would be convincing evidence that the treatments have a really small difference?"

23.3.2 Group Size for Exclusion of δ

Scientifically, the immediate answer to the latter questions is "Repeat the trial." Statistically, however, a numerical solution can be offered. If a suitable confidence interval excludes the "big" value of δ, the demonstration that

$$d_o + Z_\alpha (SED) < \delta \qquad [23.1]$$

could be reasonably assuring. It would indicate that the "small" value of d_o is probably not merely a stochastic variation from a true large value of δ.

To determine the group size required for this assurance, we first convert Formula [23.1] to $Z_\alpha(SED) < (\delta - d_o)$. Assuming equal group sizes, SED can then be calculated as $\sqrt{2\hat{\pi}(1 - \hat{\pi})/n}$. After the algebra is developed, the size of n needed in each group will be

$$n > \frac{Z_\alpha^2 2\hat{\pi}(1 - \hat{\pi})}{(\delta - d_O)^2} \qquad [23.2]$$

To illustrate the calculation, suppose we assume that d_o will be .054, as in Section 23.1.2.2.2. We determine $\hat{\pi}$ as the average of the estimated p_A and p_B, which is $(.483 + .429)/2 = .456$, so that $1 - \hat{\pi} = .544$. We set $Z_\alpha = 1.96$ and then substitute in [23.2] to get

$$n > [(1.96)^2(2)(.456)(.544)]/(.150 - .054)^2$$

which turns out to be $1.906/(.096)^2 = 206.8$.

Thus, if a trial with 207 patients in each group yields the expected $p_A = .483$, $p_B = -.429$, and $d_o = .054$, the value of $\delta = .15$ would be excluded from the confidence interval. The investigator could then be able, with 95% confidence, to conclude that Treatment A does *not* exceed Treatment B by a difference of $\delta = .15$ or more.

If things turn out almost exactly as anticipated in the preceding paragraph, the results with the larger sample size will be $p_A = 100/207 = .483$ and $p_B = 89/207 = .430$. The SED will be

$$\sqrt{[(89 + 100)(107 + 118)]/[(414)(207)(207)]} = .049$$

The 95% confidence interval will be $(.483 - .430) \pm (1.96)(.049) = .053 \pm .096$; and it will extend from $-.043$ to .149. With 0 included, the result is *not* stochastically significant; and with .150 excluded, the result offers stochastic assurance that d_o is unlikely to be as large as .150. The investigator could now conclude that the original scientific hypothesis was probably wrong. Despite the desired hope, Treatment A is not substantially better than Treatment B.

23.4 Formation of Alternative Stochastic Hypothesis

The foregoing tactics brought us into a new type of stochastic reasoning. In everything done until now, we found a "big" difference, d_o, that was scientifically expected and welcome, so we tried to confirm it stochastically. The stochastic hypothesis, symbolized as Δ, was assumed to be the opposite of what we wanted to prove. We made Δ as small as possible, i.e., $\Delta = 0$.

For the new situation, however, we want stochastic confirmation for a "small" difference, i.e., $d_o < \delta$. We therefore want to reject a different hypothesis, i.e., that $\Delta \geq \delta$. If δ is *excluded* from the corresponding confidence interval, we could conclude stochastically that the observed result, d_o, is indeed smaller than δ.

This conclusion, however, would reverse the original goal of the trial, which was done with the hope of finding $d_o \geq \delta$. The reversal is not important for the statistical procedures that follow in the next few sections, but becomes a crucial feature of the reasoning when we reach the Neyman-Pearson strategy considered in Section 23.6.

23.4.1 Statement of Alternative Hypothesis

The conventional null hypothesis places the value of Δ at 0 for increments, correlation coefficients, or slopes, and at **1** for a ratio. To avoid frequently repeating the comment about "1 for a ratio," all null hypotheses about "equivalence" or "no distinction" will hereafter be cited as **0**. The same ideas and approaches will also pertain, if expressed for a ratio, but the null hypothesis will be **1**.

With Δ representing the value of the stochastic hypothesis, the conventional "null" assumption, $\Delta = 0$, was stated (for two proportions) as $H_o: \pi_A - \pi_B = 0$. In the new procedure, however, the hypothesis to be rejected is the alternative statement that $\Delta \geq \delta$. The symbols would be $H_H: \pi_A - \pi_B \geq \delta$

23.4.1.1 *Imprecise Counter-Hypothesis* — In the logic of stochastic testing, a primary hypothesis can be rejected or conceded, but never accepted. The primary hypothesis is therefore set to be the opposite of what we would like to conclude; and when the hypothesis is rejected, we concede the counter-hypothesis. To be the direct opposite of the null hypothesis, $\Delta = 0$, the counter-hypothesis must be imprecise, without a stipulated focal point. If $\Delta = 0$, the *counter-hypothesis* can be either a two-tailed $\Delta \neq 0$, or in a one-tailed direction, $\Delta > 0$ or $\Delta < 0$; but it cannot be $\Delta = \delta$.

This logic is responsible for the "boundless significance" discussed in Section 23.1.2.3.1. Suppose $\delta = .15$ is set as the level of quantitative significance for an increment in two proportions, and suppose the results show that $p_A = 27/42 = .64$ and $p_B = 11/39 = .28$. For the *quantitatively* significant distinction of $d_o = p_A - p_B = .36$, the value of Z_o turns out to be 3.25. Although the *observed* value of d_o can now be deemed stochastically significant at a two-tailed $P < .05$, the actual *stochastic* conclusion is only that $\Delta \neq 0$. The observed $d_o = .36$ acquires its label of "stochastic significance" merely by being compatible with the stochastic conclusion. This same conclusion could have been obtained with adequately large group sizes if d_o were smaller, at .19. The observed d_o could even be stochastically significant when smaller than δ, at values of .10, .07, or .03. For example, suppose $p_A = 238/2166 = .11$ and $p_B = 80/2184 = .04$, so that $d_o = .07$. This result is substantially smaller than $\delta = .15$, but it would produce $Z_o = 2.5$, for which $2P < .05$. Despite the relatively small d_o, we can still reach the same stochastic conclusion, i.e., $\Delta \neq 0$, as with the previous big d_o.

23.4.1.2 *Precise Location for Alternative Hypothesis* — Unlike a counter-hypothesis, the alternative hypothesis has its own specific dignity and focal location. Like any other stochastic hypothesis, the alternative hypothesis can be rejected or conceded but not accepted. When considered for the possibility of being false, i.e., rejected, the alternative stochastic hypothesis must have a precisely specified location, analogous to the precision of $\Delta = 0$.

If the goal is to get stochastic confirmation that $d_o < \delta$, the precise value of the alternative hypothesis is usually set at δ. With H_H as the symbol, the alternative hypothesis becomes expressed as $H_H: \Delta = \delta$; and its counter-hypothesis becomes $\Delta \neq \delta$. For reasons to be cited shortly, the alternative hypothesis is almost always checked in a one-tailed direction. The appropriate statement would then be $H_H: \Delta \geq \delta$; and the counter-hypothesis would be $\Delta < \delta$. For simplicity of expression and calculation, however, the usual statement is simply $H_H: \Delta = \delta$. The directional issues are implicit when the results are interpreted.

In a contrast of two proportions, p_A and p_B, the parametric alternative hypothesis is $H_H: \pi_A - \pi_B = \delta$, or (if specifically two-tailed) $H_H: |\pi_A - \pi_B| = \delta$. In a contrast of two means, $\overline{X}_A$ and $\overline{X}_B$, the same principles are used, but the parameters in the hypothesis are μ_A and μ_B.

With this operating principle, we can explore what has been called "the other side of statistical significance,"[9] by considering what happens if the original null hypothesis is *false* and should have been rejected. Its falsity is explored with the alternative stochastic hypothesis, for which δ replaces the null-hypothesis value of 0. Under the alternative hypothesis, the observed value of d_o is examined as the increment of $\delta - d_o$.

23.4.2 Alternative Standard Error

Under the alternative hypothesis (as under the null hypothesis), the increment in two means or in two proportions continues to have a theoretical Gaussian (or Gossetian) sampling distribution for values of Z (or t). Figure 23.1 shows the location of the observed d_0 and the potential Gaussian distributions of increments under each of the two stochastic hypotheses.

As noted earlier, the standard error of a difference in two central indexes, symbolized as SED, is calculated differently when $\Delta = \delta$ rather than $\Delta = 0$. For contrasting two observed proportions with $\Delta = 0$, Formula [15.9] for SED is

$$SED_0 = \sqrt{NPQ/n_A n_B}$$

but for $\Delta \geq \delta$, the analogous calculation in Formula [15.12] is

$$SED_H = \sqrt{(p_A q_A/n_A) + (p_B q_B/n_B)}$$

Both calculations can be eased with the "shortcut" formulas shown earlier in Expressions [14.11] and [14.13].

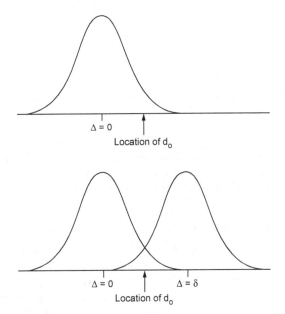

FIGURE 23.1
Location of d_0 in reference to distributions for original null hypothesis (upper drawing) and for alternative hypothesis (lower drawing).

The actual difference between the two SEDs, however, is usually small and inconsequential (see Section 14.4.2). For example, although the SED was calculated as SED_0 in Section 23.1.2.2.2, the procedure was aimed at rejecting the alternative hypothesis that $\Delta \geq \delta$. Consequently, the calculation should have used SED_H, which would have been $\sqrt{(14)(15)/29^3 + (12)(16)/28^3} = .132$. The result (at three decimal places), however, is the same as the previously calculated $SED_0 = .132$.

In many ensuing discussions in this text, the SED symbol will be used in a general way, regardless of which formula it comes from. For illustrative calculations, SED_H will be used when it is particularly pertinent, but SED_0 will often be preferred because of its greater general applicability. A single calculation for SED_0 has the advantage of letting the same confidence interval sometimes be used, as in Section 23.1.2.2.2, for checking both the null hypothesis (in the lower boundary) and the alternative hypothesis (in the upper boundary).

23.4.3 Determining Z_H and P_H Values

Using the alternative hypothesis, the symbols Z_H and P_H will correspond to the Z_0 and P_0 obtained with the ordinary null hypothesis. For comparing two groups, the alternative Z values will come from the formula

$$Z_H = (\delta - d_0)/SED \qquad [23.3]$$

With the alternative SED_H calculated for two proportions, the formula will be

$$Z_H = \frac{\delta - d_0}{\sqrt{\dfrac{p_A q_A}{n_A} + \dfrac{p_B q_B}{n_B}}} \qquad [23.4]$$

For example, in a clinical trial where $p_A = 9/18$ and $p_B = 8/17$, so that $d_o = .500 - .471 = .029$, the value of SED_H under the alternative hypothesis will be

$$\sqrt{[(9)(9)/18^3] + [(8)(9)/17^3]} = .169$$

If δ is designated as .15,

$$Z_H = \frac{.15 - .029}{.169} = .716$$

The values of Z_H are interpreted as P values in exactly the same way as under the conventional null hypothesis. At the Gaussian value of $Z_H = .716$, the two-tailed P_H is .47. Thus, there is a two-tailed chance of .47, and a one-tailed chance of .235, that the observed result of $d_o = .029$ came from a population in which the true difference was as large as .15.

23.4.4 Role of β

For the original null hypothesis, the α level establishes the boundary of *α-error* or *Type I error* for false positive conclusions if a correct hypothesis is rejected. For the alternative hypothesis, a corresponding level, called β, establishes the boundary of *β-error* or *Type II error* for the relative frequency of wrong decisions if a correct alternative hypothesis is rejected. If H_H is true, its rejection would lead to the false negative conclusion that the two groups are not substantially different, when in fact they are.

Table 23.1 shows the use of α and β levels in reasoning for the *original null-hypothesis decision*. If the null hypothesis that $\Delta = 0$ is correct, there is an α chance that rejection is wrong, and a $1 - \alpha$ chance that concession is right. If the true state of affairs is $\Delta = \delta$, however, concession of the *original null hypothesis* has a β chance of being wrong, and rejection has a $1 - \beta$ chance of being correct.

TABLE 23.1

α, β, and Accuracy of Stochastic Decisions for Null Hypothesis

Conclusion RE Stochastic Hypothesis That $\Delta = 0$	True State of Reality	
	$\Delta = \delta$	$\Delta = 0$
Reject	True Positive Conclusion $(1 - \beta)$	False Positive Conclusion (α)
Concede	False Negative Conclusion (β)	True Negative Conclusion $(1 - \alpha)$

23.4.5 Analogy to Diagnostic Marker Tests

The statistical parlance does not use the language of diagnostic marker decisions, but the concepts are almost identical. Suppose a pap smear is done as a diagnostic marker test for a cancer. If the pap smear result agrees with the definitive tissue biopsy, the pap smear conclusion is either a true positive or true negative. If the pap smear and biopsy disagree, the original conclusion is either falsely positive or falsely negative.

23.4.5.1 *False Positive Conclusions* —

If the null hypothesis is rejected with $P_o < \alpha$, there is still a probability of P_o that the rejection is wrong. The selected value of α is the upper boundary of risk for the false positive conclusion. Thus, if α is set at .05 and stochastic significance is proclaimed when $P_o = .049$, the two groups may still be truly similar, and the probability is .049 that the decision is wrong. With α set at a higher level of .1, the quantitative range of false positive conclusions is expanded. The two groups might really be similar and the decision that they are different might be wrong in .03, .06, .08, .09, or .099 of the occasions when the null hypothesis is rejected at the corresponding values of $P < .1$.

When α is set as the boundary of "risk" for a false positive decision, the level of $1 - \alpha$ is analogous to the *specificity* of a diagnostic test. In previous usage, $1 - \alpha$ helped establish the boundaries of a confidence interval. In the application here, $1 - \alpha$ helps denote the relative "confidence" attached to a stochastic decision to *concede* the null hypothesis.

23.4.5.2 *False Negative Conclusions* — If the original null hypothesis is rejected as false, we infer that the parent universe has a big distinction (at least as big as the observed d_o), rather than none. If the null hypothesis is conceded, however, and if the parent universe really does have a big distinction, the concession will be a false-negative conclusion. Because β is set as the permissible frequency of false-negative conclusions, the value of $1 - \beta$ is analogous to the *sensitivity* of a diagnostic test.

23.4.5.3 *Role of Horizontal "Gap"* — When "vertical" indexes of sensitivity and specificity are used in diagnostic decisions (see Chapter 21), we cannot immediately make "horizontal" appraisals of accuracy, because the prevalence of diseased cases will vary in different clinical situations. An analogous problem prevents horizontal conclusions in stochastic decisions, but the problem does not arise from prevalence. The stochastic problem is caused by the numerical gap that separates $\Delta = 0$ from $\Delta = \delta$ in Table 23.1. If the observed value of d_o lies in the intermediate zone where $0 < d_o < \delta$, we might have to concede (or reject) *both* the original null *and* the alternative hypotheses.

23.4.6   Choice of β

Stated as $\Delta \geq \delta$, the alternative hypothesis obviously has a clear direction and could therefore be tested with a one-tailed choice of β. Accordingly, for a .05 level of rejection, Z_β could be set at $Z_{.1} = 1.645$.

The concept becomes important if confidence intervals are used to examine both the null and the alternative hypotheses. In previous examples, this examination was done with a "single" arrangement, constructed as

$$d_o \pm Z_\alpha(\text{SED}_o)$$

A more accurate approach, however, would require two arrangements:

$$d_o - Z_\alpha(\text{SED}_o)$$

would be used to locate the lower border, and

$$d_o + Z_\beta(\text{SED}_H)$$

would indicate the upper border.

If the alternative hypothesis is $\Delta \geq \delta$, a one-tailed 95% confidence interval can be used to check the upper border, which will be enlarged if calculated with a two-tailed Z_α, rather than with a one-tailed Z_β. Unless the original *null* hypothesis was clearly expressed in advance as $\Delta > 0$ or $\Delta < 0$, however, a one-tailed calculation is not appropriate for the *lower* border of the confidence interval.

[This distinction led to a major legal battle between the U.S. tobacco industry and the Environmental Protection Agency (EPA), which had done a meta-analysis of results for lung cancer attributed to environmental tobacco exposure (i.e., "passive smoking"). Certain crucial odds ratios that were not stochastically significant in two-tailed 95% confidence intervals, calculated with $Z_\alpha = 1.96$, became "significant" when the EPA's 90% confidence intervals, calculated with $Z_\alpha = 1.645$, excluded the null value of 1 from the *lower* border. The tobacco industry contended that substituting 90% for the customary 95% criterion was a political rather than scientific decision. (The argument included other scientific disputes beyond the accusation of "rigged" confidence intervals.)]

Both the lower and upper margins of confidence intervals should be examined when investigators either claim stochastic significance in rejecting $\Delta = 0$, or argue that the upper level of "risk" might be much higher than what was found in the observed d_o. Rejection of $\Delta = 0$ is easier if the interval is calculated with a one-tailed Z_α; the converse claims of a potentially larger d_o are facilitated with a two-tailed Z_β.

23.5 The Concept of "Power"

The unfamiliar term *capacity* was used in Section 23.2 to refer to group sizes that were too small to do the desired job of rejecting the original null hypothesis when d_o was "big." *Capacity* is an unfamiliar word, because statisticians regularly use the term *power* in reference to the adequacy of group (or sample) sizes. The idea of *power*, however, refers to the ability to reject the alternative, rather than the null, stochastic hypothesis.

23.5.1   Statistical Connotation of "Power"

In the customary "test of significance," a big distinction has been observed, and the stochastic question is "How small might it have been?" If the P_o value exceeds α, or if the lower end of a $1 - \alpha$ confidence interval includes the null hypothesis value of 0, the distinction is not stable enough for its "quantitative significance" to be confirmed stochastically.

The "other side of statistical significance" is examined when the observed distinction is small, or obviously not big, i.e., $d_o < \delta$. The stochastic question is then "How large might it have been?" This question can be answered with a direct counterpart of the former reasoning. If the P_H value exceeds β, or if the upper end of a $1 - \beta$ confidence interval includes the alternative hypothesis value of δ, the quantitative "nonsignificance" is not confirmed. Although small, the observed distinction might really be big. Thus, rejection of the alternative stochastic hypothesis is intended to confirm that the observed small distinction is really small.

Although the ability of a group size to reject a stochastic hypothesis is often called "power," the statistical definition of *power* is much more constrained. When δ and β are set in advance, $1 - \beta$ is called the statistical power to reject the alternative hypothesis that $\Delta \geq \delta$. This prospective concept of power is also sometimes applied in retrospect, after a study is completed. When Z_H is determined from Formula [23.4] and converted to P_H, the value of $1 - P_H$ may be called "power."

The latter usage of "power" has been vigorously disputed,[10] however, because the strict definition requires a single boundary value of δ that was designated *before* the research began. This "prospective" boundary is often not established, however; and in its absence, the investigator or data analyst can retrospectively make various choices of δ. Each choice would yield different results for Z_H and for the $1 - P_H$ value of "power." For example, consider the clinical trial in Section 23.4.3, where $P_A = 9/18$, $P_B = 8/17$, $d_o = .029$, and $SED_H = .169$. When δ was chosen to be .15, $Z_H = .716$, and the one-tailed value of $1 - P_H$ was $1 - .235 = .765$. If δ is set at .10, $Z_H = .420$, $2P_H = .674$, and $1 - P_H = .663$. If δ is set at .20, $Z_H = 1.01$, $2P_H = .312$, and $1 - P_H = .844$. To get an impressively high value of power, we could set δ at .32. Z_H would then be 1.72, $2P_H = .085$, and $1 - P_H = .9575$.

With these arbitrary retrospective choices of δ, however, "power" would become a type of "variable," rather than a distinctive, fixed attribute of the study. The opponents of this retrospective manipulation of "power" argue that the best way to answer the retrospective question, "How big might it have been?" is with an appropriate confidence interval (or perhaps a form of Bayesian strategy). Thus, in the foregoing example, Z_β would be 1.645 for the upper end of a one-tailed 95% confidence interval, constructed around d_o as

$$.029 + (1.645)(.169) = .307.$$

With this result, we could "rule out" the possibility that d_o was as large as .32, but not that it might be as large as .30.

23.5.2   Comparison of "Capacity" and "Power"

Because *power* refers to the alternative hypothesis, the term *capacity* was introduced here for the ability of a group (or sample) size to achieve "single significance" by rejecting the original stochastic hypothesis. If the scientific goal of the research is to find something big, the original stochastic hypothesis is $\Delta = 0$;

and the proportion of capacity calculated in Section 23.2 indicates how close the group size came to what would have been needed to confirm $d_o \geq \delta$ under the original null hypothesis.

Power, however, refers to the ability to reject the alternative hypothesis that $\Delta \geq \delta$. For capacity, Z_o is converted directly to P_o under the null hypothesis; for power, Z_H is converted directly to P_H under the alternative hypothesis, and $1 - P_H$ might then be called *power*.

23.5.3 Example of Complaints and Confusion

The confusion between capacity and power was demonstrated in a fervent exchange of letters called "Statistical problems with small sample size." The original investigators[11] found that the mean volumes (per cm^3) of the fourth ventricle in magnetic resonance imaging were 1.11 in 12 autistic patients and 0.99 in 12 controls. When the t test showed P < .10, the investigators concluded that their results did not confirm earlier findings of abnormal fourth ventricles in autism. This conclusion was disputed[12] after the increment of 0.12 and common standard deviation of 0.18 were used to calculate that the effect size (~ .12/.18) had a quantitatively significant value of 0.69. The opponents then claimed that the results had low power, with only "a 37% chance of rejecting" the alternative hypothesis.

In fact, however, with only 24 patients in the study, the standard error of the observed difference is $.18/\sqrt{(12)(12)/24} = .073$, and the original Z_o for the null hypothesis is $.12/.073 = 1.633$. If the Z_α required for stochastic significance with the original null hypothesis was 1.96, then the required minimum sample size for each group, according to Formula [13.19], would have been $n = 2(1.96)^2 (.18)^2/(.12)^2 = 17.3$. With 24 patients observed and about 35 required, the study had a proportionate capacity of only about $24/35 = .69$. Thus, if the observed effect size was "large," the study was defective in its original capacity to reject the null hypothesis. The idea of "power" was not required to complain that the study was too small.

On the other hand, in responding to the complaint about too-low power, the original investigator[13] said that the sample size had been calculated in anticipation of the much higher effect-size values (0.81 and 1.21) reported in previous research. The observed increment of 0.12, with its effect size of only 0.69, was therefore dismissed as quantitatively insignificant, regarded as "not a clinically valuable result." Nevertheless, a one-tailed 95% confidence interval for the upper border of the result would yield $0.12 + (1.645)(.073)$ and would extend to .24, which would have an impressive effect size of $.24/.18 = 1.33$.

23.5.4 Reciprocity of Z_o and Z_H

Regardless of whether the aim is capacity or power, Z_H is calculated in the same way with Formula [23.3]; and Z_H has a special relationship both to Z_o and to the value of Z_δ that occurs at δ. If the three values of Z_o, Z_δ, and Z_H are respectively calculated as d_o/SED, δ/SED, and $(\delta - d_o)/SED$, Figure 23.2 shows that the values of Z_o and Z_H will be additively reciprocal in the relationship

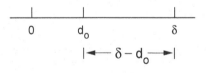

$$Z_o + Z_H = Z_\delta \qquad [23.5]$$

For fixed values of δ and Z_δ, Z_H must go down as Z_o goes up, and vice versa. This relationship between Z_o and Z_H is also analogous to diagnostic specificity and sensitivity. As one of the diagnostic indexes rises for a particular set of test results, the other must fall.

In general, large values of Z_o, which allow the null hypothesis to be rejected, will be accompanied by small values of Z_H, which allow the alternative hypothesis to be conceded. Conversely, small values of Z_o, which allow

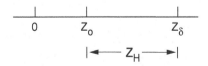

FIGURE 23.2

Relationship of the three Z values (lower line) that correspond to d_o and δ (upper line).

concession of the null hypothesis, will be accompanied by large values of Z_H, allowing rejection of the alternative hypothesis.

Statistically, because *confidence* is often used for the level of $1 - \alpha$ (or $1 - P_o$), and power for the level of $1 - \beta$ (or $1 - P_H$), we can note that confidence goes up as Z_o increases (making P_o smaller) and power goes up as Z_H increases (making P_H smaller). Because of the reciprocity of Z_o and Z_H at a fixed level of Z_δ, however, an ordinary ("single significance") sample size is likely to produce high confidence and low power, or low confidence and high power.

The goal of the "doubly significant" sample size, discussed shortly, is to produce both high confidence *and* high power.

23.6 Neyman-Pearson Strategy

Before beginning the research, an investigator hoping to show a big distinction would ordinarily calculate a stochastically significant sample size, using the formulas discussed earlier in Sections 13.9.1 and 14.5.4. If this calculation was not done and if the too small group size showed a big distinction that was not confirmed stochastically, the deficit in group size could be determined with an assessment of capacity. This strategy for assessing capacity seems scientifically straightforward and reflects the way in which most investigators might approach their quantitative challenges if uncommitted to any mathematical doctrines.

This straightforward approach has not been generally used during the past few decades, however, because of the dominance of a different strategy that is often called *Neyman-Pearson hypothesis testing*. The eponym commemorates Jerzy Neyman (a Polish statistician) and Egon S. Pearson (son of Karl Pearson), who first described[14] the principles in 1928. The Neyman-Pearson strategy uses a type of diagnostic "decision analysis," in which a single boundary value, set at δ, creates two zones. One zone contains the "big" distinction where d_o is $\geq \delta$; the other is the "small" zone where $d_o < \delta$. In the Neyman-Pearson approach, δ is statistically regarded as a perfect single boundary, separating "big" from "small."

23.6.1   Calculation of "Doubly Significant" Sample Size

With δ as a single demarcation for "big" and "small" zones, the Neyman-Pearson calculation of sample size is intended to provide a "doubly significant" stochastic confirmation, no matter which way the observed results may go. If d_o turns out to be big, i.e., $\geq \delta$, the value of P_o determined from Z_o should allow rejection of the original null hypothesis. If d_o turns out to be small, i.e., $< \delta$, the value of P_H determined from Z_H should allow rejection of the alternative hypothesis.

23.6.1.1   Z Procedures — The customary method of calculating a doubly significant sample size is to use Z procedures for P values. (The same result and the same calculational formula can be obtained with a confidence-interval approach.) To allow rejection of the null and alternative hypotheses, the sample size should let $Z_o \geq Z_\alpha$ if d_o turns out to be $\geq \delta$, and $Z_H \geq Z_\beta$ if $d_o < \delta$.

Before calculating the size of each group for a comparison of two proportions, we first consider a potential observed d_o, and the value of Z_o that will be determined under the null hypothesis as

$$Z_o = \frac{d_o}{\sqrt{2PQ/n}} \qquad [23.6]$$

For determining sample size, P is estimated as π (with the "^" hat omitted for simplicity) and Z_o is set equal to Z_α. With these designations, Formula [23.6] becomes

$$Z_\alpha = \frac{d_o}{\sqrt{2\pi(1-\pi)/n}} \qquad [23.7]$$

When the observed d_0 is tested under the alternative hypothesis, the calculation (letting $SED_H = SED_0$) will be

$$Z_H = \frac{\delta - d_0}{\sqrt{2PQ/n}} \qquad [23.8]$$

For estimating sample size, we revert to Greek parameters, and we want $Z_H \geq Z_\beta$. The result in Formula [23.8] will be stochastically significant if

$$Z_\beta \leq \frac{\delta - d_0}{\sqrt{2\pi(1-\pi)/n}} \qquad [23.9]$$

To take care of both stochastic goals, we solve Formula [23.7] for d_0, and then substitute its value into Formula [23.9]. When carried out, the algebra produces

$$Z_\beta\sqrt{2\pi(1-\pi)/n} \leq \delta - Z_\alpha\sqrt{2\pi(1-\pi)/n}$$

which becomes

$$(Z_\beta + Z_\alpha)\sqrt{2\pi(1-\pi)/n} \leq \delta$$

Squaring both sides, and solving for n leads to

$$n \geq \frac{(Z_\alpha + Z_\beta)^2[2\pi(1-\pi)]}{\delta^2} \qquad [23.10]$$

In many statistics books, Formula [23.10] is regularly cited as the method of calculating a "doubly significant" Neyman-Pearson sample size.

23.6.1.2 *Formula for Calculation with SED$_0$ and SED$_H$* —
Formula [23.10] was developed with the assumption that SED was the same for both hypotheses. For greater precision under the alternative hypothesis, however, the value of $\sqrt{2\pi(1-\pi)/n}$ in Formula [23.9] would be replaced by $\sqrt{[\pi_A(1-\pi_A) + \pi_B(1-\pi_B)]/n}$. After appropriate substitution, rearrangement, and solving for n, Formula [23.10] would be replaced by

$$n \geq \frac{\left[Z_\alpha\sqrt{2\pi(1-\pi)} + Z_\beta\sqrt{\pi_A(1-\pi_A) + \pi_B(1-\pi_B)}\right]^2}{\delta^2} \qquad [23.11]$$

This formula is preferred by many statisticians because it uses the "correct" standard error for each stochastic hypothesis.

In Formula [23.11], the value of π is usually estimated with $(\pi_A + \pi_B)/2$, not with the π_B value employed as a "compromise choice" when sample size was calculated earlier for "single significance" in Section 14.5.4.1. Probably the main reason for this custom is the esthetic mathematical appeal of symmetry. With π_A and π_B symmetrically cited in the "double significance" formula, an asymmetrical choice for π would not be "elegant." Besides, in deference to reality when the research is actually done, the common value of P that corresponds to π will be calculated not with p_B, but with $(p_A + p_B)/2$ [or with $(n_Ap_A + n_Bp_B)/N$].

23.6.2   Example of Calculations

In a forthcoming clinical trial, suppose we expect π_B to be .33, set δ at .15, and then choose a two-tailed $Z_\alpha = 1.96$ and a one-tailed $Z_\beta = 1.645$.

Because π_A is expected to be .48, we can let the anticipated π be $(.33 + .48)/2 = .405$ and $1 - \pi = .595$. Substituting into Formula [23.10], we get

$$n = \frac{(1.96 + 1.645)^2 [2(.405)(.595)]}{(.15)^2} = 278.4$$

The trial would therefore need at least 279 persons in each group, for a total sample size of 558.
     With Formula [23.11], the result would be

$$n = \frac{\left[1.96\sqrt{2(.405)(.595)} + 1.645\sqrt{(.33)(.67) + (.48)(.52)} \right]^2}{(.15)^2} = 275.4$$

If π were anticipated as π_B, the value of $(.405)(.595) = .241$ in the foregoing formula would be replaced by $(.33)(.67) = .221$. After the rest of the calculation is carried out, n would be 262.9.

23.6.3   Use of Tables

All of the cited computations can be avoided by using appropriately prepared tables, such as Table A.3 (260–280) of the textbook by Fleiss.[15] Fleiss cites values of α and "power" for $1 - \beta$, and he uses P_1 and P_2 as symbols for what have here been called π_A and π_B (or p_A and p_B). The values in the Fleiss table are slightly higher than what would be obtained with Formula [23.11] because he applies a "continuity correction." If n' is the result obtained with Formula [23.11], the continuity correction converts the final sample size to

$$n = (n'/4) \left\{ 1 + \sqrt{1 + [4/(n'\delta)]} \right\}^2 \qquad\qquad [23.12]$$

where $\delta = |\pi_A - \pi_B|$.
     For example, suppose we set $\pi_B = .30$, $\delta = .15$, $\pi_A = .45$, two-tailed $\alpha = .05$ and one-tailed $\beta = .1$. The value of π would be estimated as $(.30 + .45)/2 = .375$ and $1 - \pi$ would be .625. With Formula [23.11], we would get

$$n' = \frac{\left[1.96\sqrt{2(.375)(.625)} + 1.22\sqrt{(.30)(.70) + (.45)(.55)} \right]^2}{(.15)^2} = 216.9$$

With the continuity correction, this becomes

$$n = (216.9/4) \left\{ 1 + \sqrt{1 + [4/(216.9)(.15)]} \right\}^2 = 230$$

which is the result listed in Fleiss's Table A.3 for the values used in this example.
     Fleiss also offers a "short-cut" formula, which calculates n as $n' + (2/\delta)$. In this instance, where $\delta = .15$ and $2/\delta = 13.3$, the result would be $n = 216.9 + 13.3 = 230.2$, a value almost identical to what was found with the cumbersome Formula [23.12].

23.7 Problems in Neyman-Pearson Strategy

The *Neyman-Pearson* strategy of "double significance" has been used to calculate the size of many large-scale clinical trials during the past few decades. The strategy became particularly popular after the 1978 publication of an influential paper,[16] showing that many published clinical trials reaching a "negative" conclusion were undersized, having a high potential for "beta error" in conceding the null hypothesis and perhaps "missing an important therapeutic improvement."

Unfortunately, the authors of the influential paper did not distinguish between trials that were "singly undersized" and those that were "doubly undersized." In a singly undersized trial, the problem is low capacity. The group size may not have been large enough to reject the null hypothesis even if the observed d_0 is $\geq \delta$. This type of problem would be easily avoided by calculating an advance sample size with the simple Formula [14.19] or [14.20]. If prophylaxis of the *singly* undersized problem leads to the use of Formula [23.10] or [23.11], however, several new problems are created in mathematics, science, and pragmatic realities.

23.7.1 Mathematical Problems

The mathematical problems in the "double-significance" strategy are inflated sample sizes, declarations of stochastic significance for values of d_0 much smaller than the original goal of $d_0 \geq \delta$, and violation of the principle that pre-established decision boundaries should not be altered after the research is done.

23.7.1.1 Inflated Sample Size — Regardless of whether α has a one-tailed or two-tailed direction, the sample sizes for "double significance" are several times larger than what is ordinarily needed to reject the null hypothesis if $d_0 \geq \delta$.

For example, suppose π_B is estimated at .33 and δ is set at .15, as in Section 23.2. If only the null hypothesis is considered, the sample size for a two-tailed $Z_\alpha = 1.96$ turns out to be about 83 persons in each group. With both the null and alternative hypotheses taken into account, however, the sample size becomes between 3 and 4 times larger, at 279 persons in each group with Formula [23.10], and 276 persons with Formula [23.11].

If Formula [23.10] is divided by the earlier Formula [15.19], the result shows that sample size is enlarged by a factor of

$$\frac{(Z_\alpha + Z_\beta)^2}{Z_\alpha^2} = \left(1 + \frac{Z_\beta}{Z_\alpha}\right)^2 \qquad [23.13]$$

If $Z_\beta/Z_\alpha = 1.645/1.96 = .839$, the "doubly significant" sample will be $(1 + .839)^2 = 3.38$ times the size of the "singly significant" sample.

23.7.1.2 Deflated Boundary for Quantitative Significance — Although the trial is planned with the idea that *quantitative* significance requires $d_0 \geq \delta$, the inflated sample size will regularly allow *stochastic* significance to be attained with $d_0 < \delta$. Thus, a difference that was originally regarded as too small to be quantitatively significant may emerge as stochastically significant.

For example, consider the clinical trial discussed in Section 23.6.2, where the calculated sample-size values ranged from 263 to 279 for each group. Suppose we try to enroll more than 290 patients in each group, having added a few more people for "insurance." After the trial is done, we are chagrined that only 240 patients were obtained in each group, despite vigorous recruiting efforts. The chagrin turns to despair when we find that $p_B = 79/240 = .329$ and $p_A = 100/240 = .417$, so that $d_0 = .088$, which is substantially below the desired $\delta \geq .15$.

The despair soon turns to elation, however, after the stochastic tests work their magic. For these results, the standard error for the null hypothesis will be calculated as

$$\sqrt{(179)(301)/[(480)(240)(240)]} = .044$$

and Z_0 will be $.088/.044 = 2.00$, which exceeds the Z_α of 1.96 needed for two-tailed stochastic signifi-cance. Although the observed d_0 of .088 will be substantially smaller than $\delta = .15$, the investigators will almost surely claim to have found a "significant" result. (The term "delta wobble" has been applied[17] to the retroactive lowering of δ that allows a stochastically confirmed d_0 to be called "significant.")

If we let n_0 and n_D represent the sample sizes calculated respectively for "single" and for "double" significance, the algebraic mechanism that produces the elation was shown in Formula [23.13]. Because n_D is larger than n_0 by a factor of $[1 + (Z_\beta/Z_\alpha)]^2$, stochastic significance can be achieved with an observed difference, d_0, that is smaller than δ by a factor of $Z_\beta/(Z_\alpha + Z_\beta)$. If $Z_\alpha = 1.96$ and $Z_\beta = 1.645$, this factor will be $1.96/3.605 = .54$.

23.7.1.3 *Violation of Advance Demarcation* — When "significance" is declared despite the finding that $d_0 < \delta$, the advance demarcation of boundaries has been violated as a prime principle of stochastic testing. According to this principle, all decisional boundary values should be fixed *before* the results are observed and should not be changed afterward with a "delta wobble."

For example, to avoid manipulation of α after the research results are analyzed, many statisticians insist that α always be two-tailed, although a one-tailed direction is regularly acceptable for β. Regardless of whether α and β are one-tailed or two-tailed, however, almost everyone agrees that their pre-established level should *not* be altered afterward to fit the observed data. Nevertheless, the pre-established level of δ, which might be expected to have a similar sanctity, is frequently altered to fit the observed results. It becomes adjusted downward to comply with whatever value of d_0 turned out to be stochas-tically significant.

An example of the problems occurred when Kronmal[18] complained that a pre-established α was changed from the .01 level, used in the originally calculated sample size, to the .05 level used for interpreting results in the famous Lipid Research Clinics Coronary Primary Prevention Trial.[19] The investigators defended[20] the change of α by stating that the original level was chosen for sample size calculations "that would be desirable for ensuring greater credibility"; but that after the trial, $\alpha = .01$ was "not relevant to the issue at hand." The investigators argued that the "results" would be no more convincing "had α been set at .1 in these preliminary calculations; they would be no less convincing had α been set at .001." Because the investigators also noted, however, that "the observed reductions in ... CHD incidence ... were ... only about half as great as those assumed in the sample size computation," a sample size calculated with $\alpha = .1$ would probably not have been large enough to provide $P < .05$ in the observed results.

23.7.2 Scientific Problems

Several scientific problems in the double-significance approach will be discussed later in Chapter 24. The three main problems noted now are that the results are often reported as incomplete truths, that the observed d_0 is *forced* to be $< \delta$ in the calculations, and that the calculated results are cited in an almost inscrutable phrasing.

23.7.2.1 *"Incomplete Truth" in Reporting* — Having done all the work of conducting the trial in the belief that Treatment A is better than B, an investigator may not want to admit that the observed distinction is much smaller than desired, particularly if it is stochastically significant. Conse-quently, ignoring the originally established value of δ, the investigators will usually conclude that Treatment A is "significantly" better than B.

The report becomes an example of incomplete "truth in reporting" — the claims are correct stochas-tically but not strictly correct quantitatively. The issue is a matter of scientific taste rather than morality, however, because the investigators can usually re-express things to convince themselves (as well as reviewers and readers) that the relatively unimpressive increment is really impressive. For example, in Section 23.7.1.2, the observed direct increment of .088, although smaller than the desired $\delta = .15$, will seem much more impressive if cited as a proportionate increment of $.088/.329 = 27\%$.

The occurrence of the "incomplete-truth" phenomenon can be discerned if you review the published literature of randomized trials. Whenever the investigators report a "significant" result without citing the level of δ that was originally used for the sample-size calculations, you can suspect that the observed value of d_0 was $< \delta$.

23.7.2.2 Forcing d_0 to Be $< \delta$ —

A striking scientific oddity in calculating "doubly significant" sample sizes is that the statistical strategy forces the anticipated value of d_0 to be $< \delta$ in the calculation. Rejecting the null hypothesis requires that $d_0 - Z_\alpha \, (SED_0) \geq 0$; and rejecting the alternative hypothesis requires that $d_0 + Z_\beta \, (SED_H) \leq \delta$. Thus, d_0 must be simultaneously $\geq Z_\alpha \, (SED_0)$ and $\leq \delta - Z_\beta \, (SED_H)$. If we let $SED_0 = SED_H$, and if we ignore the unequal parts of these two Formulas, the two equations can be added and solved to show that

$$2d_0 \simeq \delta + (Z_\alpha - Z_\beta)SED$$

If $Z_\alpha = Z_\beta$, then $d_0 \simeq \delta/2$ and is forced to be half the value of δ. If $Z_\alpha = 1.96$ and $Z_\beta = 1.645$, d_0 is slightly larger, at $\delta/2 + [(.315)(SED)/2]$. For example, if $\delta = .15$ and $SED = .169$, as in Section 23.4.3, then $(.315)(.169) = .05$, and $d_0 = (.15 + .05)/2 = .10$. If $SED = .132$, as in Section 23.1.2.2.2, $d_0 = (.15 + .04)/2 = .095$. If $SED = .049$, as in Section 23.3.2, $d_0 = (.15 + .015)/2 = .083$. In each instance, the two stochastic demands can be satisfied only if d_0 is substantially smaller than δ.

This constraint on d_0 was not overtly specified earlier when we solved Formula [23.7] for d_0, and substituted it into Formula [23.9] to produce the doubly-significant sample size Formula [23.10]. A careful examination of the required location of d_0, however, shows that the "doubly significant" sample size also becomes a mechanism for getting stochastic significance *under the null hypothesis* for quantitatively nonsignificant values of $d_0 < \delta$.

The mechanism is responsible for the scientific inconsistencies of the mathematical problems cited earlier. Having originally stated in the sample-size calculation that d_0 must equal or exceed δ to be quantitatively "significant," the investigator then makes that same claim paradoxically when d_0 turns out to be $< \delta$.

23.7.2.3 Unfamiliar Numerical Statements —

After the double-significance calculations are completed, the attempt to put α, β, and δ into a single statement often produces prose that seems like an inscrutable jumble of numbers. The statement will say something like "The result will have a 90% chance of detecting a difference of .15 at the 5% level." In this statement, power is $.90 = 1 - \beta$, for a δ level of .15, tested at an α level of .05.

The statement is difficult to comprehend because it no longer resembles the language and ideas of diagnostic marker tests. In diagnostic-marker language, the results are given a single "horizontal" diagnostic summary, which is a simple statement of predictive accuracy. Whether obtained directly or with Bayesian combinations of sensitivity, specificity, and prevalence, the final diagnostic statement cites one number, not three. The statistical statement for "double significance," however, does not come out as one number. It achieves the counterpart of the "horizontal" diagnostic phrase by specifying three numbers that correspond to sensitivity (i.e., $1 - \beta$), specificity (i.e., the $1 - \alpha$ complement of α), and, instead of prevalence, the gap (δ) that separates the null and alternative hypotheses.

A clearer way to communicate this information would be first to determine the estimated level of $\hat{d}_0$ at which the null hypothesis ($\Delta = 0$) will be rejected for the calculated sample size. For example, if $\hat{d}_0 = .08$, the statement would say that "If the observed difference is $\geq .08$, stochastic significance will be confirmed by $P < .05$; otherwise, the P value will be $< .1$ for the possibility that the difference exceeds .15."

23.7.3 Additional Scientific Problems

Four other scientific problems in "double significance" and "power" will be saved for discussion in Chapter 24. These problems arise as peculiarities in calculating "power" for a goal at which the investigator is not aiming, in assuming that the investigator does not care what happens in the research as long as a stochastic hypothesis can be rejected, in using a black-and-white-but-no-gray partition that divides all quantitative magnitudes into being either **big** or **small**, and in permitting "power" to be calculated retroactively with highly arbitrary methods.

23.8 Pragmatic Problems

Despite exact precision in the mathematical formulas, sample sizes are regularly augmented prophylactically for the type of "insurance" discussed earlier in Section 14.6.5. The magnificent numerical precision produced by the formulas can then be raised arbitrarily to values that are larger by 10%, 20%, or more.

23.8.1 "Lasagna's Law" for Clinical Trials

A different sample-size problem in clinical trials arises from recruiting rather than calculating. Regardless of what the basic and "insurance-augmented" sizes may be, the trial will be unsuccessful if enough patients cannot be recruited.

As prophylaxis for this problem, the investigator usually tries to estimate how many patients might be acquired, either at the local institution alone or with a consortium of several collaborating institutions. (The latter activity has several names. It can be called a *multi-center, multi-investigator, multi-institutional*, or *cooperative* study.) As past experience and medical records are reviewed to estimate the number of available patients, the investigators regularly fall prey to a fallacy, described by the clinical pharmacologist, Louis Lasagna, that has sometimes been called *Lasagna's Law*. It states that the number of patients who are actually available for a trial is about 1/10 to 1/3 of what was originally estimated.

The reason for this problem is scientific and pragmatic, not statistical. Planning to study Disease D, the investigators usually determine how many patients with that disease were seen at their institution during an appropriate time period. When offered as the estimate of potential candidates, this number does not take into account the depletions caused by eligibility criteria or by refusals to participate.

The obvious possibility of refusals is generally considered, but optimistic investigators may underestimate the proportion of reluctant candidates. The problems of eligibility, however, are usually much greater and more complex than those of refusal. Most clinical trials admit only an eligible subset of patients, not everyone who may have Disease D. The eligibility criteria may demand certain age limits, appropriate degrees of mild or advanced disease severity, the patient's ability to avoid or receive specified treatments, the absence of co-morbid diseases that might interfere with the study, and the presence of geographic or personal attributes that facilitate cooperation with the study's protocol. These restrictions in the eligibility criteria usually remove a much greater proportion of potential candidates than refusal of eligible persons to enter the study.

Consequently, an investigator who wants to avoid the pitfalls of Lasagna's Law will try to estimate the potential availability of eligible candidates, not just persons who have Disease D.

23.8.2 Clinical Scenario

The calculation of a doubly significant sample size in real-world research is commonly altered by a scenario that resembles the events described in Section 8.8.3. The calculation requires selection of Z_α and Z_β, choice of δ, and an estimate of π_B.

When asked to indicate δ and π_B, however, the clinician may say he does not know, but wants a "significant" result. Desperate to get some numbers, the statistician offers a guess such as $\pi_B = .20$ and $\delta = .10$ (the latter determined from $\theta = .5$). When the clinician says, "Sounds good," the statistician sets a two-tailed $Z_\alpha = 1.96$, a one-tailed $Z_\beta = 1.645$, and then uses Formula [23.10] to calculate

$$n = \frac{\left[1.96\sqrt{2(.25)(.75)} + 1.645\sqrt{(.30)(.70) + (.20)(.80)}\right]^2}{(.10)^2}$$

The result is n = 485, so that 2n = 970. When this large number is mentioned, the clinician says, "No way," and goes into a state of shock.

The statistician therefore tries a one-tailed $Z_\alpha = 1.645$ and, letting $\beta = .10$, uses a one-tailed $Z_\beta = 1.28$ to recalculate

$$n = \frac{\left[1.645\sqrt{2(.25)(.75)} + 1.28\sqrt{(.30)(.70) + (.20)(.80)}\right]^2}{(.10)^2}$$

The result is n = 319, so that 2n = 638. The clinician's response is, "Still can't be done."

The statistician then asks, "How many patients do you think you can get?" The clinician says, "About 200." With this "bottom line," the statistician asks if the achieved difference in $\delta = \pi_A - \pi_B$ might be as high as .20. The clinician says, "Why not?" Letting α and β stay where they were, the statistician then uses new values of π_A and π to calculate

$$n = \frac{\left[1.645\sqrt{2(.30)(.70)} + 1.28\sqrt{(.40)(.60) + (.20)(.80)}\right]^2}{(.20)^2}$$

The result is n = 88, so that 2n = 176. If the anticipated 200 patients can actually be obtained, the additional 24 patients will be "insurance." The clinician is delighted and tells all his colleagues how wonderful the statistician is, and the grant request is approved.

Everything eventually works out splendidly, but not quite as expected. The trial accrues only 160 patients, and p_B turns out to be 14/80 = .175, with p_A = 24/80 = .325, so that d_o is .15, rather than the anticipated $\delta = .20$. Nevertheless, because the initial "double-significance" calculations made the sample size so large, the result shows

$$Z_o = \frac{(.325 - .175)}{\sqrt{2(.25)(.75)/80}} = \frac{.15}{.0685} = 2.19$$

which is "statistically significant," with $P_o < .05$ in a two-tailed interpretation.

Everyone is jubilant.

23.9   Additional Topics

Beyond all of the cited problems, six additional topics warrant further comment before this long chapter ends. These topics are: the "power" of "single significance," the dilemma of stopping trials when $d_o < \delta$, the choice of relative values assigned to α and β, the possible usefulness of making stochastic decisions with a concept called "gamma error," some generally unpublicized objections by prominent statisticians to the Neyman-Pearson strategy, and some issues that involve scientific rather than mathematical considerations.

23.9.1   The "Power" of "Single Significance"

An investigator who ignores the Neyman-Pearson doctrine and who calculates sample size only for "single significance," using a formula such as [14.19], will regularly be told that the result will have "low power." The usual value cited for the low power is .5. The reason for this value is that if δ is the anticipated value for d_o, and if Z_α is chosen to be the anticipated value at Z_δ, a trial that turns out exactly as expected, with $d_o = \delta$, will have Z_o equal Z_α. Consequently, Z_H will equal 0 when calculated from either Formula [23.3] or [23.5]. For $Z_H = 0$, $2P_H = 1$ and the single-tailed interpretation will be $P_H = .5$, for which "power" will be $1 - P_H = .5$.

Traumatized by the threat of this low power, the investigator may accept the reassurance offered by a Neyman-Pearson calculation and arrange to get a much larger sample size. If the investigator really wants to show $d_0 \geq \delta$, however, the smaller "singly-significant" sample size would have ample capacity to provide stochastic significance if d_0 turns out to be $\geq \delta$. If d_0 turns out to be disappointingly $< \delta$, the investigator will be comforted by the almost certain inclusion of δ in the upper zone of the confidence interval, for reasons shown in Section 23.1.2.2.2.

Consequently, the only reason for transferring to the Neyman-Pearson calculation is if the investigator wants to reject the alternative hypothesis and confirm "insignificance" if d_0 is $< \delta$. This stochastic goal, however, is seldom what the investigator seeks in doing the trial. Because most investigators do not understand that the Neyman-Pearson calculation is aimed at such a goal, the statistical procedure is usually proposed and accepted without an adequately "informed consent."

23.9.2   Premature Cessation of Trials with $d_0 < \delta$

To avoid ethical problems, investigators usually want to end a long-term randomized trial as soon as it shows a "significant" difference. If this achievement occurs before accrual of the previously calculated sample size, the trial is stopped prematurely. Therefore, to check for "significance," the investigators may repeatedly "peek" at the accumulating results. The multiple "peeking" then leads to the multiple-comparison problem, discussed later in Chapter 25, which has evoked diverse statistical proposals for adjusting levels of α.

Because *stochastic* significance is almost always required before a trial is prematurely ended, the early termination would be unambiguous if the accumulating results show that d_0 is $> \delta$; such results will be "significant" both quantitatively and stochastically. Dissidence will occur, however, if an inflated sample size produces stochastic significance for $d_0 < \delta$ before the entire planned group has entered (or completed) the trial.

This dissidence, as well as the multiple-comparison stochastic problem, could be avoided if the investigators always insisted on quantitative significance, so that $d_0 \geq \delta$. With this demand, the repeated "peeks" at accruing data could simply examine the value of d_0 descriptively without doing any stochastic calculations. The stochastic tests would be withheld until the results show that $d_0 \geq \delta$. In the current approaches, however, achievement of stochastic significance is given priority, regardless of the magnitude of d_0. Consequently, the multiple-peek problem will continue to occur, accompanied by incomplete "truth-in-reporting," when trials are prematurely ended and then proclaimed stochastically significant for values of d_0 smaller than what was originally regarded as quantitatively significant.

23.9.3   Choice of Relative Values for α and β

Instead of making simple choices for the one- or two-tailed levels of α and β, data analysts may try to assign relative values according to the "seriousness" of Type I and Type II errors. In this mode of reasoning, as described by Fleiss[15] and by Cohen,[21] a Type I error is less serious "if the study is aimed only at adding to the body of published knowledge concerning some theory" than if the goal is "to replace a standard form of treatment with a new one." Thus, for investigators who believe that a "typical ... Type I error is some four times as serious as a Type II error," the value of β might be set at 4α. (This idea offers justification for setting α at .05 and β at .20.) If a Type I error is regarded as "less serious," however, α might be increased to .10.

23.9.4   Gamma-Error Strategy

An interesting but extreme mathematical view is the proposal by Schwartz and Lellouch[22] that α (Type I) and β (Type II) errors are sometimes relatively unimportant, and that the most serious (Type III) error is to draw a "significant" conclusion in the *wrong* direction. Thus, if the true parametric state of affairs is a directional $(\pi_A - \pi_B) \geq \delta$, the most serious error is to proclaim stochastic significance when the actual difference, $d_0 = p_A - p_B$ goes in the opposite direction and is $\leq -\delta$.

Emphasizing only the avoidance of a Type III error, Schwartz and Lellouch are willing to assign extremely relaxed values, such as $\alpha = 1$ and $1-\beta = 0$, for the usual two stochastic boundaries, but will put a strict requirement, such as .05, on the third stochastic boundary, called γ. For a Type III error, the incremental magnitude of the observed and expected differences will exceed $\delta - (-\delta) = 2\delta$. Using the corresponding Z_γ, the sample size can then be calculated so that

$$Z_\gamma \leq \frac{2\delta}{\sqrt{2\pi(1-\pi)/n}} \qquad [23.14]$$

The value of n becomes

$$n \geq \frac{Z_\gamma^2[2\pi(1-\pi)]}{4\delta^2}$$

Because the denominator contains $4\delta^2$ rather than δ^2, the sample size will be about one fourth of what would ordinarily be required with "one-way" significance at Z_α.

The gamma strategy will strongly appeal to investigators who would like to reduce the sample sizes (and costs) of clinical trials. Unfortunately, the small group sizes may make the subsequent results fail to achieve stochastic significance for the α and β decisions that continue to be demanded by most reviewers and readers. For example, suppose Z_γ is set at 1.645 for a unidirectional .05 level of γ, with $\delta = .15$ and $\pi_A = .33$. The sample size will be

$$n \geq \frac{(1.645)^2(2)(0.405)(.595)}{4(.15)^2} = 14.5$$

Suppose the investigator, ecstatic about the small sample size, decides to double it and enroll 30 people in each group.

If emerging even better than expected (in the desired direction), the results might show $p_B = 10/30 = .33$ and $p_A = 15/30 = .50$. The pooled value for the common P will be $(10+15)/(30+30)$; and the standard error will be $\sqrt{(25/60)(35/60)(60)/(30)(30)} = .127$. With a one-tailed Z_α set at 1.645, the confidence-interval component will be $(1.645)(.127) = .209$, and the interval calculated as $.17 \pm .209$ will include both 0 and δ. Although the γ hypothesis could be rejected, the customary α and β stochastic hypotheses would have to be conceded. Despite the quantitatively impressive $d_o \geq \delta$, the stochastic claim of "significance" would probably not be accepted.

23.9.5   Prominent Statistical Dissenters

The Neyman-Pearson "double-significance" strategy, which currently dominates the calculation of sample sizes for clinical trials, has been widely promulgated and accepted despite major reservations by prominent statisticians.

According to David Salsburg,[23] "R. A. Fisher was strongly opposed to this formulation. He did not believe that one can think of scientific research in terms of type I and type II errors. This type of thinking, he said, belongs in quality control, where the type I error rate predicts the number of good items rejected and the type II error rate predicts the number of bad items accepted." Fisher himself[24] said that the Neyman-Pearson principles come from "an unrealistic formalism" and "are liable to mislead those who follow them into much wasted effort and disappointment." Lehmann[25] more recently described the conflicts in the Fisher and Neyman-Pearson disputes about testing statistical hypotheses, and has proposed a "unified approach ... that combines the best features of both."

Kendall and Stuart[26] say the "crux of the paradox" in the Neyman-Pearson strategy is that "we can only fix two of the quantities, *n*, α, and β even in testing a simple H_o against a simple [alternative hypothesis]," but "we cannot obtain an optimum combination of α, β, and n for any given problem." According to Salsburg,[23] Sir David Cox believes that "We do not choose in advance a particular p-value for decision making. Rather, we use p-values to compare a number of different possible alternative hypotheses." W. E. Deming,[27] the "guru" of quality control procedures, contended that "there is no such thing as the power of a test in an analytic problem, despite all the pages covered by the mathematics of testing hypotheses."

Egon Pearson himself,[28] reviewing the basic issues over 30 years later, pointed out that the "Neyman-Pearson contributions" should be regarded not "as some static system" but as part of "the historical process of development of thought on statistical theory." Without overtly recanting the basic strategy, Pearson nevertheless confessed that "the emphasis which we gave to certain types of situations may now seem out of balance."

Despite these caveats from prominent leaders within the statistical profession, however, the ideas seem to have thoroughly triumphed in the world of medical research.

23.9.6   Scientific Goals for δ

The calculation of a doubly-significant sample size has even entered the realm of ethics. According to D. G. Altman,[29] "a sample that is too small will be unable to detect clinically important effects ... [and is] hence unethical in its use of subjects and other resources." Advocating a Neyman-Pearson approach, Altman said it will "make clinical importance and statistical significance coincide, thus avoiding a common problem of interpretation." Arguing against this idea, however, M.R. Clarke[30] stated that clinical importance and statistical significance "are two fundamentally philosophic concepts which cannot be made to coincide."

That the two concepts do *not* coincide is demonstrated by the frequent absence of statistical attention to an investigator's *scientific* hypothesis for the research. If the investigator hoped for a big difference, i.e., $d_0 \geq \delta$, and if it was found, the next step would be to confirm it stochastically. If the stochastic result was disappointing, i.e., $P > \alpha$, the power of the "nonsignificant" result would not have to be checked against an alternative hypothesis, because the observed d_0 was already larger than δ. The problem in this case is that the group size was too small, and the numerical deficit could easily be shown with a simple check of capacity.

A test of power would also be unnecessary if the investigator, wanting a big difference, found a disappointingly small one, i.e., $d_0 < \delta$. In this situation, not seeking rejection of the alternative hypothesis, the investigator would be happy to find that δ was included in a simple confidence interval. If the actual magnitude of d_0 is ignored, and if a result is deemed "nonsignificant" merely because $P > \alpha$, the calculated confidence interval will let both the investigator and the reader see how big the "nonsignificant" difference might have been.

To calculate a specific index of "power," however, the investigator must choose a value for δ, thereby addressing the challenge of setting a boundary for *quantitative* significance. Because this challenge has not been vigorously pursued — mainly because investigators have not insisted on it — the mathematical power games are usually played with the proportional-increment values of θ. To evaluate a quantitative distinction by examining only θ, however, is as unsatisfactory as evaluating a distribution of data from its central index only, without considering spread.

Until a better set of guidelines and criteria is developed for choosing δ, calculations of "power" will remain an interesting theoretical exercise that gives a "politically correct" acknowledgment to the Neyman-Pearson mathematical dogma, without the risk of any real scientific thought. As long as the choice of δ remains an intellectually underdeveloped territory, confidence intervals have the major advantage of reasonably answering the question "How big might it have been?" without any arbitrary calculations of "power."

23.9.7   Choosing an "Honest" δ

Although the use of confidence intervals can avoid decisions about "power" after the research is done, both δ and a mathematical strategy must be chosen to calculate sample sizes before the research begins. If the goal is to show a "small" difference, as discussed in Chapter 24, the usual strategy does not involve Neyman-Pearson reasoning, which is aimed mainly at finding a "big" difference, as in most clinical trials.

If the sample always has a large enough capacity to achieve "single significance" by rejecting the null hypothesis when $d_0 \geq \delta$, the main question is then whether the investigator will want to claim "significance," "insignificance," or neither, if the observed difference goes the other way, so that $d_0 < \delta$. The Neyman-Pearson strategy seems fundamentally unsatisfactory, therefore, because it substantially inflates the sample sizes needed for "single significance" if d_0 turns out to be $\geq \delta$; and it does not suitably cope with the scope of possible decisions if d_0 turns out to be smaller than δ, as noted in Chapter 24.

The main scientific challenge is to choose an "honest" value of δ that is fixed in advance and maintained thereafter. It should be the smallest distinction that will still be regarded as quantitatively significant. Thus, if d_o is deemed impressive at a value of .08 but not at .07, the "honest" δ should be set at .08. In many doubly significant calculations, however, δ has been inflated to levels of .10 or .20 so that the sample size, although also inflated, is kept to a feasible magnitude. Nevertheless, the size may be large enough to confer stochastic significance if d_o turns out to be .08. With an honest δ set at .08, however, a singly significant sample size, calculated with Formula [14.19] rather than Formula [23.10], will provide ample capacity to do the desired job.

Nevertheless, investigators who hope to get approval for their proposed clinical trials today and who know that the proposal will be reviewed according to "mainstream" statistical principles, will probably have to continue playing the Neyman-Pearson game until a better and more suitable strategy is created. Perhaps the best guideline for the new strategy was offered by Egon Pearson[31] himself: "Hitherto the user has been accustomed to accept the function of probability laid down by the mathematicians, but it would be good if he could take a larger share in formulating himself what are the practical requirements that the theory should satisfy in application." Establishing those requirements and developing the new strategy are fascinating challenges for collaborative clinical-biostatistical research.

References

1. Jacobson, 1992; 2. Farr, 1852; 3. Elmore, 1994a; 4. Gordon, 1983; 5. Morinelli, 1984; 6. Passey, 1990; 7. Prosnitz, 1991; 8. Benedetti, 1992; 9. Feinstein, 1975; 10. Goodman, 1994; 11. Garber, 1992; 12. Baehr, 1993; 13. Garber, 1993; 14. Neyman, 1928; 15. Fleiss, 1981; 16. Freiman, 1978; 17. Fischer, 1997; 18. Kronmal, 1985; 19. Lipid Research Clinics Program, 1984; 20. Lipid Research Clinics Program, 1985; 21. Cohen, 1977; 22. Schwartz, 1967; 23. Salsburg, 1990; 24. Fisher, 1959; 25. Lehmann, 1993; 26. Kendall, 1973; 27. Deming, 1972; 28. Pearson, 1962; 29. Altman, 1980; 30. Clarke, 1981; 31. Pearson, 1976; 32. Stephen, 1966; 33. Uretsky, 1990.

Exercises

23.1. From the description offered in Section 23.1.1, what do you think produced the bias that made the *Literary Digest* political poll, despite a huge sample size, yield results dramatically opposite to those of the actual election?

23.2. In a clinical trial of medical vs. surgical therapy for coronary artery disease, the investigators expect the surgical group to achieve results that are 30% proportionately better than the medical group. Two endpoints are available for calculating sample size. The "hard" endpoint is rate of death at two years, which is expected to be 10% in the medical group. The "soft" endpoint is improvement in clinical severity of angina pectoris. This improvement is expected to occur in 70% of the medical group.

23.2.1. Using $\alpha = .05$ and $\beta = .1$ for a Neyman-Pearson calculation, what sample size is required for the "hard" endpoint?

23.2.2. Using the same arrangement as 23.2.1, what sample size is required for the "soft" endpoint?

23.2.3. In view of the smaller samples needed with the soft endpoint, why do you think the hard endpoint is so popular?

23.2.4. What sample sizes would you propose for quantitatively significant results in the hard and soft endpoints if you do not use the Neyman-Pearson approach? How do these sizes compare with what you obtained in 23.2.1 and 23.2.2?

23.3. In a multicentre trial of treatment for acute myocardial infarction,[32] the in-hospital mortality rate was 15/100 (15%) in patients receiving propranolol, and 12/95 (13%) in those receiving placebo. Aside from stating that the trial "demonstrated no difference in mortality," the authors drew no therapeutic recommendations, such as abandoning the use of propranolol for patients with acute myocardial infarction.

23.3.1.   Why do you think no recommendations were made?

23.3.2.   What is the chance that these results arose from a "parent universe" in which mortality rate with propranolol is actually 10% incrementally *below* that of placebo?

23.4. Enoximone, a phosphodiesterase inhibitor that is a derivative of imidazole, had been observed to exert an inotropic cardiac effect in hemodynamic studies of patients with moderate to moderately severe (New York Heart Association Class II or III) congestive heart failure. The manufacturers of the drug therefore sponsored a randomized placebo-controlled trial[33] to determine whether enoximone, when combined with digoxin and diuretics, improves symptoms and exercise tolerance of such patients.

The disappointing results showed that in 50 patients receiving enoximone and 52 receiving placebo, "there were no significant differences in exercise duration between groups at any time point" and the "symptom scores for dyspnea, fatigue, overall functional impairment and NYHA class were similar in both groups." In addition, "The dropout rate was significantly higher (P < .05) in the enoximone group than in the placebo group (46% enoximone, 25% placebo)." At the end of the study period, "there were 10 deaths in patients assigned to enoximone (20%)" and "three deaths (6%) in the patients assigned to placebo (P < .05)."

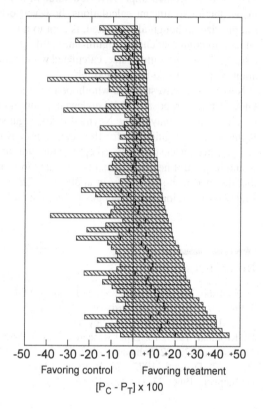

-50 -40 -30 -20 -10   0 +10 +20 +30 +40 +50
Favoring control   Favoring treatment

$[P_C - P_T] \times 100$

FIGURE E.23.5

Ninety percent confidence limits for the true percentage difference for the 71 Trials. The vertical bar at the center of each interval indicates the observed value, $\hat{P}_C - \hat{P}_T$, for each trial. [Figure taken from Chapter Reference 16.]

23.4.1.   In the discussion section of the report, the investigators considered various pharmaco-physiologic reasons why the drug had failed (dose too high, excessive response in placebo group, incomplete exercise testing, etc.) but did not mention any statistical tests for the possibility that the results were wrong.

What would you do to check the possibility that enoximone is really a superior agent and that the differences in drop-out rates and deaths were due to the stochastic fickleness of fate? Illustrate your idea with at least one calculation.

23.4.2.   In the published report, the investigators presented a graph showing the mean values of exercise duration at baseline and at 4, 8, 12, and 16 weeks for the enoximone group and for the placebo group. In the legend of that figure, the investigators make seemingly contradictory statements about exercise duration. They say that "there were no significant differences between groups at any time point," but they also state that there was "a significant (P < 0.05) increase ... compared with baseline values." Are these two statements contradictory? If not, why not? What kind of tests do you think were done to support the two statements?

23.5. When Freiman et al. concluded that 71 "negative" randomized trials were undersized, their often cited paper[16] had a major impact in promoting the current fashion of calculating "doubly significant" sample sizes for randomized trials. Figure E.23.5 shows the plot of confidence intervals for the 71 trials. Do you believe the authors distinguished between two kinds of problems: (1) a sample size too small to reject the null hypothesis for a quantitatively significant difference, and (2) a sample size too small to reject both the null and the alternative hypotheses?

24

Testing for "Equivalence"

CONTENTS

In all the stochastic discussions thus far, the investigator wanted to confirm something impressive: to show that a quantitatively "big" distinction was accompanied by a satisfactory P value or confidence interval. The ideas about "capacity," alternative hypotheses, β error, and "power" that appeared in Chapter 23 were all related to the same basic goal. They offered hope for salvaging something favorable if a trial's results were disappointingly "negative," with the desired "significance" being obtained neither quantitatively nor stochastically.

Stochastic hypotheses can also be formulated and tested, however, for at least four other goals beyond the aim of confirming something "big." For the main goal discussed in this chapter, the investigator wants to show stochastically that an observed distinction, d_o, is "small" or "insignificant," rather than "big." For example, the aim may be to confirm that the compared effects of treatments A and B are essentially similar, rather than substantially different. The other three stochastic procedures, which will be discussed in Chapter 25, involve testing multiple hypotheses.

24.1 Delineation of Equivalence

For the alternative-hypothesis procedures in Chapter 23, the investigator began the research hoping to find a large d_o, which would be either confirmed stochastically under the primary null hypothesis or at least conceded under the alternative hypothesis. The new stochastic procedures to be discussed now, however, have a diametrically opposite main goal. They are directly aimed at finding and stochastically confirming a distinction that is "small" enough to support the idea that the two compared entities are essentially equivalent.

24.1.1 Research Situations

Seeking similarity rather than a difference is the goal in many research situations. An epidemiologic investigator, concerned with "risk factors," may want to claim that a particular "exposure" is "safe," i.e., it does *not* elevate the risk of "non-exposure." For pharmaceutical "equivalence" in clinical research, the claim might be that a "generic" product has the same effect as the "brand-name" original drug; or that Agent B, which is prepared more conveniently or cheaply than Agent A, is just as effective.

In tests of efficacy for new pharmaceutical agents, the comparative agent has usually been placebo, not only because of its "standard" effect, but also because it avoids having to choose a single comparative agent from among several active competitors. In recent years, however, the use of placebo has been denounced both for ethical reasons (because the patient may be unfairly deprived of an effective agent) and for clinical reasons (because the results of a placebo comparison may not be directly applicable in patient care). Consequently, pharmaceutical efficacy may be increasingly tested in the future with the requirement that a new agent be at least as good as (i.e., equivalent to) an existing active agent.

In a non-pharmaceutical clinical situation, the aim might be to show equal efficacy for a "conservative" therapy. The investigator might want to demonstrate that simple surgery is no worse than radical surgery for treating cancer, that angioplasty gets the same results as bypass grafting for coronary disease, that most patients with acute myocardial infarction can be managed as effectively at home as in the hospital, or that nurse practitioners can work just as well as physicians in giving primary care. A policy planner proposing a new system for lowering the expense of health care may want to get clinical results that are essentially the same as with the old system, while costing less.

Kirshner[1] has written a thoughtful review of the many differences in design when the evaluation process is aimed at demonstrating small distinctions for "equivalence," rather than big ones for "efficacy." In addition to a major change in the general scheme of stochastic reasoning, the evaluation process is often beset with major sources of ambiguity or confusion in specifying the concept of *equivalence* itself.

24.1.2 Type of Equivalence

What kind of equivalence is being examined? Is it chemical/physical, therapeutic, biologic, or etiologic? The first type of equivalence refers to such issues as the chemical structure of two pharmaceutical agents or the physical properties of two materials used for surgical sutures. Questions about equivalence for chemical or physical attributes seldom require studies in people, and can usually be answered with laboratory research. The other questions, which are the main topic in this chapter, require testing human subjects.

Therapeutic equivalence refers to effects on an outcome that would be sought in a patient's clinical care. This outcome might be a laboratory entity, such as a change in antibody titer or blood glucose level, but is often something that is clinically overt, such as symptoms, functional capacity, or survival. Biological equivalence, which is usually called *bioequivalence*, refers to the bioavailability of a pharmaceutical agent, as measured by various features of its absorption, dissemination, concentration, excretion, or other aspects of pharmacokinetics in the human body. For etiologic equivalence, which can be regarded as a subdivision of biologic equivalence, a particular disease would develop at essentially the same rate in the presence or absence of exposure to a particular "risk factor."

24.1.3 Basic Design

For studies of therapeutic or biologic equivalence, the basic design of the research often involves complex decisions about population, "schedule," and crossovers. Some of the many fundamental questions that require scientific rather than mathematical answers are the following:

Population: Should the equivalence of pharmaceutical or other agents be tested in people who are sick or well? If one of those two groups is chosen, can the results be extrapolated to the other group?

Schedule: Should the dosage of agent and duration of effect be evaluated with the same criteria, regardless of whether the agent is ordinarily given once a day, twice a day, in multiple daily doses, in a sustained or "long-acting" form, or in absorption via dermal patch or subcutaneous pellet?

Crossovers: Although crossover plans can probably be routinely justified more easily in healthy than in sick people, how many agents can (or should) be crossed over in a single person? Most scientific comparisons involve two agents, but statisticians enjoy making special crossover plans to compare three or more pharmaceutical agents in each person. The crossover plans, usually called *squares*,[2] are prefixed with such names as *Latin, Graeco-Latin, Youden*, and *lattice*. These multi-crossover squares, which were conceived in the agricultural studies that fertilized much of current statistical thinking, are often taught in statistical courses devoted to "experimental design." Nevertheless, the "square" plans are seldom used in clinical research, because their mathematical elegance almost never overcomes the pragmatic difficulty of conducting, analyzing, and understanding the results of multiple crossovers in people. (A prominent biostatistician, Marvin Zelen,[3] has remarked that "the statistical design of experiments ... as taught in most schools, seems so far removed from reality, that a heavy dose may be too toxic with regard to future applications.")

24.1.4 Personal vs. Group Focus

The next basic problem is to choose a personal focus for decisions when the same persons are exposed to different agents. Are the decisions aimed at demonstrating equivalence for individual persons, for specified groups, or for a general average?

Anderson[4] has illustrated these three types of bioequivalence with the "cases" shown in Figure 24.1. In the first case, which she calls "switchability," the same person gets essentially the same result with each of two formulations. In case 2, which she calls "prescribability," the clinician does not know (and may not care) about individual responses as long as the average response is the same, without excessive

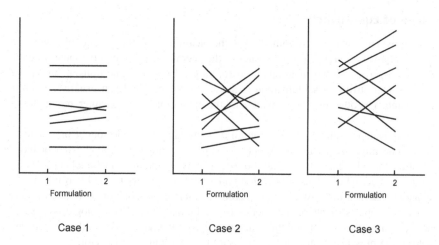

FIGURE 24.1
Levels of outcome in individual patients receiving formulation 1 vs. formulation 2. The pattern of results for equivalence, discussed further in the text, can be called "switchable" (Case 1), "prescribable" (Case 2), or "average" (Case 3). [Figure derived from Chapter Reference 4.]

variability, in the two treated groups. In case 3 of Figure 24.1, however, the variability among both individuals and groups may be too extensive for either formulation to be regarded as "switchable" or "prescribable," although the average results (such as the means) may still be close enough to allow the two compared formulations to be called "equivalent."

The statistical procedures used for evaluation, as well as the basic design of the research itself, will vary with the desired type of equivalence.

24.1.5 Mensurational Problems

Yet another problem arises in choosing the prime "outcome" variable for measuring equivalence. In most clinical trials, this choice is relatively easy. The target variable is usually either a binary event, such as survival, or the change in a ranked variable, such as blood pressure or pain. In etiologic studies, the outcome is development of a particular disease.

In pharmacologic kinetics, however, many candidate variables can be measured to assess bioavailability. The variables include area under the time curve (AUC) of blood or plasma concentration, the level of maximum concentration (C_{max}), or time to maximum concentration[5] (T_{max}), as well as such phenomena as plateau time, half-value duration, and several variants of peak-trough fluctuation.[6] For antibiotic drugs, effectiveness against specific bacteria can be checked with a minimum inhibitory concentration (MIC), with the time at which MIC is first reached, or with the duration of time for which the concentration remains above MIC.[7]

Choosing an appropriate measurement to express a drug's action or a treatment's accomplishment is an important scientific issue that is beyond the scope of the statistically oriented discourse here. For the subsequent discussion, we shall assume that an appropriate measurement has been selected, and that the results can be evaluated for their quantitative distinctions in that measurement.

24.2 Quantitative Boundary for Tolerance

Perhaps the most crucial *statistical* decision is the choice of a quantitative boundary. Because we cannot expect the two compared effects to be exactly identical, a boundary of tolerance must be set to demarcate the zone within which different effects can still be regarded as equivalent. This boundary obviously depends on scientific considerations, but its magnitude—which involves answering the question, "How big is small?"—will affect all the subsequent statistical activities.

The maximum boundary of a "small" increment corresponds to the level of ζ that was briefly considered in Chapters 10 and 23. If an increment is quantitatively small enough for two means to be regarded as "similar" or "equivalent," we would want $|\bar{X}_A - \bar{X}_B|$ to be $\leq \zeta$. For two proportions, the zone would be $|p_A - p_B| \leq \zeta$.

24.2.1 Problems and Ambiguities

The choice of ζ is a major source of quantitative ambiguity. When equivalence is statistically defined as a difference having "negligible practical interest,"[8] or being below the "minimum difference of practical interest,"[9] the boundary for this difference might be expected to have a small magnitude for ζ. For many years, however, the boundary chosen for "small" in most statistical discussions of equivalence has been the same relatively large δ that was previously used (in Chapters 10 and 23) to demarcate "big." With the statistical idea that *small* is the opposite of *big*, the values of an observed $d_0 \geq \delta$ are **big**; and the not-big values of $d_0 < \delta$ are regarded as **small** and in the zone of equivalence.

With uncommon exception, most statistical discussions do not use an additional zone to separate "small" from "big." Even when recognizing that the "traditional statistical framework does not seem appropriate" and that "the observed difference between treatments is relatively small for demonstrating equivalence,"[10] the authors may still place the main focus on confidence intervals for which the specific magnitude of a "small" boundary is *not* demarcated.

In etiologic research, where the statistical comparison is usually expressed as an odds ratio or risk ratio, the magnitude of an "incremental risk" is seldom discussed or considered. Instead, the investigators focus on elevation of the ratio above the "equivalent" value of 1. In this situation, values of δ and ζ respectively refer to the boundaries of large and tiny ratios rather than increments. No overt consensus has developed, however, about the choice of those boundaries. Some epidemiologists, referring to the additional cases of disease that might occur when a huge population is exposed to a "risk factor," may refuse to consider any elevated risk ratio as tiny or safe. Nevertheless, because of the small numbers of "exposed cases" that are found in many case-control studies of risk, and because of problems in misclassification, in detection, and in enumeration, most epidemiologists will regard ratios below 2 as unimpressive and within the limits of "noise" in the observational system.[11] Ratios of 3 or higher, however, are almost always deemed impressive. With the latter criteria, the boundaries for ratios might be set at 3 for δ and at 2 (or something between 1 and 2) for ζ.

The topic of etiologic equivalence for ratios is complex, controversial, and will not be considered further in this chapter. The rest of the discussion is devoted to decisions about increments that have clinical and/or pharmaceutical equivalence.

24.2.2 Use of Single Two-Zone Boundary

Whatever its mathematical merits, the statistical custom of forming a dichotomous two-zone "decision space," using a single boundary of δ, is a drastic departure from the realities of clinical reasoning.[12] Clinicians usually think about a three-zone "space," shown in Figure 24.2, in which anything $\geq \delta$ is big, anything $\leq \zeta$ is small or "tiny," and values between ζ and δ are intermediate or inconclusive. The clinical decisions are regularly cited in such trichomotous ordinal scales as **too high**, **normal**, or **too low; positive, uncertain,** or **negative; hyperglycemic, euglycemic,** or **hypoglycemic; tall, medium,** or **short**.

With the customary two-zone statistical scheme, however, "equivalence" would receive a relatively large upper bound-

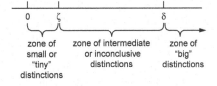

FIGURE 24.2

Two boundaries (ζ and δ) forming three categorical zones for magnitude of observed distinctions. [The zones here are for positive distinctions. A similar set of zones could be shown on the left of 0 for negative distinctions.]

ary if "small" or "equivalent" is regarded as anything less than "big." This approach would let the same big value of δ be used for deciding either that a new active treatment is more efficacious than standard therapy or, conversely, that a "conservative" or "inexpensive" treatment has essentially the same effects.[13,14]

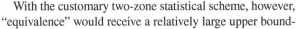

The relatively large size of the boundary for "tiny" is evident in a set of FDA guidelines[15] for bioavailability studies, which state (according to Westlake[7]) that "products whose rate and extent of absorption differ by 20% or less are generally considered bioequivalent." Although a proportionate rather than direct increment, the 20% boundary will often allow the upper level of a *small* difference to be larger than the $\delta \geq .15$ often used in Chapter 23 as the lower boundary of a *big* direct increment in two proportions.

24.2.3   Consequences of "Big" Two-Zone Boundary

When tiny distinctions are allowed big statistical boundaries, several immediate problems occur. The most obvious is that the quantitative criterion is not compatible with ordinary common sense. If someone who is ≥ 72 inches (183 cm.) is regarded as **tall**, we are forced to say that anyone whose height is <72 is **short**. If a fasting blood sugar of ≥ 140 mg/dL is regarded as **hyperglycemic**, anyone whose level is below 140 would have to be called **hypoglycemic**. If a diastolic blood pressure of ≥ 90 mm Hg demarcates **hypertension**, pressures below 90 become **hypotensive**.

24.2.4   Use of "Small" Two-Zone Boundary

In recent years, a smaller boundary has been proposed[10,16] to distinguish zones of equivalence from zones of efficacy. The authors usually employ the same symbol (such as δ), however, whether the boundary is large or small. To avoid ambiguity, the δ symbol will be reserved here for the big value and ζ will be used for the small one.

The use of a small ζ has at least two important consequences. First (as discussed later), it can substantially raise the sample sizes needed for one-boundary–two-zone calculations of stochastic significance. Second, the introduction of a small ζ also allows construction of a new three-zone approach for the calculations.

24.2.5   Directional Decisions

Regardless of whether equivalence is given a large or small boundary, the choice of a scientific direction is particularly important, because it is the source of one-tailed vs. two-tailed decisions in testing stochastic hypotheses.

Do we really want to show that Treatments A and B are similar? If so, the evaluation definitely goes in both directions. Using ζ as the boundary of a small difference, we would want to demonstrate that $|A - B| \leq \zeta$ regardless of whether the results are slightly larger or smaller for A than for B.

In many other situations, however, we may want to show mainly that A, although perhaps better, is not much more effective than B. Alternatively phrased, we want to show that B is almost as good as A. In this situation, where A might be the somewhat better "brand-name" and B the almost-as-good generic product, the goal would be to find that $A - B \leq \zeta$. If the results unexpectedly show that B seems better than A, we might be pleased, but we would probably not intend to claim stochastically that B is *more* effective. In another situation, if "active" treatment A turns out to produce a *lower* success rate than placebo, we might be happy or unhappy (according to the preceding scientific hopes); but if p_A for active treatment is lower than p_B for placebo, we probably would not do stochastic tests to confirm the higher efficacy of placebo. (Stochastic testing might be done to demonstrate that A is more *harmful* than placebo, but the "harm" would be measured with some other variable, and tested with information different from what was used stochastically to compare rates of "success.")

On the other hand, when two "active" pharmaceutical agents are compared, direction may be important for the incremental magnitude of tolerance within the zone of equivalence. For example, suppose X is the outcome variable chosen for showing equivalence, and suppose $\bar{X}_A$ and $\bar{X}_B$ are its mean values in two compared agents, A and B. Suppose further that A is the standard, "brand-name," or customary treatment, whereas B is the perhaps inferior, generic, or less costly competing agent. In the selected variable that measures bioavailability, we would expect $\bar{X}_A$ to be greater than $\bar{X}_B$. To demonstrate equivalence, we would therefore want $\bar{X}_A - \bar{X}_B$ to be less than some relatively small positive value.

Nevertheless, if $\overline{X}_B$ turns out unexpectedly to exceed $\overline{X}_A$ and if B is a generic drug, its greater availability may impair the established dosing schedule of the standard agent. [This problem arose a few decades ago when digitalis toxicity developed in patients who transferred, at apparently similar constant dosage, from a "brand name" to a generic product.[17]]

To deal with the possibility that $\overline{X}_A < \overline{X}_B$, a separate boundary can be established for the largest permissible *negative* increment in $\overline{X}_A - \overline{X}_B$. The data analysts may then demarcate two boundaries of tolerance, one for $\overline{X}_B - \overline{X}_A < \zeta_1$ and the other for $\overline{X}_A - \overline{X}_B < \zeta_2$. The extra complexity of using different positive and negative values for tolerance can be avoided, however, if we use the same value for both. (If desired, the discussions that follow can be readily adapted to encompass separate positive and negative boundaries.)

24.3 Stochastic Reasoning and Tests of Equivalence

As recently noted by Greene et al.,[18] many studies claiming that results showed equivalence did not set a boundary for its magnitude, and made the claim only after the null hypothesis was *not* rejected when stochastic significance was tested for the observed distinction. The appropriate stochastic methods for examining and confirming equivalence create a challenging and currently unresolved problem. Because stochastic conclusions are based on rejecting hypotheses, equivalence obviously cannot be tested with the goal of rejecting the conventional null hypothesis, $\Delta = 0$, which is actually the basic idea we would like to confirm. Because the customary procedure cannot be used, some other approach is needed for stochastic tests of equivalence. The discussion that follows will first describe the approach that is currently used and will then introduce a new strategy, based on conventional stochastic logic, which can be reversed for testing equivalence.

24.4 Customary Single-Boundary Approach

The customary stochastic approaches for testing equivalence rely on confidence intervals, not on tests of a specific hypothesis. The calculations and consequences will differ according to whether a big δ or small ζ is used in stating the permissible boundaries of the confidence intervals.

24.4.1 Procedure for "Big" δ

The earliest stochastic proposals for testing equivalence applied a confidence-interval strategy[19,20] in which δ for equivalence was set as the maximum "big" boundary. The confidence interval needed to stochastically confirm an observed difference, d_o, as small was

$$d_o + Z_\alpha(\text{SED}) < \delta \qquad [24.1]$$

Regardless of whether the selected Z_α is designated as Z_α or Z_β and regardless of whether the probabilities are one- or two-tailed, this confidence-interval strategy uses the same statement that appeared in Chapter 23 for rejecting the alternative stochastic hypothesis that $H_H: \Delta \geq \delta$. Furthermore, the confidence interval statement can readily be converted to an equivalence hypothesis symbolized as $H_E: \Delta \geq \delta$. The confirmatory stochastic decision would thus require either a confidence interval that excludes δ, or an appropriately small P value, determined when Z_E (for equivalence) is calculated as

$$Z_E = (\delta - d_o)/\text{SED} \qquad [24.2]$$

This formula is identical to the previous Formula [23.3] for a two-boundary arrangement.

24.4.1.1   Conventional Calculations under H_E — Because H_E is a nonzero hypothesis, the standard error of the difference, SED, is determined with the SED_H formula discussed previously. The designated value of Z can be marked as Z_α, because H_E becomes the counterpart of the primary hypothesis to be rejected. After an appropriate value of Z_α is chosen, a $1 - \alpha$ confidence interval can be constructed as in Formula [24.1]. If the hypothesis boundary of δ is excluded from the upper part of this interval, the observed "equivalence" is stochastically confirmed. For a two-tailed decision, the interval should lie between $-\delta$ and $+\delta$.

24.4.1.2   Direction of Evaluation — The decision about a one-tailed or two-tailed direction will affect the magnitude of Z_α or $Z_{2\alpha}$ used for calculating confidence intervals or advance sample sizes, as well as the interpretation of P values as being 2P or half of the 2P value. Because a firm consensus has not been reached on this matter, you might use the compromise guidelines, suggested earlier in Section 11.8.4, which propose that the decisions always be two-tailed except when a one-tailed direction has been specified in advance and is suitably justified.

24.4.1.3   Examples of Calculations — The calculations for advance sample size and for stochastic confirmation of results are similar to those done in Sections 23.4.2 and 23.4.3. An illustration for comparing two proportions, $p_A = 63/70$ and $p_B = 56/70$, with δ set at .18, would be as follows: To test stochastic significance for the "small" value of $d_0 = .90 - .80 = .10$, we first find

$$SED_H = \sqrt{[(.90)(.10)/70] + [(.80)(.20)/70]} = .060$$

The 95% confidence interval is then $.10 \pm (1.96)(.060)$, and extends from $-.018$ to .218. Because the value of .18 is contained in this interval, we cannot stochastically confirm that $d_0 = .10$ is small. Alternatively, we could have calculated $Z_E = (.18 - .10)/.060 = 1.33$, which produces a "nonsignificant" $2P_E = .184$.

If an argument is offered that the stochastic hypothesis should be unidirectional because a generic product was being tested, the foregoing 2P value would be halved to .092 with a one-tailed interpretation; and the upper end of the 95% confidence interval, calculated with a one-tailed $Z_{.1} = 1.645$, would be $.10 + (1.645)(.060) = .199$, which would still include .18. Thus, the "small" increment of .10 would be stochastically "nonsignificant" at $\alpha = .05$ for both a one-tailed and two-tailed decision.

To illustrate the procedure for dimensional data, suppose δ is set at a direct increment of 10 units in a study for which the observed means, standard deviations, and group sizes respectively are $\overline{X}_A = 100$, $s_A = 10$, and $n_A = 50$ in the standard group, with $\overline{X}_B = 95$, $s_B = 9$, and $n_B = 49$ in the test group. The value of $d_0 = |\overline{X}_A - \overline{X}_B| = 100 - 95 = 5$ seems small, and is well below the boundary of $\delta = 10$. To test the "insignificant" difference stochastically, we first find

$$SED_H = \sqrt{(10)^2/50 + [(9)^2/49]} = 1.91$$

The value of Z_E will be $(10 - 5)/1.91 = 2.62$, for which 2P =.009. With $Z_\alpha = 1.96$, the two-tailed 95% confidence interval will extend from 1.26 to 8.74, thus excluding the value of $\delta = 10$. [The upper boundary of a one-tailed 95% confidence interval, with $Z_\alpha = 1.645$, will be $5 + (1.645)(1.91)$ and will extend only to 8.14.] The observed "small" difference will therefore be stochastically confirmed as "insignificant."

24.4.1.4   Paradoxical Results — The 95% two-tailed confidence interval in the immediately preceding example (for two means) shows the kind of paradox that can sometimes occur with stochastic tests of "insignificance." The observed d_0 of 5 seemed small and is only 5% of the common mean, which is 97.5 for the two groups. [The latter value was calculated as $\{(100 \times 50) + (95 \times 49)\}/99$.] Nevertheless, because 0 is excluded from the lower end of the 2-tailed 95%-confidence interval, the observed result would also be stochastically significant for the *original* null hypothesis that $\Delta = 0$. This paradox — which allows a small difference to be stochastically confirmed as both "big" and "small" — arose from the relatively large sample size, and from d_0, at a value of 5, being equidistant from the locations of $\Delta = 10$ and $\Delta = 0$ for the two hypotheses.

24.4.2 Example of a "Classical" Study

A classical clinical study of equivalence was presented many years ago by Kramer, Rooks, and Pearson.[21] Wanting to show that childhood growth and development are *not* impaired by the sickle-cell trait, the investigators measured several indexes of physical growth and cognitive development in 50 matched pairs of black infants with either normal (AA) blood or sickle cell (AS) trait. The pairs were matched according to date of birth, sex, birth weight, gestational age, and parental socioeconomic status at the time of delivery. The follow-up measurements were done, when the children were between 39 and 63 months of age, by examiners who were "blind" to the child's genotype, and for the cognitive tests, by a black psychologist.

For each measured variable, the investigators determined the d_0 mean increments and corresponding P_0 values for members of the matched-pair groups. A value of δ was also established for each variable as a substantively "larger potential difference" in the incremental means for each group. Values of P_E were then determined for the values of $\delta - d_0$. (The symbols used by the investigators have been converted to those of the text here.) The results were small and quantitatively unimpressive for the diverse results of d_0 in 6 variables indicating physical growth and in 6 variables indicating cognitive development. In all of these comparisons P_E was $\leq .05$. In one variable, the McCarthy Perceptual-Performance subtest, d_0 for the AA–AS increment was -2.4, for which P_0 was 0.036 under the original null hypothesis. Nevertheless, for the corresponding established $\delta = +2.0$, P_E was "< 0.001." The reversed direction of d_0 and the "significant" P_0 were attributed to a chance event occurring "because of the many outcome variables under comparison."

The investigators concluded that sickle-cell-trait children have "no deficits in standard measurements of growth and development," and that previous beliefs that such children were impaired were due to methodologic flaws in the research.

24.4.3 Procedure for "Small" δ

Recognizing that the big value of δ may be too large for satisfactory appraisals of equivalence, Makuch et al.[10] and Jones et al.[16] have proposed that a smaller boundary be used in the hypothesis for H_E. If ζ symbolizes this boundary, the demand made in Formula [24.1] becomes expressed as

$$d_0 + Z_\alpha(SED) < \zeta \qquad\qquad [24.3]$$

and the primary stochastic hypothesis for equivalence of two means would be stated as

$$H_E : (\mu_A - \mu_B) > \zeta$$

If the hypothesis is symmetrically two-tailed, Formula [24.3] becomes stated as

$$|d_0 \pm Z_\alpha(SED)| < \zeta \qquad\qquad [24.4]$$

This approach produces the draconian demand that the entire confidence interval be contained between the boundaries of $-\zeta$ and $+\zeta$. The demand seems scientifically peculiar because an observed value of $d_0 < \zeta$, although small enough to be regarded as "equivalent," cannot be stochastically confirmed unless d_0 is "super-small" enough for the entire interval to be smaller than ζ.

24.4.3.1   Consequences of "Small" Value for H_E — When the increments of $\delta - d_o$ are replaced by $\zeta - d_o$, much larger sample sizes will be needed for stochastic confirmation of the small differences. For example, consider the small increment in the two means, $\overline{X}_A = 100$ and $\overline{X}_B = 95$, that was stochastically confirmed in the second part of Section 24.4.1.3. Suppose the observed d_o was still 5, with $SED_H = 1.91$, but the "small" boundary for ζ was set at 6, rather than at the previous $\delta = 10$. Z_E would then be calculated as $(6 - 5)/1.91 = .523$ and would not provide stochastic confirmation, because $2P_E$ is $> .5$.

Because the observed d_o was $< \zeta$, the failure to confirm would be caused by inadequate capacity in a too-small sample. The sample size needed to confirm the "smallness" of $d_o = 5$ could be calculated from the formula

$$n \geq Z_\alpha^2 (s_A^2 + s_B^2)/(\zeta - d_o)^2 \qquad [24.5]$$

For a one-tailed $Z_\alpha = 1.645$, with $s_A = 10$ and $s_B = 9$, the requirement would be

$$n \geq (1.645)^2(100 + 81)/(6 - 5)^2 = 489.8$$

At least 490 members would be needed in each group. Thus, the total group size of 99 members ($= 50 + 49$) had ample capacity to reject H_E when it was set at the "big" $\delta = 10$, but the capacity would be only $99/980 = .10$, if H_E were located at the "small" $\zeta = 6$. If the latter H_E were tested with $Z_\alpha = 1.96$ instead of $Z_\beta = 1.645$, the required sample size would be increased to 695.3 per group.

As an additional example, consider the comparison in the first part of Section 24.4.1.3, where "success" was achieved by 90% and by 80% of two groups that each contained 70 persons. When H_E was set at the large value of $\delta = .18$, the incremental difference of 10% was not stochastically confirmed as small. For $Z_\alpha = 1.96$, a sample size of 150 persons would have been required. If H_E were set at the smaller value of $\zeta = .12$, however, the observed increment of .10 would still have satisfied the quantitative requirement for equivalence, but the sample size needed for stochastic confirmation would have risen to $(1.96)^2(.25)/(.12 - .10)^2 = 2401$ for each group. With $Z_\alpha = 1.645$, the required sample size per group would have been 1691.3.

24.4.3.2   Advantages of "Big" Value for H_E — As shown in the foregoing calculations, when the equivalence hypothesis, H_E, is set at a relatively large value of δ, stochastic confirmation can be attained with much smaller group sizes than if H_E is placed at the small ζ. In fact, the calculations can also show the impossibility of trying to *prove* the null hypothesis that $\Delta = 0$. If the demanded $\zeta = 0$ is attained by an observed $d_o = 0$, the value of 0 would be entered in the denominator of Formula [24.5], and an infinite sample size would be required.

24.4.4   Alternative Hypothesis for Single Boundaries

As discussed earlier in Sections 11.5 and 11.9, when a stochastic hypothesis is rejected, its counter-hypothesis is conceded. In customary two-tailed procedures with the null hypothesis that $\Delta = 0$, the counter-hypothesis is $\Delta \neq 0$ and does not have a location. The *alternative* hypothesis, however, has a distinct location, which is set (for tests of efficacy) at the "large" value of δ. As shown in Chapter 23, the alternative hypothesis can offer "consolation" when the desired big d_o turns out to be disappointingly small, i.e., $d_o < \delta$.

In stochastic testing for equivalence, however, if H_E is set with only a single boundary for either δ or ζ, a specific location is not cited for an alternative hypothesis. The term "alternative hypothesis" is sometimes mentioned[16,22] in stochastic discussions of equivalence tests, but the discussed entity is really a counter-hypothesis, expressed in terms such as $|\mu_A - \mu_B| < \zeta$. A specifically located *alternative* hypothesis is not cited. Consequently, in the customary one-boundary strategy, a differently located alternative hypothesis is not available either for additional testing or for "confidence-interval consolation" if a desired small d_o turns out to be disappointingly large.

24.4.5 Double-Significance (Neyman-Pearson) Approach

As discussed in Chapter 23, the Neyman-Pearson strategy deals with two hypotheses, but has only one distinct quantitative boundary. The strategy is intended to produce stochastic significance no matter which way the results turn out. Using the big δ as a single two-zone boundary, the doubly significant sample would let the results be stochastically significant if the observed d_o is $\geq \delta$ and also if $d_o < \delta$. The analogous events would happen if the single boundary is set at a small ζ, rather than a big δ.

Among the various problems associated with the Neyman-Pearson approach, perhaps the most scientifically peculiar idea is that the investigator is passively disinterested in the outcome of the research and does not care what emerges as long as it is stochastically significant. This approach inevitably leads to excessively large sample sizes, which can often stochastically confirm, as "big," a disappointingly small quantitative value of d_o that is $< \delta$ A counterpart of this dissidence would occur if the double-hypothesis strategy were used in a trial aimed at showing equivalence. The trial might produce a value of d_o that is bigger than the boundary of a smaller ζ, but the large sample size might allow the result to be confirmed stochastically as small.

When the Neyman-Pearson two-hypothesis strategy has been proposed[16,23] with a single-δ-boundary for the challenge of testing equivalence, δ has been set at smaller boundaries than the customary "big" δ. Nevertheless, after estimates of π_1, π_2, and the common π, the advance sample size formula becomes

$$n = 2\pi(1-\pi)(Z_\alpha + Z_\beta)^2/\delta^2 \qquad [24.6]$$

which is the conventional "double significance" Formula [23.10] cited in Chapter 23.

One of the problems produced by the Neyman-Pearson strategy can be illustrated in an example offered by Jones et al.[16] for equivalence of two bronchodilator inhalers. The upper boundary for equivalence was set at 15 l/min in mean values of morning peak expiratory flow rate. The "between subject variance," i.e., s^2, was estimated as 1600 (l/min)^2. Using $Z_\alpha = 1.96$ and $Z_\beta = 1.28$, the authors then applied the Neyman-Pearson formula of $2s^2(Z_\alpha + Z_\beta)^2/\zeta^2$ to calculate a sample size of 150 patients. Suppose this sample size is used in a trial that produces $d_o = 12$ between the two groups, with $s = 40$ in each group. The value of SED will be $\sqrt{2(40)^2/150} = 4.62$, and the upper boundary of the confidence interval will be $12 + (1.96)(4.62) = 21$, thus exceeding the boundary of 15. Consequently, although the observed $d_o = 12$ was less than $\zeta = 15$, the sample size would not allow stochastic confirmation of the small difference.

24.5 Principles of Conventional Stochastic Logic

A new strategy, which can avoid the problems and dilemmas of the currently used one-boundary approach, is to identify the principles of conventional stochastic logic, and then reverse them.

24.5.1 Identification of Four Principles

When we wanted to prove that something was big, the principles of customary stochastic logic placed the primary "null" hypothesis at the opposite extreme, setting H_o at the smallest possible distinction, i.e., $\Delta = 0$. The hypothesis was rejected if the calculated value of P was below a selected value α or if Δ was excluded from the zone of an appropriately calculated $1 - \alpha$ confidence interval.

As noted earlier in Section 23.1.2.3.1, the primary hypothesis was "boundless" because it did not contain the boundary of δ (for **big**) either in its main statement or in demarcation of a confidence interval. The value of δ was used only for appraising the *quantitative* distinction of d_o. Later on, however, δ appeared as the location of the alternative secondary hypothesis, which was set at $H_H : \Delta \geq \delta$.

This reasoning, used for stochastically confirming a "big" difference, contained four crucial principles:

1. The primary stochastic hypothesis, Δ, is located at a value opposite to what we want to confirm.
2. The observed distinction, d_o, is stochastically confirmed, i.e., the primary hypothesis is rejected, if Δ is excluded from a $1 - \alpha$ confidence interval around d_o, or if the pertinent P value is $\leq \alpha$

3. The critical *quantitative* boundary (for δ) is not contained in the statement of the primary hypothesis itself and is not used to demarcate limits for confidence intervals.

4. The critical *quantitative* boundary is used to mark the location of the alternative hypothesis. For a "big" difference, this boundary is set at δ.

These principles are illustrated in Figure 24.3, which shows four ways in which the confidence intervals can stochastically confirm "efficacy." In the top two instances, d_o was $> δ$ and in the lower two, d_o was $< δ$; but in all four, the value of $\Delta = 0$ was excluded from the lower boundary of the confidence interval. Note that in Situations B and D, the value of δ was not included in the confidence interval around d_o. (Situations C and D are excellent examples of statistical dissidence, where the observed distinction is stochastically but not quantitatively significant.)

24.5.2   Reversed Symmetry for Logic of Equivalence

If applied with reverse symmetry for stochastic testing of equivalence, the four principles just cited would require the following:

1. The primary hypothesis of equivalence, H_E, should be set at a value of Δ that is large, i.e., the opposite of the small quantitative distinction that we want to confirm.

2. The observed small distinction, d_o, is stochastically confirmed if the "large" hypothesis is rejected by being excluded from a $1 - \alpha$ confidence interval around d_o, or if the pertinent P value is $\leq \alpha$.

3. The critical quantitative boundary, ζ, for the small distinction does not appear in the statement of the primary hypothesis, and is not used to demarcate limits for confidence intervals.

4. The critical boundary, ζ, is used to mark the location of the alternative hypothesis.

These principles are illustrated in Figure 24.4, which is a counterpart of Figure 24.3. In Situations A and B, the value of d_o is $<ζ$, and in C and D, d_o is $>ζ$, but in all four, the value of $\Delta = δ$ is excluded

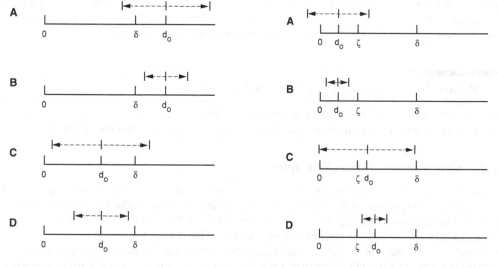

FIGURE 24.3
Dotted lines and arrows show extent of confidence intervals for the observed value of d_o and the designated boundary of δ. In all four situations, "efficacy" is confirmed because the lower end of the confidence interval exceeds 0. In situations A and B, d_o exceeds δ, but in situations C and D, d_o is $< δ$

FIGURE 24.4
Dotted lines and arrows show extent of confidence intervals for the observed value of d_o and the designated values of δ and ζ. In all four situations, equivalence is "confirmed" because the upper boundary of the confidence interval does not exceed δ. In parts A and B, d_o is $\leq ζ$; and in Parts C and D, d_o is $> ζ$. In part B, the entire confidence interval is contained between 0 and ζ, thus confirming d_o as both "big" and "small." In part D, the entire confidence interval excludes both ζ and δ.

from the upper boundary of the confidence limit. Note that in Situations B and D, the value of ζ is not included in the confidence interval around d_0. Situation D here is almost identical to Situation D in Figure 24.3 and shows the same statistical dissidence. The observed d_0, although too large to be called quantitatively "small," is nevertheless stochastically confirmed as small. (Because both 0 and ζ are excluded from the confidence intervals, the observed d_0 in Situation D in both Figures 24.3 and 24.4 is stochastically confirmed as being both large and small.)

The more common kind of statistical dissidence occurs in Situation C of both figures where a difference that fails to satisfy the quantitative requirement is stochastically confirmed for that requirement, but is not confirmed for the alternative hypothesis.

24.5.3 Applicability of Previous Logic

For testing equivalence, the four cited principles of logic cannot be applied with a single-boundary two-zone demarcation. The first principle requires that one boundary, such as δ, be set for a large value of Δ; and the third principle requires another boundary, such as ζ, to demarcate something small. If δ and ζ are used for these boundaries, they produce three zones, rather than the two zones formed when a single boundary is placed at either a big δ or a small ζ. A three-zone system has not hitherto been applied, however, for stochastic evaluations of equivalence. The analysts have regularly used only a single boundary, placed at a big δ or a small ζ, as discussed earlier throughout Section 24.4. The next section (24.6) describes the two-boundary–three-zone approach that produces symmetrical stochastic logic for testing equivalence.

24.6 Logical (Three-Zone–Two-Boundary) Approach

To evaluate equivalence with a mirror image (or reverse symmetry) of the basic stochastic logic used for evaluating efficacy, the first step is to set the primary hypothesis of equivalence at a large value, i.e.,

$$H_E : \Delta \geq \delta$$

The alternative hypothesis is set at the small value, i.e.,

$$H_S : \Delta \leq \zeta$$

The two sets of arrangements for efficacy and equivalence are shown in Table 24.1.

TABLE 24.1

Changing Location of Hypotheses for Testing Efficacy or Equivalence

		Location of	
Desired Goal	**Quantitative Criterion**	**Primary Hypothesis**	**Alternative Hypothesis**
Efficacy	$d_0 \geq \delta$	$H_0 : \Delta = 0$	$H_H : \Delta \geq \delta$
Equivalence	$d_0 \leq \zeta$	$H_E : \Delta \geq \delta$	$H_s : \Delta \leq \zeta$

24.6.1 Calculations for Advance Sample Size

With the two-boundary–three-zone arrangement, the advance calculation of a "singly significant" sample size for equivalence can be done with a confidence interval or a P value. With a confidence interval, using Z_α for the primary hypothesis, the observed maximum difference of ζ should have the attribute that $\zeta + Z_\alpha(\text{SED}) \leq \delta$.

24.6.1.1   Calculation for Two Proportions — With equal sizes in each group and with π_A and π_B as the estimated values of the two proportions, the sample size will be

$$n \geq \frac{Z_\alpha^2[\pi_A(1 - \pi_A) + \pi_B(1 - \pi_B)]}{(\delta - \zeta)^2} \qquad [24.7]$$

This same result emerges with the P value approach, if we determine n by using the formula

$$Z_E = \frac{\delta - d_o}{SED} \qquad [24.8]$$

after substituting Z_α for Z_E, ζ for d_o, and $\sqrt{[\pi_A(1 - \pi_A) + \pi_B(1 - \pi_B)]/n}$ for SED.

To demonstrate the calculations, suppose we expect that a suitable measurement of bioequivalence will be achieved by 90% of persons receiving Drug A and by 80% of persons receiving a generic product, B. If we use the FDA two-zone guideline that allows proportionate increments within 20% to be regarded as small, the boundary value of δ for this comparison will be $\delta = (.20)(.90) = .18$. We can then set the anticipated increment of .10 as the value of ζ.

Using Formula [24.7], the required sample size for each group would be

$$n \geq (1.96)^2[(.90)(.10) + (.80)(.20)]/(.18 - .10)^2 = 150.1$$

if $Z_\alpha = 1.96$, and 105.7 if $Z_\alpha = 1.645$.

24.6.1.2   Calculation for Two Means — For dimensional data, the appropriate modification of Formula [24.7] produces

$$n \geq \frac{Z_\alpha^2[\sigma_A^2 + \sigma_B^2]}{(\delta - \zeta)^2} \qquad [24.9]$$

To illustrate the calculations, suppose the large value of δ is set at 12 for a study in which the two groups are expected to differ by no more than $\zeta = 5$. We also expect that the two groups will have standard deviations of $\sigma_A = 9$ and $\sigma_B = 10$. With these expectations, and with α set at a two-tailed .05, the required sample size for each group will be $n \geq (1.96)^2 (181)/(12 - 5)^2 = 14.2$.

Note that the expected values of the two means, μ_A and μ_B, do not appear in Formula [24.9], and the sample size will depend on only the increments and variances.

24.6.2   Effect of Different Boundaries for δ and ζ

An important feature of Formula [24.7] is that the sample-size requirement enlarges if the boundaries are "relaxed" so that δ is made smaller and ζ is larger. Thus, if δ is reduced to .16 and ζ is raised to .12 in the foregoing trial, the required per-group size for $Z_\alpha = 1.96$ will be

$$n \geq (1.96)^2(.25)/(.16 - .12)^2 = 600.2$$

Conversely, the required sample size will decrease if either δ is made larger or ζ is smaller (or both).

For example, suppose the clinical trial in Section 24.6.1.1, done with 151 patients in each group, turns out to show $p_A = 136/151 = .901$ and $p_B = 125/151 = .828$. The observed d_o will be $.901 - .828 = .073$, and SED will be

$$\sqrt{(136)(15)/(151)^3 + (125)(26)/(151)^3} = .0392$$

The value of Z_E will be $(.18 - .073)/.0392 = 2.73$, for which $2P_E = 006$. Thus, a stochastically significant result (with $2P_E < .05$) could have been achieved with smaller groups.

On the other hand, suppose the study comparing two means in Section 24.6.1.2 were done with 15 persons in each group, and that the standard deviations produced the expected results of $s_A = 9$ and $s_B = 10$, but the observed difference in means turned out to be $d_o = 7$. With Formula [24.8], SED will be $\sqrt{(9^2 + 10^2)/15} = 3.47$ and Z_E will be $(12-7)/3.47 = 1.44$, which is too small to yield $P_E < .05$ with either a two-tailed or one-tailed evaluation.

24.6.3   Exploration of Alternative Hypothesis

If d_o is $< \zeta$ but the result is *not* stochastically confirmed, the main problem will be low capacity. If d_o exceeds ζ, however, symmetrical logic will allow the investigator to explore the alternative hypothesis, which will be

$$H_S : \Delta \leq \zeta$$

The investigator can then be consoled if ζ is included within the *lower* boundary of a confidence interval around the too big d_o.

For example, in the foregoing comparison of two means, with SED = 3.47, $Z_\beta = 1.645$ can be used to calculate the lower boundary of a one-tailed 95% confidence interval, which will be $7 - (1.645)(3.47) = 1.29$. Because the value includes the desired $\zeta = 5$, the result can be regarded as a compatible stochastic variation. Similarly, if ζ had been set at .04 rather than .10 in the foregoing clinical trial, and if the results still showed $d_o = .073$ with SED = .0392, the lower boundary of the one-tailed confidence interval would be $.073 - (1.645)(.0392) = .0085$, which would be stochastically compatible with the desired $\zeta = .04$.

24.6.4   Symmetry of Logic and Boundaries

The logic in Table 24.1 is "symmetrical," because each of the scientific goals — efficacy and equivalence — has a separate location for its own primary hypothesis and its alternative hypothesis. The boundary values at those locations, however, are not symmetrically reversed. The "big" value of δ does double duty in locating the alternative hypothesis for a big distinction and the primary hypothesis for a small one. The "small" value of ζ, however, does not have a mirror image when the primary hypothesis is set at 0 for a big distinction.

To achieve the attractive scientific appeal of a perfect mirror image would require changing the primary *null* hypothesis from 0 to ζ in tests of efficacy. This change would probably be anathema to most statistical theorists, because it would alter a century of statistical reasoning. All of the ordinary parametric tests (t, Z, chi-square, etc.) based on $\Delta = 0$ would have to be recalled and reconfigured, and statisticians and investigators would have to collaborate closely in choosing an appropriate value of ζ for each situation. Nevertheless, this idea may have considerable merit when parametric reasoning is eventually replaced in the new era of computer-intensive statistics; and besides, in Bayesian inference, a close clinico-statistical collaboration is needed to choose the appropriate values for prior probabilities. Furthermore, a clearly demarcated pair of boundaries, with ζ for small and δ for big, would allow tests of fragility (as discussed earlier) to be used for making stochastic decisions according to descriptive rather than probabilistic zones of reasoning.

24.7   Ramifications of Two-Boundary–Three-Zone Decision Space

The most important ramifications of a three-zone decision space extend far beyond the testing of "equivalence." The use of two boundaries and three zones can promptly help eliminate some of the prime difficulties produced by the Neyman-Pearson "double significance" method for calculating sample size. One main source of these difficulties is the choice of an unrealistically high value of δ to lower the "inflated" sample size to an attainable value. The subsequently observed d_o, although substantially smaller than the originally selected δ, may then be proclaimed "significant" after receiving stochastic confirmation for its large value.

24.7.1   Realistic Modifications for δ and ζ

With a three-zone decision space, the Neyman-Pearson calculations could be abandoned, and the investigators could set goals for values of δ and ζ that are closer to realistically acceptable boundaries for clinical decisions about quantitative magnitudes. For example, although δ could be set at .15 for an increment in two proportions, the investigator might still be willing to claim quantitative significance for smaller observed values, such as $d_0 = .14$ or even $d_0 = .10$, but not for $d_0 = .09$. If so, a new boundary for "big" can be set at δ = .10. Similarly, if ζ were originally set as an increment of .02, the investigator might still be willing to claim "equivalence" if $d_0 = .03$ or .04, but not if $d_0 = .05$. If so, a new boundary for "small" can be set at ζ = .04. With δ made smaller and ζ larger than the unrealistic previous boundaries of δ and ζ , the magnitude of the intermediate zone would be substantially reduced.

The sample-size calculation would then involve two computations: one for "single significance" under the primary null hypothesis, with $H_0 : \Delta = 0$ and δ as the boundary of big; and the other for "single significance" under the primary equivalence hypothesis, with $H_E : \Delta \geq \delta$ and with ζ as the boundary of small. The larger of these two sample-size values would then be used in the trial. Because the denominators for these calculations will have δ in the first and δ − ζ in the second, the second calculation should always produce the larger result.

24.7.2   Effects on Sample Size

Single-significance calculations with these modified boundaries for δ and ζ would be scientifically realistic and "honest," and will usually be smaller than the sample sizes that emerge with the "double significance" approach.

For example, suppose δ is set at .15 for a desired $p_A = .35$ and $p_B = .20$ in a randomized trial, so that $\hat{\pi} = (.35 + .20)/2 = .275$. If Z_α is set at a two-tailed 1.96 and Z_β is set at a one-tailed 0.84, the "double-significance" calculation with Formula [23.10] would produce

$$n \geq \frac{\left[1.96\sqrt{2(.275)(.725)} + 0.84\sqrt{(.35)(.65) + (.20)(.80)} \right]^2}{(.15)^2}$$

which is n ≥ 137.8.

For a singly significant result if $d_0 > \delta$, the sample size calculated with Formula [14.19] would be $n \geq (1.96)^2[2(.275)(.725)]/(.15)^2 = 68.1$. For a small value of d_0 with ζ set at .02, a single-significance calculation to confirm the small result would use Formula [24.7] to produce $n \geq (1.96)^2[(.35)(.65) + (.20)(.80)]/(.15 - .02)^2 = 88.1$. Thus, the trial could be done with 89 persons in each group rather than with the 138 persons needed for "double-significance."

On the other hand, if the investigators more realistically set δ = .10 and ζ = .04 as the "bottom-line" quantitative boundaries for respective claims of "big" or "small," the sample size needed to confirm single significance of the large difference (with $d_0 \geq .10$) would be $n \geq (1.96)^2[2(.275)(.725)]/(.10)^2 = 153.2$; and confirmation of the small difference (with $d_0 \leq .04$) would use Formula [24.7] to require $n \geq (1.96)^2[(.35)(.65) + (.20)(.80)]/(.10 - .04)^2 = 413.5$. Thus, the new approach might occasionally seem to enlarge rather than reduce sample sizes, because the latter number (413.5) more than triples the 137.8 that emerged from the previous "double-significance" calculation.

The investigator could now be assured, however, that stochastic confirmation for $d_0 \geq .10$ would be obtained with the sample size of 154 persons in each group, although it is larger than the 138 persons required when double-significance was determined for an unrealistically enlarged δ = .15. Furthermore, if seeking a big difference, the investigator might decide that 414 persons are not needed in each group because stochastic confirmation would not be wanted for the discouragingly small value of $d_0 \leq .04$.

Accordingly, instead of obtaining "double-significance" with 138 persons for an excessively high δ = .15, the trial could be done for single significance with 154 persons and a reasonable δ = .10. Nevertheless, if the investigator really wants to show and confirm a small difference for a realistic boundary of ζ =.04, the trial would require 414 persons in each group. This number would still be smaller, of course, than what would emerge with a "double-significance" calculation using $\delta = .10$. The latter calculation, with .10 rather than .15 in the denominator of Formula [23.10], would produce $n \geq 511.4$.

24.7.3 Choices of α and β

If realistic values for δ and ζ were set before the trial and maintained afterward, the main method for reducing sample size would be to change the values of α and β. In the foregoing double-significance calculations, Z_β was already quite relaxed at a one-tailed $\beta = .1$, but the value of Z_α was chosen for a two-tailed boundary of .05. If a one-tailed direction is accepted for α, the corresponding sample size would be smaller.

For the two separate calculations of single significance, a separate primary hypothesis is set for each calculation, and a β level need not be chosen. The foregoing calculations, however, were done with Z_α set at 1.96 for a two-tailed test at $\alpha = .05$. With each hypothesis having a clear direction, a one-tailed test could be used for each calculation, and the sample sizes would be reduced when Z_α is set at 1.645 rather than 1.96.

24.7.4 Resistance to Change

Having become thoroughly entrenched, the "double-significance" approach will probably become another instance of an outmoded paradigm that is resistant to change. The resistance will probably be aided by the reluctance of clinical investigators to accept responsibility for setting quantitative boundaries for "big" and "small." Unlike α and β, which can be designated arbitrarily regardless of what is happening in the research, the appropriate values of δ and ζ will often require ad hoc choices based on substantive content. If both the clinical investigators and statistical consultants, however, are willing to acknowledge that the prime scientific decisions depend on quantitative magnitudes rather than stochastic probabilities, the clinico-statistical collaborators can work together to set appropriate boundaries.

The consequences will be an enlightened improvement in statistical features of both the planning and reporting of medical research. Sample sizes can be determined according to what the investigator wants to show; the sizes will usually be smaller than under the "double-significance" paradigm; and readers of the published reports will be protected from possibly deceptive claims of "significance" that have been adapted to fit the observed results rather than to corroborate well-made plans. The new process would even be consistent with the recommendations (cited in Section 23.9.5) that were offered by both Ronald Fisher and Egon Pearson after they thoughtfully reconsidered and changed their original proposals, respectively, for testing "significance" and for determining "double significance."

24.8 Evaluating All Possible Outcomes

The three-zone approach would also allow development of a new statistical strategy that emphasizes what the investigator wanted to achieve when the research project was planned. With this strategy, any project can have at least eight possible outcomes, formed by two states for each of the following phenomena: the initial desire (or hope) is to find that d_o is either big ($\geq \delta$) or small ($\leq \zeta$); the observed result can be either desired or not desired; and the result can be either stochastically confirmed or not confirmed. The desired, observed, and stochastic results can then be evaluated as noted in the next two sections.

24.8.1 Large Value Desired for d_o

When a large value is desired for d_o, the possible findings and conclusions are shown in Table 24.2. In these four situations, the investigator wants or expects the observed result to be big. If the observed result comes out as expected, the stochastic tests will either confirm the scientific hypothesis or show that the study had defective capacity in group sizes. If the observed result is contrary to expectations, the disappointed investigator might be either comforted by the possibility that the result was a stochastic variation or distressed by having to reject the original *scientific* hypothesis as being probably wrong. (The wrong result, however, might have been produced by bias, rather than by an erroneous scientific hypothesis.)

TABLE 24.2

Stochastic Results and Conclusions When Large Value Is Expected for d_o

Was Result Desired?	Observed Descriptive Result	Stochastic Result for Confidence Interval	Conclusion
YES	$d_o \geq \delta$	0 excluded	Scientific hypothesis confirmed
		0 included	Defective capacity in group size
NO	$d_o < \delta$	δ excluded	Scientific hypothesis is probably wrong
		δ included	Result may be a stochastic variation

24.8.2   Small Value Desired for d_o

In a study of "equivalence," when a small value is desired for d_o, a similar set of conclusions can emerge under the different numerical circumstances shown in Table 24.3.

TABLE 24.3

Stochastic Results and Conclusions When Small Value Is Desired for d_o

Was Result Desired?	Observed Descriptive Result	Stochastic Result for Confidence Interval	Conclusion
YES	$d_o \leq \zeta$	δ excluded	Scientific hypothesis confirmed
		δ included	Defective capacity in group size
NO	$d_o > \zeta$	0 excluded	Scientific hypothesis is probably wrong
		0 included	Result may be a stochastic variation

24.8.3   Subsequent Actions

If the scientific hypothesis is confirmed, the investigator has nothing further to do, except perhaps to arrange publication for the research. If the scientific hypothesis is probably wrong, the investigator can try to find an alternative explanation by identifying cogent sources of bias. If the possibility of bias does not offer a suitable explanation, the original scientific hypothesis might have to be abandoned.

The other two conclusions are caused by statistical problems that can be solved with additional research. Defective capacity can be augmented in an ongoing project, or the research can be repeated with an adequately large sample. If the result might be a stochastic variation, a new attempt can be made to get stochastic confirmation or rejection by repeating the study with an adequate sample size.

24.8.4   Problems with Intermediate Results

The foregoing set of evaluations and conclusions will take care of all eight cited circumstances where d_o is either $\geq\delta$ or $\leq\zeta$. A different problem arises, however, if the observed value of d_o is in the intermediate zone between ζ and δ. Such results are almost always undesired and disappointing for the investigator, who usually wants to show that a distinction is either big or small, but not intermediate.

The intermediate result can be evaluated with both sets of procedures for managing unexpected findings, because data showing that $\zeta < d_0 < \delta$ will usually be unwelcome, regardless of whether the investigator had a "big" or "small" goal. The four possibilities for the intermediate situation are shown in Table 24.4. The confidence intervals will lead to conclusions that either the result is a stochastic variation or one (or both) scientific hypotheses are probably wrong. If both scientific hypotheses are discarded, the conclusion is that d_0 indeed has an intermediate location, which has been stochastically confirmed. With the latter conclusion, the investigated phenomenon has produced a distinction that is too small to be "big" and too big to be "small." If the investigator still wants something impressively big or small, some other phenomenon (or explanation) should be explored.

TABLE 24.4

Stochastic Results and Conclusions When d_0 Is in Intermediate Zone

Observed Descriptive Result	Stochastic Result for Confidence Interval	Conclusion
$\zeta < d_0 < \delta$	δ excluded	Stochastically not "big"
	δ included	Possible stochastic variation from "big"
	0 included	Possible stochastic variation from "small"
	0 excluded	Stochastically not "small"

24.9 Conflicts and Controversies

Because testing and confirming equivalence is a relatively new activity, many conflicts and controversies have arisen about almost every component of the procedures.

24.9.1 Clinical Conditions and Measurements

A major controversy erupted in 1997 when the manufacturer of a "brand name" thyroxine product provided sponsorship and then tried to suppress publication of a study in which the corresponding generic products were found to be bioequivalent and therefore "interchangeable." The controversy[24] included issues of academic freedom, financial conflicts of interest, choice of additional data released by the manufacturer, and the advertisement policy of a prominent medical journal. At the level of scientific discourse, however, the main contentions about the claim of equivalence referred to the appropriateness of patients used for the research, the reliability of area-under-the-curve (AUC) calculations, and the adequacy of serum thyrotropin measurements.

24.9.2 Quantitative Boundaries for Efficacy and Equivalence

As noted by Greene et al.,[18] many investigators have published claims of equivalence without previously establishing a quantitative boundary for ζ. Instead, equivalence has been claimed after a failed stochastic test for "efficacy." The results of such studies are defective in both quantitative and stochastic decisions about equivalence.

A different problem arises when different boundaries are established in investigations of the same phenomenon. For example, in comparisons of thrombolytic treatment for acute myocardial infarction, the investigators in the GUSTO III trial[25] claimed equivalence when an observed difference of $d_o = .53\%$ was less than the preselected $\zeta = 1\%$. In the COBALT trial,[26] however, the incremental value of $d_o = .44\%$ was even smaller than the .53% found in GUSTO, but was regarded as "inequivalent" because it exceeded the preset limit of $\zeta = .40\%$. The GUSTO investigators[25] commented on "the question of an appropriate boundary for the definition of equivalence" and expressed concern that "acceptance of broad statistical definitions of equivalence may compromise previously established benchmarks of therapy."

24.9.3   Stochastic Problems and Solutions

In the absence of well-accepted boundaries for both quantitative distinctions and stochastic locations, and without a suitably symmetric logic for the stochastic evaluations, the evaluation of "equivalence" has many uncertainties and produces many difficulties. The three main problems are outlined in Table 24.5.

TABLE 24.5

Stochastic Problems Arising from Absence of Quantitative Boundaries for "Big" and "Small"

Observed d_o to Be Stochastically Confirmed	Location of Stochastic Hypothesis to Be Rejected	Problem
"Big"	0 (Null)	Large sample may confirm small d_o as "significant"
"Small" (equivalent)	Big	Anything smaller than "big" may be confirmed as 'small'
	Small	Huge sample size needed for confirmation

The first two problems produce statistical dissidence: in a test of efficacy, a big sample may confirm a small d_O as significant; and in a test of equivalence, a relatively large difference may be confirmed as small. The third problem is the excessively large sample size needed for confirmation of equivalence if the primary stochastic hypothesis is set at a small value, such as ζ.

Table 24.6 indicates how a suitable choice of quantitative boundaries can eliminate the problems noted in Table 24.5.

TABLE 24.6

Boundary Solutions to Problems Noted in Table 24.5

Observed d_o to Be Stochastically Confirmed	Location of Quantitative Boundary	Location of Stochastic Hypothesis	Confirmatory Conclusion
"Big"	$\geq \delta$	0	Can't be "big" unless $d_o \geq \delta$
"Small"	$\leq \zeta$	δ	Can't be "small" unless $d_o \leq \zeta$
	$\leq \zeta$	ζ	Improper logic: boundary and hypothesis should not be similar

24.9.4   Retroactive Calculations of "Power"

The last topic to be considered before this chapter ends is the retroactive calculation of "power" for an observed d_o that fails to achieve stochastic significance under the original null hypothesis. Although the proposals for this calculation do not clearly separate defects in power from defects in capacity, the usual assumption is that the observed d_o is smaller than δ, which is then used as the location of a secondary hypothesis for the power calculation. As Detsky and Sackett[27] have pointed out, the location of a "rejectable" δ will vary with the group sizes, so that larger groups can increase power for smaller values of δ than otherwise.

In the Detsky-Sackett illustrations, the power of a contrast of two proportions was determined with a chi-square test, not with the customary Z procedure; and the chi-square test[28] was done with a new primary equivalence hypothesis that $\Delta \geq \delta$. The Detsky-Sackett approach, however, was later attacked by Makuch and Johnson,[10] who advocated a Neyman-Pearson technique. Both of these approaches were then denounced by Goodman and Berlin,[29] who claimed that "power" is a prospective concept and should not be calculated retroactively. Smith and Bates[30] also argued that after a study has been completed, "power calculations provide no information not available from confidence limits" and that "once an actual relative risk estimate has been obtained, it makes little sense to calculate the power of that same study to detect some other relative risk."

Until this controversial issue receives a consensus solution, the best way of estimating how large d_o might have been is to determine a suitable confidence interval around d_o, without getting into disputes about demarcating a post-hoc δ and calculating "power."

References

1. Kirshner, 1991; 2. Armitage, 1971; 3. Zelen, 1969; 4. Anderson, 1993; 5. Chow, 1992; 6. Schulz, 1991; 7. Westlake, 1979; 8. O'Quigley, 1988; 9. Blackwelder, 1984; 10. Makuch, 1986; 11. Wynder, 1987; 12. Feinstein, 1990a; 13. Blackwelder, 1982; 14. Rodda, 1980; 15. Food and Drug Administration, 1977; 16. Jones, 1996; 17. Lindenbaum, 1971; 18. Greene, 2000; 19. Westlake, 1972; 20. Metzler, 1974; 21. Kramer, 1978; 22. Roebruck, 1995; 23. Makuch, 1978; 24. "Bioequivalence," 1997; 25. GUSTO III investigators, 1997; 26. COBALT investigators, 1997; 27. Detsky, 1985; 28. Dunnett, 1977; 29. Goodman, 1994; 30. Smith, 1992; 31. Carette, 1991; 32. Steering Committee of the Physicians' Health Study Research Group, 1989; 33. Peto, 1988; 34. Oski, 1980; 35. Pascoe, 1981.

Exercises

24.1. The investigators planning the clinical trial described in Exercise 23.1 realize that their results will be most acceptable if the main endpoint is death rather than improvement in angina. They are unhappy, however, to have to get about 3000 patients to prove the point. Having heard about the potential sample-size savings discussed in Chapter 24, the investigators now want to know how much smaller the sample size might be, with death as the end point, if they ignore the conventional Neyman-Pearson calculations and if, instead, they take precautions both to avoid α error for a "big" difference and to allow stochastic significance to be confirmed if a "tiny" difference is found. For this purpose, δ is set at .02 (a 20% proportionate reduction in death rate) and $\zeta = .005$ (a 5% proportionate reduction). What does the sample size become for the new goal? If the results are somewhat disappointing, what is your explanation?

24.2. In a double-blinded randomized trial in which the control group received isotonic saline injections, the investigators concluded that "injecting methylprednisolone into the facet joints is of little value in the treatment of patients with chronic low back pain."[31] To be eligible for the trial, the participants were required first to have had low back pain, lasting at least 6 months, that was substantially relieved within 30 minutes of a lidocaine injection in the facet joint space. Two weeks later, the back pain should have returned to at least 50% of its pre-lidocaine level. Patients meeting these requirements were then entered in the trial.

    24.2.1. After deciding that "significant benefit" would be the outcome for "only patients who reported very marked or marked improvement," the investigators "calculated that a sample size of 50 patients per group would be adequate at 80 percent power to detect at the 5 percent level of significance [by one-sided test] an estimated improvement in 50 percent of the patients given corticosteroid [and in] ... 25 percent of those given placebo." Demonstrate the calculation that you think was used to obtain the estimate of "50 patients per group."

24.2.2. In the published report, very marked or marked improvement was noted as follows in the two groups:

Time	Methylprednisolone	Placebo	Difference and 95% CI
One month	42% (= 20/48)	33% (= 16/48)	9% (–11 to 28)
Six months	46% (= 22/48)	15% (= 7/47)	31% (14 to 48)

In reaching the stated conclusion, the investigators believed that the six-month differences could be ignored because the methylprednisolone group received more "concurrent interventions," and because sustained improvement from the first month to the sixth month occurred in only 11 patients in the prednisolone group and in 5 of the placebo group.

Do you agree that these results justify the conclusions that "injections of methylprednisolone...are of little value in the treatment of patients with chronic low back pain"?

24.2.3. What aspect of the clinical and statistical design and analysis of this trial suggests that the trial was not an appropriate test of the hypothesis?

24.3. Exercise 10.1 was concerned with two clinical trials devoted to the merits of prophylactically taking an aspirin tablet daily (or every other day). In Exercise 14.4.1, you concluded that the U.S. study had an excessive sample size. Can you now apply a formula and appropriate assumptions re α, β, δ, etc. that will produce the sample size used for the trial in Exercise 14.4?

24.4. In a controlled pediatric trial of gastrointestinal symptoms produced by iron-fortified formulas for infants,[34] the mothers reported cramps for 41% (= 20/49) of infants receiving formula with no iron, and for 57% (= 25/44) of those receiving iron-fortified formula. The investigators concluded that "our study failed to provide any evidence for the commonly held belief that iron-fortified formulas produce gastrointestinal side effects in infants."

In a subsequent letter to the editor, titled "Was It a Type II Error?" the writer[35] claimed that the observed difference was "clinically important" but underpowered. According to the writer, "β is > 0.5" for the observed difference, but a "larger sample (about 150 per group) would have probably ($\beta = 0.35$) generated a significant 16% difference."

24.4.1. Do you agree with the investigators' original conclusions?

24.4.2. Do you agree with the basic dissent in the letter to the editor (i.e., that the investigators haven't proved their claim)? If you agree with the dissent, do you agree with the way it has been expressed? If not, suggest a better expression.

24.4.3. Do you agree with the dissenter's claim that stochastic significance would require about 150 per group, and that such a size would be associated with $\beta = 0.35$? Show the calculations that support your answer.

25

Multiple Stochastic Testing

CONTENTS

All of the previously discussed stochastic analyses were concerned with appraising results for a single *scientific* hypothesis. The scientific goal, the observed result, and the stochastic test may or may not have been in full agreement (as discussed throughout Section 24.8), but the testing itself was aimed at a single main *scientific* hypothesis.

This chapter is concerned with three situations that involve multiple stochastic testing. It can occur for different hypotheses in the same set of data, for repeated checks of accruing data for the same hypothesis, or for new tests of aggregates of data that previously received hypothesis tests. In the first procedure, which is often called *multiple comparisons*, the results of a single study are arranged into a series of individual contrasts, each of which is tested for "significance" under a separate stochastic hypothesis. In the second procedure, often called *sequential testing*, only a single hypothesis is evaluated, but it is tested repeatedly in a set of accumulating data. In the third procedure, which occurs during an activity called *meta-analysis*, a hypothesis that has previously been checked in each of several studies is tested again after their individual results have been combined.

25.1 Formation of Multiple Comparisons

The first part of the chapter is concerned with the controversial problem of multiple comparisons, which warrants a more extensive discussion than the brief outline offered in Section 11.10.

25.1.1   Example of Problem

To illustrate one aspect of the problem, suppose four different therapeutic agents — A, B, C, and D — are tested in the same randomized clinical trial. When the trial is over, the results for a single outcome, such as "success," are compared in each pair of groups: A vs. B, A vs. C, A vs. D, B vs. C, B vs. D, and C vs. D. Because k groups can be paired in $k(k - 1)/2$ ways, 6 pairs of comparisons can be done for the 4 groups.

If α is set at .05, and if the null hypothesis is correct that all four agents in the trial are essentially similar, each "positive" comparison has a .05 chance of being a false-positive result, and a .95 chance of being truly negative. For any two comparisons, the chances are $.95 \times .95 = .90$ that both will be truly negative and $1 - .90 = .10$ that at least one of the two comparisons will be falsely positive. For six comparisons under the null hypothesis, the chance is $(.95)^6 = .735$ that all six will be negative, and $1 - .735 = .265$ that a false positive result will emerge somewhere in the group of six tests. Thus, although set at .05 for each comparison, the operational level of α for the total of six pairs of comparisons becomes elevated to .265.

If each pair in a set of k comparisons has a $1 - \alpha$ chance of being truly negative, the overall chance of getting a true negative result is $(1 - \alpha)^k$. The chance of getting a false positive result somewhere in the set becomes $1 - (1 - \alpha)^k$. Thus, with α designated at .05 for each of 20 comparisons, the chance that at least one of them will be positive by stochastic variation alone is $1 - (.95)^{20} = 1 - .358 = .642$. For 100 comparisons, $(.95)^{100} = .0059$; and the chance of getting at least one false positive result will be .9941. Therefore, even if nothing is really "significant," stochastic significance can almost surely occur by random chance alone somewhere in the set of data if enough comparative tests are done.

Because of this problem, the α level for a single stochastic comparison may no longer be pertinent if the data of a particular study are tested in a series of comparisons. The difficulty has received many names. It is most often called the *multiple-comparison* problem, because the stochastic tests are usually applied to multiple two-group contrasts; but *multiple-association* has been the label when the multiple testing occurs in correlation or regression analysis. Both of these titles are covered in Miller's generic but longer name, *simultaneous statistical inference*,[1] for which *multiple inference* might be a shorter term.

25.1.2   Architectural Sources

Often approached as a purely statistical problem, multiple comparisons can usually be "sensibly" analyzed if their scientific sources are appropriately considered. These sources are the questions asked for data arising from architectural components that can be agents, outcomes, subgroups, and time.

25.1.2.1   Multiple Agents or Maneuvers — The term *agent* or *maneuver* can be used for the entity regarded as a possible cause, risk, or impacting factor for the "effect" noted as an outcome event. The maneuver can be examined in a prospective (or "longitudinal") manner when "exposed" cohort groups are followed in observational studies or randomized trials. The maneuver can also be determined in retrospect for the "outcome" groups analyzed in case-control studies and other forms of cross-sectional research.

25.1.2.1.1   Cohort Studies.   In clinical trials or in nonrandomized cohort studies, pragmatic convenience may make the investigators examine several agents simultaneously. In the "four-arm" randomized trial discussed in Section 25.1.1, agents A, B, C, and D might have been examined concomitantly because the investigators wanted to learn all they could from the expensive complexity of arranging personnel, laboratory facilities, and other "apparatus" for the trial, without incurring the extra costs and efforts of doing separate trials to compare each pair of agents. Besides, the comparisons might be impeded if the trials were done at several locations (where the patient groups might differ) or at different periods in calendar time.

Another arrangement of multiple agents occurs when a "dose-response curve" is analyzed for parallel groups of patients receiving fixed but different doses of the same substance. A placebo may or may not be used in such studies; a small, almost homeopathic dose of the active agent is sometimes substituted for a placebo.

In the two examples just cited, the muliitple agents delineated the groups under study. In certain observational cohorts, however, specific agents have not been deliberately assigned. Instead, the investigators collect information about a series of baseline variables, which can then be analyzed as "risk factors" when pertinent events later occur as "outcomes." The pertinent outcome events may have been individually identified beforehand, such as coronary heart disease in the Framingham Study,[2,3] or may be chosen according to ad hoc topics of interest, as in the Harvard Nurses Study.[4]

25.1.2.1.2 Case-Control Studies. Retrospective case-control research is a fertile source of stochastic tests for multiple agents. After the studied groups have been assembled according to presence or absence of the outcome event, the investigative inquiries, aimed in a backward temporal direction, can seek evidence of antecedent exposure to many etiologic agents or risk factors. If the results do not incriminate the main agent(s) under suspicion, the investigators may then "screen" all the other possible agents for which information was collected.

Some 20 years ago, this type of screening led to a highly publicized but now discredited accusation that coffee drinking was causing pancreatic cancer. The accusation came from a case-control study[5] in which the main etiologic suspicions were originally directed at tobacco and alcohol. After these suspects were "exonerated" by the data, the investigators explored an unidentified number of additional agents, from which coffee emerged as having a "statistically significant" association with the cases of pancreatic cancer. The "significance" was not corrected for multiple comparisons,[6] however, and the association was refuted when the research was repeated by the original investigators.[7]

Multiple comparisons are easily and regularly arranged in case-control studies of "risk factors" for etiology of disease. The investigators can "round up the usual suspects" by collecting information about diverse features of demographic status (age, sex, education, income, social status), past medical history (childhood and other previous diseases), family medical history (diseases in relatives), environmental exposure (pets, atmospheric pollution, travel abroad, home conditions), occupational exposure (fumes, chemicals), and personal habits (smoking, alcohol, dietary components, physical activities, cosmetics, hair dyes). In the usual questionnaire for such studies, more than 100 candidate variables can readily be assembled and then checked for their statistical relationship to the occurrence (or nonoccurrence) of the selected outcome disease.

25.1.2.2 Multiple Outcomes

— Multiple outcome events will occur in any cohort study, regardless of whether the "causal" maneuvers are self-selected or assigned as part of a randomized trial. To satisfy regulatory agencies, reviewers, or readers and to provide a specific focus in design of the research, one of the many possible outcomes is usually designated as the prime target. The many other outcome events, however, are still observed, recorded, and then available as data that can be examined for purposes of confirmation, explanation, or exploration.

In a *confirmatory* examination, the desired primary outcome was achieved; and the confirmation provides additional, consistent evidence. For example, if imaging evidence shows that a thrombus dissolved or disappeared as the primary goal of treatment, additional laboratory evidence of clot-dissolution effects would be confirmatory. In an *explanatory* examination, the additional evidence would help explain why the primary effect occurred. For example, a reduction in fever and white blood count could help explain the disappearance of pain or malaise in patients with a bacterial infection.

In an *exploratory* examination, however, the desired primary outcome was not achieved. The investigator may then check the additional outcome events, hoping to find some other evidence of a beneficial (or adverse) effect. Thus, if mortality was not reduced with an anti-leukemic treatment, the investigators may search for efficacy in evidence of remission, reduction in number of white cells, or other selected targets.

25.1.2.3 Multiple Agents and Outcomes

— In a case-control study, the diverse risk-factor candidates can be explored only in relation to the specific disease chosen for the cases; but in a cohort or cross-sectional survey, a diverse collection of diseases (or other conditions) can also be available as outcome events.

An extraordinary opportunity for multiple comparisons occurs in collections of data where the investigators can check simultaneously for multiple agents and multiple outcomes. Thus, if adequate data are available for 100 candidate "risk" variables and 50 outcome diseases, 5,000 relationships can be tested. Opportunities for these "mega-comparisons" arise when information is collected in a medico-fiscal claims system or in special data banks for pharmacologic surveillance of hospitalized patients. In both types of data banks, the investigators will have information about multiple therapeutic agents that can then be explored as etiologic precursors of multiple diseases.

The exploration is sometimes called a "fishing expedition," "mining the data," or "dredging the data bank." If data are available for 200 therapeutic agents and 150 diseases, 30,000 relationships can be explored. With α set at .05 for each relationship, a "positive" result could be expected by chance alone in 1500 of the explorations, even if no true relationships exist.

25.1.2.4 *Multiple Subgroups* — If nothing exciting emerges from all the other possibilities, the relationships of agents and outcomes can be checked in different subgroups. The subgroups can be demarcated by demographic attributes such as age, sex, race, occupation, religion, and socioeconomic status; by medical attributes such as stage of disease and laboratory tests; and by geographic regions.

For example, in a large case-control study of the relationship between saccharin and bladder cancer,[8] the investigators were apparently disappointed to find an overall odds ratio of essentially 1. After multiple subgroup analyses, however, a significantly elevated odds ratio was found in two subgroups: white men who were heavy smokers and nonsmoking white women who were not exposed to certain chemical substances.

Probably the greatest opportunity to explore multiple subgroups occurs if the analyst has access to data collected for different geographic regions, such as individual nations or parts of a nation. For the United States, the nation can be divided into whatever zones the investigator wants to check: individual states (such as West Virginia), large regions (such as "the South"), counties, cities, political districts, or census tracts. If outcome events such as death or disease are available for these zones, and if exposures can also be demonstrated or inferred from concomitant data about occupation, industry, air pollution, or sales of different substances, an almost limitless number of explorations is possible, particularly because the relationships between any outcome and any exposure in any geographic zone can also be checked in multiple demographic subgroups. Explorations in search of a particular relationship have sometimes been called "data torturing,"[9] and, when zealously applied, "torturing the data until they confess."

Aside from the problem of mathematical corrections for "chance" results, the scientific interpretation of the findings is always difficult. Do the different occurrence rates of cancer reflect true differences in the zones demarcated for "cancer maps"[10] or differences in the use of diagnostic surveillance, testing, and criteria? Has a true "cluster" or mini-epidemic of disease really occurred at a particular site, or is the event attributable to chance when so many possible sites are available for the occurrence?[11,12]

25.1.2.5 *Temporal Distinctions* — Beyond all the explorations of variables for agents, outcomes, subgroups, and regions, a separate set of opportunities for multiple comparisons is presented by time, which can appear in both *secular* and *serial* manifestations.

The word *secular* is regularly used in an ecclesiastical sense to distinguish worldly or "profane" things from those that are religious or sacred; but in epidemiologic research, *secular* refers to calendar time. The word *serial* refers to time elapsed for a particular person since a selected "zero time," which might be randomization, onset of therapy, or the date of admission to an ongoing study. The two concepts appear in a single sentence if we say that the five-year survival rate (serial) has been steadily rising for a particular cancer during the past thirty years (secular).

Secular trends are regularly examined in epidemiologic studies of mortality rates, cancer incidence, etc. for the same single geographic zones. Because the trends are usually reported with a single index of association, major stochastic problems do not occur. The problem of multiple comparisons would arise, however, if an investigator compared a mortality rate for a recent year against the corresponding rate for each of a series of previous years.

The main role of time in multiple comparisons, however, usually occurs as a *serial* problem in timing of outcome measurements, discussed next, or in the sequential accrual of data, discussed in Section 25.3.

25.1.2.6 Timing of Outcome Measurement — If the outcome is a binary event, such as death or recurrences of myocardial infarction, the analysis is usually managed with the "life-table" methods, discussed in Chapter 22, that focus on time to occurrence of the "failure" event. In many other studies, however, the outcome is expressed with an ordinal or dimensional variable, such as level of pain or blood pressure, for which average magnitude (or change) in two treated groups can be checked at different serial times after onset of treatment. For pain, the intervals might be at 15 min, 30 min, 60 min, and 90 min; for blood pressure, they might be at 1, 2, 4, 6, and 8 weeks.

If stochastic significance is present at just one or two of these intervals, but not at the others, questions can arise about how (if at all) to adjust the α level for the multiple comparisons.

25.1.3 Analytic Sources

Beyond all the opportunities just cited in the architecture of the research, multiple comparisons can also be produced as a purely statistical activity when the data are analyzed. One opportunity comes when the same comparison receives alternative stochastic tests. Another opportunity arises during a "stepped" sequence for multivariable analyses.

25.1.3.1 Alternative Stochastic Procedures — A multi-comparison issue that seldom receives statistical attention occurs when the same hypothesis in the same set of data is tested with different stochastic procedures. For example, a set of dimensional results in two groups can be contrasted stochastically with a t test, a Wilcoxon-Mann-Whitney rank test, or a Pitman-Welch permutation test. [One-tailed and two-tailed interpretations cannot be regarded as more than one comparison, because they use different stochastic hypotheses. The null hypothesis would be $\Delta = 0$ for two tails, and $\Delta \geq 0$ (or ≤ 0) for one tail.]

If the alternative stochastic tests do not all lead to the same conclusion for "significance," the data analysts usually choose the results they like. This problem is probably ignored in most statistical discussions because it arises not from random chance, but from the different mathematical strategies used to evaluate the role of random chance.

25.1.3.2 Sequential Stepping in Multivariable Analysis — A more "legitimate" random-chance problem occurs in multivariable regression where the outcome event is a single dependent variable that is associated with different combinations of individual "independent" variables in sequentially stepped analyses. The stepping can go in an upward (or "forward") direction, starting with one independent variable and progressively adding others, or in a downward (or "backward") direction, starting with all the available independent variables, and progressively removing them one at a time. [The process can also go back and forth in a "stepwise" (or "zig-zag") arrangement].

Despite occasional discussion,[13] no agreement has been reached on whether the α level should be adjusted for the multiple inferences. Consequently, the problem is usually ignored, and the analysts then apply the same preset level of α without alteration during each of the successive analyses.

25.2 Management of Multiple Comparisons

The management of multiple comparisons is a complex and controversial issue. The proposals range from a purely stochastic "correction," to a "benign neglect" that imposes no adjustment at all, to decisions based on architectural and other scientific principles.

25.2.1   Stochastic Decisions

The many mathematical proposals offered for prophylactic and remedial management of the "multiple inference" problem have enriched the world of statistical eponyms with such names as Bonferroni,[14] Duncan,[15] Dunn,[16] Dunnett,[17] Newman-Keuls,[18,19] Scheffe,[20] and (of course) Tukey.[21,22] In almost all of the proposed methods, the overall level of α is "penalized" by reduction to a smaller α' for the individual comparisons (or tests). When a smaller α' is used for individual tests, the overall level of α can be kept at the desired boundary for the total set of comparisons. The diverse proposals differ in the arrangements used for planning the multiple comparisons and for setting the penalties.

25.2.1.1   Bonferroni Correction — Of the diverse penalty proposals, the most obvious and easy to understand is called the *Bonferroni correction*.[14] For k comparisons, the level of α for each test is reduced to $\alpha' = \alpha/k$. Thus, with 6 comparisons, each would be called stochastically significant only if its P value were below $\alpha' = .05/6 = .00833$. This tactic would make $1 - \alpha'$ become $1 - .00833 = .99167$ for each comparison and $(1 - \alpha')^k$ would be $(.99167)^6 = .951$ for the group. The overall $\alpha = 1 - .951 = .049$ would remain close to the desired level of .05.

For interpretation, each of the multiple P_i values is multiplied by k (i.e., the number of comparisons) and the "Bonferronied" P value is compared against the original α. For example, if 8 comparisons were done, a result that obtains P = .023 would be evaluated as though P = .184. If decisions are made with confidence intervals rather than P values, the confidence interval is constructed with α/k rather than α. Thus, for 8 comparisons at $\alpha = .05$, the value of Z_α selected for the confidence interval would be $Z_{.00625}$ rather than $Z_{.05}$. The larger adjusted value of Z would produce a larger confidence interval and a reduced chance of excluding the null value of the stochastic hypothesis.

In recent years, the Bonferroni procedure has been criticized for having low power, i.e., truly "significant" results may be declared "nonsignificant." Of alternative methods proposed by Holm,[23,24] Hochberg,[25] and Simes,[26] the Holm procedure, which requires arranging the P_i values in increasing order, has been hailed[27] as "simple to calculate, ... universally valid, ... more powerful than the Bonferroni procedure," and a preferable "first-line choice for distribution-free multiple comparisons." Nevertheless, after examining the operating characteristics of 17 methods for doing the correction, Brown and Russell[28] concluded that "the only guaranteed methods to correct for multiplicity are the Bonferroni method and (the Holm) step-down analogue."

Although each of the many multiple-comparison proposals has its own special mathematical virtues, the Bonferroni correction has the scientific advantage of remarkable simplicity. It is still probably the best correction to know, if you plan to know only one.

25.2.1.2   Other Proposals — Unlike the Bonferroni and other tactics just cited, which can be applied in almost any situation, most other proposals[29,30] for managing the multiple-comparison problem are "tailored" to the particular structure of the research. For example, when treatments A, B, C, and D are tested simultaneously in the same trial, the conventional statistical analysis might begin with an analysis of variance (discussed later in Chapter 29), which first checks for "overall significance" among the four treatments. The stochastic adjustments thereafter are aimed at the pairwise comparisons of individual treatments.

If accruing data for two treatments are checked at periodic intervals in an ongoing randomized trial, the stochastic adjustments are set at lower levels of α' for each of the sequential decisions, so that α will have an appropriate value when the trial has finished. The choices proposed for the sequentially lowered α' levels have brought an additional set of eponyms, which are discussed later in Section 25.3.3.3.

Among other purely stochastic approaches, Westfall and Young[31] have developed a compendium of bootstrap correction methods. Another strategy[32] is to split the data into two parts, of which the first is used to explore multiple hypotheses. Those that are "significant" are then tested in the second part; and attention thereafter is given to only the hypotheses that "passed" both tests.

25.2.1.3   *Problems of Intercorrelation* — When multiple factors are individually checked for their impact on an outcome event, some of them may be stochastically significant by chance alone, but their actual impact may be altered by correlations among the diverse factors. An example of this problem was noted[3] for intercorrelations among such baseline "risk factors" as blood pressure, weight, serum cholesterol, age, and pulse rate among men who did or did not develop coronary disease in the famous Framingham study.

The suitable adjustment of intervariable correlations is more of a descriptive than a stochastic challenge, however, and is managed with multivariable analytic methods. The main intervariable problems arise, as noted in Section 25.1.3.2, when multiple testing is done as individual variables are added or removed incrementally during a "stepping" process.

25.2.1.4   *Bayesian Methods*   — All of the challenges of interpreting and adjusting P values can be avoided by using the methods of Bayesian inference. For each relationship, a prior probability is specified beforehand. It then becomes transformed, with the likelihood ratio determined from the observed data, into a posterior probability that reflects belief in the observed relationship, given the data. Adjustments are not needed for multiple-null-hypothesis P values, because each relationship has its own prior probability.

Appealing as the Bayesian approach may be, it has one supreme disadvantage. The prior probabilities cannot be established *beforehand* for relationships that emerge as "significant" only in conventional P values obtained *after* the data have been explored. A second problem, which may or may not be a disadvantage, is that the selection of prior probabilities, even when possible, will depend more on scientific anticipations (discussed later in Section 25.2.4.) than on purely mathematical estimations.

25.2.2   "Permissive Neglect"

At the opposite extreme of management, the stochastic adjustments are replaced by a "permissive-neglect" argument that "no adjustments are needed for multiple comparisons."[33] Perhaps the simplest way of stating this argument is that a stochastic test is intended to demonstrate numerical stability of the results. If not stable, they need receive no further attention; if stable, their further evaluation depends on the scientific context and connotations. The stochastic criterion for stability, however, should not be altered according to whatever additional comparisons may have occurred. If the number of additional comparisons is really pertinent, perhaps "an investigator should control his 'career-wise' alpha level, or … all investigators should agree to control the 'discipline-wise' level."[32]

Proponents of the permissive-neglect argument may dismiss not only the stochastic but also the scientific approach to multiple comparisons. According to one proposal,[34] the investigator's "perspective" in deciding what data to collect and analyze is "irrelevant to assessing the validity of the product." The "motivations for including the specific items in the study and conducting the analyses has [*sic*] no independent relation to the quality of the data generated."

At the extreme of the anti-multiple-comparison-correction argument is the claim that hypotheses generated from the data need not be distinguished from those tested with the data.[34,35] Cole has proposed a theoretical hypothesis-generating machine,[35] with which "all possible cause-effect hypotheses have been generated," so that all subsequent activities can be regarded as hypothesis testing rather than generating. This approach would allow epidemiologists to use a counterpart of the "Texas sharpshooter strategy" in which someone fires a shot at a barn and then draws a target around the site where the bullet hit.

25.2.3   Scientific Validity

In contrast to the mathematical rigidity of the purely stochastic approach and the nihilistic permissiveness of the no-correction approach, multiple comparisons can be evaluated with principles, discussed elsewhere[36] and earlier in Section 11.10.3, that focus on *scientific* rather than *statistical* inference. The principles refer to the internal validity of the comparisons or associations examined in the data, and to their external validity when applied beyond the particular persons who were investigated.

For *internal validity*, the architectural components of the research should be free from four types of biased comparison: susceptibility bias in the baseline states, performance bias in the maneuvers, detection bias in the outcome events, and transfer bias in the collection of groups and data. For *external validity*, the groups and data should be suitable for the derived conclusion, and for the observed results to be extrapolated to the outside world beyond the special conditions of the study. For scientific decisions, these internal and external evaluations should always take place after (and preferably before) any statistical conclusions have been formed. If scientific validity is dubious, the statistical results can often be dismissed without further attention.

For example, when multiple-comparison analyses lead to highly publicized reports that pizza protects against prostate cancer whereas hot dogs raise the risk of brain cancer, a first step might be to determine whether the surveillance and monitoring that detected those cancers were carried out similarly in the groups who are "exposed" or "non-exposed" to the ingestion of pizza or hot dogs. In most such reports, the investigators have given no attention to the problem of "detection bias."

Without resorting to architectural appraisals, scientists who are familiar with real-world medical phenomena might even use a simple analog of Bayesian inference called "clinical common sense." For example, after the erroneous statistical association that led to coffee being widely publicized as a cause of pancreatic cancer, a distinguished Canadian scientist[37] told me, "I knew it couldn't be true. If it were, pancreatic cancer would be a major problem in Brazil." Analogous common sense might have been used to dismiss the anti- or pro-carcinogenic assertions about pizza and hot dogs, and to avoid some of the other epidemiologic embarassments produced by erroneous but highly publicized accusations about the "menace of daily life."[38]

25.2.4 Specification of Scientific Hypotheses

An additional scientific approach to the multiple-comparison problem involves appraising the timing and specificity with which the statistical hypotheses were formulated. The choice and severity of a stochastic (or other) penalty might depend on the way those hypotheses were scientifically articulated before the analyses began. This approach has been advocated even in statistical publications, with the recommendation that no corrections are needed for multiplicity when "a select number of important well-defined clinical questions are specified at the design."[39]

If the *scientific* hypotheses are stipulated in advance when the research is planned, the main mathematical challenges are to choose one- or two-tailed test directions, magnitudes for the boundaries of δ and ζ, and pertinent stochastic levels for α and β. In multiple-comparison problems, however, the scientific hypotheses may have been stipulated, vaguely anticipated, uncertain, or unknown before the data were statistically analyzed. If suitable attention is given to these previous specifications for the *scientific* hypothesis, the multiple-comparison problem might be effectively managed with substantive, rather than statistical, decisions.

25.2.4.1 Stipulated — Suppose the investigator wants to compare the virtues of a new analgesic agent, Excellitol, against a standard active agent, such as aspirin. To get approval from a regulatory agency, Excellitol must also be compared against placebo. When the randomized trial is designed with three "arms"— Excellitol, aspirin, and placebo—the main goal is to show that Excellitol is better than aspirin or at least as good. In this trial, the placebo "arm" does not really have a therapeutic role; its main job is scientific, to avoid the problem of interpretation if two allegedly active analgesic agents seem to have similar effects. The similar results may have occurred if the active agents were not adequately challenged because the patients under study had pain that was either too severe or too mild. A superiority to placebo will indicate that both active agents were indeed efficacious.

Many data analysts would readily agree that previously stipulated hypotheses should be tested without a mathematical penalty. Instead of the "three-arm" randomized trial just discussed, the investigators might have done three separate trials, testing Excellitol vs. aspirin in one study, aspirin vs. placebo in another, and Excellitol vs. placebo in a third. Because the results of each of these three studies would be appraised with the customary levels of α, a penalty imposed for research done with an efficient design would seem to be an excessive act of pedantry.

Similarly, when investigators check multiple post-therapeutic outcomes to *explain* a significant main result, no penalties seem necessary or desirable. For example, if Treatment A achieved significant improvement in the main global rating, various other individual manifestations — such as pain, mobility, or dyspnea — may then be checked to help explain other significant distinctions in the compared treatments. In these explanatory contrasts, the main role of the stochastic hypothesis is to confirm numerical stability, not to test new causal concepts.

In another situation, if cogent subgroups are defined by well-established and well-documented confounders, the examination of their results would represent the equivalent of previously stipulated hypotheses. For example, if a new chemotherapy significantly prolongs survival in a large group of patients with advanced cancer, the results can quite reasonably be checked in "well-established" subgroups that are demarcated by such well-known prognostic factors as age and severity of clinical stage. The subgroups would not be well established or well documented if they were "dredged" from data for such factors as occupation or serum sodium level. Analysis of results within clinically cogent subgroups[40] would therefore be an appropriate scientific activity, requiring no mathematical penalties. Because the explanatory tests would be done to confirm and explain the original hypothesis, not to generate new ones, the level of α need not be penalized for the tests.

25.2.4.2 *Vaguely Anticipated*

Vaguely Anticipated — Suppose 8 active analgesic agents — A, B, C, D, E, F, G, and H — are compared in the same trial, in addition to aspirin and placebo. The investigators who do such a 10-"arm" trial might check all of the 45 ($= 10 \times 9/2$) pairwise comparisons afterward, but the main focus might be only on the 8 comparisons of active agents vs. aspirin, and the 9 comparisons of active agents vs. placebo. The original scientific hypothesis was that aspirin would be inferior to at least one of the non-aspirin agents, but its identity was not stipulated. Hence, a superior individual result, if found, can be regarded as vaguely anticipated. A stochastic penalty might be imposed for the 8 tests of active agents vs. aspirin, but not for all the other comparisons.

25.2.4.3 *Uncertain*

Uncertain — Examples of multiple explorations for previously uncertain hypotheses can be found in most retrospective case-control studies. In cohort research, a counterpart example is provided by the results now published for more than 20 "cause–effect" relationships examined in a group of about 100,000 nurses who were assembled and "followed-up" by responses to mailed questionnaires.[4,41]

Because most of the "risk" information would not be collected if it were regarded as wholly unrelated to the outcome event, the investigators may argue that any positive results in the multiple comparisons were "anticipated." Furthermore, stochastic penalties are obviously not needed in certain analyses where special additional data were collected for tests of specific *scientific* hypotheses.[41] On the other hand, if the relationship between an individual risk factor and an individual outcome were not deliberately stipulated in advance as a focus of the research, the scientific hypothesis for each test can be regarded as uncertain. A stochastic penalty might be imposed, but it need not be quite as harsh as the draconian "punishment" warranted for totally unknown hypotheses discussed in the next subsection.

25.2.4.4 *Unknown*

Unknown — The data-dredging activities mentioned earlier are the most glaring example of the multiple-comparison problem, which is abetted by the modern availability of digital computers that can store and easily process huge amounts of data. With this capability, computer programs can be written to check any appropriate "risk" variable against any appropriate "outcome" variable in any suitably large collection of data. The computer can then print stars or ring bells whenever a "significant" distinction is found.

In one famous example of this type of "hypothesis-generating" adventure, previous exposures to medication were associated with hospital admission diagnoses for an estimated 200 drugs and 200 diseases in a "data bank" for a large group of patients.[42] Among the "significant" results of the explorations, which were not stochastically corrected for multiple comparisons, was a relationship suspected as causal between reserpine and breast cancer.[43] After diverse sources of bias were later revealed in the original and in two concomitantly published "confirmatory" studies,[44–45] the relationship has now become a classic teaching example of sources of error in epidemiologic research.

If the analytic procedures are pure acts of exploration, data-dredging, or other exercises in "looking for a pony" whose identity was not anticipated beforehand, some type of intervention is obviously needed to protect the investigators from their own delusions. For example, if the primary hypotheses were not supported by the main results of a clinical trial, and if the investigators then explore other outcome events (such as individual manifestations or laboratory data) hoping to find something — anything — that can be deemed "significant," the process is a counterpart of data dredging. Similarly, in various epidemiologic studies, when diverse variables are checked as "confounders" without having been previously identified as such for the relationship under investigation, the results are obviously not a product of stipulated scientific hypotheses.

In the absence of both an established strategy for "common sense" and data that allow appraisal of architectural validity, the most consistent approach is to apply a mathematical adjustment. The mathematical penalty could be harsh for previously unknown exploratory hypotheses, slightly reduced for uncertain hypotheses, and "softened" for hypotheses that were vaguely anticipated or tested repeatedly in sequential evaluations. A more powerful alternative strategy, of course, is to apply rigorous scientific standards to raise quality in designing and evaluating the architecture of the research, rather than using arbitrary mathematical methods to lower the α levels.

25.2.5   Commonsense Guidelines

Regardless of whether and how the foregoing *scientific* guidelines are applied, several non-mathematical principles of scientific common sense can always be applied.

25.2.5.1   Acceptibility of "Proof" — No hypothesis derived from statistical data can ever be regarded as proved by the same data used to generate it. At least one other study, with some other set of data, must be done to confirm the results. For example, in the previously cited erroneous accusation that reserpine was causing breast cancer, a causal claim would probably not have been accepted for publication if supported only by results of the original data-dredged study.[43] The claim was published because it had been "confirmed" (at least temporarily) by two other investigations[44,45] elsewhere.

25.2.5.2   Check for Scientific Error/Bias — Many unexpectedly "positive" relationships arise not by stochastic chance alone, but from bias and/or inaccuracy in the compared groups and data. The appropriate exploration and suitable management of these scientific errors will do much more to eliminate "false positive" results than anything provided by mathematical guidelines.

25.2.5.3   Demand for "Truthful" Reporting — Many clinical trials and other research projects today are done only after a sample size has been calculated, using selected levels of δ, α, and perhaps β. The previously set levels should preferably be maintained in the analysis and always be cited when the research is reported.

Another aspect of "truthful" reporting would be a citation of all the comparisons that were made before the analysis hit "bingo." The citation would allow readers to determine whether and how much of a stochastic or other "penalty" should be imposed. For example, in the erroneous coffee-pancreatic cancer study mentioned earlier,[5] a reader of the published report could discern that at least six relationships had been explored, but the investigators had probably checked many others before achieving "success" with coffee.

25.2.5.4   Focus on Quantitative Significance — In many reports, the boundaries set for quantitative distinctions are *not* cited, particularly when the "delta wobble" lowers the initial value of δ so that stochastic significance is claimed for a value of d_o that might not have been previously regarded as impressive. If readers and reviewers (as well as investigators) begin to focus on the quantitative importance rather than stochastic significance of the numbers, many of the existing problems can be avoided or eliminated. The dominant role of sample size should always be carefully considered when

analyses of large groups of persons (and data) produce impressive P values (or confidence intervals) for distinctions that may have little or no importance. With emphasis on the quantitative magnitude of the distinction rather than its stochastic accompaniment, many issues can be resolved on the basis of triviality in descriptive magnitude, without the need to adjust levels of α.

(The concept of quantitative magnitude will also require careful consideration if Bayesian methods are used to estimate prior probability, because both the prior and posterior probabilities will involve the "effect size" of anticipated and observed distinctions.)

If quantitative magnitude continues to receive its current neglect, however, investigators may preserve and increase the contemporary emphasis on stochastic confidence intervals and P values. An excellent example of the emphasis was presented in a guideline suggested for dealing with the problem of multiple comparisons: "Any unexpected relationships should be viewed with caution unless the P value is very extreme (say less than 0.001). However, this difficulty does not affect the relationships assessment of which would have been expected *a priori*. Paradoxically, in a study such as ours, a correlation significant at the 1 in 20 level demonstrating an expected relationship is more reliable than an unexpected correlation significant at the 1 in 200 level."[46]

The progress of science and statistics in the 21st century will depend on investigators' ability to overcome this type of stochastic infatuation.

25.3 Sequential Evaluation of Accruing Data

A different type of multiple-comparison problem, which is almost unique to long-term randomized clinical trials, occurs when the *same* hypothesis is tested repetitively as data accrue for the results of the trial.

The repetitive testing is usually motivated by both pragmatic and ethical reasons. Pragmatically, the investigators would like to keep the trial as small and short as possible, getting convincing results with a minimum of patients, duration, and costs. Ethically, the investigators worry about continuing a trial beyond the point at which the conclusions are clear.

The ethics of randomized trials are a thorny problem. Some writers[47] argue that most randomized trials are unethical because the investigators' main goal is to get convincing evidence of a superiority that they already believe. In this view, a trial is ethical only when initiated with genuine uncertainty, under the "equipoise" principle[48] that none of the compared agents has been demonstrably superior (or inferior). Most investigators, using their own concept of the term *demonstrably*, can usually justify the equipoise belief; but if the belief is altered by accruing results that show one of the agents to be unequivocally better (or worse), the investigators may want to stop the trial promptly before it reaches the scheduled ending.

25.3.1 Sequential Designs

The challenge can be approached with a *sequential design*, which makes advance plans to stop the trial as soon as a definitive conclusion emerges.

The general statistical method called *sequential analysis* was first developed during World War II by Wald[49] in the U.S. and by Barnard[50] in the U.K. The method was initially used as a quality control test in the manufacture of artillery and was later applied in other industrial circumstances. The method relied on repeated sampling, however, and the theory required suitable modification by Armitage[51] to become pertinent for the single group of people who enter a randomized clinical trial.

In the plans of a sequential design, the patients are arbitrarily arranged in pairs as they successively enter the trial. After the compared treatments, A and B, have been randomly assigned and carried out for each pair of patients, the examined results may show either a tie or that A or B is the "winner." As secular time progresses, an accruing tally of scores is kept in a graph on which the X axis is the number of entered pairs. The tally on the Y axis goes up or down for each A or B winning score. For a tie, the X axis advances by one, with no change in the level of Y.

Before the trial begins, special "outer" boundaries are statistically calculated for stopping the trial with a "significant" result when the accruing tally in favor of A or B exceeds the corresponding upper or lower boundary. The trial can also be stopped for having "insignificant" or "inconclusive" results if the tally crosses a separate "inner" boundary before reaching any of the outer boundaries of "significance." In certain drawings, the sloping outer and inner margins of the graphical pattern, shown in Figure 25.1, resemble a "pac-man" symbol.

Despite the appeal of letting a trial be stopped at the earliest possible moment with the smallest necessary sample size, the sequential-design method is seldom used. The main problem is feasibility. To find a prompt "winner" for each pair of patients, the outcome event must be something that occurs soon after treatment. The type of therapy that can be tested is therefore restricted to agents used in treating acute pain, acute insomnia, or other conditions where the outcome can be determined within a relatively short time, such as 24 hours after treatment. In the trial[52] shown in Figure 25.1, the investigators applied an unusual cross-over design to compare an active agent vs. placebo in patients with a known high attack rate of ("catamenial") epilepsy associated with the menstrual cycle.

An additional problem in sequential designs is that reliance on a single outcome event — such as relief of symptoms — may produce stochastic significance for that event, but not for associated manifestations that the investigators would also like to examine. Furthermore, unless the treated condition has a remarkably homogeneous clinical spectrum, the arbitrary pairing of consecutive accruals may produce comparisons for patients with strikingly different baseline severity of the clinical condition. Although the randomization should eventually equalize the total disparities of severity in each pair, the trial may be stopped before enough patients have been accumulated to allow either a balanced distribution of severity or an effective comparison of treatment in pertinent clinical subgroups.

25.3.2 N-of-1 Trials

An interesting variant of sequential designs is the N-of-1 trial, which was introduced[53] to help choose optimum treatment for a single patient. If the patient has a chronic condition (such as painful osteoarthritis)

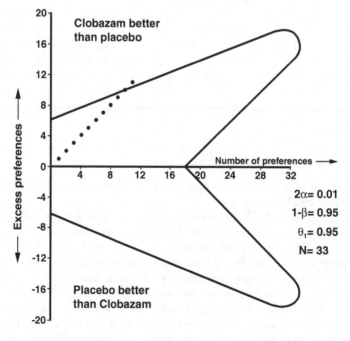

FIGURE 25.1
Sequential analysis design for comparison of clobazam and placebo in the suppression of seizures associated with menstruation. [Figure taken from Chapter Reference 52.]

or a frequently recurrent condition (such as dysmenorrhea or migraine headaches), and if several treatments are available for the condition, practicing clinicians have usually tried the treatments sequentially. Agent B was given if Agent A failed to be successful, and Agent C if Agent B failed. The N-of-1 trial provides a formal evaluative structure — with randomization, double-blinding, etc. — for appraisals that were previously done informally and sometimes inefficiently.

N-of-1 trials are limited, however, to clinical situations where the patient recurrently reaches the same baseline state before each treatment, and where the outcome does not take an inordinately long time to occur. Aside from issues in feasibility, the main statistical challenges in the trials are to choose the phenomenon that will be evaluated quantitatively as the main "outcome," and to decide whether the evaluation will depend on a simple preference for Agent A vs. Agent B, on purely descriptive evidence, or on tests of stochastic significance for the accrued data.[54]

25.3.3 Interim Analyses

Because sequential designs are seldom feasible and because N-of-1 trials are limited to individual patients, the long-term efficacy of many therapeutic agents is tested in conventionally designed randomized trials, with an advance calculation of sample size. As the trial progresses, however, the investigators then do interim analyses (often called "peeks at the data") to see what is happening.

25.3.3.1 *Quantitative and Stochastic Phenomena* — The "premature" demonstration of superiority for one of the compared treatments may involve quantitative or stochastic distinctions. The prematurity has a quantitative source if the compared difference in rates of good (or bad) outcomes is unexpectedly much greater than anticipated. With a particularly large incremental difference, the quantitative distinction between the treatments will be stochastically significant much sooner than was expected in the original plans for sample size and secular duration.

The prematurity has a stochastic source, however, when "significance" is obtained by the progressive enlargement of group sizes. With this enlargement, the same quantitative difference in the same outcome event at the same serial time (such as 6-month survival) that was "nonsignificant" in an early secular comparison may become stochastically significant in a later comparison that included many more people. This phenomenon can arise because the participating patients in long-term randomized trials are seldom admitted all at once. Instead, they are accrued over a secular period of calendar time. Thus, if the plan calls for 500 patients to be admitted, 200 may be recruited in the first calendar year of the trial, 200 more in the second year, and the last 100 in the third year. A comparison of 1-year survival rates for the treatments will therefore include enlarging groups at successive secular dates; and results for 1-year survival of all 500 patients cannot be obtained until at least the fourth calendar year of the trial.

Another source of premature "significance" is both quantitative and stochastic. As noted in Chapter 23, the Neyman-Pearson calculation for "double significance" will produce a sample size much larger than what is needed if the observed d_o exceeds the anticipated "big" δ. With the "inflated" sample size, however, a value of d_o much smaller than δ can become stochastically significant. As the group sizes accrue in the trial, stochastic significance can be reached with $d_o < \delta$, while the group size is also still smaller than the originally scheduled N.

25.3.3.2 *Problems in Interim Examinations* — To determine whether a stochastically significant difference has occurred in the accruing data, the investigators may regularly examine the interim results at sequential intervals of calendar time.[55] If the quantitative value of the observed quantitative distinction, d_o, is unexpectedly higher than the anticipated δ, stochastic testing is easily justified. On the other hand, if the original value of δ is preserved, *and* if sample size was originally calculated for "single significance," *and* if d_o is required to reach the level of δ, stochastic significance cannot be obtained until the full sample size is accrued.

The main problems arise when sample size has been calculated with the Neyman-Pearson strategy for "double" significance. Because the interim analyses are almost always done to test the original null hypothesis (which does not specify a value for δ), the "inflated" value of N can readily allow stochastic significance to occur with $d_0 < \delta$, long before the planned numbers of patients are fully accrued. The frequency of the "delta wobble" problem and the interim stochastic tests could both be substantially reduced if a preserved level of δ were demanded for any declaration of "significance." As noted in Chapter 23, however, investigators usually lower the original value of δ to correspond to whatever smaller value of d_0 produced stochastic significance. Consequently, with the prime quantitative distinction neglected, the main issue is no longer "scientific." It becomes mathematically relegated to a stochastic mechanism for adjusting the boundary of α.

25.3.3.3 *"Stopping Rules"* —

A series of current proposals for adjusting α are called "stopping rules" for clinical trials.[56,57] The rules contain limitations on the number of interim analyses, and offer boundaries for the reduced α' to be used at each analysis. With the Haybittle–Peto technique,[58,59] α' is kept at a strict constant level (such as .001) for all the interim analyses, but returns to the original α (such as .05) at the conclusion if the trial is not ended prematurely. In Pocock's proposal,[60] which resembles a Bonferroni adjustment, α' is set according to the number of interim analyses. With five analyses, α' would be 0.016 to achieve an overall α of .05 at the end of the trial. With the O'Brien–Fleming method,[61] the α' levels are stringent for the early tests and more relaxed later. Thus, the successive α' levels might be .0006 for the first, .015 for the second, and .047 for the third interim analysis.

O'Brien and Shampo[62] have offered an excellent discussion and illustrations of these different rules, while also citing some ethical (as well as scientific) reasons for continuing a trial until its originally scheduled completion, despite the "stopping rules."

25.3.3.4 *"Stochastic Curtailment"* —

In another interim-examination technique, called *stochastic curtailment*,[63,64] the analysts consider both the observed and unobserved data to decide whether the current conclusions would change if the trial continues to its scheduled completion. The focus is not merely on clear evidence of benefit or harm (as in the conventional stopping rule), but also on lack of "power" to show an effect. Common non-harm–non-benefit events that can lead to stochastic curtailment are inadequate recruitment of patients, and many fewer outcome events than originally expected.

25.3.3.5 *"Financial Curtailment"* —

A different form of curtailment occurs when a study is stopped because the sponsoring agency decides that the continuing costs will not be justified by the anticipated benefits. The early termination of the study may be quietly accepted if the sponsor is a governmental agency (as in termination of the DES cohort study[65] by the National Institutes of Health in the U.S.), but may evoke protests about ethical behavior[66] if the sponsor is a pharmaceutical company (as in the decision by Hoechst Marion Roussel to stop a European trial of Pimagedine).

25.3.3.6 *Additional Topics* —

An entire issue of *Statistics in Medicine* has been devoted to 25 papers from a workshop[67] on "early stopping rules." Beyond the phenomena already mentioned here, the papers contained the following additional topics: Bayesian approaches, a trial in which the later results took a direction opposite to that of early results, an "alpha spending" approach for interim analysis, "the case against independent monitoring committees," and a "lay person's perspective" on "stopping rules."

25.4 Meta-Analysis

In meta-analysis, the results of a series of studies on "similar" topics are pooled to enlarge the size of the group and volume of data. The enlarged aggregate is then statistically analyzed to check the same hypotheses that were tested previously, although the larger amount of data may sometimes allow new hypotheses to be tested for subsets of the original "causal maneuvers" (such as different doses of treatment) or for subgroups of patients. A major advantage of the meta-analytic procedure is the opportunity to get "significant" conclusions from research that was previously inconclusive because of small groups or nonconcordant results in individual studies.

25.4.1 Controversies and Challenges

The meta-analytic strategy is controversial, being hailed by some writers as a majestic scientific advance[68,69] and regarded by others as being statistical "tricks,"[70] "alchemy for the 21st century,"[71] or "shmeta-analysis."[72] Even the name of the process is controversial. Disliking the etymologic potential resemblance to meta-physics, some authors prefer to use "overview," "pooling," or "analytic synthesis" to label the work. Because aggregation is the basis of the statistical activities, meta-analysis should be distinguished from other types of re-appraisal, called "methodologic analyses"[73] or "best-evidence syntheses,"[74] in which the authors review the collection of literature for a particular topic, isolate the few reports that have really high scientific quality, and then draw conclusions from only those reports.

A full discussion of meta-analysis is beyond the scope of the brief "overview" here; interested readers can find many detailed accounts elsewhere.[75-77] The main problems and challenges of meta-analysis, however, do not arise from statistical sources. The prime scientific difficulties come from the imprecision produced by pooling evidence that is inevitably heterogeneous, from problems in the judgmental evaluation of acceptable quality in the *original* reports, and from the "publication bias" that may make the available literature an unsuitable representative of all the research done on the selected topic.

Many published reports of meta-analyses have come from the combined results of randomized clinical trials. The aggregating activities, although not unanimously applauded by clinical trialists,[78,79] have been more widely accepted than the increasing appearance of meta-analyses based on epidemiologic and other observational studies that were done without randomization. The value of meta-analysis for "observational" (rather than randomized-trial) research is particularly controversial, and some prominent epidemiologists[72,80] refuse to accept the procedure.

25.4.2 Statistical Problems

The main statistical challenges in meta-analysis are the choice of an appropriate index of contrast for expressing the "effect" in each study, the mechanism used for combining individual indexes that may be heterogeneous, and the construction of confidence intervals for the aggregated result.

25.4.2.1 Individual Indexes of Effect — A first step is to choose the particular outcome (or other event) that will be indexed. In some investigations, this event is the credible fact of total deaths, but many other studies use the highly flawed data (see Section 17.2.3) of "cause-specific" deaths.

In a second step, regardless of the outcome entity, its occurrence must be expressed in an index of contrast for the compared groups. In meta-analyses of data for the psychosocial sciences, from which meta-analysis originated, the customary index of contrast is the standardized increment or "effect size" that was discussed in Section 10.5.1. Being seldom used in medical research, however, this index has been supplanted by many other expressions, including the proportional increment (or "relative gain"), the relative risk (or risk ratio), the odds ratio, or the log odds ratio. The main problem in all the latter indexes is that they obliterate the basic occurrence rate to which everything is being referred. The same ratio of 4 will be obtained with the major incremental change of 0.3 in risk from .1 to .4, and with the relatively trivial change of .00003 from .00001 to .00004.

If the meta-analytic results are to be understood by clinicians or by patients giving "informed consent" to treatment, comprehension can be substantially improved if the results are cited in direct increments or in the number-needed-to-treat expressions that were discussed in Chapter 10.

25.4.2.2 Aggregation of Heterogeneous Indexes — Regardless of which indexes are chosen to express the contrasted effects, the next decision is to choose a method for aggregating the individual indexes. The problem of heterogeneity becomes particularly important here. If contradictory results are indiscriminately combined, the analysts violate both statistical and scientific principles of analysis. Statistically, the combination of opposite results may lead to unsatisfactory combinations and misleading conclusions (as discussed later in Chapter 26). Scientifically, the combination of contradictions will violate the opportunity to use Bradford Hill's well-accepted requirement of *consistency*[81]

(i.e., results of individual studies should almost all go in the same direction) to support decisions about causality.

In many meta-analyses, however, the heterogeneity of individual indexes is usually ignored, and the aggregated indexes are reported merely as means, medians, "weighted summary," or "standardized summary" statistics. In one novel approach to the problem, the investigators[82] obtained the original data for five trials. In contrast to a conventional meta-analysis, the data were pooled according to previously established "common definitions" that made the results "as homogeneous as possible." The pooled data allowed a "risk factor analysis not possible with meta-analysis techniques," although the aggregated risk ratios were essentially the same with both methods.

25.4.2.3   *Stochastic Tests and Confidence Intervals* — The idea of multiple inference or "multiple comparisons" seldom receives attention in meta-analysis, although the same hypothesis was previously tested repeatedly in the multiple studies that are combined. Nevertheless, studies that have been unequivocally positive in both quantitative and stochastic distinctions (as well as in scientific quality) may seldom require meta-analysis. If the latter procedure is confined to a set of k studies with equivocal individual results, the stochastic test of their combination could be regarded as yet another comparison, for which the Bonferroni correction would use k + 1. The combined numbers may often be large enough so that the final P value remains stochastically significant even if interpreted with $\alpha' = \alpha/(k + 1)$. The correction might be considered, however, when the final P value (or confidence interval) is quite close to the uncorrected stochastic boundary.

With the multiple-comparison problem generally ignored, perhaps the most vigorous statistical creativity in meta-analysis has been devoted to the stochastic method of reporting "significance" of the aggregated summary. The methods include the following: P value, mean P value, "consensus combined" P, Z-score, mean Z-score, t score, "meta-regression" slopes,[83,84] the "support" of a likelihood ratio,[85] and Bayesian estimates.[86]

With the current emphasis on confidence intervals rather than other expressions, new attention has focused on the stochastic aggregation of summary indexes. For the odds ratio, which is a particularly popular index, the customary method of aggregation was the Mantel–Haenszel (M-H) strategy,[87] which receives detailed discussion later in Chapter 26. In recent years, however, many statisticians have preferred the DerSimonian–Laird (D-L) strategy.[88] The main difference in the two approaches is that M-H uses a "fixed-effects," whereas D-L uses a "random-effects" model. With a fixed-effects model, we assume that the available batch of strata (i.e., individual trials) is the "universe," and the aggregated variance is calculated from individual variances in each stratum. With a random-effects model, we assume that the available strata (or trials) are a sample of a hypothetical larger universe of trials. Accordingly, variation among the strata is added to the individual variances within each stratum. (The dispute about which model to use somewhat resembles the controversy, discussed in Section 14.3.5, about calculating the chi-square test in a fourfold table with the idea of either fixed or non-fixed marginal totals.)

The net effect of the random-effects model is to enlarge the total variance, thereby making stochastic significance, i.e., rejection of the null hypothesis, more difficult to obtain. In general, however, when large numbers of studies are combined, the total group size is big enough so that most of the quantitatively impressive aggregated indexes are also stochastically significant, regardless of whether variance was calculated with a "random" or "fixed" model.

25.4.3   Current Status

Having been vigorously advocated by prominent statisticians and clinical epidemiologists, meta-analysis is becoming a well-accepted analytic procedure. The Cochrane Collaboration, a special new organization, has been established at Oxford to encourage the process and to promote activities in which clinical trialists at diverse international locations contribute their data for meta-analyses that can produce "evidence-based medicine."

Like any new procedure that becomes enthusiastically accepted, meta-analysis will doubtlessly undergo an evolutionary course that reduces the initial enthusiasm and eventually demarcates the true value of the procedure. Some of the reduced enthusiasm has already been manifested in occasional contradictions between the results of large new trials and previous meta-analyses of the same relationship. In one striking recent example, the results of at least five published meta-analyses were contradicted by a subsequent large trial,[89] which showed that calcium supplementation during pregnancy did *not* prevent pre-eclampsia, pregancy-associated hypertension, or adverse perinatal outcomes. After ascribing the differences to distinctions in dosage, patient selection, and definition of outcomes, the authors concluded that "meta-analyses cannot substitute for large, well-conducted clinical trials." In another separate analysis, Lelorier et al.[90] found that the outcomes of "12 large randomized, controlled trials ... were not predicted accurately 35 percent of the time by the meta-analyses published previously on the same topics."

Because a prime source of the problems is scientific rather than statistical, arising from the potential fallacies of heterogeneous combinations and the imprecision produced when important clinical variables are omitted from the data, the ultimate role of meta-analysis will depend more on improvements in clinical science than on better statistical methods for analyzing inadequate data.

References

1. Miller, 1966; 2. Dawber, 1980; 3. Cupples, 1984; 4. Hennekens, 1979; 5. MacMahon, 1981; 6. Feinstein, 1981; 7. Hsieh, 1986; 8. Hoover, 1980; 9. Mills, 1993; 10. Pickle, 1996; 11. Am. J. of Epidemiol., Special Issue, 1990; 12. Walter, 1993; 13. Kupper, 1976; 14. Bonferroni, 1936; 15. Duncan, 1955; 16. Dunn, 1961; 17. Dunnett, 1955; 18. Newman, 1939; 19. Keuls, 1952; 20. Scheffe, 1953; 21. Tukey, 1949; 22. Braun, 1994; 23. Holm, 1979; 24. Aickin, 1996; 25. Hochberg, 1988; 26. Simes, 1986; 27. Levin, 1996; 28. Brown, 1997; 29. Thompson, 1998; 30. Goodman, 1998; 31. Westfall, 1993; 32. Thomas, 1985; 33. Rothman, 1990; 34. Savitz, 1995; 35. Cole, 1993; 36. Feinstein, 1985; 37. Genest; 38. Feinstein, 1988a; 39. Cook, 1996; 40. Feinstein, 1998b; 41. Sanchez-Guerrero, 1995; 42. Boston Collaborative Drug Surveillance Programme, 1973; 43. Boston Collaborative Drug Surveillance Program, 1974; 44. Armstrong, 1974; 45. Heinonen, 1974; 46. Vessey, 1976; 47. Royall, 1991; 48. Freedman, 1987; 49. Wald, 1947; 50. Barnard, 1946; 51. Armitage, 1975; 52. Feely, 1982; 53. Guyatt, 1986; 54. Guyatt, 1988; 55. McPherson, 1974; 56. Freedman, 1983; 57. Pocock, 1992; 58. Haybittle, 1971; 59. Peto, 1976; 60. Pocock, 1977; 61. O'Brien, 1979; 62. O'Brien, 1988; 63. Lan, 1982; 64. Davis, 1994; 65. Jefferies, 1984; 66. Viberti, 1997; 67. Souhami, 1994; 68. Chalmers, 1993; 69. Sackett, 1995; 70. Thompson, 1991; 71. Feinstein, 1995; 72. Shapiro, 1994; 73. Gerberg, 1988; 74. Slavin, 1995; 75. Hedges, 1985; 76. Rosenthal, 1991; 77. Spitzer, 1995; 78. Ellenberg, 1988; 79. Meinert, 1989; 80. Petiti, 1993; 81. Hill, 1965; 82. Fletcher, 1993; 83. Brand, 1992; 84. Greenland, 1992; 85. Goodman, 1989; 86. Carlin, 1992; 87. Mantel, 1959; 88. DerSimonian, 1986; 89. Levine, 1997; 90. Lelorier, 1997.

Exercises

25.1. Find a report of a study in which the authors appear to have used multiple comparisons. Briefly outline the study and what was done statistically. Did the authors acknowledge the multiple-comparison problem and do anything about it (in discussion or testing)? What do you think should have been done?

25.2. The basic argument for not making corrections for multiple comparisons is that an ordinary (uncorrected) P value or confidence interval will answer the question about numerical stability of the data. As long as the results are stable, their interpretation and intellectual coordination should be a matter of scientific rather than statistical reasoning, and should not depend on how many other comparisons were done. Do you agree with this policy? How do you justify your belief? If you disagree, what is your reasoning and proposed solution to the problem?

25.3. With automated technology for measuring constituents of blood, multiple tests (such as the "SMA-52") are regularly reported for sodium, potassium, calcium, bilirubin, glucose, creatinine, etc. in a single specimen of serum. If 52 tests are done, and if the customary "zone of normal" is an inner-95-percentile range, the chance of finding an "abnormality" in a perfectly healthy person should be

$1 - (.95)^{52} = 1 - .07 = .93$. Consequently, when healthy people are increasingly "screened" with these tests, a vast number of false positive results can be expected. Nevertheless, at many medical centers that do such screening, this "epidemic" of excessive false positive tests has not occurred. What is your explanation for the *absence* of the problem?

25.4. Find a report of a randomized trial that seems to have been stopped prematurely, before the scheduled termination. Briefly outline what happened. Do you agree with the early-termination decision? Offer reasons for your conclusion.

25.5. Have you ever done or been tempted to do an N-of-1 trial, or have you read the results of one? If so, outline what happened. If you have had the opportunity to do one, but have not, indicate why not.

26

Stratifications, Matchings, and "Adjustments"

CONTENTS

Beyond the confusing array of rates, risks, and ratios discussed earlier in Chapter 17, epidemiologists use certain strategies that almost never appear in other branches of science. One of those strategies — the "adjustment" of data — is discussed in this chapter.

The adjustment process is seldom needed when an investigator arranges the experiments done with animals, biologic fragments, or inanimate substances. In the epidemiologic research called *observational studies*, however, the investigated events and data occur in groups of free-living people. Without the advantages of a planned experiment, the raw information may be inaccurate and the compared groups may be biased. The role of "adjustment" is to prevent or reduce the effects of these problems.

26.1   Problems of Confounding

A particularly prominent problem is confounding, which is easy to discuss, but difficult to define. It arises when the results of an observed relationship are distorted by an extrinsic factor. The consequence is that what you see is true, but is not what has really happened. An example of the problem appeared earlier in Section 19.6.4, when a correct statistical association was found between amyl nitrite "poppers" and AIDS. The interpretation that "poppers" were causing AIDS was wrong, however, because the relationship was confounded by an external factor: the particular sexual activity, often accompanied by use of "poppers," that transmitted the AIDS virus.

Although *confounding* is commonly used as a nonspecific name for these distortions, the source of the problem can often be identified from biases arising in specific architectural locations for the baseline states, maneuvers, outcomes and other sequential events in the alleged causal pathway for the compared groups.[1]

26.1.1   Role of "Effect-Modifiers"

The statistical relationship between an outcome and maneuver can be altered by factors called *effect modifiers*. These factors are not cited (and sometimes not recognized) when the data are merely reported as outcomes for maneuvers, such as success rates for different treatments, or mortality rates for people "exposed" to living in different regions. For example, postsurgical success can be affected by the patient's preoperative condition, concomitant anesthesia, and postoperative care, not just by the operation itself; and general-population mortality rates are affected by age, not just by region of residence. If the effect-modifiers are equally distributed in the compared groups, bias may be avoided. If the effect-modifiers have a substantially unequal distribution, however, the bias produces confounding.

The relationship between poppers and AIDS was confounded by *performance* (or *co-maneuveral*) *bias*, arising from the initially disregarded sexual activity that accompanied the "maneuver" of using poppers. *Performance bias* would also occur if results were compared for radical surgery, done with excellent anesthesia and postoperative care, versus simple surgery, done without similar excellence in the "co-therapy." Confounding can also arise from *detection bias* if the outcome events are sought and identified differently in the compared groups. "Double-blind" methods are a precaution used in randomized trials to avoid this bias.

A particularly common source of confounding is the *susceptibility bias* produced when the compared groups are prognostically different in their baseline states, before the compared "causal" maneuvers are imposed. For example, a direct comparison of "crude" mortality rates in Connecticut and Florida would be biased because Florida has a much older population than Connecticut. An analogous susceptibility bias would occur if survival rates are compared for surgical treatment, given to patients who are mainly in a favorable "operable" condition, versus nonsurgical treatment, for patients who are "inoperable."

26.1.2   Requirements for Confounding

The biases that produce confounding require the concurrence of two phenomena: (1) a particular effect-modifying factor — such as age, "operability," or certain sexual activity — has a distinct impact that alters the occurrence of the outcome event, such as death, "success," or AIDS; and (2) the factor has a substantially unequal distribution in the compared groups. If these phenomena occur together, the factor is a confounding variable or *confounder*. Thus, the relatively good clinical condition that constitutes "operability" can affect survival (regardless of whether surgery is done), but the variable is *not* a confounder if it is equally distributed in randomized groups having similar "operability." In most nonrandomized comparisons of surgical and nonsurgical groups, however, the survival rates are usually confounded by susceptibility bias, because the non-surgical group contains predominantly inoperable patients. Analogously, if the populations have similar age distributions, the general mortality rates would not be confounded in comparisons of Connecticut vs. Massachusetts, or Florida vs. Arizona. If the use of "poppers" were examined in persons who all engaged in the same kind of sexual activity, the activity might no longer be a confounder.

26.1.3 Simpson's Paradox

A particularly striking form of confounding, called *Simpson's Paradox*, occurs when the extremely unbalanced distribution of an effect-modifier makes the total results go in a direction opposite from that found in components of the compared groups.

For example, consider the success results for the two treatments shown in Table 26.1. The success rates for Treatment B are higher than for Treatment A by an increment of 6.8% (= 34.5% − 27.7%), which is a proportionate increase of 22% from the common proportion of 31.3%. The value of X^2 is 6.50, so that $2P < .025$. The results thus seem stochastically and quantitatively significant in favor of Treatment B.

In the condition being treated, however, prognostic status is an effect modifier, for which the "good risk" group is Stratum I and the "poor risk" group is Stratum II. When examined within these two strata, the results produce the surprise shown in Table 26.2. In each stratum, the results for Treatment A are significantly better than for Treatment B, both quantitatively and stochastically.

The "Simpson's-paradox" deception in the combined results of Table 26.1 arose from the markedly unbalanced distributions of treatment in the two strata. Treatment B was used predominantly for the good-risk patients of Stratum I, and Treatment A mainly for the poor-risk patients of Stratum II. This

TABLE 26.1

Illustration of Simpson's Paradox, as Demonstrated Later in Table 26.2

	Success	Failure	Total	Rate of Success
Treatment A	158	412	570	27.7%
Treatment B	221	419	640	34.5%
TOTAL	379	831	1210	31.3%
		$X^2 = 6.50; 2P < .025$		

TABLE 26.2

Results in Strata for the Simpson's Paradox of Table 26.1

	Success	Failure	Total	Rate of Success
STRATUM I				
Treatment A	10	10	20	50.0%
Treatment B	216	384	600	36.0%
TOTAL	226	394	620	36.5%
		$X^2 = 5.12; 2P < .025$		
STRATUM II				
Treatment A	148	402	550	26.9%
Treatment B	5	35	40	12.5%
TOTAL	153	437	590	25.9%
		$X^2 = 4.03; 2P < .05$		

type of imbalance might occur if Treatment B is an arduous procedure, such as "radical" therapy, that is reserved for the "healthier" patients, whereas the less arduous Treatment A is given mainly to the "sicker" patients.

26.1.4   Scientific Precautions

The main scientific approach to confounding is to avoid it with suitably planned research. The plans are designed to reduce or eliminate bias when raw data are collected and when groups are formed for comparison. The prophylactic precautions can easily be applied if the investigator, doing the research as an experiment (e.g., a randomized clinical trial), can assign the agents to be compared and can plan the collection of data. In nonexperimental circumstances — such as the work done at national bureaus of health statistics, or in any other form of "retrospective" research — the agents were already received and the data were already recorded for diverse groups before the investigation begins. The prophylactic precautions must then be replaced by remedial adjustments.

One type of adjustment, called *matching*, is discussed later in Section 26.5. Another method of adjustment is done with multivariable analytic strategies. The most common and traditional form of epidemiologic adjustment is called *standardization*, which is discussed throughout the next section.

26.2   Statistical Principles of Standardization

The procedure called *standardization* was devised by demographers to convert the "crude" rate of a group into a "standardized" rate that is adjusted for unbalanced distributions of confounders. The key elements in the adjustment are the outcome rates and constituent proportions for component strata. The group is first divided into strata of different levels for the confounding variable. For example, as an effect-modifier for general mortality, *age* might be partitioned into such strata as ≤ 29, 30–49, 50–64, 65–79, and ≥ 80. For each stratum, the outcome *rate* is the occurrence of a selected target event, such as death or success, and the constituent *proportion* is the fraction occupied by that stratum in the group's total composition. Thus, in Table 26.2, the success rate is 36.5% in Stratum I, which occupies $620/1210 = .512$ of the total population. For Stratum II, the corresponding values are 25.9% for the rate and $590/1210 = .488$ for the proportion. For the adjustment process, the rates and proportions in the component strata are given appropriate "weights" and then combined into a single "standardized" result.

In adjusting general mortality rates, we begin with the total "crude" rate, decompose it into pertinent strata, and then weight and recombine the strata suitably. In other situations, when the results are expressed in odds ratios rather than rates, the weighted adjustments and recombinations are applied to stratum components of the ratios. The standardization process can thus be regarded as a statistical form of recombinant DNA: denominator-numerator-adjustments.

26.2.1   Weighted Adjustments

The principles used in weighted adjustment are analogous to a mechanism taught in elementary school for finding the average of two rates (or proportions). For example, if you want to get the average of two rates, .34 and .20, the *wrong* approach is to add them directly as $.34 + .20 = .54$, and then divide by 2 to get .27 as the average. This tactic is wrong because the reported rates may come from groups having unbalanced denominators. Thus, if $.34 = 51/150$ and $.20 = 2/10$, the correct average result would be the much higher value of $(51 + 2) / (150 + 10) = 53/160 = .33$. Conversely if $.34 = 10/29$ and $.20 = 96/480$, the correct result is the much lower $(10 + 96)/(29 + 480) = 106/509 = .21$. To add the rates directly and then divide by 2 to produce .27 would be appropriate only if the two denominators had equal sizes, so that $.34 = 17/50$ and $.20 = 10/50$. The average would then be $(17 + 10)/(50 + 50) = 27/100 = .27$.

For the correct approach here, we added the two numerators, added the two denominators, and then divided the two sums. This basic strategy is used later to prepare "adjusted" values for *ratios*, and is also used for decomposing and then recombining *rates*.

26.2.2 Algebraic Mechanisms

To show how rates are weighted, suppose one rate is constructed as $r_1 = t_1/n_1$ and the other as $r_2 = t_2/n_2$. With the total group sizes being $N = n_1 + n_2$ in the denominators and $T = t_1 + t_2$ in the numerators, the "correct" average result is T/N.

The algebraic weighting process recapitulates this result by using the component *proportions* of the total denominator. They would be $p_1 = n_1/N$ in the first group and $p_2 = n_2/N$ in the second. The component proportions and rates for each group are then multiplied and added to produce p_1r_1 and p_2r_2. Their sum is $p_1r_1 + p_2r_2 = T/N$. [To prove this point, note that $p_1 = n_1/N$ and $r_1 = t_1/n_1$, so their product is $p_1r_1 = t_1/N$. Similarly, $p_2r_2 = t_2/N$. The sum of the products is $(t_1 + t_2)/N = T/N$.]

The general formula for constructing the average "crude" rate, R, from a series of component groups (or "strata") is

$$R = \Sigma p_i r_i = T/N$$

The values of p_i are the "weighting factors" for the rates, r_i. In the foregoing examples for two groups, the result was wrong when we ignored weighting factors and calculated R as $(r_1 + r_2)/2$, instead of $p_1r_1 + p_2r_2$. In the first example, where $N = 150 + 10 = 160$, p_1 was $150/160 = .9375$ and $p_2 = 10/160 = .0625$. In the second example, p_1 was $29/509 = .057$ and p_2 was $480/509 = .943$. In the third example, $p_1 = 50/100 = .5$ and $p_2 = 50/100 = .5$. The immediate addition of rates gave the correct answer only in the third example, where $p_1 = p_2 = .5$ was the correct weighting factor for their sum. In any other adjustment that merely adds the r_i values, the results would be wrong unless the appropriate p_i values were used as the weighting factor for each stratum.

The basic arrangement of $\Sigma p_i r_i$ is used for all the conventional epidemiologic adjustments that produce "standardized" mortality rates.

26.3 Standardized Adjustment of Rates

The customary standardization processes, discussed throughout this section, were developed to adjust the rates obtained in cohort or cross-sectional research. For the research structures, each denominator is either the "crude" total or a component stratum containing persons "at risk" for occurrence of the event cited in the numerator. The target rates are constructed as $r = t/n$ for the total group and $r_i = t_i/n_i$ for a stratum. [The entities are cited here with lower-case symbols, because capital letters will be used later for the counterpart entities in a "standard" population.]

In retrospective case-control studies, however, rates of "risk" cannot be directly determined and compared. Instead, the "risk ratio" for contrasting two groups is estimated with an odds ratio, constructed as $(a \times d)/(b \times c)$ from cross-products of cells in the 2×2 table that reflects (but does not show) the actual risks. The complexity of working with four component numbers, rather than two, in each stratum requires that odds ratios be adjusted with a process, discussed later in Section 26.4, different from what is used for rates in the subsections that follow.

26.3.1 Identification of Components

Every "target" rate in a group of people can be "decomposed" into *stratum proportions* and *stratum-specific target rates* for the components. In a particular group of people whose success rate for Treatment X was $60/200 = 30\%$, the "decomposition" for old and young persons forms the stratification shown in Table 26.3. In this table, the "crude rate" is the total success rate of 30%, or .30, before stratification. The stratum-specific rates of .40 and .27 are shown directly, but the stratum proportions are *not* immediately evident. They are determined

TABLE 26.3

Hypothetical Success Rates for Young and Old Patients

Strata	Success Rates
Young	20/50 (40%)
Old	40/150 (27%)
TOTAL	60/200 (30%)

when the *denominator*, n_i, of each stratum is divided by n, the total size of the combined strata. In this instance, $n_1 = 50$, $n_2 = 150$, and $n = 200$, so that $p_1 = 50/200 = .25$ and $p_2 = 150/200 = .75$.

In general symbols, the data for a group can be partitioned into strata identified with the subscript i, as 1, 2, 3, ..., i, ..., k, where k is the total number of strata. Each stratum contains a denominator of members, n_i, and a corresponding numerator, t_i, of focal or target events in those members. The rate of the target event in each stratum will be $r_i = t_i/n_i$. In Table 26.3, $r_1 = t_1/n_1 = 20/50 = .40$ and $r_2 = t_2/n_2 = 40/150 = .27$.

The total number of people in the group will be $\Sigma n_i = n$; the total number of target events will be $\Sigma t_i = t$; and the crude rate for the target event will be $t/n = \Sigma t_i/\Sigma n_i$. In Table 26.3, $n = \Sigma n_i = 50 + 150 = 200$; t $= \Sigma t_i = 20 + 40 = 60$, and r (the crude rate) $= t/n = 60/200 = .30$.

To avoid the sometimes ambiguous symbol, p, the stratum proportions can be symbolized with w (for "weights") and calculated as $w_i = n_i/n$. In Table 26.3, they are $w_1 = 50/200 = .25$ and $w_2 = 150/200 = .75$. Each stratum thus has a proportion, w_i, which is n_i/n. Each stratum also has a specific rate, r_i, calculated as t_i/n_i, for the target event. As shown earlier in Section 26.2.2, the crude rate is

$$r = \Sigma w_i r_i$$

Applying this formula to the data in Table 26.3 produces $(.25)(.40) + (.75)(.27) = .10 + .20 = .30$, which is the observed crude rate.

26.3.2 Principles of Direct Standardization

The w_i proportions are the main source of problems when crude rates are compared. If the compared groups have substantially different w_i values for the stratum proportions *and* if the corresponding strata have different target rates, the comparison of crude rates will be distorted by confounding. The imbalance in stratum proportions for baseline susceptibility was the source of the biased comparisons discussed earlier for the geographic regions of Connecticut vs. Florida, for surgical vs. nonsurgical treatment, and for Simpson's Paradox in Table 26.1.

Unless your cerebrum has been overwhelmed by the mathematics, you may have already thought of a solution for the problem. Because the stratum-specific target rates, r_i, are the main results and the w_i component values produce the distortion, the imbalance can be "fixed" if the two compared groups are given the *same* set of w_i values. An "adjusted" rate can then be calculated with these similar w_i values for the appropriate strata in each group. This solution is exactly what happens in the process called *direct standardization*. The next main decision is to choose appropriate values of w_i.

26.3.2.1 Choice of Standardizing Population — We could get a fair comparison by choosing the "standardizing" w_i values from either of the compared groups. Thus, we could standardize the mortality results in Florida by using w_i weights from the population of Connecticut, or standardize the Connecticut results with w_i values from Florida. To avoid an invidious choice between the two sources, however, the standardizing population is customarily selected in a neutral manner. The usual choice of the *reference* or *standard* population (in epidemiologic research) is the composition and associated death rates for an entire national population. The results of the standardizing population can be shown with capital letters of W, R, T, and N, corresponding to the lower-case values of w, r, t, and n in the observed groups.

For example, if the selected standard population contains 10% young people and 90% old people, the standardizing W_i values are $W_1 = .10$ and $W_2 = .90$. If these W_i values are applied to the r_i values in Table 26.3, the adjusted rate would be $\Sigma W_i r_i = (.10)(.40) + (.90)(.27) = .04 + .24 = .28$. With the adjustment, the previous crude level of 30% for the success rate would fall to a standardized value of 28%.

The choice of a standard population is tricky. In clinical situations (where standardization is seldom used), national data are almost never available for such important confounding factors as severity of disease. Accordingly, a standard "clinical" population is usually chosen ad hoc to be the *total* of the observed groups, irrespective of therapy or other group distinctions. Thus, for the data in Table 26.2, the standardizing weights (as noted in Section 26.2) would be $W_1 = .512$ for Stratum I, and $W_2 = $

.488 for Stratum II. Using the stratum rates in Table 26.2, we could then apply the formula $\Sigma W_i r_i$ to obtain standardized rates of $(.512)(.500) + (.488)(.269) = .387$ for Treatment A, and $(.512)(.360) + (.488)(.125) = .245$ for Treatment B. The superiority of Treatment A is now clearly apparent in the standardized rates.

26.3.2.2 Illustration of Direct Standardization — The foregoing standardization, using information for "clinical" strata, is rare. The common type of direct epidemiologic standardization is done with demographic data and can be illustrated with the following example: In 1980, the crude death rate per 1000 persons was 8.831 in Connecticut, and 10.741 in Florida. With a death rate that is proportionately higher by more than 20%, is Florida an unhealthy place to live?

To answer this question, the numbers, proportions, and rates in strata for the two regions can be examined in Table 26.4. The age-specific stratum rates show that Connecticut had lower death rates than Florida in each of the first four age strata, but that in people at age >64, the Florida mortality rate was substantially lower (43.711 vs. 52.255).

TABLE 26.4

Population, Deaths, Stratum Proportions, and Stratum Rates for Connecticut and Florida in 1980

Age Stratum (Years)	Connecticut				Florida			
	Population ($\times 10^3$)	No. of Deaths	Stratum Proportion	Stratum Rate $\times 10^{-3}$	Population ($\times 10^3$)	No. of Deaths	Stratum Proportion	Stratum Rate $\times 10^{-3}$
< 5	185.2	489	.060	2.641	567.8	2,283	.058	4.021
5–19	730.9	383	.237	0.524	2114.8	1,406	.217	0.655
20–44	1132.5	1,564	.367	1.381	3262.0	6,400	.335	1.962
45–64	674.3	5,757	.218	8.538	2109.1	20,781	.217	9.853
>64	364.9	19,066	.118	52.255	1687.6	73,765	.173	43.711
TOTAL	3087.8	27,269	1.000	8.831	9741.3	104,635	1.000	10.741

[Source of data: *Vital Statistics of the United States. 1980. Volume II. Mortality, Part A*. U.S. Dept. of Health and Human Services. Public Health Service. Natl. Center for Health Statistics. Hyattsville, MD, 1985.]

If the two populations were added to get a standard population for the comparison, Florida would dominate the results because it has so many more people than Connecticut. Accordingly, the entire U.S. population for 1980 can be used as a "neutral" standard population. The information for that year is shown in Table 26.5.

TABLE 26.5

Stratum Proportions and Death Rates for Entire U.S. Population in 1980

Age Stratum (Years)	Entire U.S. Population ($\times 10^6$)	(W_i) Stratum Proportion	(R_i) Stratum-Specific Death Rate ($\times 10^{-3}$)
< 5	16.3	.072	3.286
5–19	56.1	.248	0.560
20–44	84.0	.371	1.630
45–64	44.5	.196	9.558
65+	25.6	.113	52.524
TOTAL	226.5	1.000	8.782

[Source of data: Same as in Table 26.4.]

Using the formula

$$r_{DS} = \Sigma r_i w_i (\text{or } \Sigma w_i r_i)$$

for a direct standardized rate, the direct adjustment for Connecticut would be $(2.641)(.072) + (0.524)(.248) + \cdots + (52.255)(.113) = 8.41$ per thousand. For Florida, the corresponding direct age-standardized rate is $(4.021)(.072) + (0.665)(.248) + \cdots + (43.711)(.113) = 8.05$ per thousand. The adjusted rates for the two regions now seem relatively similar.

26.3.2.3   Interpretation of Results — The main reason for learning about the standardization process is to know what was done and what to beware when you see results that were "age-adjusted" or "age-sex-standardized" in epidemiologic or public-health reports.

The most important thing to beware is that the standardized result can be substantially altered by the W_i proportions in the particular census year and region that is arbitrarily chosen for the standardizing population. For example, in an increasingly aging U.S. population, the W_i proportions for the older age groups will be higher in 2000 than in 1980, higher in 1980 than in 1960, and so on. Because the r_i mortality rates are also higher in the older age groups, the standardized result can be made larger or smaller according to the magnitude of the W_i proportions. Thus, the standardized result for 1987 in the United States will be smaller with the 1960 rather than 1980 standard population, but will enlarge with the 1990 standard population. Unless the *same* standardizing population has been used for all comparisons, the calendar trends of rises and falls in standardized mortality rates for heart disease, cancer, etc. may be impossible to evaluate. Nevertheless, many "standardized" results are published without identification of the standardizing population, and without assurance that the same population was used throughout for all comparisons.

Another thing to beware is that the standardized rate is a completely arbitrary number, established merely for the purposes of an immediate comparison. It has no enduring value beyond the comparison itself; and the only entity that has been "standardized" is the particular factor(s), such as age and/or sex, used in the mathematical adjustment. Although aimed at reducing "confounding," the process cannot account for important factors — such as baseline state of health — that were omitted from the adjustment. Furthermore, if the outcome event is the occurrence of death from a specific disease, rather than death itself, the numerator data have all the untrustworthy attributes discussed earlier in Section 17.2.3.

26.3.3   Symbols for Components

To show the algebraic tactics more precisely, the stratum proportions, stratum-specific rates, and other pertinent results can be given the symbols shown in Table 26.6. The standardization process involves a "crossover" of components in the products $r_i w_i$ and $R_i W_i$. In the direct standardization just illustrated, the crossover used $r_i W_i$ for the adjusted components. With indirect standardization, as discussed in the next section, the crossover uses $R_i w_i$.

TABLE 26.6

Symbols for Components of Observed and Standard Populations

	Observed Population	Standard Population
Stratum Proportions	$w_i = n_i/n$	$W_i = N_i/N$
Stratum-Specific Rates	$r_i = t_i/n_i$	$R_i = T_i/N_i$
Crude Rate	$r_0 = \Sigma w_i r_i$	$R_0 = \Sigma W_i R_i$
	or	or
	$r_0 = t/n$	$R_0 = T/N$
	$(t = \Sigma t_i$	$(T = \Sigma T_i$
	$n = \Sigma n_i)$	$N = \Sigma N_i)$

26.3.4   Principles of Indirect Standardization

In many public-health situations (particularly in underdeveloped countries), we may know a group's crude total rate of mortality, r_0, but not the stratum-specific rates, r_i. From census results, however, we can find the stratum proportions, w_i, and we can get R_i values for a standard population. The values of r_0 and w_i in the observed population and the values of R_0 and R_i in the standard population can then be used for an indirect standardization.

26.3.4.1 Determining Expected Rates — The indirect standardization process begins by calculating an *expected* stratum-specific rate as R_iw_i for each stratum in the observed population. [R_iW_i would be the expected value if the rates were the same for corresponding strata of the observed group and the standard population.] The sum of the expected values, $r_e = \Sigma R_iw_i$, will be the expected crude rate in the observed group. When the group's observed crude rate, r_0, is divided by the expected rate, r_e, the ratio of r_0/r_e is called either the *standardized incidence ratio* (SIR) in reference to an "incidence" rate or the *standardized mortality ratio* (SMR) for a mortality rate.

The indirect standardized rate, r_{IS}, is produced when the SIR or SMR is multiplied by the corresponding crude rate, R_0, in the standard population.

26.3.4.2 Illustration of Indirect Standardization — Suppose we do not know the stratum-specific rates and have data for only the stratum proportions and the crude death rates, 8.831×10^{-3} and 10.741×10^{-3} in Connecticut and Florida, respectively, in Table 26.4. From the Census Bureau and National Center for Health Statistics, we learn the stratum-specific rates (R_i) and the crude rate ($R_0 = 8.782 \times 10^{-3}$) that were shown for the standard population in Table 26.5.

The expected values and remainder of the adjustment process for Connecticut produce the following: $r_e = \Sigma R_iw_i = (3.286 \times .060) + (0.560 + .237) + (1.630 \times .367) + (9.558 \times .218) + (52.520 \times .118) = 9.21$. The SMR is $r_0/r_e = 8.831/9.21 = .959$. The indirect standardized mortality rate is $r_{IS} = SMR \times R_0 = .959 \times 8.782 = 8.42$ per thousand. For Florida, the analogous calculations produce $r_e = (3.286 \times .058) + (0.560 \times .217) + (1.630 \times .335) + (9.558 \times .217) + (52.520 \times .173) = 12.02$. The SMR would be $10.741/12.02 = .894$, and the value of r_{IS} is $.894 \times 8.782 = 7.85$.

The indirect standardized results for Connecticut are almost identical to the direct standardized results found in Section 26.3.2.2, and are reasonably similar for Florida.

26.3.5 Role of "Standardization Factor"

The direct and indirect standardization processes initially seem quite different. For the direct process, values of W_i are simply substituted for w_i, and the standardized results emerge promptly. The indirect process seems much more convoluted, requiring calculation of expected values and an intervening standardized ratio, such as SMR.

Chan et al.,[2] however, after comparing the two processes, noted that they are quite symmetrical because the standardized rate in both procedures is obtained when the crude rate is multiplied by a standardizing factor. For direct standardization, this factor is R_e/r_0; for indirect standardization, the corresponding factor is R_0/r_e. The direct process seems much simpler only because of an algebraic "cancellation" of r_0 when the direct standardized rate is calculated as

$$r_{DS} = r_0 \times (R_e/r_0) = R_e = \Sigma r_iW_i$$

The "adjusted" value, $R_e = \Sigma r_iW_i$, is really the expected crude rate in the *standard* population. With the indirect procedure, the corresponding standardizing factor is R_0/r_e, but summations are needed for both R_0 and r_e. The result becomes

$$r_{IS} = r_0 \times (R_0/r_e) = (\Sigma r_iw_i)(\Sigma R_iW_i)/(\Sigma R_iw_i)$$

and seems more "convoluted" because of the additional summations.

If all we want is a single index of comparison, the complete calculation of r_{IS} for indirect standardization is unnecessary. The two populations can be compared immediately from their standardized incidence or mortality ratio, r_0/r_e, because each r_{IS} is produced when this ratio is multiplied by the same value of R_0.

Thus, in Section 26.3.4.2, Connecticut and Florida could be compared either for indirectly adjusted mortality rates of 8.42 vs. 7.85 or for standardized mortality ratios of .959 vs. .894.

26.3.6   Importance of Standardizing Population

As noted in Section 26.3.2.3, reports of "age-standardized" or "age-sex-standardized" results may not cite the standardizing population—a crucial choice that can greatly affect the outcome results. Direct standardization will be altered by different values of W_i, and indirect standardization, by the rates of R_i. With appropriate selections of a standardizing population and of direct vs. indirect methods (or vice versa), an ingenious investigator might even be able to make the adjusted rates produce a previously "desired" result. You should therefore be skeptical of any "standardized adjustment" if the investigator does not cite (1) the choice of the standard population, (2) the method of adjustment (direct or indirect), and (3) a satisfactory justification for the choices.

One way to avoid the problem is to use the same population for all standardizations. For example, after noting that direct standardization in a single epidemiologic journal had been done with eight different populations, Carson et al.[3] proposed that the Segi Standard World Population be applied for worldwide consistency. Another way to avoid the problem is to eliminate the age-stratum proportions by giving a fixed set of weights to the rates in the strata. The weights can be chosen according to a "reciprocal" pattern calculated by Yerushalmy[4] or the duration of age-intervals proposed by Abramson.[5] Nevertheless, after appraising all the available and proposed indexes, Kitagawa[6] concluded that "no single summary index can be a substitute for a detailed comparison of age-specific death rates."

Although the best approach is to avoid standardization and to compare the age-specific rates directly, the comparison in multiple strata is unappealing if you prefer the simplicity of contrasting results for just a single index. This simplicity is about to become more complex, however. For many decades in the United States, the 1940 population was used for standardization. In 1998, however, the National Center for Health statistics decided to use a new "modern" standard[7]—a projected estimate of the U.S. population for 2000. Because the later population is much older, certain standardized rates of disease may rise dramatically—merely because of the change of the reference population.

Some of the consequences are shown in Figure 26.1. The left side shows the change in distribution, with higher proportions in 2000 for each age stratum at levels of 35–44 and older. The right side shows the impact on the adjusted rates for four cause-specific rates of death.[8] Although hardly changed for HIV infection and homicide, the rates are more than doubled for heart disease and about 2/3 higher for cancer. Misinterpretation of the results will offer a splendid new opportunity for sensational stories in the media.

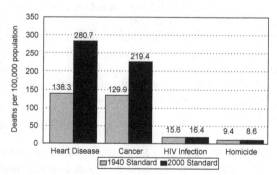

Age	1940 Standard		2000 Standard*	
	Population	Distribution	Population	Distribution
Total	131,669,275	1.000000	274,634,000	1.000000
< 1	2,020,174	0.015343	3,795,000	0.013818
1-4	8,521,350	0.064718	15,192,000	0.055317
5-14	22,430,557	0.170355	39,977,000	0.145565
15-24	23,921,358	0.181677	38,077,000	0.138646
25-34	21,339,026	0.162066	37,233,000	0.135573
35-44	18,333,220	0.139237	44,659,000	0.162613
45-54	15,512,071	0.117811	37,030,000	0.134834
55-64	10,572,205	0.080294	23,961,000	0.087247
65-74	6,376,189	0.048426	18,136,000	0.066037
75-84	2,278,373	0.017304	12,315,000	0.044842
85 +	364,752	0.002770	4,259,000	0.015508

* Projected based on population projection from Bureau of Census, P-25, No. 1130, 1996.

FIGURE 26.1

Impact of change in standardizing population from 1940 to 2000. Left side shows counts and proportions of the two populations. Right side shows cause-specific death rates of 1995 when age-adjusted for the two standard populations. [Data and figures taken from Chapter Reference 8.]

26.3.7   Choice of Method

If standardization is used at all, the direct method is usually preferred as being easier and more straightforward than the indirect approach. The indirect method is used in two circumstances: (1) absence of suitable data and (2) too-small numerators for the rates.

26.3.7.1 Absence of Suitable Data — If stratum proportions and crude rates are known for the study population, but stratum-specific rates are unknown, the results cannot be directly standardized. In this situation, the stratum proportions and target rates of a standardizing population would be used first to construct the standardized mortality ratio as an expected crude rate, and then to form the indirect standardized rate.

26.3.7.2 Excessively Small Numerators — The necessary information may be known both for stratum proportions and for stratum rates in the study population, but the numerators of rates in the strata may be quite small, such as 0/9 or 1/18, making the stratum-specific target rates too unstable to be reliable. Accordingly, the larger numbers in the denominators of those rates can be used as stratum proportions for an indirect standardization, which will rely on target rates in the standardizing population.

This virtue of the indirect method was used in a cohort survey[9] of morbidity associated with maintenance, cessation, or nonusage of oral contraceptive agents in 47,000 women. Because the morbidity data were simultaneously standardized for age (seven levels), parity (six levels), social class (seven levels), and cigarette consumption (six levels), a total of 1764 (= $7 \times 6 \times 7 \times 6$) strata were formed, so that many of the strata had small or 0 numerators for occurrence of "morbid" events. Because of small numerators, the indirect method was also used when Chan et al.[2] did an age-sex standardization for the rates of previously undetected disease found in a necropsy population.

26.3.8 Clinical Applications

Although bias is usually a more common problem in clinical rates of death than in demographic public-health mortality rates, the standardization procedure is rarely used in clinical research, because clinicians seldom want to combine everything into a single "adjusted" result. For scientific and clinical precision, they want to know the effects of compared treatments within the strata of pertinent subgroups. Clinicians would also want to know results in subgroups demarcated by clinically cogent prognostic factors, not just by age or sex.

Even when willing to accept a single adjusted result, however, clinicians may be uncertain about how to attain it. In the usual public-health standardization of general mortality rates, the adjustment is almost always done with age, sex, or other *demographic* "risk" factors. In clinical studies of therapy, however, confounded rates for the outcome (rather than occurrence) of disease usually come from biased distributions of *clinical* prognostic factors, such as extent of disease, severity of illness, and severity of co-morbidity. Accustomed to epidemiologic standardizations that rely on age and/or sex, the analysts of clinical data may not realize that adjustments can also be done, as shown near the end of Section 26.3.2.1, with clinical and para-clinical rather than demographic variables.

Another problem that discourages the use of clinical standardization is the fear of too many strata. With two categories of *sex* and perhaps as many as six for *age*, a public-health adjustment might need no more than 12 strata. With the diverse clinical variables that might be confounders, however, a much larger number of strata can be produced. Within the hordes of multivariate strata, many cells might be empty or have too few members to be used with confidence. This problem can be eliminated, however, with an appropriate composite staging system[10] that consolidates categories into smaller numbers of strata, thereby reducing or eliminating the many empty cells. Because relatively few appropriate composite staging systems have been constructed, however, clinical rates are usually "adjusted" not with the stratified standardizations used in public-health epidemiology, but with multivariable analytic methods.

Nevertheless, when not too many strata are needed and adequate numbers are available, clinical rates can receive a stratified adjustment. Concato et al.[11] used this process to evaluate a previous claim that 5-year postsurgical mortality was higher with transurethral prostatectomy (TURP) than with open-prostatectomy (OPEN). In the original study,[12] based on medico-fiscal claims data for men with benign prostatic hyperplasia, the stochastically significant crude relative risk of 1.27 for TURP vs. OPEN persisted after multivariable adjustment for differences in age, co-morbidity, and other possibly confounding variables. The published results then evoked extensive publicity about the alleged dangers of TURP. Suspecting that the severity of co-morbidity had not been suitably classified and analyzed in the original research, Concato et al. did a smaller but more detailed study, using medical records rather than claims data. The Concato group noted crude 5-year mortality rates of 13% (17/126) for OPEN and 17% (22/126) in the corresponding TURP group, thus confirming the crude risk ratio of 1.29 found in the previous investigation. With better data and classification for severity of co-morbidity, however, the Concato study found the stratified results that appear in Table 26.7. Within the co-morbidity strata, TURP seemed no more dangerous than OPEN surgery.

When directly standardized from proportions of co-morbidity strata in the total population, the 5-year mortality rates in Table 26.7 became 15.02% for OPEN and 14.38% for TURP, and the adjusted risk ratio dropped to 0.96. (An additional concomitant standardization for age brought this ratio even closer to 1).

26.3.9 Stochastic Evaluations

Back in Chapters 3 and 4, the "standard error" of a central index was used as a stochastic "estimate of uncertainty" for the observed value. The same standard-error strategy, although more complex than for a single group, is applied to the composite rates constructed with a standardization process.

TABLE 26.7

Stratified Results for Postsurgical Mortality and Grade of Co-Morbidity [Data taken from Chapter Reference 11.]

Grade of Co-Morbidity	5-Year Postsurgical Mortality		
	OPEN	TURP	TOTAL
None	6/64	1/37	7/101
	(9%)	(3%)	(7%)
Intermediate	10/59	14/75	24/134
	(17%)	(19%)	(18%)
Severe	1/3	7/14	8/17
	(33%)	(50%)	(47%)
TOTAL	17/126	22/126	39/252
	(13%)	(17%)	(15%)

Note: OPEN = Prostatectomy; TURP = Transurethral resection of prostate

For a direct standardized rate, the standard error is calculated with the actual numbers, rather than the proportions, in each stratum. If r_i is the rate in a stratum containing n_i members and N_i is the corresponding membership in the "standard" stratum, the standard error of the direct standardized rate is

$$SE(r_{DS}) = \sqrt{\Sigma(N_i^2 r_i/n_i)/\Sigma N_i}$$

Morris and Gardner[13] offer a worked example of the calculation.

For indirectly standardized rates, stochastic uncertainty is usually expressed with confidence intervals for the SMR (or SIR) ratio. The approach has not evoked universal agreement because of different beliefs about the mathematical distribution to be used for the observed number of deaths (or cases) in the study group. A formula for variance of the SMR proposed in 1971 by Armitage[14] relied on the Poisson distribution, which is used for events that occur randomly at low frequency. The Poisson distribution was also the basis for a shortcut calculation of the 95% confidence interval proposed by Vandenbroucke[15] in 1982, and for a simple formula listed in 1988 by Morris and Gardner.[13] In 1983, however, a chi-square distribution was proposed by Mulder,[16] and was later also advocated by Liddell[17] and by Ulm.[18] In 1994, Lee[19] contended that a binomial distribution was the best strategy, and in 1991, Greenland[20] proposed using an F-distribution.

Until a summit conference is held to achieve resolution or consensus, you can choose whatever confidence-interval method you think will be approved by the reviewers. No one, as yet, however, seems to have proposed that the dispute about distributions be avoided by calculating the confidence interval with bootstrap resampling.

26.3.10 Role of Proportionate Mortality Ratio (PMR)

Proportionate mortality ratios (PMR), calculated as discussed earlier in Section 17.2.6, can be "standardized" to form a cause-specific SPMR. The latter is an observed/expected ratio formed when the observed number of disease-specific deaths in the study population is divided by the corresponding number of deaths expected if the study population had the same PMR as a standard population. The use of the SPMR is controversial, with supporters contending[21] that it is often similar to a relative SMR, determined when the SMR for an individual disease is divided by the SMR for all deaths. The detractors[22] respond that PMRs can lead to biased, erroneous conclusions if large differences exist in the "overall death rates of study and comparison groups." The argument can be resolved at a scientific rather than mathematical level by noting that the basic disease-specific death rates are so untrustworthy that neither the PMR nor the SPMR data can regularly be accepted as credible.

26.4 Standardized Adjustment of Odds Ratios

Despite the apparent complexity, the foregoing adjustment of rates was a relatively simple mathematical process, because each rate came from two numbers: a numerator, t_i, and a denominator, n_i. These two numbers formed the target rate, $r_i = t_i/n_i$, and the denominator formed the stratum proportion, $n_i/n = w_i$.

The adjustment process becomes more complex when the results of case-control studies are expressed in odds-ratios rather than rates, because each odds ratio comes from four numbers, not two. If the total groups are divided into strata, the original 2×2 table that expressed the "crude" results as $\left\{\begin{smallmatrix} A & B \\ C & D \end{smallmatrix}\right\}$, becomes divided into a set of tables, constructed as $\left\{\begin{smallmatrix} a_i & b_i \\ c_i & d_i \end{smallmatrix}\right\}$ for each stratum i.

26.4.1 Weighting for 2×2 Tables

The appropriate combination of a set of 2×2 tables has been a statistical challenge for more than 40 years, ever since Cochran[23] first suggested a weighting mechanism. The results are expressed with an appropriate index of contrast, which is then appropriately weighted. The two most obvious choices for the index of contrast are the direct increment and the odds ratio.

26.4.1.1 Direct Increment — The rates of success for Treatment E and Treatment F in stratum i can be subtracted to form the increment

$$g_i = p_{E_i} - p_{F_i}$$

If the row totals in each stratum are designated as n_{1_i} (for treatment E) and n_{2_i} (for Treatment F), the total membership of the stratum will be $n_i = n_{1_i} + n_{2_i}$. If the column containing a_i and c_i represents success, the success rates will be $p_{E_i} = a_i/n_{1_i}$, and $p_{F_i} = c_i/n_{2_i}$.

Cochran proposed that each g_i increment be weighted by a factor

$$w_i = [(n_{1_i})(n_{2_i})]/n_i$$

and that a weighted mean increment be formed as

$$\bar{g} = (\Sigma w_i g_i)/\Sigma w_i$$

The process can be illustrated with the data in Table 26.2. In stratum I, $g_i = (10/20) - (216/600) = 0.140$ and $n_1 n_2/n = (20)(600)/620 = 19.35$. In stratum II, $g_i = (148/550) - (5/40) = 0.144$ and $n_1 n_2/n = (550)(40)/590 = 37.29$. The combined weighted mean increment will be $[(.140)(19.35) + (.144)(37.29)]/(19.35 + 37.29) = .143$.

This result can be compared with results of the direct standardization carried out for these data near the end of Section 26.3.2.1. The standardized rates were .387 for Treatment A and .245 for Treatment B, with an increment of .142. The two results are identical (except for rounding). In fact, if you work out the algebra for two strata, Cochran's weighted mean increment is the same as the increment in the direct standardized rates.

The approach can also be used for more than two strata. For example, in the data of Table 26.7, the results for the first (no co-morbidity) stratum are $g_i = (6/64) - (1/37) = .067$, and $(n_1 n_2)/(n_1 + n_2) = (64)(37)/101 = 23.45$. In the **intermediate** comorbidity stratum, $g_i = (10/59) - (14/75) = -.017$ and $(n_1 n_2)/(n_1 + n_2) = (59)(75)/134 = 33.02$. In the **severe** co-morbidity stratum, $g_i = (1/3) - (7/14) = -.167$, and $w_i = (3)(14)/17 = 2.47$.

The combined weighted increment will be

$$\frac{(.067)(23.45) - (.017)(33.02) - (.167)(2.47)}{23.45 + 33.02 + 2.47} = \frac{.597}{58.94} = .010$$

This result is close to the value of $.1502 - .1438 = .0064$ obtained with direct standardization at the end of Section 26.3.8.

26.4.1.2   Odds Ratio — The Cochran adjustment for an increment in rates can be applied when the stratified tables come from cohort or cross-sectional studies. The adjustment is not appropriate for case-control studies, however, because an increment cannot be used. The appropriate index of contrast for each stratum is the odds ratio, $a_i d_i / b_i c_i$.

In their original discussion of an adjustment process for odds ratios, Mantel and Haenszel[24] considered two possible approaches: to adjust the exposed group for the distribution of the unexposed group or to adjust both groups for a combined "standard" population. After pointing out the disadvantages of both methods, Mantel and Haenszel offered their "compromise formula" which produces the "weighted average" that has made their names a popular eponym in epidemiologic case-control studies.

To get an appropriate weighting factor, Mantel and Haenszel used the following reasoning. In any 2×2 table, the p_1 and p_2 rates of *exposure* for the compared groups can legitimately be contrasted with an odds ratio formed as $(p_1/p_2)/(q_1/q_2)$. For a stratum arranged as shown in Table 26.8, the corresponding rates of previous exposure will be $p_1 = a/n_1$, $q_1 = c/n_1$, $p_2 = b/n_2$, and $q_2 = d/n_2$. Thus, the ad/bc odds ratio represents $n_1 n_2 p_1 q_2 / n_1 n_2 p_2 q_1$. With an enlarging total stratum size, n, the values of n_1 and n_2 in each stratum will also enlarge. Because each numerator and denominator contains the products of two components, n_1 and n_2, the division of $n_1 n_2$ by n will produce $n_1 n_2/n$ as a standardizing factor. In fact, if $n_1 = kn$ and $n_2 = (1-k)n$, the value of $n_1 n_2/n$ becomes $(k)(1-k)n$; and the standardizing factor contains a multiplication by n, modified by $(k)(1-k)$, which reflects the distribution of n in the two groups. Therefore, if the numerators and denominators of an odds ratio are to be decomposed into strata and suitably weighted when they are additively reassembled, the adjusted values in each stratum should be $n_1 n_2 p_1 q_2/n$, which is ad/n for each numerator, and $n_1 n_2 p_2 q_1/n$, which is bc/n for each denominator.

TABLE 26.8

Symbols for Cells in 2×2 Table of Stratum in a Case-Control Study

	Cases	Controls	TOTAL
Exposed	a	b	f_1
Nonexposed	c	d	f_2
TOTAL	n_1	n_2	N

With this approach, the weighted values will be $a_i d_i / n_i$ and $b_i c_i / n_i$ for each of the i strata, and the ratio of their sum over all strata will form the adjusted odds ratio. It is named after Mantel and Haenszel and calculated as

$$O_{M-H} = \Sigma(a_i d_i / n_i)/\Sigma(b_i c_i / n_i) \tag{26.1}$$

26.4.2   Illustration of Problems in "Crude" Odds Ratio

Suppose a hypothetical case-control study of the relationship between smoking and omphalosis produces the results shown in Table 26.9. The "crude" odds ratio for these data has a reasonably impressive value of $(47 \times 46)/(23 \times 35) = 2.69$, and X^2 is also impressive at 8.66 (2P < .01).

A closer examination of additional data is troublesome, however, because smoking and occupation have the relationship shown in Table 26.10. The occupation was "dusty" for 38% (= 31/82) of the smokers but for only 14% (= 10/69) of the nonsmokers. If omphalosis is particularly likely to occur among people who work at dusty occupations, and if a much higher proportion of smokers work in dusty occupations, the "crude" odds ratio of 2.69 for smoking will be confounded.

To check this suspicion, we can examine data in Table 26.11 for the relationship between occupation and omphalosis. The results show that occupation is indeed an effect modifier. With a "crude" odds ratio of $(33 \times 73)/(8 \times 37) = 8.14$ and $X^2 = 26.4$, dusty occupation has an even more impressive effect, both quantitatively and stochastically, than the apparent result of smoking alone. Consequently, to get an unbiased estimate for the impact of smoking, the results must be adjusted for the confounding effect of occupation.

When stratified to show the effect of smoking in the two categories of occupation for the cases and controls, the data of Table 26.12 confirm the suspicion of confounding. The odds ratios for smokers have dropped to 2.23 in dusty occupations and 1.88 in non-dusty occupations; and neither one of these odds ratios is stochastically significant.

TABLE 26.9

Results in Hypothetical Case-Control Study

	Cases of Omphalosis	Controls without Omphalosis	TOTAL
Smokers	47	35	82
Nonsmokers	23	46	69
TOTAL	70	81	151

TABLE 26.10

Relationship of Occupation and Smoking for Groups in Table 26.9

Occupation	Smokers	Nonsmokers	TOTAL
Dusty	31	10	41
Non-dusty	51	59	110
TOTAL	82	69	151

TABLE 26.11

Relationship of Occupation and Disease for Groups in Table 26.9

Occupation	Cases of Omphalosis	Controls without Omphalosis	TOTAL
Dusty	33	18	41
Non-dusty	37	73	110
TOTAL	70	81	151

TABLE 26.12

Stratification of Results in Table 26.9

	Dusty Occupation			Non-Dusty Occupation		
	Cases	Controls	TOTAL	Cases	Controls	TOTAL
Smokers	26	5	31	21	30	51
Nonsmokers	7	3	10	16	43	59
TOTAL	33	8	41	37	73	110

odds ratio = 2.23   odds ratio = 1.88

X^2 (uncorrected) = 0.93 X^2 (uncorrected) = 2.42

26.4.3   Illustration of Mantel–Haenszel Adjustment

As noted in Section 26.4.1.2 and Formula [26.1], the Mantel–Haenszel process consists of choosing a component product, giving it a weight, adding the weighted components, and then dividing the two sums. The component product is the odds ratio in each stratum, and $1/n_i$ is the appropriate weight.

Thus, to get the ad numerator component of the adjusted odds ratio, we can form ad/n as a weighted component for each stratified table and then use the sum of the weighted components. For the 41 people with dusty occupation in Table 26.12, the ad weighted adjustment would be $(26 \times 3)/41 = 1.902$. For non-dusty occupation, the corresponding adjusted ad component would be $(21 \times 43)/110 = 8.209$. The total adjusted ad component would be $1.902 + 8.209 = 10.111$. The corresponding adjustment process for bc would yield a total of $[(7 \times 5)/41] + [(16 \times 30)/110] = .8537 + 4.3636 = 5.2173$. The final adjusted odds ratio would be $10.111/5.2173 = 1.94$. The adjusted value, as might be expected, lies between the two stratum values of 2.23 and 1.88.

26.4.4   Stochastic Evaluations

When a composite rate contains weighted combinations of rates in individual groups, the result can be evaluated stochastically, as discussed in Section 26.3.9, by using the individual standard errors of those rates. This tactic cannot be used with odds ratios, however, because two groups are compared in each ratio. Accordingly, both Cochran and Mantel–Haenszel proposed a stochastic strategy that determines a Z-score type of "standardized deviate" from pooled values for each 2×2 table (or stratum). The numerator of each Z-deviate is a weighted sum of the increment in each stratum divided by a weighted sum of the square root of the corresponding variance. These Z-deviates are squared, added, and interpreted with the chi-square distribution discussed in Section 14.1.3. Because the same basic strategy is used in both the Cochran and Mantel–Haenszel procedures, the results are sometimes called the *Cochran–Mantel–Haenszel chi-square test*. [For readers who are interested in the stochastic strategy, it is outlined in the next few subsections. If your quality of life does not demand this understanding, skip directly to Section 26.4.6.]

26.4.4.1   *Cochran–Armitage Approach* — Despite a similar stochastic strategy, different authorities have proposed different ways to calculate the variance and to use or avoid the Yates correction in the calculations. In Cochran's original proposal, the variance of each g_i is $p_o q_o n/n_1 n_2$ where p_o is the common value determined as $p_0 = (n_1 p_1 + n_2 p_2)/n$. The variance of $\bar{g}$ is then $\mathrm{Var}(\bar{g}) = \Sigma w_i p_{0_i} q_{0_i}/(\Sigma w_i)^2$, for the w_i values defined in Section 26.4.1.1. The Z-deviate is then formed as

$$Z = \bar{g}\sqrt{\mathrm{Var}\,(\bar{g})}$$

Armitage[14] gives an equivalent formula as

$$Z = \Sigma w_i d_i / \sqrt{\Sigma w_i p_{0_i} q_{0_i}}$$

26.4.4.2   *Mantel–Haenszel Approach* — Mantel and Haenszel also worked with a ratio of the same two weighted sums: one from the difference in proportions, $p_1 - p_2$, in each stratum and the other from the variance of each difference. The numerator of the ratio was converted, however, to an adjustment not for $p_1 - p_2$, but for its equivalent expressed as the observed-minus-expected values of a single cell in each 2×2 table.

As noted in Section 14.2.5, the observed-minus-expected value, e, will have the same absolute magnitude in each cell of a 2×2 table. Some further algebraic development, which the reader is spared, will show that

$$|p_1 - p_2| = (N/n_1 n_2)e$$

The value of e can be regarded as a sampling variation in which the sample $n_i p_i$ is taken from a "parent" population having the binomial parameter, $n_i P$. For this one-group "sample," a Z-type ratio can be constructed as:

$$\text{(observed value – parametric value)}/\sqrt{\text{variance of observation}}$$

The variance of the binomial "parametric" observation will be $n_i PQ = n_i(f_1/N)(f_2/N)$. Because of the finite "sampling," however, Mantel–Haenszel believed that the variance should be adjusted by the finite population correction factor, $(N - n_i)/(N - 1)$, whose role was discussed in Section 7.6. Accordingly, the variance becomes calculated as $[(N - n_i)/(N - 1)][n_i(f_1/N)(f_2/N)]$. Some further algebra will then show that the variance of $n_i p_i - n_i P = e$, in any cell of the 2×2 table, will be

$$n_1 n_2 f_1 f_2/N^2(N-1) \tag{26.2}$$

The square of the critical Z-type ratio for a cell will be

$$e^2/\text{variance} = \frac{n_1 n_2 (N-1)(p_1 - p_2)^2}{f_1 f_2}$$

As noted in Chapter 14, $p_1 - p_2 = (ad - bc)/n_1 n_2$. Thus, the squared critical ratio becomes

$$[(ad - bc)^2(N-1)]/(n_1 n_2 f_1 f_2) \tag{26.3}$$

This result is identical to the customary formula for X^2 except that Formula [26.3] uses $N - 1$ rather than N in the numerator. Thus, the square of the critical ratio for a cell in the 2×2 table produces essentially the same value as the X^2 calculated for the entire table. [According to Mantel–Haenszel, the conventional X^2 formula uses $(N - n_i)/N$, rather than $(N - n_i)/(N - 1)$, as the correction factor. The conventional arrangement leads to the customary chi-square formula, $(ad - bc)^2 N/(n_1 n_2 f_1 f_2)$.]

The focus of the adjusted chi-square calculation is usually the a cell, designated as a_i in each stratified table. In the first step, the sum of numerators is obtained for the single values of $(0 - E)^2$ in the a_i cells. This sum is then divided by the sum of corresponding variances.

26.4.5 Alternative Stochastic Approaches and Disputes

The strategy used to calculate the numerators and denominators, and sometimes the entire process, has evoked some of the same kinds of disputes (noted in Chapter 14) for the calculation of chi square in a 2×2 table. The disputes involve whether to use or omit Yales correction, whether the effects of the "sampling" should be analyzed with "fixed" or "random" models, and whether (or how) heterogeneous strata should be combined.

26.4.5.1 *Determination of Numerators* — The sum of the numerators can be determined in two ways. The obvious way is

$$[\Sigma(\text{observed } a_i - \text{expected } a_i)]^2$$

but advocates of Yates correction prefer that it be subtracted from the sum of the absolute increments before they are squared. With the correction, the sum that forms the "adjusted" numerator would be

$$[(\Sigma|\text{observed } a_i - \text{expected } a_i|)-0.5]^2$$

The Yates correction was used in the original M-H paper,[24] and is maintained in the M-H formulas cited by Breslow and Day,[25] Fleiss,[26] Kahn and Sempos,[27] and Schlesselman,[28] but not by Kleinbaum et al.[29] or Rothman.[30] A vigorous argument is offered in favor of the Yates correction by Breslow and Day and against it by Kleinbaum et al. In the absence of unanimity, probably the best approach is to calculate both ways. If the ultimate (P-value) results agree, there is no problem; if they do not, report both results and let the reader decide. If the adjusted X^2 value that emerges is close to the boundary needed for α = .05, honesty in reporting should compel a citation of both sets of results.

26.4.5.2 *Determination of Denominators* — The denominators of the M-H chi-square can also be calculated in two ways, according to a different type of dispute about variances. In the easy approach, which accepts the Mantel–Haenszel concept, the denominator is determined simply as Σ(variance of a_i). For each stratum, with N members having the marginal totals of n_1, n_2 and f_1, f_2, the variance of the a_i cell was shown in Formula [26.2]. With the Yates correction, the adjusted chi-square value will be

$$X^2_{MH_c} = \frac{\{[\Sigma|\text{observed } a_i - \text{expected } a_i|] - 0.5\}^2}{\Sigma \text{variance of } a_i} \qquad [26.4]$$

Without the Yates correction, the 0.5 subtraction is omitted in the numerator term. The uncorrected value can be designated as X^2_{MH}.

An alternative approach, mentioned previously, uses a "random-effects model" rather than the "fixed-effects model" employed in the customary chi-square calculations. With the "fixed-effects" model, Mantel and Haenszel regard the observed data as the "available universe," and use $N - 1$ in the calculations as a "finite population correction factor" for the "sampling process." With the random-effects model, the strata are regarded as samples from a larger undefined universe, for which variances are calculated according to the DerSimonian–Laird method.[31] (The D-L method produces larger variances, thereby reducing the eventual value of the combined X^2 result and increasing the size of confidence intervals).

Most calculations in packaged computer programs and in published literature have been done with the fixed-effect M-H model, but the D-L model is becoming increasingly popular, perhaps because it reportedly offers a better management of heterogeneous results in the strata.

26.4.5.3 *Example of Calculations* — The first stratum (for dusty occupation) in Table 26.12 has 26 as the a cell. Its expected value is (31)(33)/41 = 24.95. The corresponding variance, according to Formula [26.2], is [(33)(8)(31)(10)]/[(41)²(40)] = 1.217. The second stratum, for non-dusty occupation, has 21 as the a cell. Its expected value is (37)(51)/110 = 17.15, and the corresponding variance is [(37)(73)(51)(59)]/[(110)²(109)] = 6.162. Substituting these values into Formula [26.4], we get

$$X^2_{MH_c} = \frac{(|26 - 24.95| + |21 - 17.15| - 0.5)^2}{1.217 + 6.162} = \frac{(4.9 - 0.5)^2}{7.379} = 2.62$$

Without the Yates correction,

$$X^2_{MH} = \frac{(4.9)^2}{7.379} = 3.25$$

At one degree of freedom, neither result exceeds the 3.84 boundary value of X^2 needed for 2P < .05. Note that the adjusted M-H value of X^2 exceeds the X^2 values of 0.93 and 2.42 in the individual tables.

26.4.5.4 *Use of Confidence Intervals* — As confidence intervals have increasingly begun to replace P values, the combined results are often expressed with a confidence interval placed around the adjusted value of the odds ratio. For calculational convenience, the latter is regularly expressed as a natural logarithm, for which the standard error is used in the calculation.

Several methods, which were cited earlier (Section 17.5.5.2) for the log odds ratio in one 2 × 2 table, can be expanded to calculate the standard error of the adjusted combined ratio.

26.4.6 Caveats and Precautions

Although often proposed as a mechanism for dealing with "confounders," the Mantel–Haenszel (or analogous forms of) adjustment can produce a false sense of security if the adjusted variables do not really "confound." Three other problems which can arise are the results having opposite directions in the individual strata, the numbers in the partitioned strata becoming too small to be meaningful, or the strata being defined by a variable in which an ordinal trend is expected.

26.4.6.1 *Choice of "Confounders"* — To be regarded as a confounder, a variable must exert a confounding effect. For example, if *sex* does not affect the development of omphalosis but is the only variable used for the Mantel–Haenszel stratification, the results of smoking and nonsmoking would *not* be adjusted for confounding.

In the example here, occupation was a "legitimate" confounder because it affected both the frequency of smoking and the frequency of omphalosis. In many instances, however, the variables used to "adjust for confounding" may include diverse attributes that affect the exposure or the outcome but not both. The problem is particularly common in multivariable analysis, as discussed elsewhere.[10]

26.4.6.2 *Problems of Heterogeneity* — The results of any form of combined adjustment can be distorted if the component results, such as risk ratios, odds ratios, or gradients for target rates, go in opposite directions.

In the smoking–occupation–omphalosis example, both of the stratified odds ratios exceeded 1 and so the adjustment was justified. Consider the situation, however, for the case-control study shown in Table 26.13. When stratified, the crude odds ratio of 1.74 becomes an apparently protective value of 0.52 in women but rises to an impressive "causal" value of 11.8 in men.

TABLE 26.13

Hypothetical Case-Control Study

A. Crude Results:

	Case	Control	Total
Exposed	56	38	94
Nonexposed	104	123	227
Total	160	161	321

$$\text{odds ratio} = (56 \times 123)/(38 \times 104) = 1.74$$
$$X^2 = 5.03; 2P < .05$$

B. Stratified Results:

	Women				Men		
	Case	Control	Total		Case	Control	Total
Exposed	20	32	52	Exposed	36	6	42
Nonexposed	72	60	132	Nonexposed	32	63	95
Total	92	92	184	Total	68	69	137

odds ratio = $(20 \times 60)/(32 \times 72) = 0.52$ odds ratio = $(36 \times 63)/(6 \times 32) = 11.8$
$X^2 = 3.86; 2P < .05$ $X^2 = 31.5; 2P < .000001$

If these data receive a Mantel–Haenszel adjustment, the numerator for the odds ratio would be $[(20)(60)/184] + [(36)(63)/137] = 23.08$. The denominator would be $[(32)(72)/184] + [(6)(32)/137] = 13.92$. The Mantel–Haenszel adjusted odds ratio would be

$$O_{MH} = \frac{23.08}{13.92} = 1.66$$

This result is consistent with what might have been expected judgmentally. It is *lower* than the original crude odds ratio of 1.74, and it lies between the odds ratios of 0.52 and 11.8 in the two strata. Nevertheless, a scientific "commonsense" evaluation of the stratified results would suggest that men seem to be at risk but women are not. Because the stratification led to this apparently valuable discovery, the opposing "risk" and "no risk" results should *not* be combined into a single adjustment, which will distort what is really happening.

Heterogeneity — a problem that plagues any efforts to combine a series of results into a single adjusted value — usually receives two approaches that are reasonable but incompatible. The connoisseurs of substantive issues usually want the results to be substantively "precise," i.e., kept separate for such detailed distinctions as men vs. women, Stage I vs. Stage III cancer, severely ill vs. moderately ill patients. Connoisseurs of mathematical issues, who usually regard "precision" as an issue in statistical variance rather than biologic or clinical variation, want a combined single result that will have enhanced numerical size and that will avoid the need for inspecting and comparing results in multiple subgroups. In the mathematical approach, heterogeneity depends on the numerical values of the results; in the substantive approach, heterogeneity depends on the biologic (or other substantive) distinctions of the entities being compared. Thus, despite the obvious biologic heterogeneity, a small child, a large dog, and a huge fish might be mathematically regarded as homogeneous if they all weigh the same.

In the mathematical approach, various statistical tests are proposed for appraising heterogeneity of results in the strata that are candidates for combination. No guidelines are offered, however, for a level of heterogeneity that contra-indicates the combined "adjustment." An advantage claimed for the DerSimonian–Laird random-effects strategy[31] is that it improves the mathematical process when heterogeneous results are aggregated.

26.4.6.3   Effect of Small Numbers

— When the relationship between clear-cell vaginal carcinoma and in-utero exposure to diethystilbestrol (DES) was explored with the case-control study cited in Section 17.5.4, the original results showed the following:

	Cases	Controls
Exposed	7	0
Nonexposed	1	32

With 0.5 added to each cell, the odds ratio turned out to be $(7.5)(32.5)/(1.5)(0.5) = 325$.

From additional data reported by the investigators, however, two additional tables could be noted as follows for mothers who had had pregnancy problems (spontaneous abortions in previous pregnancies or bleeding, cramping, etc. early in current pregnancy):

Pregnancy Problems	Case	Control	Exposed	Nonexposed
Yes	7	5	7	5
No	1	27	0	28

The odds ratios in these two tables are $(7 \times 27)/(1 \times 5) = 37.8$ and $(7.5 \times 28.5)/(0.5 \times 5.5) = 77.7$, thus suggesting that pregnancy problems were a strong confounder of the observed relationship.

The results could be divided into the following stratification:

Mothers with Pregnancy Problems	Cases	Controls
Exposed to DES	7	0
Not Exposed to DES	0	5

Mothers without Pregnancy Problems	Cases	Controls
Exposed to DES	0	0
Not Exposed to DES	1	27

Calculated with 0.5 added to each cell, the odds ratios are $(7.5)(5.5)/(0.5)(0.5) = 165$ in the first stratum and $(0.5)(27.5)/(0.5)(1.5) = 18.3$ in the second. The Mantel–Haenszel adjusted odds ratio is

$$\frac{[(7.5)(5.5)/14] + [(27.5)(0.5)/30]}{[(0.5)(0.5)/14] + [(1.5)(0.5)/30]} = \frac{2.946 + .458}{.179 + .025} = \frac{3.405}{.204} = 16.69$$

This value is substantially lower than the unadjusted crude result of 325.

To calculate an M-H adjusted X^2, the second stratum will yield a value of 0 for both the observed and expected values in the a_i and b_i cells. In the other two cells, the observed-minus-expected values will be 0. In the first stratum, the expected value in the a cell is $(7 \times 7)/12 = 4.08$, and the observed-minus-expected value is $(7 - 4.08) = 2.82$.

The numerator of X_{M-H_c} might be calculated as $[|2.82| + |0| - 0.5]^2 = 5.38$, but the denominator is a problem. From Formula [26.2], the variance in the first stratum is $(7)(5)(7)(5)/[(11)(12)^2] = .773$, but the variance in the second stratum will be $(1)(27)(28)(0)/[(27)(28)^2] = 0$. If these two variances are added, the result for $X^2_{MH_c}$ would be $5.38/.773 = 6.96$. The result is still stochastically significant at $2P < .05$, but the adjustment makes X^2 much smaller than the original corrected X^2_c value, which would have been $[|(7)(32) - (1)(0)| - (40/2)]^2(40)/(8)$ $(32)(33)(7) = 28.15$.

On the other hand, a major mathematical assault occurs on scientific "common sense," when odds ratios, "expected" values, and variances are calculated for 2×2 tables with two zero values in cells, such as $\begin{Bmatrix} 7 & 0 \\ 0 & 5 \end{Bmatrix}$ or $\begin{Bmatrix} 0 & 0 \\ 1 & 27 \end{Bmatrix}$. In particular, the individual critical ratio in the second table where $0 - E = 0$ and variance $= 0$ would be an incalculable $0/0$. Furthermore, the M-H chi-square value here becomes derived essentially from only the first stratum.

Although possibly justified by diverse forms of mathematical reasoning, the results are too scientifically peculiar to be acceptable. They suggest that the basic design of the study should have been improved. Cases and controls should have been originally matched on the basis of pregnancy problems, rather than leaving the latter variable to be "adjusted" during an analysis afterward.

26.4.6.4 *Ordinal Trend in Strata* — When stratified results are combined with any of the methods discussed so far, the particular order of the strata is not considered. The standardized or adjusted descriptive summaries, and the corresponding stochastic calculations, will be the same regardless of whether age is divided as **young, medium, old** or as **old, young, medium**.

In data for "dose-response curves," however, we expect the trend in response to go progressively up or down, according to the trend in dose. For example, the odds ratios (or risk ratios) for success with active treatment vs. placebo might be expected to rise in strata with progressively increasing doses of the treatment. An analogous rise in occurrence rates of disease might be anticipated (and might help prove "causation") with higher magnitudes of exposure to a suspected etiologic agent.

These trends cannot be evaluated with the described arrangements for standardizing or adjusting. A special method of weighting, discussed in Chapter 27, is needed to allow appraisal of "linear trend" in the "dose-response" curves of the ordinal strata.

26.4.7 Extension to Cohort Data

Because cohort data can be expressed with rates and risk ratios, the cumbersome use of odds ratios is not necessary. Nevertheless, the M-H adjustment is sometimes applied to cohort data. The tactic is particularly justified when the cohort data contain many "censored" results that preclude a direct calculation and comparison of survival rates. The investigator may also want the stochastic comparison to reflect dynamic results for the entire survival curve rather than for a single time point alone.

Unlike odds-ratio data, for which the M-H adjustment provides both descriptive and stochastic indexes, the adjustment for cohort data is only stochastic and often applies to a comparison of two (or more) survival curves. The customary stochastic index is the log rank statistic, which was discussed in Chapter 22. Because this latter statistic has had so many versions, it is sometimes called the Cox-Mantel test or designated with other eponyms.

26.5 Matching and "Matched Controls"

All of the stratifications and recombinations that have been discussed so far are but one way of dealing with confounders. Another approach, not discussed here, makes use of multivariable algebraic procedures. A third approach, discussed in the rest of this section, is the use of "matching."

To match individual persons seems ideal for managing the problem of confounding. In fact, the use of cross-over trials, where the same person receives different treatments, is based on the appealing idea of letting the treated persons be their own "controls." As noted earlier, however, the idyllic hopes of the cross-over design are destroyed by the reality that severely restricts the clinical circumstances amenable to a cross-over arrangement.

In observational studies, the ideal hope would be to find a "control" whose confounder attributes exactly match those of the compared person. This hope, however, is also regularly thwarted by reality. The main confounders may not be known, or the number of different confounders may be too extensive to permit suitable matchings. Accordingly, although matchings are commonly done, they are arranged mainly for investigative convenience, not for management of confounding. Disputes may then arise about the best way to analyze the "matched" results.

26.5.1 Application in Case-Control Studies

In many case-control studies, the *cases* are chosen as an available group of people who all have the disease under consideration. The *controls* are selected from a group of people who are believed not to have the disease. Certain criteria may be applied to restrict eligibility, in either the case or control group or in both, to persons having a demarcated range of age, occupations, clinical conditions, or other possibly pertinent attributes.

The selection of a suitable control group is a complex topic about which universal agreement does not exist, and the topic has received abundant discussion elsewhere.[1] The main point to be considered now is not the paramount importance of scientific propriety in the matching process, but the pragmatic method often used for choosing controls and for doing the subsequent statistical analysis.

The process sometimes involves getting 2 or more controls for each case, but the most common tactic (which is discussed here) involves a 1-to-1 matching arrangement.

26.5.2 Choosing "Matched" Controls

In a case-control study, the investigator usually begins with a group of cases, found via some type of medical roster or registry of persons with the appropriate disease. The controls can then come from three general sources of presumably nondiseased persons: the same medical milieu (e.g., a hospital where the cases were identified); the same large cohort study from which the cases emerged; or the general community (e.g., neighbors, friends, persons found via "random-digit" telephone dialing).

Because age and sex (and sometimes race) are commonly applied for epidemiologic adjustment, these demographic variables are often used to "match" the controls chosen for the cases. The subsequent analysis is easier because the compared groups are demographically similar, but the matching process can also have a major chronologic virtue. If the two groups come from a common roster, such as a list of admissions to a hospital or to a cohort study, the controls can be matched for admission at about the same date as the cases. For example, if the cases have all been hospitalized, the controls can receive a time-age-sex matching if chosen from the chronologic roster of hospital admissions, going upward and downward from the admission date of each case to find the next ensuing or previously admitted person who is similar in sex and in age ±5 years.

26.5.3 Formation of Tables

In a 1-to-1 matching, the investigator emerges with N case-control pairs, containing 2N persons. When previous exposure to the suspected etiologic agent is ascertained for each person, each case-control pair will have one of four possible results that can be arranged as follows for the N matched pairs:

Exposure Status		Frequency of Each Cell in Matched Arrangement
Case	Control	
Yes	Yes	a
Yes	No	b
No	Yes	c
No	No	d
	TOTAL	N

Table 26.14 shows the agreement matrix for the N matched pairs, and Table 26.15 shows the "unmatched" arrangement for these data, presented in the more customary format of case-control tabulations. In the familiar unmatched arrangement, the odds ratio for the "risk" of exposure will be $(n_1 \times f_2)/(f_1 \times n_2) = [(a + b)(b + d)]/[(a + c)(c + d)]$. If you work out all the algebra, this result eventually becomes

$$\{b + [(ad - bc)/N]\}/\{c + [(ad - bc)/N]\} \qquad [26.5]$$

It can be compared with the odds ratio for the matched arrangement, which is calculated simply as b/c. The mathematical justification for the latter calculation is the topic for the rest of this discussion.

TABLE 26.14

Agreement Matrix for Matched Case-Control Pairs

Cases	Controls		Total
	Exposed	Nonexposed	
Exposed	a	b	n_1
Nonexposed	c	d	n_2
TOTAL	f_1	f_2	N

TABLE 26.15

Unmatched Arrangement of Data in Table 26.14

	Cases	Controls	Total
Exposed	n_1	f_1	$n_1 + f_1$
Nonexposed	n_2	f_2	$n_2 + f_2$
TOTAL	$n_1 + n_2$	$f_1 + f_2$	2N

26.5.4 Justification of Matched Odds Ratio

If the unmatched odds ratio is 1, ad = bc; so ad − bc = 0, thus reducing expression [26.5] to b/c. For the matched and unmatched ratios to be equal, however, b/c must also equal 1. Therefore b = c, and ad must equal $b^2 = c^2$. For example, suppose the matched agreement matrix is $\begin{Bmatrix} 20 & 10 \\ 10 & 5 \end{Bmatrix}$. In this situation b/c = 10/10 = 1 and ad − bc = 100 − 100 = 0. The 2 × 2 table for the unmatched arrangement will be $\begin{Bmatrix} 15 & 15 \\ 30 & 30 \end{Bmatrix}$, which will have an odds ratio of 1. More commonly, however, neither the unmatched nor the matched odds ratio is 1, and the process needs a mathematical justification that is provided by the Mantel–Haenszel procedure.

26.5.4.1 Stratification of Matched Pairs — If we consider each of the N matched pairs as an individual stratum in an "unmatched" arrangement, each of the strata will have one of the four possible arrangements shown in Table 26.16. Because each pair contains 2 persons, the matched pairs in Table 26.14, when displayed in Table 26.16, will contain *2a* persons in Arrangement I, *2b* in Arrangement II, *2c* in Arrangement III, and *2d* in Arrangement IV.

TABLE 26.16

Arrangements of Strata of Matched Pair Results in Case-Control Study

	Arrangement I: (Both exposed)		Arrangement II: (Case exposed, not control)		Arrangement III: (Control exposed, not case)		Arrangement IV: (Neither case nor control exposed)	
	Case	Control	Case	Control	Case	Control	Case	Control
Exposed	1	1	1	0	0	1	0	0
Nonexposed	0	0	0	1	1	0	1	1

26.5.4.2 Formation of Adjusted Odds Ratio — For the M-H summary odds ratio, each stratum adds its own "intrinsic" $a_i d_i / n_i$ term to the adjusted numerator and its own $b_i c_i / n_i$ term to the adjusted denominator. In arrangements I, III, and IV of Table 26.16, the $a_i d_i$ terms will be 0. In arrangements I, II, and IV, the $b_i c_i$ terms will be 0. The only nonzero values will occur in arrangement II, where $a_i d_i / n_i$ = (1)(1)/(1 + 1) = 1/2, and in arrangement III, where $b_i c_i / n_i$ = (1)(1)/(1 + 1) = 1/2. The number of strata will be *a* for arrangement I, *b* for II, *c* for III, and *d* for IV. Because *b* strata will have $a_i d_i / n_i$ values of 1/2, with all other strata having corresponding values of 0, $\Sigma a_i d_i / n_i$ for the M-H adjusted numerator will be b/2. For the M-H denominator, *c* strata will have $b_i c_i / n_i$ values of 1/2 and all other strata will have corresponding values of 0. Thus, $\Sigma b_i c_i / n_i$ for the M-H adjusted denominator will be c/2. The M-H adjusted odds ratio will then be (b/2)/(c/2) = b/c.

26.5.4.3 Formation of Adjusted Variance — In arrangements I and IV of Table 26.16, the variance will be 0, for reasons discussed earlier. In arrangements II and III, the variance will be nonzero and identical. The four marginal totals in each arrangement will be 1, with n_i = 2. Thus, according to Formula [26.2], the variance will be $(1)(1)(1)(1)/[(2^2)(1)]$ = 1/4 for each arrangement of the *b* strata (with arrangement II) and the *c* strata (with arrangement III). Thus, Σ (variance of a_i) will be b(1/4) + c(1/4) = (b + c)/4. The expected value in the a_i cell of arrangements II and III will be 1/2[= (1)(1)/(2)]. The observed-expected value in the a_i cell will be 1 − 1/2 = 1/2 in arrangement II and 0 − 1/2 in arrangement III. Thus, the value of Σ(observed − expected) will be b(1/2) + c(−1/2) = (b − c)/2.

26.5.5   Calculation of "Matched" X²

When the (b − c)/2 value is squared for the uncorrected calculation, we get X_{M-H}^2 = [(b − c)² /4]/(b + c)/4 = (b − c)²/(b + c), which is the same result as the formula previously cited for the uncorrected McNemar chi-square test for a matched 2 × 2 table. Consequently, when uncorrected, the McNemar and the Mantel–Haenszel procedures give identical results (and thus help justify one another) for determining X² in the matched analysis of a 2 × 2 table.

The 0.5 subtraction to "correct" the M-H results, however, becomes very tricky to apply to the matched arrangements II and III in Table 26.13, because the observed values are either 1 or 0 and the expected values are 0.5. Accordingly, if Yates correction is desired, the best stochastic approach for the matched 2 × 2 table is simply to calculate a corrected McNemar chi-square value as

$$X_M^2(\text{corrected}) = \frac{(|b - c| - 1)^2}{b + c}$$

26.5.6 Scientific Peculiarities

Despite the apparent mathematical merits, the procedure just described for getting a matched odds ratio has at least four scientific peculiarities:

26.5.6.1 *Nonconfounding "Confounders"* — The Mantel–Haenszel adjustment is intended to deal with *confounding* variables, but the matching in most case-control studies is an act of demographic convenience, not a precaution against confounding. For reasons discussed elsewhere,[1] age and sex (and perhaps race) are seldom the main confounding variables in case-control studies of etiology (or therapy).

26.5.6.2 *Neglect of Bulk of Data* — In a study where most of the data are in the matched a and d cells of Table 26.14, it seems odd to place the main emphasis on the "disagreement" in the relatively sparse b and c cells. This problem can be illustrated as follows. Suppose the matched data for 250 pairs in a case-control study are arranged in the format of Table 26.14 as follows: $\begin{Bmatrix} 150 & 20 \\ 8 & 72 \end{Bmatrix}$. The matched odds ratio will be $20/8 = 2.5$, X_M^2 (uncorrected) will be $(20-8)^2/(20+8) = 5.14$; and $2P < .05$. The unmatched results will be $\begin{Bmatrix} 170 & 158 \\ 80 & 92 \end{Bmatrix}$ so that the unmatched odds ratio is $[(170)(92)]/[(158)(80)] = 1.24$, with a stochastically nonsignificant $X^2 = 1.3$. Although the investigator might want to use the matched data to claim a "significantly" elevated risk, the claim would be contradicted by the unmatched results. The main findings in this study would seem to be the predominant similarity of exposure or nonexposure in 222 ($= 150 + 72$) of the matched pairs, rather than the dissimilarity noted in 28 pairs. To draw a conclusion from only the latter results would ignore what is found in the great bulk of all the other data.

26.5.6.3 *Results with Variance of 0* — It seems intuitively unacceptable to dismiss arrangements I and IV of Table 26.16 as having 0 variance. Although quite correct mathematically, the dismissal runs counter to the ingrained idea that all samples have variations. For example, a proportion such as $0/2$ has 0 variance according to the formula $\sqrt{pq/n}$ (for the proportion) or the formula npq (for the numerator). Nevertheless, despite the 0 variance, most evaluators would regard such a proportion as unstable. The stability might be determined by resorting to binomial distributions, but these distributions are not used in the McNemar or M-H formulas; and the Yates corrections are but arbitrary attempts to substitute for the actual distributions.

26.5.6.4 *Ambiguous Results* — Because the odds ratios and the X^2 values can become ambiguous, yielding substantially different results when calculated with the matched and unmatched methods,[32] an investigator can always do things both ways and then report the "desired" result. For this reason, reviewers, editors, and readers should always demand that both sets of results be presented. If the conclusions disagree, the decision about which set to accept will usually be controversial, depending on the professional ancestry of the person who does the deciding. For persons with a mathematical background, the preferred choice will usually be the statistical appeal of the matched analysis. For persons with a scientific background, the preferred choice—for reasons stated in the first two points here—will be the unmatched analysis. As long as both sets of results are presented, however, you can make your own choice.

26.6 Additional Statistical Procedures

If you feel mentally tired and somewhat confused after all the foregoing discussion, you are in good company. Most health professionals and scientific workers become distinctly uncomfortable (if not overtly oppressed) when confronted with the extensive mathematical reasoning used for the cited concepts. Complex as they may be, however, the concepts just discussed are but a few of the diverse mathematical strategies that have been developed for the statistical analysis of "risk" in case-control and cohort studies.

The Mantel–Haenszel and many other methods can be used to adjust the risk ratio in cohort studies as well as the odds ratio in case-control studies. The matched odds ratio can be calculated in special ways when the controls are matched as ≥ 2 to 1, rather than 1 to 1. Special confidence intervals can be calculated for these multiple matchings, as well as for 1 to 1 matchings. And all of the mathematical strategies have inspired multiple ideas and multiple pages of statistical literature.

As a reward for having come this far in the chapter, however, you will be spared an account of all the additional ideas and operational tactics. If you ever want (or need) to find out what they are, you can look them up (and try to understand them) from the accounts and cited references given in several textbooks.[25–28] After discovering that the authors do not always agree on the best way to do things, you can feel particularly grateful to have escaped the risk of the exposure here.

References

1. Feinstein, 1985; 2. Chan, 1988; 3. Carson, 1994; 4. Yerushalmy, 1951; 5. Abramson, 1995; 6. Kitagawa, 1966; 7. Anderson, 1998; 8. Sorlie, 1999; 9. Royal College of General Practitioners, 1974; 10. Feinstein, 1996; 11. Concato, 1992; 12. Roos, 1989; 13. Morris, 1988; 14. Armitage, 1971; 15. Vandenbroucke, 1982; 16. Mulder, 1983; 17. Liddell, 1984; 18. Ulm, 1990; 19. Lee, 1994; 20. Greenland, 1991; 21. Kupper, 1978; 22. Decoufle, 1980; 23. Cochran, 1954; 24. Mantel, 1959; 25. Breslow, 1980; 26. Fleiss, 1981; 27. Kahn, 1989; 28. Schlesselman, 1982; 29. Kleinbaum, 1982; 30. Rothman, 1986; 31. DerSimonian, 1986; 32. Feinstein, 1987b.

Exercises

26.1. Use your calculator to confirm the statement in the text that the direct standardized rates in Table 26.5 are 15.02% for OPEN and 14.38% for TURP. Show at least some of the component calculations.

26.2. If you did an indirect rather than direct standardized adjustment for the data in Table 26.5, what would be the standardized mortality ratios for TURP and OPEN? What would be the indirectly standardized mortality rates?

26.3. The investigators whose work was contradicted have vigorously disputed the conclusions by Concato et al.[11] What do you think is the focus of the counter-attack by the original investigators?

26.4. The five-year survival rate for breast cancer is reported to be 71% at the prestigious Almamammy Medical Center and 59% at the underfunded Caritas Municipal Hospital. The nationally reported five-year rate of survival for breast cancer is 63%. We also know the following data:

TNM Stage	Reported Number of Patients		5-Year National Survival Rates
	Almamammy	Caritas	
I	129	631	.80
II	35	266	.62
III	32	642	.54
IV	23	307	.17
TOTAL	219	1846	.63

What could you do to standardize the two sets of results for comparison? What are the standardized values?

26.5. In 1970, the crude death rate (all causes) for Guyana was 6.8 per 1000; for the United States it was 9.4 per 1000.

    26.5.1.   Can the lower crude death rate in Guyana be attributed to the fact that the United States has a larger population? Explain your answer.

    26.5.2.   Cite two other possible explanations for the lower rate in Guyana.

    26.5.3.   Additional information about these countries for the same year is as follows:

	Guyana	United States
Crude birth rate (per 1000 population)	38.1	18.2
Infant mortality rate (per 1000 live births)	38.3	19.8

    How does this additional information assist you in interpreting the difference in crude death rates?

26.6. In Figure E.26.6, curves (1) and (2) represent two ways of showing the secular trend in overall mortality in the United States between 1900 and 1960. One curve represents crude death rates; the other, age-adjusted death rates.

    26.6.1.   The United States population of what year was used as the standard for the age-adjusted rates? Explain your answer.

    26.6.2.   From your examination of the two rates, which is the crude rate and which the age-adjusted rate? Explain your answer.

    26.6.3.   Why has one curve leveled off after 1940, while the other has continued to decline?

26.7. Try to find (group cooperation permissable) a paper in which the Mantel–Haenszel adjustment was used. Do you understand what was done? Do you agree with the results and conclusions?

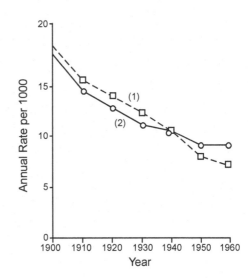

FIGURE E.26.6

Crude and age-adjusted death rates, United States (1900–1930, death registration states; 1940–1960 total, United States).

27

Indexes of Categorical Association

CONTENTS

In Chapter 26, we considered methods of adjusting and combining a set of results in which a binary variable — such as survival, success, or development of a disease — had been partitioned into a set of strata or an array of 2×2 tables. For reasons discussed in Chapter 18, the data presented in Chapter 26 can all be regarded as associations, but our main interest was in contrasting groups rather than relating variables. We wanted to examine standardized rates or adjusted odds ratios.

In this chapter, we turn to relationships, rather than contrasts, for categorical variables, and to the pertinent indexes of categorical association. These indexes appear infrequently but regularly in medical literature; and some of them may already have been thrust upon you, uninvitedly, by the computer printout of a "packaged" program (in the BMDP, SAS, or other systems) that was used merely to obtain a chi-square or Fisher exact test for a simple 2×2 table. Although the additional indexes may often be neither necessary nor useful for such tables, the computer programs may include the extra embellishment, somewhat like automated laboratory tests that report many measurements beyond the result you wanted only for glucose or electrolytes.

The discussion now is intended to acquaint you with the additional categorical indexes, mention some of their many titles or eponyms, outline their construction, and show how and where they might be useful. The operational details need not be remembered, because you can always expand the acquaintance (or even develop a friendship) if you meet or need the indexes in the future. Detailed descriptions are available in a plethora of textbooks.[1-8]

The many additional indexes are needed because of (1) difficulty in expressing results for variables cited in ordinal or nominal categories and (2) the diverse structures created when the categories of ordinal or nominal variables are related to one another or to other (dimensional or binary) variables.

27.1 Sources of Complexity in Categorical Indexes

In previous discussions of indexes of association, Chapter 18 outlined the needs created by different scales for the two variables. In Chapter 19, the most commonly used indexes were shown for bi-dimensional trends; and the many indexes of concordance appeared in Chapters 20 and 21. In the remaining indexes that have been reserved for this chapter, the associations are constructed with strategies of estimation or covariation; and at least one of the two variables in each index is categorical — expressed in binary, ordinal, or nominal data. The categorical relationships produce four complexities beyond those discussed previously.

27.1.1 Asymmetrical Orientations

In statistical jargon, the words *symmetrical* and *asymmetrical* are sometimes used respectively for the interdependent and dependent relationships of trend in two variables. In symbols, $Y \times X$ (or $X \times Y$) can indicate a general bivariate relationship; $Y \leftrightarrow X$; represents a symmetric correlation; and $Y \to X$ or Y vs. X represents an asymmetric dependence of Y on X.

The asymmetry can lead to strikingly different statistical structures and expressions. Thus, if a dimensional $\times$ binary relationship is arranged as dimensional $\to$ binary, the structure of the data will produce a contrast of two means, but if the relationship is binary $\to$ dimensional, the structure can resemble a survival curve.

27.1.2 Non-Commensurate Scales

Even if the two variables have similar types of scales, such as ordinal $\times$ ordinal, the statistical index can differ for non-commensurate scales that have different numbers of categories. For example, if each ordinal variable has 3 categories, the two-way table has a "square" 3×3 structure, as in the relationship of TNM Stage **I, II, III** for cancer vs. **young, middle,** and **old** age groups. If one ordinal variable has 3 categories and the other has 4, however, the 3×4 table may require a different "rectangular" index of association. The relationship of TNM Stage **I, II, III** to *symptoms* would be "rectangular" if the symptoms were cited in four categories as **none, mild, moderate,** and **severe.**

As a nicety of nomenclature, note that a scale "cut" into two categories is called *binary* or *dichotomous*. The latter term comes from *dicha*, which is Greek for "two," and from *tom*, which also appears in such surgical cutting as *laparotomy*. Because *tricha* is Greek for "three," a scale with three categories is *trichotomous*. Prefixed by the Greek for "many," a scale with more than three categories is *polytomous*. The latter term, however, is often mistakenly called *polychotomous* if the *dicha-* and *tricha-* prefixes lead to expectations that a "cho" should precede the "tom."

Trichotomous and *polytomous* scales will always involve either ordinal or nominal variables.

27.1.3   Tied Ranks

When ordinal categories have a limited set of grades (such as **none, mild, moderate, severe**) rather than an unlimited array of consecutive "cardinal" ranks (such as **1, 2, 3, … 39, 40, …**), the ranks in the graded categories can have many tied values, as discussed in Chapter 15. In such situations, indexes conceived with an unlimited-rank strategy will require "corrections" to account for the ties.

27.1.4   Presentation: Contingency Tables or Variables

Data expressed in categories are usually presented in a two-way contingency table, having r rows for one of the categorical variables and c columns for the other. The numbers in the cells of the $r \times c$ table represent frequency counts for the "contingent" occurrence of each bivariate category. (The most common such table is a 2×2 or "fourfold" arrangement of two binary variables.) Most of the additional indexes to be discussed here are produced by the different structures of the $r \times c$ tables. If the categories are ordinal grades, for which many tied ranks can be expected, the analysis is usually aimed directly at tied and non-tied frequencies in the tabular arrangement.

Not all ordinal data, however, are cited in frequently tied grades. An ordinal scale may sometimes have ranks that contain either unlimited cardinal counts or very few (if any) ties, because the ranks were obtained from dimensional variables. For these ordinal scales, the analysis can be approached simply as a relationship of variables. (If two unlimited-rank variables are arranged as a contingency table, each cell will often have only one member.)

27.1.5   Construction with Estimates or Trends

As noted earlier in Section 18.3.1, the association between two variables can be expressed with an index of either estimation or covariation. For the bi-dimensional data in Chapter 19, both types of indexes were obtained with a single procedure — the linear regression method, which is aimed at estimates, but also produces regression and correlation coefficients for trend (or "covariation"). This type of "two-fer" bonus is seldom possible with other forms of bivariate association, which are usually expressed with indexes of either estimation or trend, but not both. The few methods of estimation will be discussed in the next section, and the rest of the chapter thereafter is devoted to the many indexes of trend.

27.2   Indexes of Estimation

The improved accuracy achieved when one variable is estimated from values of the other can be cited as proportionate reductions in error, in variance, or in "entropy."

27.2.1   Lambda

The index called lambda was proposed by Guttman[9] and christened by Goodman and Kruskal.[10] With these origins, the eponymic designation for lambda is usually given to Guttman by psychosocial scientists[11] and to Goodman and Kruskal by statisticians.[12,13]

Having been constructed for tables with nominal categories, the lambda index can also be used for ordinal contingencies. The basic strategy was discussed, without being so labeled, in Section 18.3.1.2. If E_y is the number of errors in the estimates made with Y alone, and if E_x is the number of errors in the estimates made with X, the index for proportionate reduction in error is

$$\text{lambda} = \frac{E_y - E_x}{E_y} \qquad\qquad [27.1]$$

With this construction, lambda is analogous to r^2 in bi-dimensional associations[13], but the errors are determined from unit counts of right or wrong categorical estimates, rather than from squared deviations of measured dimensions.

For example, consider the data in Table 27.1, showing a relationship between five ordinal categories of TNM stages (X-variable in rows) and four ordinal symptom stages (Y-variable in columns) in a random sample of 200 patients with lung cancer.[14,15] To estimate a value for *symptom stage* using data from Y alone, the best estimate would be the mode, **stage 2**, which appears most often (82 times) among the 200 ratings. If estimated for all 200 ratings, this value would be wrong in 118 (= 200 −82) instances. When an associated X value is available for TNM stages, however, the respective modal values of 27, 21, 8, and 17 in each of the first four TNM rows (stages 1, 2, 3, and 4) would lead to **Stage 2** as the corresponding estimate for symptom stage in each row. These estimates would be wrong in (51 + 27 + 18 + 36) − (27 + 21 + 8 + 17) = 59 cases. In the row for TNM stage 5, however, the modal estimate of symptom **Stage 4** would be wrong in 68 − 39 = 29 cases. Thus, the total number of errors using the X variable would be 59 + 29 = 88. The proportionate reduction in errors would be

$$\text{lambda} = (118 - 88)/118 = .25$$

TABLE 27.1

Relationship of Symptom Stage and TNM Stage in Random Sample of 200 Patients with Lung Cancer*

Variable X: TNM Stage Ordinal Categories	Variable Y: Symptom Stage Ordinal Categories				
	1	2	3	4	Total
1	13	27	0	11	51
2	3	21	0	3	27
3	4	8	4	2	18
4	6	17	7	6	36
5	2	9	18	39	68
Total	28	82	29	61	200

* The full set of data is reported in Chapter Reference 14 and the random sample is further analyzed in Chapter Reference 15.

The expression for lambda is asymmetric. In this instance, it was oriented as though Y (for symptom stage) depended on X, but it can also be calculated, if desired, either with the orientation that X depends on Y or with a symmetrical expression.

Although not a particularly useful index now, lambda will be valuable later on (in Section 27.4.1.1) to describe the effects of categorical stratifications for a binary variable.

27.2.2 Eta Correlation Ratio

Despite the "correlation" in the title, eta is a descriptive index of estimation. It can be used when a dimensional variable, such as weight, is examined in a series of nominal groups A, B, C, ... This statistical arrangement commonly appears in the *analysis of variance*, and the results are usually expressed with a stochastic index, called F, which is a polytomous counterpart of the stochastic Z or t for comparing two groups. As a descriptive statistic for the dimensional → nominal arrangment, eta (η) indicates the proportionate reduction of group variance and corresponds to the roles of r^2 in simple regression and ϕ^2 (discussed later) in categorical data.

Figure 27.1 displays a set of data for which eta could be applied to summarize the total proportionate reduction in group variance when serum concentration of sCD4 cells was partitioned into four diagnostic groups of patients.[16] As shown by the p values in the figure, however, the authors preferred to do pairs of two-group analyses.

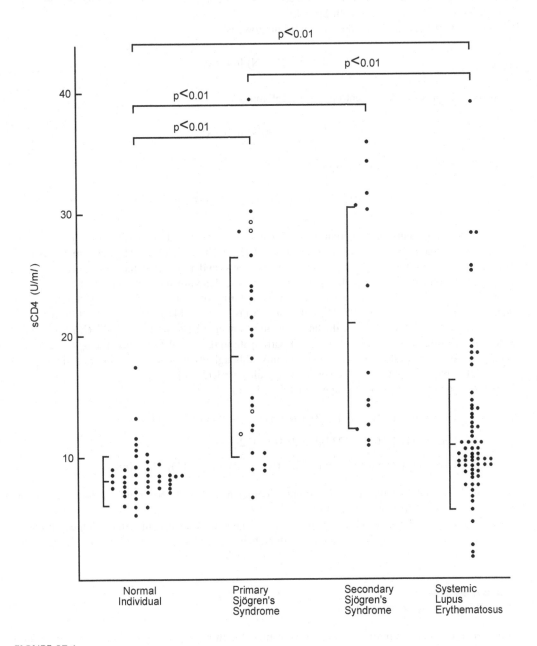

FIGURE 27.1

Serum concentrations of sCD4 in patients with primary (n = 25) and secondary (n = 13) Sjogren's syndrome, patients with SLE (n = 64), and normal individuals (n = 43). ○ =patients with sicca alone (n = 4, glandular type). Mean and standard deviation are indicated by vertical lines. [Figure and legend taken from Chapter Reference 16.]

27.2.3   "Uncertainty" Coefficient

The uncertainty coefficient is based on the idea of *entropy*, which is a concept of "information theory." According to this concept, the entropy in a proportion such as p_i is equal to p_i times its logarithm. The idea appeared (without being so labelled) when Shannon's H was presented as an index of diversity in Section 5.10.2.

The symbols in an $r \times c$ contingency table are as follows: The individual frequency counts in each cell are n_{ij}. The marginal totals of the r rows are $r_1, r_2 \ldots, r_r$, with $\Sigma r_i = N$. The marginal totals of the c columns are $c_1, c_2, \ldots, c_j, \ldots, c_c$, with $\Sigma c_j = N$.
If X represents the row variable, the entropy in the rows is

$$U(X) = \Sigma \ (r_i/N) \ \ln \ (r_i/N)$$

If Y is the column variable, the entropy in the columns is

$$U(Y) = \Sigma \ (c_j/N) \ \ln \ (c_j/N)$$

The entropy in the individual cells, n_{ij}, is

$$U(XY) = \text{sum of } [(n_{ij}/N) \ \ln \ (n_{ij}/N)]$$

From these components, the uncertainty coefficient can be calculated in an asymmetric or symmetric direction. The numerator of the coefficient is always $U(X) + U(Y) - U(XY)$. The denominator is $U(Y)$ if the column values are being established from the rows, and is $U(X)$ if the row values are being established from the columns. For the symmetric value, the denominator is $[U(X) + U(Y)]/2$.

For the data in Table 27.1, the proportions in the column totals are $28/200 = 0.14$, $82/200 = 0.41$, $29/200 = 0.145$, and $61/200 = 0.305$. The value of $U(Y)$ is $.14 \ln (0.14) + .41 (\ln .41) + .145 (\ln .145) + .305 (\ln .305) = -1.283$. Analogous calculations would show that $U(X) = -1.511$, and $U(XY) = -2.5598$. [Null cells (with frequency counts of 0) do not participate in the calculations, because $n_{ij} = 0$ before an attempt can be made to calculate $\ln n_{ij}$. Consequently, although 20 terms would be expected in the 5×4 structure of Table 27.1, only 18 cells were used to calculate $U(XY)$.]

The foregoing results can then be appropriately substituted to produce

Uncertainty $C \mid R = [(-1.283) + (-1.511) - (-2.560)]/(-1.511) = .155$.

Uncertainty $R \mid C = (-.234)/(-1.283) = .182$.

Uncertainty (symmetric) $= (-.234)/\{[(-1.283) + (-1.511)]/2\} = .168$.

Regardless of which of the three uncertainty coefficients is used, the results in this instance are reasonably close, at values of .155 to .182.

The uncertainty coefficient is mentioned here because it regularly appears in certain computer printouts of indexes of association for $r \times c$ tables. Although higher values of the coefficient denote better "estimates," the coefficient is seldom (if ever) used in medical literature.

27.3   Trend in Bi-Ordinal Data

All the remaining indexes in this chapter are constructed with principles of covariation. This section is devoted to *bi-ordinal* trends, in which both variables have mainly untied ranks. The two main indexes are Kendall's tau and Spearman's rho.

27.3.1 Kendall's Tau

In Kendall's index of association, a score is constructed with the type of sequential placement strategy used when the Mann–Whitney U index (Section 15.4.1) was calculated from the number of ranks in one group that preceded the ranks of the other. If the two ordinal variables are perfectly related and the X variable is arrayed according to its ranks, each corresponding rank of the Y variable should be successively higher than the previous rank. Each compared pair of observations is *concordant* with this expectation if the rank of Y is higher than the rank of X, and *discordant*, if the rank of Y is lower. The relationship is expressed in an index constructed from successively counting the numbers of concordant and discordant pairs (as well as ties).

27.3.1.1 Sequential-Placement Scoring System — The sequential-placement scoring strategy warrants detailed description because it is used for seven indexes discussed in this chapter.

Suppose we have ordinal values for two variables, X and Y, in each of n members of a group. There will be $(n)(n-1)/2$ pairs of comparisons for the corresponding value of Y as we go from one ranked value of X to the next. As demonstrated by Simon,[17] each paired comparison can be cited in one of five counted groups:

P = no. of pairs concordant for X and Y (i.e., the item with the higher ranked X also has a higher ranked Y)

Q = no. of pairs discordant for X and Y (i.e., the item with the higher ranked X has a lower ranked Y)

T_x = no. of pairs for which X values are similar but Y values are different (i.e., the pairs are tied on X)

T_y = no. of pairs with similar Y values but different X values (i.e., the pairs are tied on Y)

W = no. of pairs tied on both X and Y

According to this construction, with T used for total score, $T = (n)(n-1)/2 = P + Q + T_x + T_y + W$.

These symbols will be used to construct three forms of Kendall's tau, the Goodman–Kruskal gamma coefficient, and three forms of the Somers D coefficient. The rest of this main section is devoted to Kendall's tau. The other indexes are discussed in Section 27.6.

27.3.1.2 Structure of Kendall's Tau — Kendall's tau actually has three forms. It was originally[18] proposed, without attention to ties, from the decrement

$$S = P - Q$$

In a perfect concordance of all pairs, Q will be zero, and P will be $(n-1) + (n-2) + (n-3) + ... + 1$, which is $n(n-1)/2$. Kendall's tau is the ratio between the observed score S and the potentially perfect score: $T = n(n-1)/2$. Thus,

$$\text{tau} = \frac{S}{T} = \frac{S}{n(n-1)/2} = \frac{2S}{n(n-1)} \qquad [27.2]$$

For the scoring system with two ordinal variables, the ranked X values are first aligned as $X_1, X_2, ..., X_n$. The ranks of the corresponding Y values will be $Y_1, Y_2, Y_3, ..., Y_n$. To inspect the Y_i ranks, we start with Y_1. Each time the rank of $Y_2, ..., Y_n$ exceeds the rank of Y_1, a score of 1 is added to P. Whenever the rank is below Y_1, a score of 1 is added to Q. If the two ranks are tied, the score is 0. We next go to Y_2 and repeat the scoring process for ranks $Y_3, ..., Y_n$. The procedure is then reiterated for Y_3 (comparing $Y_4, ..., Y_n$); and the iterations continue until the last one, when Y_{n-1} is compared with Y_n. At the end of the procedure, $S = P - Q$.

Formula [27.2] is called *tau-a* and rests on the assumption that no values are tied. Consequently, the formula cannot be used for contingency tables (where multiple frequencies occur at the same rank). To deal with ties, Formula [27.2] is adjusted into another formula, called *tau-b*. It is listed by Simon[17] as

$$tau\text{-}b = \frac{P - Q}{\sqrt{[T - T_x][T - T_y]}} \qquad [27.3]$$

where T, T_x, and T_y (as well as P and Q) are the counts defined in Section 27.3.1.1.

27.3.1.3   *Illustration of Calculations*

To illustrate the calculations for two ordinal variables, Table 27.2 has been arranged here from the ranks of the X and Y variables that were formerly used to show covariances in Table 19.1 of Chapter 19. The X ranks are shown in ascending order, with a tied last value for persons G and H.

TABLE 27.2

Rearrangement of Table 19.1 to Show Rank Ordering and Rank Differences

Person	Rank in Variable X	Rank in Variable Y	d_i	d_i^2
A	1	1	0	0
B	2	7	−5	25
C	3	3	0	0
D	4	6	−2	4
E	5	2	+3	9
F	6	8	−2	4
G	7.5	4	3.5	12.25
H	7.5	5	2.5	6.25
SUM	36	36	0	60.5

Note: The values of d_i and d_i^2 are used in calculating Spearman's rho, but not Kendall's tau.

The first rank in Y is 1, and each of the subsequent ranks in Y (7, 3, 6, 2, 8, 4, and 5) is higher than 1. We therefore give P a score of 7 for each of these seven correctly ordered paired comparisons—1 vs. 7, 1 vs. 3, 1 vs. 6, etc.—in which the second element of the pair ranks higher than the first. The next value in the ranks of Y (corresponding to the X-rank of 2) is 7. Comparing 7 with each of the Y ranks that follow it, we find 5 pairs (7 vs. 3, 7 vs. 6, 7 vs. 2, etc.) in which the correct order is reversed, and only one (7 vs. 8) having the correct order. Thus, P is incremented by one to become 8, and Q becomes 5. The next ranked Y value, 3, has four succeeding ranks (6, 8, 4, and 5) that are higher and one (2) that is lower. P becomes 12, and Q becomes 6. For the next Y rank, 6, three succeeding ranks (2, 4, 5) are smaller, and only one (8) is larger. P becomes 13, and Q becomes 9. For the next Y rank, 2, P is incremented by 3 to become 16. For the next Y rank, 8, Q is incremented by 2 to become 11; and for the final Y rank, 4, the P score is increased by one unit to become 17. The value of S = P − Q is 17 − 11 = 6. The value of a perfect score would be T = (8 × 7)/2 = 28.

Without any ties, the tau-a index in Formula [27.2] would be (2)(6)/(8)(7) = 0.214. Because one pair of values in X was tied (with different values of Y), Formula [27.3] produces

$$tau\text{-}b = \frac{6}{\sqrt{(28 - 1)(28)}} = .218$$

In Section 19.1.3, when the data of Table 27.2 were expressed dimensionally in Table 19.1, the conventional (or "Pearson") correlation coefficient was .186.

27.3.1.4   *Interpretations and Modifications*

Interpreted the same way as r, the bi-dimensional correlation coefficient, tau, is at a maximum of +1 when all n(n − 1)/2 ranks are concordant, and at a minimum value, −1, when they are all discordant. A value of 0 indicates no association.

If the two variables do not have equal numbers of categories, the structure of tau must be modified. The modified index, called *tau-c*, is further discussed in Section 27.6.5.

27.3.2   Spearman's Rho

In Spearman's rho, which is the oldest "non-parametric" index of trend, the ordinal ranks are regarded as dimensional values; and $d_i = X_i - Y_i$ is calculated as the discrepancy between the two sets of corresponding ranks for each point in the data. (An analogous process was used for Wilcoxon's signed-rank test.)

When appropriate results are entered into the customary "Pearson formula" for $r = S_{xy}/\sqrt{S_{xx}S_{yy}}$, the quantity Σd_i^2 will equal $S_{xx} + S_{yy} - 2S_{xy}$, so that $S_{xy} = (S_{xx} + S_{yy} - \Sigma d_i^2)/2$. Consequently, using r_S as the symbol for Spearman's rho, we would have

$$r_S = \frac{S_{xx} + S_{yy} - \Sigma d_i^2}{2\sqrt{S_{xx}S_{yy}}}$$ [27.4]

For two sets of untied ordinal ranks, the values of S_{xx} and S_{yy} will be similar, producing $S_{xx} = S_{yy} = (n^3 - n)/12$. Substituting these values of S_{xx} and S_{yy} into Formula [27.4] and carrying out the rest of the algebra, we get Spearman's rho as

$$r_S = 1 - \frac{6\Sigma d_i^2}{n^3 - n}$$ [27.5]

27.3.2.1   Illustration of Calculations — For the data in Table 27.2, $\Sigma d_i^2 = 60.5$, and n = 8. With Formula [27.5], the value of r_s will be $1 - [(6)(60.5)/(8^3 - 8)] = 1 - (363/504) = .280$, which is higher than the value found earlier for Pearson's r = .186. With Formula [27.4], $S_{xx} = S_{yy} = (n^3 - n)/12 = (8^3 - 8)/12 = 42$, which produces the same result: $r_s = (42 + 42 - 60.5)/[2\sqrt{(42)(42)}] = .280$.

The value just calculated for r_s, however, does not include a correction for tied ranks in the last two values for X. The correction factor is $T = (t^3 - t)/12$, where t = number of observations tied at a particular rank. With this correction, $S_{xx} = [(n^3 - n)/12] - \Sigma T_x$, where ΣT_x is the sum of all the T values in the X variable; and $S_{yy} = [(n^3 - n)/12] - \Sigma T_y$, where ΣT_y is the corresponding value in the Y variable. In the example here, $\Sigma T_y = 0$, but $\Sigma T_x = (2^3 - 2)/12 = 6/12 = 0.5$. Thus, S_{xx} would be corrected to $[(8^3 - 8)/12] - 0.5 = 41.5$. The recalculated, corrected value of r_s would be slightly lowered to

$$r_s = \frac{41.5 + 42 - 60.5}{2\sqrt{(41.5)(42)}} = \frac{23}{83.5} = .275$$

27.3.2.2   Choice of Kendall's Tau vs. Spearman's Rho — The choice between the Kendall and Spearman coefficients will usually depend on the professional ancestry of the person making the choice. (Kendall was a mathematical statistician; Spearman, a psychologist.) Both coefficients have their advocates[19,20] and both yield results that are usually in the "same ballpark." The Spearman coefficient regularly appears in medical literature, whereas the Kendall coefficient is rare. If you do the calculations yourself, the Spearman procedure is generally easier. A suitable computer "package" program usually produces both results, and you can then choose the one you like.

Because both coefficients are used mainly for description, they are seldom tested for stochastic significance, but appropriate procedures are available if desired.

27.3.3   Application to "Eccentric" Distributions

The two "non-parametric" rank correlation statistics are particularly valuable not for ordinal data, but for dimensional data that have eccentric distributions. Such distributions will violate the principles underlying the Pearson correlation coefficient, r, where the two variables are assumed to have a straight-line relationship, and where the stochastic interpretation assumes that the data have a bivariate Gaussian distribution. These requirements cannot be satisfied if the relationship is non-rectilinear or if the distribution is "eccentric" for either (or both) of the two variables. [An "eccentric" distribution has an asymmetrical ("skew") shape, unbalanced outliers, or any other patterns (such as two or more modes) that make the data non-Gaussian.] The non-Gaussian patterns can promptly be recognized when the univariate summary is checked separately for each variable, but detection of a nonlinear relationship will require special examinations such as those discussed in Section 19.6.2.

Because relatively few sets of bivariate data meet the strict rectilinear and bi-Gaussian "eligibility" requirements, most correlations for bi-dimensional data would probably best be expressed with the "non-parametric" Kendall or Spearman coefficients, which do not make draconian demands for the pattern of distribution. Nevertheless, because Pearson's r is believed to be "robust" (i.e., not greatly affected by violations of the eligibility criteria), it is often applied almost routinely for all bi-dimensional correlations. Because the violations may sometimes distort the results, the non-parametric coefficients may often be "significant" (quantitatively, stochastically, or both) in situations where Pearson's r was not. In the simple example in Tables 19.1 and 27.2, both the Kendall and Spearman coefficients had higher values than Pearson's r.

27.3.4   Published Examples

In clinical applications, the results of a randomized, double-blind, crossover trial[21] of acetazolamide versus placebo for the prevention of acute mountain sickness were expressed with Spearman's rho and with Wilcoxon's signed rank test, because the scores for symptoms did "not conform to normal distributions." Wilcoxon's test was used to contrast differences in the two treatments, and the r_s coefficient expressed the association between symptoms and age.

Another clinical application occurred in a trial[22] checking the effect of serum interleukin-6-level on survival in patients with septic shock. The investigators elected not to use the conventional Pearson r coefficient because the interleukin results were expressed in powers of 10. Accordingly, the Spearman r_s coefficient was applied to correlate the ranks of the two variables. The results are shown in Figure 27.2. You can decide for yourself whether the data seem to have a correlation as high as the cited "r = .51."

Other examples of the Spearman r_s coefficient appeared in medical publications where the entities being correlated were lipoprotein (a) with hemoglobin A1c in diabetes mellitus,[23] collateral blood flow with cardiac wall motion score in recent myocardial infarction,[24] mean faculty income at university hospitals vs. percent of women in each subspecialty fellowship,[25] and ordinal ratings of "experiences from an imaginary cardiovascular clinical trial."[26]

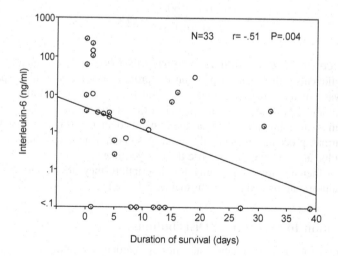

FIGURE 27.2

Correlation between the serum concentrations of IL-6 (ng/mL) measured at study entry and the duration of survival (days) in 33 nonsurvivors (Spearman rank correlation coefficient). [Figure and legend taken from Chapter Reference 22.]

27.3.5 Concerns about "Reduced Efficiency"

When non-parametric analyses were first proposed for dimensional data, many statisticians were worried about a descriptive "loss of information" (as noted in Section 15.9.1). A more substantial concern, however, was the stochastic fear that non-parametric procedures, such as the Wilcoxon–Mann–Whitney U test, were less powerful than the counterpart parametric procedures, such as the t test. The concept was checked with ratios of "power efficiency" or "asymptomatic relative efficiency" that were calculated from the sample sizes needed to give the tests the same "power" when the same null hypothesis and same alternative hypothesis were evaluated at the same level of α. As discussed earlier (Section 23.5), if test A requires n_A persons and if test B requires n_B persons to have the same power, and if n_B is larger than n_A, the reduced "power-efficiency" of test B is calculated as n_A/n_B. With this type of calculation, the relative power-efficiency of non-parametric tests was found to range from about .64 to .96 when compared with the corresponding parametric procedures.

These comparisons, however, were done under conditions that are optimal for the parametric tests, but not when eccentric distributions might handicap the parametric performance. Accordingly, the alleged superiority of the parametric tests may be due to unfair comparisons. Perhaps the best approach is to use a parametric test if it seems appropriate, but don't let the false specter of "reduced efficiency" keep you from using a non-parametric test if it does what you want or need it to do.

27.4 Trend in r × 2 Tables

Beyond the expressions of trend in bi-ordinal data, probably the most common and useful additional indexes are those that express trend in r × 2 tables. Such tables have two columns for a binary variable, which can also be cited as a proportion, and more than two rows for *r* polytomous categories of a variable that can be nominal or ordinal. (The table can also appear in a counterpart 2 × c arrangement, for 2 rows and *c* columns. Everything to be discussed here for the r × 2 format will also pertain to the alternative arrangement.)

27.4.1 General Association

To illustrate the arrangement, the r × 2 format of Table 27.3 has a row variable with A, B, and C as three polytomous categories. The column variable is a binary outcome event, such as survival. The data are easier to understand and interpret when the two-column frequency counts are rearranged and shown as proportions in Table 27.4.

TABLE 27.3

Results in a 3 × 2 Table

| Category | 5-Year Survival | | Total |
	Alive	Dead	
A	24	44	68
B	43	2	45
C	76	15	91
Total	143	61	204

TABLE 27.4

Alternative Arrangement of Table 27.3

Category	5-Year Survival Rate
A	24/68 (35%)
B	43/45 (96%)
C	76/91 (84%)
Total	143/204 (70%)

Three general indexes — lambda, ϕ^2, and ϕ — can be used to express association in any r × 2 table, regardless of whether the row categories are nominal or ordinal.

27.4.1.1 *Lambda Index of Error Reduction* — The lambda index discussed in Section 27.2.1 is a simple expression for the statistical "accomplishment" of the categories in Table 27.4. From only the "Y variable" totals, with survival rate 70%, everyone would be estimated as **alive**. The estimates would be correct in 143 instances, and wrong in 61. When the X variable is used, everyone in Category

A, with a 35% survival rate, would be estimated as **dead**. The estimates would be correct in 44 persons and wrong in 24. In categories B and C, where survival rates are 96% and 84%, everyone would be estimated as **alive**. These estimates would have 2 errors in **B** and 15 errors in **C**. The total number of errors in the three groups would be $24 + 2 + 15 = 41$.

The lambda value for proportionate reduction in errors will be

$$\text{lambda} = \frac{\text{errors for total} - \text{errors for categories}}{\text{errors for total}} \qquad [27.6]$$

which is $(61 - 41)/61 = .33$ in this instance.

27.4.1.2 ϕ^2 *for Variance Reduction* — From the customary X^2 used in the chi-square test, ϕ^2 can be calculated as X^2/N to form a descriptive index that expresses proportion of group variance reduction in an $r \times 2$ table. The mathematical justification is as follows:

Each row in the table has n_i members, of whom t_i have the target binary event, such as **alive**. The proportion in that row will be $P_i = t_i/n_i$. For the total table, $T = \Sigma t_i$, $N = \Sigma n_i$, and $P = T/N$, with $Q = 1 - P$. The original group variance, before any division into categories, is NPQ; and the group variance in each row category is $n_i p_i q_i$. The proportionate reduction in variance achieved by dividing the total group into categories will be

$$\phi^2 = \frac{NPQ - \Sigma(n_i p_i q_i)}{NPQ} \qquad [27.7]$$

After suitable substitution and carrying out the algebra, the reduction in group variance, $NPQ - \Sigma(n_i p_i q_i)$, will become

$$\Sigma(t_i^2/n_i) - T^2/N \qquad [27.8]$$

and a simple computational formula for the proportionate reduction in variance will be

$$\phi^2 = [\Sigma(t_i^2/n_i) - (T^2/N)]\{N/[T(N - T)]\} \qquad [27.9]$$

For example, in Table 27.4, $NPQ = (204)(143/204)(61/204) = 42.76$; $\Sigma n_i p_i q_i = [(24)(44)/68] + [(43)(2)/45] + [(76)(15)/91] = 29.97$; and $NPQ - \Sigma n_i p_i q_i = 42.76 - 29.97 = 12.79$. With Formula [27.8], we get $(24^2/68) + (43^2/45) + (76^2/91) - (143^2/204) = 113.03 - 100.24 = 12.79$. The value of ϕ^2 will be $12.79/42.76 = .299$ with Formula [27.7] or $12.79\{204/[(143)(61)]\} = .299$ with Formula [27.9].

These results for ϕ^2 and the preceding lambda indicate that when the total survival rate of 143/204 (70%) is divided into the three categories shown in Table 27.4, the proportionate reductions are 33% in error rate, and 30% (i.e., $\phi^2 = .299$) in group variance.

Because $X^2 = N\phi^2$, Formula [27.9], when multiplied by N, becomes exactly the same calculation of X^2 that was shown earlier for a 2×2 table with Formula [14.5]. The extension of the X^2 formula to an $r \times 2$ table is

$$X^2 = [\Sigma(t_i^2/n_i) - (T^2/N)]\{N^2/[T(N - T)]\} \qquad [27.10]$$

Formula [27.10] is particularly convenient because it avoids having to determine all the "expected" values for calculations using $\Sigma(0 - E)^2/E$. It also avoids the $n_i p_i q_i$ calculations of Formula [27.7]. With Formula [27.10], X^2 (without Yates correction) can be promptly found for any $r \times 2$ table and used as a stochastic index, interpreted with $(r - 1)(c - 1) = (r - 1)(2 - 1) = r - 1$ degrees of freedom. In

Table 27.4, where we already know that $\phi^2 = .299$, multiplication by N = 204 will produce X^2, which will have the very high value of (204)(.299) = 61, for which 2P is <.0001 at 2 d.f. If calculated first, the X^2 value in the r × 2 table can be divided by N to get ϕ^2 as a descriptive index of association, representing the proportion of reduced variance.

27.4.1.3 ϕ for Correlation — The square root of ϕ^2 yields ϕ as the counterpart of a correlation coefficient. For Table 27.4, $\phi = \sqrt{.299} = .55$.

ϕ can be justified as a correlation coefficient if you work out the algebra for the corresponding values of S_{xy}, S_{xx}, and S_{yy} in a 2 × 2 table for which the X and Y variables are each coded as 0/1. When the correlation coefficient is calculated as $S_{xy}/\sqrt{S_{xx}S_{yy}}$, the result turns out to be $\phi = \sqrt{X^2/N}$.

The ϕ index is seldom used descriptively, because a correlation coefficient intuitively seems to be a peculiar way of summarizing the results being contrasted in an r × 2 or 2 × 2 table. For larger r × c tables, however, ϕ may sometimes have the useful "screening" function described later in Section 27.8.1.

27.4.2 Problems in General Trend

Table 27.5 shows another 3 × 2 table, but the row variable contains a specifically ordinal array — **mild, moderate, severe** — rather than the unranked categories of Table 27.4. If the conventional X^2, ϕ^2, and lambda values were calculated, the results in Table 27.5 would be exactly the same as in Table 27.4. In fact, the same ϕ^2, X^2, and lambda values would also be produced for Table 27.6, where the ordinal array sequentially has exactly the same proportions as in Table 27.4.

Despite obvious differences in the results of Tables 27.5 and 27.6, the ϕ^2, X^2, and lambda values are similar because the conventional mathematical strategy and calculational formulas for the association make no provision for the *order* of the categories. The values of $\Sigma t_i^2/n_i$ in Formulas [27.8] and [27.9], $\Sigma n_i p_i q_i$ in Formula [27.7], ϕ^2 in Formula [27.9], and X^2 in Formula [27.10] remain the same regardless of whether the rows contain nominal or ordinal categories.

TABLE 27.5

Ordinal Array in a 3 × 2 Table

Severity of Clinical Condition	5-Year Survival Rate
Mild	43/45 (96%)
Moderate	76/91 (84%)
Severe	24/68 (35%)
Total	143/204 (70%)

TABLE 27.6

Another 3 × 2 Ordinal-Array Table

Severity of Clinical Condition	5-Year Survival Rate
Mild	24/68 (35%)
Moderate	43/45 (96%)
Severe	76/91 (84%)
Total	143/204 (70%)

27.4.2.1 Inadequate Descriptive Message — Nevertheless, despite the similarities in ϕ^2, X^2, and lambda, Tables 27.5 and 27.6 contain a dramatically different descriptive message. In Table 27.5, the survival rates would be expected to show their downward monotonic gradient as the categories progressively descend from the "better" to "worse" clinical conditions. In Table 27.6, however, the gradient is biologically absurd. The best survival results occurred in the **moderate** group, and patients with **severe** disease had a survival rate more than twice that of the **mild** disease group. On scientific grounds alone, these results would be rejected as bizarre. Something has gone drastically wrong in the concepts or in the data, or perhaps in the statistical index of expression.

27.4.2.2 Monotonic Gradient — The scientific message in Tables 27.5 and 27.6 was communicated from the gradient in survival rates as the ordinal categories went from **mild** to **severe**. Because the ordinal categories monotonically increase in severity and because severity of clinical condition affects survival, we would expect the survival rates to show a corresponding monotonic gradient, going pro-gressively downward.

For nominal categories, a "trend" cannot really be expected, because the categories have no ranks. Thus, if the A, B, and C categories in Table 27.4 represented different treatments or diseases, we could compare results in pairs of categories (such as A vs. B, B vs. C, or A vs. C), but a distinctive trend could not be cited. If we wanted a single descriptive index for the result in the nominal categories, it would have to be the association shown with lambda, ϕ^2, or ϕ.

With a monotonic array of ordinal categories, however, a corresponding upward (or downward) trend can be anticipated and checked. The statistical gradients can be noted from simple subtraction of the (survival) proportions in adjacent categories. In Table 27.5, the monotonic descent of gradients is indicated by the two negative values: $p_2 - p_1 = -12\% = -.12$ and $p_3 - p_2 = -.49$. Thus, the results "made sense" in Table 27.5 because it showed the expected gradient in survival. In Table 27.6, where $p_2 - p_1$ is +.61 and $p_3 - p_2 = -.12$, the results were "absurd" because the gradient had a peculiar reversal of positive and negative values.

Examining gradients in subtracted proportions is an excellent way to "screen" the data, but can be hazardous if some of the categories have small numbers that make the proportions unstable. What we would like, therefore, is a better statistical mechanism to express the gradient for an ordinal array of proportions.

27.5 Linear Trend in an r × 2 Ordinal Array

The overall gradient in proportions of an r × 2 ordinal array can be determined with a common, simple statistical approach: fitting a straight line to the data.

27.5.1 Developing a Linear Model

If appropriate dimensional coding digits are assigned to the ordinal grades, we can construct a linear regression model for the data. Despite the apparent mathematical impropriety, the procedure is prag-matically effective. The index of slope will quantitatively describe the rectilinear trend, which can then be evaluated stochastically.

The binary data, coded as **0/1**, become the Y variable in the linear regression model; and the ordinal categories become the X variable, coded with arbitrary weights, w_i. The arrangement is shown in Table 27.7. The w_i codes in this table are assigned to have equal intervals, consistent with dimensional data. The simplest approach is to code the ordinal categories in 1-unit intervals (such as **1, 2, 3, 4, ...** or **0, 1, 2, 3, ...**), and then do a conventional linear regression — with an appropriate computer program — against the **0/1** data of the Y variable.

TABLE 27.7

Arrangement and Symbols for Assigning Coded Weights in an r × 2 Ordinal Array

	Categories and Members						Totals
Identity of Ordinal Category (X variable)	1	2	3	...	i	...	
Coded Weights for X variable	w_1	w_2	w_3	...	w_i	...	
Number of Members for X-Variable Category	n_1	n_2	n_3	...	n_i	...	$N = \Sigma n_i$
Number with Codes of 1 in Y Variable	t_1	t_2	t_3	...	t_i	...	$T = \Sigma t_i$
Number with Codes of 0 in Y Variable	$n_1 - t_1$	$n_2 - t_2$	$n_3 - t_3$	...	$n_i - t_i$	...	$N - T$

27.5.2 Regression Components

For the regression analysis, the value of X_i at each category will be $n_i(w_i)$; and the mean $\overline{X}$ will be $\Sigma n_i w_i/N$. The value that corresponds to S_{xx} will be

$$\Sigma X_i^2 - N\overline{X}^2 = \Sigma n_i(w_i)^2 - N(\Sigma n_i w_i/N)^2$$

which becomes

$$S_{xx} = [N\Sigma n_i w_i^2 - (\Sigma n_i w_i)^2]/N \qquad [27.11]$$

If we let $\overline{W} = \Sigma n_i w_i/N$, Formula [27.11] can be algebraically simplified to

$$S_{xx} = \Sigma n_i w_i^2 - N\overline{W}^2 \qquad [27.12]$$

For each of the X categories, the corresponding value of Y_i will be $t_i(1) + (n_i - t_i)0 = t_i$; and for the total, $\overline{Y}$ will be $\Sigma t_i/N = T/N$. For the regression analysis, the total system variance, S_T (which corresponds to S_{yy} in ordinary regression), will be $\Sigma(Y_i - \overline{Y})^2 = \Sigma[t_1(1 - \overline{Y})^2 + (n_i - t_i)(0 - \overline{Y})^2]$, which is algebraically developed to become

$$S_T = T(N - T)/N = NPQ \qquad [27.13]$$

At each category, the value of X_iY_i will be $w_i t_i(1) + w_i(n_i - t_i)(0) = w_i t_i$. Thus, for $S_{xy} = \Sigma X_i Y_i - N\overline{X}\overline{Y}$, the result will be $\Sigma w_i t_i - [N(\Sigma n_i w_i/N)(T/N)]$, and so

$$S_{xy} = N\Sigma w_i t_i - T\Sigma n_i w_i/N \qquad [27.14]$$

Substituting $N\overline{W}$ for $\Sigma n_i w_i$, Formula [27.14] can be algebraically simplified to

$$S_{xy} = \Sigma w_i t_i - T\overline{W} \qquad [27.15]$$

27.5.3 Slope of "Trend"

With these regression concepts and symbols, the categorical data can be fitted with a straight line, and the slope of the line will indicate the average trend in the array of proportions. Using $b = S_{xy}/S_{xx}$ for the slope of the regression line, the values of N will cancel in the two denominators of [27.14] and [27.11], and the algebraic calculation will become

$$\text{Slope} = b = \frac{N\Sigma w_i t_i - T\Sigma n_i w_i}{N\Sigma n_i w_i^2 - (\Sigma n_i w_i)^2} \qquad [27.16]$$

Using the simplifications of Formulas [27.12] and [27.15], the formula for slope would become

$$b = \Sigma w_i t_i - T\overline{W}/(\Sigma n_i w_i^2 - N\overline{W}^2) \qquad [27.17]$$

27.5.3.1 Illustration for Two Categories — To illustrate the calculation, suppose we compare just two proportions t_1/n_1 vs. t_2/n_2, and suppose (for this example) we let $w_1 = 0$ and $w_2 = 1$. The components of Formula [27.16] become $N\Sigma w_i t_i = Nt_2$; $T\Sigma n_i w_i = Tn_2$; $N\Sigma n_i w_i^2 = Nn_2$; and $(\Sigma n_i w_i)^2 = n_2^2$. When all the algebra is then carried out, these components for Formula [27.16] produce $b = p_2 - p_1$. Thus, with two X categories coded as **0/1**, the slope is simply the increment in proportions, $p_2 - p_1$.

If the codes had been $w_1 = -1$ and $w_2 = +1$, the numerator of [27.16] would be $N(-t_1 + t_2) - T(-n_1 + n_2)$, which becomes $2(n_1 t_2 - n_2 t_1)$, which is twice the previous value. The denominator would be $N(n_1 + n_2) - (n_2 - n_1)^2 = 4n_1 n_2$. The slope would be $2(n_1 t_2 - n_2 t_1)/4n_1 n_2$ which reduces to $(p_2 - p_1)/2$, which is half the previous value. The halving would be expected since the $-1/+1$ coding made the slope span 2 units in the X-variable, rather than 1.

27.5.3.2   *Standardized Slope in 2 × 2 Table* — The standardized slope for a 2×2 table would be the correlation coefficient, r, which is bs_x/s_y, or $b\sqrt{S_{xx}/S_{yy}}$. With the 0,1 coding for w_1 and w_2, the value of S_{xx} in Formula [27.11] becomes $[Nn_2 - (n_1)^2]/N$, which is n_1n_2/N. The value that corresponds to S_{yy} in Formula [27.13] is $T(N - T)/N$, which becomes NPQ. Thus, with the formula $b\sqrt{S_{xx}/S_{yy}}$, the value of r can be expressed as

$$ r = (p_1 - p_2)\sqrt{\frac{n_1 n_2}{N} / NPQ} $$

which becomes $(p_1 - p_2)\sqrt{(1/N)}\sqrt{n_1 n_2/PQ}$. This value is the same as $1/\sqrt{N}$ times the Z statistic shown earlier in Formula [13.16]. Because $Z^2 = X^2$ in a 2×2 table, r becomes $(1/\sqrt{N})Z$ and $r^2 = Z^2/N = X^2/N = \phi^2$. Thus, in a 2×2 table, the values of r and ϕ are identical. (The similarity is seldom true for larger tables.)

27.5.3.3   *Illustration for Three Ordinal Categories* — For the three ordinal categories inspected in Tables 27.4 through 27.6, the simplest codes (for "hand" electronic calculation) would be $w_1 = -1$, $w_2 = 0$, and $w_3 = +1$. With these codes, Formula [27.16] becomes

$$ \text{Slope} = \frac{N(t_3 - t_1) - T(n_3 - n_1)}{N(n_3 + n_1) - (n_3 - n_1)^2} \qquad [27.18] $$

For Table 27.5, the numerator of [27.18] will be $204(24 - 43) - 143(68 - 45) = 204(-19) - 143(23) = -7165$. The denominator of [27.18] will be $204(45 + 68) (68 - 45)^2 = 204(113) - (23)^2 = 22523$. The slope will be $-7165/22523 = -.32$.

Note that this slope is just what would have been expected from a judgmental evaluation of Table 27.5. Because the gradient drops 12% (= 96% − 84%) from the first to the second category, and then drops 49% (= 84% − 35%), the "average" drop would be $-(12\% + 49\%)/2 = -30.5\%$ or $-.305$, which is consistent with the linear calculation of $-.32$. Because the trend is monotonic, another judgmental approach could have been used to determine the total gradient as 96% − 35% = 61%, going downward from the first to third categories. Because the drop of 61% is spread over two zones of change, the "average" gradient would be $-61\%/2 = -.305$.

For Table 27.6, however, judgmental examination would argue against calculating an average gradient. The gradient rises by 61% (= 96% − 35%) from the first to second category, but then falls by 12% (= 84% − 96%) from the second category to the third. With this reversal in trend, a single expression of directional gradient would be misleading. Nevertheless, if such an expression is desired, the judgmental "average" rise over the two categorical intervals would be $.49/2 = .245$. When the statistical "average" for these data is calculated with Formula [27.16], the numerator is $[204(76 - 24)] - [143(91 - 68)] = 7319$. The denominator is $[204(91 + 68)] - [(91 - 68)^2] = 31907$. The slope would be $7319/31907 = .23$, which is close to the judgmentally approximated value of $.245$.

To get standardized slopes for the three categories, we need to determine $r = b\sqrt{S_{xx}/S_{yy}}$. The value that corresponds to S_{yy} is $NPQ = T(N-T)/N$, which is $(143)(204 - 143)/204 = 42.76$ in both tables. The value of S_{xx} is $1/N$ times the denominator of Equation [27.16]. It was 22523 for Table 27.5 and 31907 for Table 27.6. Thus, for Table 27.5,

$$ r = (.32)\sqrt{22523/[(204)(42.76)]} = .51 $$

and for Table 27.6,

$$ r = (.23)\sqrt{31907/[(204)(42.76)]} = .44 $$

27.5.4   Precautions and Caveats

The linear trends calculated for Tables 27.5 and 27.6 should serve as an important warning whenever ranked data — expressed in either ordinal or dimensional values — are fitted with a straight-line regression model. The mathematical model will fit an average constant rectilinear slope to the data, regardless of whether the data do or do not have the constant monotonic trend denoted by the slope. Because the value of the constant slope may be used for conclusions such as "You live 2 years longer for every 5-point drop in Substance X," the conclusion can be misleading or grossly distorted if the data do not conform to the linear model.

For example, in Table 27.5, the slope of −.32 would denote an average drop of 32% in survival from one category to the next. This result would be misleading because the gradient is not constant. It drops 12% from the first to second category, and then drops 49% from the second to the third. In Table 27.6, the slope of .23 denotes a constant rise of 23% from one category to the next. This result is a gross distortion of the sharp rise followed by a fall in gradient for the actual data. In both instances, the statistically calculated slopes are correct as "average" values, but wrong in different zones of the data. Similarly, the standardized slopes of .51 and .44 in the two tables seem moderately impressive, although the impression is not strictly accurate in Table 27.5 and egregiously misleading in Table 27.6.

The point to remember is that fitting a linear slope is an excellent "screening" mechanism, but it cannot replace a direct examination of the data, and it should not be used for final conclusions until confirmation that the data actually conform to the linear mathematical pattern.

27.5.5 X_L^2 Test of Linear Trend

The descriptive index for trend in the linear slope is regularly checked stochastically with a chi-square test for linear trend. In the conventional simple regression discussed in Chapter 19, the stochastic procedure was a t test on either b or the correlation coefficient, r. For an ordinal $r \times 2$ table, the stochastic approach is more complex because it involves using a partition of X^2.

27.5.5.1   *Strategy for X^2 Partition* — The X^2 partition is derived from the principles of partitioning variance that were introduced in Section 19.2.1.2.

The diverse concepts and symbols are shown in Table 27.8. In the ordinary arrangement that is used for chi-square, a group of binary data, $\{Y_i\}$, having N members with mean (or summary proportion) $\overline{Y} = P$, is divided into k categories, each having p_i as its mean. The total system variance, $S_T = NPQ$, becomes partitioned as a sum of the within-category group variance, S_W, and the between-category group variance, S_B. The latter value is the numerator of the ordinary chi-square test, when X^2 is formed as $S_B/PQ = (NPQ - \Sigma n_i p_i q_i)/PQ$.

When a regression model is imposed on the same set of data, the group variance becomes partitioned into $S_T = S_r + S_M$. (The latter value is used for the calculation of r^2 as S_M/S_T.) The linear accomplishment of the model can be stochastically examined in two ways. In the first way, S_M represents the effect of a linear model for the entire set of unpartitioned data. This procedure, as discussed in Chapter 19, uses a t test on the correlation coefficient r. In the second way, the goal is to check what the linear model does for the categorical partition of data. For the latter examination, the group variance between categories, S_B, is divided, as noted by Armitage and Berry,[27] into

$$\Sigma(\overline{Y}_i - \overline{Y})^2 = \Sigma(\overline{Y}_i - \hat{Y}_i)^2 + \Sigma(\hat{Y}_i - \overline{Y})^2 \qquad [27.19]$$

In the symbols of Table 27.8, the foregoing expression is

$$S_B = S_U + S_M$$

When all terms in this expression are divided by PQ, the result is a partitioning of X^2 as

$$X^2 = X_R^2 + X_L^2 \qquad [27.20]$$

TABLE 27.8

Arrangement of Deviations and Group Variances in Tests of Ordinary X^2 and X_L^2 for Linear Trend

Symbols:	Y_j = any observed value in the data
	Y_i = any observed value in a category
	$\bar{Y}_i$ = mean, i.e., summary proportion p_i, for a category
	$\bar{Y}$ = overall mean, i.e., summary proportion P, for the data
	n_i = number of members in category
	N = total number in data
	Q = 1 − P
	$q_i = 1 - p_i$

Deviation	Group Variance for This Deviation	Name and Symbol for the Group Variance	Algebraic Formula for the Group Variance
$Y_j - \bar{Y}$	$\Sigma(Y_j - \bar{Y})^2$	S_T = total system variance	NPQ
$Y_i - \bar{Y}_i$	$\Sigma(Y_i - \bar{Y}_i)^2$	S_W = variance within categories	$\Sigma n_i p_i q_i$
$\bar{Y}_i - \bar{Y}$	$\Sigma(\bar{Y}_i - \bar{Y})^2$	S_B = variance between categories	$NPQ - \Sigma n_i p_i q_i$
$Y_i - \hat{Y}_i$	$\Sigma(Y_i - \hat{Y}_i)^2$	S_r = "regression residual" = residual variance of individual values around regression line at category	$(1 - r^2)NPQ$
$\hat{Y}_i - \bar{Y}$	$\Sigma(\hat{Y}_i - \bar{Y})^2$	S_M = "linear residuals" = model variance between estimates for regression categories and for overall mean	$r^2(NPQ)$
$\bar{Y}_i - \hat{Y}_i$	$\Sigma(\bar{Y}_i - \hat{Y}_i)^2$	$S_U = S_B - S_M$ = "nonlinear residuals" = variance between category mean and regression estimate	$NPQ - \Sigma n_i p_i q_i - r^2(NPQ)$ $= (1 - r^2)(NPQ) - \Sigma n_i p_i q_i$

In Equation [27.20], the X_L^2 component, derived from S_M, represents the linearity of the model's fit, and the X_R^2 component represents nonlinearity in the residual categories. The degrees of freedom for interpreting the partitioned chi-square values in results for the k categories are k −1 for X^2, 1 for X_L^2, and k − 2 for X_R^2.

27.5.5.2 Illustration of Calculations — If you do the calculations yourself, the easiest approach is to note that X_L^2 is determined as S_M/PQ, and that S_M was established when a regression line was fitted to the data in Sections 27.5.1 and 27.5.2. From Chapter 19, we can recall that $S_M = (r^2)$(total system variance) $= r^2(NPQ) = bS_{xy}$. We can then recognize that both b and S_{xy} have already been found. The value of b is the slope previously obtained in [27.16] (or for a three-category coding in [27.18]); and the value of NS_{xy}, as noted in [27.14], is the numerator in the formulas for b. The value of X_L^2 can then be calculated as

$$X_L^2 = bS_{xy}/PQ \qquad [27.21]$$

For example, in Tables 27.5 and 27.6, NPQ = (143)(61)/204 = 42.76. For Table 27.5, the slope was calculated as −7165/22523, which will be the value of b in Formula [27.21]. From the numerator of the previous slope calculation, we get NS_{xy} = 7165, and so S_{xy} = 7165/204. Since NPQ = 42.76, PQ = 42.76/204. The value of S_{xy}/PQ will be 7165/42.76 = 167.56. The value of X_L^2 in Formula [27.21] will be (7165)(167.56)/(22523) = 53.3. For Table 27.6, the slope was calculated as 7319/31907. Substituting NS_{xy}/NPQ for S_{xy}/PQ, the corresponding value of X_L^2 will be (7319)(7319)/(31907)(42.76) = 39.3. At 1 d.f., both these values of X_L^2 are "highly significant" with 2P < .001. The "high significance" found for the linear trend in X_L^2 values for *both* of these two tables should serve to warn against drawing conclusions by inspecting P values alone.

27.5.5.3 Relationship of r^2 and X_L^2 — An even simpler approach is to realize that $X_L^2 = S_M/PQ$ and that when a regression line is fitted to the data, $S_M = r^2(NPQ)$. Therefore,

$$X_L^2 = r^2N \qquad [27.22]$$

A linear regression computer program applied to the original results will produce a value of r^2, from which X_L^2 can promptly be found after multiplication by N.

Conversely, if a calculation has produced X_L^2, but not the value of r^2, it can be easily found as

$$r^2 = X_L^2/N \qquad [27.23]$$

Thus, $r^2 = 53.3/204 = .26$ and $r = .51$ for Table 27.5, whereas $r^2 = 39.9/204 = .19$ and $r = .44$ for Table 27.6. Table 27.6 thus continues to show a modestly high linear correlation coefficient despite the reversed gradient in the last category.

The main point conceptually is that X^2 reflects the variation that is "explained" by imposing categories on the total data, and X_L^2 reflects the further "explanation" produced when a linear trend is imposed on the categories. Because $\phi^2 = X^2/N$ and $r^2 = X_L^2/N$, the relationship can be expressed as $X_L^2/X^2 = r^2/\phi^2$. In a 2 × 2 table, as noted in Section 27.5.3.2, the difference in the two proportions $(p_1 - p_2)$ always forms a straight line, and so $\phi^2 = r^2$. Because the total system variance is NPQ and the variance within the categories is $\Sigma n_i p_i q_i$, the value of NPQ − $\Sigma n_i p_i q_i$ becomes the numerator of X^2, which can be expressed as $\Sigma(\overline{Y}_i - \overline{Y})^2$, as shown in Table 27.8. The latter value becomes partitioned into the non-linear and linear components shown in Equation [27.19]. The reason for the easy calculation of r^2 is that the S_M term is used for both the ordinary linear regression partition of variance and the subsequent partition of chi-square.

27.5.5.4 *Check of Residual Nonlinear Variance* (X_R^2) — With the ordinal linear regression arrangement, we can check the residual variance of the p_i category values around the regression line to see whether a stochastically "significant" amount of "nonlinear variance" still remains. For this purpose, the value of X_L^2 is subtracted from X^2, and the result is interpreted (using k for the number of categories) with k − 2 degrees of freedom. Thus, $X_R^2 = X^2 - X_L^2 = 61.0 - 53.3 = 7.7$ at 2 d.f. for Table 27.5, and the corresponding value is $61.0 - 39.3 = 21.7$ for Table 27.6. Both of these values are highly stochastically significant, indicating that a great deal of variance has *not* been explained by imposition of the linear model alone. The particularly high value of X_R^2 for Table 27.6 could serve as warning of linear inadequacy in that table.

27.5.6 Applications of Linear Trend Test

The linear trend in a set of ordinal proportions can serve as an alternative to the Wilcoxon–Mann–Whitney U test. It can be used to appraise ordinal staging systems, to demonstrate "significance" for ordinal partitions, or to screen for a "double gradient" before the conjunctive consolidation procedure of targeted multivariable analyses.[15]

27.5.6.1 *Alternative to Wilcoxon–Mann–Whitney U Test* — A two-group rank test, such as the Wilcoxon–Mann–Whitney U procedure, is customarily done for a 2 × c structure, such as the earlier data in Table 15.5. Such data can also be regarded, however, as an r × 2 structure, and then evaluated for linear trend.

For example, the data in Table 15.5 could be rearranged as follows:

Category of Improvement	Proportion in Placebo Group
Worse	8/10 (80%)
No change	9/17 (53%)
Improved	19/48 (40%)
Much improved	10/29 (34%)
TOTAL	46/104 (44%)

The average crude gradient of decline in the binary proportions is (80% − 34%)/3 = 15.33%. With a more formal calculation, assigning codes of **1, 2, 3, 4** to the ordinal categories, and using Formula

[27.17], the slope of the gradient is $\{104[(1 \times 8) + (2 \times 9) + (3 \times 19) + (4 \times 10)] - 46[(10 \times 1) + (17 \times 2) + (48 \times 3) + (29 \times 4)]\}/\{104[(10 \times 1) + (17 \times 4) + (48 \times 9) + (29 \times 16)] - [(10 \times 1) + (17 \times 2) + (48 \times 3) + (29 \times 4)]^2\} = (12792 - 13984)/(101296 - 92416) = -1192/8880 = -.134$. The precise linear trend, showing a decline of 13.4% per category, is similar to the crude gradient of 15.3%. This is a quantitatively impressive trend, and it is also stochastically significant, as shown in Section 27.5.6.2.

The main problem with the foregoing arrangement is that it transposes the basic variables, so that the outcome category (improvement) becomes regarded as though it were the "independent" variable, and the preceding binary treatment becomes the "dependent" variable. Despite the transposed variables, however, the quantitative evaluation of trend is easy to understand and has been vigorously preferred[28,29] over the customary statistical method[30] (discussed in Chapter 15) for analyzing ordinal data.

27.5.6.2   Comparison of X^2 vs. X_L^2

Comparison of X^2 vs. X_L^2 — The distinction between X^2, for any array of categorical data, vs. X_L^2, for an ordinal array, should be kept in mind when stochastic tests are done for an $r \times 2$ table. For example, the linear trend in proportions was used in Section 27.5.6.1 to provide a *descriptive* summary of the ordinal gradings in Table 15.5. When this result is tested stochastically, the Wilcoxon–Mann–Whitney U procedure takes account of the ordinal arrangement, but an ordinary X^2 test does not. Thus, the X_L^2 test should be used if stochastic significance is to be appraised for Table 15.5. In those results, the overall X^2 is 7.247, which has $2P = .06$ at 3 degrees of freedom. The linear regression of the data, however, shows $r^2 = .0600$ and $X_L^2 = Nr^2 = (104)(.0600) = 6.24$, which has $2P < .025$ at 1 degree of freedom. This result is more consistent with the Wilcoxon–Mann–Whitney test for the same data in Section 15.5.4, where Z was -2.25, for which $2P = .024$.

27.5.6.3   Appraisal of Ordinal Staging Systems

Appraisal of Ordinal Staging Systems — With increasing attention being given to factors that affect etiologic "risk" for disease or prognostic outcome of disease, individual variables or groups of variables are regularly arranged into the ordinal categories of a "risk stratification" or prognostic "staging" system, such as Table 27.5. When several contender candidate variables are available, the linear trend of the gradient in the outcome event can be examined to help choose a "best" candidate.

27.5.6.4   "Significance" for Ordinal Partitions

"Significance" for Ordinal Partitions — The categorical variables used in a prognostic staging system can be constructed from an ordinal partition of dimensional data (such as dividing age into categories of **<20, 21–49, 50–69,** and **70+**) or from an ordinal array (such as TNM stages **I, II, III, …**). After the variable has been constructed, stochastic significance may not always occur in results for *adjacent* categories, even though the gradient shows a distinct linear trend. Rather than compressing the categories to form larger numbers of members in a small number of groups, the analyst may be content to let the original partition remain if it shows stochastic significance in the X_L^2 test for linear trend.

27.5.6.5   Screening for "Double Gradients"

Screening for "Double Gradients" — The conjunctive-consolidation procedure[14,15] offers an easily understood multivariable-analytic method to construct prognostic staging systems. The method begins by screening for impressive "double gradients" in both the rows and columns of each conjunctive $2 \times r \times c$ table that becomes "consolidated." An inspection of linear trend in the outcome rates for cells in the r rows and c columns is a useful way to do the screening.

27.5.7   Additional Approaches

Throughout the foregoing discussion, survival was examined as the "response" to a change in the ordinal category of severity. This type of "dose-response" phenomenon frequently occurs in clinical and epidemiologic literature. The ordinal "dose" can often be levels of a pharmaceutical agent or a risk factor.

Problems can arise if the ordinal categories do not ascend in equi-interval dimensions that justify a linear coding, and if the responses do not show a linear relationship. Various alternative approaches,[31–33] including spline regression, have been proposed for dealing with these problems. Nevertheless, the linear-trend method has the advantage of being a useful "screening" procedure that is relatively simple and easy to understand (despite the length of the previous discussion).

27.6 Indexes of Ordinal Contingency

In addition to *tau-b*, other indexes for analyzing trend in the graded categories of two-way ordinal contingency tables are called *gamma*, *Somers D*, and *tau-c*. These indexes all use the basic sequential-placement scoring system described in Section 27.3.1.1 for the co-related pattern of ranks.

27.6.1 Scores for Co-Relationship of Tabular Grades

The scoring system discussed in Section 27.3.1.1 for ordinal co-relationships is not too difficult to understand, but can be tricky to apply for tabular grades. To illustrate the basic strategy, suppose we have a 3×3 ordinal contingency table, with cells designated as *a*, *b*, ... , *h*, *i* as shown in Table 27.9, which is oriented so that the X variable advances downward in the rows and the Y variable goes rightward in the columns.

The cells are compared and scored as we advance through the table, going across each row, down to the next row, and then across that row. The ranks for each pair of cells will be either tied, concordant, or discordant. Any two cells in the same row have tied ranks on the row variable, and any two cells in the same column are tied on the column variable. Between any two cells, the trend is *concordant* if the second cell has higher ranks in *both* the row and column variable. The trend is *discordant* if the second cell has a *lower* rank in the column variable while having a *higher* rank in the row variable, or vice versa.

Each score for concordances (marked P) and discordances (marked Q), and for ties, is the product of frequency counts in the two compared cells. The pattern of scoring for Table 27.9 is shown in Figure 27.3 and the scores are entered in the display of Table 27.10.

To illustrate the process, suppose we start with the *a* members of cell (1,1). The X variable is tied in cells (1,2) and (1,3) for members b and c, and the Y variable is tied in members d and g. In all other cells, i.e., e, f, h, and i, the ranks are higher for both variables. We thus enter the "scores" for cell *a* into Table 27.10 as $P = a(e + f + h + i)$, $Q = 0$; ties on X for $a(b + c)$ and ties on Y for $a(d + g)$. Going right and down from the

TABLE 27.9

Contingency Table with Two Ordinal Variables

	Variable Y		
Variable X	**(1)** **Low**	**(2)** **Medium**	**(3)** **High**
(1) Low	a	b	c
(2) Medium	d	e	f
(3) High	g	h	i

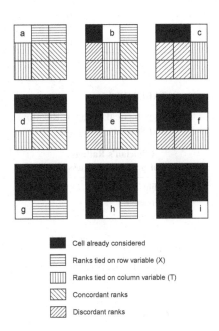

Cell already considered

Ranks tied on row variable (X)

Ranks tied on column variable (T)

Concordant ranks

Discordant ranks

FIGURE 27.3

Pattern of concordant, discordant, and tied ranks in "advancing" cells of Table 27.9.

b members of cell (1,2), there are c ties on the X variable and (e + h) ties on the Y variable. Cells (2,1) and (3,1) have discordant values because the rank of variable Y is lower than **2**, and cells (2,3) and (3,3) have concordant values because the rank of Y is higher. Thus, as shown in Table 27.10, the scores for cell (1,2) are b(f + i) for P, b(d + g) for Q, b(c) for ties in X and b(e + h) for ties in Y.

In the next step, nothing lies to the right of cell (1,3), but two downward cells are tied in the Y rank, and four cells in the next two downward rows are discordant because of lower values in the Y rank as X increases. Thus, the entries for cell (1,3) in Table 27.10 are P = 0, Q = c(d + e + g + h), X-ties = 0, and Y-ties = c(f + i). The entries for the remaining cells are shown in the rest of Table 27.10.

The scoring system can be pragmatically illustrated for Table 27.11, which has 9 cells showing hypothetical data of 150 hospitalized patients' ratings for satisfaction with care in relation to clinicians' ratings for severity of illness. The letters in parentheses of Table 27.11 correspond to the letters of Table 27.9. Table 27.12 shows the corresponding scores for P, Q, and ties. The total scores are 1339 for P, 3775 for Q, 2032 for ties in X, and 2347 for ties in Y.

The scores for P, Q, and ties in Table 27.12 become the constituents of the indexes called gamma, Somers D, tau-b, and tau-c, which differ only in the way they use these scores.

TABLE 27.10

Minding the Ps and Qs for Table 27.9

Location	Cell	Score for P	Score for Q	Score for Ties Variable X	Variable Y
(1, 1)	a	a(e + f + h + i)	0	a(b + c)	a(d + g)
(1, 2)	b	b(f + i)	b(d + g)	b(c)	b(e + h)
(1, 3)	c	0	c(d + e + g + h)	0	c(f + i)
(2, 1)	d	d(h + i)	0	d(e + f)	d(g)
(2, 2)	e	e(i)	e(g)	e(f)	e(h)
(2, 3)	f	0	f(g + h)	0	f(i)
(3, 1)	g	0	0	g(h + i)	0
(3, 2)	h	0	0	h(i)	0
(3, 3)	i	0	0	0	0

TABLE 27.11

Hypothetical Data for Relationship of Patient Satisfaction and Severity of Illness

Clinician's Ratings of Severity of Illness	Patients' Ratings of Satisfaction with Care Low	Medium	High	Total
Mild	8[a]	12[b]	25[c]	45
Moderate	17[d]	13[e]	18[f]	48
Severe	32[g]	15[h]	10[i]	57
Total	57	40	53	150

Note: Letters in parentheses correspond to the cells listed in Table 27.8.

24.6.2 Gamma

The *gamma* (or *Goodman* and *Kruskal's gamma*)[10–12] index is constructed in essentially the same way as tau-a and tau-b, except that ties are ignored. The formula is

$$\text{gamma} = \frac{P - Q}{P + Q} \qquad [27.24]$$

TABLE 27.12

Scores for P, Q, and Ties in Table 27.11

Location	Cell	Score for P	Score for Q	Score for Ties Variable X	Variable Y
(1, 1)	a	8(13 + 18 + 15 + 10)	0	8(12 + 25)	8(17 + 32)
(1, 2)	b	12(18 + 10)	12(17 + 32)	12(25)	12(13 + 15)
(1, 3)	c	0	25(17 + 13 + 32 + 15)	0	25(18 + 10)
(2, 1)	d	17(15 + 10)	0	17(13 + 18)	17(32)
(2, 2)	e	13(10)	13(32)	13(18)	13(15)
(2, 3)	f	0	18(32 + 15)	0	18(10)
(3, 1)	g	0	0	32(15 + 10)	0
(3, 2)	h	0	0	15(10)	0
(3, 3)	i	0	0	0	0
	Totals	1339	3775	2307	2347

For the data in Tables 27.11 and 27.12, gamma will be $(1339 - 3775)/(1339 + 3775) = -2436/5114 = -.48$. The moderately strong negative value, indicating an inverse trend, is consistent with the hypothesis that satisfaction with care goes down as severity of illness goes up.

27.6.3 Somers D

Somers D resembles gamma, but is asymmetric and takes ties into account. The asymmetry is expressed in two indexes. One of them, D_{yx}, accounts for the number of pairs tied on variable Y, but not on X. The expression is

$$D_{yx} = (P - Q)/(P + Q + T_y) \qquad [27.25]$$

where T_y is the score for the pairs tied on Y but not on X. The other index, D_{xy}, accounts for ties on variable X, but not on Y. The expression is

$$D_{xy} = (P - Q)/(P + Q + T_x) \qquad [27.26]$$

where T_x is the score for the corresponding tied pairs.

For the data uuder discussion, $T_y = 2347$ and $T_x = 2307$. The value of $D_{yx} = -2436/(5114 + 2347) = -.326$ and $D_{xy} = -2436/(5114 + 2307) = -.328$.

In this instance, because of the belief that satisfaction (the Y variable) depends on severity of illness (the X variable), the appropriate index is D_{yx}. Its value, somewhat analogous to a regression coefficient, is smaller than gamma because of the ties that enlarge the denominator under $P - Q$. (If someone believed that dissatisfied people are particularly likely to become or be made seriously ill, the appropriate index would D_{xy}. In this example, but not always, the values for D_{yx} and D_{xy} happen to be quite similar.)

27.6.4 Tau-b

After the values of P, Q, T_x, and T_y are obtained, tau-b can be calculated for contingency tables, using either Formula [27.3] or the alternative

$$\text{tau-b} = (P - Q)/\sqrt{(P + Q + T_y)(P + Q + T_x)} \qquad [27.27]$$

which, in the cited example, becomes $-2436/\sqrt{(7461)(7421)} = -.33$.

In Formula [27.27], the structure of tau-b uses the two Somers indexes in a way resembling the calculation of the Pearson correlation coefficient, r, as the geometric mean of the two slopes b and b′. Thus, $r = \sqrt{bb'}$ and tau-b $= \sqrt{D_{yx}D_{xy}}$. Accordingly, tau-b could have been calculated from D_{yx} and D_{xy} as $\sqrt{(-.326)(-.328)} = -.33$.

27.6.5 Tau-c

The calculation of tau-b requires a "square" table, with equal numbers of rows and columns. If the table is rectangular, rather than square, the value of tau is corrected to

$$\text{tau-c} = 2(P - Q)/\{(N^2)[(m - 1)/m]\} \qquad [27.28]$$

where N is the total number of members in the entire table, and m is the *smaller* value of either the number of rows or the number of columns. Formula [27.28] should not be used for square tables, such as Table 27.11, but if applied, the result would be

$$\text{tau-c} = 2(-2436)/\{(150)^2[(3 - 1)/31\} = 4872/15000 = -.325$$

which is almost the same as the value obtained for tau-b, while being much simpler to compute. Gamma and Somers D do not require an analogous correction for non-square tables.

27.6.6 Lambda

Table 27.11 could also be summarized with the lambda index discussed in Sections 27.2.1 and 27.4.1.1. With 57 **low** ratings for satisfaction, the modal estimation would have $150 - 57 = 93$ errors. Using the severity-of-illness ratings, the estimates of **high** satisfaction for the **mild** and **moderate** rows of illness and **low** satisfaction for **severe** illness would respectively have $(45 - 25) + (48 - 18) + (57 - 32) = 75$ errors. The lambda index would be $(93 - 75)/93 = .19$.

This result, using a method of estimation, is much lower than the range of absolute values from .32 to .48 in all of the corresponding indexes that use scores for trend — gamma, Somers D, and the two tau coefficients of association. The reason for the disparity is that lambda reflects accuracy in estimation, whereas the "score" indexes reflect trend. Lambda is thus analogous to r^2, whereas the score indexes are analogous to r.

27.7 Other Indexes of Ranked Categorical Trend

Ranked categorical trends can be determined whenever one of the variables has dimensional or ordinal data that can be ranked in relation to categories of the other variable. The diverse ways of arranging variables, categories, and tables have evoked many proposals of statistical indexes. The ones that have been cited in this chapter were chosen because they seem particularly pertinent for medical literature, or because they commonly appear in printouts of computer "package" programs for indexing associations. Beyond the bi-ordinal coefficients and contingency tables just discussed, three additional indexes are briefly outlined here. The text by Freeman[34] has particularly good worked examples of their application.

Jaspen's multiserial coefficient (dimensional × ordinal) can express the association between a dimensional variable, such as *weight*, and an ordinal variable, such as *social class*. The coefficient has been used[35] to cite the relationship between a dimensionally measured "scan artifact" in pelvic magnetic resonance imaging, and a four-grade ordinal scale of radiologist's assessment of scan quality. A computer program has been constructed[36] to do the calculations, but the index is seldom used, probably because many analysts ignore the mathematical impropriety, accept the ordinal grades as dimensional values, and then use conventional bi-dimensional regression methods.

In the *biserial coefficient* (dimensional × binary), which is a special case of the Jaspen multiserial coefficient, the ordinal scale has only two (binary) ranks. The biserial index can be pertinent when a binary variable, such as existence of *survival*, depends on a dimensional variable, such as *age* or *weight*. The coefficient would indicate the association in data showing the proportions of survivors at different ages or weights. If the dimensional variable is time and adequate data are available, the biserial coefficient might be used as an index of association for the survival curve. The association between binary and dimensional data could also be expressed with an index of linear trend in an r × 2 ranked array, as discussed in Section 27.5.

Freeman's theta (ordinal × nominal) can be used when an ordinal variable, such as *social class*, is examined in a set of nominal groups, A, B, C,.... The theta (θ) coefficient for this association was developed as a multi-group extension of the Wilcoxon signed-rank procedure.

27.8 Association in "Large" r × c Tables

The associations that have not yet been discussed occur in a "large" r × c table (where *r* and *c* are each ≥3) for two nominal variables. In such tables, which are not common, the arrangements are best called "associations," because the idea of "trend" seems inappropriate if either or both of the two variables is nominal. To ease comprehension, many analysts try to condense the big tables into a 2 × 2 structure by "collapsing" (i.e., compressing) suitable categories.

27.8.1 "Screening" with ϕ and X^2

Before the "collapse," the entire r × c table is often "screened" to see whether any "significant" findings are present. The most common screening procedure is to examine the ϕ coefficient of correlation for the two categorical variables. To determine ϕ, the expected values are first noted in each cell, and the value of X^2 for the entire table is calculated as the sum of the [(observed − expected)^2/expected] values in the cells. The value of ϕ, calculated as $\phi = \sqrt{X^2/N}$, is then interpreted like a correlation coefficient, with values ranging from 0 to |1|.

Further examination beyond the screening can be stimulated by a stochastically significant X^2 [interpreted at $(r − 1)(c − 1)$ degrees of freedom], by a quantitatively significant value of ϕ, or by both. The "significant" cells in the table will be those with individually high values of the [(observed − expected)^2/expected] ratios.

Other data analysts, however, may collapse the table immediately and omit the "screening" process. The collapsing is usually done according to "sensible" strategies derived from the biologic content of the data and/or from the quantitative need to combine cells with small frequencies.

27.8.2 Example in Medical Literature

Large r × c tables with nominal categories seldom appear in medical literature. In one example, however, a letter[37] to the editor of *The New England Journal of Medicine* reported a study of bimanual dexterity and batting "handedness" in baseball players. The players were divided into five groups: high school students, elementary school students, all recorded professional players, current major-league players (excluding pitchers), and best hitters of all time. The players' handedness was divided into 6 categories based on whether each player threw right-handed or left-handed and also batted right, left, or both ways.

The 5 ×6 table was then analyzed with a chi-square procedure, which led to the conclusion that the "professional baseball players had a significantly ... higher number of left handed batters than the (student) controls."

27.8.3 ϕ in 2 × 2 Tables

ϕ is seldom applied for indexing a 2 ×2 table, because the investigator will usually want to contrast the two proportions as an increment or ratio, not with a correlation coefficient.

If the 2 × 2 table is subjected to regression analysis, however, the slope (as shown in Section 27.5.3.1) is simply the increment, $p_2 − p_1$. Because the two proportions can be compared in two directions, as

a/n_1 vs. c/n_2 or as a/f_1 vs. b/f_2, two different increments can be determined. Appropriate algebraic activity will demonstrate that ϕ, as a correlation coefficient, is the geometric mean of these two increments.

27.8.4   Alternatives to ϕ

An ideal correlation coefficient should be able to range from values of 0 to $|1|$. In a 2×2 table, the maximum value that X^2 can attain is N; and so the largest possible value for ϕ^2 will be $N/N = 1$. (This situation occurs when diagonally opposite cells such as a, d or b, c are both empty in a table structured as $\begin{Bmatrix} a & b \\ c & d \end{Bmatrix}$.) In a larger $r \times c$ table, however, X^2 can exceed the value of N, and if so, ϕ^2 will have an inappropriate value that exceeds 1. To avoid this problem, three alternative indexes are available — all of them constructed as modifications of X^2/N.

27.8.4.1   *Pearson's C* — Pearson's "contingency coefficient," C, is calculated as

$$C^2 = X^2/(X^2 + N)$$

With this structure, C^2 will always be <1. When $X^2 = N$, C^2 will be 1/2. C is seldom used for 2×2 tables because its maximum value will be $\sqrt{1/2} = .71$ and because it does not have a good "intuitive" meaning for larger tables.

27.8.4.2   *Tschuprow's T* — To eliminate the possibility of getting a correlation coefficient that exceeds 1, Tschuprow's T^2 divides ϕ^2 by $\sqrt{(r-1)(c-1)}$. The formula is

$$T^2 = X^2 / \left[N\sqrt{(r-1)(c-1)} \right]$$

The square root of this value is Tschuprow's T. In a 2×2 table, $(r-1)(c-1) = 1$, and so the result will be identical to ϕ. For "large" tables, $(r-1)(c-1)$ will exceed 1, and its square root division will lower the value of ϕ.

27.8.4.3   *Cramer's V* — Tschuprow's T has the disadvantage of producing an overcorrection. Although kept from being >1, the correlation coefficient often cannot reach the permissible maximum value of 1. This problem is particularly likely to occur if r is much greater than c (or vice versa) in a large $r \times c$ table.

To eliminate this problem, Cramer divided X^2/N by an entity called Min $(r-1, c-1)$, which represents the smaller value of either $r-1$ or $c-1$. The formula is

$$V^2 = X^2/[N \times Min (r-1, c-1)]$$

Thus, if $r = 3$ and $c = 4$, the smaller value is $r-1 = 2$, and $V^2 = X^2/2N$. When $r = c$, Tschuprow's T and Cramer's V are identical. When either r or c is 2, V and ϕ will be identical.

This attribute of Cramer's V makes it the preferred index of association for large $r \times c$ tables. The index almost never appears in medical literature, but was used many years ago in an analysis where the investigators screened for correlations of 7 categorical variables in a study of limb sarcomas.[38] The number of categories in the variables ranged from two to four; and Cramer's V was used as the index of association because "it adjusts for ... degrees of freedom ... in a convenient manner, so that tables with differing degrees of freedom may be compared."

References

1. Siegel, 1988; 2. Bradley, 1968; 3. Ferguson, 1965; 4. Edgington, 1969; 5. Kendall, 1990; 6. Tate, 1957; 7. Conover, 1980; 8. Sprent, 1993; 9. Guttman, 1941; 10. Goodman, 1954; 11. Kohout, 1974; 12. Everitt, 1977; 13. Makuch, 1989; 14. Feinstein, 1990b; 15. Feinstein, 1996; 16. Sawada, 1992; 17. Simon, 1978; 18. Kendall, 1955; 19. Griffiths, 1980; 20. Noether, 1981; 21. Greene, 1981; 22. Calandra, 1991; 23. Ramirez, 1992; 24. Sabia, 1992; 25. Robbins, 1993; 26. Follman, 1992; 27. Armitage, 1987; 28. Poole, 1984; 29. Detsky, 1984; 30. Moses, 1984; 31. Boucher, 1998; 32. Liu, 1998; 33. Kallen, 1999; 34. Freeman, 1965; 35. Wright, 1992; 36. Cicchetti, 1982; 37. McLean, 1982; 38. Freeman, 1980.

Exercises

27.1. These questions all refer to Figure 27.2 in the text. The two verbatim descriptions here are from pertinent sections of the research report.

Methods: "Measures of association were calculated using either simple linear regression or the Spearman rank correlation coefficient, when appropriate. All reported significance levels are two-sided."

Results: "In the 33 nonsurvivors, as well as in the subgroup of 21 patients who died of irreversible septic shock, the serum concentrations of IL-6 measured at study entry correlated inversely with the duration of survival ($r = -0.51$, $p = 0.004$ and $r = -0.62$, $p = 0.005$, respectively; Spearman rank correlation coefficient). In particular, of nine patients who died of irreversible septic shock within the first 24 hours of study, all but one had a very high concentration of IL-6 (median: 64 ng/mL, range: 0.26 to 305 ng/mL) at study entry."

  27.1.1. Because the Spearman coefficient is for correlation, not regression, how do you think the apparent regression line was determined? Do you agree with the result? If not, why not?

  27.1.2. Do you like the way the graph is arranged? If not, what would you prefer?

  27.1.3. Does the graph have any obvious errors or inconsistencies? If so, what are they?

27.2. In a study of diagnostic fashions among psychiatrists, the diagnoses were compared for two groups of 145 patients each in a London and a New York hospital. In London, 51 patients were diagnosed as *schizophrenic* and 67 as *affectively ill*. The corresponding numbers of diagnoses in New York were, respectively, 82 and 24. The remaining diagnoses at each institution were classified as *miscellaneous*.

  27.2.1. What would you suggest as the best statistical index to summarize this set of results?

  27.2.2. To express concordance for these data, how should kappa be weighted?

27.3. In a study of prognostic stratification, a cohort with 5-year survival rate of $85/221 = 38\%$ could be divided into two different staging systems having the following results:

Stage	System A	System B
I	70/122 (57%)	36/50 (72%)
II	12/46 (26%)	40/85 (47%)
III	3/53 (6%)	9/86 (10%)

  27.3.1. Which of these two systems of staging would you prefer "intuitively," i.e., by judgmental inspection of the data? Why?

  27.3.2. The investigators would like some quantitative indexes to summarize and compare the results of the two systems. What are the values of the slope and chi-square test for linear trend?

  27.3.3. Give the results for at least three additional quantitative indexes that could be applied to each system.

27.3.4. Which of the indexes in 27.3.2 and 27.3.3 do you believe is best for citing these results? Has it made you change your mind about the answer to 27.3.1? Why?

27.4. Using any sources at your disposal (available journals, computerized-literature search, etc.) find a published paper that used any one of the additional indexes discussed in this chapter. Comment briefly on what was done and whether you think it was appropriate. Alternatively, find a published paper in which one of the indexes discussed in this chapter should have been used, but was not. If you choose this option, justify your reason for believing that the original procedure was "wrong" and for preferring the alternative index. With either option, enclose a copy of the selected publication (or a suitable abstract thereof).

28

Non-Targeted Analyses

CONTENT

Although this chapter is concerned mainly with "non-targeted" forms of analysis, the first section describes sources of complexity that can occur here or in any multivariable and multicategorical procedures.

28.1 Sources of Complexity

The brave new statistical world we are about to enter can be catalogued according to diversity in at least four entities that have appeared before in relatively simple arrangements. The entities that now produce additional complexities are the direction of relationships, the number (and symbols) of variables, the scales of the variables, and the patterns of combination.

28.1.1 Direction of Relationship

The distinction between targeted and non-targeted directions is a fundamental axis of classification for statistical procedures. All of the new tactics about to be discussed can be catalogued, according to their direction, as either targeted or non-targeted. In the previous discussion of targeted associations, an "independent" variable, X, was examined unidirectionally for its effect on a "dependent" target, Y. Thus, age might affect a child's height. Such an association was often called a *regression* of Y on X, but other targeted relationships were examined when we compared mean weight in two groups, when two variables formed a curve in which survival depended on time, or when stratifications (and adjustments) showed the effect of the variables (or groups) used for the stratification.

In the non-targeted bidirectional associations, the two variables were related to one another without implying that one depended on the other. The nondependent association was often called a correlation between Y and X. Thus, we might examine the correlation between hemoglobin and hematocrit or between hematocrit and serum cholesterol, without suggesting that one variable affected the other. We could also examine concordance for the agreement between two ratings, without choosing one of them as a "gold standard" for accuracy.

28.1.2   Number of Variables and Symbols

The two variables in a bivariate association could easily be symbolized as X and Y, and additional letters such as U, V, and W could be used to denote the multiple extra variables. Many alphabetical letters, however, have already been reserved for other purposes (e.g., N for sample size; P for proportions, rates, or probabilities; R for correlations or rates; Z for standardized scores or variables).

To avoid running out of available letters, the multiple available variables are identified with numerical subscripts in symbols such as $Y_1, Y_2, Y_3, \ldots$, which will represent the dependent or target variables. The general symbol for any of the independent variables is X_j; and the collection of independent variables (X_1, $X_2, X_3, X_4, \ldots$) in a particular analysis is denoted as $\{X_j\}$. These new symbols can be confusing because they differ from what was used previously when $X_1, X_2, X_3, \ldots$ showed the values of persons 1, 2, 3, ... for a single variable, X. In the new arrangements, the subscripts represent variables, not persons. To show both persons and variables, we would need double subscripts such as $X_{i,j}$ (often written as X_{ij}) to represent the value for person i in variable j. Thus, X_{26} would be the value of variable 6 for person 2; and $X_{39,18}$ would be the value of variable 18 for person 39. In most circumstances, however, the double subscripts can be avoided without ambiguity, and X_j will represent individual independent variables.

The analytic situation becomes multivariable when three or more variables are examined simultaneously. In directional orientation, the multivariable associations can have the relationships illustrated in Figure 28.1. In a *many-to-one* or uni-targeted relationship, independent variables such as X_1 = age, X_2 = sex, X_3 = smoking, X_4 = serum cholesterol, and X_5 = hematocrit are related to a single target, Y = blood pressure. *Multiple linear regression* is an example of this analytic procedure. In a *many-to-many* or multi-targeted relationship, a set of several independent variables might be related simultaneously to several target variables, such as Y_1 = duration of survival, Y_2 = functional status, Y_3 = costs of

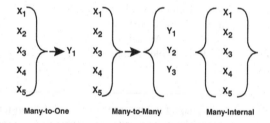

Many-to-One   Many-to-Many   Many-Internal

FIGURE 28.1

Three main types of relationships among multiple variables. On the left, the five variables X_1, X_2, X_3, X_4, and X_5 are related to a single external variable, Y_1. In the middle, they are related to several external variables, Y_1, Y_2, Y_3. On the right, the five variables are related internally to one another.

care. *Canonical analysis* is a procedure that might be used for this many-to-many association. In a *many-internal* nontargeted relationship, the variables are neither dependent nor independent. They are analyzed together for their own interrelationships with one another, not with a target variable. *Factor analysis* and *principal component analysis* are procedures applied in this manner.

28.1.3   Scales of Variables

As noted in Chapter 2, any variable can be expressed in a dimensional or categorical scale; the categorical scales can be binary or polytomous; and the polytomous categories can be ordinally ranked or nominally unranked.

Age, height, and serum cholesterol are all *dimensional* variables. Scales such as **alive/dead, success/failure, male/female** are all binary. *Severity of illness* can have an ordinally ranked polytomous scale such as **none, mild, moderate, severe**; and *religion* has an unranked nominal polytomous scale expressed (alphabetically) as **Buddhist, Catholic, Confucian, Hindu, … .**

The categorical scales are a major source of complexity, leading to different formats for the analyses. For example, if the target variable is a dimensional blood pressure, the multivariable analytic procedure will usually be multiple *linear* regression. If the target variable is a binary **alive/dead** expression, however, the analysis will usually be done with multiple *logistic* regression. In the many-internal analytic procedures that are done without a target, variables expressed in categories usually receive a procedure called *cluster analysis*, but dimensional variables usually receive *factor analysis* or *principal component analysis*. In many-to-one analyses, categorical independent variables may be examined with *recursive partitioning* or with *conjunctive consolidation* rather than with conventional regression procedures. (All of these new names are used merely to illustrate the distinctions and to give you a preview of coming attractions if you eventually go beyond the current text to learn about multivariable analysis.)

28.1.4   Patterns of Combination

Multiple variables can be combined in two fundamentally different patterns: algebraic models and decision-rule clusters.

28.1.4.1   *Algebraic Models* — With algebraic models, the variables are given coefficients, called weights, and are algebraically combined in the configuration of a geometric pattern, such as a straight or curved line. The linear regression equation $Y = a + bX$ is a rectilinear algebraic model that relates the dependent variable Y to the independent variable X, which is weighted with the coefficient b. The value of a is the intercept when $X = 0$. The expression is constructed with the assumption that the relationship between Y and X can be "modeled" with a straight line. For curved models, the format of X (or Y) is appropriately changed. For example, $Y = a + bX^2$, $Y = a + b \log X$, $\log Y = a + bX$, $Y = e^{a+bX}$, and $Y = a + bX + cX^2$ are algebraic models that form curved lines for the two variables, X and Y.

For multiple variables, the straight-line algebraic models form "hyperplanes" or "multi-dimensional surfaces." Thus, $Y = b_0 + b_1X_1 + b_2X_2$ is a plane in three dimensional space, showing the dependence of Y on the independent variables, X_1 and X_2. They are weighted with the respective coefficients, b_1 and b_2; and b_0 is the intercept. The Apgar[1] score is a multidimensional non-targeted expression that takes the form

$$V = b_1X_1 + b_2X_2 + b_3X_3 + b_4X_4 + b_5X_5$$

V is the new variable (i.e., the Apgar score) formed by the combination; each of the five constituent X_j variables is expressed in a rating scale of **0, 1,** or **2**; and each of the five b_j coefficients has a value of 1.

The formation of algebraic models is now the conventional method of statistical analysis for multiple variables or multiple categories, particularly because the availability of modern computers has eased the formidable difficulties of calculating the appropriate b_j coefficients from the data. The availability of computers, however, has also allowed development of the different approach discussed next.

28.1.4.2   *Decision-Rule Clusters* — Forming decision-rule clusters is a common (although informal) multivariable strategy in medical activities. The name *cluster* is given to a collection of categories that form a group or subgroup. The collection can be simple or compound. For example, the variable *age* can be partitioned into two simple categories, **old** and **young**. These categories form groups that can be categorically subdivided into simple subgroups such as **old men** and **tall women**. Boolean symbols such as **old ∩ male** can be used to denote categories such as **old men**. A compound categorical cluster might contain **old men** and/or **tall women**, which could be symbolized as **(old ∩ male) ∪ (tall ∩ female)**.

An analytic method that uses groups or subgroups is particularly compatible with the fundamental thought processes of biologists and clinicians, who usually think in categories, and seldom make decisions based on combinations of weighted variables. The term *clusters* is simply a formal designation for the collections of categories that form the groupings. The TNM staging system for cancer is an example of decision-rule multi-categorical clusters. The system begins with the ordinal ratings given to three variables: T, which represents features of the primary tumor; N, which represents regional lymph nodes; and M, for distant metastases. In ordinary description, the *TNM index* gives ratings for each of these variables in a tandem profile such as **T 2 N 1 M 0** or **T 4 N 0 M 2**. According to an arbitrary decision rule, these profiles are then assigned to clustered categories that are called *stages*. **Stage I** usually indicates a localized cancer. **Stage II** usually indicates a cancer that has spread to adjacent lymph nodes, but no farther. **Stages III, IV,** and **V** refer to increasingly distant degrees of spread.

Clustered categories are formed according to diverse decision rules that are determined biologically or statistically (or both), without reliance on the "model" of an algebraic configuration. The decision rule can also be expressed as an algorithm in which the sequential addition of categories leads to specified conclusions. Such algorithms now often appear as "guidelines" for clinical practice.

28.2 Basic Concepts of Non-Targeted Analyses

The multivariable procedures in this chapter contain non-targeted, "many-internal" analytic methods that have such names as *factor analysis, principal component analysis*, and *cluster analysis*. In non-targeted analyses, the selected variables are examined for their interrelationship with one another, not with a specific target variable. The goal is usually to reduce the variables into a smaller set of "factors" or other entities that contain the most cogent information.

For example, when Virginia Apgar[1] constructed the score by which she is commemorated, she wanted to form a multivariate index that would describe the "severity" of the condition of a newborn baby. The index was not intended to predict an external target, such as survival or need for special therapy. The goal was merely to specify explicitly the components of a judgment about "condition" that was formerly expressed implicitly in such general terms as **excellent, good, fair,** and **poor**.

28.2.1 "Intellectual Dissection"

Apgar's attempt to specify and reconstruct the components of an implicit global "intuition" or "judgment" has become a relatively common medical event. The initial judgment might have been singly or doubly "global." In a singly global judgment, the phenomenon under discussion is well identified, but no criteria are offered to demarcate the categories of an ordinal rating scale such as **excellent, good, fair,** or **poor**. In a doubly global judgment, neither the phenomenon nor the rating scale is clearly identified. For example, if we ask someone "How are you?," the answer is doubly global when the respondent says, "Good." The same response would be singly global, however, for the question, "How is the pain in your ankle?"

An indication of the modern non-global approach is that clinicians today seldom talk about such things as a "guarded prognosis." Instead, a duration of survival may be predicted from the specifications of an algorithm or equation containing multiple variables. In Virginia Apgar's approach, the entity she wanted to dissect and reconstruct, as *condition of newborn baby*, was a clinical pathophysiologic status, rather than such attributes as cleanliness of skin, size of limbs, or excitement of parents. After reviewing all the pathophysiologic variables that might be observed neonatally, Apgar chose five as being most important: heart rate, respiratory rate, color, muscle tone, and reflex responses. She rated each variable in a three-category ordinal scale of **0, 1,** or **2**. She then added the five ratings to form a score that ranged from **0** to **10**.

Apgar constructed the composite score entirely according to her clinical judgment, without any formal mathematical procedures. The statistical methods that are about to be discussed offer a formal approach to the analogous process.

28.2.2 Face Validity

When Apgar identified and gave rating scales to the selected five variables, she had a clear vision of what should emerge in the composite score. Her years of clinical experience had given her a substantive knowledge of the particular variables that would be most important for indicating pathophysiologic status; she could readily "dissect" her "intuition" to identify those variables; and she could examine the subsequent composite scores to determine that they were "clinically sensible" in doing the desired task. This type of "sensibility" is often called *face validity*. It cannot be discerned with any type of statistical calculation and requires a combination of "common sense" plus knowledge of the substantive issue under consideration. For example, the Apgar Score would have excellent face validity as an index of pathophysiologic condition, but not as an index of socioeconomic status.

Face validity is a particularly thorny problem in non-targeted analyses of multivariable data. If a target has been identified, it serves as a direct criterion for evaluating face validity in the analytic accomplishment. Thus, a particular prognostic index can readily be shown (with appropriate data) to be effective or ineffective in its job of predicting survival. In the absence of a target to serve as a criterion, however, the non-targeted analytic methods are constructed exclusively with mathematical principles. The constructions may then be splendidly ingenious acts of mathematics, but ultimately unsuccessful because they lack face validity.

The *factors* (or other entities) created by composite variables can be constructed in an "inside-out" or "outside-in" manner. The Apgar Score was an inside-out construction, accomplished when Apgar examined her "inside" clinical judgment to identify and recombine the cogent (i.e., "sensible") variables into a composite result. In contrast, the mathematical methods produce an outside-in approach. The available "outside" information is first processed mathematically, without any criteria for "sensibility"; and face validity of the composite result is evaluated afterward.

This distinction becomes particularly important when non-targeted analyses are used to construct and to offer a purely statistical "validation" for such composite variables as *competence, intelligence, health status, satisfaction with care,* and *quality of life.*

28.3   Algebraic Methods

The two most commonly used non-targeted algebraic methods are called *factor analysis* and *principal component analysis*. In recent years, these methods have sometimes been called "latent variable" analysis because the results are aimed at forming a separate latent idea or "construct" that is not itself directly observed. For example, Apgar's construct was the severity of the clinical condition in newborns. Other clinical constructs such as *congestive heart failure* or *hepatic decompensation* are not observed directly, but are identified or conceptually derived from such observed entities as dyspnea, edema, or jaundice. The construct called *intelligence* is the latent variable that was the incentive[2] for the early development of *factor analysis*.

In the customary factor-analytic procedure, data for a set of variables in a group of persons are examined for the intercorrelations among the variables. Those that most strongly correlate with one another have a "shared variance" that is then attributed to their presumptive correlation with the "external" latent variable. For example, students whose scores are correlated as correspondingly high (or low) values in tests of reading, writing, and arithmetic may be regarded as having a high (or low) level of a common factor, which is the latent variable called *intelligence*.

Figure 28.2, showing data for only two variables, X_1 and X_2, will give a particularly simple illustration of the ideas. The small solid square is the centroid, which is the common mean of the two variables, located at the coordinate for $(\overline{X}_1, \overline{X}_2)$. In the original axes for the two variables, the variances around the centroid would be calculated as the group variance for X_1, the group variance for X_2, and the group covariance for the two variables. To simplify the symbols, the group variances can be written as S_{11} and S_{22} for variables X_1 and X_2, respectively, and the covariance can be designated as S_{12}. Suppose we now prepare a new axis as two lines, $V_1 = a_1X_1 + a_2X_2$ and $V_2 = b_1X_1 + b_2X_2$, that pass through the centroid as shown in the figure, and suppose we cite the coordinate of each point according to its distance along the new axes. The group variance of the points will be larger along the V_1 axis, where the points are widely spread, than along the V_2 axis, where the points have smaller distances. (In an ideal situation, all of the points would fit perfectly on the V_1 line, and no deviations would remain to produce variance along the V_2 axis.) If we wanted to replace the original variables, X_1 and X_2, by a new factor that "captured" most of the common variance in their interrelationship, the line constructed as $V_1 = a_1X_1 + a_2X_2$ would be an excellent choice, and the residual variance could be ignored in the V_2 axis.

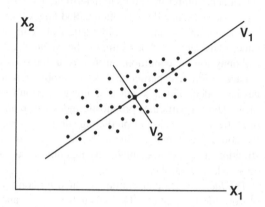

FIGURE 28.2
Data for two variables, X_1 and X_2, with V_1 and V_2 as new axes passing through the centroid. Each data point is much closer to the V_1 axis than to the V_2 axis. For further details, see text.

28.3.1   Analytic Goals and Process

The mathematical goal is to combine some or all of the existing variables into a smaller set of new variables, called factors, that best "explain" the relationships among the original variables. The new factors should ideally not be correlated with one another, but should be composed of variables having substantial inter-correlations. For example, suppose we have five variables, X_1, X_2, ..., X_5. When finished, the analytic procedure should produce four (or fewer) factors constructed as the following weighted combinations:

$$V_1 = a_1X_1 + a_2X_2 + a_3X_3 + a_4X_4 + a_5X_5$$

$$V_2 = b_1X_1 + b_2X_2 + b_3X_3 + b_4X_4 + b_5X_5$$

$$V_3 = c_1X_1 + c_2X_2 + c_3X_3 + c_4X_4 + c_5X_5$$

$$V_4 = d_1X_1 + d_2X_2 + d_3X_3 + d_4X_4 + d_5X_5$$

The second factor, V_2, is constructed to "explain" the variance that remains after the construction of V_1. Factor V_3 explains what is left after V_1 and V_2 are formed, and so on. In general, the goal is to get the desired "explanation" with no more than two factors, and the original variables need not appear in each factor. (For the Apgar Score, a large number of possible candidate variables was judgmentally reduced to five, which were then combined into a single factor in which all coefficients had a value of 1. The single Apgarian factor could be cited as $V = X_1 + X_2 + X_3 + X_4 + X_5$, with each X_j having a rating scale of **0**, **1**, or **2**.)

The analytic process begins by examining the matrix grid that is outlined with the variables cited in the rows and columns in Table 28.1. The entries in the cells of Table 28.1 can be either correlations or group variances and covariances. When each variable is related to itself, the group variances are S_{11} for X_1X_1, S_{22} for X_2X_2, etc. For intervariable relationships, the group covariances are S_{12} for X_1X_2 (or X_2X_1), S_{34} for X_3X_4 (or X_4X_3) and so on. The entries in the cells can also be correlation coefficients such as r_{12} (or r_{21}) and r_{34} (or r_{43}). In the main left-upper-to-right-lower diagonal, these coefficients will all be

TABLE 28.1

"Skeletal" Outline of Variables in a Correlation or Variance–Covariance Matrix

	X_1	X_2	X_3	X_4 ...
X_1				
X_2				
X_3				
X_4				
:				

1, when each variable is correlated with itself. Inspection of a matrix of correlation coefficients will immediately offer an idea of which variables are closely or hardly interrelated with one another.

28.3.2 Operational Strategies and Nomenclature

The procedures have complex operational strategies and a correspondingly arcane jargon of names. [The names are mentioned here so that they will not be total strangers if you meet them in a published report. A complete explanation of the concepts, however, is beyond the scope of this text. You can read more about them (and hope to find clear presentations somewhere) if you begin giving serious attention to using these methods or their results.] Equations derived from appropriate arrangements of the correlation or variance–covariance matrixes are solved to construct factors having the form of $V = a_1X_1 + a_2X_2 + a_3X_3 + a_4X_4 + \ldots$. The solutions to a special set of equations are called *eigenvalues* (or *characteristic roots*); and the "best" factors, i.e., those that "explain" the most total variance, have the highest eigenvalues. (The hope is that the eigenvalues will be large for one or two factors, and small for others.) The coefficients $(a_1, a_2, a_3, \ldots)$ indicate the variables that are most prominent in the arrangement of each factor.

After being selected, the factors can be checked for their correlation coefficients with the individual variables. For example, the Apgar scores of a group of babies could be examined for their correlation with the variables of heart rate, reflex responses, etc. These coefficients for a particular factor are usually called *factor loadings*. They represent the prominence of each variable in each factor (and vice versa). The sum of the squared factor-loading coefficients is called its *communality*. The larger the communality, the larger is the amount of shared variance that is presumably "explained" by that factor.

Because the attached coefficients indicate the impact of the component variables, factors are sometimes named according to the constituents that have high impact. For example, V_1 might be called a *body-size factor* if it has large coefficients for the variables *height* and *weight*; and V_2 might be called a *complexion factor* if it has large coefficients for variables indicating the color of *skin, hair*, and *eyes*. The *body-size factor* in the foregoing example would probably have high factor loads for *height* and *weight*, but small loads for *skin, hair*, and *eyes*.

28.3.3 Rotations

Perhaps the most complex (and controversial) part of the operating procedure occurs after the most prominent (or "principal") components have been identified. In the basic mathematical reasoning, all of the factors are regarded as orthogonal, i.e., their axes are perpendicular to one another. (This type of orthogonality cannot be visualized for four or more axes, but it is easy to assume mathematically.)

In the next step, the axes are often rotated to produce an optimum arrangement. The criteria of optimality differ with different strategies of rotation, which can keep the axes *orthogonal* or change them into *oblique* patterns. Among the many names for these rotational procedures are *varimax* and *oblique Procrustean*.

28.3.4 Factor vs. Component Analysis

Factor analysis and *principal component analysis* are mathematical "siblings" that do essentially the same thing in slightly different ways. In published literature, the investigators often begin with *principal component analysis*, but then call the results *factor analysis* after the rotations cited in the preceding section. The operations of the two methods also differ in using "standardized" Z scores, e.g., $(X - \overline{X})/s$, or the original units of expression for the variables. The methods may also work with the matrix of correlation coefficients or covariances, and may find the appropriate components (or factors) with least squares computations or with a special method called maximum-likelihood solutions. The main conceptual distinction has been described by Maurice Kendall:[3] "In component analysis we begin with the observations and look for components … [going] from the data toward a hypothetical model. In factor analysis, we work the other way round … ."

28.3.5 Published Examples

The published examples cited here were taken from literature that happened to be noted by the author, without a systematic search. The investigators almost never cite reasons for choosing between factor and principal component analysis, and probably use whatever program is conveniently available or preferred by the statistical consultant.

28.3.5.1   Factor Analysis — With factor analysis, an "index of need for health resources" was developed[4] for geographic regions of the nation of India. After the original principal components approach, applied to 7 variables, "revealed two factors" that were "not directly meaningful," the investigators applied varimax rotation to produce two other factors that had "immediate use." The first factor, called *proximate determinants*, had high "loadings" for the four variables that indicated rates of homicide, crude deaths, infant mortality, and crude births. The second factor, called *sociomedical background*, had high loadings for the other three variables, which indicated population rates or proportions of doctors, illiterates, and hospital beds. The percentage of "explained variation" was 67% for the first factor and 16% for the second.

When data for 360 patients with rheumatoid arthritis received an "iterated principal component factor analysis," the investigators[5] decided that the 9 constituents of the Arthritis Impact Measurement Scale could be reduced to a 4-factor model that accounted for 77% of the variance. After a 5th factor was added to allow better assessment of "the areas of clinical interest," the investigators concluded that the "model" containing "5 distinct components" was "preferable to 9 more highly correlated scales for use as explanatory variables."

Factor analysis was applied[6] when 428 physicians responded to a questionnaire containing 56 items intended to measure attitudes that "influence resource utilization." After various forms of matrix rotation and statistical checking, the investigators emerged with factors for "four prominent domains [that] closely corresponded with our hypothesized domains a priori. [They] were interpreted as cost-consciousness, discomfort with uncertainty, fear of malpractice, and annoyance with utilization review."

In other medical applications, factor analysis was used as follows: to reduce 28 candidate variables to four "meaningful factors" that could be used as "outcome measures" in chronic obstructive pulmonary disease[7]; to convert ten variables in patients with asthma to three factors that "provided a useful summary of asthma severity"[8]; and to produce 3 factors for 46 sociogeographic variables associated with multiple sclerosis in regions of the United States.[9]

28.3.5.2   Principal Component Analysis — After examining data from a battery of 24 audiologic tests, Henderson et al.[10] used principal component analysis to derive a composite score as the primary outcome variable in a clinical trial comparing the efficacy of three cochlear implant devices for bilateral profound hearing loss. The investigators found that "the first principal component had its largest coefficients associated with the most difficult audiologic tests" and that "changes in the composite score over time were also closely related to subjective impressions of implant performance" by the patients and clinicians.

In an ophthalmologic application,[11] principal component analysis was used to analyze 53 variables, which were the "threshold" value at visual field locations checked with the Humphrey automated perimeter. For locations in both eyes of 304 "normal" persons, the data set contained $53 \times 2 \times 304 = 32,224$ threshold measurements. The investigators found (probably to no one's surprise) that the average threshold value for each person became the first principal component in accounting for variations.

Principal component analyses have often been applied to differentiate symptom patterns in patients with schizophrenia, tested with the PANSS (Positive and Negative Syndrome Scale) inventory. A five-factor model is reported[12] to be "an interesting tool when new, selective, psychopharmacological drugs are to be evaluated." Principal component analyses have also been used to combine laboratory tests and culture conditions in melanomas grafted onto mice,[13] to reduce 6 tests of function to three principal components in pulmonary disease,[14] and to divide 61 patients receiving coronary bypass grafts into three "subtypes" formed from eight morphologic and electrocardiographic variables.[15]

28.3.6   Biplot Illustrations

If a good reduction of the variables is provided by the first two principal components, they can be used as the main axes of a bi-plot graph, which shows the relationships among different members of a group. Each member's location is plotted according to coordinates for the first and second principal component.

28.4 Cluster Analysis

Cluster analysis, which yields sets of composite categories rather than sums of weighted variables, can have an intuitive appeal to biologists concerned with challenges in taxonomic classification. Appropriate new forms of taxonomy were the basis for such major scientific advances as the Linnaean classification of animals and plants, Darwin's theory of evolution, Mendeleyev's periodic table, and the astronomic partition of "dwarf" and "giant" stars. In clinical medicine, the fundamental taxonomy used for thoughts about human ailments is a set of nosographic categories, called the International Classification of Disease, which is revised every 10 years.

During the latter half of the 20th century, as new forms of technologic and other data become available, diverse investigators wanted to eliminate the "subjective" judgments of traditional taxonomy, and to substitute new systems created by numerical methods that were presumably objective and "stable." According to an excellent text by Everitt,[16] the strategies of cluster analysis were applied in all of these methods but were given different names: *numerical taxonomy* in biology, *Q analysis* in psychology, and *unsupervised pattern recognition* in the field of artificial intelligence.

The goal of cluster analysis is to divide the persons or other entities into an appropriate set of categorical clusters; and the process begins, as in factor or component analysis, with data for multiple variables in members of an observed group.

28.4.1 Basic Structures

The clustering process can be arranged to form either *partitions* or *trees*. In a partition, each object is assigned to a single clustered location. In a tree, the hierarchical organization allows objects to belong to a "pedigreed" family of clusters.

Figure 28.3 illustrates a hierarchical family arrangement of different species of horses.[16] The hierarchy in this instance was established judgmentally. The process begins with the "parent" group and forms a "family" in successive splits of the "pedigree." When cluster analysis is done mathematically with a hierarchical method, the direction is reversed, starting with individual members that are successively combined to form the family groups. The branching pattern of construction is often called a *dendogram*. Figure 28.4 shows a dendogram developed[17] to classify the distribution of pain in 127 patients with

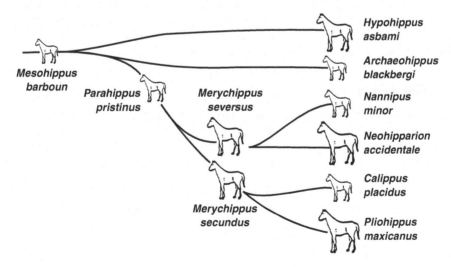

FIGURE 28.3
Hierarchical family arrangement showing an evolutionary tree for species of horses. (Figure taken from Chapter Reference 16.)

temporomandibular (TM) joint dysfunction who had indicated the locations of their pain graphically in squares of a stylized graph of the face. In the main hierarchical clusters of Figure 28.4, the pain was mainly over the TM joint for group A, involved the ramus (vertical portion) of the mandible in group B, and extended over the zygomatic arch in group C.

In nonhierarchical partitions, the members are grouped into clusters that do not overlap and that do not have "familial" relationships. Figure 28.5 illustrates a partition[18] of four clusters for 16 members.

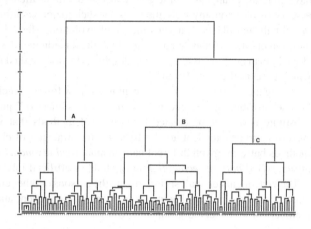

28.4.2   Operational Strategies

The main operational strategies in cluster analysis involve the choice of mechanisms for "measuring" the "similarity" or "affinity" of different objects. The different tactics used for this purpose create a complex array of strategies and nomenclatures.

FIGURE 28.4

Dendrogram showing distribution of temporomandibular pain in 127 patients, and subsequent hierarchical formation of three main groups, marked **A**, **B**, and **C**. (Figure taken from Chapter Reference 17.)

One common approach is to measure the distance between values of the variables. For example, suppose person A has values of 35 and 109, respectively, in variables 1 and 2, and person B has the corresponding values of 27 and 183. With the Pythagorean theorem, the squared Euclidean distance between the two persons is $(35 - 27)^2 + (109 - 183)^2 = 74.4$. A similar tactic can be used for Euclidean distance in more than two variables. Because the values of the variables may be correlated with one another, multivariable distance is usually measured instead with an entity called *Mahalanobis* D^2, which takes account of the covariances.

The diverse methods proposed for evaluating and joining distances have produced an extensive nomenclature, which is mentioned here just to give you an idea of the names. The measures of distance include *city block metric, genetic distance,* and *information radius.* The strategies[16] for joining distances can be called *single linkage, nearest neighbor, complete linkage, furthest neighbor, Ward's information loss, Lance and Williams' recurrence formula, monothetic* or *polythetic divisions,* and *minimizing traces* for matrixes showing dispersion of appropriate sums of squared values between and among groups.

28.4.3   Published Examples

Cluster analysis has been medically applied in various attempts to form "typologies" consisting of clustered categories that form subgroups for a particular ailment. Clinicians have formed many such subgroups judgmentally with staging systems for cancer, categories of *insulin-dependent* and *non-dependent* for diabetes mellitus, the various "non-" forms of disease nosology,[19] and many other purely clinical subclassifications. With cluster analysis methods, these judgments are replaced by a formal mathematical approach. Cluster analysis has been used to form subgroups for the clinical spectrum of back pain,[20] hepatitis,[21] chronic affective disorders,[22] insulin-dependent diabetes mellitus,[23] eating habits of obese patients,[24] and the previously illustrated partition of the temporomandibular joint syndrome.[17] Other relatively recent medical applications include efforts to categorize the geographic distribution of female cancer patterns in Belgium,[25] epidemiologic transitions in cause-specific mortality trends in The Netherlands,[26] and the resource utilization of Veterans Administration medical centers.[27]

In memorable nonmedical applications, cluster analysis was used to help identify an unknown mummy according to its craniofacial morphologic similarity with other Egyptian queens,[28] and to achieve a classification of 109 pure malt Scotch whiskies according to features of "nose, colour, body, palate and finish."[29]

In one medical application that reported use of cluster analysis, the investigators did *not* employ the customary many-internal, non-dependent-variable arrangement. After analyzing an array of variables that might be predictors of pre-term delivery, the investigators[30] divided each variable into binary categories, and then used the presence or absence of pre-term delivery to group the categories into three clusters of "risk": younger women, older women who were smokers, and nonsmoking older women. Because the grouping and clustering was done in direct relation to the outcome variable, this study is an example of the targeted multicategorical stratification procedure.

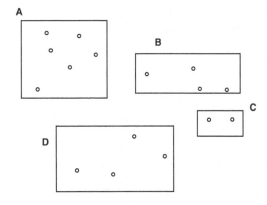

FIGURE 28.5

Illustration of a partition that forms four clusters, marked A, B, C, and D. (Figure taken from Chapter Reference 18.)

28.4.4 Epidemiologic Clusters

Beyond these statistical procedures, epidemiologists often use the word *cluster* in a quite different, nonmathematical way, referring to apparent mini-epidemics of disease. The mini-epidemic becomes noted when the scanners of vital-statistics data find a "spatial cluster," in which a particular disease seems to have an unexplainably increased occurrence either in calendar time or at a particular geographic location. The usual next step is to search for etiology of the spatial cluster by looking for correlations with suspected hazards such as contaminated water, nuclear power plants, electromagnetic radiation, or "toxic wastes." Various statistical methods have been and continue to be proposed for analyzing the geographic-temporal patterns of data[31] to find (or confirm) these clusters and their alleged causes.

Unfortunately, the investigators seldom consider checking data for the possibility that the "outbreak" is due to increased detection of the disease via increased screening, surveillance, and new diagnostic technologies in the selected spatial region. Other obvious possibilities are that the increase is a stochastic variation among the huge plethora of opportunities for "blips" when multitudes of different diseases are recorded for a multitude of geographic regions over a multitude of different points in time. After the needless fears induced by the publicity for diverse "clusters" that turned out to be etiologic "false alarms," the topic is now being approached with greater caution than formerly. Nevertheless, a media-sensitive and suitably zealous investigator can almost always get publicity for "discoveries" that can warn an already frightened public about yet another "menace" of daily life.[32]

28.5 Correspondence Analysis

In correspondence analysis, the variables are demarcated into categories (as in cluster analysis), but the operational strategy uses algebraic models, as in principal component analysis. The procedure has been advocated as a powerful method for analyzing multi-categorical contingency tables.[33]

Although seldom applied in medical activities, the correspondence analysis technique has been used[34] "to reduce the dimensions of the raw … (mainly) categorical data" in preparation for a cluster analysis that provided a "four group typology" of nonspecific low back pain, "using both organic and psychiatric symptoms and signs." In another application,[35] where the correspondence technique was combined with a Bayesian strategy, the arrays of symptoms, called *indicants*, in sets of patients with chest pain and with abdominal pain, were reduced and divided into clusters that were then "validated" for their accuracy in separating "risk groups" for various diagnoses.

28.6 Psychometric Attractions

Latent-variable analytic methods, such as factor and principal component analyses, have had substantial appeal in the world of psychometrics, where new indexes (or rating scales) are regularly prepared to "measure" such "constructs" as intelligence, social opinions, or health status, that cannot readily be cited in ordinary dimensions.

In the customary arrangement, a psychometric "instrument" contains a set of multiple items, each of which can be regarded as a variable. Each item often asks a question or makes an assertion for which the response is cited on a five-point (or other) scale that can refer to degrees of frequency (*never, ...,* *always*), agreement (*strongly disagree, ..., strongly agree*), volume (*none, ..., a lot*), or other pertinent expressions. The psychometrician usually begins with a large number of items (often more than 100) and tries to reduce them to a smaller group (perhaps 30 or fewer) that will provide a "unidimensional" representation of the selected construct.

To demonstrate that all the items refer to the same construct, i.e., the "latent variable," they are required to have the "homogeneity" shown by a high intercorrelation with one another. The index of multivariable intercorrelation is called *Cronbach's alpha*, but also receives other names (e.g., *Kuder-Richardson formula 20*) when the variables are expressed in binary categories rather than ordinal (or dimensional) scales.

The factor and principal component analyses usually produce several "constructs," rather than just one; but the individual factors are sometimes checked for the "internal reliability" demonstrated by a high value in Cronbach's alpha. (It was used in the previously cited study[12] of PANSS to support the construct "validity" of the "positive and general psychopathology scales.")

Despite the psychometric enthusiasm, the demonstration of "homogeneity" among multiple items is often contrary to clinimetric goals[36,37] in forming new indexes and rating scales. The clinician usually wants to combine *different* attributes into a single composite index (such as the Apgar Score or TNM staging system), not to join multiple items that all presumably measure the *same* attribute. If all the items express the same thing, the clinician may want to eliminate the ones that seem redundant. For example, in routinely assessing a patient's red blood status, an efficient clinician might examine the value of hematocrit or hemoglobin or red blood count, but not all three. A psychometrician, however, might combine all three into an index of erythematosity that would have a particularly high value for Cronbach's alpha. Furthermore, because Cronbach's alpha inevitably gets much higher when more items are included, an impressively high value may merely represent multiplicity of items rather than maximization of homogeneity.[38]

The psychometrician's methods may therefore be quite suitable for the goal of getting a "unidimensional construct," but ineffective (or misleading) when applied for the clinimetric goal of forming a multi-dimensional composite of different entities.

28.7 Scientific Problems and Challenges

Lacking an established criterion or a target variable to validate the results, the diverse forms of non-targeted analysis produce accomplishments that are wholly arbitrary. The approaches were at first rejected by most statisticians, but then began to gain respectability as the challenges became mathematically intriguing. For example, factor analysis was originally advocated and used exclusively in the psychosocial sciences, but is now often discussed as a statistical method. About 3 decades ago, Cormack[39] denounced the "irrelevantly and unjustifiably ... large quantities of multivariate data [summarized] by clusters, undefined *a priori* ... [as a] waste of more valuable time than any other statistical innovation." More recently, however, Hansen and Tukey[40] benevolently stated that clustering can "help with either graphical or verbal description ... [particularly] if we can avoid asking too much of clustering techniques." Hartigan[18] suggested that clustering can "be used routinely in the early stages of a data analysis in a similar way to drawing graphs or histograms," but his belief that "the classification of disease ... [is]

an important ... area of application" has not been confirmed when cluster methods were used for subsequent nosographic explorations.

Because every scientific taxonomy must have a specific purpose and function,[36] the main reason scientists do not like the various forms of non-targeted analysis is that the substantive goal of the classification may be neither identified nor overtly checked. The results depend completely on the mathematical methods used for the statistical arrangement and on the particular collection of data being analyzed. For example, *insulin-dependent diabetes mellitus*, although an important and well-recognized clinical category, might not emerge as a significant entity if the analytic data came from a clinic having very few such patients.

A separate scientific problem, particularly in nonclinical activities, is the "reification" that occurs when the factors or clusters, although constructed as acts of pure mathematics, become regarded as specific real entities. For example, a still raging controversy in the psychosocial sciences was provoked when *intelligence*, originally called a *g factor* in analyses by Spearman,[41] became advocated as a specific attribute of human biology. The initial dispute was whether the attribute was appropriately examined with "intelligence tests" and catalogued with factor-analytic gambits.[2] The more recent dispute arises from attempts[42] to separate genetic, ethnic, and environmental contributions to personal *intelligence*.

In a different application, the principal component method has been proposed for solving problems of multicollinearity in regression analysis. When multiple "independent" variables are regressed against a single target variable, efforts are often made to eliminate the independent variables that are highly correlated with one another. To avoid the sometimes invidious choice of deciding which variables are redundant, the principal component method might allow all of them to be retained when reformulated as suitably constructed new principal-component variables. Despite the theoretical attractiveness, the approach was recently shown to have major flaws and "very serious potential pitfalls" when checked in several "well-known data sets."[43]

In an intriguing investigation, Juniper et al.[44] compared "two philosophically different methods for selecting items for a disease-specific quality of life questionnaire." One method was a psychometric factor analysis. The other was an "impact approach" in which patients with asthma chose what they regarded as important. The investigators found substantial agreement in many of the selections, but also noted that the psychometric approach produced items that did not always "make clinical sense" while omitting "three items of the greatest importance to patients."

In medical applications, non-targeted analyses seem to attain face validity only when clinicians agree that the results are "sensible." For example, to avoid idiosyncratic effects from 30 individual variables that could be used in prognostic prediction for a cohort of 4226 patients receiving coronary angiography, Harrell et al.[45] tried the "parsimonious approach" of grouping the variables into more "simple indices." The approach depended on clusters formed after a principal component analysis, but the actual clinical index for each group was created only after the variables were "further grouped" by "two cardiologists." The 5 indexes that emerged referred to pain, myocardial damage, vascular disease, risk factors, and conduction defects; and 5 of the original variables were left "standing alone." These 10 entities then gave a better prognostic performance than the original 30 variables alone and were just as effective (but more comprehensible) than the results of the original principal component analysis. The authors recommended use of the "clustering method for clinical prediction problems when the number of potential predictor variables is large" but also stated that "the more clinical insight one injects into the analysis at any point, the better is the end result."

If clinical "insight" is indeed valuable, however, clinicians might be urged more often to take the incentive in creating suitable classifications by working from "inside-out" in the manner used by Virginia Apgar and other clinical taxonomists. The need for mathematical approaches, working from "outside-in," seems to arise only when clinicians have been delinquent in meeting their own intellectual responsibilities.[36,46,47] If connoisseurs of the substantive phenomena have not made suitable taxonomic efforts, the mathematical procedures will obviously seem more attractive than nothing. On the other hand, if non-targeted analytic methods are not guided by a substantive direction or orientation, the approach can perhaps be best summarized with the waggish remark once made to me by the late Donald Mainland: "If you don't know what you're doing, factor analysis is a great way to do it."

References

1. Apgar, 1953; 2. Gould, 1981; 3. Kendall, 1968; 4. Chandra Sekhar, 1991; 5. Mason, 1988; 6. Goold, 1994; 7. Ries, 1991; 8. Bailey, 1992; 9. Lauer, 1993; 10. Henderson, 1990; 11. Oden, 1992; 12. von Knorring, 1995; 13. Aubert, 1990; 14. Cowie, 1985; 15. Flameng, 1984; 16. Everitt, 1993; 17. Wastell, 1987; 18. Hartigan, 1973; 19. Ellman, 1985; 20. Heinrich, 1985; 21. Persico, 1993; 22. Furukawa, 1992; 23. Ciampi, 1990; 24. Schlundt, 1991; 25. Thielemans, 1988; 26. Wolleswinkel-van den Bosch, 1997; 27. Krim, 1987; 28. Harris, 1978; 29. Lapointe, 1994; 30. Peacock, 1995; 31. Waller, 1995; 32. Feinstein, 1988a; 33. Hill, 1974; 34. Coste, 1991; 35. Crichton, 1989; 36. Feinstein, 1987a; 37. Wright, 1992; 38. Steiner, 1995; 39. Cormack, 1971; 40. Hansen, 1992; 41. Spearman, 1904; 42. Herrnstein, 1994; 43. Hadi, 1998; 44. Juniper, 1997; 45. Harrell, 1984; 46. Feinstein, 1967a; 47. Feinstein, 1994.

29

Analysis of Variance

CONTENTS

The targeted analytic method called *analysis of variance*, sometimes cited acronymically as ANOVA, was devised (like so many other procedures in statistics) by Sir Ronald A. Fisher. Although often marking the conceptual boundary between elementary and advanced statistics, or between amateur "fan" and professional connoisseur, ANOVA is sometimes regarded and taught as "elementary" enough to be used for deriving subsequent simple procedures, such as the t test. Nevertheless, ANOVA is used much less often today than formerly, for reasons to be noted in the discussions that follow.

29.1 Conceptual Background

The main distinguishing feature of ANOVA is that the independent variable contains polytomous categories, which are analyzed simultaneously in relation to a dimensional or ordinal dependent (outcome) variable.

Suppose treatments A, B, and C are tested for effects on blood pressure in a randomized trial. When the results are examined, we want to determine whether one of the treatments differs significantly from the others. With the statistical methods available thus far, the only way to answer this question would be to do multiple comparisons for pairs of groups, contrasting results in group A vs. B, A vs. C, and B vs. C. If more ambitious, we could compare A vs. the combined results of B and C, or group B vs. the combined results of A and C, and so on. We could work out various other arrangements, but in each instance, the comparison would rely on contrasting two collected groups, because we currently know no other strategy.

The analysis of variance allows a single *simultaneous* "comparison" for three or more groups. The result becomes a type of screening test that indicates whether at least one group differs significantly from the others, but further examination is needed to find the distinctive group(s). Despite this disadvantage, ANOVA has been a widely used procedure, particularly by professional statisticians, who often like to apply it even when simpler tactics are available. For example, when data are compared for only two groups, a t test or Z test is simpler, and, as noted later, produces exactly the same results as ANOVA. Nevertheless, many persons will do the two-group comparison (and report the results) with an analysis of variance.

29.1.1 Clinical Illustration

Although applicable in experimental trials, ANOVA has been most often used for observational studies. A real-world example, shown in Figure 29.1, contains data for the survival times, in months, of a random sample of 60 patients with lung cancer,[1,2] having one of the four histologic categories of WELL (well-differentiated), SMALL (small cell), ANAP (anaplastic), and CYTOL (cytology only). The other variable (the five categories of TNM stage) listed in Figure 29.1 will be considered later. The main analytic question now is whether histology in any of these groups has significantly different effects on survival.

29.1.1.1 *Direct Examination* — The best thing to do with these data, before any formal statistical analyses begin, is to examine the results directly. In this instance, we can readily determine the group sizes, means, and standard deviations for each of the four histologic categories and for the total. The results, shown in Table 29.1, immediately suggest that the data do not have Gaussian distributions, because the standard deviations are almost all larger than the means. Nevertheless, to allow the illustration to proceed, the results can be further appraised. They show that the well-differentiated and small-cell groups, as expected clinically, have the highest and lowest mean survival times, respectively. Because of relatively small group sizes and non-Gaussian distributions, however, the distinctions may not be stochastically significant.

TABLE 29.1

Summary of Survival Times in Four Histologic Groups
of Patients with Lung Cancer in Figure 29.1

Histologic Category	Group Size	Mean Survival	Standard Deviation
WELL	22	24.43	26.56
SMALL	11	4.45	3.77
ANAP	18	10.87	23.39
CYTOL	9	11.54	13.47
Total	60	14.77	22.29

Again before applying any advanced statistics, we can check these results stochastically by using simple t tests. For the most obvious comparison of WELL vs. SMALL, we can use the components of Formula [13.7] to calculate $s_p = \sqrt{[21(26.56)^2 + 10(3.77)^2]/(21 + 10)} = 21.96$; $(1/n_A) + (1/n_B) = (1/22) + (1/11) = .369$; and $\overline{X}_A - \overline{X}_B = 24.43 - 4.45 = 19.98$. These data could then be entered into Formula [13.7] to produce $t = 9.98/[(21.96)(.369)] = 2.47$. At 31 d.f., the associated 2P value is about .02. From this distinction, we might also expect that all the other paired comparisons will *not* be stochastically significant. (If you check the calculations, you will find that the appropriate 2P values are all >.05.)

29.1.1.2 *"Holistic" and Multiple-Comparison Problems* — The foregoing comparison indicates a "significant" difference in mean survival between the WELL and SMALL groups, but does not answer the "holistically" phrased analytic question, which asked whether histology has significant effects in *any* of the four groups in the entire collection. Besides, an argument could be made, using

distinctions discussed in Section 25.2.1.1, that the contrast of WELL vs. SMALL was only one of the six ($4 \times 3/2$) possible paired comparisons for the four histologic categories. With the Bonferroni correction, the working level of α' for each of the six comparisons would be $.05/6 = .008$. With the latter criterion, the 2P value of about .02 for WELL vs. SMALL would no longer be stochastically significant.

We therefore need a new method to answer the original question. Instead of examining six pairs of contrasted means, we can use a holistic approach by finding the grand mean of the data, determining the deviations of each group of data from that mean, and analyzing those deviations appropriately.

OBS	ID	HISTOL	TNMSTAGE	SURVIVE
1	62	WELL	I	82.3
2	107	WELL	II	5.3
3	110	WELL	IIIA	29.6
4	157	WELL	I	20.3
5	163	WELL	I	54.9
6	246	SMALL	I	10.3
7	271	WELL	IIIB	1.6
8	282	ANAP	IIIA	7.6
9	302	WELL	I	28.0
10	337	CYTOL	I	12.8
11	344	WELL	II	4.0
12	352	ANAP	IIIA	1.3
13	371	WELL	IIIB	14.1
14	387	SMALL	IIIA	0.2
15	428	SMALL	II	6.8
16	466	ANAP	IIIB	1.4
17	513	ANAP	I	0.1
18	548	ANAP	IV	1.8
19	581	ANAP	IV	6.0
20	605	CYTOL	IV	1.0
21	609	CYTOL	IV	6.2
22	628	SMALL	IV	4.4
23	671	SMALL	IV	5.5
24	764	SMALL	IV	0.3
25	784	ANAP	IV	1.6
26	804	WELL	I	12.2
27	806	ANAP	IIIB	6.5
28	815	WELL	I	39.9
29	852	WELL	IIIB	4.5
30	855	WELL	II	1.6
31	891	CYTOL	IIIB	8.1
32	892	WELL	IIIB	62.0
33	931	CYTOL	IIIB	8.8
34	998	WELL	IIIB	0.2
35	1039	SMALL	IV	0.6
36	1044	ANAP	II	19.3
37	1054	WELL	IIIB	0.6
38	1057	ANAP	I	10.9
39	1155	ANAP	I	0.2
40	1192	SMALL	IV	11.2
41	1223	ANAP	IV	0.9
42	1228	ANAP	II	27.9
43	1303	ANAP	IIIB	2.9
44	1309	ANAP	II	99.9
45	1317	ANAP	IV	4.7
46	1355	CYTOL	IIIB	1.8
47	1361	WELL	IV	1.0
48	1380	CYTOL	IV	10.6
49	1405	SMALL	IV	3.7
50	1444	WELL	II	55.9
51	1509	SMALL	IV	3.4
52	1515	WELL	I	79.7
53	1521	ANAP	IV	1.9
54	1556	ANAP	IIIB	0.8
55	1567	SMALL	IV	2.5
56	1608	CYTOL	I	8.6
57	1612	WELL	IIIA	13.3
58	1666	CYTOL	IV	46.0
59	1702	WELL	II	23.9
60	1738	WELL	II	2.6

FIGURE 29.1

Printout of data on histologic type, TNM Stage, and months of survival in a random sample of 60 patients with primary cancer of the lung. [OBS = observation number in sample; ID = original indentification number; HISTOL = histology type; TNMSTAGE = one of five ordinal anatomic TNM stages for lung cancer; SURVIVE = survival time (mos.); WELL = well-differentiated; SMALL = small cell; ANAP = anaplastic; CYTOL = cytology only.]

Many different symbols have been used to indicate the entities that are involved. In the illustration here, Y_{ij} will represent the target variable (survival time) for person i in group j. For example, if WELL is the first group in Figure 29.1, the eighth person in the group has $Y_{8,1} = 4.0$. The mean of the values in group j will be $\overline{Y}_j = \Sigma Y_{ij}/n_j$, where n_j is the number of members in the group. Thus, for the last group (cytology) in Table 29.1, $n_4 = 9$, $\Sigma Y_{i,4} = 103.9$, and $\overline{Y}_4 = 103.9/9 = 11.54$. The grand mean, $\overline{G}$, will be $\Sigma (n_j\overline{Y}_j)/N$, where $N = \Sigma n_j = $ size of the total group under analysis. From the data in Table 29.1, $G = [(22 \times 24.43) + (11 \times 4.45) + (18 \times 10.87) + (9 \times 11.54)]/60 = 885.93/60 = 14.77$.

We can now determine the distance, $\overline{Y}_j - \overline{G}$, between each group's mean and the grand mean. For the ANAP group, the distance is $10.87 - 14.77 = -3.90$. For the other three groups, the distances are -3.23 for CYTOL, -10.32 for SMALL, and $+9.66$ for WELL. This inspection confirms that the means of the SMALL and WELL groups are most different from the grand mean, but the results contain no attention to stochastic variation in the data.

29.1.2   Analytic Principles

To solve the stochastic challenge, we can use ANOVA, which like many other classical statistical strategies, expresses real world phenomena with mathematical models. We have already used such models both implicitly and explicitly. In univariate statistics, the mean, $\overline{Y}$, was an *implicit* "model" for fitting a group of data from only the values in the single set of data. The measured deviations from that model, $Y_i - \overline{Y}$, were then converted to the group's basic variance, $\Sigma(Y_i - \overline{Y})^2$.

In bivariate statistics for the associations in Chapters 18 and 19, we used an explicit model based on an additional variable, expressed algebraically as $\hat{Y}_i = a + bX_i$. We then compared variances for three sets of deviations: $Y_i - \hat{Y}_i$, between the items of data and the explicit model; $Y_i - \overline{Y}$, between the items of data and the implicit model; and $\hat{Y}_i - \overline{Y}$, between the explicit and implicit models. The group variances or sums of squares associated with these deviations were called *residual* (or "error") for $\Sigma(Y_i - \hat{Y}_i)^2$, *basic* for $\Sigma(Y_i - \overline{Y})^2$, and *model* for $\Sigma(\hat{Y}_i - \overline{Y})^2$.

29.1.2.1   Distinctions in Nomenclature — The foregoing symbols and nomenclature have been simplified for the sake of clarity. In strict statistical reasoning, any set of observed data is regarded as a sample from an unobserved population whose parameters are being estimated from the data. If "modeled" with a straight line, the parametric population would be cited as $Y = \alpha + \beta X$. When the results for the observed data are expressed as $\hat{Y}_i = a + bX_i$, the coefficients a and b are estimates of the corresponding α and β parameters.

Also in strict reasoning, *variance* is an attribute of the parametric population. Terms such as $\Sigma(Y_i - \overline{Y})^2$ or $\Sigma(\hat{Y}_i - \overline{Y})^2$, which are used to estimate the parametric variances, should be called sums of squares, not group variances. The linguistic propriety has been violated here for two reasons: (1) the distinctions are more easily understood when called *variance*, and (2) the violations constantly appear in both published literature and computer print-outs. The usage here, although a departure from strict formalism, is probably better than in many discussions elsewhere where the sums of squares are called *variances* instead of *group variances*.

Another issue in nomenclature is syntactical rather than mathematical. In most English prose, *between* is used for a distinction of two objects, and *among* for more than two. Nevertheless, in the original description of the analysis of variance, R. A. Fisher used the preposition *between* rather than *among* when more than two groups or classes were involved. The term *between groups* has been perpetuated by subsequent writers, much to the delight of English-prose pedants who may denounce the absence of literacy in mathematical technocracy. Nevertheless, Fisher and his successors have been quite correct in maintaining *between*. Its use for the cited purpose is approved by diverse high-echelon authorities, including the *Oxford English Dictionary*, which states that "*between* has been, from its earliest appearance, extended to more than two."[3] [As one of the potential pedants, I was ready to use *among* in this text until I checked the dictionary and became enlightened.]

29.1.2.2   Partition of Group Variance — The same type of partitioning that was used for group variance in linear regression is also applied in ANOVA. Conceptually, however, the models are expressed differently. Symbolically, each observation can be labelled Y_{ij}, with j representing the group and i, the person (or other observed entity) within the group. The grand mean, $\overline{G}$, is used for the "implicit model" when the basic group or system variance, $\Sigma(Y_i - \overline{G})^2$, is summed for the individual values of Y_i in all of the groups. The individual group means, $\overline{Y}_j$, become the explicit models when the total system is partitioned into groups. The residual group variance is the sum of the values of $\Sigma(Y_i - \overline{Y}_j)^2$ within each of the groups. [In more accurate symbolism, the two cited group variances would be written with double subscripts and summations as $\Sigma\Sigma(Y_{ij} - \overline{G})^2$ and $\Sigma\Sigma(Y_{ij} - \overline{Y}_j)^2$.] The model group variance, summed for each group of n_j members with group mean $\overline{Y}_j$, is $\Sigma n_j(\overline{Y}_j - \overline{G})^2$. These results for data in the four groups of Figure 29.1 and Table 29.1 are shown in Table 29.2.

TABLE 29.2

Group-Variance Partitions of Sums of Squares for the Four Histologic Groups in Figure 29.1 and Table 29.1

Group	Basic (Total System)	Model (Between Groups)	Residual (Within Groups)
WELL	16866.67	$22(24.43 - 14.77)^2 = 2052.94$	14813.73
SMALL	1313.52	$11(4.45 - 14.77)^2 = 1171.53$	141.99
ANAP	9576.88	$18(10.87 - 14.77)^2 = 273.78$	9303.10
CYTOL	1546.32	$9(11.54 - 14.77)^2 = 93.90$	1452.42
Total	29304.61*	3593.38*	25711.24

* These are the correct totals. They differ slightly from the sum of the collection of individual values, calculated with rounding, in each column.

Except for minor differences due to rounding, the components of Table 29.2 have the same structure noted earlier for simple linear regression in Section 19.2.2. The structure is as follows:

{Basic Group Variance} = {Model Variance between Groups} + { Residual Variance within Groups}

or $S_{yy} = S_M + S_R$.

The structure is similar to that of the deviations

Total Deviation = Model Deviation + Residual Deviation

which arises when each individual deviation is expressed in the algebraic identity

$$Y_{ij} - \overline{G} = (\overline{Y}_j - \overline{G}) + (Y_{ij} - \overline{Y}_j)$$

If $\overline{G}$ is moved to the first part of the right side, the equation becomes

$$Y_{ij} = \overline{G} + (\overline{Y}_j - \overline{G}) + (Y_{ij} - \overline{Y}_j)$$

and is consistent with a parametric algebraic model that has the form

$$Y_{ij} = \mu + \gamma_j + \varepsilon_{ij}$$

In this model, each person's value of Y_{ij} consists of three contributions: (1) from the grand parametric mean, μ (which is estimated by $\overline{G}$); (2) from the parametric increment, γ_j (estimated by $\overline{Y}_j - \overline{G}$), between the grand mean and group mean; and (3) from an error term, ε_{ij} (estimated by $Y_{ij} - \overline{Y}_j$), for the increment between the observed value of Y_{ij} and the group mean.

For stochastic appraisal of results, the null hypothesis assumption is that the m groups have the same parametric mean, i.e., $\gamma_1 = \gamma_2 = \ldots = \gamma_j = \ldots = \gamma_m$.

29.1.2.3   Mean Variances and Degrees of Freedom — When divided by the associated degrees of freedom, each of the foregoing group variances is converted to a mean value. For the basic group variance, the total system contains $N = \Sigma n_j$ members, and d.f. $= N - 1$. For the model variance, the m groups have $m - 1$ degrees of freedom. For the residual variance, each group has $n_j - 1$ degrees of freedom, and the total d.f. for m groups is $\Sigma(n_j - 1) = N - m$.

The degrees of freedom are thus partitioned, like the group variances, into an expression that indicates their sum as

$$N - 1 = (m - 1) + (N - m)$$

The mean variances, however, no longer form an equal partition. Their symbols, and the associated values in the example here, are as follows:

$$\text{Mean Group Variance} = S_{yy}/(N - 1) = 29304.61/59 = 496.69$$

$$\text{Mean Model Variance} = S_M/(m - 1) = 3593.38/3 = 1197.79$$
$$\text{(between groups)}$$

$$\text{Mean Residual Variance} = S_R/(N - m) = 25711.24/56 = 459.13$$
$$\text{(within groups)}$$

29.2   Fisher's F Ratio

Under the null hypothesis of no real difference between the groups—i.e., the assumption that they have the same parametric mean—each of the foregoing three mean variances can be regarded as a separate estimate of the true parametric variance. Within the limits of stochastic variation in random sampling, the three mean variances should equal one another.

To test stochastic significance, R. A. Fisher constructed a variance ratio, later designated as F, that is expressed as

$$\frac{\text{Mean variance between groups}}{\text{Mean variance within groups}}$$

It can be cited symbolically as

$$F = \frac{S_M/(m-1)}{S_R/(N-m)} \qquad [29.1]$$

If only two groups are being compared, some simple algebra will show that Formula [29.1] becomes the square of the earlier Formula [13.7] for the calculation of t (or Z). This distinction is the reason why the F ratio is sometimes used, instead of t (or Z), for contrasting two groups, as noted earlier in Section 13.3.6.

The Fisher ratio has a sampling distribution in which the associated 2P value is found for the values of F at the two sets of degrees of freedom in values of $m - 1$ and $N - m$. The three components make the distribution difficult to tabulate completely; and it is usually cited according to values for F for each degree of freedom simultaneously at fixed values of 2P such as .1, .05, .01.

In the example under discussion here, the F ratio is $1197.79/459.13 = 2.61$. In the Geigy tables[4] available for the combination of 3 and 56 degrees of freedom, the required F values are 2.184 for 2P = .1, 2.769 for 2P = .05, and 3.359 for 2P = .025. If only the Geigy values were available, the result would be written as $.05 < 2P < .1$. In an appropriate computer program, however, the actual 2P value is usually calculated and displayed directly. In this instance, it was .0605.

If 2P is small enough to lead to rejection of the null hypothesis, the stochastic conclusion is that at least one of the groups has a mean significantly different from the others. Because the counter-hypothesis for the F test is always that the mean variance is larger between groups than within them, the null hypothesis can promptly be conceded if the F ratio is < 1. In this instance, because the null hypothesis cannot be rejected at $\alpha = .05$, we cannot conclude that a significant difference in survival has been stochastically confirmed for the histologic categories. The observed quantitative distinctions seem impressive, however, and would probably attain stochastic significance if the group sizes were larger.

29.3 Analysis-of-Variance Table

The results of an analysis of variance are commonly presented, in both published literature and computer printouts, with a tabular arrangement that warrants special attention because it is used not only for ANOVA but also for multivariable regression procedures that involve partitioning the sums of squared deviations (SS) that form group variances.

In each situation, the results show the partition for the sums of squares of three entities: (1) the total SS before imposition of an explicit model, (2) the SS between the explicit model and the original implicit grand mean, and (3) the residual SS for the explicit model. The last of these entities is often called the "unexplained" or "error" variance. Both of these terms are unfortunate because the mathematical "explanation" is a statistical phenomenon that may have nothing to do with biologic mechanisms of explanation and the "error" represents deviations between observed and estimated values, not mistakes or inaccuracies in the basic data. In certain special arrangements, to be discussed shortly, the deviations receive an additionally improved "explanation" when the model is enhanced with subdivisions of the main variable or with the incorporation of additional variables.

Figure 29.2 shows the conventional headings for the ANOVA table of the histology example in Figure 29.1. For this "one-way" analysis, the total results are divided into two rows of components. The number of rows is appropriately expanded when more subgroups are formed (as discussed later) via such mechanisms as subdivisions or inclusion of additional variables.

Dependent Variable: SURVIVE

Source	DF	Sum of Squares	Mean Square	F Value	Pr > F
Model	3	3593.3800000	1197.7933333	2.61	0.0605
Error	56	25711.2333333	459.1291667		
Corrected Total	59	29304.6133333			

R-Square	C.V.	Root MSE	SURVIVE Mean
0.122622	145.1059	21.427300	14.766667

FIGURE 29.2
Printout of analysis-of-variance table for survival time in the four histologic groups of Figure 29.1.

29.4 Problems in Performance

The mathematical reasoning used in many ANOVA arrangements was developed for an ideal experimental world in which all the compared groups or subgroups had the same size. If four groups were being compared, each group had the same number of members, so that $n_1 = n_2 = n_3 = n_4$. If the groups were further divided into subgroups—such as **men** and **women** or **young**, **middle-aged**, and **old**—the subgroups had the same sizes within each group.

These equi-sized arrangements were easily attained for experiments in the world of agriculture, where R. A. Fisher worked and developed his ideas about ANOVA. Equally sized groups and subgroups are seldom achieved, however, in the realities of clinical and epidemiologic research. The absence of equal sizes may then create a major problem in the operation of computer programs that rely on equal sizes, and that may be unable to manage data for other circumstances. For the latter situations, the computer programs may divert ANOVA into the format of a "general linear model," which is essentially a method of multiple regression. One main reason, therefore, why regression methods are replacing ANOVA methods today is that the automated regression methods can more easily process data for unequal-sized groups and subgroups.

29.5 Problems of Interpretation

The results of an analysis of variance are often difficult to interpret for both quantitative and stochastic reasons, as well as for substantive decisions.

29.5.1 Quantitative Distinctions

The results of ANOVA are almost always cited with F ratios and P values that indicate stochastic accomplishments but not quantitative descriptive distinctions. The reader is thus left without a mechanism to decide what has been accomplished quantitatively, while worrying that "significant" P values may arise mainly from large group sizes.

Although not commonly used, a simple statistical index can provide a quantitative description of the results. The index, called *eta squared*, was previously discussed in Section 27.2.2 as a counterpart of r^2 for proportionate reduction of group variance in linear regression. Labeled "R-square" in the printout of Figure 29.2, the expression is

$$\eta^2 = \frac{\text{Model (between-group) variance}}{\text{Total system (basic) variance}} = \frac{S_M}{S_{yy}}$$

For the histologic data in Figure 29.2, this index is $3593.38/29304.61 = 0.12$, representing a modest achievement, which barely exceeds the 10% noted earlier (see Section 19.3.3) as a minimum level for "quantitative significance" in variance reduction.

29.5.2 Stochastic "Nonsignificance"

Another important issue is what to do when a result is *not* stochastically significant, i.e., $P > \alpha$. In previous analytic methods, a confidence interval could be calculated around the "nonsignificant" increment, ratio, or coefficient that described the observed d_O distinction in the results. If the upper end of this confidence interval excluded a quantitatively significant value (such as δ), the result could be called stochastically *nonsignificant*. If the confidence interval included δ, the investigator might be reluctant to concede the null hypothesis of "no difference."

This type of reasoning would be equally pertinent for ANOVA, but is rarely used because the results seldom receive a descriptive citation. Confidence intervals, although sometimes calculated for the mean of each group, are almost never determined to give the value of eta the same type of upper and lower confidence boundaries that can be calculated around a correlation coefficient in simple linear regression.

In the absence of a confidence interval for eta, the main available descriptive approach is to examine results in individual groups or in paired comparisons. If any of the results seem quantitatively significant, the investigator, although still conceding the null hypothesis (because $P > \alpha$), can remain suspicious that a "significant" difference exists, but has not been confirmed stochastically. For example, in Figure 29.2, the P value of 0.06 would not allow rejection of the null hypothesis that all group means are equal. Nevertheless, the modestly impressive value of 0.12 for eta squared and the large increment noted earlier between the WELL and SMALL group means suggest that the group sizes were too small for stochastic confirmation of what is probably a quantitatively "significant" distinction.

29.5.3 Stochastic "Significance"

If $P < \alpha$, the analysis has identified something that is stochastically significant, and the next step is to find where it is located. As noted earlier, the search involves a series of paired comparisons. A system containing m groups will allow $m(m - 1)/2$ paired comparisons when each group's mean is contrasted against the mean of every other group. With m additional paired comparisons between each group and the total of the others, the total number of paired comparisons will be $m(m + 1)/2$. For example, the small-cell histologic group in Table 29.1 could be compared against each of the three other groups and also against their total. A particularly ingenious (or desperate) investigator might compare a single group or paired groups against pairs (or yet other combinations) of the others.

This plethora of activities produces the multiple comparison problem discussed in Chapter 25, as well as the multiple eponymous and striking titles (such as Tukey's *honestly significant difference*[5]) that have been given to the procedures proposed for examining and solving the problem.

29.5.4   Substantive Decisions

Because the foregoing solutions all depend on arbitrary mathematical mechanisms, investigators who are familiar with the substantive content of the data usually prefer to avoid the polytomous structure of the analysis of variance. For example, a knowledgeable investigator might want to compare only the SMALL vs. WELL groups with a direct 2-group contrast (such as a t test) in the histologic data, avoiding the entire ANOVA process. An even more knowledgeable investigator, recognizing that survival can be affected by many factors (such as *TNM stage* and *age*) other than histologic category, might not want to do any type of histologic appraisal unless the other cogent variables have been suitably accounted for.

For all these reasons, ANOVA is a magnificent method of analyzing data if you are unfamiliar with what the data really mean or represent. If you know the substantive content of the research, however, and if you have specific ideas to be examined, you may want to use a simpler and more direct way of examining them.

29.6   Additional Applications of ANOVA

From a series of mathematical models and diverse arrangements, the analysis of variance has a versatility, analogous to that discussed earlier for chi square, that for many years made ANOVA the most commonly used statistical procedure for analyzing complex data. In recent years, however, the ubiquitous availability of computers has led to the frequent replacement of ANOVA by multiple regression procedures, whose results are often easier to understand. Besides, ANOVA can mathematically be regarded as a subdivision of the general-linear-model strategies used in multivariable regression analysis.

Accordingly, four of the many other applications of ANOVA are outlined here only briefly, mainly so that you will have heard of them in case you meet them (particularly in older literature). Details can be found in many statistical textbooks. The four procedures to be discussed are multi-factor arrangements, nested analyses, the analysis of covariance (ANCOVA), and repeated-measures arrangements (including the intraclass correlation coefficient).

29.6.1   Multi-Factor Arrangements

The procedures discussed so far are called *one-way* analyses of variance, because only a single independent variable (i.e., histologic category) was examined in relation to survival time. In many circumstances, however, two or more independent variables can be regarded as "factors" affecting the dependent variable. When these additional factors are included, the analysis is called *two-way* (or *two-factor*), *three-way* (or *three-factor*), etc.

For example, if the two factors of histologic category and TNM stage are considered simultaneously, the data for the 60 patients in Figure 29.1 would be arranged as shown in Table 29.3. The identification of individual survival times would require triple subscripts: i for the person, j for the row, and k for the column.

TABLE 29.3

Two-Way Arrangement of Individual Data for Survival Time (in Months)
of Patients with Lung Cancer

Histologic Category	TNM Stage					Mean for Total Row Category
	I	**II**	**IIIA**	**IIIB**	**IV**	
Well	82.3	5.3	29.6	1.6	1.0	
	20.3	4.0	13.3	14.1		
	54.9	1.6		4.5		
	28.0	55.9		62.0		24.43
	12.2	23.9		0.2		
	39.9	2.6		0.6		
	79.7					
Small	10.3	6.8	0.2	—	4.4	
					5.5	
					0.3	
					0.6	
					11.2	4.45
					3.7	
					3.4	
					2.5	
Anap	0.1	19.3	7.6	1.4	1.8	
	10.9	27.9	1.3	6.5	6.0	
	0.2	99.9		2.9	1.6	10.87
				0.8	0.9	
					4.7	
					1.9	
Cytol	12.8	—	—	8.1	1.0	
	8.6			8.8	6.2	11.54
				1.8	10.6	
					46.0	
Mean for Total Column Category	27.7	24.72	10.40	8.72	5.96	14.77

29.6.1.1 "Main Effects"

— In the mathematical model of the two-way arrangement, the categorical mean for each factor—Histology and TNM Stage—makes a separate contribution, called the "main effect," beyond the grand mean. The remainder (or unexplained) deviation for each person is called the residual error. Thus, a two-factor model for the two independent variables would express the observed results as

$$Y_{ijk} = \overline{G} + (\overline{Y}_j - \overline{G}) + (\overline{Y}_k - \overline{G}) + (Y_{ijk} - \overline{Y}_j - \overline{Y}_k + \overline{G}) \qquad [29.2]$$

The $\overline{G}$ term here represents the grand mean. The next two terms represent the respective deviations of each row mean ($\overline{Y}_j$) and each column mean ($\overline{Y}_k$) from the grand mean. The four components in the last term for the residual deviation of each person are constructed as "residuals" that maintain the algebraic identity. The total sum of squares in the system will be $\Sigma(Y_{ijk} - \overline{G})^2$, with $N - 1$ degrees of freedom. There will be two sums of squares for the model, cited as $\Sigma n_j(\overline{Y}_j - \overline{G})^2$ for the row factor, and as $\Sigma n_k(\overline{Y}_k - \overline{G})^2$ for the column factor. The residual sum of squares will be the sum of all the values of $(Y_{ijk} - \overline{Y}_j - \overline{Y}_k + \overline{G})^2$.

Figure 29.3 shows the printout of pertinent calculations for the data in Table 29.3. In the lower half of Figure 29.3, the 4-category histologic variable has 3 degrees of freedom and its "Type I SS" (sum of squares) and mean square, respectively, are the same 3593.38 and 1197.79 shown earlier. The 5-category TNM-stage variable has 4 degrees of freedom and corresponding values of 3116.39 and 779.10. The residual error group variance in the upper part of the table is now calculated differently—as the "corrected

Dependent Variable: SURVIVE

Source	DF	Sum of Squares	Mean Square	F Value	Pr > F
Model	7	6709.7729638	958.5389948	2.21	0.0486
Error	52	22594.8403695	434.5161610		
Corrected Total	59	29304.6133333			

	R-Square	C.V.	Root MSE	SURVIVE Mean
	0.228966	141.1629	20.845051	14.766667

Source	DF	Type I SS	Mean Square	F Value	Pr > F
HISTOL	3	3593.3800000	1197.7933333	2.76	0.0515
TNMSTAGE	4	3116.3929638	779.0982410	1.79	0.1443

FIGURE 29.3
Printout for 2-way ANOVA of data in Figure 29.1 and Table 29.3.

total" sum of squares minus the sum of Type I squares, which is a total of 6709.77 for the two factors in the model. Since those two factors have 7 (=3 + 4) degrees of freedom, the mean square for the model is 6709.77/7 = 958.54, and the d.f. in the error variance is 59 − 7 = 52. The mean square for the error variance becomes 22594.84/52 = 434.52. When calculated for this two-factor model, the F ratio of mean squares is 2.21, which now achieves a P value (marked "Pr > F") just below .05. If the α level is set at .05, this result is "significant," whereas it was not so in the previous analysis for histology alone.

The label "Type I SS" is used because ANOVA calculations can also produce three other types of sums of squares (marked II, III, and IV when presented) that vary with the order in which factors are entered or removed in a model, and with consideration of the interactions discussed in the next section. As shown in the lower section of Figure 29.3, an F-ratio value can be calculated for each factor when its mean square is divided by the "error" mean square. For histology, this ratio is 1197.79/434.52 = 2.76. For TNM stage, the corresponding value in the printout is 1.79. The corresponding 2P values are just above .05 for histology and .14 for TNM stage.

29.6.1.2   Interactions

29.6.1.2   Interactions — In linear models, each factor is assumed to have its own separate additive effect. In biologic reality, however, the conjunction of two factors may have an antagonistic or synergistic effect beyond their individual actions, so that the whole differs from the sum of the parts. For example, increasing weight and increasing blood pressure may each lead to increasing mortality, but their combined effect may be particularly pronounced in persons who are at the extremes of obesity and hypertension. Statisticians use the term *interactions* for these conjunctive effects; and the potential for interactions is often considered whenever an analysis contains two or more factors.

To examine these effects in a two-factor analysis, the model for Y_{ijk} is expanded to contain an interaction term. It is calculated, for the mean of each cell of the conjoined categories, as the deviation from the product of mean values of the pertinent row and column variables for each cell. In the expression of the equation for Y_{ijk}, the first three terms of Equation [29.2] are the same: $\overline{G}$, for the grand mean; $\overline{Y}_j - \overline{G}$ for each row; and $\overline{Y}_k - \overline{G}$ for each column. Because the observed mean in each cell will be $\overline{Y}_{jk}$, the interaction effect will be the deviation estimated as $\overline{Y}_{jk} - \overline{Y}_j - \overline{Y}_k + \overline{G}$. The remaining residual effect, used for calculating the residual sum of squares, is $Y_{ijk} - \overline{Y}_{jk}$. For each sum of squares, the degrees of freedom are determined appropriately for the calculations of mean squares and F ratios.

The calculation of interaction effects can be illustrated with an example from the data of Table 29.3 for the 7-member cell in the first row, first column. The grand mean is 14.77; the entire WELL histologic category has a mean of 24.43; and TNM stage I has a mean of 27.71. The mean of the seven values in the cited cell is (82.3 + 20.3 + ⋯ + 79.7)/7 = 45.33. According to the algebraic equation, $\overline{G}$ = 14.77; in the first row, $(\overline{Y}_j - \overline{G})$ = 24.43 − 14.77 = 9.66; and in the first column, $(\overline{Y}_k - \overline{G})$ = 27.71 − 14.77 = 12.94. The interaction effect in the cited cell will be estimated as 45.33 − 24.43 − 27.71 + 14.77 = 7.96. The estimated value of the residual for each of the seven Y_{ijk} values in the cited cell will be $Y_{ijk} - 7.96$.

Figure 29.4 shows the printout of the ANOVA table when an interaction model is used for the two-factor data in Table 29.3. In Figure 29.4, the sums of squares (marked Type I SS) and mean squares for histology and TNM stage are the same as in Table 29.3, and they also have the same degrees of freedom. The degrees of freedom for the interaction are tricky to calculate, however. In this instance, because some of the cells of Table 29.3 are empty or have only 1 member, we first calculate degrees for freedom for the residual sum of squares, $\Sigma (Y_{ijk} - \overline{Y}_{jk})^2$. In each pertinent cell, located at (j, k) coordinates in the table, the degrees of freedom will be $n_{jk} - 1$. Working across and then downward through the cells in Table 29.3, the sum of the $n_{jk} - 1$ values will be $6 + 5 + 1 + 5 + 7 + 2 + 2 + 1 + 3 + 5 + 1 + 2 + 3$ = 43. (The values are 0 for the four cells with one member each and also for the 3 cells with no members.) This calculation shows that the model accounts for $59 - 43 = 16$ d.f.; and as the two main factors have a total of 7 d.f., the interaction factor contributes 9 d.f. to the model, as shown in the last row of Figure 29.4.

Source	DF	Sum of Squares	Mean Square	F Value	Pr > F
Model	16	13835.482381	864.717649	2.40	0.0114
Error	43	15469.130952	359.747231		
Corrected Total	59	29304.613333			

	R-Square	C.V.	Root MSE	SURVIVE Mean
	0.472126	128.4447	18.967004	14.766667

Source	DF	Type I SS	Mean Square	F Value	Pr > F
HISTOL	3	3593.3800000	1197.7933333	3.33	0.0282
TNMSTAGE	4	3116.3929638	779.0982410	2.17	0.0890
HISTOL*TNMSTAGE	9	7125.7094171	791.7454908	2.20	0.0408

FIGURE 29.4
Two-way ANOVA, with interaction component, for results in Table 29.3 and Figure 29.3. [Printout from SAS PROC GLM computer program.]

Calculated with the new mean square error term in Figure 29.4, the F values produce 2P values below <.05 for the model, for the histology factor, and for the histology-TNM-stage interaction. The 2P value is about .09 for the TNM-stage main effect.

The difficult challenge of interpreting three-way and more complex interactions are considered elsewhere[2] in discussions of multivariable analysis.

29.6.2   Nested Analyses

The groups of a single factor in ANOVA can sometimes be divided into pertinent subgroups. For example, the three treatments A, B, and C might each have been given in two sets of doses, low and high, so that six subgroups could be analyzed, two for each treatment. The results can then be evaluated with a procedure called a *hierarchical* or *nested* analysis. The variations in the total sum of squares would arise for the six subgroups and the three main groups, and the analysis is planned accordingly.

29.6.3   Analysis of Covariance

An analysis of covariance (acronymically designated as ANCOVA) can be done for at least two reasons. The first is to adjust for the action of a second factor suspected of being as a confounder in affecting both the dependent variable and the other factor under analysis.

The second reason is to allow appropriate analyses of a ranked *independent* variable that is expressed in either a dimensional or ordinal scale. This ranking is ignored when the ordinary ANOVA procedure relies on nominal categories for the independent variable. Thus, in the analyses shown in Figs. 29.3 and 29.4, the polytomous categories of TNM stage were managed as though they were nominal. To allow maintenance of the ranks, TNM stage could be declared a covariate, which would then be analyzed as though it had a dimensional scale.

The results of the covariance analysis are shown in Figure 29.5. Note that TNM stage now has only 1 degree of freedom, thus giving the model a total of 4 D.F., an F value of 3.61 and a P value of 0.0111, despite a decline of R-square from .229 in Figure 29.3 to .208 in Figure 29.5. The histology variable, which had P = .052 in Figure 29.3 now has P = .428; and TNM stage, with P = .144 in Figure 29.3, has now become highly significant at P = .0012. These dramatic changes indicate what can happen when the rank sequence is either ignored or appropriately analyzed for polytomous variables.

Source	DF	Sum of Squares	Mean Square	F Value	Pr > F
Model	4	6087.9081999	1521.9770500	3.61	0.0111
Error	55	23216.7051334	422.1219115		
Corrected Total	59	29304.6133333			

	R-Square	C.V.	Root MSE	SURVIVE Mean
	0.207746	139.1350	20.545606	14.766667

Source	DF	Type I SS	Mean Square	F Value	Pr > F
TNMSTAGE	1	4897.3897453	4897.3897453	11.60	0.0012
HISTOL	3	1190.5184546	396.8394849	0.94	0.4276

FIGURE 29.5
Printout of Analysis of Covariance for data in Figure 29.3, with TNM stage used as ranked variable.

In past years, the effect of confounding or ranked covariates was often formally "adjusted" in an analysis of covariance, using a complex set of computations and symbols. Today, however, the same adjustment is almost always done with a multiple regression procedure. The adjustment process in ANCOVA is actually a form of regression analysis in which the related effects of the covariate are determined by regression and then removed from the error variance. The group means of the main factor are also "adjusted" to correspond to a common value of the covariate. The subsequent analysis is presumably more "powerful" in detecting the effects of the main factor, because the confounding effects have presumably been "removed." The process and results are usually much easier to understand, however, when done with multiple linear regression.[2]

29.6.4   Repeated-Measures Arrangements

Repeated measures is the name given to analyses in which the same entity has been observed repeatedly. The repetitions can occur with changes over time, perhaps after interventions such as treatment, or with examinations of the same (unchanged) entity by different observers or systems of measurement.

29.6.4.1   Temporal Changes — The most common repeated-measures situation is an ordinary crossover study, where the same patients receive treatments A and B. The effects of treatment A vs. treatment B in each person can be subtracted and thereby reduced to a single group of increments, which can be analyzed with a paired t test, as discussed in Section 7.8.2.2. The same analysis of increments can be used for the before-and-after measurements of the effect in patients receiving a particular treatment, such as the results shown earlier for blood glucose in Table 7.4.

Because the situations just described can easily be managed with paired t tests, the repeated-measures form of ANOVA is usually reserved for situations in which the same entity has been measured at three or more time points. The variables that become the main factors in the analysis are the times and the groups (such as treatment). Interaction terms can be added for the effects of groups × times.

Four major problems, for which consensus solutions do not yet exist, arise when the same entity is measured repeatedly over time:

1. *Independence.* The first problem is violation of the assumption that the measurements are independent. The paired t test manages this problem by reducing the pair of measurements to their increment, which becomes a simple "new" variable. This distinction may not always be suitably employed with more than two sets of repeated measurements.

2. *Incremental components.* A second problem is the choice of components for calculating incremental changes for each person. Suppose t_0 is an individual baseline value, and the subsequent values are t_1, t_2, and t_3. Do we always measure increments from the baseline value, i.e., $t_1 - t_0$, $t_2 - t_0$, and $t_3 - t_0$, or should the increments be listed successively as $t_1 - t_0$, $t_2 - t_1$, $t_3 - t_2$?

3. *Summary index of response.* If a treatment is imposed after the baseline value at t_0, what is the best single index for summarizing the post-therapeutic response? Should it be the mean of the post-treatment values, the increment between t_0 and the last measurement, or a regression line for the set of values?

4. *Neglect of trend.* This problem is discussed further in Section 29.8. As noted earlier, an ordinary analysis of variance does not distinguish between unranked nominal and ranked ordinal categories in the independent polytomous variable. If the variable represents serial points in time, their ranking may produce a trend, but it will be neglected unless special arrangements are used in the calculations.

29.6.4.2 Intraclass Correlations — Studies of observer or instrument variability can also be regarded as a type of repeated measures, for which the results are commonly cited with an *intraclass correlation coefficient (ICC).*

As noted in Section 20.7.3, the basic concept was developed as a way of assessing agreement for measurements of a dimensional variable, such as height or weight, between members of the same class, such as brothers in a family. To avoid the inadequacy of a correlation coefficient, the data were appraised with a repeated-measures analysis-of-variance. To avoid decisions about which member of a pair should be listed as the first or second measurements, all possible pairs were listed twice, with each member as the first measurement and then as the second. The total sums of squares could be partitioned into one sum for variability between the individuals being rated, i.e., the subjects (SSS), and another sum of squares due to residual error (SSE). The intraclass correlation was then calculated as

$$R_I = \frac{SSS - SSE}{SSS + SSE}$$

The approach was later adapted for psychometric definitions of *reliability.* The appropriate *means* for the sums of squares were symbolized as s_c^2 for variance in the subjects and s_e^2 for the corresponding residual errors. *Reliability* was then defined as

$$R_I = s_c^2/(s_c^2 + s_e^2)$$

Using the foregoing symbols, when each of a set of n persons is measured by each of a set of r raters, the variance of a single observation, s, can be partitioned as

$$s^2 = s_c^2 + s_r^2 + s_e^2$$

where s_r^2 is the mean of the appropriate sums of squares for the raters.

These variances can be arranged into several formulas for calculating R_I. The different arrangements depend on the models used for the "sampling" and the interpretation.[6] In a worked example cited by Everitt,[7] vital capacity was measured by four raters for each of 20 patients. The total sum of squares for the 80 observations, with d.f. = 79, was divided into three sets of sums of squares: (1) for the four observers with d.f. = 3; (2) for the 20 patients with d.f. = 19; and (3) for the residual "error" with d.f. = $3 \times 19 = 57$. The formula used by Everitt for calculating the intraclass correlation coefficient was

$$R_I = \frac{n(s_c^2 - s_e^2)}{ns_c^2 + rs_r^2 + (nr - n - r)s_e^2}$$

A counterpart formula, using SSR to represent sums of squares for raters, is

$$R_I = \frac{SSS - SSE}{SSS + SSE + 2(SSR)}$$

The intraclass correlation coefficient (ICC) can be used when laboratory measurements of "instrument" variability are expressed in dimensional data. Nevertheless, as discussed in Chapter 20, most laboratories prefer to use simpler pair-wise and other straightforward statistical approaches that are easier to understand and interpret than the ICC.

The simpler approaches may also have mathematical advantages that have been cited by Bland and Altman,[8] who contend that the ICC, although appropriate for repetitions of the same measurement, is unsatisfactory "when dealing with measurements by two different methods" where "there is no ordering of the repeated measures and hence no obvious choice of X or Y." Other disadvantages ascribed to the ICC are that it depends "on the range of measurement and ... is not related to the actual scale of measurement or to the size of error which might be clinically allowable." Instead, Bland and Altman recommend their "limits of agreement" method, which was discussed throughout Section 20.7.1. The method relies on examining the increments in measurement for each subject. The mean difference then indicates bias, and the standard deviation is used to calculate a 95% descriptive zone for the "limits of agreement." A plot of the differences against the mean value of each pair will indicate whether the discrepancies in measurement diverge as the measured values increase.

For categorical data, concordance is usually expressed (see Chapter 20) with other indexes of variability, such as kappa, which yields the same results as the intraclass coefficient in pertinent situations.

29.7 Non-Parametric Methods of Analysis

The mathematical models of ANOVA require diverse assumptions about Gaussian distributions and homoscedastic (i.e., similar) variances. These assumptions can be avoided by converting the dimensional data to ranks and analyzing the values of the ranks. The *Kruskal-Wallis* procedure, which is the eponym for a one-way ANOVA using ranked data, corresponds to a Wilcoxon–Mann–Whitney U test for 3 or more groups. The *Friedman* procedure, which refers to a two-way analysis of ranked data, was proposed almost 60 years ago by Milton Friedman, who later become more famous in economics than in statistics.

29.8 Problems in Analysis of Trends

If a variable has ordinal grades, the customary ANOVA procedure will regard the ranked categories merely as nominal, and will not make provision for the possible or anticipated trend associated with different ranks. The problem occurs with an ordinal variable, such as TNM stage in Figure 29.1, because the effect of an increasing stage is ignored. The neglect of a ranked effect can be particularly important when the independent variable (or "factor") is *time*, for which the effects might be expected to occur in a distinct temporal sequence. This problem in repeated-measures ANOVA evoked a denunciation by Sheiner,[9] who contended that the customary ANOVA methods were wholly inappropriate for many studies of the time effects of pharmacologic agents.

The appropriate form of analysis can be carried out, somewhat in the manner of the chi-square test for linear trend in an array of proportions (see Chapter 27), by assigning arbitrary coding values (such as **1, 2, 3, 4**) to the ordinal categories. The process is usually done more easily and simply, however, as a linear regression analysis.

29.9 Use of ANOVA in Published Literature

To find examples of ANOVA in published medical literature, the automated Colleague Medical Database was searched for papers, in English, of human-subject research that appeared in medical journals during 1991–95, and in which analysis of variance was mentioned in the abstract-summary. From the list of possibilities, 15 were selected to cover a wide array of journals and topics. The discussion that follows is a summary of results in those 15 articles.

A one-way analysis of variance was used to check the rate of disappearance of ethanol from venous blood in 12 subjects who drank the same dose of alcohol in orange juice on four occasions.[10] The authors concluded that the variation between subjects exceeded the variations within subjects. Another classical one-way ANOVA was done to examine values of intestinal calcium absorption and serum parathyroid hormone levels in three groups of people: normal controls and asthmatic patients receiving either oral or inhaled steroid therapy.[11] A one-way ANOVA compared diverse aspects of functional status in two groups of patients receiving either fluorouracil or saline infusions for head and neck cancer.[12] In a complex but essentially one-way ANOVA, several dependent variables (intervention points, days of monitoring, final cardiovascular function) were related to subgroups defined by APACHE II severity scores in a surgical intensive care unit.[13] (The results were also examined in a regression analysis.) In another one-way analysis of variance, preference ratings for six different modes of teaching and learning were evaluated[14] among three groups, comprising first-year, second-year, and fourth-year medical students in the United Arab Emirates. The results were also examined for the preferences of male vs. female students.

In a two-way ANOVA, neurologic dysfunction at age four years was related[15] to two main factors: birth weight and location of birth in newborn intensive care units of either Copenhagen or Dublin. Multifactor ANOVAs were applied,[16] in 20 patients with conjunctival malignant melanoma, to the relationship between 5-year survival and the counts of cells positive for proliferating cell nuclear antigen, predominant cell type, maximum tumor depth, and site of tumor. The result, showing that patients with low counts had better prognoses, was then "confirmed" with a Cox proportional hazards regression analysis. (The latter approach would probably have been best used directly.)

Repeated measures ANOVA was used in the following studies: to check the effect of oat bran consumption on serum cholesterol levels at four time points;[17] to compare various effects (including blood pressure levels and markers of alcohol consumption) in hypertensive men randomized to either a control group or to receive special "advice" about methods of reducing alcohol consumption;[18] to assess the time trend of blood pressure during a 24-hour monitoring period in patients receiving placebo or an active antihypertensive agent;[19] and to monitor changes at three time points over 6 months in four indexes (body weight, serum osmolality, serum sodium, and blood urea nitrogen/creatinine ratios) for residents of a nursing home.[19]

The intraclass correlation coefficient was used in three other studies concerned with reliability (or reproducibility) of the measurements performed in neuropathic tests,[21] a brief psychiatric rating scale,[22] and a method of grading photoageing in skin casts.[23]

References

1. Feinstein, 1990d; 2. Feinstein, 1996; 3. Oxford English Dictionary, 1971; 4. Lentner, 1982; 5. Tukey, 1968; 6. Shrout, 1979; 7. Everitt, 1989; 8. Bland, 1990; 9. Sheiner, 1992; 10. Jones, 1994; 11. Luengo, 1991; 12. Browman, 1993; 13. Civetta, 1992; 14. Paul, 1994; 15. Ellison, 1992; 16. Seregard, 1993; 17. Saudia, 1992; 18. Maheswaran, 1992; 19. Tomei, 1992; 20. Weinberg, 1994; 21. Dyck, 1991; 22. Hafkenscheid, 1993; 23. Fritschi, 1995.

References

[Numbers in brackets indicate chapter(s) where reference was cited]

Abbe, E. Gesammelte Abhandlungen. Vol. II. Jena, Germany: Gustav Fischer Verlag, 1906. [14]

Abramson, J.H. Age-standardization in epidemiological data (Letter to editor). Int. J. Epidemiol. 1995; 24:238–239. [26]

Adams, W.J. The Life and Times of the Central Limit Theorem. New York: Kaedmon Publishing Co., 1974. [7]

Agocs, M.M., White, M.C., Ursica, G., Olson, D.R., and Vamon, A. A longitudinal study of ambient air pollutants and the lung peak expiratory flow rates among asthmatic children in Hungary. Int. J. Epidemiol. 1997; 26:1272–1280. [22]

Aickin, M. and Gensler, H. Adjusting for multiple testing when reporting research results: the Bonferroni vs. Holm methods. Am. J. Public Health 1996; 86:726–728. [25]

Aitken, R.C.B. Measurement of feelings using visual analogue scales. Proc. Roy. Soc. Med. 1969; 62:989–993. [15]

Albert, J. Exploring baseball hitting data: What about those breakdown statistics? J. Am. Stat. Assn. 1994; 89:1066–1074. [8]

Allman, R.M., Goode, P.S., Patrick, M.M., Burst, N., and Bartolucci, A.A. Pressure ulcer risk factors among hospitalized patients with activity limitation. JAMA 1995; 273:865–870. [15]

Allred, E.N., Bleecker, E.R., Chaitman, B.R. et al. Short-term effects of carbon monoxide exposure on the exercise performance of subjects with coronary artery disease. N. Engl. J. Med. 1989; 321:1426–1432. [19]

Altman, D.G. Statistics and ethics in medical research. III. How large a sample? Br. Med. J. 1980; 281:1336–1338. [23]

Altman, D.G. and Gardner, M.J. Presentation of variability (Letter to editor). Lancet 1986; 2:639. [9]

Altman, D.G. and Gardner, M.J. Calculating confidence intervals for regression and correlation. Br. Med. J. 1988; 296:1238–1242. [19]

American Journal of Epidemiology. Special issue on National Conference on Clustering of Health Events, Atlanta. Am. J. Epidemiol. 1990; 132:Sl–S202. [25]

Anderson, R.N. and Rosenberg, H.M. Age Standardization of Death Rates: Implementation of the Year 2000 Standard. National Vital Statistics Reports, v. 47, n. 3. Hyattsville, MD: National Center for Health Statistics, 1998. [26]

Anderson, S. Individual bioequivalence: A problem of switchability. Biopharm. Rep. 1993; 2:1–5. [24]

Anscombe, F.J. Graphs in statistical analysis. Am. Statist. 1973; 27:17–21. [19]

Apgar, V. A proposal for a new method of evaluation of the newborn infant. Anesth. Analg. 1953; 32:260–267. [28]

Armitage, P. Statistical Methods in Medical Research. New York: John Wiley & Sons, 1971, 239–250 [24]; 389. [26]

Armitage, P. Sequential Medical Trials. 2nd ed. New York: John Wiley and Sons, 1975. [25]

Armitage, P. and Berry, G. Statistical Methods in Medical Research. 2nd ed. Oxford: Blackwell 1987. [27]

Armitage, P. and Hills, M. The two-period crossover trial. Statistician 1982; 31:119–131. [15]

Armstrong, B., Stevens, N., and Doll, R. Retrospective study of the association between use of rauwolfia derivatives and breast cancer in English women. Lancet 1974; 2:672–675. [25]

Ashby, D. (Guest Ed.). Conference on methodological and ethical issues in clinical trials. Stat. in Med. 1993; 12:1373–1534. [11]

Aubert, C., Rouge, F., and Voulot, C. New variants of the B16 melanoma: tumorigenicity and metastatic properties under different culture conditions. J. Natl. Cancer Inst. 1990; 82:952–958. [28]

Avis, N.E., Brambilla, D., McKinlay, S.M., and Vass, K. A longitudinal analysis of the association between menopause and depression. Results from the Massachusetts Women's Health Study. Ann. Epidemiol. 1994; 4:214–220. [22]

Avvisati, G., Ten Cate, J.W., Buller, H.R., and Mandelli, F. Tranexamic acid for control of haemorrhage in acute promyelocytic leukaemia. Lancet 1989; 2:122–124. [15]

Bab bage, C. Quoted in Moroney, M.J. The World of Mathematics. Vol. 3. New York: Simon and Schuster, 1956, p. 1487. [6]

Baehr, L. and Ahern, D.K. Statistical problems with small sample size (Letter to editor). Am. J. Psychiatry 1993; 150:356. [23]

Baer, F.M., Smolarz, K., Jungehulsing, M. et al. Chronic myocardial infarction: Assessment of morphology, function, and perfusion by gradient echo magnetic resonance imaging and ^{9m}Tc-methoxyisobutyl-isonitrile SPECT. Am. Heart J. 1992; 123:1636–1645. [16]

Bailar, B.A. Just what do I get for my ASA dues? Amstat News 1992; 185:4. [9]

Bailey, W.C., Higgins, D.M., Richards, B.M., and Richards, J.M., Jr. Asthma severity: a factor analytic investigation. Am. J. Med. 1992; 93:263–269. [28]

Bale, S.J., Dracopoli, N.C., Tucker, M.A. et al. Mapping the gene for hereditary cutaneous malignant melanoma-dysplastic nevus to chromosome 1_p. N. Engl. J. Med. 1989; 320:1367–1372. [17]

Bao, W., Srinivasan, S.R., Valdez, R., Greenlund, K.J., Wattigney, W.A., and Berenson, G.S. Longitudinal changes in cardiovascular risk from childhood to young adulthood in offspring of parents with coronary artery disease. JAMA 1997; 278:1749–1754. [22]

Barnard, G.A. Sequential tests in industrial statistics. J. Roy. Statist. Soc. 1946; 8(Suppl):1–26. [25]

Barnett, R.N. with contributions by I.M. Weisbrot. Clinical Laboratory Statistics. 2nd ed. Boston: Little Brown & Co., 1979. [20,21]

Baron, J.A., Bulbrook, R.D., Wang, D.Y., and Kwa, H.G. Cigarette smoking and prolactin in women. Br. J. Med. 1986; 293:482–483. [3]

Baxt, W.G. Use of an artificial neural network for the diagnosis of myocardial infarction. Ann. Intern. Med. 1991; 115:843–848. [21]

Beckmann, M.L., Gerber, J.G., Byyny, R.L., LoVerde, M., and Nies, A.S. Propranolol increases prostacyclin synthesis in patients with essential hypertension. Hypertension 1988; 12:582–588. [19]

Begg, C.B. Advances in statistical methodology for diagnostic medicine in the 1980's. Stat. Med. 1991; 10:1887–1895. [21]

Benedetti, T.J. Treatment of pre-term labor with the beta-adrenergic agonist ritodrine. Letter to editor. N. Engl. J. Med. 1992; 327:1758–1760. [23]

Berkman, P.L. Life stress and psychological well-being: A replication of Langner's analysis of midtown Manhattan society. J. Health Soc. Behav. 1971; 23:35–45. [15]

Berkson, J. and Gage, R.P. Calculation of survival rates for cancer. Proc. Staff Meetings Mayo Clin. 1950; 25:270–286. [22]

Berry, D.A. A case for Bayesianism in clinical trials. Stat. in Med. 1993; 12:1377–1393. [11]

Bierman, E.L. Law of the initial value (Letter to editor). Lancet 1976; 323:1076–1077. [19]

Bioequivalence of levothyroxine preparations: Issues of science, publication, and advertising (Letter to editor). JAMA 1997; 278:895–900. [24]

Birkelo, C.C., Chamberlain, W.E., Phelps, P.S., Schools, P.E., Zacks, D., and Yerushalmy, J. Tuberculosis case finding. A comparison of the effectiveness of various roentgenographic and photofluorographic methods. JAMA 1947; 133:359–365. [21]

Blackwelder, W.C. "Proving the null hypothesis" in clinical trials. Controlled Clin. Trials 1982; 3:345–353. [24]

Blackwelder, W.C. and Chang, M.A. Sample size graphs for "proving the null hypothesis." Controlled Clin. Trials 1984; 5:97–105. [24]

Bland, J.M. and Altman, D.G. Statistical methods for assessing agreement between two methods of clinical measurement. Lancet 1986; 1:307–310. [20]

Bland, J.M. and Altman, D.G. A note on the use of the intraclass correlation coefficient in the evaluation of agreement between two methods of measurement. Computations Biol. Med. 1990; 20:337–340. [20,29]

Blankenhorn, D.H., Brooks, S.H., Selzer, R.H., and Barndt, R., Jr. On the relative importance of Ps and rs (Letter to editor). Circulation 1978; 57:1232. [19]

Blyth, C.R. and Still, H.A. Binomial confidence intervals. J. Am. Stat. Assn. 1983; 78:108–116. [8]

Bobbio, M., Demichelis, B., and Giustetto, G. Completeness of reporting trial results: effect on physicians' willingness to prescribe. Lancet 1994; 343:1209–1211. [10]

Boffey, P.M. Anatomy of a decision. How the nation declared war on swine flu. Science 1976; 192:636–641. [6]

Bogardus, S.T., Concato, J., Feinstein, A.R. Clinical epidemiological quality in molecular genetic research. The need for methodological standards. JAMA 1999; 281:1919–1926. [21]

Boneau, C.A. The effects of violations of assumptions underlying the t test. Psychol. Bull. 1960; 57:49–64. [13]

Bonferroni, C.E. (The original publication, in a 1936 Italian economics journal, is not available. The strategy is well discussed in Miller, R.G. Simultaneous Statistical Inference. New York: McGraw-Hill, 1966.) [25]

Borenstein, M. Planning for precision in survival studies. J. Clin. Epidemiol. 1994; 47:1277–1285. [22]

Boston Collaborative Drug Surveillance Program. Oral contraceptives and venous thromboembolic disease, surgically confirmed gallbladder disease, breast tumours. Lancet 1973; 1:1399–1404. [25]

Boston Collaborative Drug Surveillance Program. Reserpine and breast cancer. Lancet 1974; 2:669–671. [10,25]

Boucher, K.M., Slattery, M.L., Berry, T.D., Quesenberry, C. and Anderson, K. Statistical methods in epidemiology: A comparison of statistical methods to analyze dose-response and trend analysis in epidemiologic studies. J. Clin. Epidemiol. 1998; 51:1223–1233. [27]

Box G.E., Hunter, W.G., and Hunter, J.S. Statistics for Experiments. New York: John Wiley and Sons, 1978. [19]

Box, J.F. and Fisher, R.A. The Life of a Scientist. New York: John Wiley and Sons, 1978. [11]

Bradley, J.V. Distribution-free statistical tests. Englewood Cliffs, NJ: Prentice-Hall, Inc., 1968. [14,15,27]

Brand, D.A., Frazier, W.H., Kohlhepp, W.C. et al. A protocol for selecting patients with injured extremities who need X-rays. N. Engl. J. Med. 1982; 306:333–339. [21]

Brand, R. and Kragt, H. Importance of trends in the interpretation of an overall odds ratio in the meta-analysis of clinical trials. Stat. Med. 1992; 11:2077–2082. [25]

Braun, H.I. (Ed.). The Collected Works of John W. Tukey: Vol. VIII, Multiple Comparisons: 1948–1983. London: Chapman and Hall, 1994. [25]

Brenner, H. and Gefeller, O. Chance-corrected measures of the validity of a binary diagnostic test. J. Clin. Epidemiol. 1994; 47:627–633. [21]

Breslow, N. Comparison of survival curves. In Buyse, M.E., Staquet, M.J., and Sylvester, R.J. (Eds.). Cancer Clinical Trials Methods and Practice. London: Oxford University Press, 1984. [22]

Breslow, N.E. and Day, N.E. Statistical Methods in Cancer Research. Vol. I. The Analysis of Case-Control Studies. Lyon: International Agency for Research on Cancer, 1980. [17,26]

Brook, R.H. Practice guidelines and practicing medicine. JAMA 1989; 262:3027–3030. [21]

Brophy, J.M. and Joseph, L. Placing trials in context using Bayesian analysis. GUSTO revisited by Reverend Bayes. JAMA 1995; 273:871–875. [11]

Bross, I.D.J. How to use ridit analysis. Biometrics 1958; 14:18–38. [15]

Browman, G.P., Levine, M.N., Hodson, D.I., Sathya, J., Russell, R., Skingley, P., Cripps, C., Eapen, L., and Girard, A. The head and neck radiotherapy questionnaire: A morbidity/quality-of-life instrument for clinical trials of radiation therapy in locally advanced head and neck cancer. J. Clin. Oncol. 1993; 11:863–872. [29]

Brown, B.W. and Russell, K. Methods correcting for multiple testing: operating characteristics. Stat. Med. 1997; 16:2511–2528. [25]

Brown, C.C. The validity of approximation methods for interval estimation of the odds ratio. Am. J. Epidemiol. 1981; 113:474–480. [17]

Brown, S.M., Selvin, S., and Winkelstein, W., Jr. The association of economic status with the occurrence of lung cancer. Cancer 1975; 36:1903–1911. [15]

Bryant, G.D. and Norman, G.R. Expressions of probability: Words and numbers (Letter to the editor). N. Engl. J. Med. 1980; 302:411. [6]

Bucher, H.C., Weinbacher, M., and Gyr, K. Influence of method of reporting study results on decision of physicians to prescribe drugs to lower cholesterol concentration. Br. Med. J. 1994; 309:761–764. [10]

Burnand, B. and Feinstein, A.R. The role of diagnostic inconsistency in changing rates of occurrence for coronary heart disease. J. Clin. Epidemiol. 1992; 45:929–940. [17]

Burnand, B., Kernan, W., and Feinstein, A.R. Indexes and boundaries for "quantitative significance" in statistical decisions. J. Clin. Epidemiol. 1990; 43:1273–1284. [10,16,17,19,20]

Calandra, T., Gerain, J., Heumann, D., Baumgartner, J-D., Glauser, M.P., and the Swiss-Dutch J5 Immunoglobulin Study Group. High circulating levels of Interleukin-6 in patients with septic shock: Evolution during sepsis, prognostic value, and interplay with other cytokines. Am. J. Med. 1991; 91:23–29. [27]

Campbell, M.J. and Gardner, M.J. Calculating confidence intervals for some non-parametric analyses. Br. Med. J. 1988; 296:1454–1456. [15]

Cancer Letters. 1994; 77:139–211 (These pages contain a series of pertinent papers on the cited topics). [21]

Capdevila, J.A., Almirante, B., Pahissa, A., Planes, A.M., Ribera, E., and Martinez-Vazquez, J.M. Incidence and risk factors of recurrent episodes of bacteremia in adults. Arch. Intern. Med. 1994; 154:411–415. [22]

Cappuccio, F.P., Strazzullo, P., Farinaro, E., and Trevisan, M. Uric acid metabolism and tubular sodium handling. Results from a population-based study. JAMA 1993; 270:354–359. [16]

Carette, S., Marcoux, S., Truchon, R., Grondin, C., Gagnon, J., Allard, Y., and Latulippe, M. A controlled trial of corticosteroid injections into facet joints for chronic low back pain. Nnew Engl. J. Med. 1991; 325:1002–1007. [24]

Carlin, J.B. Meta-analysis for 2 × 2 tables: A Bayesian approach. Stat. Med. 1992; 11:141–158. [25]

Carpenter, J. and Bithell, J. Bootstrap confidence intervals: When, which, what? A practical guide for medical statisticians. Statist. Med. 2000; 19:1141–1164. [7]

Carson, C.A., Taylor, H.R., McCarty, D.J., and Zimmet, P. Age-standardization in epidemiological data (Letter to editor). Int. J. Epidemiol. 1994; 23:643–644. [26]

Chalmers, T.C. Meta-analytic stimulus for changes in clinical trials. Stat. Methods Med. Res. 1993; 2:161–172. [25]

Chambers, J.M., Cleveland, W.S., Kleiner, B., and Tukey, P.A. Graphical Methods for Data Analysis. Boston: Duxbury Press, 1983, 60. [16]

Chan, C.K., Feinstein, A.R., Jekel, J.K., and Wells, C.K. The value and hazards of standardization in clinical epidemiologic research. J. Clin. Epidemiol. 1988; 41:1125–1134. [26]

Chandra Sekhar, C., Indrayan, A., and Gupta, S.M. Development of an index of need for health resources for Indian states using factor analysis. Int. J. Epidemiol. 1991; 20:246–250. [28]

Chappell, R. and Branch, L.G. The Goldilocks dilemma in survey design and its solution. J. Clin. Epidemiol. 1993; 46:309–312. [22]

Cherfas, J. University restructuring based on false premise? Recent studies contest the British government's argument that big science departments are better than small ones. Science 1990; 247:278. [19]

Chiang, C.L. A stochastic study of the life table and its application. III. The follow-up study with the consideration of competing risks. Biometrics 1961; 17:57–78. [22]

Chow, S.C. and Liu, J.P. Statistical consideration in bioequivalence trials. Biometric Bull. 1992; 9:19 (Abstract). [24]

Ciampi, A., Schiffrin, A., Thiffault, Q.H., Weitzner, G., Poussier, P., and Lalla, D. Cluster analysis of an insul-dependent diabetic cohort towards the definition of clinical subtypes. J. Clin. Epidemiol. 1990; 43:701–714. [28]

Cicchetti, D.V. Assessing inter-rater reliability for rating scales: Resolving some basic issues. Br. J. Psychiatry 1976; 129:452–456. [20]

Cicchetti, D.V., Lyons, N.S., Heavens, R., Jr., and Horwitz, R. A computer program for correlating pairs of variables when one is measured on an ordinal scale and the other on a continuous scale of measurement. Educ. Psych. Meas. 1982; 42:209–213. [27]

Civetta, J.M., Hudson-Civetta, J.A., Kirton, O., Aragon, C., and Salas, C. Further appraisal of Apache II limitations and potential. Surg. Gynecol. Obstet. 1992; 175:195–203. [29]

Clark, H.H. Comment on "Quantifying probabilistic expressions." Statist. Sci. 1990; 5:12–16. [6]

Clarke, M.R. Statistics and ethics in medical research (Letter to editor). Br. Med. J. 1981; 282:480. [23]

Clarke, P.R.F. and Spear, F.G. Reliability and sensitivity in the self-assessment of well-being. Bull. Brit. Psychol. Soc. 1964; 17:18A. [15]

Cleveland, W.S. Elements of Graphing Data. 2nd ed. Summit, NJ: Hobart Press, 1994. [5]

Cleveland, W.S. and McGill, R. Graphical perception: Theory, experimentation, and application to the development of graphical methods. J. Am. Statist. Assn. 1984; 79:531–554. [16]

Cliff, N. Comment on "quantifying probabilistic expressions." Statist. Sci. 1990; 5:16–18. [6]

Clopper, C.J. and Pearson, E.S. The use of confidence or fiducial limits illustrated in the case of the binomial. Biometrika 1934; 26:404–413. [8]

COBALT Investigators. Continuous infusion versus double-bolus administration of alteplace. A comparison of continuous infusion of alteplace with double-bolus administration for acute myocardial infarction. N. Engl. J. Med. 1997; 337:1124–1130. [24]

Cochran, W.G. Some methods of strengthening the common χ^2 tests. Biometrics 1954; 10:417–451. [14,26]

Cochran, W.G. and Cox, G.M. Experimental Designs. New York: John Wiley and Sons, 1950. [11]

Cohen, J. A coefficient of agreement for nominal scales. Educ. Psychol. Meas. 1960; 20:37–46. [20]

Cohen, J. Statistical Power Analysis for the Behavioral Sciences. Rev. ed. New York: Academic Press, 1977. [10,19,20,23]

Coldman, A.J. and Elwood, J.M. Examining survival data. Canad. Med. Assn. J. 1979; 121:1065–1071. [22]

Cole, P. The hypothesis generating machine. Epidemiology 1993; 4:271–273. [25]

Cole, P. and MacMahon, B. Attributable risk percent in case-control studies. Brit. J. Prev. Soc. Med. 1971; 25:242–244. [17]

Colquhoun, D. Re-analysis of clinical trial of homoeopathic treatment of fibrositis (Letter to editor). Lancet 1990; 336:441–442. [15]

Concato, J., Feinstein, A.R., and Holford, T.R. The risk of determining risk with multivariable models. Ann. Intern. Med. 1993; 118:201–210. [8,19]

Concato, J., Horwitz, R.I., Feinstein, A.R., Elmore, J.G., and Schiff, S.F. Problems of comorbidity in mortality after prostatectomy. JAMA 1992; 267:1077–1082. [26]

Conover, W.J. Practical Non-Parametric Statistics. New York: John Wiley and Sons, 1980. [27]

Cook, R.J. and Farewell, V.T. Multiplicity considerations in the design and analysis of clinical trials. J. R. Statist. Soc. A. 1996; 159:93–110. [25]

Copas, J. (Letter to editor). The Prof. Statist. 1990; 9:3. [9]

Cormack, R.M. A review of classification. J. Roy. Statist. Soc., A. 1971; 134:321–367. [28]

Cormack, R.S. and Mantel, N. Fisher's exact test: The marginal totals as seen from two different angles. Statistician 1991; 40:27–34. [14]

Cornbleet, P.J. and Shea, M.C. Comparison of product moment and rank correlation coefficients in the assessment of laboratory method-comparison data. Clin. Chem. 1978; 24:857–861. [21]

Cornfield, J. Quoted in Wynder, E.L. Workshop on guidelines to the epidemiology of weak associations. Prev. Med. 1987; 16:139–141. [17]

Cornfield, J. A method of estimating comparative rates from clinical data. Applications to cancer of the lung, breast and cervix. J. Natl. Cancer Inst. 1951; 11:1269–1275. [10]

Cornfield, J. A statistical problem arising from retrospective studies. In Neyman, J. (Ed.). Proceedings of the Third Berkeley Symposium, IV. 133–148. Berkeley: University of California Press, 1956. [17]

Coste, J., Spira, A., Ducimetiere, P., and Paolaggi, J-B. Clinical and psychological diversity of non-specific low-back pain. A new approach towards the classification of clinical subgroups. J. Clin. Epidemiol. 1991; 44:1233–1245. [28]

Coughlin, S.S., Trock, B., Criqui, M.H., Pickle, L.W., Browner, D., and Tefft, M.C. The logistic modeling of sensitivity, specificity, and predictive value of a diagnostic test. J. Clin. Epidemiol. 1992; 45:1–7. [21]

Cowie, H., Lloyd, M.H., and Soutar, C.A. Study of lung function data by principal components analysis. Thorax 1985; 40:438–443. [28]

Cox, D.R. Regression models and life tables (with discussion). J. Roy. Statist. Soc. Series B Metho. 1972; 34:187–220. [22]

Crichton, N.J. and Hinde, J.P. Correspondence analysis as a screening method for indicants for clinical diagnosis. Stat. Med. 1989; 8:1351–1362. [28]

Cupples, L.A., Heeren, T., Schatzkin, A., and Colton, T. Multiple testing of hypotheses in comparing two groups. Ann. Intern. Med. 1984; 100:122–129. [25]

Daniel, C. Quoted in Noether, G.E. Non-parametrics: The early years—impressions and recollections. Am. Statist. 1984; 38:173–178. [15]

Davis, B.R. and Hardy, R.J. Data monitoring in clinical trials: The case for stochastic curtailment. J. Clin. Epidemiol. 1994; 47:1033–1042. [25]

Davis, C.E. The effect of regression to the mean in epidemiologic and clinical studies. Am. J. Epidemiol. 1976; 104:493–498. [18]

Dawber, T.R. The Framingham Study: The Epidemiology of Atherosclerotic Disease. Cambridge: Harvard University Press (Commonwealth Fund Series), 1980. [25]

Dean, A.G., Dean, J.A., Burton, A.H., and Dicker, R.C. Epi Info, Version 5: A word processing, database, and statistics program for epidemiology and microcomputers. Stone Mountain, GA: USD, Incorporated, 1990. [17]

Decoufle, P., Thomas, T.L., and Pickle, L.W. Comparison of the proportionate mortality ratio and standardized mortality ratio risk measures. Am. J. Epidemiol. 1980; 111:263–269. [26]

De Leeuw, J. Review of Exploratory and multivariate data analysis by Michel Jambu. J. Am. Statist. Assn. 1993; 88:696–697. [6]

Deming, W.E. Review of Statistical papers in honor of Professor George W. Snedecor. New York Statistician 1972; 25(Nov.–Dec.):1–2. [23]

DerSimonian, R. and Laird, N. Meta-analysis in clinical trials. Contr. Clin. Trials 1986; 7:177–188. [25,26]

Detsky, A.S. and Baker, J.P. Analyzing data from ordered categories (Letter to editor). N. Engl. J. Med. 1984; 311:1382–1383. [27]

Detsky A.S. and Sackett, D.L. When was a "negative" clinical trial big enough? How many patients you needed depends on what you found. Arch. Intern. Med. 1985; 145:709–712. [24]

Diamond, G.A., Hirsch, M., Forrester, J.S., Staniloff, H.M., Vas, R., Halpern, S.W., and Swan, H.J.C. Application of information theory to clinical diagnostic testing. Circulation 1981; 63:915. [21]

Diggle, P.J., Liang, K-Y., and Zeger, S.L. Analysis of Longitudinal Data. New York: Oxford University Press, 1994. [22]

Dines, D.E., Elveback, L.R., and McCall, J.T. Zinc, copper, and iron contents of pleural fluid in benign and neoplastic disease. Mayo Clin. Proc. 1974; 49:102–106. [19]

Doll, R. and Hill, A.B. Mortality in relation to smoking: Ten years' observations of British doctors. Br. Med. J. 1964; 1:1399–1410, 1460–1467. [10]

Dorn, H.F. Methods of analysis for follow-up studies. Hum. Biol. 1950; 22:238–248. [22]

Duncan, D.B. Multiple range and multiple F-tests. Biometrics 1955; 11:1–42. [25]

Dunn, O.J. Multiple comparisons among means. J. Am. Stat. A. 1961; 56:52–64. [25]

Dunnett, C.W. A multiple comparison procedure for comparing several treatments with a control. J. Am. Stat. A. 1955; 50:1096–1121. [25]

Dunnett, C.W. and Gent, M. Significance testing to establish equivalence between treatments, with special reference to data in the form of 2 × 2 tables. Biometrics 1977; 33:593–602. [24]

Dwyer, J.H., Feinleib, M., Lippert, P., and Hoffmeister, H. (Eds.), Statistical Models for Longitudinal Studies of Health. New York: Oxford University Press, 1992. [22]

Dyck, P.J., Kratz, K.M., Lehman, K.A. et al. The Rochester Diabetic Neuropathy Study: Design, criteria for types of neuropathy, selection bias, and reproducibility of neuropathic tests. Neurology. 1991; 41:799–807. [29]

Dyer, A.R., Shipley, M., and Elliott, P. for the INTERSALT Cooperative Research Group. Urinary electrolyte excretion in 24 hours and blood pressure in the INTERSALT Study. I. Estimates of reliability. Am. J. Epidemiol. 1994; 139:927–939. [20]

Eagles, J.M., Beattie, J.A.G., Restall, D.B., Rawlinson, F., Hagen, S., and Ashcroft, G.W. Relation between cognitive impairment and early death in the elderly. Br. Med. J. 1990; 300:239–240. [17]

Eddy, D.M. A Manual for Assessing Health Practices and Designing Practice Policies (DRAFT). Lake Forest, IL: John A. Hartford Foundation and the Council of Medical Specialty Societies, 1990. [21]

Ederer, F., Axtell, L.M., and Cutler, S.J. The Relative Survival Rate: A Statistical Methodology. National Cancer Institute Monograph No. 6, Cancer: End Results and Mortality Trends, 1961. [22]

Edgington, E.S. Statistical Inference. The Distribution-Free Approach. New York: McGraw-Hill, 1969. [27]

Edmunds, L.H., Jr., Stephenson, L.W., Edie, R.N., and Ratcliffe, M.B. Open-heart surgery in octogenarians. N. Engl. J. Med. 1988; 319:131–136. [20]

Efron, B. Bootstrap methods: Another look at the jackknife. Ann. Statist. 1979; 7:1–26. [6]

Efron, B. and Diaconis, P. Computer-intensive methods in statistics. Sci. Am. 1983 (May):116–130. [6]

Ehrenberg, A.S.C. Data Reduction. Analyzing and Interpreting Statistical Data. London: John Wiley and Sons, 1975. [2]

Eisenberg, J.M., Schumacher, H.R., Davidson, P.K., and Kaufmann, L. Usefulness of synovial fluid analysis in the evaluation of joint effusions. Use of threshold analysis and likelihood ratios to assess a diagnostic test. Arch. Intern. Med. 1984; 144:715–719. [21]

Elandt-Johnson, R.C. Definition of rates: Some remarks on their use and misuse. Am. J. Epidemiol. 1975; 102:267–271. [17]

Ellenberg, S.S. Meta-analysis: The quantitative approach to research review. Semin. Oncol. 1988; 15:472–481. [25]

Ellison, P.H., Petersen, M.B., Gorman, W.A., and Sharpsteen, D. A comparison of neurological assessment scores from two cohorts of low-birthweight children evaluated at age four years: Dublin and Copenhagen: Neuropediatrics 1992; 23:68–71. [29]

Ellman, M.S. and Feinstein, A.R. Clinical reasoning and the new "non-" nosology. J. Clin. Epidemiol. 1993; 46:577–579. [28]

Elmore, J.G. and Feinstein, A.R. A bibliography of publications on observer variability (final installment). J. Clin. Epidemiol. 1992; 45:567–580. [20,21]

Elmore, J.G. and Feinstein, A.R. Joseph Goldberger: An unsung hero of American clinical epidemiology. Ann. Intern. Med. 1994a; 121:372–375. [23]

Elmore, J.G., Wells, C.K., Howard, D.H., and Feinstein, A.R. The impact of clinical history on mammographic interpretations. JAMA 1997; 277:49–52. [20]

Elmore, J.G., Wells, C.K., Lee, C.H., Howard, D.H., and Feinstein, A.R. Variability of radiologists' interpretations of mammograms. N. Engl. J. Med. 1994b; 331:1493–1499. [20,21]

Ericksen, E.P. and Kadane, J.B. Estimating the population in a census year. 1980 and beyond (with discussion). J. Am. Statist. Assn. 1985; 80:98–131. [17]

Esdaile, J.M., Horwitz, R.I., Levinton, C., Clemens, J.D., Amatruda, J.G., and Feinstein, A.R. Response to initial therapy and new onset as predictors of prognosis in patients hospitalized with congestive heart failure. Clin. Invest. Med. 1992; 15:122–131. [22]

Everitt, B.S. The Analysis of Contingency Tables. New York: John Wiley and Sons, 1977. [14,27]

Everitt, B.S. Statistical Methods for Medical Investigations. New York. Oxford University Press. 1989. pages 25–26. [29]

Everitt, B.S. Cluster Analysis. 3rd ed. London: Edward Arnold, 1993. [28]

Farr, W. Influence of elevation on the fatality of cholera. J. Stat. Soc. 1852; 15:155–183. [23]

Feely, M., Calvert, R., and Gibson, J. Clobazam in catamenial epilepsy. A model for evaluating anticonvulsants. Lancet 1982; 2:71–73. [25]

Feinstein, A.R. Clinical Judgment. Baltimore: Williams and Wilkins Co., 1967a. [21,28]

Feinstein, A.R. Clinical biostatistics: XVI. The process of prognostic stratification (Part 2). Clin. Pharmacol. Ther. 1972; 13:609–624. [5]

Feinstein, A.R Clinical biostatistics: XX. The epidemiologic trohoc, the abalative risk ratio, and "retrospective" research. Clin. Pharmacol. Ther. 1973; 14:291–307. [17]

Feinstein, A.R. Clinical biostatistics: XXXIV. The other side of "statistical significance": Alpha, beta, delta, and the calculation of sample size. Clin. Pharmacol. Ther. 1975; 18:491–505. [23]

Feinstein, A.R. Clinical Epidemiology. The Architecture of Clinical Research. Philadelphia: W.B. Saunders, 1985. [1,10,13,17,21,22,25,26]

Feinstein, A.R. The bias caused by high values of incidence of p_1 in the odds ratio assumption that $1 - p_1 \approx 1$. J. Chronic Dis. 1986; 39:485–487. [10]

Feinstein, A.R. Clinimetrics. New Haven: Yale University Press, 1987a. [6,28]

Feinstein, A.R. Quantitative ambiguities in matched versus unmatched analyses of the 2×2 table for a case-control study. Int. J. Epidemiol. 1987b; 16 (March):128–134. [26]

Feinstein, A.R. Scientific standards in epidemiologic studies of the menace of daily life. Science 1988a; 242:1257–1263. [25,28]

Feinstein, A.R. The inadequacy of binary models for the clinical reality of three-zone diagnostic decisions. J. Clin. Epidemiol. 1990a; 43:109–113. [21,24]

Feinstein, A.R. The unit fragility index: an additional appraisal of "statistical significance" for a contrast of two proportions. J. Clin. Epidemiol. 1990b; 43:201–209. [11]

Feinstein, A.R. Invidious comparisons and unmet clinical challenges (Editorial). Am. J. Med. 1992; 92:117–124. [10]

Feinstein, A.R. "Clinical judgment" revisited: The distraction of quantitative models. Ann. Intern. Med. 1994; 120:799–805. [6,28]

Feinstein, A.R. Meta-analysis: Statistical alchemy for the 21st century. J. Clin. Epidemiol. 1995; 48:71–79. [25]

Feinstein, A.R. Multivariable Analysis. An Introduction. New Haven: Yale University Press. 1996. [11,18,21,26,27,29]

Feinstein, A.R. P-values and confidence intervals: Two sides of the same unsatisfactory coin. J. Clin. Epidemiol. 1998a; 51:355–360. [13]

Feinstein, A.R. The problem of cogent subgroups: A clinicostatistical tragedy (Commentary) . J. Clin. Epidemiol. 1998b; 51:297–299. [25]

Feinstein, A.R. and Cicchetti, D.V. High agreement but low kappa: I. The problems of two paradoxes. J. Clin. Epidemiol. 1990c; 43:543–549. [20]

Feinstein, A.R. and Esdaile, J.M. Incidence, prevalence, and evidence. Scientific problems in epidemiologic statistics for the occurrence of cancer. Am. J. Med. 1987c; 82:113–123. [22]

Feinstein, A.R. and Kwoh, C.K. A box-graph method for illustrating relative-size relationships in a 2×2 table. Int. J. Epidemiol. 1988b; 17:222–224. [16]

einstein, A.R. and Stern, E.K. Clinical effects of recurrent attacks of acute rheumatic fever: A prospective epidemiologic study of 105 episodes. J. Chronic Dis. 1967b; 20:13–27. [9]

Feinstein, A.R. and Wells, C.K. A clinical-severity staging system for patients with lung cancer. Medicine 1990d; 69:1–33. [6,27,29]

Feinstein, A.R., Gelfman, N.A., and Yesner, R., with the collaboration of Auerbach, O., Hackel, D.B., and Pratt, P.C. Observer variability in histopathologic diagnosis of lung cancer. Am. Rev. Resp. Dis. 1970; 101:671–684. [20]

Feinstein, A.R., Horwitz, R.I., Spitzer, W.O., and Battista, R.N. Coffee and pancreatic cancer. The problems of etiologic science and epidemiologic case-control research. JAMA 1981; 246:957–961. [25]

Fendrich, M. Inconsistent coding of race and ethnicity in infants (Letter to editor). JAMA 1992; 267:3151–3152. [20]

Ferguson, G.A. Nonparametric Trend Analysis. Montreal: McGill University Press, 1965. [27]

Fetter, R.B., Shin, Y., Freeman, J.L., Averill, R.F., and Thompson, J.D. Case mix definition by diagnosis-related groups. Med. Care 1980; 18(Suppl 2):1–53. [21]

Finney, D.J. Whither biometry? In Hoppe, F.M., (Ed.). Multiple Comparisons, Selection, and Applications in Biometry. New York: Marcel Dekker, Inc. 1993. [21]

Fischer, M.A. and Feinstein, A.R. Excess sample size in randomized controlled trials. J. Invest. Med. 1997; 45:198A. [23]

Fisher, P., Greenwood, A., Huskisson, E.C., Turner, P., and Belon, P. Effect of homoeopathic treatment on fibrositis (primary fibromyalgia). Br. Med. J. 1989; 299:365–366. [15]

Fisher, R.A. Statistical Methods for Research Workers. Edinburgh: Oliver and Boyd, 1925. [6,11]

Fisher, R.A. Statistical Methods for Research Workers. 5th ed. Edinburgh: Oliver and Boyd, 1934. [12,17]

Fisher, R.A. Statistical Methods for Research Workers. 8th ed. Edinburgh: Oliver and Boyd, 1941. [20]

Fisher, R.A. Statistical Methods and Scientific Inference. Edinburgh: Oliver and Boyd, 1959. [11,23]

Flameng, W., Wouters, L., Sergeant, P., Lewi, P., Borgers, M., Thone, F., and Suy, R. Multivariate analysis of angiographic, histologic, and electrocardiographic data in patients with coronary heart disease. Circulation 1984; 70:7–17. [28]

Fleiss, J.L. Statistical Methods for Rates and Proportions. 2nd ed. New York: John Wiley and Sons, 1981. (15,17,19,20,23,26]

Fleiss, J.L. Confidence intervals vs. significance tests: Quantitative interpretation (Letter to editor). Am. J. Public Health 1986; 76:587. [13,14]

Fletcher, K.A. on behalf of the Atrial Fibrillation investigators. Pooling data from five stroke prevention clinical trials versus performing a meta-analysis. Controlled Clin. Trials 1993; 14(abstract P 90). [25]

Follman, D., Wittes, J., and Cutler, J.A. The use of subjective rankings in clinical trials with an application to cardiovascular disease. Stat. Med. 1992; 11:427–437. [27]

Food and Drug Administration. The Bioavailability Protocol Guideline for ANDA and NDA Submission. Division of Biopharmaceutics. Rockville, MD:Drug Monographs/Bureau of Drugs, Food and Drug Administration, 1977. [24]

Forrow, L., Taylor, W.C., and Arnold, R.M. Absolutely relative: How research results are summarized can affect treatment decisions. Am. J. Med. 1992; 92:121–124. [10]

Forsythe, A.B. and Frey, H.S. Tests of significance from survival data. Comput. Biomed. Res. 1970; 3:124–132. [22]

Freedman, B. Equipoise and the ethics of clinical research. N. Eng. J. Med. 1987; 317:141–145. [25]

Freedman, D.A. Adjusting the 1990 census. Science 1991; 252:1233–1236. [17]

Freedman, L.S. Tables of the number of patients required in clinical trials using the logrank test. Stat. Med. 1982; 1:121–129. [22]

Freedman, L.S. and Spiegelhalter, D.J. The assessment of subjective opinion and its use in relation to stopping rules for clinical trials. Statistician 1983; 32:153–160. [25]

Freeman, D.H. and Jekel, J.F. Table selection and log linear models. J. Chronic Dis. 1980; 33:513–524. [27]

Freeman, L.C. Elementary Applied Statistics: For Students in Behavioral Science. New York: John Wiley and Sons, 1965. [27]

Freiman, J.A., Chalmers, T.C., Smith, H., Jr. et al. The importance of beta, the Type II error and sample size in the design and interpretation of the randomized control trial: Survey of 71 'negative' trials. N. Engl. J. Med. 1978; 229:690–694. [23]

Friederici, H.H.R. and Sebastian, M. The concordance score. Correlation of clinical and autopsy findings. Arch. Pathol. Lab. Med. 1984; 108:515–517. [20]

Fritschi, L., Battistutta, D., Strutton, G., and Green, A. A non-invasive measure of photoageing. Int. J. Epidemiol. 1995; 24:150–154. [29]

Fulton, M., Raab, G., Thomson, G., Laxen, D., Hunter, R., and Hepburn, W. Influence of blood lead on the ability and attainment of children in Edinburgh. Lancet 1987; 1:1221–1225. [3]

Furukawa, T. and Sumita, Y. A cluster-analytically derived subtyping of chronic affective disorders. Acta. Psychiatr. Scand. 1992; 85:177–182. [28]

Galton, F. Regression towards mediocrity in hereditary stature. J. Anthropol. Instit. 1885; 15:246–263. [18]

Galton, F. Natural Inheritance. London: Macmillan, 1889. [4,17]

Garber, H.J. Response to Letter to editor. Am. J. Psychiatry 1993; 150:356–357. [23]

Garber, H.J. and Ritvo, E.R. Magnetic resonance imaging of the posterior fossa in autistic adults. Am. J. Psychiatry 1992; 149:245–247. [23]

Gardner, M.J. and Altman, D.G. Confidence intervals rather than P values: Estimation rather than hypothesis testing. Br. Med. J. 1986; 292:746–750. [16]

Gardner, M.J. and Altman, D.G. (Eds.). Statistics with Confidence — Confidence Intervals and Statistical Guidelines. London: British Medical Journal, 1989. [8]

Gart, J.J. The comparison of proportions: A review of significance tests, confidence intervals, and adjustments for stratification. Rev. Int. Statist. Instit. 1971; 39:148–169. [14]

Gart, J.J. and Thomas, D.G. Numerical results on approximate confidence limits for the odds ratio. J. Roy. Statist. Soc. Series B 1972; 34:441–447. [17]

Gart, J.J. and Thomas, D.G. The performance of three approximate confidence limit methods for the odds ratio. Am. J. Epidemiol. 1982; 115:453–470. [17]

Geary, R.C. Moments of the ratio of the mean deviation to the standard deviation for normal samples. Biometrika 1936; 28:295. [5]

Gehan, E.A. A generalized Wilcoxon test for comparing arbitrarily singly-censored samples. Biometrika 1965; 52:203–223. [22]

Gehan, E.A. Discussion on the paper by R. and J. Peto. J. Roy. Statist. Soc. Series A Stat. 1972; 135:204–205. [22]

Genest, J. Personal communication, 1981. [25]

Gentleman, R. and Crowley, J. Graphical methods for censored data. J. Am. Statist. Assn. 1991; 86:678–683. [22]

Gerbarg, Z.B. and Horwitz, R.I. Resolving conflicting clinical trials: Guidelines for meta-analysis. J. Clin. Epidemiol. 1988; 41:504–509. [25]

Gittlesohn, A. and Royston, P.N. Annotated Bibliography of Cause-of-Death Validation Studies 1958–1980. Washington, DC: U.S. Government Printing Office, 1982. (Vital and health statistics. Series 2: No. 89)(DHHS publication no. [PHS] 82–1363). [17,22]

Glass, G.V., McGaw, B., and Smith, M.L. Meta-Analysis in Social Research. Beverly Hills, CA: Sage Publications, 1981. [10]

Glindmeyer, H.W., Diem, J.E., Jones, R.N., and Weill, H. Noncomparability of longitudinally and cross-sectionally determined annual change in spirometry. Am. Rev. Respir. 1982; 125:544–548. [22]

Godfrey, K. Simple linear regression in medical reserach. N. Engl. J. Med. 1985; 313:1629–1636. [19]

Goldman, L. Electrophysiological testing after myocardial infarction. A paradigm for assessing the incremental value of a diagnostic test. Circulation 1991; 83:1090–1092. [21]

Gonzalez, E.R., Bahal, N., Hansen, L.A., Ware, D., Bull, D.S., Ornato, J.P., and Lehman, M.E. Intermittent injection vs. patient-controlled analgesia for sickle cell crisis pain. Arch. Intern. Med. 1991; 151:1373–1378. [15]

Goodman, L.A. and Kruskal, W.H. Measures of association for cross classifications. J. Am. Statist. Assn. 1954; 49:732–764. [27]

Goodman, S.N. Meta-analysis and evidence. Controlled Clin. Trials 1989; 10:188–204. [25]

Goodman, S.N. Multiple comparisons, explained. Am. J. Epidemiol. 1998; 147:807–812. [25]

Goodman, S.N. and Berlin, J.A. The use of predicted confidence intervals when planning experiments and the misuse of power when interpreting results. Ann. Intern. Med. 1994; 121:200–206. [23,24]

Goold, S.D., Hofer, T., Zimmerman, M., Hayward, R.A. Measuring physician attitudes toward cost, uncertainty, malpractice, and utilization review. J. Gen. Intern. Med. 1994; 9:544–549. [28]

Gordon, R.S., Jr. Minimizing medical costs (Letter to editor). Arch. Intern. Med. 1983; 143:845. [23]

Gould, S.G. The Mismeasure of Man. New York: W.W. Norton, 1981. [28]

Greene, M.K., Kerr, A.M., McIntosh, I.B., and Prescott, R.J. Acetazolamide in prevention of acute mountain sickness: A double-blind controlled cross-over study. Br. Med. J. 1981; 282:811–813. [27]

Greene, W.L., Feinstein, A.R., and Concato, J. Claims of equivalence in medical research: Are they supported by evidence? Ann. Int. Med. 2000; 132:715–722. [24]

Greenland, S. RE: "A simple method to calculate the confidence interval of a standardized mortality ratio (SMR)" (Letter to editor). Am. J. Epidemiol. 1991; 133:212–213. [26]

Greenland, S. and Longnecker, M.P. Methods for trend estimation from summarized dose-response data, with applications to meta-analysis. Am. J. Epidemiol. 1992; 125:1301–1309. [25]

Greenwald, P., Barlow, J.J., Nasca, P.C. et al. Vaginal cancer after maternal treatment with synthetic estrogens. N. Engl. J. Med. 1971; 285:390–392. [17]

Greenwood, M. The "errors of sampling" of the survivorship tables. In Reports on Public Health and Medical Subjects, No. 33, App. 1, London: H.M. Stationery Office, 1926. [22]

Griffiths, D. A pragmatic approach to Spearman's rank correlation coefficient. Teach. Statist. 1980; 2:10–13. [27]

Griner, P.F., Mayewski, R.J., Mushlin, A.I., and Greenland, P. Selection and interpretation of diagnostic tests and procedures. Principles and applications. Ann. Intern. Med. 1981; 94:553–600. [21]

Guilford, J.P. Fundamental Statistics in Psychology and Education. New York: McGraw-Hill, 1956. [19]

GUSTO III Investigators. Global use of strategies to open occluded coronary arteries. A comparison of reteplase with alteplase for acute myocardial infarction. N. Engl. J. Med. 1997; 337:1118–1123. [24]

Guttman, L. An outline of the statistical theory of prediction. In Horst, P. (Ed.). The Prediction of Personal Adjustment. New York. Social Science Research Council 1941. [27]

Guyatt, G., Sackett, D., Adachi, J., Roberts, R., Chong, J., Rosenbloom, D., and Keller, J. A clinician's guide for conducting randomized trials in individual patients. Can. Med. Assoc. J. 1988; 139:497–503. [25]

Guyatt, G., Sackett, D., Taylor, D.W., Chong, J., Roberts, R., and Pugsley, S. Determining optimal therapy: Randomized trials in individual patients. N. Engl. J. Med. 1986; 314:889–892. [25]

Hadi, A.S. and Ling, R.F. Some cautionary notes on the use of principal components regression. Am. Stat. 1998; 52:15–19. [28]

Hafkenscheid, A. Reliability of a standardized and expanded Brief Psychiatric Rating Scale: a replication study. Acta Psychiatr. Scand. 1993; 88:305–310. [29]

Hall, G., Chowdhury, S., and Bloem, M. Use of mid-upper-arm circumference Z scores in nutritional assessment (Letter to editor). Lancet 1993; 341:1481. [4]

Hamilton, D.P. Census adjustment battle heats up. Science 1990; 248:807–808. [17]

Hammond, E.C. and Horn, D. Smoking and death rates—Report on forty-four months of follow-up of 187,783 men. JAMA 1958; I. Total mortality 166:1159–1172. II. Death rates by cause 166:1294–1308. [13]

Hansen, K.M. and Tukey, J.W. Tuning a major part of a clustering algorithm. Int. Stat. Rev. 1992; 60:21–44. [28]

Harrell, F.E., Jr., Lee, K.L., Califf, R.M., Pryor, D.B., and Rosati, R.A. Regression modelling strategies for improved prognostic prediction. Stat. Med. 1984; 3:143–152. [28]

Harrell, F.E., Jr., Lee, K.L., Matchar, D.B., and Reichert, T.A. Regression models for prognostic prediction: advantages, problems, and suggested solutions. Cancer Treat. Rep. 1985; 69:1071–1077. [8]

Harris, J.E., Wente, E.F., Cox, C.F., Nawaway, I.E., Kowalski, C.J., Storey, A.T., Russell, W.R., Pointz, P.V., and Walter, G.F. Mummy of the "elder lady" in the tomb of Amenhotep II: Egyptian Museum catalog number 61070. Science 1978; 200:1149–1151. [28]

Hartigan, J.A. Clustering. Annu. Rev. Biophys. 1973; 2:81–101. [28]

Harvey, M., Horwitz, R.I., and Feinstein, A.R. Diagnostic bias and toxic shock syndrome. Am. J. Med. 1984; 76:351–360. [20]

Haybittle, J.L. Repeated assessment of results in clinical trials of cancer treatment. Br. J. Radiol. 1971; 44:793–797. [25]

Haybittle, J.L. and Freedman, L.S. Some comments on the logrank test statistic in clinical trial applications. Statistician 1979; 28:199–208. [22]

Healy, M.J.R. and Goldstein, H. Regression to the mean. Ann. Hum. Biol. 1978; 5:277–280. [18]

Hedges, L.V. and Olkin, I. Statistical Methods for Meta-Analysis. San Diego: Academic Press, Inc., 1985. [25]

Heinonen, O.P. , Shapiro, S., Tuominen, L. et al. Reserpine use in relation to breast cancer. Lancet 1974; 2:675–677. [25]

Heinrich, I., O'Hara, H., Sweetman, B., and Anderson, J.A.D. Validation aspects of an empirically derived classification for non-specific low back pain. Statistician 1985; 34:215–230. [28]

Henderson, W.G., Fisher, S.G., Cohen, N., Waltzman, S., Weber, L., and the VA Cooperative Study Group on Cochlear Implantation. Use of principal components analysis to develop a composite score as a primary outcome variable in a clinical trial. Controlled Clin. Trials. 1990; 11:199–214. [28]

Hennekens, C.H., Speizer, F.E., Rosner, B., Bain, C.J., Belanger, C., and Peto, R. Use of permanent hair dyes and cancer among registered nurses. Lancet 1979; 1:1390–1393. [25]

Herbst, A.L., Kurman, R.J., Scully, R.E., and Poskanzer, D.C. Clear cell adenocarcinoma of the genital tract in young females: Registry report. N. Engl. J. Med. 1972; 287:1259–1264. [17]

Herrnstein, R.J. and Murray, C. The Bell Curve: Intelligence and Class Structure in American Life. New York: Free Press, 1994. [28]

Hill, A.B. The environment and disease: Association or causation. Proc. R. Soc. Med. 1965; 58:295–300. [25]

Hill, M.O. Correspondence analysis: A neglected multivariate method. Appl. Statist. 1974; 23:340–354. [28]

Hlatky, M.A., Pryor, D.B., Harrell, F.E. Jr. et al. Factors affecting the sensitivity and specificity of the exercise electrocardiogram: A multivariable analysis. Am. J. Med. 1984; 77:64–71. [21]

Hochberg, Y. A sharper Bonferroni procedure for multiple tests of significance. Biometrika 1988; 75:800–802. [25]

Hogue, C. and Gaylor, D. Case-exposure studies: A new, simplified approach to relative risk. Am. J. Epidemiol. 1981; 114:427 (Abstract). [17]

Hogue, C.J.R., Gaylor, D.W., and Schulz, K.F. Estimators of relative risk for case-control studies. Am. J. Epidemiol. 1983; 118:396–407. [17]

Holford, T.R. The estimation of age, period, and cohort effects for vital rates. Biometrics 1983; 39:311–324. [22]

Holford, T.R. An alterative approach to statistical age-period-cohort analysis. J. Chronic Dis. 1985; 38:831–836. [22]

Hollander, J. Types of Shape. New Haven: Yale University Press, 1991. [9]

Holm, S. A simple sequentially rejective multiple test procedure. Scand. J. Stat. 1979; 6:65–70. [25]

Hoover, D.R., Extension of the life table to repeating and changing events. Am. J. Epidemiol. 1996; 143:1266–1276. [22]

Hoover, R.N. and Strasser, P.H. Artificial sweetners and human bladder cancer: Preliminary results. Lancet 1980; 1:837–840. [25]

Horwitz, R.I. and Feinstein, A.R. Estrogens and endometrial cancer. Responses to arguments and current status of an epidemiologic controversy. Am. J. Med. 1986; 81:503–507. [19]

Hospital Association of New York State. Compendium of Clinical Protocols, Criteria and Efficacy Research — Guidelines and Ongoing Research. Albany, NY: Hospital Association of New York State; October 1989. [21]

Hourani, L.L., Jakowatz, J., Goodman, M., Mueller, G., Brodie, G., and Jaffery, A. Concordance of hospital cancer registry- and physician-collected data for patients with melanoma. J. Natl. Cancer Instit. 1992; 84:1749–1750. [20]

Howell, E.M. and Blondel, B. International infant mortality rates: Bias from reporting differences. Am. J. Public Health. 1994; 84:850–852. [17]

Hsieh, C.C., MacMahon, B., Yen, S., Trichopoulus, D., Warren, K., and Nardi, G. Coffee and pancreatic cancer. Chapter 2 (Letter to editor). N. Engl. J. Med. 1986; 315:587–589. [25]

Hsieh, H-K. Chinese tally mark. Am. Statist. 1981; 35:174. [2]

Hull, R., Hirsh, J., and Sackett, D. The use of long-term outcome to validate diagnostic approaches to patients with clinically suspected recurrent deep venous thrombosis. Clin. Res. 1983; 31:234A (Abstract). [21]

Hulley, S.B., Cummings, S.R., Browner, W.S., Grady, D., Hearst, N., and Newman, T.B. Designing Clinical Research. 2nd ed. Philadelphia: Lippincott Williams & Wilkens, 2000. [1]

Huskisson, E.C. Measurement of pain. Lancet 1974; 2:1127–1131. [15]

Irwin, J.O. Tests of significance for differences between percentages based on small numbers. Metron 1935; 12:83–94. [12]

Jacobsen, S.J., Girman, C.J., Guess, H.A., Oesterling, J.E., and Lieber, M.M. A population-based study of aging and prostatism: Do longitudinal changes in urinary symptom frequency match cross-sectional estimates? J. Gen. Int. Med. 1995; 10:44 (Abstract). [22]

Jacobson, R.M. and Feinstein, A.R. Oxygen as a cause of blindness in premature infants: "Autopsy" of a decade of errors in clinical epidemiologic research. J. Clin. Epidemiol. 1992; 45:1265–1287. [23]

Jaeschke, R., Guyatt, G.H., and Sackett, D.L. User's guide to the medical literature III. How to use an article about a diagnostic test. A. Are the results of the study valid? JAMA 1994; 271:389–391. B. What are the results and will they help me in caring for my patients? JAMA 1994; 271:703–707. [21]

Jeffries, J.A., Robboy, S.J., O'Brien, P.C. et al. Structural anomalies of the cervix and vagina in women enrolled in the Diethylstilbestrol Adenosis (DESAD) Project. Am. J. Obstet. Gynecol. 1984; 148:59–66. [25]

Jenkins, J. Investigations: How to get from guidelines to protocols (Editorial). Br. Med. J. 1991; 303:323–324. [21]

Jones, A.W. and Jonsson, K.A. Between-subject and within-subject variations in the pharmacokinetics of ethanol. Br. J. Clin. Pharmac. 1994; 42:427–431. [29]

Jones, B., Jarvis, P., Lewis, J.A., and Ebbutt, A.F. Trials to assess equivalence: The importance of rigorous methods. Br. Med. J. 1996; 313:36–39. [24]

Jones, C.P. Living beyond our "means": New methods for comparing distributions. Am. J. Epidemiol. 1997; 146:1056–1066. [16]

Juniper, E.F., Guyatt, G.H., Streiner, D.L., and King, D.R. Clinical impact versus factor analysis for quality of life questionnaire construction. J. Clin. Epidemiol. 1997; 50:233–238. [28]

Kadel, C., Vallbracht, C., Buss, F., Kober, G., and Kaltenbach, M. Long-term follow-up after percutaneous transluminal coronary angioplasty in patients with single-vessel disease. Am. Heart J. 1992; 124:1159–1169. [22]

Kahaleh, M.B. and LeRoy, E.C. Interleukin-2 in scleroderma: Correlation of serum level with extent of skin involvement and disease duration. Ann. Intern. Med. 1989; 110:446–450. [19]

Kahn, H.A. and Dawber, T.R. The development of coronary heart disease in relation to sequential biennial measures of cholesterol in the Framingham Heart Study. J. Chronic Dis. 1966; 19:61–620. [22]

Kahn, H.A. and Sempos, C.T. Statistical Methods in Epidemiology. New York: Oxford University Press, 1989. [26]

Kallen, A and Larsson, P. Dose response studies: How do we make them conclusive? Statist. Med. 1999; 18:629–641. [27]

Kantor, S., Winkelstein, W., Jr., Sackett, D.L. et al. A method for classifying blood pressure: An empirical approach to reduction of misclassification due to response instability. Am. J. Epidemiol. 1966; 84:510–523. [15]

Kaplan, E.L. This week's citation classic. Current Contents 1983; No. 24 (June 13):14. [22]

Kaplan, E.L. and Meier, P. Non-parametric estimation from incomplete observations. J. Am. Statist. Assn. 1958; 53:457–481. [22]

Katz, D., Baptista, J., Azen, S.P., and Pike, M.C. Obtaining confidence intervals for the risk ratio in cohort studies. Biometrics 1978; 34:469–474. [17]

Katz, J. and Sommer, A. Reliability indexes of automated perimetric tests. Arch. Ophthalmol. 1988; 106:1252–1254. [21]

Kauffman, G.R., Wenk, M., Taeschner, W. et al. N-acetyltransferase 2 polymorphism in patients infected with human immunodeficiency virus. Clin. Pharm. Therap. 1996; 60:62–67. [9]

Keelan, P. Double-blind trial of propranolol (Inderal) in angina pectoris. Br. Med. J. 1965; 1:897–898. [15]

Kempthorne, O. Inference from experiments and randomization. In Srivasta, J.N. (Ed.). A Survey of Statistical Design and Linear Models. North Holland: Amsterdam, 1975. [21]

Kendall, M.G. Rank Correlation Methods. 2nd ed. London: Charles W. Griffin & Co., 1955. [27]

Kendall, M.G. A Course in Multivariate Analysis. London: C. Griffin & Co., 1968. [28]

Kendall, M.G. and Buckland, W.R. A Dictionary of Statistical Terms. 3rd ed. New York: Hafner Publishing Co., 1971. [2]

Kendall, M.G. and Gibbons, J.D. Rank Correlation Methods. 5th ed. London: Oxford, 1990. [27]

Kendall, M.G. and Stuart, A. Advanced Theory of Statistics. Vol. 2. Inference and Relationship. 3rd ed. London: Griffin, 1973. [11,23]

Kernan, W.N., Feinstein, A.R., and Brass, L.M. A methodological appraisal of research on prognosis after transient ischemic attacks. Stroke 1991; 22:1108–1116. [22]

Keuls, M. The use of the studentized range in connection with the analysis of variance. Euphytica 1952; 1:112–122. [25]

Kirshner, B. Methodological standards for assessing therapeutic equivalence. J. Clin. Epidemiol. 1991; 44:839–849. [24]

Kitagawa, E.M. Theoretical considerations in the selection of a mortality index, and some empirical comparisons. Human Biol. 1966; 38:293–308. [26]

Kleinbaum, D.G., Kupper, L.L., and Morgenstern, H. Epidemiologic Research. Principles and Quantitative Methods. Belmont, CA: Lifetime Learning Publications, 1982. [26]

Klinkenberg-Knol, E., Festen, H.P., Jansen, J.B. et al. Long term treatment with omeprazole for refractory reflux esophagitis: efficacy and safety. Ann. Intern. Med. 1994:121:161–167. [15]

Knapen, M.H.J., Hamulyak, K., and Vermeer, C. The effect of vitamin K supplementation on circulating osteocalcin (bone gla protein) and urinary calcium excretion. Ann. Intern. Med. 1989; 111:1001–1005. [19]

Knaus, W.A., Wagner, D.P., Draper, E.A., Zimmerman, J.E., Bergner, M., Bastros, P.G. et al. The APACHE III prognostic system. Risk prediction of hospital mortality for critically ill hospitalized adults. Chest 1991; 100:1619–1636. [21]

Knottnerus, J.A. and Leffers, P. The influence of referral patterns on the characteristics of diagnostic tests. J. Clin. Epidemiol. 1992; 45:1143–1154. [21]

Kochanek, K.D., Maurer, J.D., and Rosenberg, H.M. Why did black life expectancy decline from 1984 through 1989 in the United States? Am. J. Public Health 1994; 84:938–944. [22]

Kodlin, D. and Collen, M.F. Automated diagnosis in multiphasic screening. In Lacam, L.M., Neyman, J., and Scott, E.L. (Eds.). Proceedings of the Sixth Berkeley Symposium on Mathematical Statistics and Probability. Vol. IV: Biology and Health. Berkeley, CA: University of California Press, 1971. [21]

Kohout, F.J. Statistics for Social Scientists. A Coordinated Learning System. New York: John Wiley and Sons, 1974. [27]

Koivisto, P. and Miettinen, T.A. Long-term effects of ileal bypass on lipoproteins in patients with familial hypercholesterolemia. Circulation 1984; 70:290–296. [17]

Kolmogorov, A.N. Confidence limits for an unknown distribution function. Ann. Math. Statist. 1941; 12:461–463. [14]

Kong, A., Barnett, O., Mosteller, F., and Youtz, C. How medical professionals evaluate expressions of probability. N. Engl. J. Med. 1986; 315:740–744. [6]

Kraemer, H.C. Ramifications of a population model for κ as a coefficient of reliability. Psychometrika 1979; 44:461–472. [20]

Kramer, M.S. and Feinstein, A.R. Clinical biostatistics: LIV. The biostatistics of concordance. Clin. Pharmacol. Ther. 1981; 29:111–123. [20]

Kramer, M.S., Rooks, Y., and Pearson, H.A. Growth and development in children with sickle-cell trait. N. Engl. J. Med. 1978; 299:686–689. [24]

Krieger, K., Krieger, S., Jansen, O., Gass, P., Theilmann, L., and Lichtnecker, H. Manganese and chronic hepatic encephalopathy. Lancet 1995; 346:270–274. [15]

Krim, J. and Thomas, K. Resource utilization: A medical center cluster model. VA Practitioner 1987; 4:100–108. [28]

Kronmal, R.A. Commentary on the published results of the Lipid Research Clinics Coronary Primary Prevention Trial. J. Am. Med. Assn. 1985; 253:2091–2093. [23]

Kupper, L.L., Janis, J.M., Karmous, A., and Greenberg, B.G. Statistical age-period-cohort analysis: A review and critique. J. Chronic Dis. 1985; 38:811–830. [22]

Kupper, L.L., McMichael, A.J., Symons, M.J., and Most, B.M. On the utility of proportional mortality analysis. J. Chron. Dis. 1978; 31:15–22. [26]

Kupper, L.L., Stewart, J.R., and Williams, K.A. A note on controlling significance levels in stepwise regression. Am. J. Epidemiol. 1976; 103:13–15. [25]

Kurtzke, J.F. On estimating survival; A tale of two censors. J. Clin. Epidemiol. 1989; 42:169–175. [22]

Labarthe, D., Adam, E., Noller, K.L. et al. Design and preliminary observations on National Cooperative Diethylstilbestrol Adenosis (DESAD) project. Obstet. Gynecol. 1978; 51:453–458. [17]

Lachin, J.M. On a stepwise procedure for two population Bayes decision rules using discrete variables. Biometrics 1973; 29:551–564. [21]

Lachs, M.S., Nachamkin, I., Edelstein, P., Goldman, J., Feinstein, A.R., and Schwartz, J.S. Spectrum bias in the evaluation of diagnostic tests: Lessons from the rapid dipstick test for urinary tract infection. Ann. Intern. Med. 1992; 117:135–140. [21]

Ladenheim, M.L., Kotler, T.S., Pollock, B.H., Berman, D.S., and Diamond, G.A. Incremental prognostic power of clinical history, exercise electrocardiography and myocardial perfusion scintigraphy in suspected coronary artery disease. Am. J. Cardiol. 1987; 59:270–277. [21]

Lan, K.K.G., Simon, R., and Halperin, M. Stochastically curtailed tests in long-term clinical trials. Commun. Stat-Sequential Analysis 1982; 1:207–219. [25]

Landis, J.R. and Koch, G.G. The measurement of observer agreement for categorical data. Biometrics 1977; 33:159–174. [20]

Lapedes, D.N. (Ed.). Dictionary of Scientific and Technical Terms. New York: McGraw-Hill, 1974. [2]

Lapointe, F.J. and Legendre, P. A classification of pure malt Scotch whiskies. Appl. Statist. 1994; 43:237–257. [28]

Last, J.M. (Ed.). A Dictionary of Epidemiology. 2nd ed. New York: Oxford University Press, 1988. [17]

Lauer, K. The risk of multiple sclerosis in the U.S.A. in relation to sociogeographic features: a factor-analytic study. J. Clin Epidemiol. 1993; 47:43–48. [28]

Laupacis, A., Sackett, D.L., and Roberts, R.S. An assessment of clinically useful measures of the consequences of treatment. N. Engl. J. Med. 1988; 318:1728–1733. [10]

Lee, J. Exact confidence interval of the SMR based on prevalence data (Letter to editor). Int. J. Epidemiol. 1994; 23:428–429. [26]

Lehmann, E.L. The Fisher, Neyman-Pearson theories of testing hypotheses: one theory or two? J. Am. Stat. Soc. 1993; 88:1242–1249. [23]

Leibovici, L., Samra, Z., Konigsberger, H., Drucker, M., Ashkenazi, S., and Pitlik, S. Long-term survival following bacteremia or fungemia. JAMA 1995; 274:807–812. [15]

Lelorier, J. et al, Discrepancies between meta-analysis and subsequent large randomized, controlled trials. N. Engl. J. Med. 1997; 337:536–542. [25]

Lemna, W.K., Feldman, G.L., Kerem, B. et al. Mutation analysis for heterozygote detection and the prenatal diagnosis of cystic fibrosis. N. Engl. J. Med. 1990; 322:291–296. [21]

Lentner, C. (Ed.). Geigy Scientific Tables. Vol. 2. 8th ed. Basle, Switzerland: Ciba-Geigy, 1982. [8,29]

Levin, B. Annotation on the Holm, Simes and Hochberg multiple test procedures. Am. J. Public Health 1996; 86:628–629. [25]

Levine, R.J., Hauth, J.C., Curet, L.B., Sibai, B.M., Catalano, P.M. et al. Trial of calcium to prevent preeclampsia. N. Engl. J. Med. 1997; 337:69–76. [25]

Lichtenstein, J.L., Feinstein, A.R., Suzio, K.D., DeLuca, V.A., Jr., and Spiro, H.M. The effectiveness of panendoscopy on diagnostic and therapeutic decisions about chronic abdominal pain. J. Clin. Gastroenterol. 1980; 2:31–36. [21]

Liddell, F.D.K. Simple exact analysis of the standardized mortality ratio. J. Epidemiol. Comm. Health 1984; 38:85–88. [26]

Lieberman, J., Schleissner, L.A., Nosal, A., Sastre, A., and Mishkin, F.S. Clinical correlations of serum angiotensin-converting enzyme (ACE) in sarcoidosis. A longitudinal study of serum ACE, ^{67}gallium scans, chest roentgenograms, and pulmonary function. Chest 1983; 84:522–528. [22]

Lindenbaum, J., Mellow, M.H., Blackstone. M.O., and Butler, V.P., Jr. Variation in biologic availability of digoxin from four preparations. N. Engl. J. Med. 1971; 285:1344–1347. [24]

Lipid Research Clinics Program. The Lipid Research Clinics Coronary Primary Prevention Trial results. JAMA, 1984; I. Reduction in incidence of coronary heart disease 251:351–364. II. The relationship of reduction in incidence of coronary heart disease to cholesterol lowering. JAMA 1984; 365–374. [23]

Lipid Research Clinics Program. Reply to commentary by Richard Kronmal. JAMA 1985; 254:263–264. [23]

Liu, Q. An ordered-directed score test for trend in ordered $2 \times K$ tables. Biometrics 1998; 54:1147–1154. [27]

Loewenson, R.B., Bearman, J.E., and Resch, J.A. Reliability of measurements for studies of cerebrovascular atherosclerosis. Biometrics 1972; 28:557–569. [20]

Lorenz, W., Duda, D., Dick, W. et al. Incidence and clinical importance of perioperative histamine release: Randomised study of volume loading and antihistamines after induction of anaesthesia. Lancet 1994; 343:933–940. [20]

Luengo, M., Picado, C., Piera, C., Guanabens, N., Montserrat, J.M., Rivera, J., and Setoain, J. Intestinal calcium absorption and parathyroid hormone secretion in asthmatic patients on prolonged oral or inhaled steroid treatment. Eur. Respir. J. 1991; 4:441–444. [29]

Machin, D. and Gardner, M.J. Calculating confidence intervals for survival time analyses. Br. Med. J. 1988; 296:1369–1371. [22]

Maclure, M. and Willett, W.C. Misinterpretation and misuse of the kappa statistic. Am. J. Epidemiol. 1987; 126:161–169. [20]

MacMahon, B., Yen, S., Trichopoulos, D. et al. Coffee and cancer of the pancreas. N. Engl. J. Med. 1981; 304:630–633. [25]

Mahalanobis, P.C. Errors of observation in physician measurements. Sci. Cult. 1940; 7:443–445. [20]

Maheswaran, R., Beevers, M., and Beevers, D.G. Effectiveness of advice to reduce alcohol consumption in hypertensive patients. Hypertension 1992; 19:79–84. [29]

Makuch, R. and Simon, R. Sample size requirements for evaluating a conservative therapy. Cancer Treat. Rep. 1978; 62:1037–1040. [24]

Makuch, R.W. and Johnson, M.F. Some issues in the design and interpretation of "negative" clinical studies. Arch. Int. Med. 1986; 146:986–989. [24]

Makuch, R.W., Rosenberg, P.S., and Scott, G. Goodman and Kruskal's λ: A new look at an old measure of association. Stat. Med. 1989; 8:619–631. [27]

Malkin, D., Li, F.P., Strong, L.C. et al. Germ line p53 mutations in a familial syndrome of breast cancer, sarcomas, and other neoplasms. Science 1990; 250:1233–1238. [21]

Mann, H.B. and Whitney, D.R. On a test of whether one of two random variables is stochastically larger than the other. Ann. Math. Statist. 1947; 18:50–60. [15]

Mann, J., Holdstock, G., Harman, M., Machin, D., and Loehry, C.A. Scoring system in improve cost effectiveness of open access endoscopy. Br. Med. J. 1983; 287:937–940. [21]

Mantel, N. Evaluation of survival data and two new rank order statistics arising in its consideration. Cancer Chemother. Rep. 1966; 50:163–170. [22]

Mantel, N. Ridit analysis and related ranking procedures—Use at your own risk. Am. J. Epidemiol. 1979; 109:25–29. [15]

Mantel, N. and Haenszel, W. Statistical aspects of the analysis of data from retrospective studies of disease. J. Natl. Cancer Inst. 1959; 22:719–748. [25,26]

Manton, K.G., Patrick, C.H., and Stallard, E. Population impact of mortality reduction: The effects of elimination of major causes of death on the "saved" population. Int. J. Epidemiol. 1980; 9:111–120. [22]

Mapes, R.E.A. Verbal and numerical estimates of probability in therapeutic contexts. Soc. Sci. Med. 1979; 13A:277–282. [6]

Margolick, J.B., Munoz, A., Vlahov, D. et al. Direct comparison of the relationship between clinical outcome and change in CD4+ lymphocytes in human immunodeficiency virus-positive homosexual men and injecting drug users. Arch. Intern. Med. 1994; 154:869–875. [16]

Margolis, J.R., Gillum, R.F., Feinleib, M., Brasch, R.C., and Fabsitz, R.R. Community surveillance for coronary heart disease: The Framingham Cardiovascular Disease Survey. Methods and preliminary results. Am. J. Epidemiol. 1974; 100:425–436. [22]

Mason, J.H., Anderson, J.J., and Meenan, R.F. A model of health status for rheumatoid arthritis. A factor analysis of the arthritis impact measurement scales. Arthritis Rheum. 1988; 31:714–720. [28]

Matthews, D.E. and Farewell, V.T. Using and Understanding Medical Statistics. 2nd ed. New York: Karger, 1988. [22]

Matthews, J.N.S., Altman, D.G., Campbell, M.J., and Royston, P. Analysis of serial measurements in medical research. Br. Med. J. 1990; 300:230–235. [22]

Mazur, D.J. and Merz, J.F. How age, outcome severity, and scale influence general medicine clinic patients' interpretations of verbal probability terms. J. Gen. Intern. Med. 1994; 9:268–271. [6]

McFarlane, M.J., Feinstein, A.R., and Horwitz, R.I. Diethylstilbestrol and clear cell vaginal carcinoma. Reappraisal of the epidemiologic evidence. Am. J. Med. 1986; 81:855–863. [17]

McFarlane, M.J., Feinstein, A.R., Wells, C.K., and Chan, C.K. The "epidemiologic necropsy." Unexpected detections, demographic selections, and changing rates of lung cancer. J. Am. Med. Assn. 1987; 258:331–338. [17]

McGill, R., Tukey, J.W., and Larsen, W.A. Variations of box plots. Am. Statist. 1978; 32:12–16. [5,16]

McLean, J., Ciurczak, F. Bimanual dexterity in major league baseball players: A statistical study (Letter to editor). New Engl. J. Med. 1982; 307:1278–1279. [27]

McNeil, B.J., Keeler, E., and Adelstein, S.J. Primer on certain elements of medical decision making. N. Engl. J. Med. 1975; 293:211–215. [21]

McNemar, Q. Note on the sampling error of the difference between correlated proportions or percentages. Psychometrika 1947; 12:153–157. [20]

McNemar, Q. Psychological Statistics. New York: John Wiley and Sons, 1955. [20]

McPherson, K. Statistics: The problem of examining accumulating data more than once. N. Engl. J. Med. 1974; 290:501–502. [25]

Meinert, C.L. Meta-analysis: Science or religion? Controlled Clin. Trials. 1989; 10:257S–263S. [25]

Merrell, M. Time-specific life tables contrasted with observed survivorship. Biometrics 1947; 3:129–136. [22]

Metz, C.E., Goodenough, D.J., and Rossmann, K. Evaluation of receiver operating characteristic curve data in terms of information theory, with applications in radiography. Radiology 1973; 109:297–303. [21]

Metzler, C.M. Bioavailability—A problem in equivalence. Biometrics 1974; 30:309–317. [24]

Micceri, T. The unicorn, the normal curve, and other improbable creatures. Psychol. Bull. 1989; 105:156–166. [6]

Miettinen, O. Estimability and estimation in case-referent studies. Am. J. Epidemiol. 1976; 103:226–235. [14,17]

Miller, J.N. Outliers in experimental data and their treatment. Analyst 1993; 118:455–461. [5]

Miller, R.G. Simultaneous Statistical Inference. New York: McGraw-Hill, 1966. [25]

Mills, J.L. Data torturing. N. Engl. J. Med. 1993; 329:1196–1199. [25]

Mohr, R., Smolinsky, A., and Goor, D. Treatment of nocturnal angina with 10° reverse trendelenburg bed position. Lancet 1982; 1:1325–1327. [13]

Moller-Petersen, J. Nomogram for predictive values and efficiencies of tests (Letter to editor). Lancet 1985; 1:348. [21]

Moorman, P.W., Siersema, P.D., de Ridder, M.A.J., and van Ginneken, A.M. How often is large smaller than small? (Letter to editor). Lancet 1995; 345:865. [6]

Morinelli, D., Levine, M.S., and Young, M. Importance of sample size for statistical significance (Letter to editor). Am. J. Radiol. 1984; 143:923–924. [23]

Mormor, M., Friedman-Kien, A., Laubenstein, L. et al. Risk factors for Kaposil's sarcoma in homosexual men. Lancet 1982; 1:1083–1086. [19]

Morris, J.A. and Gardner, M.J. Calculating confidence intervals for relative risks (odds ratios) and standardised ratios and rates. Br. Med. J. 1988; 296:1313–1316. [26]

Morrison, D.E. and Henkel, R.E. The Significance Test Controversy. Chicago: Aldine Publishing Co., 1970. [11]

Moses, L.E., Emerson, J.D., and Hosseini, H. Analyzing data from ordered categories. N. Engl. J. Med. 1984; 311:442–448. [15,27]

Mosteller, F. and Youtz, C. Quantifying probabilistic expressions. Statist. Sci. 1990; 5:2–12. [6]

Mulder, P.G.H. An exact method for calculating a confidence interval of a Poisson parameter (Letter to editor). Am. J. Epidemiol. 1983; 117:377. [26]

Mulvihill, J.J., Myers, M.H., Connelly, R.R. et al. Cancer in offspring of long-term survivors of childhood and adolescent cancer. Lancet 1987; 3:813–817. [15]

Nakao, M.A and Axelrod, S. Numbers are better than words. Verbal specifications of frequency have no place in medicine. Am. J. Med. 1983; 74:1061–1065. [6]

Naylor, C.D., Chen, E., and Strauss, B. Measured enthusiasm: Does the method of reporting trial results alter perceptions of therapeutic effectiveness? Ann. Intern. Med. 1992; 117:916–921. [10]

Nelson, D.E., Sacks, J.J., and Chorba, T.L. Required vision testing for older drivers (Letter to editor). N. Engl. J. Med. 1992; 326:1784–1785. [16]

Newman, D. The distribution of the range in samples from a normal population in terms of an independent estimate of standard deviation. Biometrika 1939; 31:20–30. [25]

Newman, L.G., Waller, J., Palestro, C.J. et al. Unsuspected osteomyelitis in diabetic foot ulcers. Diagnosis and monitoring by leukocyte scanning with Indium in 111 Oxyquinoline. JAMA 1991; 266:1246–1251. [9]

New Yorker Magazine, 1991. [16]

Neyman, J. and Pearson, E.S. On the use and interpretation of certain test criteria for the purposes of statistical inference. Biometrika 1928; 20:175–240. [23]

Nickol, K. and Wade, A.J. Radiographic heart size and cardiothoracic ratio in three ethnic groups: a basis for a simple screening test for cardiac enlargement in men. Br. J. Radiol. 1982; 55:399–403. [16]

Noether, G.E. Why Kendall tau? Teach. Statist. 1981; 3:41–43. [27]

The Norwegian Multicenter Study Group. Timolol-induced reduction in mortality and reinfarction in patients surviving acute myocardial infarction. N. Engl. J. Med. 1981; 304:801–807. [14]

O'Brien, P.C. and Fleming, T.R. A multiple testing procedure for clinical trials. Biometrics 1979; 35:549–556. [25]

O'Brien, P.C. and Shampo, M.A. Statistical considerations for performing multiple tests in a single experiment. 6. Testing accumulating data repeatedly over time. Mayo Clin. Proc. 1988; 63:1245–1249. [25]

Oden, N. Morphology of the normal visual field in a population-based random sample: Principal components analysis. Stat. Med. 1992; 11:1131–1150. [28]

O'Quigley, J. and Baudoin, C. General approaches to the problem of bioequivalence. Statistician 1988; 37:51–58. [24]

Oski, F. et al. Iron-fortified formulas and gastrointestinal symptoms in infants: A controlled study. Pediatrics 1980; 66:168–170. [24]

Osterziel. K.J., Dietz, R., Schmid, W., Mikulaschek, K., Manthey, J., and Kubler, W. ACE inhibition improves vagal reactivity in patients with heart failure. Am. Heart J. 1990; 120:1120–1129. [19]

Oxford English Dictionary, Compact Edition. Micrographic reproduction. 1971. Oxford: Clarendon Press, 835. [29]

Pascoe, J.M. Was it a type II error? (Letter to editor). Pediatrics 1981; 68:149. [24]

Passey, M.M. The effects of polyunsaturated fat vs. monounsaturated fat on plasma lipoproteins: The power of a study (Letter to editor). JAMA 1990; 264:2071. [23]

Paul, S., Bojanczyk, M., and Lanphear, J.H. Learning preferences of medical students. Med. Educ. 1994; 28:180–186. [29]

Peacock, J.L., Bland, J.M., and Anderson, H.R. Preterm delivery: Effects of socioeconomic factors, psychological stress, smoking, alcohol, and caffeine. Br. Med. J. 1995; 311:531–536. [28]

Pearson, E.S. Some thoughts on statistical inference. Ann. Math. Statist. 1962; 33:394–403. [23]

Pearson, E.S. Quoted in Edwards, A.W.F. Likelihood. Cambridge: Cambridge University Press, 1976, v. [23]

Peduzzi, P., Concato, J., Feinstein, A.R., and Holford, T.R. Importance of "events per independent variable" in proportional hazards regression analysis. II. Accuracy and precision of regression estimates. J. Clin. Epidemiol. 1995; 48:1503–1510. [8]

Persico, M., Luzar, V., Saporaso, N., and Coltorti, M. Histologic reclassification of chronic viral hepatitis. A cluster analysis. Medic 1993; 1:23–27. [28]

Petersen, E.A., Alling, D.W., and Kirkpatrick, C.H. Treatment of chronic mucocutaneous candidiasis with ketoconazole. Ann. Intern. Med. 1980; 93:791–795. [14]

Petiti, D.D. Meta-analysis of non-experimental studies: Problems and prospects. Am. J. Epidemiol. 1993; 138:672 (Abstract). [25]

Peto, R., Gray, R., Collins, R. et al. Randomized trial of prophylactic daily aspirin in British male doctors. Br. Med. J. 1988; 296:13–16. [10,24]

Peto, R. and Peto, J. Asymptomatically efficient rank invariant test procedures. J. Roy. Statist. Soc. Series A Stat. 1972; 135:185–206. [22]

Peto, R., Pike, M.C., Armitage, P. et al. Design and analysis of randomized clinical trials requiring prolonged observation of each patient. II. Analysis and examples. Br. J. Cancer 1977; 35:1–39. [22]

Peto, R., Pike, M.C., Armitage, P., Breslow, N.E., Cox, D.R. et al. Design and analysis of randomized clinical trials requiring prolonged observation of each patient. I. Introduction and design. Br. J. Cancer 1976; 34:585–612. [25]

Pickle, L.W. (Ed.). Atlas of United States Mortality. DHHS pub. no. (PHS) 97–1015. Washington, DC: U.S. Printing Office, 1996. [25]

Pillo-Blocka, F., Jurimae, K., Khoshoo, V., and Zlotkin, S. How much is "a lot" of emesis? (Letter to editor). Lancet 1991; 337:311–312. [6]

Pitman, E.J.G. Significance tests which may be applied to samples from any population. J. Roy. Statist. Soc. Series B Metho. 1937; 4:119–130. [12]

Plewis, II. Analysing Change: Measurement and Explanation Using Longitudinal Data. New York: John Wiley and Sons, 1985. [22]

Pocock, S.J. Group sequential methods in the design and analysis of clinical trials. Biometrika 1977; 64:191–199. [25]

Pocock, S.J. When to stop a clinical trial. Br. Med. J. 1992; 305:235–240. [25]

Pocock, S.J., Gore, S.M., and Kerr, G.R. Long term survival analysis: The curability of breast cancer. Stat. Med. 1982; 1:93–104. [22]

Poole, C., Lanes, S., and Rothman, K.J. Analyzing data from ordered categories (Letter to editor). N. Engl. J. Med. 1984; 311:1382. [27]

Prentice, R.L. and Marek, P. A qualitative discrepancy between censored data rank tests. Biometrics 1979; 35:861–867. [22]

Prosnitz, L.R. Radiotherapy for lung cancer (Letter to editor). Ann. Intern. Med. 1991; 114:95–96. [23]

Quenouille, M.H. Approximate tests of correlation in time series. J. Roy. Statist. Soc. Ser. B. Metho. 1949; 11:18–84. [6]

Raju, T.N.K., Langenberg, P., and Sen, A. Treatment effect size in clinical trials: An example from surfactant trials. Controlled Clin. Trials 1993; 14:467–470. [10]

Ramirez, L., Arauz-Pacheco, C., Lackner, C., Albright, G., Adams, B., and Raskin, P. Lipoprotein (a) levels in diabetes mellitus: Relationship to metabolic control. Ann. Intern. Med. 1992; 117:42–47. [27]

Ransohoff, D.F. and Feinstein, A.R. Problems of spectrum and bias in evaluating the efficacy of diagnostic tests. N. Engl. J. Med. 1978; 299:926–930. [21]

Reaven, G.M. and Chen, Y-D.I. Role of abnormal free fatty acid metabolism in the development of non-insulin-dependent diabetes mellitus. Am. J. Med. 1988; 85:106–112. [19]

Reger, R.B., Petersen, M.R., and Morgan, W.K. Variation in the interpretation of radiographic change in pulmonary disease. Lancet 1974; 1:111–113. [20]

Reid, M.C., Lachs, M.S., and Feinstein, A.R. Use of methodological standards in diagnostic test research. JAMA 1995; 274:645–651. [21]

Reid, M.C., Lane, D.A., and Feinstein, A.R. Academic calculations versus clinical judgments: Practicing physicians' use of quantitative measures of test accuracy. Am. J. Med. 1998; 104:374–380. [21]

Resseguie, L.J. Comparison of longitudinal and cross-sectional analysis: Maternal age and stillbirth ratio. Am. J. Epidemiol. 1976; 103:551–559. [22]

Reynolds, T., Nix, B., and Dunstan, F. Use of MoMs in medical statistics (Letter to editor). Lancet 1993; 341:359. [5]

Ries, A.L., Kaplan, R.M., and Blumberg, E. Use of factor analysis to consolidate multiple outcome measures in chronic obstructive pulmonary disease. J. Clin. Epidemiol. 1991; 44:497–503. [28]

Risch, N. Genetic linkage: Interpreting lod scores. Science 1992; 255:803–804. [17]

Robbins, J.A. Subspecialty choice and faculty income (Letter to editor). J. Gen. Intern. Med. 1993; 8:401. [27]

Roberts, C.J. and Powell, R.G. Interrelation of the common congenital malformations. Lancet 1975; 2:849. [9]

Robertson, W.O. Quantifying the meanings of words. J. Am. Med. Assn. 1983; 249:2631–2632. [6]

Robinson, W.B. The statistical measurement of agreement. Amer. Sociol. Rev. 1957; 22:17–25. [20]

Rodda, B.E. and Davis, R.L. Determining the probability of an important difference in bioavailability. Clin. Pharmacol. Ther. 1980; 28:247–252. [24]

Rodriguez, B.L., Masaki, K., Burchfiel, C., Curb, J.D., Fong, K-O, Chyou, P-H, and Marcus, E.B. Pulmonary function decline and 17-year total mortality: The Honolulu heart program. Am. J. Epidemiol. 1994; 140:398–408. [22]

Roebruck, P. and Kuhn, A. Comparison of tests and sample size formulae for proving therapeutic equivalence based on the difference of binomial probabilities. Stat. Med. 1995; 14:1583–1594. [24]

Roos, N.P., Wennberg, J.E., Malenka, D.J., et al. Mortality and reoperation after open and transurethral resection of the prostate for benign prostatic hyperplasia. N. Engl. J. Med. 1989; 320:1120–1124. [26]

Rosenthal, R. Meta-Analytic Procedures for Social Research. (Rev. ed.) Newbury Park: Sage Publications, 1991. [25]

Rossen, R.M., Goodman, D.J., Ingham, R.E., and Popp, R.L. Ventricular systolic septal thickening and excursion in idiopathic hypertrophic subaortic stenosis. N. Engl. J. Med. 1974; 291:317–319. [10]

Rosvoll, R.V., Mengason, A.P., Smith, L., Patel, H.J., Maynard, J., and Connor, F. Visual and automated differential leukocyte counts. A comparison study of three instruments. Am. J. Clin. Path. 1979; 71:695–703. [21]

Rothman, K.J. Modern Epidemiology. Boston: Little, Brown & Co., 1986. [26]

Rothman, K.J. No adjustments are needed for multiple comparisons. Epidemiology 1990; 1:43–46. [25]

Royal College of General Practitioners. Oral Contraceptives and Health: An Interim Report from the Oral Contraception Study. London: Pitman Medical, 1974. [26]

Royall, R.M. Ethics and statistics in randomized clinical trials (with discussion). Statist. Science 1991; 12:277–292. [25]

Royston, P. A toolkit for testing non-normality in complete and censored samples. Statistician 1993a; 42:37–43. [5]

Royston, P. Graphical detection of non-normality by using Michael's statistic. Appl. Statist. 1993b; 42:153–158. [5]

Rozanski, A., Diamond, G.A., Berman, D. et al. The declining specificity of exercise radionuclide ventriculography. N. Engl. J. Med. 1983; 309:518–522. [21]

Ruel, M.T., Habicht, J.-P., Pinstrup-Andersen, P., and Grohn, Y. The mediating effect of maternal nutrition knowledge on the association between maternal schooling and child nutritional status in Lesotho. Am. J. Epidemiol. 1992; 135:904–914. [4]

Rumke, C.L. Implications of the statement: No side effects were observed (Letter to editor). N. Engl. J. Med. 1975; 292:372–373. [8]

Runyon, B.A., Montano, A.A., Akriviadis, E.A., Antillon, M.R., Irving, M.A., and McHutchison, J.G. The serum-ascites albumin gradient is superior to the exudate-transudate concept in the differential diagnosis of ascites. Ann. Intern. Med. 1992; 117:215–220. [16]

Saad, M.F., Lillioja, S., Nyomba, B.L. et al. Racial differences in the relation between blood pressure and insulin resistance. N. Engl. J. Med. 1991; 324:733–739. [19]

Sabia, P., Powers, E., Ragosta, M., Sarembock, I., Burwell, L., and Kaul, S. An association between collateral blood flow and myocardial viability in patients with recent myocardial infarction. N. Engl. J. Med. 1992; 327:1825–1831. [27]

Sackett, D.L. Applying overviews and meta-analyses at the bedside. J. Clin. Epidemiol. 1995; 48:61–66. [25]

Sackett, D.L. and Cook, R.J. Understanding clinical trials. What measures of efficacy should journal articles provide busy clinicians? Brit. Med. J. 1994; 309:755–756. [10]

Sackett, D.L, Haynes, R.B., Guyatt, G.H., and Tugwell, P. Clinical Epidemiology. A Basic Science for Clinical Medicine. 2nd. ed. Boston: Little, Brown and Co., 1991. [1,21]

Sakia, R.M. The Box-Cox transformation technique: A review. Statistician 1992; 41:169–178. [3]

Salsburg, D. Hypothesis versus significance testing for controlled clinical trials: A dialogue. Statist. Med. 1990; 9:201–211. [23]

Sanchez-Guerrero, J., Colditz, G.A., Karlson, E.W., Hunter, D.J., Speizer, F.E., and Liang, M.H. Silicone breast implants and the risk of connective-tissue diseases and symptoms. N. Engl. J. Med. 1995; 332:1666–1670. [25]

Sanderson, C. and McKee, M. Commentary: How robust are rankings? The implications of confidence intervals. Br. Med. J. 1998; 316:1705. [7]

SAS Procedures Guide. Chapter 42, The Univariate Procedure. Ver. 6, 3rd ed. Cary, NC: SAS Institute, Inc., 1990, 617–634. [5]

Saudia, T.L., Barfield, B.R., and Barger, J. Effect of oat bran consumption on total serum cholesterol levels in healthy adults. Milit. Med. 1992; 157:567–568. [29]

Saunders, J., Baron, M.D., Shenouda, F.S., and Sonksen, P.H. Measuring glycosylated haemoglobin concentrations in a diabetic clinic. Br. Med. J. 1980; 281:1394. [20]

Savage, I.R. Contributions to the theory of rank order statistics—The two-sample case. Ann. Math. Statist. 1956; 27:590–615. [22]

Savitz, D.A. and Olshan, A.F. Multiple comparisons and related issues in the interpretation of epidemiologic data. Am. J. Epidemiol. 1995; 142:904–908. [25]

Sawada, S, Sugai, S., Iijima, S. et al. Increased soluble CD4 and decreased soluble CD8 molecules in patients with Sjogren's Syndrome. Am. J. Med. 1992; 92:134–140. [27]

Schacker, T.W., Hughes, J.P., Shea, T., Coombs, R.W., and Corey, L. Biological and virologic characteristics of primary HIV infection. Ann. Intern. Med. 1998; 128:613–620. [19]

Scheffe, H. A method of judging all contrasts in the analysis of variance. Biometrika 1953; 40:87–104. [25]

Schlesselman, J.J. Case-Control Studies. New York: Oxford University Press, 1982. [26]

Schlundt, D.G., Taylor, D., Hill, J.O., Sbrocco, T., Pope-Cordle, J., Kasser, T., and Arnold, D. A behavioral taxonomy of obese female participants in a weight-loss program. Am. J. Clin. Nutr. 1991; 53:1151–1158. [28]

Schulz, H.-U. and Steinijans, V.W. Striving for standards in bioequivalence assessment: A review. Int. J. Clin. Ther. Toxicol. 1991; 29:293–298. [24]

Schulze, R.A., Jr., Rouleau, J., Rigo, P., Bowers, S., Strauss, H.W., and Pitt, B. Ventricular arrhythmias in the late hospital phase of acute myocardial infarction. Relation to left ventricular function detected by gated cardiac blood pool scanning. Circulation 1975; 52:1006:1011. [9]

Schulzer, M., Anderson, D.R., and Drance, S.M. Sensitivity and specificity of a diagnostic test determined by repeated observations. J. Clin. Epidemiol. 1991; 44:1167–1179. [21]

Schwartz, D. and Lellouch, J. Exploratory and pragmatic attitudes in therapeutic trials. J. Chron. Dis. 1967; 20:637–648. [23]

Sechi, L.A., Zingaro, L., DeCarli, S., Sechi, G., Catena, C., Falleti, E., Dell'Anna, E., and Bartoli, E. Increased serum lipoprotein(a) levels in patients with early renal failure. Ann. Intern. Med. 1998; 129:456–461. [19]

Seregard, S. Cell proliferation as a prognostic indicator in conjunctival malignant melanoma. Am. J. Ophthalmol. 1993; 116:93–97. [29]

Shann, F. Nutritional indices: Z, centile, or percent? Lancet 1993; 341:526–527. [4]

Shannon, C.E. A mathematical theory of communication. Bell Syst. Tech. J. 1948; 27:379–423, 623–656. [5]

Shapiro, S. Meta-analysis/Shmeta-analysis. Am. J. Epidemiol. 1994; 140:771–778. [25]

Sheikh, K.H., Bengtson, J.R., Rankin, J.S., de Bruijn, N.P., and Kisslo, J. Intraoperative transesophageal Doppler color flow imaging used to guide patient selection and operative treatment of ischemic mitral regurgitation. Circulation 1991; 84:594–604. [20]

Sheiner, L.B. The intellectual health of clinical drug evaluation. Clin. Pharmacol. Ther. 1992; 52:104–106. [29]

Sheppard, H., Winkelstein, W., Lang, W., and Charlebois, E. CD4+ T-lymphocytopenia without HIV infection (Letter to editor). N. Engl. J. Med. 1993; 328:1847–1848. [16]

Sheps, M.C. Shall we count the living or the dead. N. Engl. J. Med. 1958; 259:1210–1214. [10]

Sherrill, D.L., Lebowitz, M.D., Knudson, R.J., and Burrows, B. Longitudinal methods for describing the relationship between pulmonary function, respiratory symptoms and smoking in elderly subjects: The Tucson Study. Eur. Respir. J. 1993; 6:342–348. [22]

Shrout, P.E. and Fleiss, J.L. Intraclass correlations: Uses in assessing rater reliability. Psychol. Bull. 1979; 86:420–428. [29]

Siegel, S, and Castellan, N.J., Jr. Non-Parametric Statistics for the Behavioral Sciences. 2nd ed. New York: McGraw-Hill Book Co., 1988. [15,20,27]

Simel, D.L., Samsa, G.P., and Matchar, D.B. Likelihood ratios for continuous test results— Making the clinicians' job easier or harder? J. Clin. Epidemiol. 1993; 46:85–93. [21]

Simes, R.J. An improved Bonferroni procedure for multiple tests of significance. Biometrika 1986; 73:751–754. [25]

Simon, G.A. Efficacies of measures of association for ordinal contingency tables. J. Am. Statist. Assn. 1978; 73:545–551. [27]

Simon, G.E. and VonKorff, M. Reevaluation of secular trends in depression rates. Am. J. Epidemiol. 1992; 135:1411–1422. [22]

Simon, J.L. Basic Research Methods in Social Science. New York: Random House. 1969. [6]

Sinclair, J.C. and Bracken, M.B. Clinically useful measures of effect in binary analyses of randomized trials. J. Clin. Epidemiol. 1994; 47:881–889. [10]

Singer, P.A. and Feinstein, A.R. Graphical display of categorical data. J. Clin. Epidemiol. 1993; 46:231–236. [9,16]

Slavin, R.E. Best evidence synthesis: An intelligent alternative to meta-analysis. J. Clin. Epidemiol. 1995; 48:9–18. [25]

Smirnov, N.V. Tables for estimating the goodness of fit of empirical distributions. Ann. Math. Statist. 1948; 19:279–281. [14]

Smith, A.H. and Bates, M.N. Confidence limit analyses should replace power calculations in the interpretation of epidemiologic studies. Epidemiology 1992; 3:449–452. [24]

Smith, D.E., Lewis, C.E., Caveny, J.L., Perkins, L.L., Burke, G.L., and Bild, D.E. Longitudinal changes in adiposity associated with pregnancy. J. Am. Med. Assn. 1994; 271:1747–1751. [22]

Snedecor, G.W. and Cochran, W.G. Statistical Methods. 7th ed. Ames, Iowa: Iowa State University Press, 1980 (5th ed., 1956). [5,19]

Sorlie, P.D., Thom, T.J., Manolio, T., Rosenberg, H.M, Anderson, R.N., and Burke, G.L. Age-adjusted death rates: Consequences of the year 2000 standard. Ann. Epidemiol. 1999; 9:93–100. [26]

Souhami, R.L. and Whitehead, J. (Eds.). Workshop on early stopping rules in cancer clinical trials. Statist. Med. 1994; 13:1289–1499. [25]

Sox, H. (Ed.). Common Diagnostic Tests: Use and Interpretation. Philadelphia: American College of Physicians, 1987. [21]

Spear, M. Charting Statistics. New York: McGraw-Hill Book Co., Inc., 1952. [5]

Spearman, C. General intelligence objectively determined and measured. Am. J. Psychol. 1904; 15:201–293. [28]

Special Writing Group of the Committee on Rheumatic Fever, Endocarditis, and Kawasaki Disease of the Council on Cardiovascular Disease in the Young of the American Heart Association. Guidelines for the diagnosis of rheumatic fever. Jones Criteria, 1992 update. JAMA 1993; 269:476. [21]

Spitzer, R.L., Fleiss, J.L., Kernohan, W., Lee, J., and Baldwin, I.T. The Mental Status Schedule: Comparing Kentucky and New York schizophrenics. Arch. Gen. Psychiatry 1965; 12:448–455. [15]

Spitzer, W.O. (Ed.). Potsdam International Consultation on Meta-Analysis. (Special issue) J. Clin. Epidemiol. 1995; 48:1–171. [25]

Sprent, P. Applied Nonparametric Statistical Methods. 2nd ed. London: Chapman and Hall, 1993. [15,20,27]

SPSS^X User's Guide. 2nd ed. Chapter 28, General linear models. Chicago, IL: SPSS Inc., 1986, 477–552. [5]

Stacpoole, P.W., Wright, E.C., Baumgartner, T.G. et al. A controlled clinical trial of dichloroacetate for treatment of lactic acidosis in adults. N. Engl. J. Med. 1992; 327:1564–1569. [10]

Staniloff, H.M., Diamond, G.A., Forrester, J.S., Pollock, B.H., Berman, D.S., and Swan, H.J.C. The incremental information boondoggle: When a test result seems powerful but is not. Circulation 1982; 66:184 (Abstract). [21]

Stead, E.A., Jr. Response to Letter to editor. Circulation 1978; 57:1232. [19]

Steen, P.M., Brewster, A.C., Bradbury, R.C., Estabrook, E., and Young, J.A. Predicted probabilities of hospital death as admission severity of illness. Inquiry 1993; 30:128–141. [21]

Steering Committee of the Physicians' Health Study Research Group. Final report on the aspirin component of the ongoing Physicians' Health Study. N. Engl. J. Med. 1989; 321:129–1135. [10,14,24]

Steiner, D.L. and Norman, G.R. Health Measurement Scales. A Practical Guide to Their Development and Use. 2nd ed. Oxford: Oxford University Press. 1995. [28]

Stephen, S.A. et al. Propranolol in acute myocardial infarction. Lancet 1966; 2:1435–1438. [23]

Stevens, S.S. On the theory of scales of measurement. Science 1946; 103:677–680. [2]

Student. The probable error of a mean. Biometrika 1908; 6:1. [6,7]

Stukel, T.A. Comparison of methods for the analysis of longitudinal interval count data. Stat. Med. 1993; 12:1339–1351. [22]

Sulmasy, D.P., Haller, K., and Terry, P.B. More talk, less paper: Predicting the accuracy of substituted judgments. Am. J. Med. 1994; 96:432–438. [20]

Surgeon General's Advisory Committee On Smoking and Health. Smoking and Health 1964. United States Department of Health, Education and Welfare, Public Health Service Publication No. 1103. [13]

Tasaki, T., Ohto, H., Hashimoto, C., Abe, R., Saitoh, A., and Kikuchi, S. Recombinant human erythropoietin for autologous blood donation: Effects on perioperative red-blood-cell and serum erythropoietin production. Lancet 1992; 339:773–775. [19]

Tate, M.W. and Clelland, R.C. Non-Parametric and Shortcut Statistics. Danville, IL: Interstate Printers and Publishers, 1957. [27]

Teigen, K.H. Studies in subjective probability. III: The unimportance of alternatives. Scand. J. Psychol. 1983; 24:97–105. [6]

Thielemans, A., Hopke, P.K., De Quint, P., Depoorter, A.M., Thiers, G., and Massart, D.L. Investigation of the geographical distribution of female cancer patterns in Belgium using pattern recognition techiniques. Int. J. Epidemiol. 1988; 17:724–731. [28]

Thomas, D.C., Siemiatycki, J., Dewar, R., Robins, J., Goldberg, M., and Armstrong, B.G. The problem of multiple inference in studies designed to generate hypotheses. Am. J. Epidemiol. 1985; 122:1080–1095. [25]

Thompson, J.D., Fetter, R.B., and Mross, C.D. Case mix and resource use. Inquiry 1975; 12:300–312. [21]

Thompson, J.R. Invited Commentary: Re: Multiple comparisons and related issues in the interpretation of epidemiologic data. Am. J. Epidemiol. 1998; 147:801–806. [25]

Thompson, S.G. and Pocock, S.J. Can meta-analyses be trusted? Lancet 1991; 338:1127–1130. [25]

Tibshirani, R. A plain man's guide to the proportional hazards model. Clin. Invest. Med. 1982; 5:63–68. [22]

Tomei, R., Rossi, L., Carbonieri, E., Franceschini, L., Molon, G., and Zardini, P. Antihypertensive effect of lisinopril assessed by 24-hour ambulatory monitoring: A double-blind, placebo-controlled, cross-over study. J. Cardiovasc. Pharmacol. 1992; 19:911–914. [29]

Trentham, D.E., Dynesius-Trentham, R.A., Orav, E.J. et al. Effects of oral administration of Type II collagen on rheumatoid arthritis. Science 1993; 261:1727–1730. [15]

Tsai, S.P., Lee, E.S., and Kautz, J.A. Changes in life expectancy in the United States due to declines in mortality, 1968–1975. Am. J. Epidemiol. 1982; 116:376–384. [22]

Tufte, E.R. The Visual Display of Quantitative Information. Cheshire, CT: Graphics Press, 1983. [16]

Tufte, E.R. Envisioning Information. Cheshire, CT: Graphics Press, 1990. [16]

Tukey, J.W. Comparing individual means in the analysis of variance. Biometrics 1949; 5:99–114. [25]

Tukey, J.W. Bias and confidence in not-quite large samples. Ann. Math. Statist. 1958; 29:614. [6]

Tukey, J.W. The problem of multiple comparisons. Unpublished notes. Princeton University, 1953. [Discussed in Bancroft, T.A. Topics in Intermediate Statistical Methods. Vol. 1. Ames: Iowa State University Press. 1968, 100–112.] [29]

Tukey, J.W. Some graphic and semigraphic displays. Chapter 18, pgs. 295–296. In Bancroft, T.A. (Ed.). Statistical Papers in Honor of George W. Snedecor. Ames, Iowa: Iowa State University Press, 1972. [3]

Tukey, J.W. Exploratory Data Analysis. Reading, MA: Addison-Wesley, 1977. [2,3,5]

Twisk, J.W.R., Kemper, H.C.G., and Mellenbergh, G.J. Mathematical and analytical aspects of tracking. Epidemiol. Rev. 1994; 16:165–183. [22]

Ulm, K. A simple method to calculate the confidence interval of a standardized mortality ratio (SMR). Am. J. Epidemiol. 1990; 131:373–375. [26]

Uretsky, B.F., Jessup, M., Konstam, M.A. et al. Multicenter trial of oral enoximone in patients with moderate to moderately severe congestive heart failure. Circulation 1990; 82:774–780. [23]

Vandenbroucke, J.P. A shortcut method for calculating the 95 per cent confidence interval of the standardized mortality ratio (Letter to editor). Am. J. Epidemiol. 1982; 115:303–304. [26]

Vandenbroucke, J.P. and Pardoel, V.P.A.M. An autopsy of epidemiologic methods: the case of "poppers" in the early epidemic of the acquired immunodeficiency syndrome (AIDS). Am. J. Epidemiol. 1989; 129:455–457. [19]

Vessey, M., Doll, R., Peto, R., Johnson, B., and Wiggins, P. A long-term follow-up study of women using different methods of contraception—An interim report. J. Biosoc. Sci. 1976; 8:373–427. [25]

Viberti, G. et al. Early closure of European Pimagedine trial (Letter to editor). Lancet 1997; 350:214–215. [25]

Vollset, S.E. Confidence intervals for a binomial proportion. Stat. Med. 1993; 12:809–824. [8]

von Knorring, L. and Lindstrom, E. Principal components and further possibilities with the PANSS. Acta Psychiatr. Scand. 1995; 91(Suppl 388): 5–10. [28]

Wagner, G.S., Cebe, B., and Rozen, M.P. (Eds.). E.A. Stead, Jr.: What This Patient Needs Is a Doctor. Durham, NC: Academic Press, 1978. [19]

Wald, A. Sequential Analysis. New York: John Wiley and Sons, 1947. [25]

Wald, N. Use of MoMs (Letter to the editor). Lancet 1993; 341:440. [5]

Waller, L.A. and Turnbull, B.W. Probability plotting with censored data. Am. Statist. 1992; 46:5–12. [22]

Waller, L.A., Turnbull, B.W., Gustafsson, G., Hjalmars, U., and Andersson, B. Detection and assessment of clusters of disease: An application to nuclear power plant facilities and childhood leukemia in Sweden. Stat. Med. 1995; 14:3–16. [28]

Wallis, W.A. and Roberts, H.V. Statistics: A New Approach. New York: The Free Press, 1956. [5,14]

Wallsten, T.S. and Budescu, D.V. Comment on "Quantifying probabilistic expressions." Statist. Sci. 1990; 5:23–26. [6]

Walravens, P.A., Chakar, A., Mokni, R., Denise, J., and Lemonnier, D. Zinc supplements in breastfed infants. Lancet 1992; 340:683–685. [4]

Walter, S.D. Statistical significance and fragility criteria for assessing a difference of two proportions. J. Clin. Epidemiol. 1991; 44:1373–1378. [11]

Walter, S.D. Visual and statistical assessment of spatial clustering in mapped data. Statist. Med. 1993; 12:1275–1291. [25]

Wastell, D.G. and Gray, R. The numerical approach to classification: A medical application to develop a typology for facial pain. Statist. Med. 1987; 6:137–146. [28]

Weinberg, A.D., Pals, J.K., McGlinchey-Berroth, R., and Minaker, K.L. Indices of dehydration among frail nursing home patients: Highly variable but stable over time. J. Am. Geriat. Soc. 1994; 42:1070–1073. [29]

Weinstein, M.C. and Fineberg, H.V. Clinical Decision Analysis. Philadelphia: Saunders, 1980. [21]

Weiss, J.S., Ellis, C.N., Headington, J.T., Tincoff, T., Hamilton, T.A., and Voorhees, J.J. Topical tretinoin improves photoaged skin. A double-blind vehicle-controlled study. JAMA 1988; 259:527–532. [15]

Welch, B.L. On the Z test in randomized blocks and Latin squares. Biometrika 1937; 29:21–52. [12]

Westfall, P.H. and Young, S.S. Resampling-Based Muiltiple Testing: Examples and Methods for p-Values Adjustment. John Wiley and Sons, New York, 1993. [25]

Westlake, W.J. Use of confidence intervals in analysis of comparative bioavailability trials. J. Pharm. Sci. 1972; 61:1340–1341. [24]

Westlake, W.J. Statistical aspects of comparative bioavailability trials. Biometrics 1979; 35:273–280. [24]

Whitehead, J. The case for frequentism in clinical trials. Statist. Med. 1993; 12:1405–1413. [11]

WHO Working Group. Use and interpretation of anthropometric indicators of nutritional status. Bull. WHO 1986; 64:929–941. [4]

Wiggs, J., Nordenskjold, M., Yandell, D. et al. Prediction of the risk of hereditary retinoblastoma, using DNA polymorphisms within the retinoblastoma gene. N. Engl. J. Med. 1988; 318:151–157. [21]

Wilcoxon, F. Individual comparisons by ranking methods. Biometrics Bull. 1945; 1:80–82. [15]

Wilk, M.B. and Gnanadesikan, R. Probability plotting methods for the analysis of data. Biometrika 1968; 55:1–17. [16]

Williams, K. The failure of Pearson's goodness of fit statistic. Statistician 1976; 25:49. [14]

Wintemute, G.J. Handgun availability and firearm mortality (Letter to editor). Lancet 1988; 335:1136–1137. [19]

Wolleswinkel-van den Bosch, J.H., Looman, C.W., van Poppel, F.W., and Mackenbach, J.P. Cause-specific mortality trends in the Netherlands, 1875–1992: A formal analysis of the epidemiologic transition. Int. J. Epidemiol. 1997; 26:772–779. [28]

Wolthius, R.A., Froelicher, V.F., Jr., Fischer, J., and Triebwasser, J.H. The response of healthy men to treadmill exercise. Circulation 1977; 55:153–157. [16]

Woolf, B. On estimating the relation between blood group and disease. Ann. Hum. Genet. 1955; 19:251–253. [17]

Woolf, B. The log likelihood ratio test (the G-test). Methods and tables for tests of heterogeneity in contingency tables. Ann. Hum. Genetics 1957; 21:397–409. [14]

Wright, J.G. and Feinstein, A.R. A comparative contrast of clinimetric and psychometric methods for constructing indexes and rating scales. J. Clin. Epidemiol. 1992; 45:1201–1218. [28]

Wright, J.G., McCauley, T.R., Bell, S.M., and McCarthy, S. The reliability of radiologists' quality assessment of MR pelvic scans. J. Comput. Assist. Tomogr. 1992; 16:592–596. [27]

Wulff, H.R. Rational Diagnosis and Treatment. 2nd ed. Oxford: Blackwell Scientific, 1981. [4,21]

Wynder, E.L. Workshop on guidelines to the epidemiology of weak associations. Prev. Med. 1987; 16:139–141. [17,24]

Wynder, E.L., Bross, I.D.J., and Hiroyama, T. A study of the epidemiology of cancer of the breast. Cancer 1960; 13:559–601. [15]

Yates, F. Contingency tables involving small numbers and the χ^2 test. J. Roy. Statist. Soc. Suppl. 1934; 1:217–235. [14]

Yates, F. Tests of significance for 2×2 contingency tables. J. Roy. Statist. Soc. Series A 1984; 147:426–463. [14]

Yerushalmy, J. Statistical problems in assessing methods of medical diagnosis, with special reference to X-ray techniques. Public Health Rep. 1947; 62:1432–1449. [21]

Yerushalmy, J. A mortality index for use in place of the age-adjusted death rate. Am. J. Public Health 1951; 41:907–922. [26]

Yerushalmy, J. The statistical assessment of the variability in observer perception and description of roentgenographic pulmonary shadows. Radiol. Clin. North Am. 1969; 7:381–392. [20]

Youden, W.J. Quoted in Tufte, E.R. The Visual Display of Quantitative Information. Cheshire, CT: Graphics Press, 1983. [9]

Zeger, S.L. and Liang, K-Y. An overview of methods for the analysis of longitudinal data. Stat. Med. 1992; 11:1825–1839. [22]

Zelen, M. The education of biometricians. Am. Statist. 1969; 23:14–15. [24]

Zerbe, G.O., Wu, M.C., and Zucker, D.M. Studying the relationship between change and initial value in longitudinal studies. Stat. Med. 1994; 13:759–768. [22]

Zmuda, J.M., Cauley, J.A., Kriska, A., Glynn, N.W., Gutai, J.P., and Kuller, L.H. Longitudinal relation between endogenous testosterone and cardiovascular disease risk factors in middle-aged men. Am. J. Eidemiol. 1997; 146:609–617. [22]

Index

Answers to Exercises

The following "official" answers are for Exercises that have an odd second number. Answers to the even-numbered Exercises are contained in an Instructor's Manual.

Chapter 1

1.1. 4. (Architecture)
1.3. 3. (Stochastic)
1.5. 1. (A descriptive summary, expressed in nonquantitative terms.)
1.7. 5. (A decision about classifying the raw data. If you cited 6 as the answer, you can also be justified, although data processing usually refers to the conversion of *sick* into a coded category, such as "1 in column 37 of card 6," rather than the data acquisition process that converts raw data, such as "Apgar ≤ 6," into a designated category, such as "sick." Because the distinctions are somewhat blurred, either answer is acceptable.)
1.9. 5, if you think the research was done to demonstrate the quality of the raw data; 4, if you think the research has an architectural role with respect to biased observations. Either answer is acceptable.
1.11. 4. (Architecture)

Chapter 2

2.1.

2.1.1. Age, height, and each blood pressure measurement are dimensional. Sex is binary. Diagnosis is nominal. Treatment is nominal, if different agents are used; dimensional, if different dosages of the same agent are given in the same schedule; ordinal, if the dosages of the same agent can be ranked but cannot be arranged in exact dimensions because of the different schedules.

2.1.2. To analyze blood pressure responses, some of the following changes might be examined:

Ultimate Effect: Increment of *before* and *after* values.

Immediate Effect: Increment of *before* and *during* values.

Therapeutic Trend: Rating of **rise, stable, fall, up-and-down, down-and-up,** etc. for trend observed in the three consecutive BP values

Ultimate Success: Deciding if the blood pressure after treatment is normal or abnormal.

2.3. *Examples*

"How do you feel today compared with yesterday?"
"What has happened to your pain since you received the medication?"
"What sort of change has occurred in your child's temperature?"
"How much heavier have you gotten since your last birthday?"

2.5. The TNM index expressions are composite "profiles" that contain three single-state variables. They are nominal and cannot be readily ranked because they do not have an aggregated expression. In the TNM *staging* system, each TNM profile index is assigned to an ordinal stage such as **I, II, III, ...** If desired, the TNM indexes could be ordinally ranked according to their locations in the staging system.

2.7. There are no real advantages. The trivial saving of effort in citing one rather than two digits when the data are extracted will be followed by massive disadvantages when the data are later analyzed. The investigator will be unable to determine any averages (such as means or medians), unable to find any trends within the same decade, and unable to find distinctions that cross decades (such as the age group **35–54**). The moral of the story is: *Always* enter dimensional data in their original dimensions or in direct transformations (such as **kg ↔lb**) that preserve the original dimensions. *Never* compress dimensional data for their original citation; the compression can always be done later, during the analyses.

2.9. Individual answers.

Chapter 3

3.1. The median is probably the best choice for this right-skewed distribution.

3.3. Mean $= \overline{X} = 120.10$. For these 20 numbers, the median is between ranks 10 and 11. The actual values at these ranks are 91 and 96; and so median $= (91 + 96)/2 = 93.5$. Mode is 97. Geometric mean is $(3.198952738 \times 10^{40})^{1/20} = (3.198952738 \times 10^{40})^{.05} = 105.99$.

Chapter 4

4.1. The data set contains 56 members.

    4.1.1. For lower quartile, $(.25)(56) = 14$, and the rank is between 14 and 15. The values of **17** appear at both the 14th and 15th rank, and so $Q_L = \mathbf{17}$. For upper quartile, $(.75)(56) = 42$, and rank is between 42 and 43. $Q_U = \mathbf{28}$, which occupies ranks 41–44. [With the $r = P(n + 1)$ formula, $(.25)(57) = 14.25$ and so Q_L is at **17** between 14th and 15th rank. For Q_U, $(.75)(57) = 42.75$, which is again between rank 42 and 43.]

    4.1.2. $(.025)(56) = 1.4$, which will become rank 2, at which the value is **12** for $P_{.025}$. For $P_{.975}$, $(.975)(56) = 54.6$, which will become rank 55, at which the value is **41**. [With the $r = P(n + 1)$ formula, $(.025)(57) = 1.4$, which would put the 2.5 percentile value at **11.5**, between ranks 1 and 2. Since $(.975)(57) = 55.6$, the 97.5 percentile value is at **42** between the 55th and 56th ranks.]

    4.1.3. The value of 30 in Table 3.1 is at the 48th rank. At rank 47, $47/56 = .839$; and at rank 48, the cumulative proportion is $48/56 = .857$. Therefore **30** occupies both the 84th and 85th percentiles. [With the formula $P = r/(n + 1)$, we get $48/57 = .842$, which would be the 84th percentile.]

4.3. If the data were Gaussian, the positive and negative Z-scores would be symmetrically distributed around the mean. They are *not*.

4.5. Let each candidate's raw score be X_i. From the array of candidate raw scores, calculate $\overline{X}$ and s and then calculate $Z_i = (X_i - \overline{X})/s$ for each candidate. These results will have a mean of zero and s.d. of 1. To make the s.d. 100, multiply each Z_i by 100, to get $100Z_i$. The results will have a mean of zero and s.d. of 100. Then add 500 to each $100Z_i$. The results will have a mean of 500 and s.d. of 100. Thus, the formula is: Final Score $= [100(X_i - \overline{X})/s] + 500$.

Practical Demonstration of the Formula:

    Three candidates get 75, 83, and 92 in the raw scores. For these data, $\overline{X} = 83.33$ and $s = 8.50$. The original Z_i scores for the three candidates will be $(75 - 83.33)/8.50 = -0.98$, $(83 - 83.33)/8.50 = -0.04$ and $(92 - 83.33)/8.50 = 1.02$. Multiplied by 100, these scores become -98, -4, and 102. When 500 is added, the scores become 402, 496, and 602. For these three values, a check on your calculator will confirm that $\overline{X} = 500$ and $s = 100$.

4.7.

    4.7.1. False. The percentile reflects a ranking among candidates, not the actual score on the test.

    4.7.2. False. If the actual results have a Gaussian or near-Gaussian distribution, only a small change is needed to go from the 50th to 59th percentile. A much larger change is needed to go from the 90th to 99th percentile. Thus, Mary made comparatively more progress than John.

    4.7.3. False. Same problem as 4.7.2. Percentiles give ranks, not scores, and may distort the magnitudes of differences in actual scores. The three cited percentiles (84, 98, and 99.9) are roughly about l, 2, and 3 standard deviations above the mean in a Gaussian distribution, so that the actual magnitudes of scores are about equidistant.

4.7.4. False. In this "middle" zone of the distribution, where data are usually most abundant, a small change in actual score can produce large changes in percentiles.

4.7.5. Uncertain. The overall percentile scores for each student last year represent a comparative ranking among all students who took the test last year. The percentile rating averaged for different students will not be a meaningful number. On the other hand, if percentiles (rather than actual test scores) are the only information available to the dean, he has no other option if he wants to compare this year's results.

4.9. As Joe's lawyer, you argue that "grading on a curve" is an abominable way to assess competence. If you give the exam exclusively to an assembled collection of the most superb omphalologists in the country, some of them will nevertheless fail if "graded on a curve." Why should Joe, whose actual score of 72% is usually accepted as passing in most events, be failed because of the performance of other people? As lawyer for the Board, you argue that it is impossible to determine an *absolute* passing score for the complex examination. Accordingly, the passing score is determined from a point on the curve of scores obtained by a reference group of Joe's peers. He failed because his performance was worse than that of other people with presumably similar backgrounds and training. (This approach has been used, and successfully defended despite legal attacks, by almost all certification Boards in the U.S.)

Chapter 5

5.1. It seems peculiar to assemble a group of people who have been deliberately chosen for all being "healthy," and then to exclude 5% of them arbitrarily as being outside the "range of normal." Why not include the full range of data in the healthy, i.e. "normal," people?

5.3. Individual answers.

5.5.

5.5.1   Let $s = \sqrt{v/n - 1}$ and $s' = \sqrt{v/n}$. Since $s^2 = v/(n-1)$, we can substitute $s^2(n-1)$ for v, to get $s' = \sqrt{s^2(n-1)/n}$. Accordingly, in the 56-item data set, $s' = \sqrt{(7.693)^2(55)/56} = 7.624$.

5.5.2. $cv = s/\overline{X} = 7.693/22.732 = .388$.

5.5.3. The lower quartile is at rank $(.25)(56) = 14 \rightarrow$ between 14 and 15. The upper quartile is at rank $(.75)(56) = 42 \rightarrow$ between 42 and 43. In Table 3.1, the value of **17** occupies ranks 12–16. The value **28** occupies ranks 41–44. The quartile coefficient of variation will be $(28 - 17)/(28 + 17) = 11/45 = .24$.

5.7. Individual answers.

Chapter 6

6.1.

6.1.1. Since each tossed coin can emerge as a head or tail, there are four possibilities: HH, HT, TH, and TT. The chance is 1/4 for getting two heads or two tails. The chance is 2/4 = 1/2 for getting a head and a tail.

6.1.2. Each of the two dice has six sides marked 1, 2,..., 6. When tossed, the pair can have 36 possible outcomes, ranging from 1-1 to 6-6. A value of **7** occurs on six occasions: 1–6, 2–5, 3–4, 4–3, 5–2, and 6–1. Thus, the probability of a **7** is 6/36 = 1/6.

6.1.3. Common things occur commonly, but uncommon things can also occur if given enough opportunity. A pair of consecutive **7**'s can be expected about once in 36 pairs of tosses. If you stay at the dice table long enough to observe 72 or more tosses, two of them could yield consecutive **7**'s under ordinary circumstances. If the consecutive pairs of **7**'s appear with substantially greater frequency than .03, you might suspect that the dice are "loaded".

6.1.4. The 5 possible ways of tossing a **6** are 1–5, 2–4, 3–3, 4–2, and 5–1. Thus, the probability of getting a 6 on a single roll is 5/36. The fact that a 6 was just tossed is irrelevant, since each toss is a new or "independent" event. (If you were considering, in advance, whether two consecutive sixes might be tossed, the probability would be $(5/36)(5/36) = .019$.)

6.1.5. Although effectively balanced on its pivot, no roulette wheel is ever perfectly balanced. Accordingly, the roulette ball is more likely to fall in slots for certain numbers than for others. If you prepare a frequency count of the consecutive outcomes of each rotation, you can begin to see the pattern of the higher-probability outcomes for each wheel on its particular pivot. This "histogram" can then guide you into successful betting. Changing the wheels at regular intervals will destroy the characteristics of the histograms.

6.3. If $\bar{X}$ is the mean, a zone of 1.96 standard deviations around the mean should include 95% of the data. Conversely, a zone of 1.96 standard deviations around the observed value of 40 should have a 95% chance of including the mean. Thus, if we calculate $40 \pm (1.96)(12.3) = 40 \pm 24.1$, the mean can be expected, with 95% chance or confidence, to lie within the zone of 15.9 to 64.1. (This principle will be used more formally in Chapter 7 for determining confidence intervals.)

6.5.

6.5.1. As noted in Section 4.9.3., the standard deviation of a proportion P is $\sqrt{pq}$. For the cited data, the result will be $\sqrt{(6/9)(3/9)} = \sqrt{18}/9$. The standard error, estimated as $s/\sqrt{n}$, will be $(\sqrt{18}/9)/3 = \sqrt{18}/27$. The coefficient of stability will be $(s/\sqrt{n})/p$. Substituting 6/9 for P, we get $(\sqrt{18})/27)/(6/9)$, which becomes $(\sqrt{18}/27)(9/6) = (\sqrt{18}/3)(1/6) = \sqrt{18}/18 = 1/\sqrt{18}$. Since $\sqrt{18}$ lies between 4 and 5, this result lies between $1/5 = .20$ and $1/4 = .25$, and is obviously much larger than the smaller value (e.g. .1 or .05) needed for a stable central index. (If you actually did the calculation, c.s. $= .24$.)

6.5.2. The result is now stable because $\sqrt{900} = 30$; and the standard error and c.s. will be 1/10 of their previous values. The main "non-statistical" question is whether the poll was taken from a random sample of all potential voters. If the 900 people were a "convenience sample"—comprising casual passers-by in a single neighborhood, all members of the same club, or respondents to a mailed questionnaire--the sample may be highly biased and unrepresentative, regardless of the stable result. Also, are the sampled people actually likely to vote?

6.7. Individual answers.

Chapter 7

7.1.

7.1.1. The two-tailed value for $t_{7,.05}$ is 2.365. The 95% confidence interval is $34 \pm (2.365)(5.18/\sqrt{8}) = 34 \pm 4.33$, and extends from 29.67 to 38.33.

7.1.2. For a one-tailed confidence interval of 90%, we want to use $t_{7,.20}$ which is 1.415. The lower border for the interval would be $34 - (1.415)(5.18/\sqrt{8})$, which is $34 - 2.59 = 31.41$.

7.1.3. The extreme values in the data are **28** and **42**. Removal of these values reduces the respective means to **34.86** and **32.86**. The maximum proportional variation is $(34 - 32.86)/34 = .03$, which does not seem excessive.

7.1.4. The median is **36** with removal of any item from **28–31**, and **31** with removal of any item from **36–40**. For the original median of **33.5**, the maximum proportional variation is $2.5/33.5 = .07$.

7.1.5. According to the jackknife procedure, the coefficients of potential variation for the mean are a maximum of .03 (as noted in Answer 7.1.3). The analogous coefficient (as noted in Answer 7.1.4) for the median is .07. According to the parametric procedure, the standard error of the mean is $5.18/\sqrt{8} = 1.83$ and so its coefficient of potential variation is $1.83/34 = .05$. With either the empirical or parametric procedure, the mean seems more stable than the median, perhaps because the median in this data set comes from the two middlemost values, **31** and **36**, which are more widely separated than any two other adjacent members of the data. Without knowing more about the source of the data or what one intends to do with the mean, its stability is difficult to evaluate.

Using the parametric result (.05) for the coefficient of potential variation would in general produce a more cautious decision than the jackknife results. In this instance, if we accept the parametric coefficient of .05 as indicating stability, the mean might be regarded as stable.

7.3. The laboratory is trying to indicate a 95% interval for the range of the observed data, but the phrase "95% confidence interval" refers to dispersion around an estimate of the mean, not to dispersion of the data. The correct phrase should be simply "range of normal" or "customary inner 95% range." The word *confidence* should be used only in reference to the location of a *mean* (or proportion or other central index of a group).

Chapter 8

8.1. The value of .40 is relatively unstable since the standard error is $\sqrt{(.40)(.60)/30} = .089$ and $.089/.40 = .22$. To answer the policy question, one approach is to put a 95% Gaussian confidence interval around the observed proportion. The interval would be $.40 \pm 1.96 \times .089 = .40 \pm .175$; it extends from .225 to .575. Because the confidence interval does *not* include the hypothesized value of .10, the result is probably not compatible with the 10% policy. A second approach is to do a one-sample Z test for the hypothesized parameter of .10. The calculation would be $Z = (.40 - .10)/\sqrt{(.40)(.60)/30} = .30/.089 = 3.37$, for which $2P \le .001$.

An entirely different approach is to jackknife 12/30 into 12/29 = .41 or 11/29 = .38. This range of maximum difference is $.41 - .38 = .03$, which is proportionately $.03/.40 = .075$. Because the ratio exceeds .05, it immediately shows that the original proportion (.40) is unstable. The jackknife approach, however, does not answer the policy question.

8.3. With an 80% failure rate, the usual rate of success is 20% or .20. The chance of getting three consecutive successes is $.2 \times .2 \times .2 = .008$. Unless you think that the clinician is a wizard or that his patients have unusually good prognoses, this low probability seems hard to believe.

8.5.

8.5.1. Since 95% confidence intervals are regularly accepted, use $Z_\alpha = Z_{.05} = 1.96$. If the proportion of dementia is unknown, use $p = q = .5$. With a 1% tolerance, $e = .01$. Then solve $n \ge (.5)(.5)(1.96)^2/(.01)^2$ to get $n \ge 9604$.

8.5.2. With .20 as the estimated proportion, solve $n \ge (.20)(.80)(1.96)^2/(.01)^2$ to get $n \ge 6147$.

8.5.3. When the commissioner is distressed by the large sample sizes, offer to raise the tolerance level to 5%. The sample size will then be $n \ge (.20)(.80)(1.96)^2/(.05)^2$, which reduces the sample to $n \ge 246$, which is within the specified limit of 300.

8.7. Individual answers.

Chapter 9

9.1 ⎱
9.3 ⎰ Individual answers.

Chapter 10

10.1. Like beauty, the concept of what is *cogent* is in the eye of the beholder. For the investigators, the most important issue seems to have been myocardial infarction. If this is your choice, do you also want to focus on *all* myocardial infarctions, or just the associated deaths? Would you prefer to focus, instead, on total deaths? And how about strokes, which seemed more common in the aspirin group?

Another major decision here is whether to express the risks as events per "subject," i.e., patient, or events per subject year. The investigators went to great effort to calculate and list subject years, so these are presumably the preferred units of analysis. They will be used in the first set of analyses here. The second set of analyses will use patients as the denominators of "risk."

The figures in the following tables will provide results used in answers to 10.1.1, 10.1.2, and 10.1.3, as well as 10.1.4 and 10.1.5.

	Rates per Subject Year, U.S. Study				Rates per Subject Year, U.K. Study			
	Aspirin	Placebo	Increment in Rates	Ratio of Higher to Lower Rate	Aspirin	No Aspirin	Increment in Rates	Ratio of Higher to Lower Rate
Total deaths	.00398	.00418	.000196	1.050	.0143	.0159	.0016	1.112
Fatal MI	.000183	.000478	.000295	2.612	.00473	.00496	.00023	1.049
Total rate for MI	.00255	.00440	.00185	1.725	.00898	.00929	.00031	1.035
Fatal stroke	.000165	.000110	.0000546	1.500	.00159	.000106	.00043	1.500
Total rate for stroke	.00218	.00180	.000377	1.211	.00484	.00412	.00072	1.175

Rate	Rates per Subject, U.S. Study				Rates per Subject, U.K. Study			
	Aspirin	Placebo	Increment in Rates	Ratio of Higher to Lower Rate	Aspirin	No Aspirin	Increment in Rates	Ratio of Higher to Lower Rate
Total deaths	.0197	.0206	.000873	1.046	.0787	.0883	.0096	1.122
Fatal MI	.000906	.002356	.00145	2.600	.02596	.02749	.00153	1.059
Total rate for MI	.0126	.0217	.0091	1.722	.0493	.0515	.00216	1.045
Fatal stroke	.000816	.000544	.000272	1.500	.00875	.00702	.00173	1.246
Total rate for stroke	.0108	.00888	.00192	1.216	.0265	.0228	.0037	1.162

Note: The ratios of rates are essentially identical, whether the denominators are subject years or subjects. The increments in rates are higher with subjects than with subject years and will be used here for calculations of the number needed to treat.

10.1.1. In the U.S. trial, the total death rate ratios, at values of ~1.05, were not impressively higher in the placebo group. The NNT would be $1/.000873 = 1145$ persons to prevent one death. The MI rate ratios were impressive, at 2.6 for fatal MI and 1.7 for total MI. The corresponding values of NNT, however, were less impressive, at $1/.00145 = 690$ and $1/.0091 = 110$. The rate ratios for stroke were elevated for aspirin, but less impressively (at 1.5 for fatal and 1.2 for total stroke). The corresponding NNT values were $1/.000272 = 3676$ and $1/.00192 = 521$.

10.1.2. The most impressive rate ratios in the U.K. trial were the elevated values for the risk of stroke with aspirin. The total death rate ratios in favor of aspirin, however, were more impressive in the U.K. than in the U.S. trial, but the U.K. rate ratio effects for MI were unimpressive. Nevertheless, the NNT values in the U.K. trial were more impressive, in each respect, than in the U.S. trial. The NNT results were $1/.0096 = 104$ for total deaths, $1/.00153 = 654$ for fatal MI, $1/.00216 = 463$ for total MI, $1/.00173 = 578$ for fatal stroke, and $1/.0037 = 270$ for total stroke.

10.1.3. Risk of myocardial infarction was sum of deaths + nonfatal MIs. Per subject years, the proportionate increment in aspirin vs. placebo was $-.00185/.00440 = -42\%$. Per subjects, the corresponding result was $-.0091/.0217 = -42\%$. Both of these values are close to but not exactly 44%, which may have been calculated with a statistical adjustment for age. The corresponding relative risks are $.00255/.00440 = .58$ per subject year and $.0126/.0217 = .58$ per subject.

10.1.4. Even though the U.K. subjects were "healthy," they were probably older than the U.S. group.

10.1.5. In the U.S. trial, the NNT values were 110 for total MI and 521 for total stroke. Thus, for the one stroke created in about 500 patients in the U.S., about 5 MIs would have been prevented. In the U.K. trial, the NNT values were 463 for total MI and 270 for total stroke. Thus, in the U.K., while one MI was being prevented in about 500 patients, about 2 strokes were being created. Your decision about whether the aspirin is worth taking may depend on whether you live in the U.S. or the U.K., and whether you prefer a stroke-free or MI-free existence.

10.1.6. Individual answers.

10.3. This was another trap question. If you fell in, please be enlightened as you emerge:

10.3.1. The actual risks cannot be calculated for users and nonusers of reserpine because this was not a forward-directed cohort study. If any "rates" are to be calculated, they would have to be antecedent rates of exposure to reserpine. These rates would be .073(= 11/150) in the cases and .022 (= 26/1200) in the controls. A formation of increments or ratios for these two rates, however, would not be particularly informative. If the idea is to determine the relative risk of breast cancer in users and nonusers of reserpine, the best index would be the odds ratio, which is $(11 \times 1174)/(26 \times 139) = 3.57$.

10.3.2. Because the actual risks cannot be determined for users and nonusers, an incremental risk cannot be calculated. One of the prime disadvantages of the etiologic case-control study is that it provides only a ratio, i.e., the odds ratio (which approximates the relative risk ratio). This type of study, however, cannot produce an increment in risks.

10.5. Individual answers, but ARF's gut reactions are as follows:

10.5.1. Look for an increment of at least 10% and a ratio of at least 1.25. This is achieved if the success rate is 56% for active treatment.

10.5.2. Because mortality is already so low, much of this decision will depend on the risks and inconvenience of the active treatment. However, on a purely quantitative basis, the mortality rate should be lowered to at least 50% of its previous value. Hence, the active treatment should have a mortality of 4% or less.

10.5.3. The active treatment should be proportionately at least 50% better, so that its mean should be $(1.5) \times (1.3) = 1.95$.

10.5.4. If the risk ratio is as high as 10, the absolute risk of getting endometrial cancer with estrogens is only .01. For a chance of only one in a hundred, the woman might be told the risk and allowed to make up her own mind. (If the risk ratio is lower than 10, the actual risk is even smaller than .01). Besides, the prognosis of estrogen-associated endometrial cancer is extraordinarily favorable compared with cancers that were not estrogen-associated.

10.7. Individual answers. Note that the investigators often fail to report (and editors fail to demand citation of) the values of δ or θ that were anticipated for the trial.

Chapter 11

11.1. In a "unit-fragility" type of procedure, do an "extreme" relocation by exchanging the *lowest* member of Group A and the *highest* member of Group B. Group A would become 12, 14, 16, 17, 17, 125. Group B would become 1, 19, 29, 31, 33, 34. For a purely "mental" approach, without any calculations, compare the two sets of medians. In medians, the original comparison was 15 vs. 32; after the exchange, the comparison is 16.5 vs. 30; and the latter comparison still seems highly impressive. [On the other hand, if you use a calculator, the "new" means become $\overline{X}_A = 33.5$ and $\overline{X}_B = 24.5$, so that the direction of the increment is reversed. Better ways to handle this problem are discussed in Chapters 12 and 16.]

11.3. If the observed "nonsignificant" difference is $\overline{X}_A - \overline{X}_B = -5$, a more extreme difference in the same direction will be more negative and, hence, at the lower end of the interval.

11.5.

11.5.1. Answers to be supplied by readers. (ARF is not happy with it for reasons discussed in the text, but has nothing better to offer unless we shift completely to the idea of descriptive boundaries.)

11.5.2. (a) When sample sizes are unavoidably small, a too strict value of α will prevent any conclusions. Rather than discard everything as "nonsignificant," the value of α might be made more lenient. The "significant" conclusions can then be regarded as tentative—to be confirmed in future research.

(b) In certain types of "data-dredging" procedures the information is being "screened" in search of anything that might be "significant." The material caught in this type of "fishing expedition" would then have to be evaluated *scientifically* as being viable fish or decayed auto tires.

11.5.3. Before any *conclusion* is drawn for a difference that emerged from multiple comparisons in a data-dredged screening examination.

11.5.4. Raising α to more lenient levels would reduce the sample sizes needed to attain "significance." The research costs would be reduced. Lowering α to stricter levels would have the opposite effects. Since the credibility of the research depends mainly on its scientific structure rather than the stochastic hypotheses, the scientific credibility of the research might be unaffected. The purely statistical effect depends on how you feel mathematically about the old and new α levels. As noted later, however, a stricter level of α will reduce the possibility of "false positive" conclusions, but will raise the possibility of "false negatives." A more lenient level of α will have opposite effects: more false positives but fewer false negatives.

11.7. The chance of getting two consecutive **7**'s requires a **7** on each toss. The probability of this event is the product of $(1/6)(1/6) = .03$. It would also be possible, however, to get a **7** on one toss, but not the other. This event could occur as **yes/no** with a probability of $(1/6)(5/6) = .14$, or as **no/yes** with a probability of $(5/6)(1/6) = .14$. The total probability for the **yes/yes, yes/no, no/yes,** and **no/no** events would be $.03 + .14 + .14 + .69 = 1.00$.

Chapter 12

12.1. The remaining untested tables are

$$\left\{\begin{array}{cc} 2 & 3 \\ 3 & 3 \end{array}\right\} \quad \text{and} \quad \left\{\begin{array}{cc} 3 & 2 \\ 2 & 4 \end{array}\right\}$$

$$\text{(40\% vs. 50\%)} \qquad \text{(60\% vs. 33\%)}$$

using $k = 1.870129870 \times 10^2$, the p value for the first table is $k/2!3!3!3! = .433$ and for the second table is $k/3!2!2!4! = .325$. The sum of these two p values is 0.758, which, when added to .242 (the two-tailed p value noted in Section 12.6.1) gives 1.

12.3. Observed difference in means is 5.17, which is $34/4 = 8.50$ for Treatment X and $10/3 = 3.33$ for Treatment Y. This difference is exceeded by only the following four arrangements.

X	Y	Mean X	Mean Y	Difference, $\bar{X} - \bar{Y}$
3,8,11,13	1,2,6	8.75	3	5.75
6,8,11,13	1,2,3	9.5	2	7.5
1,2,3,6	8,11,13	3	10.6	−7.6
1,2,3,8	6,11,13	3.5	10	−6.5

The seven items in the trial can be divided into one group of four and one group of three in 35 ways $[= 7!/(4!)(3!)]$. Of these arrangements, three yield mean differences that are as great or greater than 5.17; and two yield mean differences that are negatively as large or larger than 5.17. The two-tailed P value is thus $3/35 + 2/35 = 5/35 = .143$.

Chapter 13

13.1. For Group A, $\overline{X} = 12.833$ and $s = 6.113$. For Group B, $\overline{X} = 45.167$ and $s = 39.479$. The value of s_p becomes 28.25, and $t = (32.334/28.25)\sqrt{(6)(6)/12} = 1.98$. At 10 d.f., this result falls below the required $t_{.05} = 2.23$ and so $2P > .05$. A major source of the problem is the high variability in both groups, particularly in Group B, where the coefficient of variation is 0.8. The standardized increment, which is $(32.334/28.25) = 1.145$, seems impressive despite the large value for s_p, but the group size factor is not quite big enough to get t across the necessary threshold.

13.3

Group A	Group B
$\Sigma X_A = 66$	$\Sigma X_B = 49$
$n_A = 9$	$n_B = 6$
$\overline{X}_A = 7.33$ lbs	$\overline{X}_B = 8.17$ lbs
$\Sigma X_A^2 = 504$	$\Sigma X_B^2 = 411$
$(\Sigma X_A)^2/n_A = 484$	$(\Sigma X_B)^2/n_B = 400.17$
$\Sigma X_A^2 - (\Sigma X_A)^2/n_A = 20$	$\Sigma X_B^2 - (\Sigma X_B)^2/n_B = 10.83$
$s_A^2 = 2.50$	$s_B^2 = 2.17$
$s_A = 1.58$	$s_B = 1.47$
$s_{\overline{X}_A} = .527$	$s_{\overline{X}_B} = .601$

13.3.1. For Group A: $t_{8,.05} = 2.306$ $t_{8,.01} = 3.355$

95% Conf. Interval: $7.33 \pm 2.306\,(.527) = 7.33 \pm 1.22 = 6.11$ to 8.55 lbs
99% Conf. Interval: $7.33 \pm 3.355\,(.527) = 7.33 \pm 1.77 = 5.56$ to 9.10 lbs.

For Group B: $t_{5,.05} = 2.571$ $t_{5,.01} = 4.032$

95% Conf. Interval: $8.17 \pm 2.571\,(.601) = 8.17 \pm 1.55 = 6.62$ to 9.72 lbs
99% Conf. Interval: $8.17 \pm 4.032\,(.601) = 8.17 \pm 2.42 = 5.75$ to 10.59 lbs

13.3.2. Using the formula $t = (\overline{X} - \mu)/[s/\sqrt{n}]$, we get

$$t_A = \frac{7.33 - 6.7}{.527} = 1.195. \quad \text{At 8 d.f., } .20 < 2P < .40$$

$$t_B = \frac{8.17 - 6.7}{.601} = \frac{1.47}{.601} = 2.45. \quad \text{At 5 d.f., } .05 < 2P < 0.1$$

13.3.3.

For t test, $t = \dfrac{\overline{X}_A - \overline{X}_B}{\text{s.e.}_{(\overline{X}_A - \overline{X}_B)}}$, and $\text{s.e.}_{(\overline{X}_A - \overline{X}_B)} = \sqrt{s_p^2\left(\dfrac{1}{n_A} + \dfrac{1}{n_B}\right)}$. Because

$$s_p^2 = \frac{(n_A - 1)s_A^2 + (n_B - 1)s_B^2}{n_A + n_B - 2} = \frac{30.85}{13} = 2.3731, \text{ and } \text{s.e.}_{(\overline{X}_A - \overline{X}_B)} = \sqrt{(2.3731)\left(\frac{1}{9} + \frac{1}{6}\right)}$$

$$= \sqrt{.6595} = .812, \quad t = \frac{-.84}{812} = -1.034. \text{ At 13 d.f., the 2P value for this t is } > 0.2.$$

For *confidence interval* calculations, a 97.5% confidence interval around $\overline{X}_A - \overline{X}_B$ is $\overline{X}_A - \overline{X}_B \pm (t_{13,.025})(\text{standard error}) = (-.84) \pm (2.553)(.812) = -.84 \pm 2.06$, which spans from -2.90 to $+1.22$. Since this interval includes 0 (the assumed mean of the populational difference), we cannot conclude that a remarkable event has occurred.

13.3.4. If this is a single Gaussian population, its mean, μ, is 7.67 and its standard deviation, σ, is estimated as $\sqrt{S_{XX}/n} = \sqrt{33.333/15} = 1.491$. We would expect to find 95% of the cases within $\mu \pm 1.96\sigma$. This interval is $7.67 \pm 1.96(1.491) = 4.75$ to 10.59. Because this interval includes 5, there is nothing peculiar about the baby who gained only 5 lbs. (The baby becomes "peculiar" only if you erroneously determine a 95% confidence interval around the *mean* and find that the baby does not fit into that interval. But why should it?)

13.5.

13.5.1. Adding the two standard errors mentally, the commentator got $6 + 4 = 10$. The doubled value, 20, was more than twice the incremental difference in means, which was $25 - 16 = 9$. At this magnitude for the crude approximation, the commentator felt reasonably sure that the 95% confidence interval around 9 would include the null hypothesis value of 0.

13.5.2. To do a t test with the pooled variance Formula [13.13] requires converting the standard errors back to standard deviations. With a slightly less accurate but much simpler approach, you can use Formula [13.15], calculating the denominator as $\sqrt{4^2 + 6^2} = 7.21$. The value of Z (or t) is then $9/7.21 = 1.25$. With the large sample sizes here, you can refer to a Z distribution, and note (from the Geigy tables or the computer printout) that the corresponding 2P value is .21. If you used the pooled-variance method, the standard deviations are $s_A = 4\sqrt{81} = 36$ and $s_B = 6\sqrt{64} = 48$. The value of s_p becomes

$$\sqrt{[(80)(36)^2 + (63)(48)^2]/(81 + 64 - 2)} = \sqrt{1740} = 41.71$$

and

$$t = (9/41.71)(\sqrt{(81)(64)/145}) = 1.29$$

In the Geigy tables, for $v = N - 2 = 143$, the two-tailed P value is 0.2 when $t = 1.29$ and 0.1 when $t = 1.66$. (The result is the same as what was obtained with Z.)

13.5.3. The commentator easily calculated the standard deviations by first taking square roots of the group sizes as $\sqrt{n_A} = \sqrt{81} = 9$ and $\sqrt{n_B} = \sqrt{64} = 8$. Mentally multiplying these values times the cited standard errors produced the respective standard deviations of $s_A = 36$ and $s_B = 48$. These values are so much larger than the corresponding means of $\overline{X}_A = 16$ and $\overline{X}_B = 25$ that both distributions must be greatly eccentric and unsuitable for summarization with means.

13.5.4. The distibutions should be examined for shape before any decisions are made. Without any further information, however, a good approach might be to compare medians and do a Pitman-Welch test on the medians.

13.7. All of the answers are available in previous discussions that can be summarized as follows:

13.7.1. The subtraction of means is direct, easy, and conventional. Alternative stochastic tests can be arranged, however, with ratios or other indexes of contrast.

13.7.2. Not necessarily. The discrepancies may be misleading if the data greatly depart from a Gaussian distribution. (In such circumstances, a better approach may be to use percentile and other "distribution-free" tactics.)

13.7.3. If deviations from the mean are added directly, the sum of $\Sigma(X_i - \overline{X})$ will always be zero.

13.7.4. Division by $n - 1$ offers a better estimate, on average, of the corresponding (and presumably larger) standard deviation in the larger parametric population from which the observed results are a "sample."

13.7.5. The *standard error* is a purely analytic (and poorly labeled) term, denoting the standard deviation in a sampled series of means. The term has nothing to do with the original process of measurement.

13.7.6. Division produces a standardized result in a manner analogous to converting the number of deaths in a group to a rate of death.

13.7.7. When a parameter is estimated from n members of an observed group of data, the same parameter is presumably estimated from all subsequent theoretical samplings. To produce the same parametric value, the samplings lose a degree of freedom from the original n degrees. The term *degree* is an arbitrary label for n − k, where k is the number of parameters being estimated.

13.7.8. Under the null hypothesis that two groups are similar, the P value represents the random stochastic chance of getting a result that is at least as large as the observed difference. (Other types of P values, discussed in later chapters, have other meanings for other hypotheses.) The P value has become dominant because of intellectual inertia and professional conformity, and because investigators have not given suitable attention to the more important quantitative descriptive issues in "significance."

13.7.9. In repeated theoretical parametric samplings, we can be confident that the true value of the parameter will appear in $1 - \alpha$ (e.g., 95%) of the intervals constructed around the observed estimate, using the corresponding value of Z_α or t_α. The confidence is statistically unjustified if the samples are small, if they widely depart from a Gaussian distribution, or if the parameter is a binary proportion with values near 0 or 1, far from the meridian value of .5. The confidence is also unjustified, for substantive rather than statistical reasons, if the sample is biased, i.e., not adequately representative of what it allegedly represents.

13.7.10. If we reject the null hypothesis whenever $P \leq \alpha$, the hypothesis can be true for an α proportions of rejections, leading to false positive conclusions that a distinction is "significant" when, in fact, it is not. The P value is often, although not always, determined from standard errors, but has nothing to do with errors in the measurement process. The value of α is regularly set at .05 because of (again) intellectual inertia and professional conformity.

Chapter 14

14.1. For evaluating "clinical significance," the death rates were .104 (or 10.4%) for timolol and .162 (or 16.2%) for placebo. This is an absolute reduction of $16.2 - 10.4 = 5.8\%$ in deaths, and a proportionate reduction of $5.8\%/16.2\% = 36\%$. Many people would regard this as a quantitatively significant improvement. On the other hand, the survival rates were 89.6% and 83.8%, respectively. The proportionate improvement in survival was $5.8\%/83.8\% = 7\%$, which may not seem so impressive (unless you were one of the survivors). Another way of expressing the quantitative contrast is with the number needed to treat, discussed in Chapter 10. For the direct increment of $.162 - .104 = .058$, NNT = 1/.058 $\cong 17$. Thus, about 1 extra person survived for every 17 actively treated.

For statistical significance, X^2 can be calculated as

$$\left[\frac{(98)^2}{945} + \frac{(152)^2}{939} - \frac{(250)^2}{1884} \right] \left[\frac{(1884)^2}{(250)(1634)} \right] = 13.85$$

Alternatively, since the fourfold table will be

98	847	945
152	787	939
250	1634	1884

the calculation can be

$$\frac{[(98 \times 787) - (847 \times 152)]^2 \, 1884}{(250)(1634)(945)(939)} = 13.85$$

At 1 degree of freedom, this value of X^2 has an associated 2P < .001. The authors seem justified in claiming "statistical significance."

14.3. What Mendel observed was 74% (= 787/1064) and 26% in his proportions. Intuitively, this seems quite consistent with the proposed ratios. If we want mathematical confirmation for this intuition, we can proceed as follows.

At a ratio of 3:1, the expected values for 1064 crosses are (3/4)(1064) and (1/4)(1064), i.e, 798 and 266. Using the observed-expected formula, we have

$$X^2 = \frac{(787 - 798)^2}{798} + \frac{(277 - 266)^2}{266} = \frac{(-11)^2}{798} + \frac{(11)^2}{266}$$

$$= \frac{121}{798} + \frac{121}{266} = .152 + .455 = .607$$

At 1 d.f., this is not stochastically significant (P > .3). Therefore, the result is consistent with the hypothesis.

14.5. To use the mental calculation approach with Formula [14.8], note that we must get .001 multiplied by something that will make the result exceed 2. Since $.001 = 1 \times 10^{-3}$, the multiplier must be 2×10^3 or 2000. The latter is the square root of N, which should therefore be 4×10^6, or about 4 million. Consequently, each player should have batted about 2 million times.

For a more formal calculation, let $Z_\alpha = 1.96$. Let $\pi = (.333 + .332)/2 = .3325$. Then $1 - \pi = .6675$. Substitute in Formula [14.19] to get $n = (2)(.3325)(.6675) (1.96)^2/(.001)^2 = 1,705,238.2$ as the number of times at bat for each player. [To check the accuracy of this calculation, assume that $N = 2n = 3,410,478$ and apply Formula [14.7] with $k = .5$. The result is $[.001 / \sqrt{(.3325)(.6675)}] \times (.5) \times \sqrt{3,410,478} = 1.96$, which is the Z needed for 2P < .05.]

Chapter 15

15.1. Like the common cold, "fibrositis" is often a self-limited condition that gradually improves with time. Patients could therefore be expected to be generally "better" in the second month of treatment than in the first. Unless the "fibrositis" was distinctly chronic and stable, it was not a suitable condition for a crossover trial. In the entry criteria, however, the investigators made no demands for a minimum duration of symptoms.

15.3.

15.3.1. The data are "perfectly" aligned, so that the first 6 ranks are in Group A, and the next 6 ranks are in Group B. The sum of the first 6 ranks is (6)(7)/2 = 21. The total sum of ranks is (12)(13)/2 = 78. For the U test, the lower value will be 21 − [(6)(7)/2] = 0. In Table 15.4, for $n_1 = n_2 = 6$, a U value of ≤5 will have 2P ≤.05.

15.3.2. The data are not matched, but we could arbitrarily form sets of 6 matched pairs in which each of the 6 values in Group A is matched with each of the 6 values in Group B. We could determine the total number of possible matchings and then check results for all the associated sign tests. An enormously simpler approach, however, is to recognize that the value in Group B will always be larger than the value in Group A, no matter how the matching is done. Thus, the six matched pairs will always have 6 positive signs for B − A. For a "null hypothesis" probability of 1/2, this result has a P value of $(1/2)^6 = 1/64 = .016$.

15.3.3. The median for the total data set is at 18 (between 17 and 19). For the 2 × 2 table, we get

	Below Median	Above Median	TOTAL
Group A	6	0	6
Group B	0	6	6
TOTAL	6	6	12

The Fisher test requires only 1 calculation, because the table is at the "extreme" value; and the calculation is quite simple (because 2 sets of values cancel for 6!). Thus, the P value for the table can be calculated as $(6!)(6!)/12! = .001$. For two tails, this is doubled to a 2P value of .002.

Note that in this instance, the Fisher test on the median gave a more "powerful," i.e. lower, P value than the two other tests. Its result in this instance is also the same as the Pitman-Welch P value, which was obtained as $2/[12!/(6!)(6!)]$.

15.5. Of the 19 paired comparisons, 11 are tied and 8 favor propranolol. Ignoring the 11 ties, we can do a sign test to get a P value for $(1/2)^8$. Because $(1/2)^5 = 1/32 = .03$ and $(1/2)^8$ will be even smaller, we can state that P < .05. With greater mental effort, we can calculate $(1/2)^8 = 1/256$, which is P < .01. (The authors reported "P < 0.04" for the comparison, but did not say which test was used.)

Chapter 16

16.1.

16.1.1. Since the symmetrical confidence-interval component is $10.9 - 6.0 = 4.9$, and since $Z_\alpha = 1.96$ for a 95% C.I., the value of SED must have been $4.9/1.96 = 2.5$. The coefficient of potential variation for SED/$d_o = 2.5/6.0 = .42$, which is below .5. If you use .5 as a boundary, you can be impressed.

16.1.2. Since the two groups have equal size, SED was calculated as $\sqrt{(s_A^2 + s_B^2)/n}$. If we assume $s_A = s_B = s$, SED = $\sqrt{2s^2/n}$, and $s = (SED)\sqrt{n/2}$. For SED = 2.5 and n = 100, s = 17.7. The respective ratios for C.V., which are $17.7/140.4 = .13$ and $17.7/146.4 = .12$, are not large enough to suggest that the means misrepresent the data.

16.1.3. In Figure 16.7, the, confidence interval component is $13.0 - 6.0 = 7.0$, and so SED = $7.0/1.96 = 3.57$. Using the same reasoning as in 14.1.2, and with n = 50, we now calculate s = $(SED)\sqrt{n/2} = 3.57\sqrt{50/2} = 17.8$, which is close enough to 17.7 to confirm the authors' statement.

16.1.4. The diabetic group in Figure 16.7 contains a value >190 and the non-diabetic group contains a value >180. Neither of these values appeared in Figure 16.6. Therefore, the groups in Figure 16.7 could not have been sampled from those in Figure 16.6. Another suspicion of "different sources" could be evoked by the statement that the means and standard deviations in Figure 16.7 are the same as in Figure 16.6. This exact similarity is unlikely if the groups in Figure 16.7 were each randomly sampled from those in Figure 16.6. What probably happened is that the data in both figures were obtained via a "Monte Carlo" construction, using the assigned means of 146.4 and 140.4, the assigned standard deviation of ~17.7, the assumption that both groups were Gaussian, and then doing random sampling from the theoretical Gaussian curve for each group. Alternatively, both groups could have been sampled from a much larger population.

16.3. If ±2 is a standard deviation, the value of 2 SD is about 4, and 95% of the data on the right side should extend as 4 ± 4, or from about 0 to 8, which corresponds roughly to what is shown in the graph. If ±2 is a standard error, the value of SD is about 18, since $\sqrt{88} \sim 9$. The data would extend as $4 \pm 2(18)$, which they do not. Therefore, the ± values are SDs.

16.5. The lower quartile, median, and upper quartile points are connected with a solid line in Figure AE 16.1. Dotted lines show the extensions to the "0th" and "100th" percentiles at the extremes of the data for age in the African and Caucasian groups of Figure 16.12. The three quartile points show that Africans are older than Caucasians in the mid-zone of the data (although not at the extremes). The "bend" in the quantile-quantile line shows that the two groups have unequal variance (which could have been readily noted from the asymmetrical box for Caucasians in Figure 16.12).

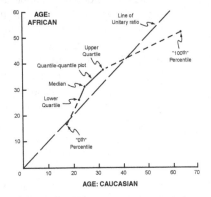

FIGURE AE 16.1
Quantile-quantile plot for Exercise 16.1

16.7. Individual answers. As for the Supreme Court, as might be expected, it did not take a clear stand on the scientific issue. Instead, after acknowledging that the Frye rule might be too rigid, the Court said that local judges could use their own wisdom to evaluate scientific evidence and to decide what might be admissible, even if it did not comply with the Frye rule. Because the Court offered no guidelines for the local decisions, judges may have to start enrolling in appropriate courses of instruction.

Chapter 17

17.1.

17.1.1. With increased use of screening tests (such as cervical pap smears, mammography, and routine white blood counts) and more definitive technologic tests (such as ultrasound, CT scans, and MRI), many cancers are now detected that would formerly have been unidentified during the life of the patients. If incidence rates are determined not from death certificates, but from tumor registries or other special repositories of diagnostic data, the incidence rates will inevitably increase. The cancers that would formerly be found only as "surprise discoveries" at necropsy (if necropsy was done) will now be found and counted among the "vital statistics."

17.1.2. Many of the cancers identified with the new screening and technologic procedures will be relatively asymptomatic and slow-growing. They will usually have better prognoses, even if left untreated, than the cancers that formerly were diagnosed because they had produced symptoms. Because the customary morphologic classifications do not distinguish these functional behaviors of cancer, the survival rates will rise because the relatively "benign" cancers are now included in the numerators and denominators. The relatively "malignant" cancers, however, may continue to be just as lethal as before. When referred to a community denominator, the cancer death rates may seem unchanged.

17.1.3. Because no unequivocal data (about nutrition, life style, smoking, alcohol, etc.) exist about risk factors for these cancers, it is difficult to choose a suitable public-health intervention that offers the prospect of more good than harm. Many nonmedical scientists — if professionally uncommitted to a particular "cause" or viewpoint — might therefore conclude that basic biomedical research has a better potential for preventing these cancers than any *currently* known public-health intervention.

17.3.

17.3.1. The denominator is 300, and 4 cases existed on July 1. Prevalence is $4/300 = .0133$.

17.3.2. The incidence rate depends on whom you count as the eligible people and what you count as incidence. Three new episodes occurred during the cited time period. If we regard everyone as eligible, the denominator is 300, and the incidence of new episodes will be $3/300 = .01$. If you insist that the eligible people are those who are free of the disease on July 1, the eligible group consists of $300 - 4 = 296$ people. If you insist on counting only new instances of disease, the recurrence in case #3 is not counted as an episode. The incidence would be $2/296 = .0068$. If you allow the denominator to include anyone who becomes disease-free during the interval, only case 1 is excluded. If the numerator includes any new episode of disease, there are 3 such episodes in the interval. Incidence would be $3/299 = .01$.

17.3.3. Numerator depends on whether you count 7 episodes or 6 diseased people. Denominator is 300.

17.5.

17.5.1. Adding 0.5 to each cell produces $(5.5)(8.5)/(0.5)(.05) = 187$.

17.5.2. The main arguments were (1) the control groups were improperly chosen and should have contained women with the same pregnancy problems (threatened abortion, etc.) that might have evoked DES therapy in the exposed group; (2) the ascertainment of previous DES exposure may have been biased; (3) the Connecticut Tumor Registry shows an apparently unchanged annual incidence of clear-cell cancer despite little or no usage of DES for pregnancies of the past few decades.

17.5.3. If the occurrence rate of CCVC is very small, perhaps 1×10^{-5} in non-exposed women, the cohorts of 2000 people were too small to pick up any cases. On the other hand, if the rate is 1×10^{-4} (as some epidemiologists believe) and if the case-control odds ratios of 325 or 187 are correct, we should expect about 32.5 or 18.7 cases per thousand in the exposed group. This number is large enough for at least several cases to be detected in a cohort of 2000 people. Accordingly, either the odds ratios are wrong or the occurrence rate of CCVC is much smaller than currently believed. Either way, the cancerophobic terror seems unjustified.

17.7.

1.   What were the four numbers from which the odds ratio was calculated? (If they are small enough to make the result sufficiently unstable, i.e., far from stochastic significance, you can dismiss the study without any further questions. You can also get an idea, from the control group data, of the exposure rate in the general population.)

2.   What *is* the particular adverse event? (If it is a relatively trivial phenomenon, major public-policy action may not be needed.)

3.   What is the customary rate of occurrence of the adverse event? (If it has a relatively high rate, e.g., > .1, the odds ratio may be deceptively high. If it has a particularly low rate, e.g., ≤ .0001, the high odds ratio (or risk ratio) might be deceptively frightening. Examination of the NNE or some other index of contrast might give a better idea of how "impressive" the distinction may be.

4.   What is the particular "exposure"? (If it is sufficiently beneficial, such as a useful vaccination or surgical procedure, you can consider whether an alternative beneficial exposure is available if the current agent is "indicted" or "removed" from general usage.)

Chapter 18

18.1.

18.1.1. The simplest approach is to note that the intercept is 1.6 for the displayed formula $Y = 1.07X + 1.6$. This stated intercept appears to be the correct location of the point where the line crosses the Y axis when $X = 0$. (Note that the artist's statement of "+1.6" for the intercept disagrees with the "+0.02" listed in the caption.) A more complicated, but still relatively simple approach, is to note that the vertical extent of the Y points is from about 2 to 86 units and the horizontal extent of X is from 0 to 80. Thus, the crude slope is $(86 - 2)/(80 - 0) \sim 1$, consistent with the stated slope of 1.07.

18.1.2. The abscissa has a break and does not begin at 0. The intervals can be measured by eye and ruler, however. When 0 is reached, the line seems to intersect at about $Y = -0.9$. At $X = 50$, the value of Y is roughly 1, so that it covers 2 units (from -1 to $+1$) of Y during an X-span of 50 units. The value of $2/50 = .04$, which is the cited slope of the line. About 19 points are above the line and 12 points are below it, but the latter points have larger distances from the line. Thus, although the numbers of points are unequal above and below the line, the sum of values for $\hat{Y}_i - Y_i$ is probably equal and the line fits properly.

19.3. Individual answers.

Chapter 19

19.1.

19.1.1. The statistician first drew the graph for the 11 points shown in Figure AE.19.1. Drawing a new visual axis through the point containing both median values (**10,45**), the statistician noted that all other points were in the positive covariance zones of Quadrants I or III. The range of points, from 1 to 19 on the X-axis and from 10 to 80 on the Y-axis, suggested a slope of about 70/18, which is about 4. Because the points seemed about equally distributed around the median

values on both axes, the statistician guessed that the standard deviations for X and Y would each be about one fourth the corresponding range, i.e., $s_x \sim 18/4 = 4.5$ and $s_y \sim 70/4 = 17.5$, and so s_x/s_y was guessed as about 4.5/17.5, which is the inverse of the estimated slope, 70/18. Because $r = bs_x/s_y$, the guesswork implies that r will roughly be $(70/18)[(18/4)/(70/4)] \cong 1$ if the slope is as high as 4. From the dispersion of points, the statistician knows that the slope will not be as high as 4 and that r will not be as high as 1, but the statistician also knows, from Table 19.3, that for 11 points of data, with $n = 11$, P will be $< .05$ if $r > .6$. Believing that r will be close to or exceed .6, the statistician then guessed that the result will be stochastically significant. [A simpler approach is to note that the bi-median split produces a 2×2 table that is $\left\{\begin{smallmatrix} 0 & 5 \\ 5 & 0 \end{smallmatrix}\right\}$. This is at the extreme of a Fisher test for $10!/(5!\ 5!) = 252$ possibilities. The two-tailed P will be $2/252 = .008$.]
19.1.2.

$$\Sigma X = 110;\ \bar{X} = 10;\ \Sigma X^2 = 1430;\ S_{xx} = 1430 - (110^2/11) = 330$$

$$\Sigma Y = 490;\ \bar{Y} = 44.55;\ \Sigma Y^2 = 26700;\ S_{yy} = 26700 - (490)^2/11 = 4872.73$$

$$\Sigma XY = 5635;\ (\Sigma X \Sigma Y)/N = 4900;\ S_{xy} = 735;\ b = S_{xy}/S_{xx} = 2.23$$

$$a = \bar{Y} - b\bar{X} = 44.55 - (2.23)(10) = 22.28$$

The graph of points is shown in Fig. AE19.1, and the line passes through (0, 22.28) and (10, 44.55). If you plotted the alternative line, $b' = S_{xy}/S_{yy} = 735/4872.73 = .151$; $a' = 10 - (.151)(44.55) = 3.28$. The line passes through (3.28, 0) and (10, 44.55).

$$r^2 = S_{xy}^2/(S_{xx}S_{yy})(735)^2/[(330)(4872.73)] = .336;\ \text{and } r = .58$$

$$t = (r/\sqrt{1-r^2})\sqrt{n-2} = (.58/\sqrt{1-.336})\sqrt{9} = 2.14$$

Because the required $t_{.05}$ is 2.26 for $P \le .05$ at $\nu = 9$, the result just misses being stochastically significant. On the other hand, because the investigator clearly specified an advance direction for the co-relationship, an argument can be offered that a one-tailed P value is warranted. If so, t_1 is 1.833, and "significance" is attained.

The visual guess of 4 for the slope was too high because the lowest and highest values for Y do not occur at the extreme ends of the range for X. The guess of $1/4 = .25$ for the estimated s_x/s_y was quite good, however, because $S_{xx}/S_{yy} = 330/4872.73 = .068$ and $s_x/s_y = \sqrt{S_{xx}/S_{yy}} = .26$.

19.3. Official Answer: YES. If one-tailed P values are permissible for comparisons of two groups, they should also be permissible for comparisons of two variables.

19.5.

19.5.1. The top figure (for firearm homicide) shows too much scatter to have a correlation as high as .913. The lower figure (for firearm suicide) looks like its data could be fit well with two horizontal lines, one at about 5.5 for low values of X, and the other at about 6.5 for higher values of X. In fact, the upper figure might also be relatively well fit with two horizontal lines, one through the lower values of X and the other through higher values.

19.5.2. Neither of the two graphs shows a relationship "strong enough" to suggest that the correlations have r values as high as .64 and .74.

19.5.3. An excellent example of a correlation that got $r = -.789$ and $P < .05$ for only 7 data points. In view of what happens for values beyond $x \ge 120$, however, the relationship doesn't seem convincing.

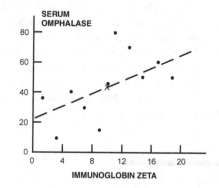

FIGURE AE.19.1

Graph (and regression line) for data in Exercise 19.1.

19.5.4. Does this look like a good correlation? Nevertheless, it achieved $r = .45$.

19.7.

19.7.1. The graph has too much scatter for the relationship to be biologically meaningful; also r is too low.

19.7.2. Each regression line seems to intersect the Y-axis at the stated intercepts of ~ 130, ~ 48, and ~ 120.

Chapter 20

20.1.

TABLE AE.20.1

Answer to Exercise 20.1.1

Subject	Incremental Differences between 1st and 2nd		Mean of Two First Readings	Increment First Wright and First Mini-Wright Heading
	Wright	Mini-Wright		
1	4	−13	503	−18
2	−2	15	412.5	−35
3	4	12	518	−4
4	33	−16	431	6
5	6	0	488	−24
6	−54	−25	578.5	−43
7	−2	−96	388.5	49
8	11	−10	411	62
9	12	−16	654	-8
10	4	13	439	−12
11	−3	12	424.5	−15
12	23	21	641	30
13	−8	33	263.5	7
14	−14	10	477.5	1
15	13	−9	218.5	−81
16	51	−20	386.5	73
17	6	8	439	−24
ΣX^2	7966	13479		$\bar{d} = -1.88$
$\Sigma X^2/17$	468.59	792.88		$\sqrt{\Sigma d^2/17} =$
$\sqrt{\Sigma X^2/17}$	21.64	28.16		$\sqrt{24120/17} =$ 37.67

20.1.1. (See Table AE.20.1.) The mini-Wright seems more inconsistent. Its average squared increment in the two readings is 28.2 vs. 21.6 for the Wright.

20.1.2. (a) No, r shows good correlation, but not necessarily good agreement, and some points seem substantially discrepant from the line of "unity."

(b) Check mean square increment of the two readings. Table AE.20.1 shows it is 37.67. Thus, the two sets of readings agree better with themselves than across readings with each other.

(c) Check mean increment. It is −1.88 (see Table AE.20.1) and thus not very biased. Check plot of increments vs. average magnitudes. A suitable graph will show that no major pattern is evident.

20.3.

20.3.1. (NYHA IV) + (CCS IV) − BOTH = 51 + 50 − 11 = 90. Seems correct.

20.3.2. Wide disagreements in Groups I–IV and IV–I are disconcerting. They suggest that many patients without angina are disabled, and many patients with severe angina had no functional problems. This is either an odd clinical situation or a major disagreement in the two scales.

20.3.3. Not a useful table prognostically. It shows *current* status of patients after operation, but does not indicate pre-op status of those who lived or died. For predictions, we need to know outcome in relation to pre-op status.

20.5.

20.5.1.

(a)   Value of X^2 for "agreement" seems to be $[(19 \times 12) - (5 \times 1)]^2 (37)/(24 \times 13 \times 20 \times 17) = 17.345$, which is an *ordinary* chi-square calculation. This is an inappropriate approach to these data.

(b)   Value of X^2 for "change" seems to be $(5 - 1)^2/(5 + 1) = 16/6 = 2.67$. This is the McNemar formula and would be appropriate for indexing disagreement, but these small numbers probably need a correction factor so that $X_M^2 = (|5 - 1| - 1)^2/6 = 9/6 = 1.5$, not 2.67.

(c)   Better citations would be $p_o = (19 + 12)/37 = 31/37 = .84$, or kappa. Because $p_e = [(20 \times 24) + (13 \times 17)]/37^2 = .512$, kappa $=(.84 - .512)/(1 - .512) = .672$.

20.5.2.   McNemar index of bias here is $(5-1)/(5+1) = 4/6 = .67$, suggesting that the therapists are more likely to make "satisfactory" ratings than the patients. Because of the small numbers, this index would have to be checked stochastically. The McNemar chi-square values in 20.5.1.(b), however, are too small (even without the correction factor) to exceed the boundary of 3.84 (= 1.96^2) needed for stochastic significance of X^2 at 1 d.f.

Chapter 21

21.1. If we start with 10,000 school-aged children, of whom 4% are physically abused, the fourfold table will show

Physical Exam	Confirmed Condition		Total
	Abused	Not Abused	
Positive	384	768	1152
Negative	16	8832	8848
TOTAL	400	9600	10000

Of the 400 abused children, 96% (384) are detected by the physical exam; of the 9600 nonabused, 8% (768) have false-positive exams. Consequently, nosologic sensitivity = 96% (384/400), nosologic specificity = 92% (8832/9600), and diagnostic sensitivity (positive predictive accuracy) = 33% (384/1152).

21.3. Results from nomogram table show:

Value of +LR	Value of P(D)	Value of P(D|T)
10	2%	~17%
10	20%	~75%
5	2%	~8%
5	20%	~53%
20	2%	~35%
20	20%	~83%

Usefulness of test cannot be determined without knowing its negative predictive accuracy. The nomogram technique, however, does not seem easy to use, and many clinicians might prefer to do a direct calculation, if a suitable program were available to ease the work. For example, recall that posterior odds = prior odds × LR. For P(D) = .02, prior odds = .02/.98 = .0196. For LR = 10, posterior odds = 10 × .0196 = .196. Because probability = odds/(1 + odds), posterior probability = .196/(1 + .196) = .16. This is close to the ~17% estimated from the nomogram. For a working formula, convert P(D) to prior odds of P(D)/[1 − P(D)]; multiply it by LR to yield posterior odds, and convert the latter to posterior probability as LR[P(D)/{1 − P(D)}]/(1 + LR[P(D)/{(1 − P(D))}]). The latter algebra simplifies to P(D|T) = LR[P(D)]/{1 − P(D) + LR[P(D)]}. Thus, for LR = 20 and P(D) = 20%, P(D|T) = [20(.20)]/[1 − .2 + (20)(.20)] = .83, as shown in the foregoing table.

21.5. Prevalence depends on total group size, N, which is not used when likelihood ratios are calculated from the components T and S in N = T + S.
21.7. Individual answers.
21.9. Individual answers.

Chapter 22

22.1.

22.1.1. Calculations for fixed-interval method:

Interval	Alive at Beginning	Died during Interval	Lost to Follow-Up	Withdrawn Alive	Adjusted Denominator	Proportion Dying	Proportion Surviving	Cumulative Survival Rate
0–1	126	47	4	15	116.5	0.403	0.597	0.597
1–2	60	5	6	11	51.5	0.097	0.903	0.539
2–3	38	2	0	15	30.5	0.066	0.934	0.503
3–4	21	2	2	7	16.5	0.121	0.879	0.443
4–5	10	0	0	6	7.0	0.000	1.000	0.443

22.1.2. Calculations for direct method:

Interval	Censored People Removed	Cumulative Mortality Rate	Cumulative Survival Rate
0–1	19	47/107 = 0.439	0.561
1–2	17	52/90 = 0.578	0.422
2–3	15	54/75 = 0.720	0.280
3–4	9	56/66 = 0.848	0.151
4–5	6	56/60 = 0.933	0.067

22.1.3. The distinctions clearly illustrate the differences between analyses in which the censored people do or do not contribute to the intervening denominators. At the end of the fifth year of follow-up in this cohort of 126 people, we clinically know only two things for sure: 56 people have died and 60 people have actually been followed for at least 5 years. Everyone else in the cohort is either lost or in the stage of censored suspended animation called withdrawn alive. Assuming that the 12 (= 4 + 6 +0 + 2) lost people are irretrievably lost, we still have 54 people (= 15 + 11 + 15 + 7 + 6) who are percolating through the follow-up process at various stages of continuing observation before 5 years. The cumulative survival rate of 0.067 in the direct method is based on the two clearly known items of clinical information at 5 years. The cumulative survival rate of 0.443 in the fixed-interval method is based on the interval contributions made by all the censored people. In fact, if you take 33 as half the number of the 66 (= 12 + 54) censored people and add 33 to the direct numerator and denominator at 5 years, the cumulative survival becomes 0.398; and the two methods agree more closely.

Rather than dispute the merits of the two methods, we might focus our intellectual energy on the basic scientific policy here. Why are 5-year survival rates being reported at all when the 5-year status is yet to be determined for almost as many people (54) as the 60 for whom the status is known? Why not restrict the results to what was known at a 1-year or at most a 2-year period, for which the fate of the unknown group has much less of an impact? A clinician predicting a patient's 5-year chances of survival from these data might be excessively cautious in giving the direct estimate of 0.067. On the other hand, the clinician would have a hard time pragmatically defending an actuarial estimate of 0.443, when the only real facts are that four people of a potential 60 have actually survived for 5 years.

22.3. See Figure EA.22.3.

22.5. Individual answers.

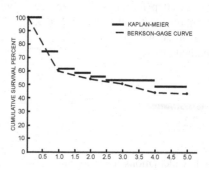

FIGURE EA.22.3

Graph showing answer to Exercise 22.3. The Kaplan-Meier "curve" is shown as a step-function, without vertical connections.

Chapter 23

23.1. In 1936, telephones were not yet relatively inexpensive and ubiquitous in the U.S. Owners of telephones were particularly likely to be in higher socioeconomic classes and, therefore, Republicans. In addition, readers of the "upscale" literary magazine were likely to be college graduates, a status which, in 1936, was also commonly held by Republicans. The use of these two "sampling frames," despite the random selection of telephone owners, produced an overwhelmingly Republican response.

23.3.

23.3.1. Authors did not indicate why they made no recommendations. Perhaps they were worried about "β error" because the confidence interval around the observed result goes from –0.120 to +.070. [Observed mortality rates were $15/100 = .150$ for propranolol and $12/95 = .126$ for placebo, so that result was lower in placebo by $.126 - .150 = -.024$. Standard error under H_0 is $\sqrt{(27)(168)/[195(100)(95)]} = .049$ and two-tailed 95% C.I. would be $-.024 \pm (1.96)(.049) = -.024 \pm .096$, which extends from –0.12 to +.072. Thus, the result might be regarded as a stochastic variation for the possibility that propranolol was 7.2% better. The authors also state that their population was unusually "mild" in prognosis. [Perhaps propranolol works better in patients with worse prognoses.]

23.3.2. The most direct, simple approach is as follows. If mortality rate with propranolol is 10% below that of placebo, the true propranolol mortality rate is $12.6\% - 10\% = 2.6\%$. In the 100 patients treated with propranolol, we would expect 2.6 deaths and 97.4 survivors. Applying a chi-square goodness-of-fit test to this "model," we would have

$$X^2 = \frac{(15 - 2.6)^2}{2.6} + \frac{(85 - 97.4)^2}{97.4} = 59.14 + 1.58 = 60.72 \text{ and } P < .001$$

The chance is therefore tiny that the observed results arose by chance from such a population.

In a more "conventional" way, we can use the formula

$$Z_H = \frac{\delta - d_o}{\sqrt{[p_A q_A / n_A] + [p_A q_A / n_B]}}$$

where $\delta - d_o$ would be $.10 - (-.024) = .124$, and

$$\sqrt{[(.15)(.85)/100] + [(12/95)(83/95)/95]} = .04936$$

so that $Z_H = .124/.04936 = 2.51$, $P < .025$. We can reject the alternative hypothesis that propranolol mortality was 10% below that of placebo.

23.5. Figure E.23.5 shows that the values of d_o (labeled $P_C - P_T$) ranged from –.20 to +.20, with negative values favoring treatment. Without knowing the actual values of P_C and P_T, we cannot decide how large δ should be for quantitative significance. Most investigators would probably accept $d_o = .10$ as quantitatively significant, regardless of magnitudes for P_C and P_T. Using the principle that $\delta = \theta P_C$ and letting $\theta = .5$, we would have $\delta \geq .1$ for $P_C \geq .2$, $\delta \geq .05$ for $P_C \geq .1$, and $\delta \geq .025$ for $P_C \geq .05$. With these boundaries, most of the "positive" trials that favored treatment in Figure E.23.5 seemed to have $d_O > \delta$ and certainly had upper confidence limits that exceeded δ, although the lower confidence interval included 0. Accordingly, the main defect in these trials was capacity, not power. A recommendation to use the Neyman-Pearson approach would needlessly inflate the sample sizes. Conversely, the top eight negative trials, favoring the control group would seem to have their quantitative "nonsignificance" confirmed by upper confidence limits that were $< \delta$. The other "negative" trials in Figure E.23.5 seemed to have upper confidence limits that included δ and lower limits that included 0. The investigator would thus have to concede both the original null and the alternative hypothesis. An appropriate sample size for the latter trials would depend on which hypothesis the investigator wanted to reject, i.e., to confirm a big or small difference.

Thus, although a Neyman-Pearson calculation would probably have been unnecessary for any of the cited trials, Freiman et al. recommended that the "determination of sample size" should be done as cited in two references[9,15] that presented the Neyman-Pearson approach.

Chapter 24

24.1. For the big difference, set Z_α at 1.645 for a one-tailed $P_o < .05$. With $\pi_A = .08$ and $\pi_B = .10$, $\pi = .09$ and so

$$n \geq [1/(.02)^2][1.645]^2 [2(.09)(.91)] = 1068$$

and 2n would be 2136.

For the tiny difference, Z_α can also be set at 1.645 for a one-tailed $P_E < .05$. The calculation will be

$$n \geq [1/(.02 - .005)^2] [1.645]^2[(.08)(.92) + (.10)(.90)] = 1968$$

and 2n would be 3935 — which is larger than the 2958 calculated previously in Exercise 23.2.

The main reason why sample size for the big difference did not become much smaller than before is the shift from $\delta = .03$ to $\delta = .02$. These values are quite small for a "big" difference, and the "gain" of having only one Z_α term in the numerator of the calculation is offset by the loss of having to divide by the square of a smaller value of δ.

24.3. Using the data employed in Exercise 14.4, we can assume that the rate of total myocardial infarction is .02 per person in the placebo group, and will be reduced by 25% to a value of .015 in the aspirin group, so that $\delta = .005$. The anticipated value for π will be $(.02 + .015)/2 = .0175$. If we choose a two-tailed $\alpha = .05$, so that $Z_\alpha = 1.96$, and a one-tailed $\beta = .2$, so that $Z_\beta = 0.84$, the Neyman-Pearson calculation becomes

$$n \geq [1/(.005)^2][1.96 + 0.84]^2[2(.0175)(.9825)] = 10783.9$$

This result is close to the actual sample size of about 11,000 in each group.

According to the original grant request, which was kindly sent to me by Dr. Charles Hennekens, the investigators expected that aspirin would produce "a 20% decrease in cardiovascular mortality" and a "10% decrease in total mortality" during "the proposed study period of four and one-half years." The expected $4\frac{1}{2}$ yr CVD mortality among male physicians was estimated (from population data and the anticipated "age distribution of respondents") as .048746. With a 20% relative reduction, $\delta = .009749$ and the aspirin CV mortality would be .038997. The estimate for π would be $(0.48746 + .038997)/2 = .043871$. The α level was a one-tailed .05 so that $Z_\alpha = 1.645$ and β was also a one-tailed .05 so that $Z_\beta = 1.645$. With these assumptions, $n \geq [1/(.009749)^2] [1.645 + 1.645]^2 [2(.043871) (.956129)] = 9554.2$. The increase to about 11,000 per group was presumably done for "insurance."

An important thing to note in the published "final report" of the U.S. study (see Exercise 10.1) is that neither of the planned reductions was obtained. The total cardiovascular death rate and the total death rate in the two groups were almost the same (with relative risks of .96 and .96, respectively). The significant reduction in myocardial infarction (which had not been previously designated as a principal endpoint) was the main finding that led to premature termination of the trial.

Chapter 25

25.1. Individual answers.

25.3. The stochastic calculations rely on the idea that each comparison is "independent." Thus, if treatments A, B, and C are each given independently and if the effects of the agents are not interrelated, the three comparisons are independent for A vs. B, A vs. C, and B vs. C. In a person's body, however, the values of different chemical constituents are usually interrelated by underlying "homeostatic" mechanisms. Consequently, the different chemical values are not independent and cannot be evaluated with the $[1 - (1 - \alpha)^k]$ formula used for independent stochastic comparisons. Another possible (but less likely) explanation is that the originally designated normal zones were expanded, after a plethora of "false positives" were found, to encompass a much larger range that would include more values in healthy people.

25.5. Individual answers.

Chapter 26

26.1. Stratum proportions in the total population are $W_1 = 101/252$, $W_2 = 134/252$, and $W_3 = 17/252$. Direct adjusted rate for OPEN would be $(W_1)(6/64) + (W_2)(10/59) + (W_3)(1/3) = .1502$. Analogous calculation for TURP yields .1438. [To avoid problems in rounding, the original fractions should be used for each calculation.]

26.3. Concato et al. used two different taxonomic classifications (Kaplan–Feinstein and Charlson et al.) for severity of co-morbidity, and three different statistical methods (standardization, composite-staging, and Cox regression) for adjusting the "crude" results. With each of the six approaches, the adjusted risk ratio was about 1. Nevertheless, despite the agreement found with these diverse methods, the relatively small groups in the Concato study led to 95% confidence intervals that reached substantially higher (and lower) values around the adjusted ratios. For example, with the Cox regression method in the Concato study the 95% confidence limits for the adjusted risk ratio of 0.91 extended from 0.47 to 1.75. The original investigators contended that this wide spread made the Concato result unreliable, and besides, it included the higher RR values, ranging from 1.27 to 1.45, that had been found in the previous claims-data study.

26.5.

    26.5.1. No. Crude death rate is "standardized" by the division of numerator deaths and denominator population.

    26.5.2. (1) Guyana rates may be truly lower in each age-specific stratum; (2) many of the deaths in Guyana may not be officially reported; (3) Guyana rates may be the same or higher than U.S. in each age-specific stratum, but Guyana may have a much younger population.

    26.5.3. The third conjecture in 26.5.2 is supported by the additional data. Despite the high infant mortality, if we subtract infant deaths from births, we find that Guyana increments its youth at a much higher rate than the U.S. The annual birth increment per thousand population is $38.1(1 - .0383) = 36.6$ for Guyana and $18.2(1 - .0198) = 17.8$ for U.S.

26.7. Individual answers.

Chapter 27

27.1.

    27.1.1. By ordinary linear regression for the two variables in Figure 27.2. The tactic seems inappropriate. If a Pearson correlation coefficient is not justified, the results do not warrant use of an ordinary regression model.

27.1.2. No. Duration of survival, which is the outcome (dependent) variable, has been put on the X rather than Y axis. Furthermore, the log scale makes values of interleukin < .1 look as though they were zero. If the X-axis data are divided essentially at tertiles and the Y data dichotomously at an interleukin level of 1, the tabular data that match the graph become

Duration of Survival	Proportion of Interleukin Levels ≥ 1
< 4	10/11 (91%)
4–13	4/11 (36%)
≥ 14	5/8 (63%)

The declining trend is not at all as constant as implied by "r = −.51." In fact, the trend is reversed in the high survival group.

A better way to show the results would be to orient the data properly and to divide interleukin roughly at the tertiles to get

Interleukin Level	Proportion Who Survived < 10 days
< 1	6/11 (55%)
< 10	5/10 (50%)
≥ 10	7/9 (78%)

This result is also inconsistent with the constantly declining trend implied by the value of r = −.51 for interleukin vs. survival in the graph.

27.1.3. The graph says "N = 33," but only 30 points are shown — as discovered in 27.1.2. The legend does not mention any hidden or overlapping points. What happened to the missing 3 people?

27.3.

27.3.1. System B seems preferable. It has a larger overall gradient (72 − 10 = 62% vs. 57 − 6 = 51%) and patients seem more equally distributed in the three stages.

27.3.2. Coding the three categories as −1, 0, +1, we can calculate slope with Formula [27.19]. For System A, the numerator is 221(3 − 70) − 85(53 − 122) = −14807 + 5865 = −8942. For System B, the numerator is 221(9 − 36) − 85(86 − 50) = −5967 − 3060 = −9027. Denominators are 221(122 + 53) − (122 − 53)² = 33914 for System A and 221(50 + 86) − (86 − 50)² = 28760 for System B. Slope is −8942/33914 = −.264 for A, and −9027/28760 = −.314 for B. Note that results are consistent with the "judgmental" evaluation (in AE27.3.1) that average gradient = .51/2 = .255 in A and .62/2 = .31 in B. X_L^2 can be calculated, as discussed in Section 27.5.5.2 (just after Equation [27.19]), from (numerator of slope)(slope)/NPQ, where NPQ = (221)(85)(221 − 85)/(221)² = (85)(136)/221 = 52.307. In System A, X_L^2 = (−8942)(−.264)/52.307 = 45.13. In System B, X_L^2 = (−9027)(−.314)/52.307 = 54.44. The result is highly stochastically significant in both, but is bigger in System B.

27.3.3. Note that overall X² = 45.5 in System A, so that the residual X_R^2 is X² − X_L^2 = 45.51 − 45.13 = 0.38. In System B, the overall X² is 54.89. The residual is 54.89 − 54.44 = 0.45.

27.3.3. Overall gradient (51% vs. 62%) has already been cited. Another index here could be lambda. Total errors would be 85. With System A, errors are (122 − 70) + 12 + 3 = 67. With system B, errors are (50 − 36) + 40 + 9 = 63. Thus, lambda is (85 − 67)/85 = .21 for System A, and (85 − 63)/85 = .26 for System B. Overall chi-square is 45.5 for System A and 54.9 for System B. Finally, to quantify the hunch about "better" distribution, we can use Shannon's H (recall Section 5.10.2). The proportions of data in each category of the denominator are .552, .208, and .240 in System A and .226, .385, and .389 in system B. Shannon's H is .433 for System A and .465 for System B. Thus, System B gets better scores with all four methods.

27.3.4. In each system, each stratum has "stable" numbers, the gradient is monotonic, and the gradient is relatively "evenly" distributed (31% and 20% in System A; 25% and 37% in System B). Therefore, the overall gradients of 51% vs. 62% are probably the best simple comparison. If the strata had unstable numbers and/or dramatically uneven gradients, the best summary would probably be the linear slope.